HEALTH ASSESSMENT

&PHYSICAL EXAMINATION

About the
ONLINE COMPANION™

Delmar Publishers offers a series of Online Companions.™ Through the Delmar site on the World Wide Web, the Online Companions™ let readers access online companions that update the information in the books.

To access the *Health Assessment & Physical Examination* site simply point your browser to:

http://www.DelmarNursing.com

Online Services

Delmar Online
To access a wide variety of Delmar products and services on the World Wide Web, point your browser to:
　　http://www.DelmarNursing.com
　　or email: info@delmar.com

thomson.com
To access International Thomson Publishing's home site for information on more than 34 publishers and 20,000 products, point your browser to:
　　http://www.thomson.com
　　or email: findit@kiosk.thomson.com

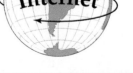

A service of I(T)P®

HEALTH ASSESSMENT

&Physical Examination

Mary Ellen Zator Estes, RN, MSN, CCRN

**Assistant Professor
School of Nursing
Marymount University
Arlington, Virginia
and
Former Critical Care Nursing Education Coordinator
The George Washington University Medical Center
Washington, D.C.**

Consulting Editors

Holly Skodol Wilson, RN, PhD, FAAN
San Francisco, California

Lynn Keegan, RN, PhD
San Antonio, Texas

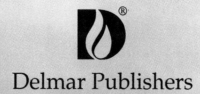

Delmar Publishers

an International Thomson Publishing company I(T)P®

Albany • Bonn • Boston • Cincinnati • Detroit • London • Madrid
Melbourne • Mexico City • New York • Pacific Grove • Paris • San Francisco
Singapore • Tokyo • Toronto • Washington

NOTICE TO THE READER

Cover Design: Brucie Rosch

The cover photograph illustrates the assessment for Tinel's sign, a test for carpal tunnel syndrome.

Delmar Staff

Publisher: William Brottmiller
Acquisitions Editor: Cathy L. Esperti
Developmental Editor: Elisabeth F. Williams
Senior Project Editor: Judith Boyd Nelson *and* Patricia Gillivan
Production Coordinator: Barbara A. Bullock
Art and Design Coordinator: Timothy J. Conners

COPYRIGHT © 1998
By Delmar Publishers
a division of International Thomson Publishing Inc.

The ITP logo is a trademark under license.

Printed in the United States of America

For more information, contact:

Delmar Publishers
3 Columbia Circle, Box 15015
Albany, New York 12212-5015

International Thomson Publishing
   Europe
Berkshire House 168-173
High Holborn
London, WC1V 7AA
England

Thomas Nelson Australia
102 Dodds Street
South Melbourne, 3205
Victoria, Australia

Nelson Canada
1120 Birchmount Road
Scarborough, Ontario
Canada, M1K 5G4

International Thomson Editores
Campos Eliseos 385, Piso 7
Col Polanco
11560 Mexico D F Mexico

International Thomson Publishing
   GmbH
Konigswinterer Strasse 418
53227 Bonn
Germany

International Thomson Publishing Asia
221 Henderson Road
#05-10 Henderson Building
Singapore 0315

International Thomson Publishing—
   Japan
Hirakawacho Kyowa Building, 3F
2-2-1 Hirakawacho
Chiyoda-ku, Tokyo 102
Japan

Library of Congress Cataloging-in-Publication Data

Health assessment & physical examination / Mary Ellen
   Zator Estes; consulting editors, Holly Skodol Wilson, Lynn Keegan.
      p.   cm.
   Includes bibliographical references and index.
   ISBN 0-8273-7147-0
   1. Nursing assessment.   2. Physical diagnosis.   I. Estes, Mary
Ellen Zator.   II. Wilson, Holly Skodol.   III. Keegan, Lynn.
   [DNLM: 1. Nursing Assessment.   2. Physical Examination—nursing.
WY 100.4 H433 1997]
RT48.H425   1997
616.07'5—dc21
DNLM/DLC
for Library of Congress   97-13500
                                                                        CIP

To Matthew, Katie, and Andrew

I love you more today than yesterday . . .
. . . but not as much as tomorrow.

Spiral Staircase

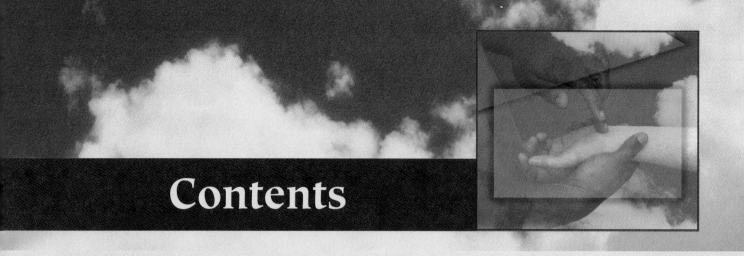

Contents

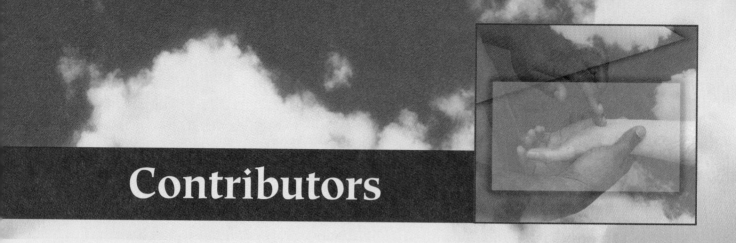

Contributors

Evelyn B. Blaemire, MS, CRNP
Certified Adult Nurse Practitioner
Instructor, Graduate Faculty
Johns Hopkins University
Baltimore, Maryland
Chapter 20: Male Genitalia

Mitzi Boilanger, RN-C, MS
Perinatal Clinical Nurse Specialist
Former Charge Nurse and Education Coordinator
Providence Birth Place
Providence Medford Medical Center
Medford, Oregon
Chapter 22: Pregnant Patient

Barbara Brown Bonheur, MS, RN
School Nurse/Health Educator
Cape Henry Collegiate School
Virginia Beach, Virginia
Chapter 9: General Assessment and Vital Signs

Theresa Perfetta Cappello, PhD, RN, Ct Hy
Acting Associate Dean
School of Nursing
Marymount University
Arlington, Virginia
Chapter 2: The Patient Interview

Eileen V. Caulfield, MA, RN-C
Education Coordinator
Fairfax Hospital
Falls Church, Virginia
Chapter 16: Abdomen

Tamera Cauthorne-Burnette, RN, MSN, FNP, CS
Adjunct Faculty
University of Virginia
Charlottesville, Virginia
and
Women's Healthcare Provider
Planned Parenthood of Virginia
Richmond, Virginia
and
Private Consultant
Richmond, Virginia
Chapter 10: Skin, Hair, and Nails

Chapter 13: Breasts and Regional Nodes
Chapter 19: Female Genitalia

Jean Urban Coleman, EdD, RN, CS
Adjunct Professor
Virginia Polytechnic Institute and State University
Falls Church, Virginia
and
Nurse Psychotherapist
Vienna, Virginia
Chapter 2: The Patient Interview

Patricia A. Connor, RN, CS, OCN, MSN
Nursing Staff
Decamp Burn Center and Wound Healing Unit
University of Virginia Medical Center
Charlottesville, Virginia
and
Lieutenant Commander
Nurse Corps, United States Naval Reserve
Naval Reserve Naval Hospital Portsmouth
Naval and Marine Corps Reserve Readiness Center
Norfolk, Virginia
and
Doctoral Student
School of Nursing
The University of Virginia
Charlottesville, Virginia
Chapter 17: Musculoskeletal System

Catherine Wilson Cox, RN, MSN, CCRN, CEN
Commander
Nurse Corps, United States Naval Reserve
Naval Reserve Naval Hospital Pensacola 108
Naval Reserve Center
Pensacola, Florida
Chapter 15: Heart and Peripheral Vasculature

Jane L. Echols, PhD, RN
Associate Professor
School of Nursing
Marymount University
Arlington, Virginia
Chapter 4: Developmental Assessment
Chapter 5: Cultural Assessment

Barbara Springer Edwards, RN, CCRN, MTS
Director
Cardiac Surgical Unit
Alexandria Hospital
Alexandria, Virginia
   Chapter 6: Spiritual Assessment

Susan P. Gardella, MSN, RN, CPNP
Clinical Instructor
Pediatric Nurse Practitioner Program
School of Nursing
University of Maryland at Baltimore
Baltimore, Maryland
   Chapter 7: Nutritional Assessment

Mary Jordheim Gokey, RN, MSN
Former Neurology Clinical Nurse Specialist
The National Institutes of Health
Bethesda, Maryland
   Chapter 18: Mental Status and Neurological Techniques

Marjorie A. Maddox, EdD, ARNP, ANP-C
Associate Professor
Coordinator of the Adult Nurse Practitioner Option
School of Nursing
University of Louisville
Louisville, Kentucky
   Chapter 4: Developmental Assessment

Randie R. McLaughlin, MS, CRNP
Certified Adult and Geriatric Nurse Practitioner
Urology Private Practice and Internal Medicine Practice
Frederick, Maryland
   Chapter 20: Male Genitalia
   Chapter 21: Anus, Rectum, and Prostate

Kathy A. Murphy, MSN, RN-C, CS
Cardiology Clinical Nurse Specialist
Egleston Children's Hospital and Emory Clinic
Atlanta, Georgia
   Chapter 23: Pediatric Patient

Jo Anne H. Peach, RN, MSN, FNP-C
Assistant Professor
School of Nursing
University of Virginia
Charlottesville, Virginia
   Chapter 11: Head and Neck
   Chapter 12: Eyes, Ears, Nose, Mouth, and Throat

Susan Abbott Rogge, RN, OB/GYN NP
Private Practice
Sacramento, California
and
Clinical Research Nurse
Kaiser Permanente
Sacramento, California
and
Clinical and Research Nurse Practitioner
Department of Obstetrics and Gynecology
University of California, Davis
Sacramento, California
   Chapter 22: Pregnant Patient

Bonnie R. Sakallaris, RN, MSN, CCRN
Patient Care Director — CV ICU
Fairfax Hospital
Falls Church, Virginia
   Chapter 18: Mental Status and Neurological Techniques

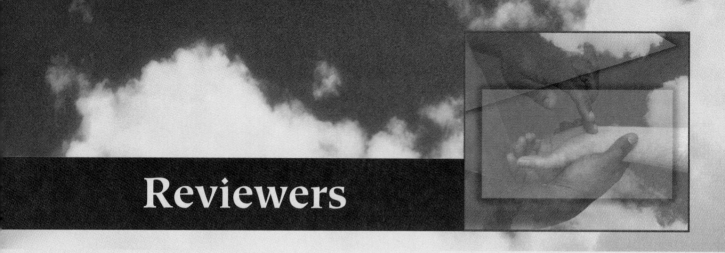

Reviewers

Jo Ann C. Abegglen, APRN, PhD
Assistant Professor
College of Nursing
Brigham Young University
Provo, Utah

Vicki Agyekum, RN, BSN, MSN
Nursing Faculty
Savannah Technical Institute
Savannah, Georgia

Emily Oubre Bond, PhD, RN
Associate Professor
Southeastern Louisiana University
Hammond, Louisiana

Heather G. Boyd-Monk, SRN, BSN, CRNO
Assistant Director of Nursing for Ophthalmic Education
    Programs
Wills Eye Hospital
Philadelphia, Pennsylvania

Frances W. Brown, PhD, RN, C
Acting Dean
Valdosta State University
Valdosta, Georgia

Brenda L. Cameron, RN, BScN, MScN, PhD Candidate
Assistant Professor
Faculty of Nursing
University of Alberta
Edmonton, Alberta, Canada

Sally Chatfield Dunn, RN, MN
Associate Librarian
Director
Nursing Educational Resources Learning Resource
    Center
College of Nursing and Health
University of Cincinnati
Cincinnati, Ohio

Annette C. Frauman, RN, PhD, FAAN
Professor and Chair
Nell Hodgson Woodruff School of Nursing
Emory University
Atlanta, Georgia

Bonnie C. Glass, RN, MSN
Level I Instructor
Jefferson State Community College
Birmingham, Alabama

Anne Hummer, RN, PhD
Associate Professor of Nursing
McAuley School of Nursing
University of Detroit Mercy
Detroit, Michigan

Elizabeth Miller Jenkins, RN, MS
College of Nursing
University of Delaware
Newark, Delaware

Sharon Jensen, RN, MN
Lecturer
Seattle University
Seattle, Washington

Barbara C. Kuper, RN, MN
Assistant Professor of Clinical Nursing
Baccalaureate Degree Program
School of Nursing
Louisiana State University Medical Center
New Orleans, Louisiana

Denise LeBlanc, RN, BScN
Professor
Humber College
Toronto, Ontario
Canada

Thom J. Mansen, PhD, RN
Associate Professor
College of Nursing
University of Utah
Salt Lake City, Utah

Cheryl McKenzie, RN, CS, MN, FNP
Associate Professor of Nursing
Northern Kentucky University
Highland Heights, Kentucky

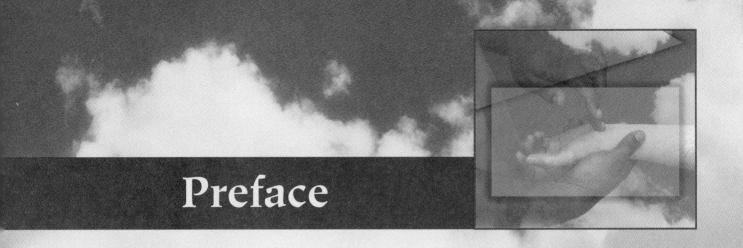

Preface

Health assessment forms the foundation of all nursing care. Whether the patient is young or old, well or ill, assessment is an ongoing process that evaluates the whole person as a physical, psychosocial, functional being. *Health Assessment & Physical Examination* provides a fresh and innovative, superbly illustrated approach to the process of holistic assessment, including physical assessment skills, clinical examination techniques, and patient teaching guidelines. Nursing students will welcome the text's clear presentation as they learn the basic skills of health assessment. Practicing nurses will find the book helpful as a review of the pathophysiological basis for abnormal findings to update their health assessment knowledge base.

CONCEPTUAL APPROACH

The concept for *Health Assessment & Physical Examination* arose from a need identified by the author for straightforward, well-organized assessment information that could be easily read and assimilated. Empowering readers as educated decision makers and developing skills of analysis and critical thinking, while encouraging excellent clinical and nursing skills, are all goals forming the foundation for this text.

Health Assessment & Physical Examination embraces a dual focus, based on nursing as the art and science of caring. Strong emphasis on science encompasses all the technical aspects of anatomy, physiology, and assessment, while highlighting clinically relevant information. The emphasis on caring is displayed through themes of assessment of the whole person; cultural, spiritual, familial, and environmental considerations; patient dignity; and health promotion. Such an approach encourages nurses to think about and care for themselves as well as for their patients.

Health Assessment & Physical Examination offers a user-friendly approach that delivers a wealth of information. The consistent, easy-to-follow format with recurring pedagogical features is based on two frameworks:

1. The **IPPA** method of examination (Inspection, Palpation, Percussion, Auscultation) is applied to body systems for a complete, detailed physical assessment.

2. The **ENAP** format (Examination, Normal Findings, Abnormal Findings, Pathophysiology) is followed for every IPPA technique, providing a useful, valuable fund of information. Pathophysiology is included for each abnormal finding, acknowledging that nurses' clinical decisions need to be based on scientific rationale.

Readers of *Health Assessment & Physical Examination* will need an understanding of anatomy and physiology, as well as a familiarity with basic nursing skills and the nursing process.

ORGANIZATION

Health Assessment & Physical Examination comprises 24 chapters organized into five units. **Unit I** lays the foundation for the entire assessment process by guiding the reader through the nursing process, the patient interview, and the health history. Specific tips on professionalism, approaching patients, and discussing sensitive topics help the reader understand the importance of the nurse/patient partnership in the assessment process.

Unit II highlights developmental, cultural, spiritual, and nutritional areas of assessment, emphasizing the holistic nature of the assessment process. These chapters are key in encouraging the reader to be aware of personal feelings and biases and how they may affect interactions with patients and coworkers.

Unit III opens with a description of fundamental assessment techniques, including measuring vital signs, then details assessment procedures and findings for specific body systems. The format used for all applicable physical assessment chapters in this unit is:

1. Anatomy and physiology overview
2. Health history
3. Equipment
4. Physical assessment
   a. Inspection
   b. Palpation
   c. Percussion
   d. Auscultation
5. Gerontological variations
6. Case study

The examination techniques presented are related primarily to adult patients. Gerontological considerations are included for each body system chapter, with a focus on identifying normal age-related variations. Because assessment techniques and findings may differ in pregnant women and children, these populations are discussed in separate chapters in **Unit IV**. The chapter on the pregnant patient includes variations in examination techniques and special techniques used only on pregnant patients, as well as normal and abnormal findings related to pregnancy. The chapter on the pediatric patient presents physical differences in the examination and explains special techniques used only with children.

Unit V helps the reader assimilate and synthesize the wealth of information presented in the text in order to perform a thorough, accurate, and efficient health assessment. Specific guidelines and reminders on gaining patient cooperation, being sensitive to legal and ethical considerations, and documenting accurately make this unit a complete health assessment resource tool.

SPECIAL FEATURES

Innovative features in *Health Assessment & Physical Examination* stimulate critical thinking and self-reflection, develop technical expertise, and encourage readers to synthesize and apply information presented in the text:

Think About It boxes introduce ethical controversies and clinical situations readers are likely to encounter, stimulating critical thinking, effective decision making, and active problem solving.

Ask Yourself features encourage readers to examine their own views on particular issues so they can understand the varying viewpoints they may encounter in patients and coworkers. These boxes encourage reflection on issues in a personal context, raise awareness of the diversity of opinions, and foster empowerment.

Nursing Checklists offer an organizing framework for the assessment of each body system or for approaching a certain task. Certain **Nursing Checklists** outline specific questions or points to consider when caring for patients with assistive devices.

Nursing Tips help the reader to apply basic knowledge to real-life situations and offer hints and shortcuts useful to both new and experienced nurses.

Nursing Alerts highlight serious or life-threatening signs or critical assessment findings that need immediate attention.

Case Studies present realistic scenarios, offering opportunities for the reader to apply the chapter material, thereby encouraging extrapolation and intuitive thinking. Case studies list normal and abnormal assessment findings in the context of a clinical scenario. Each case study includes a sample patient history, physical assessment findings, and laboratory data in documentation format, emphasizing the nurse's responsibilities in correct charting. The case studies are written in abbreviated format to simulate real clinical documentation, and deliberately have different charting styles to reflect the wide variety of norms in actual clinical practice. Nursing diagnoses and nursing care plans are included in the **Instructor's Resource Kit** for each case study in the text.

PEDAGOGICAL FEATURES

Health Assessment & Physical Examination also includes many pedagogical features that promote learning and accessibility of information:

Outstanding photographs and drawings highlight assessment techniques and procedures, anatomy and physiology, and normal and abnormal findings.

Competencies open each chapter and introduce the main areas targeted for mastery in each chapter, providing a checkpoint for study and tie-in to crucial assessment skills.

Nursing Checklists concluding each chapter offer a conceptual framework for chapter review, highlighting main points. Other **Nursing Checklists** offer step-by-step approaches to certain problems or situations, and serve as excellent resources for quick review.

Review Questions and Activities offer readers an opportunity to assess their understanding of the content and better define areas needing additional study. All chapters include self-quizzes on key information and short activities to test knowledge. Many chapters also include short scenarios with related questions.

Key Terms are boldfaced and defined in the text the first time they are used.

References and Bibliography at the end of the text document the theoretical basis of each chapter and provide additional resources for continued study.

Glossary at the end of the book defines all key terms used in the text and serves as a comprehensive resource for study and review.

Index facilitates access to material and includes special entries for tables and illustrations.

List of Abbreviations on the inside back cover includes abbreviations frequently used in charting, along with their definitions.

EXTENSIVE TEACHING/ LEARNING PACKAGE

The complete Supplements Package was developed to achieve two goals:

1. To assist students in learning the essential skills and information needed to secure a career in the area of nursing
2. To assist instructors in planning and implementing their programs for the most efficient use of time and other resources

The Pocket Companion

Order # 0-8273-8243-X

Clinical Companion for Health Assessment and Physical Examination by Tamera Cauthorne-Burnette, RN, MSN, FNP, CS, and Mary Ellen Zator Estes, RN, MSN, CCRN is a pocket-sized clinical guide. The content mirrors that of the main text, focusing on easy access and rapid retrieval of information.

Instructor's Resource Kit

Order # 0-8273-7148-9

A must-have for all instructors, this comprehensive and resource packed three-ring binder includes:

Instructor's Guide

- **Key Terms** — list the key terms for each chapter alphabetically, with corresponding definitions.
- **Helpful Hints and Exercises** — offer tips for laboratory exercises, clinical skill building, small group work, and classroom discussion.
- **Skills Checklists** — outline physical assessment techniques to be evaluated for each body system; pregnant patient and pediatric techniques; and comprehensive head-to-toe assessment outlines.

- **Care Plans** — correspond to the case studies presented in the text.

Computerized and Printed Testbank with Electronic Gradebook

- **Testbank** — both computerized (IBM format) and printed testbanks include approximately 950 multiple choice questions with answers and text page references.
- **Electronic Gradebook** — enables the instructor to create and administer on-line tests while automatically grading exams and calculating and tracking class as well as individual student performance.
- **On-line Testing** — allows exams to be administered on-line via a school network or stand-alone PC. Site license is included.

CD-ROM Image Library

The Image Library is a software tool that includes an organized digital library of approximately 600 illustrations and photographs from the text. A Windows™ 3.1 and Windows™ 95 application, it can be used with the most common graphics file formats (BMP, TIFF, GIF). This allows the instructor and/or student to add new images.

With the Image Library you can:
- Create additional libraries
- Set up electronic pointers to actual image files or collections
- Sort art by desired categories
- Print selected pieces

The Image Library will work in combination with:
- Microsoft® PowerPoint™ for Windows™ 95 version 7.0 and higher.
- Other Delmar Image Collections.

Color Transparencies

Approximately 95 images from the text provide the instructor with yet another means of promoting student understanding of skills and concepts.

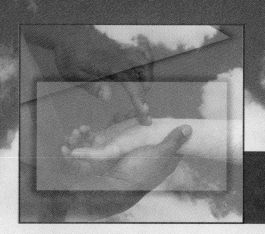

Acknowledgments

This textbook is the product of many dedicated, knowledgeable, and hard-working individuals. First, I would like to thank all the contributors who persevered to produce an outstanding contribution to the nursing literature. Few assessment skills change, but the approach and critical thinking skills highlight the development of the nursing profession. Your technical expertise radiates from cover to cover.

Likewise, I need to thank all the reviewers who thoughtfully read and commented on the manuscript. Your attention to detail and suggestions strengthened the text.

My family, friends, and professional colleagues proved incredibly supportive and encouraging. The daily heard phrase, "How is THE book going?" came to be an opportunity to reflect on the many accomplishments of the talented people who worked so hard to produce this text.

A few of the individuals and establishments that I would like to single out for their tremendous assistance include: Joe Chovan, illustrator; Tom Stock, photographer; models Hal Gerow, Reed Sutherland, Thompson Herrick, Ann Usher, Joylin Namie, Neville Woods, and the many Delmar employees and families and friends who participated in photo shoots; Michael Reppert of John B. Garrett, Inc.; Dr. Robert Silverman; Dr. Mark Dougherty; Dr. Joseph Konzelman; Dr. Alice Mandanis; John Barrat; Pete Read; Susan Steiner; Linda Shaw; Danya Plotsky; and Uniform Village of Albany.

Lastly, my sincere thanks go to the entire Delmar staff who assisted in turning this manuscript into a first-rate text. They have proven on a daily basis that they are committed to manufacturing quality nursing textbooks that will prepare today's sophisticated nurses for the 21st century. My special thanks go to Tim Conners, Barb Bullock, Judith Boyd Nelson, and Pat Gillivan. Most especially, my appreciation goes to Beth Williams, my Editor. Beth is and was the pivot around which the project revolved. With her assistance, I persevered and learned, laughed, and survived!

Mary Ellen Zator Estes

About the Author

Mary Ellen Zator Estes obtained her Baccalaureate and Master's degrees in Nursing from the University of Virginia. She has taught at the University of Virginia, Marymount University, Northern Virginia Community College, and The George Washington University Medical Center.

With over 15 years as a clinician and academician, Ms. Estes has taught physical assessment courses to nurses and nursing students from a variety of backgrounds. Her hands-on approach in the classroom, laboratory, and clinical setting has consistently led to positive learning experiences for her students.

Ms. Estes' professional development is well demonstrated at the local, regional, and national levels. She has delivered numerous presentations throughout the country. She maintains membership and has been actively involved in Sigma Theta Tau, American Nurses Association, and the American Association of Critical-Care Nurses. Ms. Estes has many journal, textbook, and abstract publications to her credit. She also serves as an expert reviewer for various journals.

Ms. Estes has been listed in *Who's Who in American Nursing* and *Who's Who in American Education*. She is currently an Assistant Professor of Nursing at Marymount University and a Critical Care Consultant.

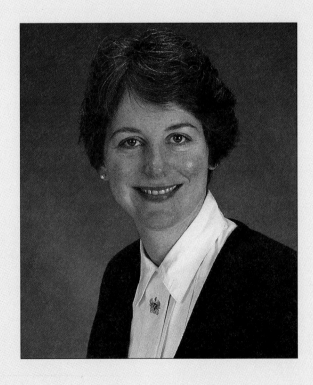

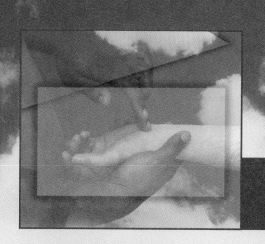

Boxed Features

Nursing Checklist

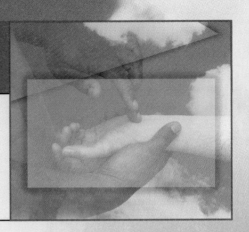

How to Use This Text

Suggestions for how you can use the features of this text to gain competence and confidence in your assessment and nursing skills follow.

ENAP format: In order for the assessment process to become "instinctual" for you as a nurse, we have highlighted each step of the "ENAP" process:

Examination sequences show you the step-by-step process of performing an assessment.

Normal Findings, highlighted in blue, describe what you will find in a normal assessment.

Abnormal Findings outline the variations from normal you may see in pathological states.

Pathophysiology explains the scientific rationale for abnormal conditions; many are illustrated.

ENAP reminder boxes repeat on assessment pages for easy reference.

Supraclavicular and Infraclavicular Lymph Nodes

E
1. Have patient seated and uncovered to the waist.
2. Encourage the patient to relax the muscles of the head and neck because this pulls the clavicles down and allows a thorough exploration of the supraclavicular area.
3. Flex the patient's head to relax the sternocleidomastoid muscle.
4. Standing in front of the patient, in a bilateral and simultaneous motion, place the finger pads over the patient's clavicles, lateral to the tendinous portion of the sternocleidomastoid muscles.
5. Using a rotary motion of the palmar surfaces of the fingers, probe deeply into the scalene triangles in order to palpate the supraclavicular lymph nodes (see Figure 13-20).
6. Palpate the infraclavicular nodes using the same rotary motion of the palmar surfaces of the fingers (see Figure 13-21).

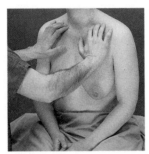

Figure 13-20 Palpation of Supraclavicular Nodes

N *Palpable lymph nodes less than 1 cm in diameter are usually considered normal and clinically insignificant provided that there are no additional enlarged lymph nodes found in other regions such as the axilla. Palpation should not elicit pain.*

A Fixed, firm, immobile, irregular lymph nodes more than 1 cm in diameter are considered abnormal.

P These nodes are considered suspicious for metastasis from a variety of sources or primary lymphoma.

A Enlarged, painful, or tender nodes that are matted together are abnormal.

P Tender, enlarged nodes may indicate systemic infection or carcinoma.

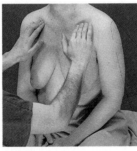

Figure 13-21 Palpation of Infraclavicular Nodes

Breasts: Patient in Sitting Position

E
1. Place the patient in a sitting position with arms at sides.
2. Stand to the patient's right side, facing the patient.
3. Using the palmar surfaces of the fingers of the dominant hand, begin the palpation at the outer quadrant of the patient's right breast.
4. Use the other hand to support the inferior aspect of the breast.
5. In small-breasted patients, the dominant hand can palpate the tissue against the chest wall, but if the breasts are pendulous, use a bimanual technique of palpation as shown in Figure 13-22.
6. Palpate in a downward fashion, sweeping from the outer quadrants to the sternal boarder of each breast.
7. Repeat this sequence on the other breast.
8. Repeat the entire assessment with the patient's arms raised over her head to enhance any potential retraction.

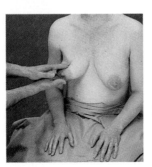

Figure 13-22 Bimanual Palpation of the Breasts While Patient Is Sitting

E	Examination
N	Normal Findings
A	Abnormal Findings
P	Pathophysiology

N *The consistency of the breasts is widely variable, depending on age, time in menstrual cycle, and proportion of adipose tissue. The breasts may have a nodular or granular consistency that may be enhanced prior to the onset of menses. The inferior aspect of the breast will be somewhat firmer due to a transverse inframammary ridge. Palpation should not elicit significant tenderness, although the breasts and especially the nipples may become full and slightly tender premenstrually. Breasts that feel fluid filled or firm throughout with accompanying inferior suture-line scars are indicative of breast augmentation.*

A The presence of any lump, mass, thickening, or unilateral granulation that is noticeably different from the rest of the breast tissue should be considered suspicious and abnormal.

P For a description of breast masses and their pathologies, refer to Table 13-2.

A Significant breast tenderness is abnormal and may indicate mammary duct ectasia.

P This is a benign condition in which lactiferous ducts become inflamed.

ANATOMY AND PHYSIOLOGY

Heart

In a resting, healthy adult, the heart contracts 60 to 100 times while pumping 4 to 5 liters of blood per minute. An individual's heart is only about the size of his or her clenched fist. The human heart is remarkably efficient considering its size in relation to the rest of the body.

The heart is located in the thoracic cavity between the lungs and above the diaphragm in an area known as the mediastinum (refer to Figure 15-1). The **base** of the heart is the uppermost portion, which includes the left and right atria as well as the aorta, pulmonary arteries, and the superior and inferior venae cavae. These structures lie behind the upper portion of the sternum. The **apex**, or lower portion of the heart, extends into the left thoracic cavity, causing the heart to appear as if it is lying on its right ventricle.

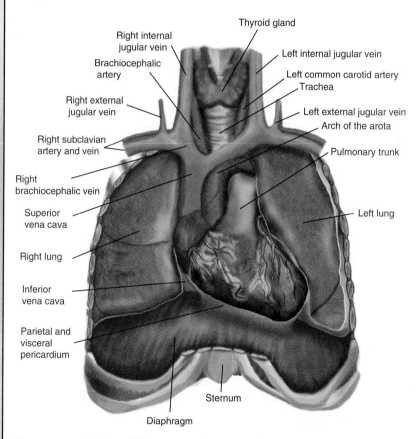

Figure 15-1   Position of the Heart in the Thoracic Cavity

Anatomy and Physiology: Understanding the function of the body systems is an important component of completing an accurate assessment. The information that is necessary for a complete and accurate assessment is highlighted, and detailed illustrations help you visualize anatomy in the context of an actual patient.

☯ THINK ABOUT IT

The Patient with Silicone Breast Implants

How would you deal with a patient who has silicone breasts implants? Would you feel differently about her if she had implants after surgery for breast cancer versus surgery for cosmetic reasons? Would you warn her to remove her implants? If you had a patient who wanted breast augmentation and she asked for your opinion, how would you respond?

Think About It: As you read in the Preface, this feature helps you to develop sensitivity to ethical and moral issues, and guides you to think critically in clinical situations and be active in problem solving. You may choose to read through each one and explore the issues *before* reading the chapter. Then as you read through the chapter, readdress each Think About It and reevaluate your original thoughts. If you choose to read them as you go through the chapter, perhaps write your thoughts down, then go back and look at them at a later time.

❖ HEALTH HISTORY

The head and neck health history provides insight into the link between a patient's life/lifestyle and head and neck information and pathology.

PATIENT PROFILE	*Diseases that are age- and sex-specific for the head and neck are listed.*
Age	Lymphadenopathies related to Hodgkin's disease (11–29) Cervical spine trauma (young adults) Hyperthyroidism (reproductive years in young women) Temporal arteritis (elderly) Decreased mobility of the cervical spine related to an inflammatory or degenerative process (elderly)
Sex	
Female	Hypo- or hyperthyroidism, thyroid cancer Degenerative cervical bone disease
Male	Lymphadenopathy related to Hodgkin's disease Trauma-related cervical spine injury
CHIEF COMPLAINT	*Common chief complaints for the head and neck are defined, and information on the characteristics of each sign/symptom is provided.*
Stiff Neck	Painful movement of the neck that restricts range of motion
Quality	Limited range of motion, either passive or active
Associated Manifestations	Headache, neck tenderness, swelling, fever, numbness and tingling in arms or hands
Aggravating Factors	Position (sitting, standing, lying down), mobility, stress, weather
Alleviating Factors	Immobility or rest, certain position, analgesics, heat
Setting	Work, driving

Health History sections give you an outline of all areas of assessment related to each body system. The standard format used throughout the text teaches you the importance of consistency and organization when discussing topics with patients during the health history interview. It provides information that guides your interview related to each body system. This enables you to link health history clues with the patient's history and clinical status.

CASE STUDY

The case study illustrates the application and objective documentation of the head and neck assessment.

The Patient with Thyromegaly

Bob is a 38-year-old high school physical education teacher. For the past week he has been aware of a tenderness and fullness in his neck. At first he thought he was coming down with a cold, but his symptoms haven't changed and he has no fever. Because the problem hasn't gone away, he made an appointment with his nurse practitioner to find out what is wrong.

❖ HEALTH HISTORY

PATIENT PROFILE	38 yo SWM
CHIEF COMPLAINT	"My neck has been sore for a week."
HISTORY OF PRESENT ILLNESS	Pt in usual state of good health until 1 wk PTA when he noticed soreness & swelling in lower front of neck; pt dismissed as a "cold"; mild discomfort at all times but aggravated by mvt & buttoned shirt collars. Pain doesn't disturb sleep or interfere c̄ eating. Pt concerned that he might have "cancer in his lymph glands." More tired recently, gained 4 lb due to lack of energy, c/o mild constipation. Denies unusual stress, irritability, frequent infections, fever, thirst, urination, hunger, heat or cold intoierance, hx of DM.
PAST HEALTH HISTORY	
Medical	Denies past problems
Surgical	Uncomplicated appendectomy at City General Hospital 12 yo; uncomplicated removal of wisdom teeth 20 yo in local oral surgeon's office
Medications	Occasional acetaminophen for H/A

Case Studies: Appearing in each body system chapter, this feature helps you to practice performing a complete assessment with an actual patient. Documentation-style entries teach you correct charting, and the variations in styles reflect real-life situations you will ultimately encounter in practice.

⟳ NURSING ALERT

Gaping Lacerations

Gaping lacerations of the scalp require emergency treatment under aseptic conditions because of their access to the brain and potential to threaten the patient's life.

Nursing Alert: As a professional, you will need to be able to react immediately in some situations in order to ensure the health and safety of your patients. Pay careful attention to this feature as it will help you to begin to identify and respond to critical situations on your own, both efficiently and effectively.

Nursing Checklist boxes outline important points for you to consider prior to beginning an assessment. Checklists are your reference guide to reviewing procedural steps and to summarizing the assessment process.

✓ NURSING CHECKLIST
General Approach to Abdominal Assessment

1. Greet the patient and explain the assessment technique.
2. Ensure that the room is at a warm, comfortable temperature to prevent patient chilling and shivering.
3. Use a quiet room that will be free from interruptions.
4. Utilize an adequate light source. This includes both a bright overhead light and a freestanding lamp for tangential lighting.
5. Ask the patient to urinate before the exam.
6. Drape the patient from the xiphoid process to the symphysis pubis, then expose the patient's abdomen.

...fortably in a supine position with knees flexed ...h the patient so that the arms are either folded ...e sides to ensure abdominal relaxation.
...g abdominal structures during the assessment ...rately describe the location of any pathology.
...to tender areas; assess these last. Mark these ...dings (scars, dullness, etc.) on the body dia-

✓ NURSING CHECKLIST
Assessing Patients with Abdominal Tubes and Drains

For all tubes, drains, and intestinal and urinary diversions, note color, odor, amount, consistency, and the presence of blood in any drainage. Check for an obstruction if there is no drainage. The skin around the device should be intact without excoriation.

Tubes
1. Enteral Tubes
   - Nasogastric, nasoduodenal, or nasojejunal.
   - Check the residual amount on a frequent basis. If greater than 100 cc, stop the feeding; restart the feeding based on further inspection of residual amounts.
2. Nasogastric Suction Tubes
   - Levin or Salem sump.
   - Ensure that the suction setting (intermittent or continuous) is set at the appropriate suction level.
3. Intestinal Tubes
   - Miller-Abbott, Cantor, Johnston, or Baker.
   - Ensure that tube is advancing with peristalsis as expected.
   - Ensure that the suction setting is at the appropriate suction level.
4. Gastrostomy
   - Continuous versus intermittent feeding.
   - With intermittent feedings, clamp is applied when not in use.
   - Tube should be secured to abdomen.
   - Check that dressing is applied.

Drains
1. Abdominal Cavity Drain (Jackson-Pratt, Hemovac)
   - To self-suction or wall suction; if wall suction, ensure that it is set at appropriate level.
2. Biliary Drain (T-Tube)
   - Tube is below insertion site.

Assistive Devices are covered in **Nursing Checklists** as part of the assessment process. These checklists help you understand the impact assistive devices can have on a patient's overall health, and also remind you that a complete physical assessment extends to the patient's immediate environment.

Special Techniques help you identify examination sequences that are performed in selected clinical scenarios based on the patient's clinical presentation and history.

✸ SPECIAL TECHNIQUE
Murphy's Sign

E 1. With the patient supine, stand at the patient's right side.
2. Palpate below the liver margin at the lateral border of the rectus muscle.
3. Have the patient take a deep breath.
N *No pain is elicited.*
A Pain is present with palpation. The patient may stop inhaling to guard against the pain. This is known as **Murphy's sign**.
P Murphy's sign is positive in inflammatory processes of the gallbladder, such as cholecystitis.

258   UNIT III   Physical Assessment

Skin Scraping for Mycelia

1. Scrape the roof of suspected vesicle or scales or take a sample of hair follicle.
2. Place a drop of 10% KOH on the sample to clear it of other organisms.
3. Warm it gently over a lighter or alcohol burner.
4. Examine the slide under a microscope for mycelia.

GERONTOLOGICAL VARIATIONS

The most visible signs of aging are manifested in the skin and hair. These changes include wrinkles, sagging skin folds, graying hair, and hair loss. Also, skin disorders are more likely to occur as a person ages. Light-skinned individuals appear to manifest the changes of aging more rapidly than do dark-skinned individuals, and these changes are accelerated by sun exposure.

With aging, the epidermis thins and elastic fibers that provide support to the dermis degenerate and lead to sagging skin folds. The number of sweat and sebaceous glands diminishes as does the vascularity of the skin, which affects thermoregulation. There is increased incidence of hypothermia due to decreased vasodilation and vasoconstriction of the dermal arterioles, and loss of subcutaneous fat.

In elderly individuals, diminished inflammatory response and diminished perception of pain increase the risk of adverse effects from noxious stimuli. The elderly are at a greater risk for frostbite and burns because of diminished pain perception. Their injuries are more serious because of the thinning epidermis and prolonged wound healing. Reepithelialization takes approximately twice as long in patients over the age of 75 than in those who are 25 years of age.

Wrinkling is the change most associated with aging. Wrinkles are most prominent on the face and neck because these areas have the greatest sun exposure. Other factors leading to wrinkling are loss of subcutaneous fat and diminished elasticity of the skin.

Another obvious, early skin change associated with aging is hyperpigmentation. Senile **lentigo**, or liver spots (see Figure 10-20A), are the result of the inability of the melanocytes to produce even pigmentation of the skin. Larger areas of hyperpigmentation are lentigines. These are generally seen on the backs of the hands and wrists of light-skinned individuals and are related to the degree of sun exposure.

Senile pruritus is the most common skin affliction in elderly individuals. Pruritus is due to a decrease in water content of the skin and atrophy of the sweat glands. Dryness and itching are exacerbated during the winter months when humidity is low, indoor temperatures are high, and drying winds are present. The condition is aggravated by frequent bathing in hot water, which robs the skin of moisture. Generalized itching is also associated with systemic diseases such as diabetes mellitus, atherosclerosis, and liver disease. Thus, prolonged itching should receive medical attention.

Keratosis, lesions on the epidermis and characterized by overgrowth of the horny layer, is prevalent among the elderly population. Actinic keratosis, also known as solar keratosis, occurs in those areas where sun exposure has been greatest (neck, ears, bald scalp, hands, forearms). Actinic keratosis is premalignant; seborrheic keratosis is usually not premalignant. However, if either is the precursor of skin cancer, the cancer is usually basal cell carcinoma (see Figure 10-20B). The lesions of seborrheic keratosis are found on the trunk, face, and scalp and are covered with greasy, velvety textured scales.

Although cancer of the skin is common among the elderly population, it is not usual... males. Fac... to sunlig... acne. Squ... than bas...

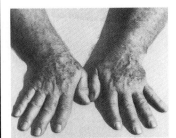

A. Senile Lentigo   *Courtesy of Delmar Publishers, Albany, NY*

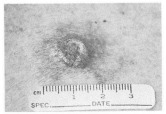

B. Basal Cell Carcinoma   *Courtesy of Robert A. Silverman, M.D., Clinical Associate Professor, Department of Pediatrics, Georgetown University*

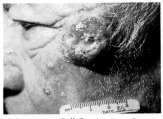

C. Squamous Cell Carcinoma   *Courtesy of Robert A. Silverman, M.D., Clinical Associate Professor, Department of Pediatrics, Georgetown University*

Figure 10-20   Skin Changes in the Elderly

Gerontological Variations: These sections are in each body system chapter to teach you about the normal physiological changes that occur with aging, so you can offer sensitive and appropriate care to your older patients. Understanding and being able to communicate these changes is crucial, as the percentage of our older population increases and our health care delivery systems change.

Ask Yourself: Since these boxes deal with self-reflection and opinions on various topics, it would be useful to keep a journal where you write down your immediate responses to each Ask Yourself on a chapter-by-chapter basis. At the end of each chapter, go back and ask yourself how your values will affect your nursing care.

❖ ASK YOURSELF

Dealing with a Chemical-Dependent Patient

What would you do if during an assessment of a patient you found signs of IV drug use? Would you confront the patient regarding substance use and practices? How would you feel about providing care to this patient? Should drug users receive the same care and treatment as other individuals? Should they receive Medicaid if their addictions are disabling?

NURSING TIP

Pericardial Friction Rub Versus Pleural Friction Rub

- A pericardial friction rub produces a *high*-pitched, multiphasic, and scratchy (may be leathery or grating) sound that *does not* change with respiration. It is a sign of pericardial inflammation.
- A pleural friction rub produces a *low*-pitched, coarse, and grating sound that *does* change with respiration. When the patient holds his or her breath, the sound disappears. The patient may also complain of pain upon breathing. It is a sign of visceral and parietal pleurae inflammation.

Nursing Tips: In any profession there are many helpful hints that assist you in performing more efficiently. In nursing, you need to be able to practice sensitivity in the process. The wide variety of hints, tips, and strategies presented here will help you as you work toward professional advancement. Study, share, and discuss them with your colleagues.

Review Questions and Activities in each chapter present exercises to assist you with the learning process and help you assimilate the information presented in the text. Many chapters contain short case scenarios with related questions, which lead you to apply the information you have learned to actual clinical cases.

REVIEW QUESTIONS AND ACTIVITIES

1. Your patient is complaining of chest pain. What questions should you ask?
2. Distinguish the risk factors that are fixed versus those that are both major and minor modifiable for cardiovascular disease.
3. When assessing the precordium, what are the five cardiac landmarks you should use? Does it matter whether you start at the base or the apex?
4. Whenever you hear a colleague state that his or her patient has an extra heart sound or murmur, ask if you can listen to it. Also, always ask the patient whether you can listen. Try to take advantage of any opportunity you can to identify heart sounds when you are working with patients.
5. Your patient has a grade III/VI systolic murmur heard best at the fifth ICS, left midclavicular line. What could be some causes of the murmur?
6. What are at least four characteristics to look for when evaluating pulses?

Questions 7–9 refer to the following situation:

Mr. Henry is admitted to your critical care unit with chest pain, DOE, and pitting edema. His chest x-ray confirms a diagnosis of heart failure.

7. What heart sound is a common finding in the patient with heart failure?
   a. S_3
   b. S_4
   c. Pericardial friction rub
   d. Pleural friction rub

The correct answer is (a).

8. While auscultating Mr. Henry's heart sounds, you detect a murmur at the patient's fifth ICS, left midclavicular line. You would suspect this to be:
   a. An aortic valve murmur
   b. A pulmonic valve murmur
   c. A tricuspid valve murmur
   d. A mitral valve murmur

The correct answer is (d).

9. The murmur that you have auscultated has a moderate intensity and you do not palpate a thrill. You would grade this murmur as a:
   a. Grade I/VI
   b. Grade II/VI
   c. Grade III/VI
   d. Grade VI/VI

The correct answer is (c).

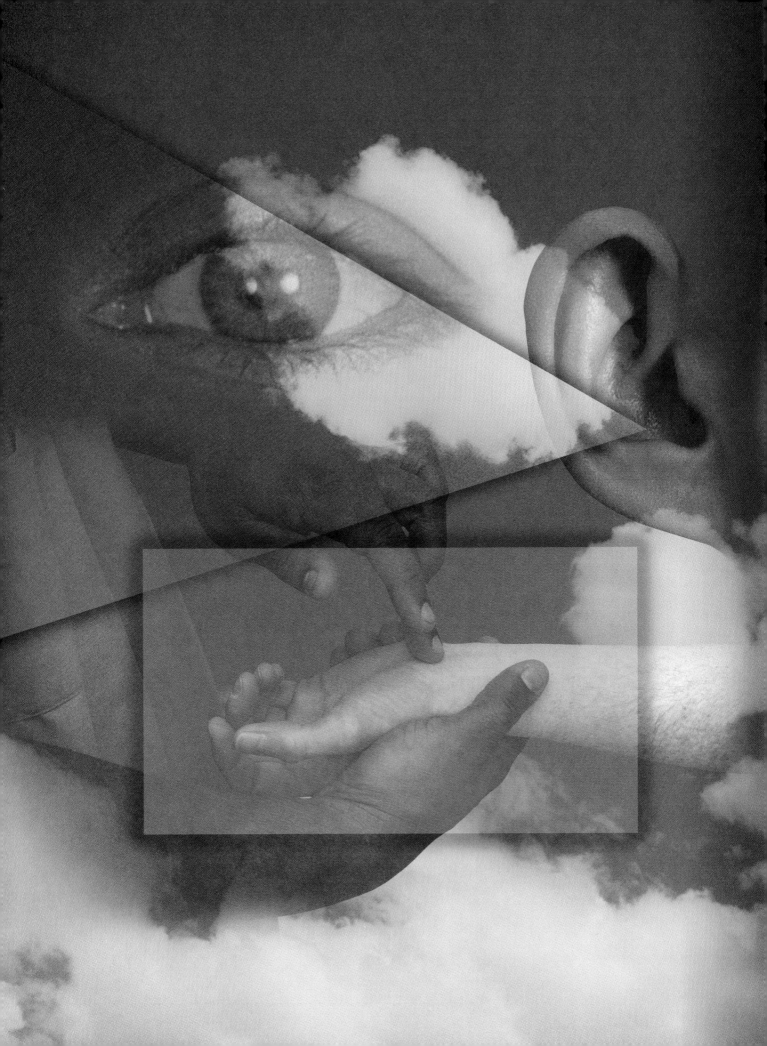

Laying the Foundation

UNIT I

The most important practical lesson that can be given to nurses is to teach them what to observe, how to observe, what are of importance...

Florence Nightingale

1

The Nursing Process

COMPETENCIES

1. Define the nursing process.
2. Describe the five steps of the nursing process.
3. Explain the distinction among actual, risk, and wellness nursing diagnoses.
4. Differentiate nursing diagnoses from collaborative problems.
5. Formulate correctly stated nursing diagnoses.
6. Devise nursing care plans for select patient scenarios.

Reprinted with permission from Standards of Clinical Nursing Practice, © 1991, American Nurses Association, Washington, DC.

Table 1-1   ANA Standards of Clinical Nursing Practice

STANDARD I. ASSESSMENT
The nurse collects [patient] health data.

STANDARD II. DIAGNOSIS
The nurse analyzes the assessment data in determining diagnoses.

STANDARD III. OUTCOME IDENTIFICATION
The nurse identifies expected outcomes individualized to the [patient].

STANDARD IV. PLANNING
The nurse develops a plan of care that prescribes interventions to attain expected outcomes.

STANDARD V. IMPLEMENTATION
The nurse implements the interventions identified in the plan of care.

STANDARD VI. EVALUATION
The nurse evaluates the [patient's] progress toward attainment of outcomes.

"As the professional society for nursing in the United States, the American Nurses Association (ANA) is responsible for defining and establishing the scope of nursing practice" (ANA, 1980, p. 1). The ANA did just that in 1991 with the publication of *Standards of Clinical Nursing Practice*. These standards provide the framework for the nursing process and give the profession broad guidelines to which nurses can be held accountable in their practices. These nursing standards are the tenets on which the entire health and physical assessments of the patient are conducted. Table 1-1 contains the ANA Standards of Clinical Nursing Practice.

The **nursing process** includes five phases: assessment, nursing diagnosis, planning/outcome formulation, implementation, and evaluation. It is a dynamic process that uses information in a meaningful way through problem solving strategies to place the patient, family, or community in an optimal health state. The primary focus of this text is assessment. The physical, emotional, mental, developmental, spiritual, and cultural assessments provide the foundation for the other steps of the nursing process. The sample nursing care plan on pages 13–15 demonstrates how the assessment data are the basis for the planning, implementation, and evaluation of patient care.

ASSESSMENT

Assessment is the first step of the nursing process. It is the orderly collection of information concerning the patient's health status. The assessment process aims to identify the patient's current health status, actual and potential health problems, and areas for health promotion. The sources of information for the assessment include the health history, the physical assessment, and diagnostic and laboratory data. Collectively, these data constitute the nursing database from which the nurse will develop a plan of care for the patient, and they serve as a baseline against which future comparisons can be made.

Health History

The health history interview is a means of gathering **subjective data**, usually from the patient. These data are subjective in that they cannot always be verified by an independent observer. In some instances, however, this information can be validated during the physical assessment; for instance, the existence of a patient-reported breast lump can be confirmed through palpation.

The health history can also be obtained from sources other than the patient. Relatives, neighbors, and friends of the patient can provide insightful data for the health history. In some instances, total strangers may be the only source of information, as in the case of a severe accident where the patient is rendered unconscious. The patient's old charts or medical records are additional sources of information, as are health care colleagues. The nurse can and should use every available medium to gather as much information about the patient as possible. The health history is further discussed in Chapter 3.

Physical Assessment Findings

Physical assessment findings constitute a second source of information that is used in the assessment phase of the nursing process. Physical assessment findings constitute **objective data**, or information that is observable and measurable, and can be verified by more than one person. These data are obtained using the senses of smell, touch, vision, and hearing (taste is not used in physical assessment because of its limited use and the danger it presents to the

Table 1-2 Body System Assessment

1. General assessment
2. Skin, hair, and nails
3. Head and neck
4. Eyes, ears, nose, mouth, and throat
5. Breasts and regional nodes
6. Thorax and lungs
7. Heart and peripheral vasculature
8. Abdomen
9. Musculoskeletal system
10. Mental status and neurological techniques
11. Female genitalia
12. Male genitalia
13. Rectum and prostate

Table 1-3 Functional Health Patterns

1. Health perception–health management pattern
2. Nutritional-metabolic pattern
3. Elimination pattern
4. Activity-exercise pattern
5. Sleep-rest pattern
6. Cognitive-perceptual pattern
7. Self-perception–self-concept pattern
8. Role-relationship pattern
9. Sexuality-reproductive pattern
10. Coping-stress-tolerance pattern
11. Value-belief pattern

From Gordon, M. (1997). Manual of Nursing Diagnosis: 1997–1998. St. Louis: Mosby-Yearbook, Inc.

❖ ASK YOURSELF

Are Nursing and Medicine Distinct?

Florence Nightingale stated over 100 years ago: "Nursing and medicine must never be mixed . . . it spoils both." Do you think this statement reflects your philosophy on the use of nursing diagnoses?

nurse). This text describes the systematic and comprehensive physical assessment techniques that will elicit this data (Chapters 8–23).

The physical assessment data can be obtained in a body system or head-to-toe approach. Table 1-2 lists the body systems that are assessed. Another approach to physical assessment is the use of Gordon's **Functional Health Patterns**, which group human behaviors into 11 patterns that facilitate nursing care (Gordon, 1994). Table 1-3 lists the Functional Health Patterns. This text uses the head-to-toe approach for physical assessment.

Diagnostic and Laboratory Data

The final element that contributes to the gathering of information in the assessment phase of the nursing process is diagnostic and laboratory data. Results of blood and urine studies, cultures, x-rays, and diagnostic procedures constitute objective data about the patient's status.

It is imperative for the nurse to document all assessment findings. The written record is a legal tool used to chart the patient's current health status. Chapter 24 discusses documentation and the legal issues of the written patient record. The documented patient assessment also serves as a means of communicating information to other health care colleagues.

Remember that the assessment phase of the nursing process is dynamic. The nurse is continuously adding to the database, validating the data, and interpreting the data. With this data the nurse is ready to progress to the second phase of the nursing process, the nursing diagnosis.

NURSING DIAGNOSIS

The National Conference Group for Classification of Nursing Diagnoses convened in 1973 to establish a nomenclature to describe conditions treated by nurses. Since that time this group has met biannually. In 1982 the organization changed its name to the North American Nursing Diagnosis Association (**NANDA**). NANDA is the recognized leader in the formulation, classification, and testing of nursing diagnoses. NANDA (1996, p. 8) defines a **nursing diagnosis** as "a clinical judgment about individual, family, or community responses to actual and potential health problems/life processes. Nursing diagnoses provide the basis for selection of nursing interventions to achieve outcomes for which the nurse is accountable."

Nursing diagnoses are holistic in nature. Nurses diagnose and treat "human responses to actual or potential health problems" (ANA, 1980, p. 9). Nurses are licensed to treat patients based on nursing diagnoses and by virtue of their educational and clinical preparation. Nursing diagnoses increase nurses' accountability for the services they render.

Nursing Diagnosis Formulation

The nursing diagnosis is formulated after the assessment data are analyzed. The process involves four steps as identified by Gordon (1994): collecting information, interpreting information, clustering information, and naming a cluster or problem formulation. Collecting information refers to the data collected in the assessment phase of the nursing process. This process is a continuous means to gain as much information about the patient as possible.

In step 2, the data are interpreted. "Collecting information is pointless if the meaning behind it is not derived. Interpretation of cues to a [patient's] health status allows one to predict or explain the findings" (Gordon, 1994, p. 29). The data, or cues, are evaluated against the standards for a patient population. Using inferential reasoning, the nurse begins to see patterns or clusters of data.

Clustering of the information is performed in the third step of nursing diagnosis development. The data are sorted into meaningful groups, usually according to Gordon's Functional Health Patterns or NANDA's **Human Response Patterns** (refer to Table 1-3 for a list of Gordon's Functional Health Patterns). All of the accepted NANDA nursing diagnoses can be organized under either of these two patterns to create nursing diagnosis **taxonomies**, or classification systems. User preference usually dictates the choice of clustering information pattern and taxonomy.

Naming the cluster is the final step in the formulation of the nursing diagnosis. This is the phase when the actual NANDA diagnostic label (NANDA approved nursing diagnosis) is used. Patterns can surface that lead to the development of more than one nursing diagnosis. Conversely, the cues may seem unrelated and no nursing diagnosis is derived from the data. In this case, the nurse needs to review the accuracy of the data. Table 1-4 lists the NANDA nursing diagnoses according to human response patterns from the 1996 conference.

Types of Nursing Diagnoses

There are three types of nursing diagnoses: actual, risk, and wellness. **Actual nursing diagnoses** are typically problem oriented and describe human responses that have been validated by the nurse, such as *Total incontinence* and *Impaired memory*. The second type of diagnosis is the **risk nursing diagnosis**. NANDA (1996, p. 89) defines the risk nursing diagnosis as "human response to health conditions/life processes which may develop in a vulnerable individual, family or community. It is supported by risk factors that contribute to increased vulnerability." Examples of risk nursing diagnoses

Table 1-4 NANDA Approved Nursing Diagnoses by Human Response Patterns

PATTERN 1: EXCHANGING

1.1.2.1	Altered Nutrition: More Than Body Requirements
1.1.2.2	Altered Nutrition: Less Than Body Requirements
1.1.2.3	Altered Nutrition: Risk for More Than Body Requirements
1.2.1.1	Risk for Infection
1.2.2.1	Risk for Altered Body Temperature
1.2.2.2	Hypothermia
1.2.2.3	Hyperthermia
1.2.2.4	Ineffective Thermoregulation
1.2.3.1	Dysreflexia
1.3.1.1	Constipation
1.3.1.1.1	Perceived Constipation
1.3.1.1.2	Colonic Constipation
1.3.1.2	Diarrhea
1.3.1.3	Bowel Incontinence
1.3.2	Altered Urinary Elimination
1.3.2.1.1	Stress Incontinence
1.3.2.1.2	Reflex Incontinence
1.3.2.1.3	Urge Incontinence
1.3.2.1.4	Functional Incontinence
1.3.2.1.5	Total Incontinence
1.3.2.2	Urinary Retention
1.4.1.1	Altered (Specify Type) Tissue Perfusion (Renal, cerebral, cardiopulmonary, gastrointestinal, peripheral)
# 1.4.1.2.1	Fluid Volume Excess
# 1.4.1.2.2.1	Fluid Volume Deficit
1.4.1.2.2.2	Risk for Fluid Volume Deficit
# 1.4.2.1	Decreased Cardiac Output
1.5.1.1	Impaired Gas Exchange
1.5.1.2	Ineffective Airway Clearance
# 1.5.1.3	Ineffective Breathing Pattern
1.5.1.3.1	Inability to Sustain Spontaneous Ventilation
1.5.1.3.2	Dysfunctional Ventilatory Weaning Response (DVWR)
1.6.1	Risk for Injury
1.6.1.1	Risk for Suffocation
1.6.1.2	Risk for Poisoning
1.6.1.3	Risk for Trauma
1.6.1.4	Risk for Aspiration
1.6.1.5	Risk for Disuse Syndrome
1.6.2	Altered Protection
1.6.2.1	Impaired Tissue Integrity
1.6.2.1.1	Altered Oral Mucous Membrane
1.6.2.1.2.1	Impaired Skin Integrity
1.6.2.1.2.2	Risk for Impaired Skin Integrity
1.7.1	Decreased Adaptive Capacity: Intracranial
1.8	Energy Field Disturbance

continued

Table 1-4   NANDA Approved Nursing Diagnoses by Human Response Patterns *continued*

PATTERN 2: COMMUNICATING

2.1.1.1	Impaired Verbal Communication

PATTERN 3: RELATING

3.1.1	Impaired Social Interaction
3.1.2	Social Isolation
3.1.3	Risk for Loneliness
3.2.1	Altered Role Performance
3.2.1.1.1	Altered Parenting
3.2.1.1.2	Risk for Altered Parenting
3.2.1.1.2.1	Risk for Altered Parent/Infant/Child Attachment
3.2.1.2.1	Sexual Dysfunction
3.2.2	Altered Family Processes
3.2.2.1	Caregiver Role Strain
3.2.2.2	Risk for Caregiver Role Strain
3.2.2.3.1	Altered Family Process: Alcoholism
3.2.3.1	Parental Role Conflict
3.3	Altered Sexuality Patterns

PATTERN 4: VALUING

4.1.1	Spiritual Distress (Distress of the Human Spirit)
4.2	Potential for Enhanced Spiritual Well-Being

PATTERN 5: CHOOSING

# 5.1.1.1	Ineffective Individual Coping
5.1.1.1.1	Impaired Adjustment
5.1.1.1.2	Defensive Coping
5.1.1.1.3	Ineffective Denial
# 5.1.2.1.1	Ineffective Family Coping: Disabling
# 5.1.2.1.2	Ineffective Family Coping: Compromised
5.1.2.2	Family Coping: Potential for Growth
5.1.3.1	Potential for Enhanced Community Coping
5.1.3.2	Ineffective Community Coping
5.2.1	Ineffective Management of Therapeutic Regimen (Individuals)
5.2.1.1	Noncompliance (Specify)
5.2.2	Ineffective Management of Therapeutic Regimen: Families
5.2.3	Ineffective Management of Therapeutic Regimen: Community
5.2.4	Effective Management of Therapeutic Regimen: Individual
5.3.1.1	Decisional Conflict (Specify)
5.4	Health Seeking Behaviors (Specify)

PATTERN 6: MOVING

6.1.1.1	Impaired Physical Mobility
6.1.1.1.1	Risk for Peripheral Neurovascular Dysfunction
6.1.1.1.2	Risk for Perioperative Positioning Injury
6.1.1.2	Activity Intolerance
6.1.1.2.1	Fatigue
6.1.1.3	Risk for Activity Intolerance
6.2.1	Sleep Pattern Disturbance
6.3.1.1	Diversional Activity Deficit
6.4.1.1	Impaired Home Maintenance Management
6.4.2	Altered Health Maintenance
6.5.1	Feeding Self-Care Deficit

6.5.1.1	Impaired Swallowing
6.5.1.2	Ineffective Breastfeeding
6.5.1.2.1	Interrupted Breastfeeding
6.5.1.3	Effective Breastfeeding
6.5.1.4	Ineffective Infant Feeding Pattern
6.5.2	Bathing/Hygiene Self-Care Deficit
6.5.3	Dressing/Grooming Self-Care Deficit
6.5.4	Toileting Self-Care Deficit
6.6	Altered Growth and Development
6.7	Relocation Stress Syndrome
6.8.1	Risk for Disorganized Infant Behavior
6.8.2	Disorganized Infant Behavior
6.8.3	Potential for Enhanced Organized Infant Behavior

PATTERN 7: PERCEIVING

7.1.1	Body Image Disturbance
# 7.1.2	Self-Esteem Disturbance
# 7.1.2.1	Chronic Low Self-Esteem
# 7.1.2.2	Situational Low Self-Esteem
7.1.3	Personal Identity Disturbance
7.2	Sensory/Perceptual Alterations (Specify) (Visual, Auditory, Kinesthetic, Gustatory, Tactile, Olfactory)
7.2.1.1	Unilateral Neglect
7.3.1	Hopelessness
7.3.2	Powerlessness

PATTERN 8: KNOWING

# 8.1.1	Knowledge Deficit (Specify)
8.2.1	Impaired Environmental Interpretation Syndrome
8.2.2	Acute Confusion
8.2.3	Chronic Confusion
# 8.3	Altered Thought Processes
8.3.1	Impaired Memory

PATTERN 9: FEELING

# 9.1.1	Pain
# 9.1.1.1	Chronic Pain
# 9.2.1.1	Dysfunctional Grieving
# 9.2.1.2	Anticipatory Grieving
# 9.2.2	Risk for Violence: Self-Directed or Directed at Others
9.2.2.1	Risk for Self-Mutilation
9.2.3	Post-Trauma Response
9.2.3.1	Rape-Trauma Syndrome
9.2.3.1.1	Rape-Trauma Syndrome: Compound Reaction
9.2.3.1.2	Rape-Trauma Syndrome: Silent Reaction
9.3.1	Anxiety
9.3.2	Fear

#Diagnosis revised by small work groups at the 1994 Biennial Conference on the Classification of Nursing Diagnoses; changes approved and added in 1996.

Reprinted with permission from NANDA (1996). Nursing diagnoses: Definitions & classification 1997–1998. Philadelphia: Author.

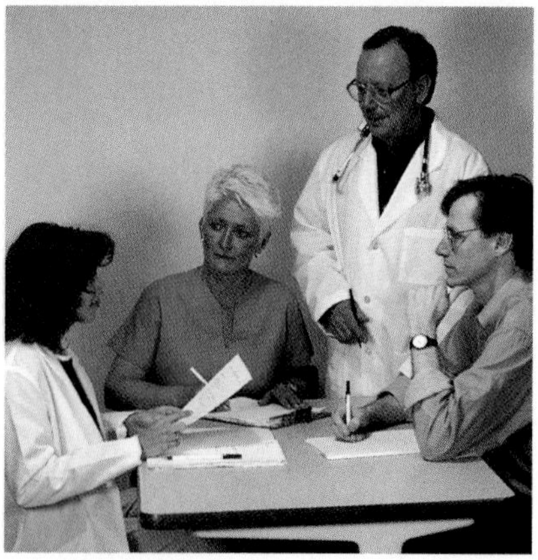

Figure 1-1 Nurses work collaboratively with health care team members.

include *risk for suffocation* and *risk for trauma*. The **wellness nursing diagnosis** represents the patient's striving for a higher level of health and wellness. It focuses on the strengths of a patient. *Potential of enhanced spiritual well-being*, and *Family coping: potential for growth* are two examples of wellness nursing diagnoses.

Some patient problems are not completely within the domain of the nurse's scope of practice and require the nurse to look beyond the nursing diagnosis. For instance, the patient experiencing cardiac tamponade (medical diagnosis) with decreased cardiac output and anxiety (nursing diagnosis) needs immediate nursing and medical attention. The nurse is not ethically or legally permitted to do all that the situation requires to alleviate the tamponade; the nurse, physician, and health care team will work collaboratively to relieve the problem. Thus, a **collaborative problem** is a patient problem that requires the nurse to work jointly with the physician and other health care workers in monitoring, planning, and implementing the patient care (refer to Figure 1-1).

Writing the Nursing Diagnosis

A nursing diagnosis can have up to four components: the descriptor, the human response, the related factors, and the defining characteristics. The **descriptor** or **qualifier** is an adjective that describes or qualifies the human response. Examples of NANDA approved descriptors are *altered, impaired, ineffective, increased, decreased,* and *potential for enhanced.*

The human response is the actual or potential health problem or wellness factors that the nurse has synthesized from the clustered data. The NANDA approved nursing diagnostic labels are the human responses that form the basis for the complete nursing diagnosis. Examples of human responses are hypothermia, pain, and social isolation. The human responses are amenable to nursing interventions (refer to Table 1-4).

Related factors are the third component of the nursing diagnosis. They are the "conditions/circumstances that contribute to the development/maintenance of a nursing diagnosis" (NANDA, 1996, p. 90). They are the origin of the patient's health problem and can be changed with nursing interventions. In the nursing diagnosis, the human response and related factors are joined by the words "related to." Examples include *Ineffective breathing pattern related to pain* and *Altered oral mucous membrane related to ineffective oral hygiene.* Frequently, the related factors are secondary to another condition and this is noted in the nursing diagnosis; e.g., *Fatigue related to anemia secondary to pregnancy.*

Defining characteristics are the final component of a nursing diagnosis. They are signs, symptoms, and/or statements made by the patient that validate the existence of the problem. There are major and minor defining characteristics. Clinical research or expert consensus specifies the percentage of **major defining characteristics** that must be present in order to use a specific nursing diagnosis. **Minor defining characteristics** represent signs and symptoms that may be present in a patient; they need not be present to use nursing diagnoses but they do provide more evidence that the correct nursing diagnosis was applied. According to NANDA (1996, p. 13), "major defining characteristics are present in 80% to 100% of the [patients] experiencing the diagnosis and minor are present in 50% to 79% of the [patients] experiencing the diagnosis." In the nursing diagnosis, the related factors and defining characteristics are joined by the words, "as evidenced by." Examples are *Social isolation related to perception of inability to engage in satisfying personal relationships as evidenced by sad dull affect, lack of eye contact, and patient verbalization;* and *Anxiety related to threat of death as evidenced by patient verbalization, restlessness, hand tremors, facial tension, and quivering voice.*

Another approach to writing a nursing diagnosis is the **PES** method. In this practical approach, *P* is the problem, *E* is the etiology, and *S* is the signs and

Common Errors in Writing Nursing Diagnoses

1. Writing in legally inadvisable terms.
   Incorrect: *Impaired skin integrity related to decreased turning*
   Correct: *Impaired skin integrity related to pressure*
2. Using value judgments.
   Incorrect: *Caregiver role strain related to laziness*
   Correct: *Caregiver role strain related to inexperience with caregiving*
3. Using medical diagnoses.
   Incorrect: *Guillain-Barré syndrome*
   Correct: *Self-care deficit related to decreased physical mobility secondary to Guillain-Barré syndrome*
4. Formulating a nursing diagnosis based on insufficient data.
   A 2-year-old presents to the ER for the first time with a broken tibia.
   Incorrect: *Risk for violence: directed at others related to child abuse*
   Discussion: The nurse may suspect child abuse but further assessment is warranted. One admission for a traumatic injury does not necessarily constitute child abuse. If the child had presented frequently to the ER with accidental injuries, the nursing diagnosis may be accurate, but the nurse would need to gather additional data to validate the diagnosis.
5. Formulating a nursing diagnosis based on incorrect data.
   The nurse walks into a patient's room and observes that the breastfeeding mother is unable to latch-on her newborn.
   Incorrect: *Ineffective breastfeeding related to maternal anxiety as evidenced by unsatisfactory breastfeeding process*
   Discussion: If the nurse formulates this nursing diagnosis after this brief patient encounter, it would be erroneous. The baby had difficulty with latch-on because it was just fed a bottle in the nursery. The nurse needs to assess all data prior to formulating nursing diagnoses.

symptoms. The PES method of writing nursing diagnoses arrives at the same nursing diagnosis as in the above theoretical approach. Table 1-5 lists the characteristics of the three types of nursing diagnoses and provides examples for each.

Writing a correct nursing diagnosis is a skill that requires knowledge and practice. Even experienced nurses need to refer to expert sources to validate information. The Nursing Tip box at left describes common errors that are made when writing nursing diagnoses.

Table 1-5 Components of Nursing Diagnoses with Examples			
		TYPE OF DIAGNOSIS	
COMPONENT	**ACTUAL**	**RISK**	**WELLNESS**
Descriptor	Can be used, i.e., altered, increased, decreased, etc.	Yes, i.e., risk for	Yes, i.e., potential for enhanced
Human response	Yes	Yes	Yes
Related factors	Yes	Yes	No
Defining characteristics	Yes	No	No

Examples

Actual Nursing Diagnoses

1. *Ineffective airway clearance related to decreased energy as evidenced by crackles, tachypnea, and ineffective cough with thick sputum*
2. *Hopelessness related to perception of terminal state as evidenced by patient's verbalizations, lack of energy, and increased sleep*

Risk Nursing Diagnoses

1. *Risk for trauma related to lack of safety education*
2. *Risk for poisoning related to medicines stored in unlocked cabinets accessible to small children*

Wellness Nursing Diagnoses

1. *Effective breastfeeding*
2. *Potential for enhanced community coping*

PLANNING

Planning is the third step in the nursing process. It involves the prioritization of nursing diagnoses, the formulation of patient outcomes, and the selection of nursing interventions.

Prioritization

The nurse formulates all of the nursing diagnoses that are derived from the clustering of data. When there is more than one nursing diagnosis, the nurse needs to determine which problem(s) are the most vital to the patient's well-being at that particular time. It is necessary to **prioritize**, or rank, the importance of each nursing diagnosis. When possible, the patient should assist the nurse with the prioritization of needs. Patients who are actively involved with the decision-making process are more likely to be amenable to nursing care, to assist with their care, and to be compliant with the plan of care.

A theoretical framework that can be used to prioritize nursing diagnoses is Maslow's Hierarchy of Needs. According to Maslow, basic needs such as food

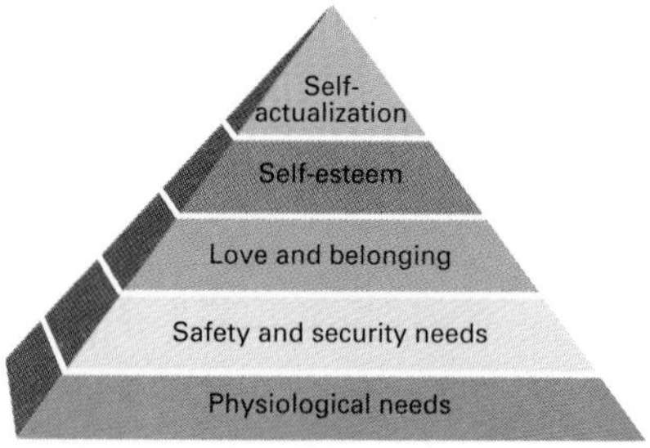

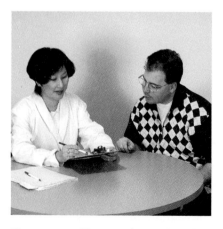

Figure 1-2 Maslow's Hierarchy of Needs

and oxygen take priority over all other issues. For example, the patient experiencing a myocardial infarction must have her physiological needs met before safety needs are attended to. In some instances, though, patients' needs may not follow Maslow's hierarchy, or they may change over time, requiring reprioritization of nursing diagnoses. The terminal breast cancer patient may be more concerned with playing with her children than staying well hydrated. Some nursing diagnoses are equally important and can be prioritized together at the same level. Figure 1-2 illustrates the progression of needs according to Maslow. The nurse, in conjunction with the patient and family, is continually reevaluating and revising the priority of the nursing diagnoses.

Patient Goals

After the nursing diagnoses have been prioritized, patient goals are established. The **patient goal** is directed toward the removal of related factors or patient response to an adverse condition. Goals are broad statements that are not measurable. For example, if a nursing diagnosis is *Anxiety related to knowledge deficit of renal failure*, the patient goal might be: The patient will experience a reduction in anxiety.

> **THINK ABOUT IT**
>
> ***Prioritizing Nursing Diagnoses***
>
> The home health nurse is meeting with Mr. S. for the first time. Mr. S. is a 44-year-old male with acute cardiomyopathy waiting for a heart transplantation. The nurse performs a health and physical assessment on Mr. S., then discusses the plan of care with him. Mr. S. and the nurse disagree on the current priorities of care.
>
> - What nursing interventions would you implement in this situation?
> - Is there additional information that you would attempt to elicit from the patient?
> - How can you align nursing priorities with patient priorities to deliver efficient and necessary care?

Patient Outcome Formulation

A **patient outcome** is a statement of the expected change in patient behavior denoting progress toward resolution of the altered human response over a specific period of time. These are written after the patient goals. Patient outcomes indicate the progression toward goal achievement. Realistic and measurable patient outcomes are written by the nurse to ensure continuity in the patient's care. Adjectives such as *more, less, increased,* and *decreased,* and verbs such as *know* and *understand* are avoided because they are subjective and not measurable. Quantitative phrases such as "walk 15 feet" and "lose 8 pounds" are used as appropriate. Measurable verbs such as *state, identify,* and *list* are used.

Every patient outcome must include a time frame that designates the time by which the patient outcome should be met. The time frame can be short or long term. **Short-term outcomes** denote a time frame over a relatively short period of time, such as 1 hour, 1 day, or 1 week. **Long-term outcomes** usually extend over weeks or months. Each nursing diagnosis can have more than one patient outcome. The complexity of the patient's problem and the type of problem dictate the number of patient outcomes that are required to develop a comprehensive plan of care. Figure 1-3 illustrates the patient and the nurse discussing outcomes.

Figure 1-3 Nurse and patient review outcomes.

Intervention Selection

Interventions are planned strategies, based on scientific rationale, devised by the nurse to assist the patient in meeting the patient outcomes. When appropriate, the patient, family, and significant others can assist in planning the interventions. As with nursing diagnosis prioritization, patients are more likely to be motivated and follow the interventions if they have been involved in the decision-making process.

Every patient outcome has its own nursing interventions. When appropriate, a frequency is included in each intervention, such as "turn every 2 hours." The number of interventions per patient outcome varies. What is essential is that the plan of care is comprehensive to ensure that the patient can meet the outcome. The interventions can be independent and collaborative nursing actions. **Independent nursing interventions** are those that the nurse is legally capable of implementing based on education and experience. **Collaborative inter-**

ventions are physician prescribed and nurse implemented. With all interventions, sound nursing judgment is required. The hypertensive patient on a sodium nitroprusside infusion who has a blood pressure of 74/49 needs immediate nursing action. The nurse, using sound judgment, turns the infusion off and consults with the physician about a new plan of care.

IMPLEMENTATION

The fourth step in the nursing process is **implementation**. In this phase the nurse executes the interventions that were devised during the planning stage to help the patient meet predetermined outcomes. The time frame of the implementation phase varies from patient to patient and from nursing diagnosis to nursing diagnosis. Remember that the nurse usually simultaneously implements the interventions from multiple nursing diagnoses for a patient at any given time. The patient may achieve the outcome for one nursing diagnosis while progressing toward the outcome for another.

Implementation is a dynamic process. The nurse is continually interacting with the patient, the family, and other health care colleagues, obtaining new data and making new judgments. Plans of care can be changed or eliminated altogether based on the continuous flow of information.

EVALUATION

Evaluation is the final phase of the nursing process. During evaluation, the patient's progress in achieving the outcomes is determined. Even before the time frame for assessing outcomes is reached, the nurse is continually assessing the patient's progress toward the outcomes, making evaluation a continual and dynamic process.

The nurse, in conjunction with the patient and the family, evaluates the status of the plan of care. One of two conclusions can be made about the patient outcome: it was met, or it was not met. When the patient outcome has been met, the nurse documents this information and then periodically reevaluates the patient's need for knowledge on the health matter.

If the outcome was not met, this should be documented. Some factors to consider are: Was the diagnosis appropriate? Was the time frame adequate? Were the interventions accurate and comprehensive? Was the patient outcome accurate? Has the patient's condition changed sufficiently that the outcome was no longer appropriate? After considering these factors, the nurse and the patient can decide to revise the patient outcome and nursing interventions or to eliminate them. Based on the ongoing assessment and evaluation, new nursing diagnoses may be formulated that warrant nursing intervention. These will be added to the patient's plan of care.

Each outcome is evaluated separately. A frequent mistake is the practice of evaluating the interventions rather than the outcomes; the outcome should be evaluated, not the mechanics of achieving it.

CRITICAL PATHWAYS

In the United States, managed care via case management is being introduced and used as a cost-effective, high-quality patient care delivery system in many institutions across the country. Critical pathways are at the core of the case management approach. **Critical pathways**, or maps, show the outcome of predetermined patient goals over a period of time, i.e., they state what activity the patient should be capable of performing daily based on the patient's Diagnostic Related Grouping (DRG). The critical incidents, or most crucial nursing interventions for each step of the pathway, are delineated.

One of the advantages of critical pathways is the early recognition of variances from the path. Once the variance is identified, the nurse, in collaboration with other members of the health care team, plans and implements specific interventions to deal with the variance. Evaluation is performed on a daily basis by the case manager, the primary nurse, or other designee.

Although the terminology is different, critical pathways incorporate the assessment, planning, implementation, and evaluation phases of the nursing process. Nursing diagnoses are not usually incorporated into critical pathways. Mention is made of this managed care delivery system because of its increasing popularity in inpatient, outpatient, and community settings, where critical pathways are replacing the nursing care plan as a documentation tool.

DOCUMENTING THE NURSING PROCESS

There are many methods that nurses use to document the nursing process, including the progress note and the nursing care plan. The progress note documents the patient's progress toward achieving stated outcomes. There are many different progress note charting systems in use such as SOAPIE (subjective data, objective data, analysis of data stated as a nursing diagnosis, plan, intervention/implementation, evaluation), PIO (problem, intervention, outcome), DAR (data, action, response/revision), and PIE (problem, intervention, evaluation). Each charting method has advantages and disadvantages. Check your institution's policy on charting directives.

The **nursing care plan** combines the elements of the nursing process to document the progress of patient care in a standardized fashion. Nursing care plans serve as a means of communicating patient progress with other health care colleagues and ensuring continuity of care among the nursing staff.

✓ **NURSING CHECKLIST**
Nursing Process Review

1. Apply all five phases of the nursing process to address different patient problems.

2. Begin with a thorough assessment of the patient, using a health history, physical assessment, and laboratory data and diagnostic procedures. Document findings.

3. Formulate and prioritize nursing diagnoses according to the patient's status. Record on the patient's clinical record.

4. Work with the patient to develop mutually agreeable and achievable outcomes and interventions.

5. Implement actions in conjunction with other members of the health care team.

6. Evaluate patient progress toward achieving outcomes.

7. Continually reassess and reprioritize diagnoses and outcomes as the patient's status changes in order to provide the best patient care.

8. Document the patient's progress toward outcomes.

SAMPLE CASE STUDY AND NURSING CARE PLAN

Health History

10/7/__(yr)

E.B. is a 24-year-old paraplegic male admitted for treatment of sacral decubitus. Fifteen months ago, E.B. fell off of a balcony; blood alcohol level was 170 mg/dl; suffered spinal cord laceration at eighth cervical nerve; spent 2 months at rehabilitation center then discharged to home in wheelchair; mother moved to a wheelchair-accessible house; today, mother noted large decubitus on E.B.'s sacrum; she contacted home health nurse who examined E.B. and recommended hospitalization; mother states "he has not coped well with his paraplegia; he refuses to eat and drinks heavily. He may not leave his bedroom for days and then he goes out and does not return for days. He refuses to associate with his friends. I've done everything I can think of for him. He has never recovered from the shock of his accident. Please, help him, help us." Upon admission, E.B. stated "I don't want to be here. I can't deal with this anymore! I'm worthless. Just let me alone. If you can't make me walk, then get out of here!" (E.B. threw a water pitcher at the nurse after this comment.)

Physical Assessment Data

General appearance: dirty, torn, malodorous clothing; hair straggly and knotted; face and hands dirty
Vital signs: temperature: 100.5°F orally; pulse: 88 and regular; respirations: 24 and regular; blood pressure: 104/72
Height: 69 inches (175 cm)
Weight: 111 pounds (50 kg)
Skin: 4-inch red circular decubitus on midsacral area; small area of purulent drainage at 5:00 position

Laboratory Data

Pending

Nursing Diagnoses

Some of the nursing diagnoses (in order of priority) for E.B. include:

1. *Impaired Skin Integrity related to lack of pressure releases by patient as evidenced by sacral decubitus.*
2. *Altered nutrition: Less than body requirements related to refusal to eat as evidenced by being 30 pounds less than ideal body weight.*
3. *Situational low self-esteem related to perception of lack of self-worth secondary to paraplegia as evidenced by verbalizations.*
4. *Caregiver role strain (mother) related to family member with significant home care needs as evidenced by mother's verbalizations.*

NURSING CARE PLAN

The top three nursing diagnoses are developed into a nursing care plan to demonstrate appropriate documentation.

Nursing Diagnosis #1
10/7
Impaired skin integrity related to lack of pressure releases by patient as evidenced by sacral decubitus.

Short-Term Outcome
E.B.'s sacral decubitus will be 3½ inches in diameter by 10/21.

continued

Nursing Interventions

1. Turn the patient every 2 hours (side to side).
   Rationale: Prolonged pressure on a body part decreases capillary blood flow to that portion of the body that can result in skin breakdown.

2. Massage the back and bony prominences every 2 hours.
   Rationale: These techniques improve blood circulation to the skin.

3. Apply an egg crate mattress to the bed.
   Rationale: Therapeutic mattresses help to equally distribute the weight of the body to decrease the likelihood of excessive pressure in one area.

4. Clean and dress decubitus every 8 hours.
   Rationale: Debridement of the wound enhances healing. The use of aseptic technique during dressing changes decreases the risk of infection.

5. Maintain clean sheets without wrinkles.
   Rationale: Clean sheets decrease the risk of infecting the decubitus. Wrinkled sheets exert more pressure on the body and lead to skin breakdown.

6. Remind the patient to perform pressure releases every hour (when in bed use trapeze).
   Rationale: Pressure releases restore capillary flow to affected areas. Having the patient actively participate is essential to ensure that the patient understands and has some control over his care.

7. Assess and record the appearance of the decubitus every shift.
   Rationale: The nurse and other members of the health care team will be able to follow the healing/nonhealing status of the decubitus.

8. Consult enterostomal therapist or skin specialist.
   Rationale: These professionals are educated in the prevention and treatment of skin pathology.

Evaluation

10/21

E.B.'s sacral decubitus now measures 3¾ inches with no purulent drainage. Continue plan of care and reevaluate in 1 week.

Nursing Diagnosis #2

10/7

Altered nutrition: Less than body requirements related to refusal to eat as evidenced by being 30 pounds less than ideal body weight.

Short-Term Outcome

Patient will gain 1 pound by 10/14.

Nursing Interventions

1. Record intake of food.
   Rationale: An accurate description of the types and quantities of ingested food will allow the nurse to calculate daily caloric intake.

2. Assess the patient's food likes and dislikes; obtain the patient's desired food.
   Rationale: E.B. is more likely to eat foods that he likes.

3. Encourage the patient to complete the daily menu.
   Rationale: The patient is more likely to eat food that was requested. It also involves E.B. in his own care.

4. Encourage E.B.'s mother to bring in her son's favorite foods when possible.
   Rationale: E.B. is more likely to eat foods that he enjoys. It also involves his mother in his care.

5. Provide a pleasant eating environment.
   Rationale: A pleasant environment provides an appropriate atmosphere for eating.

6. If possible, have the patient eat with others.
   Rationale: Eating serves a social as well as a nutritional function.

7. Weigh the patient today and every 3 days on the same scale at the same time with the same clothes.
   Rationale: Consistency in these factors provides a more accurate body weight.

continued

Evaluation

10/14

E.B. gained ½ lb (0.23 kg) after 1 week; consult a nutritional specialist and continue plan as written.

Nursing Diagnosis # 3

10/7

Situational low self-esteem related to perception of lack of self-worth secondary to paraplegia as evidenced by verbalizations.

Short-Term Outcome

Patient will identify two positive attributes about himself by 10/10.

Nursing Interventions

1. Use a nonjudgmental attitude.
   Rationale: E.B. is less likely to feel threatened by the nurse if he feels that the nurse is not judging him.

2. Use active listening.
   Rationale: In active listening, the nurse hears what the patient is saying and processes this information to give it meaning in the clinical context.

3. Talk with the patient for 5 minutes twice during each shift.
   Rationale: The nurse's therapeutic use of self will convey trust and a caring attitude to the patient.

4. Praise the patient for his accomplishments.
   Rationale: E.B. may begin to feel more positive about himself if he realizes that others see positive attributes in him.

5. Investigate self-help/support group availability.
   Rationale: Self-help and support groups may empower E.B. to assume responsibility for his actions and his life.

6. Provide for social interaction with other patients if feasible.
   Rationale: Allowing E.B. to interact with other patients may provide him with the opportunity to express his feelings to other individuals.

7. Encourage verbalization of feelings; discuss coping strategies.
   Rationale: E.B. needs to have the opportunity to express his feelings so he can recognize his emotions and learn to deal with them in a constructive manner. The nurse is in a position to discuss appropriate coping strategies to deal with these emotions.

Evaluation

10/10

E.B. refuses to talk about his condition and his future. Continue interventions and consult with a mental health clinical nurse specialist.

REVIEW QUESTIONS AND ACTIVITIES

1. Each of the following nursing diagnoses is stated incorrectly. Rewrite the nursing diagnoses so they are worded correctly.
   a. Appendectomy
   b. Poor gas exchange because of pneumonia
   c. Altered nutrition due to chemotherapy
   d. Decrease in cardiac output as evidenced by loss of 1200 cc from chest tubes in 1 hour
   e. High risk for aspiration due to patient's supine position
   f. High risk for poisoning related to parent's poor child rearing
   g. Knowledge deficit of breastfeeding

2. Each of the following patient outcomes is stated incorrectly. Rewrite the patient outcomes so they are worded correctly.
   a. Nurse should suction the patient frequently.
   b. Patient will understand how to administer insulin.
   c. Patient will have fewer outbursts.
   d. Patient will gain 2 pounds.
   e. Communicate clearly to the patient.

3. Each of the following interventions is stated incorrectly. Rewrite the interventions so they are worded correctly.
   a. Record patient's weight.
   b. Administer pain medication frequently.
   c. Patient will be able to walk 5 feet by the end of the week.
   d. Talk about patient's diet.

4. A.Z. is an 87-year-old female who was admitted with a left hip fracture after falling down the stairs at home today. A.Z. states that she got up in the middle of the night to go to the bathroom, tripped on the throw rug, and fell down 15 steps. After gaining consciousness, she crawled to the phone to call for help (she lives alone). She has a history of hypertension, myocardial infarction, diabetes mellitus, cataracts, and glaucoma. A.Z. admits to taking medications for her health problems but is unsure of the doses. "I take them when I remember."
   a. Formulate all of the nursing diagnoses for A.Z.
   b. Prioritize the nursing diagnoses according to Maslow's hierarchy.
   c. Write a nursing care plan for A.Z.

5. Formulate additional nursing diagnoses for the patient E.B. from the sample nursing care plan on pages 13–15.

6. Which of the following statements best describes an actual nursing diagnosis?
   a. Problem oriented; describes human responses that have been validated
   b. Human response to health conditions/life processes which may develop in a vulnerable individual, family, or community
   c. Focuses on the strengths of a patient
   d. None of the above
   The correct answer is (a).

7. Which of the following patient outcomes is stated correctly?
   a. Nurse should plan a multidisciplinary patient conference.
   b. Patient will understand etiology of multiple sclerosis.
   c. Record patient intake and output.
   d. Patient's oxygen saturation will be greater than 95% by the end of the shift.
   The correct answer is (d).

8. Which of the following series shows the correct progression of Maslow's hierarchy?
   a. Self-actualization, self-esteem, safety and security needs, love and belonging, physiological needs
   b. Physiological needs, safety and security needs, self-actualization, self-esteem, love and belonging
   c. Self-actualization, love and belonging, safety and security needs, self-esteem, physiological needs
   d. Physiological needs, safety and security needs, love and belonging, self-esteem, self-actualization
   The correct answer is (d).

2

The Patient Interview

The nursing health assessment interview is a purposeful, time-limited verbal interaction between the nurse and the patient. It is initiated to collect specific information regarding the patient and the patient's health status. Other purposes include validating appropriate health and illness information presented by the patient or found in the patient's record, and identifying the patient's knowledge of personal health and illness status. Accurate and complete information about the patient serves as a foundation for subsequent nurse-patient interactions and for medical and nursing interventions. The nurse-patient interaction requires skill in interviewing techniques, which the nurse can learn and refine.

THE PATIENT INTERVIEW

The nursing assessment interview can be differentiated from the more traditional medically oriented interview. The medical interview typically focuses on the patient's physical or emotional state, while the nursing interview is more holistic in nature and includes information about the total patient. The nursing interview includes an assessment of physical, mental, emotional, social, cultural, and spiritual aspects of the patient. Data are collected concerning the patient's present and past states of health, including the patient's family status and relationships, cultural background, lifestyle preferences, and developmental level. Other factors considered in data collection are the patient's self-concept, religious affiliation, social supports, sexuality, and reproductive processes.

The Role of the Nurse

The nurse is often the first person from the health care team to interact with the patient. The nurse frequently assumes the role of intermediary for the patient to the larger health care system. A critical role of the nurse is to assist the patient in effectively utilizing the system. The climate and tone of the initial patient interview may influence all future interactions the patient has in the health care setting. The nurse's attitude and expectations, both positive and negative, set the stage for the interview.

First impressions of individuals are important and imprint long-lasting thoughts and feelings. The personal appearances of both the patient and the nurse contribute significantly to the formation of first impressions. In American culture, health care providers who present a professional appearance that is appropriate for the particular setting in which they work are more readily accepted. Likewise, the manner in which the patient physically presents to the nurse may influence the nurse's perceptions of the patient.

The nurse is the facilitator of the interview and thus collaborates with the patient in establishing a mutually respectful dialogue. Encouraging the patient to speak freely and expressing concern for the patient are essential in this process. For example, if the patient thinks that no one in the health care setting can understand what is said, the patient will likely say very little. Because accurate data collection is the primary purpose of the interview, the patient must feel comfortable and safe enough to provide information, to ask questions, and to express fears or concerns. You can foster an atmosphere of safety and comfort by approaching each patient with an accepting, respectful, nonjudgmental attitude.

The Role of the Patient

The patient is an active and equal participant in the interview process and should feel free to openly communicate thoughts, feelings, perceptions, and

ꙮ THINK ABOUT IT

Being Nonjudgmental

You just landed a job in a clinic. This is your first day on the job and your second patient is an elderly woman. In assisting her to disrobe, you notice a roach on her undergarment. How do you respond?

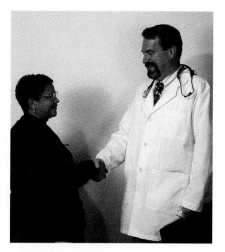

Figure 2-1 Beginning the interview with a friendly introduction will help the patient to feel at ease.

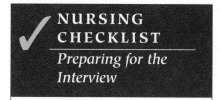

✓ **NURSING CHECKLIST**

Preparing for the Interview

1. Gather all available patient information.
2. Seek out an appropriate setting for the interview.
3. Set aside a block of time for the interview.
4. Assess yourself for possible problematic thoughts or feelings.
5. Begin the interview with a friendly introduction.
   - Introduce yourself by name and title.
   - Call the patient by formal name, i.e., Mrs. Adams.

factual information. Most patients possess previous knowledge of or experience with the health care system that influences their current perceptions and behavior. Understanding how patients see their role in this system is vital to the successful completion of any health interview. In some cultures, passivity in health care matters is the norm (see Chapter 5). However, powerlessness is contrary to the active participation required of the patient in the interview process.

In today's health care arena, patients are taking a more active role in both their own health care and in health care decisions. Patients are much more apt to question health care providers, to treat themselves, and to demand a role in decision making than patients of 10 years ago (Bradley & Edinberg, 1990). Frequently, patients actively seek health care providers who possess clinical competence as well as a willingness to provide individualized attention in a genuine, caring relationship (see Figure 2-1).

FACTORS INFLUENCING THE INTERVIEW

Approach

Prior to approaching the patient, gather all available patient information. Admission data and past medical records are often available and may significantly reduce the time needed for the interview.

Begin the interview with an introduction including your name and title. Initially call the patient by his or her formal name and ask how the patient prefers to be addressed. Simple communication utilizing appropriate names is respectful and helps identify patients as unique persons at a time when they may be feeling quite anxious. Giving recognition helps to lower patient anxiety and increase patient comfort level.

Examples of approaches you can use:
  "Good morning, Mrs. Harris."
  "Hello, Mr. Carpenter, it has been a long time since you were last here."

Providing the patient with an explanation of what is to follow and an approximate time frame for the interview helps in establishing trust. This information also helps to increase the patient's feeling of control. The more effective you are in establishing trust, the easier it will be to obtain information from the patient, for example: "Good morning, Mr. Rapt, my name is Susan Hosta. I'm a registered nurse. I am going to ask you some questions about why you are here today."

Environment

The setting for the interview has a direct influence on the amount and quality of information gathered. Time and effort spent in seeking out an appropriate setting for the interview indicates concern for the patient and for the quality and quantity of information collected. Whenever possible, the interview should be conducted in a private room with controlled lighting and temperature. When a private setting is impossible, control the environment to minimize distractions and interruptions and to increase the comfort level of the patient. Utilize any physical barriers available in the room to provide as much privacy as possible. When all efforts to ensure even minimal privacy fail, conduct a shortened interview to gather only immediately pertinent information. Defer the complete interview until a later time when privacy can be ensured.

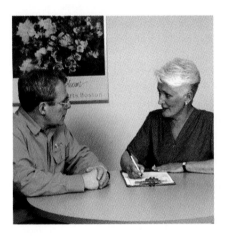

Figure 2-2 Write down important information during the interview, while maintaining your focus on the patient.

Confidentiality

Confidentiality is essential in developing trust between nurse and patient. The patient's willingness to communicate private and personal information is predicated on the assumption that this information will be used with discretion and for the benefit of the patient. Your verbal assurance of confidentiality often eases the patient's concerns and fosters trust in the relationship. In practice, there are certain exceptions to absolute confidentiality. For example, in a teaching institution where a team approach is used, information must be shared. Another important reason for sharing confidential information is when the patient is a danger to self or others. Nurses need to be familiar with institutional policy on patient confidentiality and the consequences of not adhering to it. It is essential to inform the patient prior to the interview when information will be shared with others.

Note Taking

Although it is advisable to jot down information during the interview, the simple act of writing down what the patient says may cause some patient discomfort. Early in the interview, explain the necessity of jotting down pertinent information and show the patient the form you will be using. You will become adept in skills that expedite charting information. Frequently, the patient will lead the interview or discuss sensitive issues. When this occurs, give full attention to the patient and defer formal recording of information. Jot down short phrases, words and dates that can be used to complete formal data recording following the interview (refer to Figure 2-2).

Time, Length, Duration

In order to become fully involved with the patient, enough time must be set aside for the interview. When scheduling an interview, look at the patient's daily activities, then select a block of time for the interview that does not conflict with the patient's mealtime or other planned activities.

Biases and Preconceptions

Personal belief and value systems, attitudes, biases, and preconceptions of both nurse and patient influence the sending and receiving of messages. The cultural and family contexts of each serve as a lens for interpreting societal views on ethnicity, gender, and health care. Nurses' and patients' views of themselves as cultured and gendered beings are highly influential in how they think and feel about health and illness and have an impact on how they respond to different clinical situations. For example, the nurse may unintentionally treat male and female patients differently, even in something as simple as addressing the patient (i.e., "Mr. Johnson" versus "Jessie"). The nurse must be sensitive to personal as well as patient contexts in order to treat all patients fairly and respectfully.

The nurse's subjective impressions of the patient may lead to faulty assumptions about patient abilities or illnesses. For example, a patient who appears thin and frail may be viewed by the nurse as seriously ill or unable to participate in activities of daily living when, in fact, this patient may not be seriously ill or incapacitated in any way. To counter faulty assumptions, biases, and preconceptions, continually validate information and personal impressions through the use of careful data gathering and effective interviewing techniques.

Generally, the nurse's subjective feelings during the interview are an indication of the climate of the interview and can be used to provide additional assessment information. For example, the nurse's feelings of anxiety during an

Gender-Biased Expectations

Feminist nursing leaders have asserted that the health care delivery system is patriarchal and that the health care needs of women are frequently overlooked. In addition, traditional sex-role beliefs support the idea that women bear primary responsibility for family well-being.

- How might gender-biased expectations of both nurse and patient affect the health assessment?
- Do you have any gender-biased expectations of women either as patients or as care providers?
- What measures could you take to deliver gender-conscious nursing care?

Decreasing Anxiety

Remember the last time that you were anxious. How did you demonstrate that anxiety (behaviorally, physically, etc.)? What did you do that helped you to calm down? Identify some specific actions you might take to decrease a patient's anxiety during the joining phase of the interview process.

Encouraging Active Listening

Remember the last time that you attempted to talk with someone who didn't appear to be listening. How did that make you feel? What kind of things did you do to get your message across? How many times have you listened to patients with "half an ear"? What might cause you to do this? Identify some specific actions that you might take to ensure that your patients feel heard.

interview may be an indication or a reflection of the patient's feelings of fear, anxiety, or anger. Careful attention to these feelings may direct you to change the interview format (to lower patient anxiety) or to refocus the questions (to gather specific data).

STAGES OF THE INTERVIEW PROCESS

There are three stages in the interview process: the introduction or the joining stage, the working stage, and the termination stage.

Stage I

The **joining stage** is the introduction or first stage of the interview process during which the nurse and the patient establish trust and get to know one another. Work with the patient to define the relationship and establish goals for this and any subsequent interactions.

Stage II

The **working stage** of the interview process is the time during which the bulk of the patient data is collected. It is a nursing responsibility to keep the interview goal directed, including refocusing the patient and redefining the goals established in the joining stage.

Stage III

The **termination stage** is the last stage of the interview process, during which information is summarized and validated. During this stage, give the patient an indication of the amount of time left in the interview, and allow the patient the opportunity to give additional information and make comments or statements. For example, "We have about 5 minutes more, Mr. Raferty, is there anything else you would like to add or mention?" Other important steps in the termination stage are summarizing and validating information and planning for future interviews.

FACTORS AFFECTING COMMUNICATION

Listening

Active listening, or the act of perceiving what is said both verbally and nonverbally, is a critical factor in conducting a successful health assessment interview. According to Bradley and Edinberg (1990), the primary goal of active listening is to decode patient messages in order to understand the situation or problem as the other person sees it. Pay careful attention to all sensory data to make sense of the patient's message and formulate an appropriate response. Beware of how personal characteristics, choice of communication techniques, and the manner and timing of their use can all affect communication.

Nonverbal Cues

Nonverbal communication is communicating a message without words. Nonverbal behaviors effectively supplement the spoken word and provide information about both nurse and patient. These behaviors can provide insight into the patient's cultural expectations, current physical and emotional states, and perceived self-image. Nonverbal cues such as body position, nervous repetitive movements of the hands or legs, rapid blinking, lack of eye contact, yawning, fidgeting, excessive smiling or frowning, and repetitive clearing of the throat may be indications of the patient's health and/or feelings that the patient may not feel comfortable expressing verbally.

Health care settings often evoke a great deal of anxiety, uncertainty, and/or fear in patients. Loss of personal control is a major obstacle confronting patients in health care settings, whether they are seriously ill or not (Northouse & Northouse, 1992). In an attempt to maintain some control in unfamiliar circumstances and to decrease anxiety, patients frequently look to nurses for cues on how to behave or how to respond to questions. Nonverbal acts by the nurse can indicate empathy and attention or indifference and inattention. Such behaviors powerfully influence patient comfort levels, feelings of control, and willingness to share information. Because of this, nurses need to continuously monitor their own nonverbal behaviors.

Distance

The amount of space a person considers appropriate for interaction is a significant factor in the interview process and is determined in part by cultural influences. In the United States, distances are generally categorized as follows:

- Personal distance is approximately 1.5 to 4 feet.
- Social distance is approximately 4 to 12 feet.
- Public distance is approximately 12 feet or more.

Personal distance is the most intimate and often involves some touching or physical contact. Personal distance may provide for ease of communication such as in cases of hearing impairment. But in some cases, personal distance may be threatening or invasive to the patient. Social distance is considered appropriate for the interview process because it allows for good eye contact and for ease in hearing and in seeing the patient's nonverbal cues (see Figure 2-3). Public distance is usually used in formal settings such as in a classroom where the teacher stands in front of the class. It is not considered appropriate for an interview.

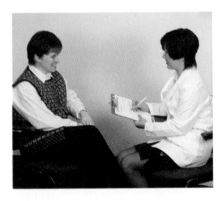

Figure 2-3 Appropriate distance between the nurse and the patient during the interview will facilitate the information-gathering process.

Territory

Territory can be defined as the space over which a person claims ownership. In an inpatient health care agency, the patient's hospital room and bathroom are considered the patient's territory. The patient may be very protective of this space and consider unauthorized use of it as an invasion of privacy.

EFFECTIVE INTERVIEWING TECHNIQUES

Effective interviewing techniques facilitate and/or support interactions between the nurse and the patient and foster their continuation. These techniques encompass both verbal and nonverbal approaches. The more skilled you can become in understanding the communication process, the more effectively you can use it in a purposeful, goal-directed manner to meet your needs for information and the patient's need for attention to health concerns or problems. Because individuals who come to a health care provider are frequently anxious, effectively communicating your interest and concern greatly enhances the interview/interaction.

Certain specific verbal communication techniques are available to help you facilitate this interaction. The effectiveness of these techniques will vary from

♣ ASK YOURSELF

Personal Territory

When was the last time you invited someone to sit on your bed? Who was this person? What would you think if a stranger sat on your bed? How would you feel about this? What would your reaction be?

individual to individual. At first, these techniques may feel awkward, stilted, or forced; keep in mind that communicating effectively is a learned skill (similar to other nursing skills) and, as such, improves with practice.

Open-Ended Questions

Open-ended questions encourage the patient to provide general rather than more focused information. Beginning the health assessment interview with open-ended questions provides the patient with a sense of control, leaving the choice of what to say, how much to say, and how to say it up to the patient. These questions indicate respect for the patient's ability to articulate important or pressing health concerns and therefore to help set priorities.

Examples of open-ended questions:

"What are some of your concerns about caring for your mother at home?"

"How do you typically deal with an asthma attack?"

"What caused you to believe that you might be drinking too much?"

Open-ended questions that begin with the words *how, what, where, when,* and *who* are usually more effective in eliciting the maximum amount of information than those that begin with the word *why. Why* questions can cause patients to become defensive and feel the need to somehow explain or defend their ideas and behaviors, thus setting up an adversarial relationship between nurse and patient. While open-ended questions are quite helpful in the health assessment interview, they can be time-consuming andmay not be appropriate in situations requiring rapid access to information and rapid response by health care providers. Overuse of this type of question, especially with the patient who is confused, vague in his or her responses, or just extremely talkative can cause the nurse to miss important information.

In certain situations, perhaps due to anxiety or unfamiliarity with the health care system, patients may attempt to ascertain what answers the nurse wants and what areas the nurse seems to feel are important. The patient will then focus on those, rather than on areas that are most important to the patient. With open-ended questions, you can encourage the patient to define what is important.

Closed Questions

Closed questions are those that somehow regulate or restrict patient response. They can frequently be answered with a "yes" or a "no." Closed questions can be used to focus the interview, pinpoint specific areas of concern, and elicit valuable information quickly and efficiently.

Examples of effective closed questions:

"Are you thinking of hurting yourself?"

"Has this type of allergic reaction ever happened to you before?"

"Are your contractions getting stronger?"

However, if used too frequently, closed questions can disrupt communication because they limit patient responses and interaction. Even well-directed closed questions may take the initiative away from the patient (Ivey, 1994), implying that the nurse is in charge of the interview, does most of the work, often knows the answer to the question asked, and is directing the patient's response.

Examples of ineffective closed questions:

> "Is your breathing better than the last time you were here?"
> "Do you still feel sad and depressed?"
> "Are you afraid to tell your parents that you are sexually active?"
> "Does being sick upset you?"

Encouraging Talking

Once the health assessment interview has started, there may be periods when patients stop talking due to anxiety, uncertainty, or embarrassment. You can use a variety of both verbal and nonverbal means to encourage patients to continue talking. Phrases such as "go on" or "uh-huh," the simple repetition of key words the patient has spoken, or even head nods prompt the patient to resume speaking and also indicate your continued interest and attention.

Silence

Silence, too, has its place in the assessment interview. Understood and used effectively by the nurse, periods of silence can help structure and pace the interview, convey respect and acceptance, and, in many cases, provide additional patient data. Silence on the part of the patient may indicate feelings of anxiety, confusion, or embarrassment, or simply a lack of understanding about the question asked or an inability to speak English. Nonverbal data such as these are often lost if the nurse is a persistent talker. Conversely, if overused, silence can contribute to an awkward, disjointed interview providing minimal structure or direction for the patient and little helpful data for the nurse.

Using silence effectively may seem like a difficult skill to master. Frequently, silences seem longer than they actually are. When silences occur, you may feel discomfort and pressure to speak in order to be actually "doing" something therapeutic; instead, handle silences by being quiet and observing the patient's behavior for what is not being said verbally (Greenstone & Leviton, 1993).

Grouping Communication Techniques

Communication techniques often seem mechanical and artificial to the beginning nurse; one way to make them less so is to group or cluster them according to their primary purposes. Grouping communication strategies based on purpose helps to clarify the intent of each communication response (Cormier & Cormier, 1991) and indicate when in the assessment interview its use might be helpful. One simple way to group interview techniques is to divide them into two groups: listening responses and action responses.

Listening Responses

Listening responses are attempts made by the nurse to accurately receive, process, and then respond to patient messages. They provide one way for the nurse to communicate empathy, concern, and attentiveness. Patients "need to know that the interviewer has heard what they have been saying, seen their point of view, and felt their world as they experience it" (Ivey, 1994, p. 99). In order to "listen" to what the patient says, the nurse must not only process the words spoken by the patient but also understand the context of the patient's experience.

Listening responses provide the nurse with a vehicle for understanding the patient's perspective. Patients will realize that they are heard and that you are working for and with them to elicit and clarify health concerns. Listening responses include: making observations, restating, reflecting, clarifying, sequencing, encouraging comparisons, and summarizing.

Making Observations When making observations, the nurse verbalizes perceptions about the patient's behavior, then shares them with the patient. Calling to attention personal behavior about which the patient might be unaware may prove insightful and help increase the patient's conscious awareness of his or her behavior. Sharing observations is also a way to reinforce patient competency and sense of control in an environment or situation where a patient often feels out of control, uncertain, or overwhelmed.

Examples of making observations:

"Speaking about these symptoms seems to make you tense. I notice that you are clenching your fists and grimacing."

"I notice that each time you've been confronted with that particular problem, you've known how to handle it appropriately."

Restating Restating involves repeating or rephrasing the main idea expressed by the patient and lets the patient know that you are paying attention. It promotes further dialogue and provides the patient with an opportunity to explain or elaborate on an issue or concern.

Examples of restating:

Patient: I don't sleep well anymore. I find myself waking up frequently at night.
Nurse: You're having difficulty sleeping? **or**
Nurse: You don't sleep well?

Reflecting Reflection is another listening response; it focuses on the content of the patient's message as well as the patient's feelings. In reflecting, the nurse directs the patient's own questions, feelings, and ideas back to the patient and provides an opportunity for the patient to reconsider and/or expand on what was just said. The patient's point of view is given value, and the nurse, although indicating an interest in what the patient has to say, refrains from giving advice, passing judgment, or assuming responsibility for the patient's thoughts or feelings.

Examples of reflecting:

Patient: Do you think I should tell the doctor I stopped taking my medication?
Nurse: What do you think about that?
Patient: Well, yes, I think that I probably should. Not taking my medication could be one of the reasons I'm feeling so run-down. But that medication just makes me so teary and agitated.
Nurse: You sound a bit agitated now. It seems as if you've been thinking about this a lot.
Patient: I told that young doctor that I had problems with this medication and he just didn't listen.
Nurse: Sounds as if you are pretty angry with him.

Clarifying Clarifying is a communication technique used by the nurse to make clear something the patient says or to pinpoint the message when the patients' words and nonverbal behavior do not agree. Be sure you understand exactly what the patient means before continuing, because communication may stop if the patient feels misunderstood or not heard. Distortions or misunderstandings about patient data can occur if the nurse interprets patient statements using only personal experiences and/or perceptions. Even more crucial is the fact that making assumptions may cause the interviewer to proceed from a faulty database.

Example of a clarifying response:

Patient: During certain activities, I have the most awful pain in my back.
Nurse: Tell me what you mean by awful. **or**
Nurse: I'm not sure that I follow you — when does this pain occur?

Example of a problematic response, involving an assumption:

Patient: We hardly have any time for exercise in our family. We are so busy.
Nurse: I know what you mean!

Sequencing To effectively assess patient needs, the nurse often requires knowledge of a time frame within which symptoms and/or problems developed or occurred. One way of getting at this information involves asking the patient to place a symptom, a problem, or an event in its proper sequence. Sequencing also helps both patient and nurse become aware of any patterns in the patient's behavior that might indicate recurring themes. They can relate to feelings (depression or anxiety), behavior (refusal to take appropriate medications, consistently putting self in risky situations), or experiences (being beaten, being hurt, being misunderstood by health care providers). Pattern identification provides the nurse with clues for further focus.

Examples of sequencing:

Nurse: Did this sharp pain occur each time you had sexual intercourse or only when you didn't empty your bladder first? **or**
Nurse: What specific events led you to feel overwhelmed and suicidal?

Encouraging Comparisons Encouraging comparisons is a technique that enables both participants in the health assessment interview to become more aware of patterns, themes, or specific symptomatology in the patient's life. It also helps the patient to deal more effectively with unfamiliar situations by placing the symptoms or problems in the context of something else that is familiar and therefore more comfortable to the patient. Often, an awareness of successful prior dealings with similar situations increases patient confidence levels and self-care potentials.

Examples of encouraging comparisons:

Nurse: Have you had similar experiences? **or**
In what way was this allergy attack different from or the same as your previous ones? **or**
In what way was your reaction to this medication similar to or different from your reaction to other antibiotics you've taken before?

Summarizing Summarizations help patients to organize their thinking (Ivey, 1994). Because of this, summarizing is a communication technique that is especially useful at the end of the health assessment interview. A brief, concise review of the important points covered helps the patient identify anything that has been left out and provides the nurse with an opportunity to make sure that what he/she understood the patient to say is actually what was said. In addition, summarizing indicates interest and concern that the patient feels heard as well as finished.

Example of summarizing:

Nurse: During this past hour, you have shared with me several health concerns of which the most vexing to you is your difficulty in losing weight. Is that correct?

Summarizing also provides a means of smoothly transitioning to a new topic or section of the health assessment.

Example of transitioning:

Nurse: You talked about your past experience with diabetes and what happened to you yesterday, now let's talk about why you came in today.

Action Responses

Action responses are the second group of effective interviewing techniques. These responses stimulate patients to make some change in their thinking and behavior. Action responses include such communication techniques as: focusing, exploring, presenting reality, confronting, informing, collaborating, limit setting, and normalizing.

Focusing Focusing allows the nurse to concentrate on or "track" a specific point the patient has made. This technique is particularly useful with patients whose heightened anxiety level causes increased confusion, altered concentration, or jumping from topic to topic. With the nurse's assistance in focusing, the patient is able to proceed with the health history in a clearer, more organized, thoughtful, thorough manner.

Examples of focusing:

"Tell me more about the chest pain you experience when you begin to exercise." **or**
"You've mentioned several times that your wife is concerned about your smoking. Let's go back to that."

Exploring In exploring, the nurse is attempting to develop, in more detail, a specific area of content or patient concern. The purpose of exploring is to identify patterns or themes in symptom presentation or in the way patients handle problems or health concerns.

Examples of exploring:

"Tell me more about how you feel when you do not take your medication."
"Could you describe for me how you handle those periods in your life when you feel out of control?"

Presenting Reality This technique, while typically used with psychiatric or confused patients, is also useful in the health assessment interview when the nurse is confronted with a patient who exaggerates or makes grandiose statements. Presenting reality, when done in a nonargumentative way, encourages the patient to rethink a statement and perhaps modify it.

Example of presenting reality:

Patient: I can never get an appointment at this clinic.
Nurse: But Mr. Jasper, I've seen you several times in the past 4 months.
Patient: Well, yes, but I can never get an appointment at a time that is convenient for me.

Confronting Confronting is a verbal response that the nurse makes to some perceived discrepancy or incongruency in the patient's thoughts, feelings, or behaviors. Gently challenging an incongruency can help the patient reframe a situation in order to see things differently. Confrontation can be used to focus the patient's attention on some aspect of personal perception or behavior that, if changed, could lead to more effective or adaptive functioning (Cormier & Cormier, 1991). When confronting is used in a caring, empathetic manner, rather than a critical or accusatory one, patients feel encouraged to see themselves as competent and effective individuals.

Example of confronting:

Patient: I never know exactly which of my symptoms to pay attention to. I think I'm such a hypochondriac.

Nurse: You say that you're not sure which symptoms are important and yet it seems that you are very clear about those symptoms you thought were serious enough for you to seek medical care and which ones you felt comfortable managing on your own.

Informing Providing the patient with needed information, such as explaining the nature of and/or the reasons for any necessary tests or procedures, is a nursing action that can help build trust and decrease patient anxiety. In addition to providing patients with needed facts or details, information giving is appropriate when trying to help patients become aware of possible choices and then evaluate those choices correctly.

Example of informing:

Patient: Dr. Jones told me that I need to have my gallbladder taken out.

Nurse: Did you understand what Dr. Jones told you about your gallbladder surgery?

Patient: No, I didn't understand what he said about the new technique. He said something about a tube.

Nurse: There is a new technique where the surgeon inserts a tube in your abdomen to remove the gallbladder rather than making a cut, which is the usual procedure.

Patient: Yes, that was it, please tell me more about that.

Collaborating In collaboration, the patient is offered a relationship in which both nurse and patient work together, rather than one in which the nurse is in total control of the interaction. Use of this technique conveys the message that the patient has important personal knowledge and information to share. Collaboration provides a respectful way for the nurse to encourage patients' active involvement in their own health care, in setting goals, in gathering information, and in problem solving.

Example of collaborating:

Nurse: Perhaps you and I can talk further about your asthma and discover what specifically is making you so anxious.

Limit Setting During the interview with a seductive, hostile, or talkative patient, the nurse may find it necessary to set specific limits on patient behavior. If, for example, the patient persists in asking the nurse personal questions or rambles despite frequent attempts by the nurse to focus, it will be difficult to obtain information needed for task completion. This patient behavior may be a manifestation of stress produced by the interview situation itself or simply a characteristic specific to that particular patient. In such situations, patients may require some direction as to how to behave; provide guidance by calmly, clearly, and respectfully telling the patient what behavior is expected. Limit only the behavior that is problematic or detrimental to the purpose of the interview and avoid making a "big issue" of whatever it is that the patient is doing. When limit setting, do not argue or use empty threats or promises, but do offer the patient alternatives.

Example of ineffective limit setting:

"If you don't start answering my questions, we'll never finish and you'll never get to see the nurse-practitioner."

Example of appropriate limit setting:

Nurse: You know, it seems that you are feeling pretty unsure of how to behave now.

Patient: What do you mean?

Nurse: Well, you're asking me a lot of personal questions and generally making it difficult for me to find out what is bothering you. The reason you are here is because you have some health concerns. How can I help you more clearly tell me what brought you to the clinic?

Normalizing Very often, individuals faced with unexpected and/or life-threatening illnesses or possible surgeries respond in ways that seem extreme or out of the ordinary (i.e., becoming depressed or overly tearful, etc.). Normalizing allows the nurse to offer appropriate reassurance that their response may be quite common for this situation. This helps to decrease patient anxiety and encourages patients to share thoughts and feelings they might otherwise keep to themselves for fear of being judged or misunderstood. However, if used inappropriately or out of context, normalizing may give false reassurance.

Example of normalizing:

"It is no wonder that you've been feeling shocked and overwhelmed since you first found that lump in your breast. Most women who have that experience react in a similar way."

Nontherapeutic Interviewing Techniques

Just as there are certain communication techniques that facilitate communication between nurse and patient, there are also some interviewing techniques that change, distort, or block communication and should be avoided. Verbal and nonverbal behaviors that involve inattentiveness, imposition of values, judgment, lack of interest, or an "I know what's best for you" attitude hinder communication by creating distance rather than connection. Patients on the receiving end of these behaviors can feel angry, defensive, or incompetent and may refuse to actively participate. Such ineffective techniques include: requesting an explanation, probing, false reassuring, giving approval/disapproval, defending, and advising.

Requesting An Explanation Questions that begin with "why" are often perceived by the patient as challenging or threatening. Such questions ask the patient to provide a reason or justification for personal beliefs, feelings, thoughts, and behaviors and imply criticism (Aromando, 1995). If or when patients are unable to provide these answers, either from lack of sufficient knowledge or because the answer is not known to the patient (some questions are really unanswerable in that individuals are frequently unaware of why they do things), patients can feel inadequate, defensive, or angry. Asking the patient to describe the belief, feeling, or behavior is preferable to asking why. Providing a description about what happened often helps the patient elaborate. Enlarging the context provides opportunities for the patient to increase self-awareness and for the nurse to increase the store of relevant information.

Example #1 of requesting an explanation:

Patient: I guess I drink two or three six-packs of beer a weekend.

Nurse: Why do you drink that much?

Patient: That's not very much, every one of my friends drinks the same amount.

A more appropriate response in the preceding example might be:

Nurse: It sounds as if you might be concerned about the amount of beer you drink. (reflection)

Example #2 of requesting an explanation:
Patient: I'm not sure why I came to the clinic today; I just feel miserable. I don't want to see anyone. I just want to stay in bed with the covers pulled over my head.
Nurse: Why do you feel that way?
Patient: I don't know.

A more effective response would be: "What happened that caused you to feel so miserable?" (clarification) or "It sounds as if you are feeling rather overwhelmed today." (reflection)

Probing Repeated or persistent questioning of the patient about a statement or a behavior increases patient anxiety and can cause confusion, hostility, and a tendency to withdraw from the interaction. This patient withdrawal and the increasing periods of silence resulting from it can escalate the nurse's anxiety. Anxious nurses tend to become more active and more directive in the interview. The patient's unwillingness or hesitancy to discuss a certain event or health concern may indicate patient misunderstanding, misinformation, or a major problem area that needs further clarification or exploration.

A helpful rule of thumb for nurses to use in identifying probing is to pay particular attention to their own behavior and feelings. If, in attempting to gather information, nurses feel frustrated or irritated, feel that they are pursuing the patient, or have become involved in a verbal tug of war with the patient, then they are most likely probing. More useful responses may include going on to the next part of the health assessment interview, asking the patient's permission to return to this subject later if it seems likely that more information will be needed, or just sitting quietly until the patient begins to speak.

Examples of probing:
1. *Nurse:* What makes you drink a six-pack of beer after dinner each night?
   Patient: I'm not sure.
   Nurse: Well, are there things going on in your life right now that would cause you to drink that much?
   Patient: Not really.
   Nurse: I don't really think that you would drink that much if things weren't happening in your life right now.
2. *Nurse:* What makes you think that you have arthritis?
   Patient: I'm not sure, I just think I do. It just seems like I have the same health problems as my mother and she had arthritis.
   Nurse: Well, do you have pain?
   Patient: Yes. (pause)
   Nurse: Why do you think the pain is arthritis pain?

If nurses can be patient, identify and manage their own anxiety, and allow silences, useful discussion usually ensues.

False Reassurance False reassurances are vague and simplistic responses that question the patient's judgment, devalue and block patient feelings, and communicate a lack of understanding and sensitivity on the part of the nurse. The impulse to provide false reassurance typically originates in the nurse's own feelings of helplessness. Giving false reassurance is an attempt by the nurse to take care of herself or himself rather than the patient and to relieve personal feelings of anxiety. This behavior often increases patient anxiety. A more valuable nursing response would be to first acknowledge personal feelings of anxiety and then to acknowledge the patient's feelings.

Examples of false reassurance:

"Everything will be fine."
"I wouldn't worry about that."
"There are hardly any problems with that type of surgery."

Example of an appropriate response:

"It must be frightening to think about the possibility of surgery."

Giving Approval or Disapproval During the health assessment interview, nurses can feel pressured to comment judgmentally on a patient's statement, feeling, or behavior, especially if these contradict the nurse's personal beliefs or feelings. Telling a patient what's right or wrong is moralizing. This may limit the patient's freedom to verbalize or behave in certain ways that might not please the nurse. Comments such as "What a good idea" or "You shouldn't feel that way," or "That is bad" hinder the nurse's attempts to establish rapport, support patient competence, and facilitate communication. When there is concern that the patient's expressed beliefs or personal behaviors are ill-informed, harmful, or destructive, the nurse might more effectively explore the source of the belief or the impact of the patient's behavior on others.

Examples of effective responses:

"What made you come to that conclusion?"
"What do you think the consequences will be if you continue to keep your illness from your wife?"
"How do you feel about withholding this information from your children?"

Defending Occasionally, patients who have had previous stressful or unpleasant experiences with physicians, hospitals, or other agents of the health care system will engage in criticism or verbal attack. It is not helpful for the nurse to defend the object of the attack. Defending implies that the patient has neither the right to hold such opinions or feelings nor the right to express them, especially if they are hostile or angry. The nurse will not be able to change the patient's opinions or feelings by defending the individual or the object attacked. Rather, deflection or criticism of patient feelings more often either blocks expression of these feelings or reinforces them. Defending is not therapeutic because it requires the nurse to speak not just for herself or himself, but for others, something that nurses truthfully and realistically are not able to do.

Examples of inappropriate responses:

"This hospital has an excellent reputation. I'm sure that if you were kept waiting as long as you say, there was a good reason."
"No one here would lie to you."
"I know that Dr. Cooke had your welfare in mind when she provided this information to social services."

It is more respectful and more useful to accept and support patients' rights to feel as they do and the right to express those feelings. The nurse can do this without agreeing with the expressed feelings. This empathetic behavior defuses any antagonism and minimizes patient resistance to the continued interaction.

Examples of appropriate responses:

Nurse: You sound pretty angry about your previous experiences in this hospital.

Patient: Of course I am. Wouldn't you be upset if no one ever told you what was going on and no one answered your call bell?

Nurse: I guess I'd be pretty upset if I thought people were not treating me respectfully. Have you told your doctor how you feel?

Advising Consistently telling a patient what to do does not foster competence. Advising encourages patients to look to others for answers, deprives them of the opportunity to learn from past mistakes, and discourages independent judgment. Because some patients may resort to dependent, passive behavior when faced with illness, it is important that the nurse not reinforce such dependence, but rather support the patient's healthy functioning as much as possible.

Example of ineffective responses:

Patient: Do you think that I should have an abortion?

Nurse: Well, if I were you, I'd certainly think long and hard before I'd have another child. You are having difficulty feeding the one you have now. **or**

Nurse: No, I think you should continue the pregnancy. Abortion is never the answer.

A more helpful response would be for the nurse to support the patient's own problem-solving ability through the use of therapeutic communication techniques such as exploring or reflection.

Examples of exploring:

"Tell me more about what made you consider an abortion."
"What other alternatives have you considered?"

Examples of reflection:

"Do you think you should?"
"How would you feel about having the abortion?"

Problematic Questioning Techniques

Experienced nurses as well as neophyte interviewers will find themselves, on occasion, feeling nervous and perhaps unsure of how to proceed at times during the health assessment interview. This anxiety can lead to the use of questioning techniques and interviewing responses that, while not specifically identified as nontherapeutic, are potentially problematic. Such techniques increase patient anxiety, decrease the flow of needed information, and have the potential to provide the nurse with irrelevant data. The following are several examples of problematic interviewing techniques.

Leading Questions Leading questions may indicate to the patient that the nurse already has a certain answer in mind. Their use can be intimidating to the patient and curtail further communication. This is especially true if these leading questions concern topics that the patient perceives as sensitive or possible sources of anxiety.

Examples of leading questions:

"You've never had any type of sexually transmitted diseases, have you, Miss Jenkins?" **or**
"Of course, you've told your daughter that her smoking really bothers you, Mr. Talbott, isn't that correct?"

Interrupting the Patient Changing the subject or interrupting the patient prevents completion of a thought or idea and introduces a new focus. Such behavior may ease the nurse's discomfort, but it shows a lack of respect and often just confuses or irritates the patient. Questions should focus on one particular topic until all relevant data have been collected and the patient feels finished. Changing the subject or interrupting cuts off the flow of ideas and communicates the message that whatever the patient was addressing is not as important as what the nurse wants to discuss next.

Talkativeness Extreme talkativeness may indicate nervousness and uncertainty on the part of the interviewer. Attempts to maintain control of the interview and ease personal anxiety can cause the nurse to talk more than necessary. Increased verbal activity minimizes patient spontaneity and can increase patient passivity, causing the nurse to work even harder at obtaining necessary information. The message to the patient is that what the nurse thinks is more important than what the patient thinks and feels.

Multiple Questions Nurses may confuse their patients by asking several questions at once. Too many questions may put patients on the defensive, minimizing patient participation and impeding the flow of necessary information.

Use of Medical Jargon The use of medical jargon or slang can be quite anxiety provoking for the patient. Nurses who belong to the larger health care system, which has its own culture and language, frequently use medical jargon; patients who may feel frightened and powerless in this unfamiliar environment are further disadvantaged by any perceived language barrier. The use of medical jargon can be seen by the patient as unwillingness to share or attempts to hide information, or it can give the impression that the nurse feels superior to the patient and is unwilling to engage in collaboration or mutual problem solving. Conduct the health assessment interview in language that is common to both participants and check periodically with the patient as to clarity; this will indicate an interest in the patient's perspective and a desire to work collaboratively.

INTERVIEWING THE PATIENT WITH SPECIAL NEEDS

Patients with special needs offer a particular challenge to the nurse during the interview. Although the goal of the interview and specific interviewing techniques remain the same, the process differs according to the patient's impairment. Conducting a successful assessment interview with the patient with special needs may require more time and effort than usual and often requires the help of an intermediary such as a family member or a friend of the patient.

The Hearing-Impaired Patient

Often, hearing-impaired patients will read lips, so it is important to remain within sight of the patient and face the patient when talking. When working with a hearing-impaired patient, ensure that background noise is at a minimum because noise can be very distracting to the patient with a hearing aid. Even if an **intermediary**, or an individual who is a liaison between the patient and a member of the health care team, is with the patient to assist in communication, always face the patient and direct all communication to the patient (see Figure 2-4). It is common for those speaking to a hearing-impaired person to speak loudly or slowly; both of these well-intentioned acts detract from the patient's ability to read lips. Tone and inflection of voice are lost to the hearing-impaired patient. However, other nonverbal cues such as facial expression and body movements can be used to convey the meaning of what is said.

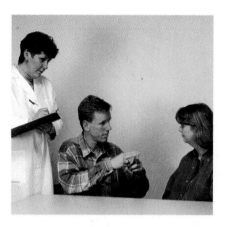

Figure 2-4 When using an interpreter during the interview, always direct your questions and attention to the patient.

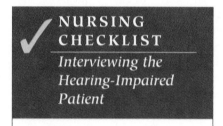

✓ **NURSING CHECKLIST**
Interviewing the Hearing-Impaired Patient

1. Check to see whether the patient wears a hearing aid. Be sure it is in working order and turned on.
2. Make every effort to move the patient to a setting with minimal background noise.
3. Always face the patient.
4. Speak in a normal tone and at a normal pace.
5. Determine whether or not the patient uses sign language. If signing is used, enlist the assistance of an interpreter.
6. Pay particular attention to nonverbal cues of the patient and to your own nonverbal behavior.
7. Provide a pen and paper to facilitate communication, if necessary.

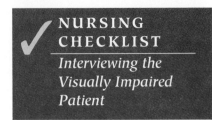

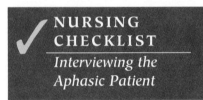

Patients who have never had the ability to hear and those who have not heard for a long time may have speech that is difficult to understand. Often, the best approach to interviewing these patients is to allow additional time with them and to use a written form for gathering data. When communicating through writing, always remain with the patient to clarify questions and answers.

The Visually Impaired Patient

When interviewing a patient with a visual impairment, always look directly at the patient as if the patient were sighted. Because they cannot rely on visual cues, voice intonation, volume, and inflection are important to the visually impaired. It is common for those speaking to a visually impaired patient to speak loudly; this is insulting and can hinder communication.

Touch is especially important to the visually impaired; however, an unanticipated touch can be frightening. Before touching the patient, be certain to inform the patient and ask permission to touch. Those patients who are partially sighted may cling to the independence that their limited vision allows; offer assistance to the partially sighted and follow their cues or responses.

The Speech-Impaired and Aphasic Patient

When interviewing the speech-impaired patient, ask simple questions that require yes and no answers. This allows the patient to give information quickly and competently. Using this technique, it is often necessary to convert open-ended questions such as "How are you today?" to closed questions such as "Are you feeling well now?" If you are unable to understand the patient's responses, use a written interview format, letter boards, or yes/no cards.

Even when all questions in the interview are asked and answered using closed questions, allow the aphasic patient the opportunity to contribute to the information gathering. For example, "I have asked all the questions I have to ask you for now. Would you like to tell me anything related to any of the questions I have asked?" then continue with, "Would you like to say anything else before we conclude the interview?"

When someone else is speaking for the patient, the nurse should speak and direct questions to the patient, not to the intermediary. If you ask the aphasic patient to complete a written format of the interview, remain with the patient to clarify questions and to explain data requirements.

The Non-English-Speaking Patient

Interviewing patients who do not speak English requires the assistance of an interpreter. Most health care agencies have a register of interpreters available. Sometimes the patient will bring a translator to the agency. The nurse should not assume that the translator can answer questions for the patient. It is important to direct interview questions to the patient and not to the interpreter.

Remember that pure translation from one language to another does not take into account dialects or **colloquialisms** (words and phrases particular to a community), which have the potential to offend someone. For example, the question "Are you pregnant?" when translated without taking into account colloquialisms may mean "Do you have intercourse outside of marriage?"

Pay special attention to nonverbal cues, especially facial expressions and body movements. Often, information that is lost in the translation to English can be gained through nonverbal cues. The use of signs, such as pointing, can be helpful in an emergency situation; however, a more complete interview should be deferred until an interpreter is present.

The Patient with Low IQ

Interviewing the patient with a low IQ requires time and patience, because the patient may require time to process questions and to formulate answers and may need clarification of the meaning or intent of questions. Hurrying may cause the patient to become confused, lose concentration, or to refuse to answer. It may be necessary to interview the patient's family or caregiver for supplemental information. Request permission from the patient to speak to someone else and respect the patient's right to be present during all phases of the interview. Always direct interview questions to the patient and allow the patient to request assistance from family members or the caregiver. Observe the interaction between the patient and the family or caregivers, because nonverbal communication can provide valuable information about the patient's present health/illness state as well as about the relationship between the patient and the family member or primary caregiver.

The Emotional Patient

Patients and those who are speaking for patients in health care settings are frequently emotionally upset. For example, the parent of a sick child may be overwhelmed by events that led to the child's hospitalization. Emotional outbursts and crying are often the result of such stress. Allow the patient, family member, or significant other to express emotions. If it is obvious that the person being interviewed is holding back tears, give permission to express emotion with a simple statement such as, "I can see that you are upset; it's ok to cry."

When interviewing an obviously angry person, recognize and acknowledge the emotion. A natural instinct is to personalize the anger and become angry in return; instead, recognize the emotion and bring it to the patient's attention. "You appear very angry about something. Before we continue with the interview, please tell me about your feelings." Avoid statements such as "take a moment to get hold of yourself," because this directive implies that the patient's feelings are not appropriate and should not be expressed. Acknowledging patients' emotions and giving them permission to express feelings will convey respect and enhance genuine communication.

The Very Ill Patient

Patients who are very sick may not have the strength or ability to go through the entire interview process. Collect pertinent data from the patient and defer the remainder of the interview until later. If a patient is very sick, it may be necessary to interview a family member or significant other. Show respect for the patient by asking permission to do this and by allowing the patient to be present during the interview. Allow the patient to participate as much as possible in answering questions and giving information.

The Sexually Aggressive Patient

A sexually aggressive patient may act out during the interview. For example, the patient may stand very close to the nurse and say, "You have been so nice to me, I would like the chance to be nice to you." The nurse may counter this behavior by defining appropriate boundaries, sharing personal reactions, and refocusing the patient, for example, stating, "It makes me feel very uncomfortable when you stand this close to me. I'm not sure what this has to do with the task at hand; let's get back to getting information to assist in your health care needs." It is important to set limits and to focus on tasks when dealing with sexually aggressive patients.

☺☺ THINK ABOUT IT

Handling Emotions

You are talking to the father of a child with a terminal disease. You feel very badly about the family situation and offer your assistance. The father says, "What do you want? You can't help us." or "It's too late for your help." How does this make you feel? What do you do or say next?

NURSING CHECKLIST
Interviewing the Hostile Patient

1. Before you begin the interview, review any available documentation that might alert you to potential problems. Be especially cautious of those patients with a history of past violence or poor impulse control.

2. Understand that patients use violence or aggressive behavior because it works to get them what they want (Morrison, 1992).

3. When interviewing patients with a potential for violence, do not position yourself in a corner from which you cannot easily exit if necessary. Arrange seating so that the patient is never between you and the door. Do not turn your back on the patient. Do not allow the patient to walk behind you.

4. Attend to patients' body language; notice anything unusual about their behavior, words, or dress.

5. Assess the risk for physical aggression. Watch for signs of increasing tension, i.e., clenched fists, loud, angry tone of voice, narrowed eyes, etc.

6. Remember that hostility tends to be contagious. Do not reciprocate anger and hostility.

7. Minimize the risk of aggression through nonthreatening interventions, such as limit-setting and refocusing.

8. Continually monitor your own reactions and feelings and respond in ways that meet your patient's emotional needs rather than your own.

9. If anxious, alert a colleague to your location and leave the door to the interview room open. This will provide you with an added sense of security and the patient with an added deterrent.

10. Respect the patient's feelings and the right to have those feelings. However, do not encourage excessive expression of feelings.

11. Remove yourself from potentially threatening situations and call for assistance, if necessary.

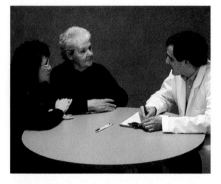

Figure 2-5 Family members, such as adult children or spouses, can provide valuable assistance during the interview process.

The Older Adult

Interviewing the older person may require additional time for question interpretation and patient responses. It is frequently necessary to schedule more than one interview for older patients because they may have multisystem changes and/or complaints, a weakened physical condition, or a cognitive impairment. It may be necessary to interview an older patient's family member or caregiver to assess the patient's past and present health/illness status. As in any interview situation when the patient is assisted by another individual, include the patient and assess the quality of interaction between the two (see Figure 2-5).

NURSING CHECKLIST
Effective Interviewing

- Be aware of personal beliefs and how these were acquired. Avoid imposing your beliefs on those you interview.

- Listen and observe. Attend to verbal and affective content as well as to nonverbal cues.

- Keep your attention focused on the patient. Do not listen with "half an ear." Do not think about other things when you are interviewing.

- Maintain eye contact with the patient.

- Notice the patient's speech patterns and any recurring themes. Note any extra emphasis that the patient places on certain words or topics.

- Do not assume that you understand the meaning of all patient communications. Clarify frequently.

- Paraphrase and summarize occasionally to help patients organize their thinking, clarify issues, and begin to explore specific concerns more deeply.

- Allow for periods of silence.

- Remember that attitudes and feelings may be conveyed nonverbally.

- Consistently monitor your reactions to the patient's verbal and nonverbal messages.

- Avoid being judgmental or critical. Avoid preaching.

- Avoid the use of nontherapeutic interview techniques.

REVIEW QUESTIONS AND ACTIVITIES

1. Conduct a patient interview on a colleague that is videotaped. Ask your colleague to critique your use of interviewing techniques, sensitivity, and style. Assess your own performance.

2. Review the videotape a second time and identify the nonverbal behaviors of both participants and the effects these behaviors have on communication.

3. During the interview, your patient says, "I don't feel good, I can't answer all these questions." What would an appropriate response be?

4. Your hearing-impaired patient has a hearing aid in the drawer. During the interview, the patient has difficulty hearing your questions. How would you handle this situation?

5. Your patient does not speak English and does not have anyone to interpret during the interview. You request that a hospital interpreter work with you. List some ways you would adapt the interview process in this situation.

6. Explain how you would adapt the interview process to meet the communication needs of the elderly patient.

7. For each of the following statements, identify which nontherapeutic techniques are used and suggest ways to transform the statements into more effective ones.
   a. "You know you are only hurting yourself when you stop taking your medication."
   b. "I'm glad that you decided not to have that surgery."
   c. "Why do you smoke so much when you know it is bad for you?"
   d. "I wouldn't worry about those sad feelings you have had for the past few months. Everyone has them occasionally and I'm sure that they will pass soon."
   e. "You shouldn't get so upset over little things like that. It really raises your blood pressure."

8. Identify each of the following therapeutic communication techniques.
   a. "You say you want to get your strength back, to feel better, and get on with your life, but you are not doing the things that would help that happen, like taking your medication."
   b. "I'm not sure exactly what you mean. Would you describe that situation again, please?"
   c. "I think that you need to know more about how your medication works and its common side effects."
   d. "You say that your injuries are self-inflicted."
   e. "A few minutes ago, you mentioned that your husband's angry outbursts seem to get especially bad each time you become pregnant. Could you tell me some more about that, please?"

9. In which stage of the interview process does the nurse obtain the majority of patient data?
   a. Introductory stage
   b. Joining stage
   c. Working stage
   d. Termination stage

   The correct answer is (c).

10. The nurse and patient are sitting 6 feet apart at a table during the patient interview. This distance is called:
    a. Personal distance
    b. Social distance
    c. Public distance
    d. None of the above

    The correct answer is (b).

11. Which interviewing technique is used in the following statement: "Tell me more about the abdominal pain you experience during intercourse?"
    a. Clarifying
    b. Confronting
    c. Informing
    d. Focusing

    The correct answer is (d).

3

The Complete Health History

1. State the purpose of the four different types of health history and provide an example of when each is used.
2. Identify the components of the complete health history.
3. Describe how to assess the nine characteristics of a chief complaint.
4. Diagram a patient's genogram correctly.
5. Demonstrate sensitivity to patients of different races, religions, ethnic backgrounds, sexual orientations, and socioeconomic status when conducting a health history.
6. Conduct a complete health history and record the data.

The health history is usually the first step of patient assessment. It is the collection of subjective information on the patient's health status from the well or ill patient and from other sources. This information is combined with the physical assessment findings to guide the nurse in formulating nursing diagnoses, which serve as the foundation for the plan of care for the patient.

The health history interview provides the mutual opportunity for the nurse and patient to become more comfortable with each other. The patient usually feels more at ease with the collection of health history data than with the physical contact necessary for the assessment. For this reason, the health history is usually performed prior to the physical assessment. Analysis of the information from the patient in the health history provides the basis for planning health care education needed by the patient and indicates areas needing attention in the physical assessment. The written health history also serves as part of the legal documentation of the patient's health status and is a means of communicating information to other health care team members.

Refer to Chapter 2 for communication techniques and strategies for dealing with patients who have special needs.

TYPES OF HEALTH HISTORY

There are four types of health history: complete, episodic, interval or follow-up, and emergency. The **complete health history**, described in this text, is a comprehensive history of the patient's past and present health status and covers many facets of a patient's life. It is usually gathered during a patient's initial visit to a health care facility on a nonemergency basis. The **episodic health history** is shorter and is specific to the patient's current reason for seeking health care. For example, the patient who seeks care for a sore throat and fever would have an episodic health history taken. The **interval** or **follow-up health history** builds on a preceding visit to a health care facility. It documents the patient's recovery from illness, such as the sore throat and fever, or progress from a prior visit. Finally, the **emergency health history** is elicited from the patient and other sources in an emergency situation. Only information required immediately to treat the emergent need of the patient is gathered; after the life-threatening condition is no longer present, the nurse may elicit a more comprehensive history from the patient.

PREPARING FOR THE HEALTH HISTORY

Taking a complete health history with a patient may require 30 to 60 minutes; inform the patient before the interview starts of the amount of time that will be required. If the health history is not completed within the allotted time, it may be best to continue it later to avoid fatiguing the patient. If the patient will be spending some time in the health care facility, then additional information can be obtained during routine nursing tasks such as bathing or assessing vital signs. Some health care agencies request that the literate patient complete detailed health history forms prior to the interview; in this instance, the nurse can validate the responses during the health history and save valuable time. In addition, information can often be obtained from prior medical records, then updated during the interview.

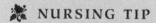

THINK ABOUT IT

Problems Encountered During History Taking

- What would you do if you were conducting a complete health history and the patient stated, "I don't feel like talking right now"?
- What would you do if the patient said, "These questions are all too personal! Why are you asking me all of this?"
- The young teenager seeking birth control tells you, "I hope you won't tell my mother about the abortion I had." How would you respond to this patient?

NURSING TIP

Tracking Care Provided to the Homeless

Homeless people frequently reside at shelter facilities. The shelter staff follows their health needs, when possible, and ensures appropriate care. If a homeless person does not reside at a shelter but lives on the street, it may be difficult to ensure appropriate follow-up care. If follow-up is essential, as in tuberculosis, you may need to initiate actions to locate the person. Law enforcement officials or social service workers may be called upon to help locate seriously ill homeless people so that their illnesses do not pose public health risks.

COMPUTERIZED HEALTH HISTORY

Some health care facilities are using computerized health histories. These can be of two types: patient generated and health care provider generated. In patient-generated health histories, the patient responds on the computer to various questions, and then reviews information with the nurse for completeness. When using a health care provider-generated health history, the nurse completes the information on screen after the patient interview. Frequently, these programs are user-friendly and save the nurse time.

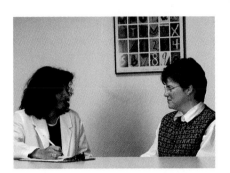

Figure 3-1 The Health History Interview

✓ **NURSING CHECKLIST**
General Approach to the Health History

1. Present with a professional appearance. Avoid extremes in dress so that your appearance does not become a hindrance to information gathering.
2. Ensure an appropriate environment, i.e., good lighting, comfortable temperature, lack of noise and distractions, adequate privacy. Refer to Chapter 2 for additional information.
3. Sit facing the patient at eye level, with the patient in a chair or on a bed. Ensure that the patient is as comfortable as possible because obtaining the health history is a lengthy process. Figure 3-1 illustrates an appropriate setting.
4. Ask the patient whether there are any questions about the interview before it is started.
5. Avoid the use of medical jargon. Use terms the patient can understand.
6. Reserve asking intimate and personal questions for when rapport is established.
7. Remain flexible in obtaining the health history. It does not have to be obtained in the exact order it is presented in this chapter or on institutional forms.
8. Remind the patient that all information will be treated confidentially.

IDENTIFYING INFORMATION

Today's Date

Record the month, date, year, and time that the health history is recorded. If the health history is not written immediately, document the time that the health history was taken and the time when it is recorded.

Biographical Data

The patient usually completes the identifying information prior to the actual physical examination.

Patient name	Occupation
Address	Insurance
Phone number	Usual source of health care
Date of birth	Source of referral
Birthplace	Emergency contact
Social security number	

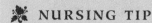
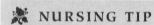
THE COMPLETE HEALTH HISTORY ASSESSMENT TOOL

Source and Reliability of Information

Usually the adult patient is the historian. However, in some instances, such as trauma, the historian may be someone other than the patient. Note the name of the historian as well as the relationship between the historian and the patient.

In addition, assess the reliability of the historian. Consider the mental state of the historian because emotions and certain medical conditions can influence the retelling of events. For example, the information provided by a patient with severe Alzheimer's disease may not be accurate.

Patient Profile

The **patient profile** provides demographics that may be linked to health status.

Age, Sex, Race

Note the patient's age, sex, and race because many diseases are linked to these characteristics.

Marital Status

A patient's marital status may provide clues to support systems.

Reason for Seeking Health Care and Chief Complaint

The **reason for seeking health care** is the reason for the patient's visit and is usually focused on health promotion. The **chief complaint** (CC) is the **sign** (objective finding) or **symptom** (subjective finding) that causes the patient to seek health care. The reason for seeking health care and the CC should be recorded as direct quotes from the patient.

"What brings you here today?" **or**
"What caused you to seek health care today?"
"How long has this condition been concerning you?"

Present Health and History of the Present Illness

If the patient is seeking health promotion, the present health states the patient's current health status.

The **history of the present illness** (HPI) is a chronological account of the patient's CC and the events surrounding it. The chronology can be taken in one of two ways: from the current state of the problem back to its origin (reverse chronology), or from the origin of the symptom leading to the current status (forward chronology). Either approach is acceptable as long as it is consistent with subsequent documentation of chronological events. Usually the patient describes one or two signs/symptoms that are abnormal and their progression. Allow the patient to give the detailed HPI without interruption, then ask questions if information is incomplete.

"Describe the condition that you are experiencing from the earliest time that it occurred to the present." (forward chronology)

Nine characteristics of each CC can be ascertained for a complete HPI:

1. Location
2. Radiation
3. Quality
4. Quantity
5. Associated manifestations
6. Aggravating factors
7. Alleviating factors
8. Setting
9. Timing

Note that all CCs may not have all nine qualifiers; hoarseness, for example, may not be characterized by quantity. The CC of chest pain will be used to demonstrate the use of these nine characteristics. Note that not all of the questions would be asked of the patient while experiencing acute chest pain, but they would be asked after the pain episode.

Location

Location refers to the primary area where the symptom occurs or originates.

"Where are you feeling the chest pain? Can you point to it?"
"Is it spread out or in one location (diffuse or localized)?"
"Have you ever experienced this type of chest pain before? When?"
"Does this current pain differ from pain you have had in the past?"

Radiation

Radiation is the spreading of the symptom or other CC from its original location to another part of the body. The areas of radiation can be diagnostic for specific pathologies. Chest pain associated with a myocardial infarction, for example, often radiates to the neck and down the left arm.

"Does the chest pain radiate or move to another part of your body? If so, where?"
"Is the pain presently radiating?"
"Describe how the pain feels in the area to which it radiated."

Quality

The quality of the CC describes the way it feels to the patient. Use the patient's own terms to describe the quality of the CC. If the patient is having difficulty describing pain, for example, suggest some quality terms such as *gnawing*, *burning*, *stabbing*, *pinching*, *aching*, *throbbing*, and *crushing*.

"What does the chest pain feel like?"
"What word would you use to describe it?"
"Is the pain deep or closer to the skin (superficial)?"

Quantity

Quantity depicts the severity, volume, number, or extent of the CC. The patient may refer to the CC with such terms as *minor*, *moderate*, or *severe*, and *small*, *medium*, or *large*. While this terminology is important to the HPI, this information is subjective and is therefore difficult to quantify. If the patient consistently uses the same terms, then a relative scale can be used to assess whether the CC is improving or becoming worse as reported by the patient.

Another mechanism that can be used to assess the quantity of pain is a numerical scale, known as the **Visual Analog Scale**, which rates pain from 0 to 10.

"Using a scale of 0 to 10, where 0 represents no chest pain and 10 is the worst chest pain that you can imagine, rate the pain that you are having now."

"When was the last time that your chest pain was at this level?"

"Has the severity of the chest pain changed? In what way?"

"Has the chest pain interfered with your normal daily activities? How?"

Associated Manifestations

The signs and symptoms that accompany the CC are termed **associated manifestations**. Rarely does a CC occur without affecting other components of the involved system or another body system. Positive findings are those associated manifestations that the patient has experienced along with the CC. Negative findings, also called **pertinent negatives**, are those manifestations expected in the patient with a suspected pathology but which are denied by the patient. If the patient does not mention specific signs or symptoms that might be present with a given disease, ask whether they are present. Document both positive findings and pertinent negatives because both give clues to the patient's condition. For example, a patient with chest pain may have nausea, diaphoresis, and anxiety as positive associated manifestations. Vomiting, fatigue, and restlessness are pertinent negatives because they might be present in a patient with chest pain; lack of these associated manifestations may lead to a different diagnosis.

"Besides your chest pain, are you experiencing any additional symptoms? Describe them."

"Have these symptoms occurred before? Are they always related to the problem that you are having now?"

Aggravating Factors

Those factors that worsen the severity of the CC are the **aggravating factors**.

"Have you done anything that makes your chest pain worse? What?"

"When you stopped this activity, did the chest pain lessen?"

Alleviating Factors

Alleviating factors are events that decrease the severity of the CC.

"Have you done anything that decreases the severity of the pain? What?"

"Has this worked in the past?"

"When you stopped this activity, did your chest pain become more severe?"

Setting

The setting in which the CC occurs can provide valuable information about the course of the HPI. The setting can be the actual physical environment in which the patient is located, the mental state of the patient, or some activity in which the patient was involved. The patient may or may not be aware of any link between the setting and the occurrence of the CC. For instance, the actual physical setting in which chest pain occurs can be a hot or a cold environment. If a patient is very anxious or excited, this mental state can precipitate chest pain. Also, an activity such as exercise can be associated with the onset of the chest pain.

"What were you doing when the chest pain started? Where were you?"

"Has this activity precipitated the pain on other occasions?"

"Has the pain occurred before in that setting? How many times?"

"What were you thinking about when the chest pain occurred?"

"Has the chest pain occurred before when you were feeling this way?"

Timing

The timing used to describe a CC has three elements: onset, duration, and frequency. Onset refers to the time at which the CC begins and is usually described as gradual or sudden. For instance, jogging may cause a sudden onset of chest pain. Duration depicts the amount of time in which the CC is present. _Continuous_ and _intermittent_ are terms that can be used to describe the duration of a CC. When possible, the duration of the CC should be stated in specific time increments, such as minutes, hours, or days. Frequency describes the number of times the CC occurs and how often it develops (i.e., number of times per day, season of year).

> "When did the chest pain first start? How long did the pain last?"
>
> "Did the pain come on suddenly or gradually?"
>
> "Is the pain continuous or intermittent? If intermittent, how much time elapsed between episodes?"
>
> "When was the last time you experienced the chest pain? Is the pain different in any way from the first time that you experienced it?"
>
> "How often does the chest pain occur in a day? In a week?"
>
> "Have you detected a pattern to the chest pain's occurrence?"

Meaning and Impact

The last two pieces of information needed in the HPI are the meaning or significance of the CC to the patient, and the impact that the CC has on the patient. For example, the patient with chest pain that leads to a myocardial infarction may require surgery for coronary revascularization. While the morbidity and mortality rates for this procedure are low, the patient may have had a relative who died during the same procedure and therefore perceives the surgery as being fatal.

Secondly, the impact that the CC has on the patient's lifestyle should be investigated. For example, consider the elderly patient who complains of minor pain but admits to canceling routine activities; in this case, the condition is presented as mild but its effects are serious.

> "What does it mean to you to have this condition (chest pain)?"
>
> "How do you see the chest pain affecting your lifestyle?"

Past Health History

The **past health history** (PHH) provides information on the patient's health status from birth to the present. The patient may think you are ignoring the reason for seeking health care. The following statements can ease the transition:

> "I will get back to the reason for your visit today in a few minutes. Now I would like to ask some questions related to your health in the past."
>
> "Sometimes the reason for an illness is connected with your past health. For this reason, let's discuss your health in the past."

Medical History

The medical history comprises all medical problems that the patient has experienced during adulthood and their **sequelae**, or aftermath. Chronic illnesses as well as episodic illnesses are included. Forward or reverse chronology can be used to describe the medical history as long as the approach is consistent with the chronological format in the HPI. If the patient denies medical illnesses, suspect that the patient may have misunderstood some questions. Some patients may overlook "a little high blood pressure" and not see this as a problem.

"Are you presently under the supervision of a health care provider for any medical illness? **or**

"Have you ever been diagnosed as having an illness? What was it?"

"When was the illness diagnosed?"

"Who diagnosed this problem?"

"What is the current treatment for this problem?"

"Do you follow the prescribed treatment? Do you have any difficulty following the prescribed treatment?"

"Have you ever been hospitalized for this illness? Where? When? For what period of time? What was the treatment? What was your condition after the treatment?"

"Have you ever experienced any complications (sequelae) from this disease? What were they? How were they treated?"

Surgical History

Record a complete account of each surgical procedure, both major and minor, including the year performed, hospital, physician, and sequelae, if known.

"Have you ever had surgery? What type?"

"Who was your physician at the time?"

"When, where, and by whom was the surgery performed?"

"Were you hospitalized? For what period of time?"

"Were there any complications? How were they treated?"

"Are you currently receiving any treatment related to this surgery?"

"Have you ever had an adverse effect from anesthesia?"

Medications

Past and present consumption of medications, both prescription and over the counter (OTC), can affect the patient's current health status.

Prescription Medication

"What prescription medications are you currently taking? Who prescribed them?" **and**

"What prescription medications have you taken in the past? Who prescribed them?"

"What is the dose? How often do you take this medication?"

"How do you take this medication (e.g., pills, drops, inhaler, ointment)?"

"How long have you been taking this medication?"

"Have you ever experienced any side effects with this medication?"

"Have you ever had an allergic reaction to this medication? What happened?"

"Tell me the purpose of these medications."

Over-the-Counter Medication

"Do you currently take any over-the-counter medications? Which ones?"

"Why do you take this medication?"

"Do you take any home remedies? Which ones? For what purpose?"

Repeat all but the first and last questions from the *Prescription Medication* section.

"Do you ever take aspirin, acetaminophen, ibuprofen, antacids, vitamins? Do you douche? Administer enemas? Do you take allergy pills or cold medications?" (If yes, repeat all but the first and last questions of the previous section.)

General Questions

"How long do you save unused drugs?"

NURSING TIP

Obtaining an Accurate Medication History

Frequently, the patient discounts OTC medications such as aspirin, acetaminophen, ibuprofen, vitamins, cathartics, enemas, douches, cold remedies, and antacids. Ask the patient whether such products are used because they can adversely interact with prescribed medications and with one another. Also, women frequently overlook birth control pills; keep this in mind when interviewing women of childbearing age.

The outcome of the medication history may point to a need for patient teaching. If contact is made with the patient prior to the health care visit, ask the patient to bring in all medications currently being taken.

NURSING TIP

Expired Medications

Many patients keep unused medications past their expiration date. This presents a potential health hazard because some medications lose their potency after a period of time and others become toxic. You should inform the patient to discard any unused portion of medication by the stated date. Encourage patients to check their medicine cabinets at the same time every year so it becomes a routine practice.

"Do you ever share medications or needles with another person? Who? For what reason? What drug do you share?"
"Do you have any questions concerning your medications?"

Communicable Diseases

Communicable diseases can have a grave impact on the individual as well as on society. Some communicable diseases generate enough of a concern to the community that they are reportable to the public health department. The most talked about communicable disease at present is human immunodeficiency virus (HIV), the virus responsible for acquired immune deficiency syndrome (AIDS). There is substantial value in asking the patient about possible exposure to communicable diseases because pathology may not manifest itself until many years after exposure.

"Have you ever been diagnosed with an infectious or communicable disease? Which one(s)?"
"What were your symptoms?"
"How were you treated?"
"Did you have any complications? What were they? Were there any permanent consequences?"
"Have you ever had gonorrhea, syphilis, chlamydia, or other venereal diseases?"
"Have you ever had measles, mumps, rubella, German measles, herpes, chicken pox, pertussis (whooping cough), tuberculosis, scarlet fever, rheumatic fever?" (If yes, repeat the second, third, and fourth questions from above.)
"Have you ever had hepatitis?" (If yes, repeat the second, third, and fourth questions.)
"Have you ever been told that you were HIV-positive?" (If yes, repeat the second, third, and fourth questions.)
"Have you ever been told that you have AIDS?" (If yes, repeat the second, third, and fourth questions.)
"Have you ever been exposed to someone who had a communicable disease? Which one(s)?"

Allergies

Carefully explore all patient allergies, which may include medications, animals, foods, and environmental allergens. Allergies are usually written in a conspicuous location in red ink on the patient's chart in order to stand out.

"Are you allergic to any medications? Animals? Foods? Bee stings?"
"Are you allergic to anything in the environment?"
"Are you allergic to anything that you touch?"
"What symptoms do you get when you are exposed to this substance?"
"What treatment do you use? Is it effective?"
"Have you experienced any complications from the allergies? Which?"
"Have you ever seen an allergist for this problem? What happened?"

Injuries/Accidents

A patient's injury/accident history can reveal a pattern that is amenable to health promotion. For example, an elderly woman who sustains an injury from slipping on throw rugs in the home would be a candidate for health teaching on maintaining a safe home environment.

"Have you ever been involved in an accident?" **or** "Have you ever been injured in any way?"

"What occurred? Did you lose consciousness?"
"Did you take any precautionary measures? What were they?"
"Were you hospitalized? For how long?"
"Were there any complications? What were they?"
"Were there any long-term effects from this injury/accident?"
"Have you ever sustained an injury in a car accident? Describe."
"Have you ever had a broken bone? Stitches? Burns?"
"Have you ever been assaulted? Raped? Shot? Stabbed?"

Disabilities/Handicaps

The awareness of any cognitive, physical, or psychosocial disability/handicap is essential to providing individualized health care to a patient. A patient with Down syndrome, a paraplegic, and a sociopathic patient all have unique needs. These patients may receive less than optimal health care if their particular limitations are not identified and considered when planning treatment.

"Do you have any disability or handicap? Describe."
"What type of limitations does this disability/handicap place on you?"
"What strategies do you use to limit the effect the disability/handicap has on your lifestyle?"
"What support systems help you cope with this disability/handicap?"
"Does your disability/handicap place an extra financial burden on you? How do you handle that?"

Blood Transfusions

According to the American Red Cross, the nation's blood supply is as safe as it can be (Dodd, 1992). Still, with every transfusion, the recipient does assume some risk. The chance of contracting AIDS or hepatitis is greatest in patients who receive a large number of transfusions, such as hemophiliacs and trauma victims. Individuals who received blood transfusions before 1981 when the HIV blood test was developed are at a higher risk for developing AIDS.

"Have you ever received a blood transfusion (whole blood or any of its components)? When?"
"Why did you receive this blood product?"
"What quantity did you receive?"
"Did you experience any reaction to this blood product? What was it?"

Childhood Illnesses

Rarely are adults familiar with a complete history of their childhood illnesses. Ask the patient about specific childhood diseases by name.

"Have you ever had any of the following illnesses: chickenpox, diphtheria, measles, mumps, rubella, pertussis (whooping cough), polio, rheumatic fever, scarlet fever, or smallpox?" (This question is eliminated if previously asked during the communicable disease section.)
"How old were you when the illness occurred?"
"Was an actual diagnosis made? By whom?"
"Were there any complications? What were they?"
"What other childhood illnesses did you have?"

Immunizations

The history of immunizations is closely tied to childhood illnesses. Most immunizations are received in childhood, though a few may be given in the

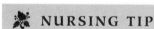

NURSING TIP

Varying Immunization Schedules

Routine vaccinations can vary among different age groups. Some immunizations have been eliminated while others have been added to the vaccination schedule as recommended by the American Academy of Pediatrics (AAP) and the Centers for Disease Control and Prevention (CDC). For example, the smallpox vaccination was discontinued in 1977. In the 1990s, the AAP added the Hib and hepatitis B vaccine to its recommended immunization schedule. Be alert to these changes in immunization schedules when interviewing patients to ensure they have received what is/was appropriate for them.

♣ ASK YOURSELF

Keeping Track of Immunizations

- Can you remember when you received vaccinations as a child? As an adult?
- Do you remember the purpose of each?
- What tips can you offer patients to keep track of their immunizations?

adult years. As with childhood illnesses, the adult patient may not recall the exact dates when the immunizations were given but will be aware that "I received everything that I should have." Routine immunizations are also associated with different groups. Health care workers are frequently given the hepatitis B vaccine. Every winter the adult population, especially those over age 65 and those with chronic diseases, are encouraged to receive the flu vaccine. In addition, travelers to underdeveloped areas of the world receive numerous vaccines prior to visiting specific regions.

"What immunizations have you received since birth? When?"

"Did you experience any reactions to the immunizations? What were they? Were there any complications?"

"As a child, did you receive the following immunizations: measles mumps rubella (MMR), polio, smallpox, diphtheria pertussis tetanus (DPT), Haemophilus influenza type b (Hib), hepatitis B?"

"Have you received any immunizations as an adult: varicella, hepatitis B, influenza, tetanus, pneumonia?"

"When was your last TB test and what was the result?"

"Have you ever received any other immunizations, perhaps prior to visiting a specific geographical region (cholera, typhoid fever, yellow fever)?"

Family Health History

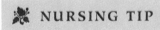

🌿 NURSING TIP

Drawing the Genogram

Draw the FHH genogram as the patient describes the family's history to you. It can be completed much more quickly than narrative documentation. Practice drawing the genograms of colleagues as they relate their FHHs to you.

The family health history (FHH) records the health status of the patient as well as immediate blood relatives. At a minimum, the history needs to contain the age and health status of the patient, spouse, children, siblings, and the patient's parents. Ideally, the patient's grandparents, aunts, and uncles should be incorporated into the history as well. Documentation of this information is done in two parts: the genogram, or family tree, and a list of familial diseases. Figure 3-2 demonstrates the appropriate method for constructing the **genogram**.

The second component of the family health history is the report of occurrences of familial or genetic diseases. Such information is crucial to the patient and may not have been revealed previously because many familial illnesses do not occur in every generation. The positive and pertinent negative findings are documented in the family health history below the genogram. Refer to Figure 3-2.

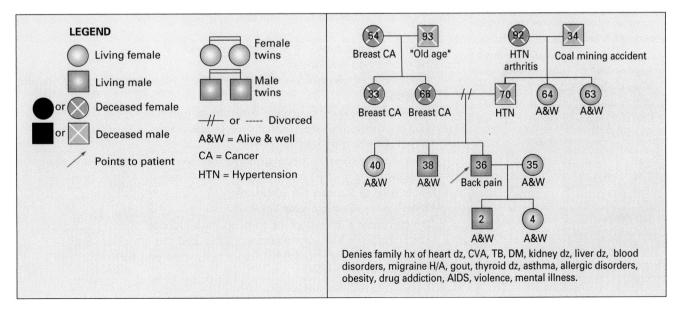

Figure 3-2 Family Health History and Genogram

NURSING TIP

Family Health History for a Patient Who Was Adopted

Patients who were adopted have varying degrees of information about their biological parents. Encourage adopted patients to be frank about their FHH. If the FHH of the biological parents is unknown, this is documented. It is not uncommon for patients to seek out their birth parents to learn more about their FHHs.

Likewise, the FHH of adoptive parents can be equally important. Certain environmental factors (smoking, drug and alcohol use, sanitation, etc.) may influence the health of the adopted child.

NURSING TIP

Family Health History and Cultural Restraints

In some cultures (e.g., Chinese and some American Indians), it is disrespectful to speak of the dead. Thus, the patient may be reluctant to provide detailed information on the family health history of dead relatives. In these cases, you can ask the patient whether there is any history of specific diseases in the family, rather than focusing on any specific deceased individual. The patient may be willing to share in which previous generation and on which side of the family the condition existed. If these approaches are unsuccessful, explain to the patient the importance of this information because it may provide clues to current health conditions.

You may want to preface the FHH questions with the following statement:

"Different diseases tend to run in families. I would like to ask you about your family and their health to gain a better understanding of your background."

You can then continue with questions about the FHH:

"Tell me about the members of your family: spouse, children, siblings, and parents. How old are they?"
"Do any of these individuals have any medical illnesses or diseases? What are they?"
"Have there been any deaths in your immediate family? What was the cause of death? How old was this person at the time of death?"
"What is the current age of each of the following members of your extended family: maternal and paternal grandparents, aunts, uncles?"
Repeat questions 2 and 3.
"Has anyone in your family ever had any of the following illnesses: heart disease, hypertension, stroke, tuberculosis, diabetes mellitus, cancer, kidney disease, blood disorders, sickle cell anemia, arthritis, epilepsy, migraine headaches, gout, thyroid disease, liver disease, asthma, allergic disorders, obesity, alcoholism, mental illness (schizophrenia, depression), drug addiction, AIDS, HIV infection, violent reactions? Who?"

Social History

The **social history** (SH) explores information about the patient's lifestyle that can affect health. Introduce this area of questioning with statements similar to the following:

"Now I would like to ask you some questions about your lifestyle. This information is important because of the effects that different practices can have on your health."

Alcohol Use

The intermittent and prolonged use of alcohol can interfere with normal metabolism and normal body function.

"How much alcohol do you drink per week?"
"How often do you drink?"
"What type of alcohol do you prefer (beer, wine, wine coolers, liquor, spirits)?"
"What quantity do you usually consume at one time?"
"Has your drinking pattern changed? In what way?"
"When did you first start to drink?"
"How long have you been drinking the amount that you are currently consuming?"
"What time of the day do you drink?"
"Where do you obtain your drinks?"
"Do you have a special place to keep your alcohol?"
"Have you ever lost consciousness or blacked out after drinking?"
"Have you ever forgotten what happened when you were drinking?"
"Do you drink alone?"
"Do you drive after drinking?"
"Did you ever drink during pregnancy? How much?" (for women)
"Do you think you have a drinking problem?"

Dealing with Sensitive Topics

Alcohol, drug use, and sexual practices are some of the most sensitive areas that are addressed in the health history. Some tips for dealing with these sensitive topics are:

- Ask these questions in the later stages of the interview after rapport has been established.
- Use direct eye contact; this demonstrates the importance of the topic to the patient and your lack of embarrassment.
- Pose questions in a matter-of-fact tone.
- Adopt a nonjudgmental demeanor.
- Use the communication technique of normalizing when appropriate (i.e., "Many high school students drink alcohol/use drugs/engage in sexual relationships on a regular basis. Does this happen at your school? With you?").
- Observe an experienced nurse elicit sensitive information from patients; note the nurse's verbal and nonverbal behavior.
- Critique your verbal and non-verbal behavior when eliciting sensitive information on a video-taped practice health history.

Tobacco Use

When assessing tobacco use, consider tobacco use other than cigarettes, such as cigar and pipe smoking, chewing tobacco, and snuff.

The quantity of cigarette smoking is usually described in **pack/year history**. To calculate the patient's pack/year history, multiply the number of packs of cigarettes smoked on a daily basis by the number of years that the patient has smoked. For example, to calculate the pack/year history for a patient who has smoked 2½ packs a day for 30 years:

$$\text{pack/year history} = 2\tfrac{1}{2} \times 30 = 75$$

"Do you use or have you ever used tobacco (cigarettes [filtered or nonfiltered], pipe, cigars, chewing tobacco, snuff)?"
"At what age did you start to use tobacco?"
"What quantity do you use on a daily basis?"
"Has this amount changed? In what way?"
"Have you ever tried to kick this habit? What method(s) did you use? What was the outcome?"
"Do you think you have a smoking (tobacco) problem?"

Drug Use

The questions about use of drugs in the social history section of the complete health history are not to be confused with the medication section under the past health history. The latter includes the use and abuse of OTC and prescription medications whereas the former refers to the use of illegal substances. You may feel uncomfortable asking the patient if there has been drug use; remind the patient that the information will be kept confidential and the withholding of information may delay necessary treatment.

"Do you use or have you ever used marijuana, amphetamines, uppers, downers, cocaine, crack, heroin, PCP, or other recreational/street drugs?"
"When did you first start to use drugs?"
"What amount do you use?"
"How often do you use this drug?"
"Has this amount changed? In what way?"
"In what form do you use the drug (pill, needle, snort, other)?"

Abused Substances

- What is your personal philosophy on the use of alcohol, tobacco, and drugs?
- What biases (if any) influence your feelings on the use of these substances?
- How do you feel about others who use these substances? Does it make a difference how much is used?
- Think back to the last time you interviewed a patient who had a problem dealing with excessive alcohol, tobacco, or drugs. Did you treat that patient any differently from your other patients?

Nursing Care for Drug Users

Twelve-year-old Barbara is brought to the Emergency Department by her mother, who explains that she heard a loud noise in the bathroom and ran upstairs to find her daughter unconscious on the floor. Barbara was unconscious for approximately 2 minutes. When Barbara awoke, she had no memory of the blackout. Barbara's mother believed that her daughter needed treatment for the multiple cuts to her forehead that she suffered when she fell. Barbara's mother excuses herself to go to the restroom. While she is out of the room, Barbara tells you that she takes LSD occasionally. Then she asks, "Do you think that has anything to do with my blackout?"

- How would you respond to Barbara's question?
- Do you exhibit any biases when working with people who take street drugs? Do these biases interfere with your nursing care? If so, what actions do you take to control your bias?
- Explore the legal ramifications of working with patients who take illegal drugs in your city/state. Are there special provisions if the patient is a minor?

"Describe how you inject the drug."
"Do you share needles? Do you clean the needles between uses? How?"
"Have you experienced any health problems from the drug use?"
"Have you ever overdosed? What happened?"
"Have you ever been through a drug rehab program? What was the outcome?"
"Do you think you have a drug problem?"

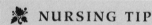

ASK YOURSELF

Intimate Questions

- How would you feel if someone asked you intimate questions about your sexual practices?
- What skills would you like to see in the interviewer to put you at ease?

NURSING TIP

Eliciting the Sexual History

Be aware that patients may refuse to answer questions pertaining to sexual history; try returning to these questions later. Ask the patient if a nurse of a different gender would make the patient more comfortable in discussing sexual practice.

The adolescent patient may refuse to answer these questions or may provide false answers if the parent or caregiver is in the room. It may be advisable to ask the caregiver to leave the room at the completion of the health history so you can ask the patient if there is anything else that he or she would like to say.

Be alert for cues that demonstrate the patient's desire for sexual education, such as questions or requests for written information. Answer the patient's questions and refer to a specialist when indicated.

Sexual Practice

Sexual practices are related to the transmission of communicable diseases. Various medications can affect sexual function.

Questioning a patient about sexual practices may be uncomfortable for both patient and nurse. The patient may notice your uneasiness with this topic and may feel embarrassed to answer the questions. Examine your personal feelings on human sexuality and attain a comfort level that will allow ease in questioning. The health histories in Chapters 19 and 20 provide additional information about female and male reproductive health.

"What term would you use to describe your sexual orientation (heterosexual, homosexual, bisexual)?"
"Does your current sexual orientation represent your past sexual practice? If not, how has it changed?"
"With how many partners are you currently involved? Has this changed?"
"What method of birth control do you use? Do you have any questions about it? Would you like additional information on other methods of birth control?" (for heterosexuals and bisexuals)
"What measures do you use to prevent exchange of body fluids during sexual activity?"
"Do you engage in oral or anal intercourse?"
"Have you ever had a sexual partner who had a sexually transmitted disease?"
"Are you satisfied with your sexual performance?"

Travel History

Endemic illnesses may be endogenous to specific regions in the world or to a single country. Patients present with symptoms that cannot or may not be attributed to routine illnesses. For these reasons, a complete travel history is warranted when obtaining a health history.

"Where within the United States have you traveled? Was this a rural or an urban environment? When?"
"Have you ever traveled outside of the United States? Where? When?"
"For what period of time were you within this region?"
"Did you receive any immunizations before you visited that area?"
"Were you ill when you were there?"
"Was a diagnosis made? By whom? What was it?"
"What treatment did you receive? Were there any complications?"
"Since returning from this area, have you been ill or not feeling normal?"

Work Environment

The work environment can be hazardous. The nature of employment itself may present health hazards whether or not safety measures are used. Carpentry, for example, is viewed as a relatively safe employment, though over time, carpenters are prone to ischemia of their fingers from repeated exposure to hand-held vibrating tools. Exposure to toxic substances in the work environment, such as asbestos and lead, is an additional factor to consider.

"Describe the work that you do. Is it physically demanding? Is it mentally or emotionally demanding?"

"How many hours a day do you normally work? How long have you been in this position?"

"Do you spend the majority of your work day sitting, standing, walking, running, lifting, or biking?"

"Do you work with any chemicals? Raw materials?"

"Are you exposed to radiation? Toxic fumes? Hazardous conditions?"

"What safety measures do you practice at work?"

"What is the noise level at your place of employment?"

"Have you noticed that you are sick on the weekend or on your days off?"

"Have you had any work-related accidents or injuries?"

"Do you enjoy your work?"

"What other jobs have you held in your lifetime?"

Home Environment

When assessing the patient's home environment, consider both the physical and psychosocial aspects. The physical assessment encompasses a broad spectrum of topics: physical condition of the house, safety from toxic substances, and the presence of modern conveniences such as a refrigerator, furnace, telephones, and electricity. Older houses may have been painted with lead-based paint, which poses a health threat to a young child who eats the paint chips. The presence of radon gas in the home has been a recent health concern.

The psychosocial component of the home environment identifies the relative safety of the neighborhood.

Physical Environment

"How old are your living quarters (i.e., house or apartment building)?"

"In what condition are your living quarters?"

"Is your home cleaned regularly?"

"Do you have heat, air conditioning, and electricity? What type of heat do you have? Do you use space heaters?"

"Do you have running water? Do you have a toilet, tub, or shower?"

"Do you have a working telephone?"

"Do you have smoke detectors? Where? Do you inspect the batteries on a regular basis? Do you have a carbon monoxide detector?"

"How many steps separate each floor? Is there a railing?"

"Do you have any throw rugs? Are they taped to the floor?"

"Do you use a nightlight when it is dark?"

"Have you adapted your living quarters to fit any special needs?"

"Do you think your living space is adequate for the number of people that live with you?"

"Have you ever had your living quarters tested for the presence of radon? What was the result?"

"How often do you have your fireplace cleaned?"

"How often do you replace the filter in your ventilation system?"

"What pets do you have? Do they live inside or outside?"

"What type of transportation do you use?"

"Who does your shopping?"

"Do you have easy access to a grocery store? Drug store? Health care facility?"

"Where do you store your medications, cleaning supplies, and other toxic substances? How are they secured?" (if children live in the living quarters)

"Where do you store gasoline and automotive supplies?"

Psychosocial Environment

"Do you feel safe in your neighborhood?"

"Does your neighborhood have a crime watch prevention program?"

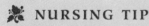

NURSING TIP

Guidelines for Assessing the Home Environment

Not all of the questions for the home environment assessment need to be asked of every patient. You need to be attentive to clues that signal the necessity of performing an in-depth home environment assessment. Some clues include, but are not limited to, poor hygiene, frequent infections, smoke inhalation, burns, malnutrition, and falls (especially among the elderly).

NURSING TIP

Assessing the Home Environment of the Homeless

Respect the dignity of the homeless patient. Modify the home environment questions for the homeless patient; not all questions will be applicable, depending on the patient's circumstances. It is vital to pursue information about the patient's living quarters to assess the conditions in which a homeless patient lives. A social services consultation may be initiated if the situation warrants it.

Hobbies/Leisure Activities

Acquiring information on patients' hobbies and leisure activities is necessary because some activities can pose health risks. For example, repeated exposure to glue used in constructing model cars and planes can lead to respiratory ailments.

"What hobbies do you have?" **or** "What do you like to do in your spare time?"

"During or after this activity, have you ever felt sick? What happened?"

"Have you ever given up some leisure activity because of the effect it had on your health? What happened?"

"Are the hobbies/leisure activities relaxing?"

Stress

Stress is a physiologically defined response to changes that disrupt the resting equilibrium of an individual. **Distress** is negative stress, or stress that is harmful and unpleasant. **Eustress** is positive stress, that which challenges the individual, provides motivation, and prevents stagnation.

"What are the current stressors in your life?"

"What do you feel is your greatest stress at the present time?"

"Are there recurring themes with the stress that you experience?"

"Have you ever progressed from the point of being stressed to panic? What were the circumstances? How did you handle it?"

"Are you able to recognize when you become stressed? What happens?"

Education

Elicit information on the patient's ability to read and write and tailor your questions and information to this level.

"What was the highest grade level that you completed?"

"Describe the type of student that you were."

"Have you completed a GED certification?"

Economic Status

Patients and nurses may be equally uncomfortable discussing financial status. The essence of the information needed is how the patient lives on the income. Patients who lack adequate financial resources may be referred to social services.

"What are the sources of your income?"

"How would you describe your economic status?"

"Are you able to meet food, medication, housing, clothing, and personal expenses for you and your family?"

"Are you able to save any money?"

"Do you hesitate seeking health care because of the cost? What is your insurance coverage?"

"Are you satisfied with your current economic status?"

Military Service

Knowledge of overseas tours of duty may provide a vital link to current health status; a patient may not reveal this information during the travel history because it is work rather than leisure travel. For instance, those military personnel who served in Operation Desert Storm may have been exposed to

---

🌺 NURSING TIP

Caring for the Illiterate Patient

The illiterate patient is unable to complete or verify written assessment data. Therefore, alternative strategies are used when caring for the illiterate patient to ensure that education on treatment and follow-up is simple and clear. Some strategies to use include:

- Illustrated charts to describe procedures and treatments
- A picture of a clock to illustrate time
- Color-coded medications
- Patient recall on instructions to double-check accuracy
- Follow-up with home health care agency when indicated to ensure appropriate care

many chemical agents. Many of them now have a variety of signs and symptoms collectively called Gulf War syndrome (Brown, 1994).

> "Are you or have you ever been in the military? What branch?"
> "How long have you been in the military? Are you on active duty or reserve?"
> "In what regions have you been assigned? How long were you there? When?"

Religion

Religion and spirituality can be powerful forces in a patient's life. You need to be aware of and sensitive to implications that spirituality or religious beliefs may have on the patient's health status and health care practices. Chapter 6 provides a more detailed assessment on religion and spiritual practices.

> "Are you affiliated with a specific religion?"
> "Do you currently practice your faith?"
> "Do your religious beliefs affect your health status? In what way?"
> "Are there any beliefs that you feel are compromised by seeking health care?"
> "Are there any religious practices that you may need assistance with?"

Ethnic Background

Closely associated with religious practices is the patient's culture or ethnic background, which can penetrate all facets of a patient's life. Integrate familiarity with various cultures into your knowledge base so you will be sensitive to and more completely understand the patient's ethnic heritage. Chapter 5 discusses the cultural assessment in greater detail.

> "With what culture or ethnic group do you identify yourself?"

Roles/Relationships

Family role(s), work role(s), and interpersonal relationships provide clues about possible stressors, areas for health promotion, support systems, and sources of altered psychosocial patterns.

> "Who lives with you?"
> "What type of relationship do you have with these individuals?"
> "What is your role within your family (i.e., caregiver, breadwinner, child, student)?"
> "What responsibilities go along with this role?"
> "Who do you turn to for support?"
> "Describe the relationship that you have with your friends/neighbors."

Characteristic Patterns of Daily Living

Questions about a patient's usual lifestyle, or **characteristic patterns of daily living**, reveal information about the patient's normal daily timetable: meal, work, and sleep schedules and social interactions.

> "Describe a typical day for you, starting from the time you wake up to the time you go to bed."
> "Do you need assistance with any activities of daily living? (If yes) Is assistance readily available?"
> "Do you socialize, meet, or talk with people outside your house on a daily basis?"
> "Does your schedule change on certain days or on the weekend? Describe."

Health Maintenance Activities

Health maintenance activities (HMA) are practices a person incorporates into his or her lifestyle to promote healthy living. You can make the transition from the social history to HMA with the following statements:

"Now I would like to discuss things that you do that promote health."
"There are many things you can do to promote healthy living. I would like us to discuss some of those practices."

Sleep

"At what time do you usually go to bed? What time do you usually awake?"
"Is this an adequate amount of sleep for you? How do you feel when you awaken?"
"Is the sleep undisturbed? Do you have difficulty staying asleep? If you awaken, is it easy for you to fall back to sleep?"
"Describe the environment in which you sleep (noise level, amount of light, temperature of the room, sleeping arrangement)."
"Are there any bedtime rituals that you practice?"
"What strategies do you use to fall asleep if you are having difficulty (medication, warm milk, other)? How many times per week do you do this?"
"What is your usual emotional state/mental condition when you go to bed? When you awaken?"
"Do you ever have difficulty falling asleep? Have you ever been told that you have insomnia?"
"Do you ever have difficulty staying awake? Have you ever been told that you have sleep apnea or narcolepsy?"
"Does the usual time of your sleep/awake cycle change (working rotating shifts)?"
"Do you take a nap during the day? For how long?"
"Do you have nightmares? How frequent are they?"
"Do you walk in your sleep?"
"Do you experience bedwetting?"
"Do you often wake up with dark circles under your eyes? Puffy eyelids? Bloodshot eyes?"

Diet

Refer to Chapter 7 for a more thorough discussion of nutrition and diet history.

"Are you on any special therapeutic diet (low salt, low cholesterol, low fat, etc.)?"
"Do you follow any particular diet plan (vegetarian, liquid, commercially available diet food, rice diet, Scarsdale diet, etc.)?"
"How many meals a day do you eat? At what times do you eat? Do you snack? When?"
"Has your weight fluctuated in the past year? Explain."

Exercise

Aerobic exercise appropriate to the patient's age and physical condition leads to cardiovascular, respiratory, and musculoskeletal fitness as well as mental alertness. Combining aerobic exercise with weight lifting (which increases strength) and calisthenics (which enhances flexibility) establishes a complete physical fitness regimen. Nonaerobic activity also has beneficial effects on the body, even though the target heart rate may not be attained.

Stress Management Counseling

D.G. is a 42-year-old woman who presents with a gastrointestinal bleed secondary to increased caffeine, alcohol, and aspirin intake. She is transferred from the critical care area to your unit. As soon as D.G. arrives, she asks for a telephone so she can call her office. Suddenly she bursts into tears and sobs, "I can't handle one more thing! I need to get a handle on life." She asks for your advice.

- How would you respond to D.G.'s statement?
- Is this the appropriate time to conduct a stress management assessment?
- What stress management resources are available in your area/institution?
- What is your bias (if any) with stress management techniques that you do not espouse? How can you become more comfortable in discussing these practices with patients to overcome your bias?

Consistent Use of Safety Devices

How would you respond in the following situations?

- J.V. is a 45-year-old police officer who admits that he never wears a seat belt. "I'm a good driver and I need to have the ability to get out of my car quickly."
- B.F. is a 31-year-old radiology technician. She states, "With the number of x-rays I perform, by the end of the day I'm tired of putting on my lead apron."
- M.E. is a 23-year-old who rides his bike through busy downtown traffic everyday on his way to work. He denies wearing a helmet, saying, "It's not cool!"

"Do you participate in a formal or informal exercise program?"
"What type of exercise do you do?"
"How many times per week do you exercise?"
"How long do you exercise (in minutes)?"
"What type of warm-up and cool-down exercises do you do?"
"What is your resting heart rate?"
"What is your heart rate at the most intense time of your exercise?"
"For what period of time do you maintain this elevated heart rate?"
"Have you ever experienced any injuries from your exercise regimen? What type?"
"How long have you been involved with this exercise program?"
"Does your health pose any restrictions on your ability to exercise?"

Stress Management

The assessment of stress management practices is vital. Some commonly used stress management techniques are exercise, eating, biofeedback, yoga, imagery, massages, verbalization, praying, humor, pet therapy, music therapy, support groups, and transcendental meditation. For others, stress management techniques include smoking, drinking, drugs, and violence.

"What do you do when you become stressed to help alleviate the stress?"
"When do you use this skill? Is it effective for you?"
"How do you evaluate the effectiveness of this technique?"
"How long do you need to perform this technique before your stress is reduced?"
"How many times per day do you use this technique? Per week?"
"Have you tried other stress management skills? How did they work?"

Use of Safety Devices

The patient's use or lack of use of safety devices on the job, in the home, and in the environment provide a source for teaching health promotion skills.

"Do you wear a seat belt when you are in an automobile?"
"Do you wear a helmet when riding a motorcycle?"
"Do your hobbies/leisure activities (e.g., cycling) require the use of safety devices (e.g., helmets)? Do you use them?"
"What precautions do you take when using pesticides or fertilizers?"

Health Check-ups

Health check-up information demonstrates patterns of health care practices by the patient during illness and health, and provides potential sources of health education.

"When was the last time you had the following performed: pulse and blood pressure, complete physical examination, chest x-ray, TB test, EKG, urinalysis, complete blood count, blood chemistry? What were the results?"
"How often do you see a dentist? For what reason?"
"How often do you see an eye doctor? Is this an ophthalmologist or an optometrist? For what reason? Have you been checked for glaucoma?"
"How often do you have a gynecological check-up? By whom? What was the date and result of your last Pap smear?" (for women)
"Do you know how to perform a breast self-examination? Who taught you? How often do you perform it? Do you have any questions about it?" (for women)
"What was the date and the result of your last mammogram?" (for women)

"Do you know how to perform a testicular self-examination? Who taught you? How often do you perform it? Do you have any questions about it?" (for men)

"How often do you have a prostate examination? What was the date and result of your last exam?" (for men)

"Do you have any other health care providers (psychiatrist, psychologist, occupational or physical therapist, chiropractor, etc.)? For what reason? How often do you see this person?"

Review of Systems

The **review of systems** (ROS) is the patient's subjective response to a series of body system-related questions, and serves as a double-check that vital information is not overlooked. The ROS covers a broad base of clinical states, but it is by no means exhaustive. The ROS follows a head-to-toe or **cephalocaudal** approach and includes two types of questions: sign/symptom related and disease related. The sign/symptoms and diseases are grouped according to physiological body parts and systems. Some of the diseases may have been discussed earlier in the interview.

Both positive and pertinent negative findings are documented in the ROS. When a response is positive, ask the patient to describe it as completely as possible. Refer to the nine characteristics of a chief complaint when gathering more information about positive responses. Table 3-1 lists the symptoms and diseases that can be ascertained during the ROS. Many institutions have preprinted ROS sheets. These are convenient to use because positive findings can be circled and noted. Negative responses are not circled.

Remember to ask the questions in terms that are understood by the patient. An appropriate statement to make the transition from the HMA to the ROS would be:

"Now I would like to ask you if you have experienced a variety of conditions. Most of the questions can be answered with 'yes' or 'no'."

Pose the same question for each item in the ROS:

"Have you ever had . . . ?"

After completing the ROS, ask the patient if there is any additional information to discuss. At the conclusion of the interview, thank the patient for the time spent in gathering the health history. Inform the patient what the next step will be, e.g., physical assessment, diagnostic tests, treatment, and when to expect it.

Table 3-1 Review of Systems

GENERAL
Patient's perception of general state of health at the present, difference from usual state, vitality and energy levels

NEUROLOGICAL
Headache, change in balance, incoordination, loss of movement, change in sensory perception/feeling in an extremity, change in speech, change in smell, fainting (syncope), loss of memory, tremors, involuntary movement, loss of consciousness, seizures, weakness, head injury

PSYCHOLOGICAL
Irritability, nervousness, tension, increased stress, difficulty concentrating, mood changes, suicidal thoughts, depression

SKIN
Rashes, itching, changes in skin pigmentation, black and blue marks (ecchymoses), change in color or size of mole, sores, lumps, change in skin texture, odors, excessive sweating, acne, loss of hair (alopecia), excessive growth of hair or growth of hair in unusual locations (hirsutism), change in nails, amount of time spent in the sun

continued

Table 3-1 Review of Systems *continued*

EYES
Blurred vision, visual acuity, glasses, contacts, sensitivity to light (photophobia), excessive tearing, night blindness, double vision (diplopia), drainage, bloodshot eyes, pain, blind spots, flashing lights, halos around objects, glaucoma, cataracts

EARS
Hearing deficits, hearing aid, pain, discharge, lightheadedness (vertigo), ringing in the ears (tinnitus), earaches, infection

NOSE AND SINUSES
Frequent colds, discharge, itching, hay fever, postnasal drip, stuffiness, sinus pain, polyps, obstruction, nosebleed (epistaxis), change in sense of smell

MOUTH
Toothache, tooth abscess, dentures, bleeding/swollen gums, difficulty chewing, sore tongue, change in taste, lesions, change in salivation, bad breath

THROAT/NECK
Hoarseness, change in voice, frequent sore throats, difficulty swallowing, pain/stiffness, enlarged thyroid (goiter)

RESPIRATORY
Shortness of breath (dyspnea), shortness of breath on exertion, phlegm (sputum), cough, sneezing, wheezing, coughing up blood (hemoptysis), frequent upper respiratory tract infections, pneumonia, emphysema, asthma, tuberculosis

CARDIOVASCULAR
Shortness of breath that wakes you up in the night (paroxysmal nocturnal dyspnea), chest pain, heart murmur, palpitations, fainting (syncope), sleep on pillows to breathe better (orthopnea; state number of pillows used), swelling (edema), cold hands/feet, leg cramps, myocardial infarction, hypertension, valvular disease, pain in calf when walking (intermittent claudication), varicose veins, inflammation of a vein (thrombophlebitis), blood clot in leg (deep vein thrombosis), anemia

BREASTS
Pain, tenderness, discharge, lumps, change in size, dimpling

GASTROINTESTINAL
Change in appetite, nausea, vomiting, diarrhea, constipation, usual bowel habits, black tarry stools (melena), vomiting blood (hematemesis), change in stool color, excessive gas (flatulence), belching, regurgitation, heartburn, difficulty swallowing (dysphagia), abdominal pain, jaundice, hemorrhoids, hepatitis, peptic ulcers, gallstones

URINARY
Change in urine color, voiding habits, painful urination (dysuria), hesitancy, urgency, frequency, excessive urination at night (nocturia), increased urine volume (polyuria), dribbling, loss in force of stream, bedwetting, change in urine volume, incontinence, pain in lower abdomen (suprapubic pain), kidney stones, urinary tract infections

MUSCULOSKELETAL
Joint stiffness, muscle pain, back pain, limitation of movement, redness, swelling, weakness, bony deformity, broken bones, dislocations, sprains, gout, arthritis, osteoporosis, herniated disc

FEMALE REPRODUCTIVE
Vaginal discharge, change in libido, infertility, sterility, pain during intercourse, menses: last menstrual period (LMP), age period started (menarche), regularity, duration, amount of bleeding, premenstrual symptoms, intermenstrual bleeding, painful periods (dysmenorrhea), menopause: age of onset, duration, symptoms, bleeding, obstetrical: number of pregnancies, number of miscarriages/abortions, number of children, type of delivery, complications, type of birth control, estrogen therapy

MALE REPRODUCTIVE
Change in libido, infertility, sterility, impotence, pain during intercourse, age at onset of puberty, testicular pain, penile discharge, erections, emissions, hernias, enlarged prostate, type of birth control

NUTRITION
Present weight, usual weight, food intolerances, food likes/dislikes, where meals are eaten

ENDOCRINE
Bulging eyes, fatigue, change in size of head, hands, or feet, weight change, heat/cold intolerances, excessive sweating, increased thirst, increased hunger, change in body hair distribution, swelling in the anterior neck, diabetes mellitus

LYMPH NODES
Enlargement, tenderness

HEMATOLOGICAL
Easy bruising/bleeding, anemia, sickle cell anemia, blood type

DOCUMENTING THE COMPLETE HEALTH HISTORY

Many health care facilities have preprinted health history forms that are checklists and require few narrative notes. Other facilities require the nurse to document the health history in its entirety. The health history that follows illustrates how to document the complete health history of an ill patient.

Black ink is preferred at most health care facilities. For each entry, write the complete date and time, and sign it with your full legal name and credentials unless institutional policy states otherwise. Use each line of the document. If a line is accidentally skipped, place a line through it. If an error in recording is made, do not cross it out or attempt to erase it. Simply place a single line through the error, initial it, and date it.

Remember that full sentences are not necessary when documenting the complete health history. Standard medical abbreviations should be used. The inside back book cover lists abbreviations that are commonly used in health care facilities. Use objective statements when documenting. Refer to page 784 for more information on documentation.

THE SYSTEM-SPECIFIC HEALTH HISTORY

This text uses a system-specific health history in each body system chapter (refer to Chapters 10–21). The system-specific health history provides detailed information that guides questioning and provides clues of related pathology. Not every item in the complete health history is addressed in every body system history. Only those sections relevant to the body system being assessed are addressed, and this can differ from chapter to chapter due to the nature of the material.

❖ COMPLETE HEALTH HISTORY: ILL PATIENT

Today's Date	July 22, _____ (yr)
BIOGRAPHICAL DATA	
Patient Name	Alvin Basmadjian
Address	1843 Pinehurst Road Arlington, VA 22209
Phone Number	(H) (703) 555-3533 (W) (703) 555-1234
Date of Birth	May 21, 1955
Birthplace	Philadelphia, PA
Social Security Number	123-45-6789
Occupation	Construction worker × 24 yr
Insurance	Blue Cross/Blue Shield #123-45-6789, Group No. 0123

continued

Usual Source of Health Care	Dr. Abolhassem Noorbakhsh × 10 yr Healthcare, Inc. 55 Azalea Drive Arlington, VA
Source of Referral	Pt's MD is out of town; wife suggested urgent care center
Emergency Contact	Mrs. Mary Basmadjian (wife) same
Source and Reliability of Information	Self; reliable historian

PATIENT PROFILE

Age	42
Sex	Male
Race	Caucasian
Marital Status	Married × 22 yr

CHIEF COMPLAINT	"I've been having chest pain at work for the past week & it's not getting better."
HISTORY OF THE PRESENT ILLNESS	Pt was in usual state of good health until 1 wk ago when experienced chest pain at work; $\bar{p}$ eating lunch, was doing heavy lifting when suddenly lost his breath & started to have mild chest discomfort (2/10 intensity). Attributing this to the heat (90°F), rested for 5 min & continued to work. Approximately 30 min later while again lifting, experienced more SOB & severe "deep, crushing" chest pain (7/10 intensity); became nauseated & diaphoretic; denies vomiting & radiation of pain to Ⓛ arm; immediately sat down & when pain subsided 10 min later, went to car & turned on air conditioner; 15 min later the episode subsided & left work for the day. Was off from work for next 2 d; no episodes of chest pain; 3 d ago returned to work, temperature in high 70°s. Shortly after starting work, experienced chest pain (3/10 intensity) similar to that experienced 3 d earlier, & "brought on by hammering"; lasted 5 min & was alleviated by rest. Then took the rest of the day off. Today, while mowing lawn, experienced substernal chest pain that left him breathless. After 1 hr still had pain & grew concerned; could not reach his usual MD, wife convinced him to go to urgent care center; denies radiation, nausea, vomiting. Pt is "concerned" about chest pain as it interferes $\bar{c}$ employment; has little sick time remaining this yr; wife currently unemployed; loss of salary "would have a devastating financial effect" on family. Wishes to get chest pain resolved so he can return to work ASAP.

PAST HEALTH HISTORY

Medical History	1992: HTN dx by Dr. Noorbakhsh; follows low-sodium diet 1996: ↑ cholesterol per Dr. Noorbakhsh; prescribed low-cholesterol diet, not followed; frontal H/A about 1 × wk; tx $\bar{c}$ Tylenol for past "few yr"

continued

Surgical History	1960: Tonsillectomy at St. Agnes Hospital, Philadelphia; hospitalized × 4 d; no complications
Medications	
Prescription	Denies
OTC	Vitamins 1 tab po q AM × 10 yr Tylenol 650 mg po for H/A per medical hx
Communicable Diseases	1972: Gonorrhea; sx: penile d/c & tender penis; treated at health dept c̄ Atb; took all of Atb but didn't return for follow-up care Never tested for HIV Denies hx rheumatic fever, TB, syphilis, hepatitis, AIDS
Allergies	Allergic to erythromycin since 1970; took it for URI & "had spots all over"; MD told him never to take med again Denies allergies to foods, animals, or environmental elements
Injuries/Accidents	1962: Broke Ⓡ arm when fell off patio deck; cast × 2 mo, no complications 1972: MVA; minor bruises; drinking beer ā driving home; severe H/A for few wks; tx c̄ Tylenol 1996: Construction accident: fell 10 ft off scaffolding & broke "lower" Ⓡ leg; cast × 8 wks; physical therapy × 4 wks; leg "gets stiff on rainy days"
Disabilities/Handicaps	dx in grade school c̄ dyslexia; attended special classes × 1 yr; still has difficulty reading
Blood Transfusions	Denies receiving blood or blood products
Childhood Illnesses	Recalls having had chicken pox, measles, & mumps (dates unknown); no complications Denies having diphtheria, pertussis, polio, rheumatic fever, rubella, scarlet fever, smallpox
Immunizations	States "I had all the right immunizations as a child"; no complications Tetanus booster last yr

FAMILY HEALTH HISTORY

LEGEND

- Living female
- Living male
- Deceased female
- Deceased male
- Points to patient

A&W = Alive & well
Chol = Cholesterol
CP = Chest pain
H/A = Headache
HTN = Hypertension
MI = Myocardial infarction

68 A&W — 50 MI Gout   57 MI

39 A&W — 42 CP H/A HTN ↑Chol   42 MI HTN   41 MI   45 MI

15 A&W   10 A&W

Denies family hx of TB, DM, CA, kidney dz, liver dz, blood disorders, arthritis, epilepsy, migraine H/A, thyroid dz, asthma, allergic disorders, obesity, alcoholism, drug addiction, mental illness, AIDS.

continued

SOCIAL HISTORY

Alcohol Use
2 beers $\bar{a}$ dinner (at home) × 19 yr
1–2 six-packs q Saturday PM $\bar{c}$ friends during poker game × 19 yr; drives home afterwards by self
Denies drinking on the job or having hiding place for beer
Denies drinking problem, but admits wife wants him to quit

Tobacco Use
21 pack/yr hx (low-tar filtered cigarettes)
Never tried to quit smoking & has no desire to quit
Denies use of pipe, cigars, chewing tobacco, & snuff

Drug Use
Experimented $\bar{c}$ drugs as teenager (ages 15–19); tried marijuana, PCP, amphetamines, & other unknown substances; used them on weekends only; denies long-lasting effects
Denies ever injecting drugs
Refuses to elaborate on any other information

Sexual Practice
States that he has "always been a heterosexual"
As teenager involved $\bar{c}$ multiple partners
Currently sexually active $\bar{c}$ wife; monogamous sexual partner × 17 yr
Refuses to elaborate on other details

Travel History
Denies travel outside the country
Vacations at the VA beaches q summer

Work Environment
Construction worker: builds houses
Wears hard helmet when at work; denies major work-related accidents $\bar{x}$ broken leg
Physically demanding job
Exposed to all types of building materials
Denies exposure to radiation, toxic fumes, & chemicals

Home Environment

Physical Environment
Urban 30 yo house that is complete $\bar{c}$ all modern conveniences (phone, gas heat, running water, electricity)
"It's too small for a family of four."
Never tested house for radon
Never uses fireplace
Smoke detector in kitchen; disconnects it when it beeps
House is cleaned regularly by wife
Dog stays outside
All cleaning supplies are kept under kitchen sink; extra gasoline is kept in garage
8 yo car, no difficulty getting around

Psychosocial Environment
"Neighborhood is usually safe"

Hobbies/Leisure Activities
Plays softball on summer weekends in work-related league
Poker q Saturday PM $\bar{c}$ work buddies
"Watch sports & drink beer all weekend long"

Stress
Biggest source of stress is chest pain
Additional sources of stress: oldest child not doing well in school; wife "nagging" him to stop drinking & smoking so much
Does not recognize stress until he becomes very nervous $\bar{c}$ SOB, trembling hands
Denies having a "nervous breakdown"

continued

Education	"Barely passed high school"
Economic Status	Describes family as "self-sufficient" Lives "paycheck to paycheck"
Military Service	Denies any military service: "I just missed the draft"
Religion	Inactive Russian Orthodox Denies religion interferes $\bar{c}$ hl care practices
Ethnic Background	Describes self as Armenian American Denies any effect of ethnicity on hl care practices
Roles/Relationships	Sole wage earner in family Lives $\bar{c}$ wife, 2 children; describes relationships as being "OK" Socializes $\bar{c}$ work buddies & next-door neighbor; not involved $\bar{c}$ rest of neighborhood
Characteristic Patterns of Daily Living	Wakes at 0430, showers, shaves, & dresses. Smokes cigarette; breakfast at 0500 & leaves for work at 0515. Starts work at 0600 (construction site differs depending on the job); break at 0900, eats snack obtained from vendor. Smokes q 30–60 min. Noon lunch break: sandwiches from home. Leaves work at 1500 unless works overtime (averages 8 hr of overtime per wk). Arrives home approximately 1600. Plays $\bar{o}$ dog for 15–20 min. Before dinner relaxes, watches TV, & drinks 1–2 beers. Family dinner at 1730. Watches sports on TV $\bar{p}$ dinner. Goes to bed between 2100 & 2200.
HEALTH MAINTENANCE ACTIVITIES	
Sleep	During wk bedtime is between 2100 & 2200; awakes at 0430 On wkend, bedtime is between 2300 & 0200; sleeps until 9–10 AM; takes 1 hr nap during day on wkends Bedroom environment is quiet, completely dark Difficulty falling asleep $\cong$ 1 × wk, usually $\bar{p}$ a big game; drinks beer to help fall asleep Denies insomnia, sleepwalking, nightmares
Diet	Doesn't add salt to food to adhere to low-sodium diet; wife doesn't add salt to food while cooking Doesn't follow low-cholesterol diet: "It's too bland" Prefers fried foods & prepared foods Denies difficulty in tasting, chewing, swallowing food
Exercise	Recreational exercise q Saturday playing softball "Works up a sweat at work" when lifting heavy materials Not involved in exercise program: "I don't have time"
Stress Management	Beer drinking; smokes when feels uptight "Not interested in learning any other techniques"
Use of Safety Devices	Wears seat belt on occasion Wears hard helmet at construction site; other restrictions as required by employer

continued

Health Check-ups	Visits Dr. Noorbakhsh only when sick ($\cong$ 1 × yr) Last yr (when broke leg) had physical, c̄ blood work & u/a Sees dentist only when something bothers him; can't remember last visit No vision check since grade school Denies having prostate exam Denies testicular self-examination; doesn't know how to perform it & "doesn't want to know"

REVIEW OF SYSTEMS

General	Well-developed, well-nourished male in usual state of good hl until
	   1 wk ago; more tired in past wk & has no energy. He feels that he
	   "may be seriously ill."

Neurological	H/A per PHH
	Denies change in balance, incoordination, loss of movement, change in
	   sensory perception, change in speech, change in smell, tremors,
	   syncope, loss of memory, involuntary movement, loss of consciousness,
	   sz, weakness

Psychological	Been more irritable past 2 wks due to deadlines at work & heat Denies nervousness, difficulty concentrating, mood changes, depression, suicidal thoughts

Skin	Excessive sweating per HPI
	Denies rashes, itching, changes in skin pigmentation, ecchymoses,
	   change in moles, sores, lumps, change in skin texture, body odors,
	   acne, alopecia, hirsutism, change in nails

Eyes	20/20 vision at last eye exam in grade school
	Difficulty seeing at night
	Denies blurry vision, photophobia, ↑ tearing, diplopia, eye drainage,
	   bloodshot eyes, pain, blind spots, flashing lights, halos around objects,
	   glaucoma, cataracts

Ears	Denies hearing deficits, hearing aid, pain, d/c, vertigo, tinnitus, earaches, infection
Nose and Sinuses	Denies frequent colds, d/c, itching, hay fever, postnasal drip, sinus pain, polyps, obstruction, epistaxis, change in sense of smell

Mouth	Denies toothache, tooth abscess, dentures, bleeding/swollen gums, sore
	   tongue, change in taste, lesions, change in salivation, bad breath,
	   difficulty chewing

Throat/Neck	Denies hoarseness, change in voice, frequent sore throats, difficulty swallowing, pain/stiffness, goiter

Respiratory	SOB & DOE per HPI
	URI q winter (congestion, cough, fever, chills); treated by Dr.
	   Noorbakhsh c̄ "some medication"
	Denies sputum, sneezing, wheezing, hemoptysis, pneumonia,
	   emphysema, asthma, TB

continued

Cardiovascular	Chest pain per HPI; HTN per PHH Denies paroxysmal nocturnal dyspnea, heart murmur, palpitations, syncope, edema, orthopnea, cold hands/feet, leg cramps, MI, intermittent claudication, varicose veins, thrombophlebitis, anemia, rheumatic heart disease
Breasts	Denies change in size, pain, tenderness, d/c, lumps
Gastrointestinal	Nausea per HPI Regular bowel habit: BM q AM, soft & brown During past wk hasn't been as hungry as usual; attributes to hot weather Denies vomiting, diarrhea, constipation, melena, change in stool color, hematemesis; ↑ flatulence, belching, heartburn, regurgitation; dysphagia, abdominal pain, jaundice, peptic ulcers, hemorrhoids, hepatitis, gallstones
Urinary	Denies change in urine color, voiding habits, hesitancy, urgency, frequency, nocturia, polyuria, dribbling, loss in force of stream, bedwetting, suprapubic pain, kidney stones, incontinence
Musculoskeletal	Broken leg & arm per PHH Right foot becomes sore if stands in one location for too long; position change & rest relieve this Denies bony deformity, weakness, swelling, sprains, dislocations, gout, arthritis, herniated disc, back pain
Male Reproductive	Penile discharge per PHH Puberty at age 14 Became sexually active at age 17 Denies use of birth control: "my wife does that" Denies change in libido, impotence, pain during intercourse, testicular pain, difficulty $\bar{c}$ erections, hernias
Nutrition	Usual weight 85 kg (187 lbs), present weight 82 kg (180 lbs) Food preferences: fried chicken, pork chops, spaghetti Food dislikes: most vegetables, liver, fish Likes to eat in front of TV Denies food intolerances
Endocrine	Fatigue × 1 wk Denies bulging eyes, change in size of head, hands, or feet, cold intolerance, ↑ thirst, ↑ hunger, change in body hair distribution, swelling in anterior neck
Lymph Nodes	Denies enlargement or tenderness
Hematological	Denies easy bruising/bleeding, anemia, blood type unknown

REVIEW QUESTIONS
AND ACTIVITIES

1. A patient presents with a complaint of severe migraine headaches. Write a sample HPI for this patient. Remember to include all nine characteristics of a chief complaint.

2. Record a complete health history on yourself. Have a colleague critique the written record.

3. Conduct a complete health history with a colleague. Have the colleague critique your approach, questioning skills, and content.

4. Identify sources for health promotion in the sample complete health history of the ill patient.

5. Identify in which section of the health history each of the following statements belongs:
   a. Grandmother died at 63 from liver CA, grandfather age 72 A&W.
   b. Smokes ½ pack cigarettes a day.
   c. Denies toothache, tooth abscess, bleeding/swollen gums.
   d. 1995 TURP, 1993 excision basal cell carcinoma on nose.
   e. Visits dentist annually for check-up & cleaning.
   f. "I hurt my knee playing basketball today."
   g. Pt is a 35-yo Hispanic male.

6. A health history that is specific to the patient's current reason for seeking health care best describes the:
   a. Complete health history
   b. Episodic health history
   c. Interval health history
   d. Follow-up health history

   The correct answer is (b).

7. Your patient is describing her abdominal pain to you. She tells you that an antacid temporarily decreased the severity of the pain. Which characteristic of a chief complaint best describes the action of the antacid?
   a. Quality
   b. Associated manifestation
   c. Alleviating factor
   d. Timing

   The correct answer is (c).

8. In which section of the health history would the following statement belong: "osteoporosis diagnosed 5 years ago"?
   a. Chief complaint
   b. History of present illness
   c. Past health history
   d. Social history

   The correct answer is (c).

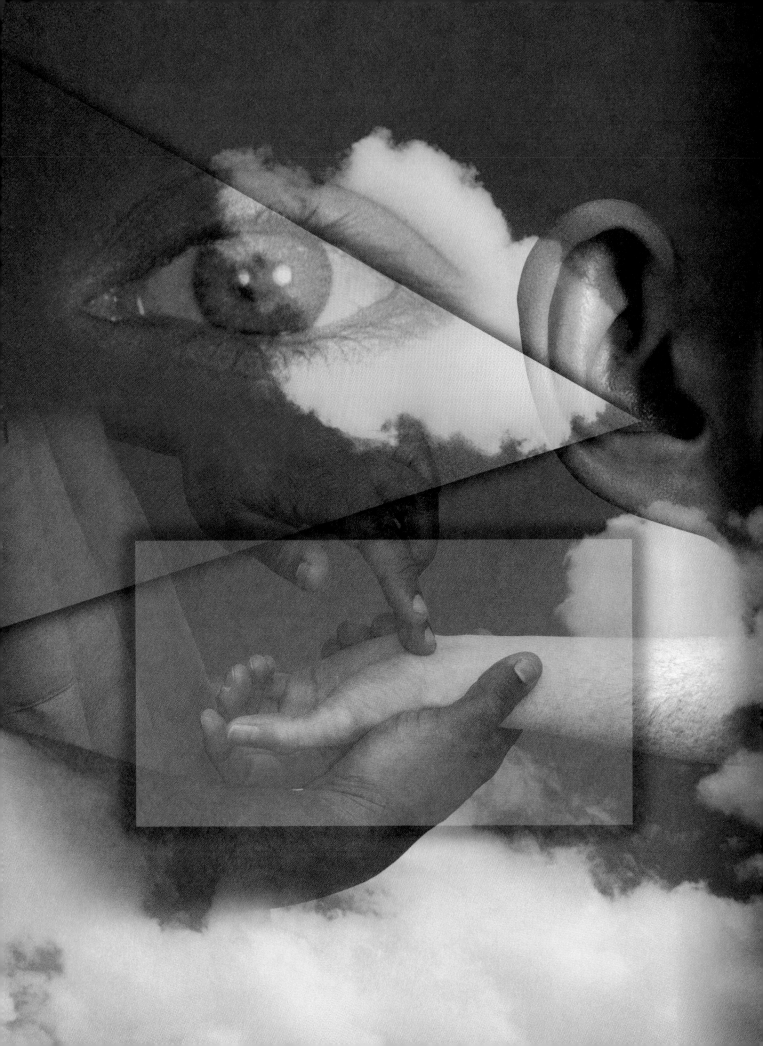

Special Assessments

UNIT II

But if you cannot get the habit of observation one way or other, you had better give up the being a nurse, for it is not your calling.

Florence Nightingale

Developmental Assessment

COMPETENCIES

1. Identify the defining concepts and principles of major developmental theories.
2. Select appropriate developmental assessment tools for use in screening a patient for developmental difficulties.
3. Incorporate appropriate developmental tasks associated with each life stage into a patient's assessment.
4. Incorporate meaningful life events in relation to a patient's current developmental state into the patient's assessment.

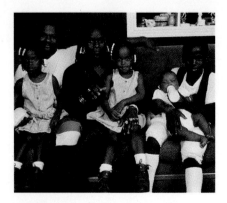

Figure 4-1   All individuals pass through identifiable growth and development stages.

$\mathbf{A}$ll individuals, from birth to death, pass through identifiable, cyclical stages of growth and development that determine who and what they are and can become (see Figure 4-1). **Growth** refers to an increase in body size and function to the point of optimum maturity. **Development** refers to patterned and predictable increases in the physical, cognitive, socioemotional, and moral capacities of individuals that enable them to successfully adapt to their environments.

Assessing the growth and development status of patients, adults as well as children, is an integral part of patient assessment. It must be noted, however, that although most development is patterned and predictable, you should not impose these expected patterns on a particular patient; assess instead the individual patient's unique development as compared to these general guidelines.

DEVELOPMENTAL THEORIES

A variety of theories have been developed that depict and predict growth and development. The theories most widely used for clinical assessment of patients are the "ages and stages" theories of Piaget (1952), Freud (1946), Erickson (1974), and Kohlberg (1981). The **ages and stages developmental theories** are based on the premise that individuals experience similar sequential physical, cognitive, socioemotional, and moral changes during the same age periods, each of which is termed a **developmental stage**. During each developmental stage there are specific physical and psychosocial skills known as **developmental tasks** that must be achieved. An individual's readiness for each new developmental task is dependent on success in achieving prior developmental tasks and on the presence of environmental opportunities to develop the new skills. If prior developmental tasks have been insufficiently achieved and/or appropriate environments in which the tasks can be achieved are not available, mastery of subsequent developmental skills may not occur, may be delayed, or may occur in a defective way, thereby decreasing the individual's capacity to successfully adapt to the environment during his or her life span. A key nursing role in assessment is to help identify areas of deficiency and then develop a plan of care designed to address the patient's needs.

A second group of theories include the life events or transitional theories of development. **Life event/transitional developmental theories** are based on the premise that development occurs in response to specific events, such as new roles (e.g., parenthood) and life transitions (e.g., career changes). Life events and transitions require adaptive, coping behavior as well as often significant changes in an individual's life patterns. Each of these events, which can occur singly or together and may be positively or negatively stressful, are not tied to a specific time or stage in the life span. Each event, however, does have certain tasks associated with it that must be achieved. For example, getting married is associated with specific developmental tasks that must be achieved regardless of the age of the individual at the time of marriage. The degree of success or failure with these tasks influences the individual's potential for success with concurrent and subsequent developmental tasks that occur in response to any other life events. A variety of factors have been found to affect how an individual responds to life events: biological status, personality, cultural orientation, socioeconomic status, interpersonal support systems, number and intensity of life events, and orientation to life (Lazarus & Folkman, 1984; Antonovsky, 1987; Aldwin, 1992). Although the stress associated with each life event or transition can serve as an impetus for growth, excessive stress can disrupt the individual's equilibrium and lead to a variety of physical and psychological health problems (Wykle, Kahana, & Kowal, 1992; Grey, 1993; Aguilera, 1994). In identifying life events and stressors, nurses can play a critical role in helping patients maintain health and control stress.

Ages and Stages Developmental Theories
Piaget's Theory of Cognitive Development

Jean Piaget's (1952) (b. 1896–d. 1980) theory of cognitive development depicts age-related, sequential stages through which all developing children must progress to learn to think, reason, and exercise judgment and to learn the cognitive life skills (e.g., language development, problem solving, decision making, critical thinking, and oral and written communication) needed to successfully adapt to their environments. The individual's cognitive development is influenced by innate intellectual capacity, maturation of the nervous and endocrine systems, and varied interactions with the environment during which sensory and motor input is experienced and processed. Piaget divides cognitive development into four periods: sensorimotor stage, preoperational stage, concrete operations stage, and formal operational stage.

Sensorimotor Stage   During the sensorimotor stage (birth to 2 years), the developing child perceives the world primarily through sensation and action response. The primary cognitive developmental task for this stage is to learn **object permanence**, i.e., to form a mental image of an object and to recognize that although the object is removed from view, it still exists. Object permanence is usually achieved by the eighth month of life and facilitates the achievement of the second cognitive task, the development of a sense of self separate from one's environment. Beginning to use language and mental representations to think about events before and/or after they occur is an additional cognitive task that must be achieved during this stage.

Preoperational Stage   The second cognitive development period is the preoperational stage (2 to 7 years), which is characterized by **egocentrism**, i.e., viewing the world in terms of self only and interpreting actions and all other events in terms of the consequences they have for self. Learning during this stage usually occurs through imitation of others, physical and cognitive exploration of the environment, and asking numerous questions. Thinking is concrete and reasoning is intuitive and based on the observable, i.e., what is directly seen, heard, or personally experienced. The major cognitive developmental task for this stage is to use language and mental representations to think and communicate about objects and events in the environment.

Concrete Operations Stage   During the third cognitive development period, the concrete operations stage (7 to 12 years), thinking becomes socialized in that thought becomes less self-oriented and others' points of view are given consideration. Thinking becomes increasingly logical and coherent, facts are organized through sorting, ordering, and classifying, the concept of time evolves, different aspects of situations are dealt with simultaneously, reasoning is inductive, problems are solved concretely and systematically, and communication is enhanced through expanding oral skills and learning to read and write. The major developmental tasks are mastering the concept of **conservation** (understanding that altering the physical state of an object does not change the basic properties of the object) and **reversibility** (understanding that an action does not need to be experienced before one can anticipate the results or consequences of the action).

Formal Operational Stage   The fourth cognitive development period is the formal operational stage (12 years to adulthood) in which thinking becomes increasingly abstract, logical, analytical, and creative. Ideas are combined to form concepts and concepts are combined to form constructs, hypotheses and theories are developed and beginning to be tested, alternate solutions for problems are generated and examined, and the antecedents, moderators, and outcomes of ideas, concepts, situations, and actions are recognized and incorporated into the individual's worldview. The primary cognitive developmental task for this stage is to develop a workable philosophy of life.

Freud's Psychoanalytic Theory of Personality Development

Sigmund Freud (1946) (b. 1856–d. 1939) contended that human behavior is motivated by psychodynamic forces within an individual's unconscious mind. Driven to act by these internal forces, individuals repeatedly interact with the external environment. The individual's personality and psychosexual identity are developed through the accumulation of these interactional experiences.

Personality   Personality, according to Freud, consists of three components with distinctly separate functions: id, ego, and superego. The **id**, evident at birth, is inborn, unconscious, and is driven by biological instincts and urges to seek immediate gratification of needs such as hunger, thirst, and physical comfort. The **ego** is conscious, rational, and emerges during the first year of life as infants begin to test the limits of the world around them. The ego seeks realistic and acceptable ways to meet needs. The **superego**, appearing in early childhood, is the internalization of the moral values formed as children interact with their parents and significant others. The superego acts as a moral arbitrator by blocking unacceptable behavior generated by the id that could threaten the social order, creating feelings of guilt when the internalized moral code is compromised, and generating feelings of pride when the moral code is upheld.

Freud believed individuals experience an ongoing struggle among the id, ego, and superego. Achieving a balance among the three, however, is prerequisite to the development of socially acceptable behavior and an integrated personality. To assist the personality to achieve this balance and to protect itself from excess anxiety created by the ongoing struggle, the ego uses unconscious defense mechanisms such as repression, denial, projection, and rationalization.

Psychosexual Stages   Freud perceived the desire to satisfy biological needs, primarily sexual, as the major drive governing human behavior. At different psychosexual developmental stages, individuals experience tension associated with a specific body region that prompts them to seek gratification of the needs and conflicts thereby engendered. Each developmental stage is centered on a specific body region and the associated conflicts. If an individual's needs are met during a given stage and conflicts are resolved, development will proceed normally to the next stage, and the developing personality will be integrated in a healthy way. If resolution of the conflict does not occur, however, the individual will become fixated at that stage, and personality and psychosexual identity will be arrested or impaired. Freud identified five psychosexual stages of development: oral, anal, phallic, latency, and genital.

Oral Stage.   The oral psychosexual stage (birth to 1 year) is focused on the sensory area of the mouth, lips, and tongue. Sucking, biting, chewing, swallowing, and vocalizing provide pleasure and reduce tension. The major conflict during this stage centers around weaning. Oral personality traits that begin to emerge are optimism versus pessimism, cockiness versus self-belittlement, admiration versus envy, determinism versus submission, and gullibility versus suspiciousness.

Anal Stage.   In the anal psychosexual stage (1 to 3 years), the focus is on the anal and urethral sensory areas. Expulsion and retention of body wastes provide pleasure and reduce tension. The major conflict centers around toilet training. Anal personality traits that begin to emerge during this period are orderliness versus messiness, acquiescence versus stubbornness, overgenerosity versus stinginess, rigid punctuality versus tardiness, and expansiveness versus constrictedness.

Phallic Stage. The phallic psychosexual stage (3 to 6 years) is focused on the sensory areas of the genitals. Pleasure is provided and tension is reduced through penile and clitoral exploration and stimulation. The major conflicts center around the controversial **Oedipus** (young boys' sexual attraction toward their mothers and feelings of rivalry toward their fathers) and **Electra** (young girls' sexual attraction toward their fathers and rivalry with their mothers for their fathers' attention) **complexes**, **castration anxiety** (young boys' fear of having their penis cut off or mutilated), and **penis envy** (young girls' desire to have a penis). Phallic personality traits that begin to emerge are gaiety versus sadness, gregariousness versus isolationism, stylishness versus plainness, blind courage versus timidity, and brashness versus bashfulness.

Latency Stage. During the latency psychosexual stage (6 to 12 years), the focus is on the exploration and discovery of the total body's relatedness, coordination, and uses rather than on a specific body region. Channeling generalized psychic and physical activity into knowledge acquisition and vigorous play provides pleasure and reduces tension. The major conflict during this stage centers around identifying with the same sex parent, learning and testing mental and physical capabilities, and comparing one's capabilities with peer norms.

Genital Stage. The genital psychosexual stage (12 years to adulthood) is focused on full sexual maturity and function. Self and mutual sexual stimulation and the formation of friendships and sexual relationships provide pleasure and reduce tension. The major conflicts during this period center around becoming sexually desirable to others and establishing meaningful relationships in preparation for lifelong pairing.

Erikson's Epigenetic Theory of Personality

The most frequently used theory of personality development is Erikson's (1974) (b. 1902–d. 1994) epigenetic theory, which is based on the biological concept that all growing organisms have an inherent plan of growth for all parts of the entity. Each part of a growing entity has a designated time of ascendancy and forms the basis for growth of the next part until the functional whole is fully developed. Erikson's theory was built on Freud's theory of personality but goes beyond it by depicting personality development as a passage through eight sequential stages of ego development from infancy through old age.

According to Erikson, developing individuals must master and resolve, to some extent, a core conflict/crisis during each stage by integrating their personal needs and skills with the social and cultural demands and expectations of their environment. Passage to each developmental stage is dependent on the resolution of the core conflict of the preceding stage. No core conflict is ever completely mastered, however. Rather, in each new life situation, the conflict can be present in a new form that can then be resolved more readily if the conflict was initially resolved favorably. If the conflict was initially resolved unfavorably, subsequent encounters with new forms of the core conflict can provide opportunities to try again to resolve it favorably. Thus the potential for further development and refinement always exists. For each of the eight core conflicts/crises, there is an associated central process for resolving the conflict, a key socializing agent, and an ego quality that results from the favorable resolution of the core conflict.

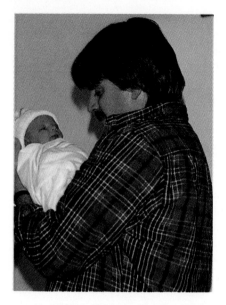

Figure 4-2 Strong parental bonding and attention to needs help the infant develop trust.

Trust versus Mistrust Stage   The core conflict/crisis for the first developmental stage (birth to 1 year) is trust versus mistrust. Through the central process of mutuality with mothering persons, the key socializing agents, the ego quality of hope is developed, resulting in faith and optimism. Thus when developing infants' basic needs are met by prompt, consistent, predictable, loving parent figures, basic, relative trust evolves (see Figure 4-2). If infants' needs are intermittently, inadequately, or perfunctorily met, mistrust results.

Autonomy versus Shame and Doubt Stage   The second developmental stage (1 to 3 years) is focused on the autonomy versus shame and doubt core conflict/crisis. Developing toddlers achieve autonomy through the central process of imitation of their parents, who are their key socializing agents during this stage. The ego qualities of self-control and willpower are the favorable results of the parental encouragement and approval children receive while they are learning to use their increasing physical and mental abilities to control their bodies (walking, climbing, toileting), to exert independence in making decisions, and to conform to social rules. If parental figures overprotect their children and overly criticize and punish their attempts to explore and control their environments and body activities, as well as their attempts to make independent decisions, then shame, doubt, and uncertainty about their abilities and themselves will result.

Initiative versus Guilt Stage   During the third developmental stage (3 to 6 years), the core conflict/crisis is initiative versus guilt. Through the central process of identification and with parents serving as the key socializing agents, preschoolers develop initiative that results in the ego qualities of direction, purpose, and, ultimately, conscience. When children are encouraged to explore their environments and to plan and work toward goals that do not infringe on the rights of others, they develop initiative and moral responsibility. In contrast, if children are restricted from exploration of their environments or are made to feel that their enterprise and active imaginations are bad, they will experience guilt and lose the courage to conceive of and pursue valued goals.

Industry versus Inferiority Stage   The central conflict/crisis for the fourth developmental stage (6 to 12 years) is industry versus inferiority. Developing school-age children achieve a sense of accomplishment, self-assurance, and self-esteem through the central process of education when teachers and peers are their key socializing agents. The ego quality of competence is the favorable result of being encouraged to and successfully engaging in achievable tasks and activities, competing and cooperating with others, and learning the rules and norms of a widening social and cultural environment. If children are not given sufficient opportunities or encouragement to develop their abilities or are pushed to achieve beyond their present abilities and thus repeatedly fail, feelings of inadequacy and inferiority result and new learning activities will be increasingly avoided.

Identity versus Role Confusion Stage   The fifth stage of development (12 to 18 years) is focused on the identity versus role confusion core conflict/crisis. Through the central processes of peer pressure and role experimentation, and with the society of peers serving as the key socializing agents, adolescents must make the transition from childhood to adulthood, redefine themselves in terms of the roles they hope to play in society, explore life work possibilities, and integrate self-concept and values with those of their peers and society. Supportive, understanding interactions with peers and adult role models help clarify self-identity and lead to the ego quality of fidelity and devotion to others as well as personal and sociocultural values and ideologies. Unfavorable interactions and/or overidentification with popular teen fads and peer culture heroes can result in role confusion and difficulty clarifying personal identity.

Intimacy versus Isolation Stage Intimacy versus isolation is the core conflict/crisis associated with the sixth developmental stage (18 to 30 years). The central process through which young adults establish a sense of intimacy is mutuality among peers, and the key socializing agents are close friends, partners, lovers, and spouses. The capacity for intimate affiliation with and the love of significant others is the ego quality that results from the favorable resolution of this core conflict. Feelings of aloneness and social isolation are the result of unsuccessful resolution.

Generativity versus Stagnation Stage The seventh developmental stage (30 to 65 years) is focused on the core conflict of generativity versus stagnation. Generativity is when one's focus on meeting the needs of others is of equal concern to that of providing for oneself. The central processes are creativity and person-environment fit (the individual's basic interests and abilities are well matched with the demands of the environment). Children, spouses, partners, and sociocultural norms become the key socializing agents during this stage. The ego qualities of productivity, perseverance, charity, and consideration result from the development of generativity. Generative young and middle-aged adults nourish and nurture the products of their creativity at home, at work, and in their communities. Individuals who are unsuccessful in resolving the core conflict during this stage of development become self-absorbed and feel chronically unfulfilled.

Ego Integrity versus Despair Stage During the eighth and last stage of development (65 years to death), the core conflict/crisis is ego integrity versus despair. The central process is introspection, which leads to the ego quality of wisdom. Supportive and accepting significant others (often including caregivers during the period of declining ability to independently perform activities of daily living) serve as the key socializing agents who can assist introspective elderly persons in the maintenance of an active concern with life while facing the inevitability of death. After reviewing one's life in its entirety, acceptance of what has passed and satisfaction with the present results in a sense of integrity. In contrast, remorse for the past and what might have been results in despair.

Kohlberg's Theory of Moral Development

The basic premise of Kohlberg's (1981) (b. 1927–d. 1987) theory of moral development is that when a conflict occurs among any of several universal values (e.g., punishment, affection, authority, truth, law, life, liberty, and justice), the moral choice that must be made and justified requires cognitive capabilities, including systematic problem solving, which constitute moral reasoning. Thus the development of the individual's moral reasoning and associated behaviors parallel the development of cognitive behavior primarily. According to Kohlberg, moral development is contingent upon children's ability to learn and internalize parental and societal rules and standards, develop the ability to empathize with others' responses, and form their own personal standards of conduct. Moral development progresses through three levels with two distinct stages per level for a total of six stages. Keep in mind that Kohlberg's theory of moral development has fallen under heavy criticism because an all-male population was studied.

Preconventional Level The first level of moral development, the preconventional level, parallels Piaget's preoperational level of cognitive development and is divided into two stages. In stage 1, the morality stage, individuals have an egocentric point of view and avoid breaking rules and damaging persons and property in order to avoid being punished by authority figures with superior power. In stage 2 — the individualism, instrumental purpose, and exchange stage — individuals have a concrete individualistic perspective and follow rules only when doing so is primarily in their own or sometimes in someone else's immediate interest, and because "right" is relative or what is "fair" and represents an equal exchange.

Conventional Level   The second level of moral development, the conventional level, parallels Piaget's concrete operational stage and the beginning of the formal operations stage of cognitive development. This level is divided into two stages: stage 3, mutual interpersonal expectations, relationships, and interpersonal conformity, in which individuals can envision the perspective of another and try to live up to the expectations of self and others through conformity to moral norms, have "good" motives, are concerned about others, believe in rules and regulations, and maintain relationships by being trustworthy, loyal, respectful, and appropriately grateful; and stage 4, social system and conscience, in which individuals can differentiate societal points of view from interpersonal agreements and motives and avoid the breakdown of the social system by recognizing and supporting how the system defines roles and rules, by fulfilling the duties to which they have agreed, and by upholding laws because they are fixed social duties. According to Kohlberg, most adults in the United States have not progressed beyond this stage of moral judgment.

Postconventional Level   The third level of moral development, the postconventional level, which parallels the latter phase of Piaget's formal operations stage of cognitive development, is also divided into two stages: stage 5, social contract or utility and individual rights, in which adult individuals recognize that there are moral and legal points of view that may sometimes be in conflict and that although most rules are relative to the group that makes them, they warrant being upheld in the interest of the greatest good for the greatest number. Individuals in this stage recognize that as people's needs change, laws may need to be changed by working through the system to do so. Nonetheless, laws that protect some universal rights such as life and liberty must be upheld regardless of people's changing opinions or desires; and stage 6, universal ethical principles, in which some middle-aged or older adults develop a rational, universal moral perspective and a commitment to laws and social agreements based on universal moral principles of justice, equal rights, and respect for human dignity. When laws violate these moral principles, the principle rather than the law must be followed regardless of the price that must be paid for doing so. Kohlberg contends that few people attain and even fewer maintain this state of moral development.

See Table 4-1 for a summary of the developmental theories discussed.

DEVELOPMENTAL STAGES, TASKS, AND LIFE EVENTS

As evident from a review of the preceding theories of development, there is no complete agreement about the age associated with each developmental stage. In addition, improved nutrition, medical advances, and healthier lifestyles have contributed to greater longevity in the United States and other Western countries. As a result, what was once considered to be the beginning of late adulthood (55 to 70 years) is now a part of middle adulthood, and what was considered to be the latter part of late adulthood (70+ years) is now recognized as the beginning rather than the end of this period. The developmental assessment process presented in this text, therefore, will be presented using the following stages:

Stage 1:	Infancy (birth to 1 year)
Stage 2:	Toddler (1 to 3 years)
Stage 3:	Preschooler (3 to 6 years)
Stage 4:	School-age child (6 to 12 years)
Stage 5:	Adolescence (12 to 18 years)
Stage 6:	Young adulthood (18 to 30 years)

❖ ASK YOURSELF

Evaluating Developmental Theories

- Do you agree with the major premises of the developmental theories presented in this chapter?
- Conduct a personal investigation into the research methodologies used by the theorists. Consider the following questions after your research is concluded:
  - What populations did the theorists study when drawing the conclusions upon which their theories are based?
  - Were the appropriate conclusions made on the research data?
  - Would you have approached the study in a different manner? How?
  - Think critically about the research. What conclusions would you draw?

Stage 7:   Early middle adulthood (30 to 50 years)
Stage 8:   Late middle adulthood (50 to 70 years)
Stage 9:   Late adulthood (70 years to death)

The following section combines the developmental tasks and life events and transitions from each major theory of development, thereby giving a composite of the developmental tasks and possible life events that characterize each developmental stage. The lists of tasks for each stage are not exhaustive nor do they reflect all the tasks facing the full range of normal human conditions and circumstances. Generally, ask yourself if the individual's overall development seems consistent with the tasks usually associated with the person's chronological age. In addition, the life events included in each stage are not restricted to that stage but may occur or reoccur during several developmental stages. Failure to meet tasks in one area does not always indicate abnormal development. It is expected that the following will form a general framework on which you can base your assessment of a patient's growth and development. Remember to consider each individual as a whole entity, not just a collection of tasks met or not met.

Developmental Tasks of Infancy (Birth to 1 Year)

Infancy is a period of dramatic and rapid physical, motor, cognitive, emotional, and social growth, which marks it as one of the most critical periods of growth and development. During the first year of life infants change from totally helpless, dependent newborns to unique individuals who actively interact with their environments and form meaningful relationships with significant others (see Figure 4-3). A list of key gross and fine motor, language, and sensory milestones associated with this period can be found in Table 4-2.

One of the major tasks of infancy is weaning, which requires children to give up the breast or bottle, which has been a major source of gratification, and learn to use a cup (Jackson & Saunders, 1993). Readiness for weaning usually occurs between 6 months and 12 to 14 months, when the child has learned that good things also come from a spoon, when more motor control has been developed so a cup can be grasped and brought to the mouth, and when the desire for freedom of movement begins to lessen the desire to be held while eating.

Conducting a comprehensive assessment of an infant requires evaluation of the degree to which the infant has achieved the developmental tasks of infancy. It is important to remember that although individuals experience similar sequential physical, cognitive, socioemotional, and moral changes during the same age periods, there is still a degree of normal variability from one child to another. Developmental tasks that must be achieved during the infancy stage are to:

1. Develop a basic, relative sense of trust.

2. Develop a sense of self as dependent but separate from others, particularly the mother.

3. Develop and desire affection for and response from others, particularly the mother.

4. Develop a preverbal communication system, including emotional expression, to communicate needs and desires.

5. Begin to develop conceptual abilities and a language system.

6. Begin to learn purposeful fine and gross motor skills, particularly eye-hand coordination and balance.

7. Begin to explore and recognize the immediate environment.

8. Develop object permanence.

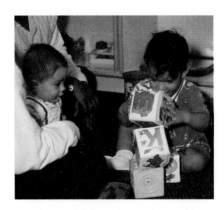

Figure 4-3 Dramatic and rapid growth and development are hallmarks of the first year of life.

◉ THINK ABOUT IT

Helping Parents Understand Development

Caregivers are often nervous about their infants and have many questions. Consider how you would respond to each of these questions:

• "My sister's baby was already holding his bottle at 6 months, but my little boy doesn't seem to be able to do that . . . and he's 2 weeks older than my sister's baby! Is there something wrong with him?"

• "I want to be sure I buy just the right toy for my little Mary. What do you suggest for her? She will be having her first birthday next week."

Table 4-1   Summary of Ages and Stages Developmental Theories

STAGE/AGE	PIAGET'S COGNITIVE STAGES	FREUD'S PSYCHOSEXUAL STAGES	ERIKSON'S PSYCHOSOCIAL STAGES	KOHLBERG'S MORAL JUDGMENT STAGES
1. Infancy Birth to 1 year	**Sensorimotor** (birth to 2 years): begins to acquire language. Task: Object permanence	**Oral:** pleasure from exploration with mouth and through sucking. Task: Weaning	**Trust vs. Mistrust** Task: Trust. Socializing agent: Mothering person. Central process: Mutuality. Ego quality: Hope	**Preconventional Level:** **1. Morality Stage:** Avoid punishment by not breaking rules of authority figures
2. Toddler 1 to 3 years	**Sensorimotor** continues. **Preoperational** (2 to 7 years) begins: use of representational thought. Task: Use language and mental images to think and communicate	**Anal:** control of elimination. Task: Toilet training	**Autonomy vs. Shame and Doubt** Task: Autonomy. Socializing agent: Parents. Central process: Imitation. Ego quality: Self-control and willpower	
3. Preschool 3 to 6 years	**Preoperational** continues	**Phallic:** attracted to opposite-sex parent. Task: Resolve Oedipus/Electra complex	**Initiative vs. Guilt** Task: Initiative and moral responsibility. Socializing agents: Parents. Central process: Identification. Ego quality: Direction, purpose, and conscience	**2. Individualism, Instrumental Purpose, and Exchange Stage:** "Right" is relative, follow rules when in own interest
4. School Age 6 to 12 years	**Preoperational** continues. **Concrete Operations** (7 to 12 years) begins: engage in inductive reasoning and concrete problem solving. Task: Learn concepts of conservation and reversibility	**Latency:** identification with same-sex parent. Task: Identify with same-sex parent and test and compare own capabilities with peer norms	**Industry vs. Inferiority** Task: Industry, self-assurance, self-esteem. Socializing agents: Teachers and peers. Central process: Education. Ego quality: Competence	**Conventional Level:** **3. Mutual Expectations, Relationships, and Conformity to Moral Norms Stage:** Need to be "good" in own and others' eyes, believe in rules and regulations
5. Adolescence 12 to 18 years	**Formal Operations** (12 years to adulthood): engage in abstract reasoning and analytical problem solving. Task: Develop a workable philosophy of life	**Genital:** develop sexual relationships. Task: Establish meaningful relationship for lifelong pairing	**Identity vs. Role Confusion** Task: Self-identity/concept. Socializing agents: Society of peers. Central process: Role experimentation and peer pressure. Ego quality: Fidelity and devotion to others, personal and sociocultural values	**4. Social System and Conscience Stage:** Uphold laws because they are fixed social duties

continued

STAGE/AGE	PIAGET'S COGNITIVE STAGES	FREUD'S PSYCHOSEXUAL STAGES	ERIKSON'S PSYCHOSOCIAL STAGES	KOHLBERG'S MORAL JUDGMENT STAGES
6. Young Adult 18 to 30 years	**Formal Operations** continues		**Intimacy vs. Isolation** Task: Intimacy Socializing agent: Close friends, partners, lovers, spouse Central process: Mutuality among peers Ego quality: Intimate affiliation and love	**Postconventional Level:** **5. Social Contract or Utility and Individual Rights Stage:** Uphold laws in the interest of the greatest good for the greatest number; uphold laws that protect universal rights
7. Early Middle Age 30 to 50 years			**Generativity vs. Stagnation** (30 to 65 years) Task: Generativity Socializing agent: Spouse, partner, children, sociocultural norms Central process: Creativity and person-environment fit Ego quality: Productivity, perseverence, charity, and consideration	
8. Late Middle Age 50 to 70 years			**Generativity vs. Stagnation** continues	**6. Universal Ethical Principles Stage:** Support universal moral principles regardless of the price for doing so
9. Late Adult 70 years to death			**Ego Integrity vs. Despair** (65 years to death) Task: Ego integrity Socializing agent: Significant others Central process: Introspection Ego quality: Wisdom	

Table 4-2   Growth and Development During Infancy

AGE	GROSS MOTOR	FINE MOTOR	LANGUAGE	SENSORY
Birth to 1 Month	• Assumes tonic neck posture • When prone lifts and turns head	• Holds hands in fist • Draws arms and legs to body	• Cries	• Comforts with holding and touch • Looks at faces • Follows objects when in line of vision • Alert to high-pitched voices • Smiles
2 to 4 Months	• Can raise head and shoulders when prone to 45°–90°; supports self on forearms • Rolls from back to side	• Hands mostly open • Looks at and plays with fingers • Grasps and tries to reach objects	• Vocalizes when talked to; coos, babbles • Laughs aloud • Squeals	• Smiles • Follows objects 180° • Turns head when hears voices or sounds
4 to 6 Months	• Turns from stomach to back and then back to stomach • When pulled to sitting almost no head lag • By 6 months can sit on floor with hands forward for support	• Can hold feet and put in mouth • Can hold bottle • Can grasp rattle and other small objects • Puts objects in mouth	• Squeals	• Watches a falling object • Responds to sounds
6 to 8 Months	• Puts full weight on legs when held in standing position • Can sit without support • Bounces when held in a standing position	• Transfers objects from one hand to the other • Can feed self a cookie • Can bang two objects together	• Babbles vowel-like sounds, "ooh" or "aah" • Imitation of speech sounds ("mama," "dada") beginning • Laughs aloud	• Responds by looking and smiling • Recognizes own name
8 to 10 Months	• Crawls on all fours or uses arms to pull body along floor • Can pull self to sitting • Can pull self to standing	• Beginning to use thumb-finger grasp • Dominant hand use • Has good hand-mouth coordination	• Responds to verbal commands • May say one word in addition to "mama" and "dada"	• Recognizes sounds
10 to 12 Months	• Can sit down from standing • Walks around room holding onto objects • Can stand alone	• Picks up and drops objects • Can put small objects into toys or containers through holes • Turns many pages in a book at one time • Picks up small objects	• Understands "no" and other simple commands • Learns one or two other words • Imitates speech sounds • Speaks gibberish	• Follows fast-moving objects • Indicates wants • Likes to play imitative games such as patty cake and peek-a-boo

Courtesy of Delmar Publishers, Albany, NY

Developmental Tasks of Toddlers (1 to 3 Years)

The toddler period is one of steadily increasing motor development and control, intense activity and discovery, rapid language development, increasingly independent behaviors, and marked personality development (see Figure 4-4). Key gross and fine motor, language, and sensory milestones associated with the toddler period can be found in Table 4-3.

An individual's readiness for each new developmental task is dependent on physical and mental maturation, success with achieving prior psychosocial developmental tasks, and on the presence of environmental opportunities to develop the new skills associated with each task. One of the major developmental tasks for toddlers is toilet training (Wong, 1995). Readiness for toilet training is usually evident by the ages of 18 to 24 months (girls tend to be ready to toilet train earlier than boys) when the following are present: voluntary control of the anal and urethral sphincters; motor skills of sitting, walking, and squatting; fine motor skills needed to remove clothing; cognitive skills of recognizing the urge to defecate or urinate and verbalizing the urge to do so; and willingness and ability to please the parents by sitting on the toilet for 5 to 10 minutes. Parental recognition of the child's level of readiness

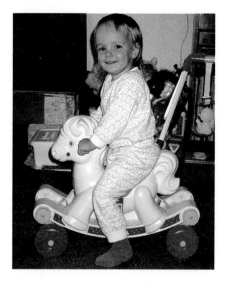

Figure 4-4 Refinement of skills as well as language development and a growing sense of independence are most noted in toddlers.

Table 4-3 Growth and Development During Toddlerhood				
AGE	**GROSS MOTOR**	**FINE MOTOR**	**LANGUAGE**	**SENSORY**
12 to 15 Months	• Can walk alone well • Can crawl up stairs	• Can feed self with cup and spoon • Puts raisins into a bottle • May hold crayon or pencil and scribble • Builds a tower of two cubes	• Says four to six words	• Binocular vision developed
18 Months	• Runs, falling often • Can jump in place • Can walk up stairs holding on • Plays with push and pull toys	• Can build a tower of three to four cubes • Can use a spoon	• Says 10 or more words • Points to objects or body parts when asked	• Visual acuity 20/40
24 Months	• Can walk up and down stairs • Can kick a ball • Can ride a tricycle	• Can draw a circle • Tries to dress self	• Talks a lot • Approximately 300-word vocabulary • Understands commands • Knows first name, refers to self • Verbalizes toilet needs	
30 Months	• Throws a ball • Jumps with both feet • Can stand on one foot for a few minutes	• Can build a tower of eight blocks • Can use crayons • Learning to use scissors	• Knows first and last name • Knows the name of one color • Can sing • Expresses needs • Uses pronouns appropriately	

Courtesy of Delmar Publishers, Albany, NY

Understanding Toilet Training

Parents often have difficulty with "potty training" their child and become frustrated when their first attempts are not successful. What suggestions could you give the caregiver who has been trying unsuccessfully for the past two months with her 15-month-old son? She comments that she had absolutely no problems with her first child, a daughter, at this age and cannot understand what the problem is this time.

and willingness to invest the necessary time for toilet training are also essential for the toddler's successful mastery of this task.

A variety of life events and transitions may produce stress in the toddler. Among the most stressful are personal injury or illness and death of a parent or loss through separation or divorce.

Children who have been successful in accomplishing the developmental tasks of infancy enter the toddler period with the basic relative trust needed for the achievement of the next tasks. The principal developmental tasks that must be mastered during the toddler stage are to:

1. Interact with others less egocentrically.
2. Acquire socially acceptable behaviors.
3. Differentiate self from others.
4. Tolerate separation from key socializing agents (mother/parents).
5. Develop increasing verbal communication skills.
6. Tolerate delayed gratification of wants and desires.
7. Control bodily functions (toilet training) and begin self-care (feed and dress self almost completely).

Developmental Tasks of Preschoolers (3 to 6 Years)

During the preschooler period, children are focused on developing initiative and purpose. Play provides the means for physical, mental, and social development and becomes the "work" of children as they use it to understand, adjust to, and work out experiences with their environment. As shown in Figure 4-5, preschoolers demonstrate an active imagination and an ability to invent and imitate. They constantly seek to discover the why, what, and how of objects and events around them, are literal in their thinking, are increasingly sociable with other children and adults other than their parents, and are increasingly aware of their places and roles in their families. Key gross and fine motor, language, and sensory milestones associated with the toddler period can be found in Table 4-4.

The preschooler stage of development is characterized by the refinement of many of the tasks that were achieved during the toddler stage and the development of the skills and abilities that prepare children for the significant

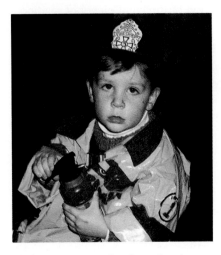

Figure 4-5 Preschoolers often have very active imaginations and enjoy imitating adult roles.

Table 4-4 Growth and Development During Preschool Years

AGE	GROSS MOTOR	FINE MOTOR	LANGUAGE	SENSORY
3 to 6 Years	• Can ride a bike with training wheels • Can throw a ball overhand • Skips and hops on one foot • Can climb well • Can jump rope	• Can draw a six-part person • Can use a scissors • Can draw circle, square, or cross • Likes art projects, likes to paste and string beads • Can button • Learns to tie and buckle shoes • Can brush teeth	• Language skills are well developed with the child able to understand and speak clearly • Vocabulary grows to over 2,000 words • Talks endlessly and asks questions	• Visual acuity well-developed • Focused on learning letters and numbers

Courtesy of Delmar Publishers, Albany, NY

lifestyle change of starting school (Wong, 1995). Readiness for school is demonstrated by increased attention span and memory, ability to interact cooperatively, ability to tolerate prolonged periods of separation from family, and independence in performing basic self-care activities. Among the principal developmental tasks that must be mastered during the preschooler stage are to:

1. Develop a sense of separateness as an individual.
2. Develop a sense of initiative.
3. Use language for increasing social interaction.
4. Interact in socially acceptable ways with others.
5. Develop a conscience.
6. Identify sex role and function.
7. Develop readiness for school.

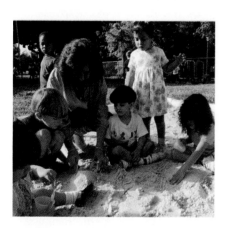

Figure 4-6 School-age children have well-developed motor skills and often play games in peer groups.

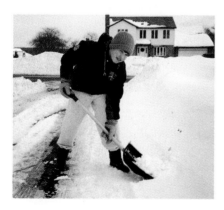

Figure 4-7 Older children can be active in sharing family responsibilities.

Developmental Tasks of School-Age Children (6 to 12 Years)

With a well-developed sense of trust, autonomy, and initiative, school-age children increasingly reduce their dependency on the family as their primary socializing agents and move to the broader world of peers (primarily same-sex peers) in their neighborhoods and schools, as well as to teachers and adult leaders of social, sports, and religious groups (Jackson & Saunders, 1993). They are increasingly exposed to the views and seek approval from people outside the home. School-age children become industrious workers as they develop significant physical, social, and intellectual skills needed to operate in the broader and more diverse environment. They strive to be a part of a peer group and to achieve a variety of skills that are approved by others; in so doing, they become competent and confident in their own eyes (see Figure 4-6). Key gross and fine motor, language, and sensory milestones associated with this period can be found in Table 4-5.

Because inherent ability, level of maturation, and opportunities to learn are variable, some children may be more successful in achieving the developmental tasks of this period earlier or more completely than others. The principal developmental tasks that must be mastered during the school-age stage are to:

1. Become a more active, cooperative, and responsible family member (refer to Figure 4-7).
2. Learn the rules and norms of a widening social, religious, and cultural environment.
3. Increase psychomotor and cognitive skills needed for participation in games and working with others.
4. Master concepts of time, conservation, and reversibility as well as master oral and written communication skills.
5. Win approval from peers and adults.
6. Obtain a place in a peer group.
7. Build a sense of industry, accomplishment, self-assurance, and self-esteem.
8. Develop a positive self-concept.
9. Exchange affection with family and friends without seeking an immediate payback.
10. Adopt moral standards for behavior.

Table 4-5 Growth and Development During School-Age Years				
AGE	**GROSS MOTOR**	**FINE MOTOR**	**LANGUAGE**	**SENSORY**
6 to 12 Years	• Can use rollerblades or ice skates • Able to ride two-wheeler • Plays baseball	• Can put models together • Likes crafts • Enjoys board games, plays cards	• Vocabulary increases • Language abilities continue to develop	• Reading • Able to concentrate on activities for longer periods

Courtesy of Delmar Publishers, Albany, NY

⊚⊚ THINK ABOUT IT

Friendship in School-Age Children

Ten-year-old Consuela, who recently emigrated to the United States and speaks broken English, presents with a sore throat. As you are assessing her, she bursts into tears and cries, "Me lonely, me have no friends." What is your response to Consuela?

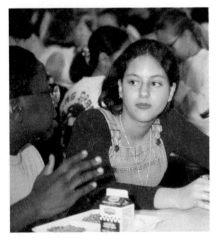

Figure 4-8 During adolescence, friendships and associations with peers are especially important.

Developmental Tasks of Adolescence (12 to 18 Years)

The adolescent period is one of struggle and sometimes turmoil as the adolescent strives to develop a personal identity and achieve a successful transition from childhood to adulthood (see Figure 4-8). The biological, social, cognitive, and psychological changes associated with adolescence are the most complex and profound of any developmental period (Neinstein, 1991). For example, physical and sexual maturity are reached during adolescence, with girls tending to experience both puberty and a growth spurt earlier than boys. In addition, adolescents develop increasingly sophisticated cognitive and interpersonal skills, test out adult roles and behaviors, and begin to explore educational and occupational opportunities that will significantly influence future adult work life and socioeconomic status. Key gross and fine motor, language, and sensory milestones associated with this period can be found in Table 4-6.

Adolescents who have the support and trust of their families as they tackle the developmental tasks of this period are more likely to have a smoother and successful transition from the dependency of childhood to the independence of adulthood. If their parents, however, have been too controlling, too permissive, or too confrontational during this period, adolescents will experience difficulty in judging the appropriateness of their behavior and in forming self-identity as competent, worthwhile individuals. If adolescents are able to find sufficient acceptance in a desired peer group or receive more positive than negative responses from the objects of their growing sexual and/or friendship interest, they will be able to work through feelings of inadequacy and insecurity and become increasingly self-assured and competent in forming and maintaining adult relationships. The principal developmental tasks that must be mastered during the adolescent stage are to:

Table 4-6 Growth and Development During Adolescence				
AGE	**GROSS MOTOR**	**FINE MOTOR**	**LANGUAGE**	**SENSORY**
12 to 19 Years	• Muscles continue to develop • At times awkward, with some lack of coordination	• Well-developed skills	• Vocabulary fully developed	• Development complete

Courtesy of Delmar Publishers, Albany, NY

⊚⊚ THINK ABOUT IT

Adolescents' Reactions to Physical Changes

As the school nurse, you are presenting sexual education classes to all students in the junior high school. While you are explaining sexually transmitted diseases, a few of the girls begin to giggle. You overhear one girl saying, "Opal doesn't have to worry about getting that. She's so flat-chested that no guy will even look at her." How would you handle this situation?

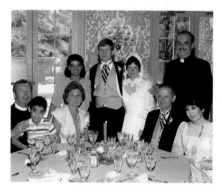

Figure 4-9 Young adulthood often means separating from the family and embracing new commitments and responsibilities.

⊚⊚ THINK ABOUT IT

Young Adult Experiencing Conflict Concerning a Developmental Task

Inger is a 27-year-old astrophysicist. After undergoing her annual gynecological check-up, she tells you that her friends are having babies. Her husband wants children soon. "I'm not ready for kids. I want my career to be first. Maybe I won't ever want kids. My husband is pressuring me, my parents, my in-laws, everybody!" How would you proceed?

1. Develop self-identity and appreciate own achievements and worth.
2. Form close relationships with peers.
3. Gradually grow independent from parents.
4. Evolve own value system and integrate self-concept and values with those of peers and society.
5. Develop academic and vocational skills and related social, work, and civic sensitivities.
6. Develop analytic thinking.
7. Adjust to rapid physical and sexual changes.
8. Develop a sexual identity and role.
9. Develop skill in relating to people from different backgrounds.
10. Consider and possibly choose a career.

Developmental Tasks of Young Adults (18 to 30 Years)

Young adulthood is a time of separation and independence from the family and of new commitments, responsibilities, and accountability in social, work, and home relationships and roles (see Figure 4-9). It is also a period when individuals are exposed to more diverse people, situations, and values and, in recent decades, to a more rapidly changing socioeconomic and technological environment than ever before. For example, the movement, particularly in the Western world, from an industrial to an information era has made extended education and a need to delay complete emancipation from the family, as well as to delay commitment to a lifelong partner, an increasing norm for young adults. Socioeconomic and cultural changes have also legitimized the entry of young adult women into the professional career work force. Although more young adult women are preparing for and launching lifelong careers outside the home, Leidy and Darling-Fisher's (1995) research indicates that young adult women continue to place a greater focus on intimacy while young men place a greater focus on autonomy, a gender difference in psychosocial development noted in previous research by Gilligan (1982) and Schiedel and Marcia (1985).

When parents and young adult offspring are able to resolve normal generational differences in philosophy and lifestyles, mastery of the young adult developmental tasks is greatly facilitated. Among the developmental tasks that the young adult must achieve are to:

1. Establish friendships and a social group.
2. Grow independent of parental care and home.
3. Set up and manage one's own household.
4. Form an intimate affiliation with another and choose a mate.
5. Learn to love, cooperate with, and commit to a life partner.
6. Develop a personal style of living (e.g., shared or single).
7. Choose and begin to establish a career or vocation.
8. Assume social, work, and civic responsibility and roles in social, professional, political, religious, and civic organizations.
9. Learn to manage life stresses accompanying change.
10. Develop a realistic outlook and acceptance of cultural, religious, social, and political diversity.
11. Form a meaningful philosophy of life and implement it in home, employment, and community settings.
12. Begin a parental role for own or life partner's children or for young people in a broader social framework, e.g., teaching, health care, volunteer work.

Developmental Tasks of Early Middle Adulthood (30 to 50 Years)

Middle age, spanning the ages of 30 to 70 years, is the longest stage of the life cycle and is now often divided into early and late middle adulthood. During early middle adulthood, individuals experience relatively good physical and mental health; settle into their chosen careers, socioeconomic lifestyles, patterns of relationships (married, parental, partnered, single), political, civic, social, professional, and religious affiliations and activities; and achieve maximum productivity in work and in influence over themselves and their environments (Murray & Zentner, 1993). It is also a period when individuals experience a need to contribute to the next generation; to raise children and/or produce something that will be socially useful to others. The generativity that characterizes this period consists of giving, sharing, facilitating the growth of others, and making a contribution that is lasting.

Many who choose to express their generativity through the parental role may, during this period, achieve both the successful launching of their children into responsible adult roles and the associated increase in leisure time and financial resources needed to pursue enjoyable, nonparental goals and activities. Others, following divorce and remarriage, may see a merging of offspring into new family groupings and the return to previous parental cycles. An increasing number of others, during or shortly after launching their young adult children, may find themselves having to take on the responsibility of chronically ill aging parents. Each such life event can generate stress and disruption in individuals' lives with which they must cope. Developing effective coping strategies to manage the stress of life events or role transitions is a developmental task facing individuals in all life stages.

Among the developmental tasks that must be achieved during early middle adulthood are to:

1. Attain a desired level of achievement and status in career.
2. Review, evaluate, refine, and redirect career goals consistent with one's personal value system.
3. Continue to learn and refine competencies in areas of personal and career interests.
4. Manage life stresses accompanying change.
5. Continue developing mature relationships with life partner and significant others.
6. Participate in social, professional, political, religious, and civic activities.
7. Cope with an empty nest and possibly a refilled nest.
8. Adjust to aging parents and help plan for when they will need assistance.
9. Continue currently enjoyable hobbies and leisure activities and begin to develop ones for post retirement.
10. Begin to plan for personal, financial, and social aspects of retirement.

Developmental Tasks of Late Middle Adulthood (50 to 70 Years)

Many individuals during late middle adulthood may be diagnosed for the first time with a chronic health problem, such as arthritis, cardiovascular disease, cancer, diabetes, or asthma. In addition, women generally experience a decrease in estrogen and progesterone production and undergo menopause during their late 40s or early 50s, with ultimate cessation of menses but generally no diminution of sexual drive or intensity of orgasms. Men experience decreased testosterone production accompanied by increased time to achieve

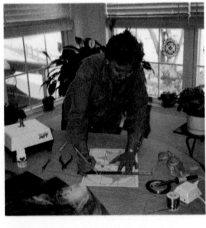

Figure 4-10 Middle-aged adults often develop new interests, such as crafts or travel.

When an Elderly Parent Needs Special Care

Jean and Don Allen, 48 and 54 years of age, had finally helped the last of their four children move into his own apartment in another city and had been looking forward to having more time together when Jean's mother, 69 years old and recently widowed, was diagnosed with cancer. Because Jean's mother lives alone, will be receiving chemotherapy on an outpatient basis, and will need a great deal of help during this period, Jean and Don have agreed to have her live with them until the chemotherapy is completed.

- What developmental needs would you anticipate Jean, Don, and Jean's mother might experience?
- What anticipatory counseling would you provide related to these needs?

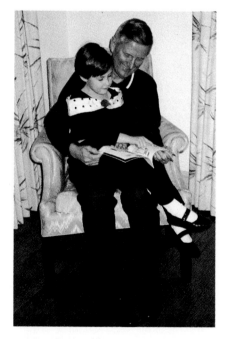

Figure 4-11 The free time that may accompany the late adulthood years can be particularly satisfying and enjoyable.

erection, less intense orgasms, and decreased sperm production during their late 50s through 60s.

Changes also occur during late middle adulthood in work, family, social, and civic areas. In many areas of the work world, for example, individuals have advanced as far as they will or have achieved as much as they can by late middle adulthood. In certain professions, however, such as law, medicine, business, religion, and government, this period may actually be the prime years of achievement and leadership. As the nuclear family contracts, parents rediscover being a couple and acquire new roles such as becoming grandparents. In addition, the gender developmental differences related to intimacy and autonomy seen in early adulthood begin to converge during late middle adulthood as men and women tend to take on similar life roles (Leidy & Darling-Fisher, 1995). Women generally become more involved and assume leadership roles in activities outside the home and work, such as politics and other civic activities, while men tend to become more aware and accepting of their nurturing and caring tendencies.

A variety of development tasks must be achieved by individuals during late middle adulthood. Among these tasks are to:

1. Manage life stresses accompanying change.
2. Maintain interest in current political, cultural, and scientific advances, trends, and issues.
3. Maintain affiliation with selected social, religious, professional, civic, and political organizations.
4. Adapt to physical and mental changes and health status accompanying aging.
5. Continue current activities and develop new interests and leisure activities that can be pursued consistent with changing abilities (see Figure 4-10).
6. Adjust to more interaction and time spent with life partner without the presence of children.
7. Develop supportive, interdependent relationships with adult children.
8. Help elderly parents and relatives cope with lifestyle changes (may include providing a home for them).
9. Adjust to possible or actual loss of parents, life partner, elder family members, and friends through death or their decreasing abilities to maintain independent living and self-care.
10. Prepare for and adjust to role changes, changing finances, and changing lifestyle resulting from retirement.

Developmental Tasks of Late Adulthood (70 Years to Death)

How individuals during late adulthood physically and emotionally age and how they confront and adjust to the changes associated with this stage are widely divergent. For those who have achieved the developmental tasks of middle adulthood and are comfortable with the life goals they have achieved, independence from the workplace and time to pursue more leisure activities are welcomed. Although a loss of work-related status and social outlets, reduced income, decline in physical and some cognitive capabilities, decreased resistance to illness, and decreased recuperative powers are inevitable during late adulthood, they are often adjusted to with equanimity. Indeed, a high percentage of individuals will live out their lives managing their activities of daily living independently and in their own homes, enjoying new roles, giving requested advice and moral support to members of younger generations (see Figure 4-11), and sharing leisure activities with new or old friends in their own age group (Carnevali & Patrick, 1993).

One of the most important developmental tasks during late adulthood is conducting a life review (Levinson, Darrow, & Klein, 1986). A **life review** entails reviewing the experiences, relationships, and events of one's life as a whole, viewing successes and failures from the perspective of age, and accepting one's life and accompanying life choices and outcomes in their entirety. Successful completion of the life review task provides a sense of having been a meaningful part of human history, provides a sense of integrity, and enables one to face death with equanimity. If, however, one is unsuccessful in achieving the life review developmental task, a sense of hopelessness, resentment, futility, despair, fear of death, and clinical depression may result.

Among the developmental tasks that must be achieved during late adulthood are to:

1. Maintain and develop new activities that help retain functional capacities.
2. Accept and adjust to changes in mental and physical strength and agility and health status.
3. Maintain and develop activities that contribute to a continuing sense of usefulness and self-worth and enhance self-image.
4. Develop new roles in family as eldest member.
5. Establish affiliation with own age group.
6. Accept and adjust to changing, possibly restricted circumstances — social, financial, and lifestyle.
7. Adapt to loss of life partner, family members, and friends.
8. Work on life review.
9. Prepare for inevitability of own death.

DEVELOPMENTAL ASSESSMENT TOOLS

A variety of developmental assessment tools are available for use by the nurse. Some of the most commonly used tools, presented in this chapter, assess mental, physical, emotional, and social functional status. It should be noted that use of some of these tools requires special training.

Brazelton Neonatal Behavioral Assessment Scale (BNBAS)

The BNBAS measures many newborn temperament characteristics: state of arousal, orienting responses to stimuli, ability to deal with disturbing stimuli, social behavior, and motor skills (Brazelton, 1996). When the assessment results are shared with parents to acquaint them with the unique aspects of their child's responsiveness and behavior, increased and improved infant-parent interactions have been subsequently noted.

Denver II

The Denver II, the most widely used screening tool, provides a developmental profile of children 1 month to 6 years of age in four areas: personal-social, fine motor-adaptive, language, and gross motor skills (see Chapter 23). A series of developmental tasks is used to assess whether a child is developmentally within the normal range for the child's age. The Denver II has been standardized for Euro Americans, African Americans, and Hispanic Americans.

Revised Prescreening Developmental Questionnaire (R-PDQ)

The R-PDQ is a quick, easily administered test that can be answered by a parent to identify children from 1 month to 6 years of age who need a more complete screening with the Denver II. The tool assesses the same four developmental areas as those included in the Denver II.

Early Language Milestones Scale (ELM)

The ELM is a simple screening tool that can be used in any office or clinical setting to assess early language development and identify children from 1 month to 3 years of age with potential language problems (Coplan, 1983). The ELM tests auditory visual, auditory receptive, and expressive language areas in greater depth than the Denver II.

Carey Infant and Child Temperament Questionnaires

Three separate questionnaires have been developed by Carey and his associates (Carey & McDevitt, 1978; Hegvik, McDevitt, & Carey, 1982; Fullard, McDevitt, & Carey, 1984) to determine the pattern of temperamental attributes of infants (4 to 8 months), toddlers, and preschoolers, respectively. Parental input is obtained about the child's patterns of eating, playing, eliminating, sleeping, and responses to different situations to determine influences on the child's relationships with parents and other caregivers.

Washington Guide to Promoting Development in the Young Child

The Washington Guide serves as a developmental assessment framework for directly observing a child's behavior on a systematic basis from birth to 5 years of age in eight areas: play, motor activities, language, feeding, dressing, toilet training, discipline, and sleep (Powell, 1981). The guide includes expected tasks for each age group as well as a list of suggested activities that provide the parent with suggestions about appropriate child-rearing practices when variations in development are noted.

ACTeRS Scale (ADD-H: Comprehensive Teachers Rating Scale)

The ACTeRS scale, which has been normed separately for boys and girls, is easily used by teachers and school health nurses in a school setting to identify problems in the areas of attention, hyperactivity, social skills, and oppositional behavior (Ullmann, Sleator, & Sprague, 1991). In addition to identifying school-age children with an attention deficit disorder-hyperactivity, the tool also is useful for assessing the degree and amount of prosocial behavior.

HEADSS (Home, Education, Activities, Drugs, Sex, and Suicide) Adolescent Risk Profile

The HEADSS interview guide is used to obtain a psychosocial, lifestyle history from adolescents in the following areas: home; education; activities, including peers, drugs, and sexuality; and suicide (Neinstein, 1991). In addition to identifying those adolescents who are at high risk, the guide provides opportunities for anticipatory guidance about health-compromising behaviors and practices.

Modified Erikson Psychosocial Stage Inventory (MEPSI)

The MEPSI is a survey measure that operationalizes Erikson's eight stages of development in the adult (Darling-Fisher & Leidy, 1988). Respondents indicate the degree to which each psychosocial attribute statement associated with each stage of development is true for them. A total score for each attribute (trust, autonomy, initiative, industry, identity, intimacy, generativity, and integrity) is obtained and serves as a basis for anticipatory guidance and counseling.

Life Experiences Survey (LES)

The LES is a self-administered tool for adults that includes events that can create change in the lives of those who experience them and necessitate some degree of social readjustment (Sarason, Johnson, & Siegal, 1978). The respondent indicates events that have occurred over the last year and the type and extent of impact the event had. A total change score is obtained that identifies respondents at risk for high stress and in need of stress and coping counseling. The LES is more appropriate for use with young and middle-age adults than with elderly adults because the content of the LES addresses more of the developmental tasks associated with young and middle-age adults.

Everyday Hassles Scale (EHS)

The EHS rank orders everyday irritants that contribute significantly to one's stress level, as well as behaviors and feelings that promote well-being (Lazarus, 1981). Studies have suggested that day-to-day hassles are more strongly correlated with physical and psychosocial problems and outcomes than are life events (Lazarus & Folkman, 1984; Weinberger, Hiner, & Tierney, 1987).

Sense of Coherence (SOC) Scale

The SOC, also known as the Orientation to Life Questionnaire, is an easily administered 29-item questionnaire that obtains measures of the respondent's sense of coherence (Antonovsky, 1993). A total SOC score as well as subscores representing the three SOC components (comprehensibility, manageability, and meaningfulness) are obtained. The tool has been used worldwide with respondents from school age through late adulthood and appears to be gender, culturally, and socioeconomically neutral. Thus the SOC is useful for individuals from diverse socioeconomic and cultural backgrounds. Results can be used as a basis for anticipatory guidance and counseling.

Stress Audit

The Stress Audit is a self-administered questionnaire that assesses experienced and anticipated stressful events, stress symptoms, responses to stress, and overall vulnerability to stress (Miller, Smith, & Mehler, 1991). The Stress Audit assists in identifying an individual's stress profile and provides a more complete basis for anticipatory guidance and counseling than most life-event tools.

Functional Activities Questionnaire (FAQ)

The FAQ is a screening tool for assessing the level of independence demonstrated in the performance of activities of daily living (McDowell & Newell, 1987). It measures universal skills among older adults (managing finances, completing government and business forms, shopping, playing games of skill and working on hobbies, using electrical appliances, preparing a balanced meal, keeping track of current events, attending to and following the plot of a TV program, movie, or book, remembering appointments and timed events such as medications, and traveling outside the home) and can be completed by a significant other or a caregiver. The tool is easy to understand and can be quickly completed.

Functional Assessment Screening in the Elderly (FASE)

Resnick (1994) developed the FASE procedure to screen for functional disability in elderly patients. The tool identifies 11 target areas for assessment and specific assessment questions and/or procedures to use for each area, indicates what would constitute an abnormal result, and lists suggested interventions when abnormal results are present. The tool is comprehensive yet practical and easily used in any clinical setting.

Minimum Data Set (MDS) for Nursing Facility Resident Assessment and Care Screening

The MDS is required by federal law for all patients residing in nursing homes (Carnevali & Patrick, 1993). Areas assessed and recorded include cognitive patterns, communication/hearing patterns, vision patterns, physical functioning and structural problems, psychosocial well-being, mood and behavior patterns, activity pursuit patterns, bowel and bladder status, disease diagnoses, health conditions, oral nutritional status, oral/dental status, skin condition, medication use, treatments and procedures, and customary activities of daily living routines. The MDS facilitates accurate and precise diagnostic and prognostic statements that can serve as a basis for anticipatory guidance and treatment interventions.

Folstein Mini-Mental State Examination (MMSE)

The MMSE is the most widely used test of cognitive function of the elderly (Resnick, 1994). The MMSE consists of two parts: part 1 is verbal and assesses orientation, memory, and attention; part 2 evaluates the ability to follow verbal and written commands, name objects, write a sentence, and copy a complex polygon design (Folstein, Folstein, & McHugh, 1975; Tombaugh & McIntyre, 1992). This tool can be easily administered in any clinical setting. A telephone version is also available for use in special situations (Brandt, Spencer, & Folstein, 1988). Results of this examination assist in determining the need for anticipatory counseling versus referral for a more definitive neurological assessment.

Beck Depression Inventory (BDI)

The BDI consists of questions on 21 characteristics associated with depression: mood, pessimism, sense of failure, dissatisfaction, guilt, sense of punishment, disappointment in oneself, self-accusations, self-punitive wishes, crying spells, irritability, social withdrawal, indecisiveness, body image, function at work, sleep disturbance, fatigue, appetite disturbance, weight loss, preoccupation with health, and loss of libido (Gallagher, 1986). A score indicating depression warrants referral to a mental health specialist for therapeutic counseling and possible pharmacological intervention.

Recent Life Changes Questionnaire

Developed for use with adults in all developmental stages, the Recent Life Changes Questionnaire is self-administered and requires the respondent to indicate which desirable and undesirable life events were experienced within the last 6 months to 2 years and the amount of adjustment that was needed to handle the events (Rahe, 1975). When the amount of social readjustment indicated by a total life stress score is high, the probability of developing health problems is also high. The questionnaire is easy to understand, quick to administer, useful with individuals in all adult stages, and provides a basis for predicting a respondent's susceptibility to stress-related illness and need for associated stress and coping counseling (see Table 4-7). A children's version of the recent life changes questionnaire, the Stress Scale for Children, is also available (Saunders & Remsberg, 1984).

😊 THINK ABOUT IT

Evaluating the Recent Life Changes Questionnaire

Self-administer the Recent Life Changes Questionnaire.
- What was your reaction to the questionnaire?
- Did you detect any inaccuracies or biases? If you answered "yes," can you suggest modifications to the questionnaire?

Table 4-7   Recent Life Changes Questionnaire

I. INSTRUCTIONS FOR MARKING YOUR RECENT LIFE CHANGES

To answer the questions below, mark an "X" in one or more of the columns to the right of each question. If the event in question has occurred to you within the past 2 years, indicate when it occurred by marking the appropriate column: 0–6 months ago, 7–12 months ago, etc. It may be the case with some of the events below that you experienced them over more than one of the time periods listed for the past 2 years. If so, mark all the appropriate columns. If the event has not occurred to you during the last 2 years (or has never occurred to you), leave all the columns empty.

Now go through the questionnaire and mark your recent life changes. The column marked "Your Adjustment Score" will be explained at the end of the questionnaire.

	19 to 24 mo. ago	13 to 18 mo. ago	7 to 12 mo. ago	0 to 6 mo. ago	Your Adjust. Score
A. Health					
Within the time periods listed, have you experienced:					
1. an illness or injury which:					
(a) kept you in bed a week or more, or took you to the hospital?	____	____	____	____	____
(b) was less serious than described above?	____	____	____	____	____
2. a major change in eating habits?	____	____	____	____	____
3. a major change in sleeping habits?	____	____	____	____	____
4. a change in your usual type and/or amount of recreation?	____	____	____	____	____
5. major dental work?	____	____	____	____	____
B. Work					
Within the time periods listed, have you:					
6. changed to a new type of work?	____	____	____	____	____
7. changed your work hours or conditions?	____	____	____	____	____
8. had a change in your responsibilities at work?					
(a) more responsibilities?	____	____	____	____	____
(b) less responsibilities?	____	____	____	____	____
(c) promotion?	____	____	____	____	____
(d) demotion?	____	____	____	____	____
(e) transfer?	____	____	____	____	____

continued

Table 4-7   Recent Life Changes Questionnaire *continued*

	19 to 24 mo. ago	13 to 18 mo. ago	7 to 12 mo. ago	0 to 6 mo. ago	Your Adjust. Score
9. experienced troubles at work?					
(a) with your boss?	____	____	____	____	____
(b) with coworkers?	____	____	____	____	____
(c) with persons under your supervision?	____	____	____	____	____
(d) other work troubles?	____	____	____	____	____
10. experienced a major business readjustment?	____	____	____	____	____
11. retired?	____	____	____	____	____
12. experienced being:					
(a) fired from work?	____	____	____	____	____
(b) laid off from work?	____	____	____	____	____
13. taken courses by mail or studied at home to help you in your work?	____	____	____	____	____

C. Home and Family

Within the time periods listed, have you experienced:

	19 to 24 mo. ago	13 to 18 mo. ago	7 to 12 mo. ago	0 to 6 mo. ago	Your Adjust. Score
14. a change in residence:					
(a) a move within the same town or city?	____	____	____	____	____
(b) a move to a different town, city, or state?	____	____	____	____	____
15. a change in family "get-togethers"?	____	____	____	____	____
16. a major change in the health or behavior of a family member (illnesses, accidents, drug, or disciplinary problems, etc.)?	____	____	____	____	____
17. major change in your living conditions (home improvements or a decline in your home or neighborhood)?	____	____	____	____	____
18. the death of a spouse?	____	____	____	____	____
19. the death of a:					
(a) child?	____	____	____	____	____
(b) brother or sister?	____	____	____	____	____
(c) parent?	____	____	____	____	____
(d) other close family member?	____	____	____	____	____
20. the death of a close friend?	____	____	____	____	____
21. a change in the marital status of your parents:					
(a) divorce?	____	____	____	____	____
(b) remarriage?	____	____	____	____	____

NOTE: (Questions 22–33 concern marriage. For persons never married, go to Item 34)

	19 to 24 mo. ago	13 to 18 mo. ago	7 to 12 mo. ago	0 to 6 mo. ago	Your Adjust. Score
22. marriage?	____	____	____	____	____
23. a change in arguments with your spouse?	____	____	____	____	____
24. in-law problems?	____	____	____	____	____
25. a separation from spouse?					
(a) due to work?	____	____	____	____	____
(b) due to marital problems?	____	____	____	____	____
26. a reconciliation with spouse?	____	____	____	____	____
27. a divorce?	____	____	____	____	____
28. a gain of a new family member?					
(a) birth of a child?	____	____	____	____	____
(b) adoption of a child?	____	____	____	____	____
(c) a relative moving in with you?	____	____	____	____	____

continued

Table 4-7   Recent Life Changes Questionnaire   *continued*

	19 to 24 mo. ago	13 to 18 mo. ago	7 to 12 mo. ago	0 to 6 mo. ago	Your Adjust. Score
29. wife beginning or ceasing work outside the home?	___	___	___	___	___
30. wife becoming pregnant?	___	___	___	___	___
31. a child leaving home:					
(a) due to marriage?	___	___	___	___	___
(b) to attend college?	___	___	___	___	___
(c) for other reasons?	___	___	___	___	___
32. wife having a miscarriage or abortion?	___	___	___	___	___
33. birth of a grandchild?	___	___	___	___	___

D. Personal and Social

Within the time periods listed, have you experienced:

	19 to 24 mo. ago	13 to 18 mo. ago	7 to 12 mo. ago	0 to 6 mo. ago	Your Adjust. Score
34. a major personal achievement?	___	___	___	___	___
35. a change in your personal habits (your dress, friends, lifestyle, etc.)?	___	___	___	___	___
36. sexual difficulties?	___	___	___	___	___
37. beginning or ceasing school or college?	___	___	___	___	___
38. a change of school or college?	___	___	___	___	___
39. a vacation?	___	___	___	___	___
40. a change in your religious beliefs?	___	___	___	___	___
41. a change in your social activities (clubs, movies, visiting)?	___	___	___	___	___
42. a minor violation of the law?	___	___	___	___	___
43. legal troubles resulting in your being held in jail?	___	___	___	___	___
44. a change in your political beliefs?	___	___	___	___	___
45. a new, close, personal relationship?	___	___	___	___	___
46. an engagement to marry?	___	___	___	___	___
47. a "falling out" in a close personal relationship?	___	___	___	___	___
48. girlfriend (or boyfriend) problems?	___	___	___	___	___
49. a loss or damage of personal property?	___	___	___	___	___
50. an accident?	___	___	___	___	___
51. a major decision regarding your immediate future?	___	___	___	___	___

E. Financial

Within the time periods listed, have you:

	19 to 24 mo. ago	13 to 18 mo. ago	7 to 12 mo. ago	0 to 6 mo. ago	Your Adjust. Score
52. taken on a moderate purchase, such as a TV, car, freezer, etc.?	___	___	___	___	___
53. taken on a major purchase or a mortgage loan, such as a home, business, property, etc.?	___	___	___	___	___
54. experienced a foreclosure on a mortgage or loan?	___	___	___	___	___
55. experienced a major change in finances:					
(a) increased income?	___	___	___	___	___
(b) decreased income?	___	___	___	___	___
(c) credit rating difficulties?	___	___	___	___	___
6-month LCU totals	___	___	___	___	
6-month SLCU totals	___	___	___	___	

continued

Table 4-7 **Recent Life Changes Questionnaire** *continued*

II. INSTRUCTIONS FOR SCORING YOUR ADJUSTMENT TO YOUR RECENT LIFE CHANGES

Persons adapt to their recent life changes in different ways. Some people find the adjustment to a residential move, for example, to be enormous, while others find very little life adjustment necessary. You are now requested to "score" each of the recent life changes that you marked with an "X" as to the amount of adjustment you needed to handle this event.

Your scores can range from 1 to 100 "points." If, for example, you experienced a recent residential move but felt it required very little life adjustment, you would choose a low number and place it in the blank to the right of the question's boxes. On the other hand, if you recently changed residence and felt it required a near maximal life adjustment, you would place a high number, toward 100, in the blank to the right of that question's boxes. For intermediate life adjustment scores, you would choose intermediate numbers between 1 and 100.

Please go back through your questionnaire and for each recent life change you indicated with an "X," choose your personal life change adjustment score (between 1 and 100) which reflects what you saw to be the amount of life adjustment necessary to cope with or handle the event. Use both your estimates of the intensity of the life change and its duration to arrive at your scores.

LCU = life change units; SLCU = subjective life change units.

Reprinted with permission from Rahe, R. H. (1975). Recent life changes questionnaire: Epidemiological studies of life change and illness. Int J Psychiatry Med, 6(1/2), 133–146.

CASE STUDY

The case study illustrates the application and objective documentation of the developmental assessment.

The Patient with Recent Physical Limitations Related to Growth and Development

Mr. Waite is an 80 yo African-American male living in the same 3 bedroom home × 48 yr. Three wk ago, fell down front steps, sustained a Ⓛ subtrochanteric fracture. Neighbor called 911. Underwent simple hip nailing. Discharged home 2 wk ago after demonstrating proficiency using a 4 point cane and an understanding of his home care management plan.

Mental Functional Status

Oriented, no recent history of recent memory loss or confusion.

Physical Functional Status

Until his accident 3 wk ago, walked at least 2 miles/d to his church 2 blocks away & to do his shopping. Voluntarily stopped driving 2 yr ago when his "reflexes got a bit too slow for the safety of me *and* the other folks on the road."

Since d/c, walks short distances using his 4-point cane for balance but has ↓ endurance, tiring easily. Able to do all his self-care activities but more slowly c̄ frequent rest periods.

Emotional Functional Status

Five yr ago when his wife died, Mr. Waite's daughter & her family urged him to move in with them. He said he was not ready to leave his "own castle" yet & that he could manage the domestic chores c̄ the help of the housekeeper 3 d/wk. Mr. Waite feels that "life has been very good to me over the yrs."

Although his physical recuperation since his sgy is progressing normally for his age, he has expressed ↑ frustration c̄ his dependence on others & his inability to walk s̄ the assistance of the cane. His housekeeper is temporarily living in & available to help him as needed. "She says I don't ask for help when I need it."

continued

Social Functional Status

Prior to retirement, Mr. Waite worked as the branch manager of a major bank. "My work was a source of great satisfaction." Mr. Waite has stayed in touch by phone c̄ many of his friends from work but has seen them less often since he quit driving. He visits his daughter & her family 2×/mo.

"My church is everything to me." He is a retired church school teacher & past leader of the men's organization. "It's annoying that I can't walk to church. I depend on church members for rides to services. I don't feel like visitors. I don't feel like talking to friends on the phone. I just don't feel like myself anymore."

✓ **NURSING CHECKLIST**
Developmental Assessment

- Note the patient's stated chronological age.
- Tailor your questions to the patient's expected level of ability according to developmental parameters until you can accurately assess the actual developmental level.
- When assessing small children, verify information with the caregiver.
- If a third party is assisting in the interview (for an elderly or handicapped patient), address all questions to the patient, not the intermediary.

REVIEW QUESTIONS AND ACTIVITIES

1. Considering the unique characteristics of individuals during each stage of development, describe how you would establish a positive rapport during the assessment process with someone in these different age groups: toddler, early childhood, school age, adolescence, middle age, and late adulthood.

2. Over the next week, observe and interview, if possible, individuals in each developmental stage. What is the status of each individual's developmental crisis/task mastery? Provide specific behaviors exhibited and statements made that support your conclusions.

3. Identify how our society views individuals in each stage of development. What stereotypes or biases are associated with each stage?

4. Carlos Ramero, a 35-year-old sales manager, has come to the medical clinic complaining of increasing epigastric discomfort, intermittent nausea, and frequent headaches. There is no evidence of intestinal bleeding, palpable masses, or specific food intolerances. His headaches usually start in the early afternoon and get worse as the day progresses. He has recently been notified that there will be another workforce reduction in his office, that his wife is pregnant with their third child, and that his rent will be raised significantly next month.

   Which developmental theory will provide the most useful base for understanding Mr. Ramero's current situation?
   a. An age and stage theory
   b. A cognitive development theory
   c. A life events theory
   d. A temperament theory

   The correct answer is (c).

5. In which age group would you first expect a child to build a tower of three or four blocks?
   a. Infancy
   b. Toddler
   c. Preschooler
   d. School age

   The correct answer is (b).

6. All of the following factors have been found to affect how an individual responds to life events except:
   a. Racial characteristics
   b. Interpersonal support systems and orientation to life
   c. Cultural orientation and socioeconomic status
   d. Number and intensity of life events

   The correct answer is (a).

5

Cultural Assessment

1. Describe the process for providing culturally competent nursing care.
2. Assess own cultural values, beliefs, and behaviors.
3. Identify increased health risks and genetic traits, and disorders prevalent in selected ethnic, racial, and population groups.
4. Identify health-seeking behaviors and health practices influenced by cultural values, beliefs, customs, and norms.
5. Identify potential areas of cultural conflict between the values and customs of patients and their families and those of health care providers.
6. Conduct a comprehensive cultural assessment.

The racial, ethnic, and cultural diversification of American society is accelerating at an unprecedented rate. In 1990, approximately 75% of the United States population were Euro-Americans (predicted to be only 53% by the year 2020) and 25% were members of ethnic and cultural minority groups, with 12.3% African American, 9.0% Hispanic (the fastest-growing minority in the United States), 2.8% Asian, and 0.7% American Indians (U.S. Department of Commerce, Bureau of the Census, 1992). It has been predicted that by the year 2010, nurses in the United States will be interacting with patients from virtually every cultural and ethnic group in the world (Leininger, 1994). These changes in the demographic and ethnic composition of the population make it imperative that nurses are able to communicate effectively with a culturally diverse group of patients, can make accurate cultural assessments, and can plan, provide, and evaluate culturally competent care. Such care must be based on an awareness of, and utilization of, knowledge and theories that explain patients' situations and responses within the context of their cultural, ethnic, gender, and sexual orientations (The American Academy of Nursing [AAN] Expert Panel on Culturally Competent Health Care, 1992; Burk, Wieser, & Keegan, 1995).

CULTURALLY COMPETENT NURSING CARE

The American health care system is now one of **cultural diversity** in that it consists of patients and health care providers from different combinations of ethnic (e.g., Hispanic), racial (e.g., Caucasian), national (e.g., Swiss), religious (e.g., Buddhist), generational (e.g., grandparent), marital status (e.g., single), socioeconomic (e.g., middle class), occupational (e.g., nurse), preference in life partner (e.g., heterosexual), health status (e.g., handicapped), and cultural orientations coexisting in a given location. Kreps and Kunimoto (1994) believe that this cultural diversity should be viewed as an opportunity for health care professionals to experience the benefits of exchange and cooperation across cultures. They note that:

> . . . the exploration of different cultures can help us learn about new ways of interpreting reality and increase our understanding of other people, their experiences, and the world they live in. The demonstration of respect and interest in the cultural perspectives of others can also serve as a foundation for developing supportive and cooperative relationships with people from different cultures. The expression of respect and interest validates the legitimacy and worth of others' cultural backgrounds, encourages their reciprocal interest in our cultural orientation, and provides a basis for communication. (pp. 10–11)

In 1990, almost half (48%) of the children in the United States were from racial or ethnic minority groups (Thomas, 1993). They and their parents, particularly those recent immigrants from countries such as Vietnam, Ethiopia, Haiti, Mexico, Lebanon, and the former countries of the Union of the Soviet Socialist Republics, may have very different attitudes toward the health care system, different health behavior patterns, and different types of health problems (see Figure 5-1). Even after these new immigrants undergo **acculturation**, an informal process of adaptation through which the beliefs, values, norms, and practices of a dominant culture are learned by new members born into a different culture, many of their beliefs and attitudes may be an amalgam of their original practices and those of the dominant Euro-American culture. Furthermore, the socioeconomic level of members within a given ethnic and cultural group may influence their health beliefs, attitudes, and customs

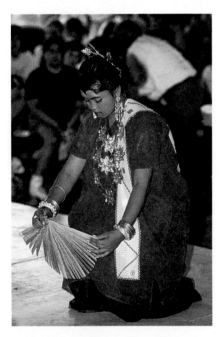

Figure 5-1 Respect and interest in cultural background will provide a strong basis for communication.
Photo courtesy of Smithsonian Institution

(Schensul & Guest, 1994). Nurses must develop a perspective of cultural relativity by viewing health beliefs and behaviors within the context of each patient's culture and by working to deliver culturally competent health care.

Culturally competent nursing care is provided by nurses who use **cross-cultural nursing care** models (nursing care provided within the cultural context of patients who are members of a culture or subculture different from that of the nurse) and research to identify health care needs and to plan and evaluate the care provided within the cultural context of patients. Culturally competent nursing care is care provided to patients who are considered to be a minority because of their racial, ethnic, cultural, gender, or sexual orientation. The process of culturally competent nursing care consists of: (1) eliciting statements of cultural values and beliefs so that culturally sensitive approaches to care based on mutual respect can be provided; (2) recognizing and understanding the normal behaviors of different cultural groups and their unique behavioral responses to health and illness; (3) obtaining information on ethnic variations and on normal racial growth patterns to assist in identifying abnormal patterns and designing appropriate interventions; and (4) using an ethic of **cultural relativism** to provide nursing services, i.e., the belief that no culture is either inferior or superior to another, that behavior must be evaluated in relation to the cultural context in which it occurs, and that respect, equality, and justice are basic rights for all racial, ethnic, subcultural, and cultural groups.

To provide culturally competent nursing care, the nurse first must be willing and able to confront his or her own cultural biases, or **ethnocentrism** (a condition that occurs when individuals or groups of people perceive their own cultural group and cultural values, beliefs, norms, and customs to be superior to all others and have disdain for the expression and expressor of any way of life but their own), and stereotyping, to whatever extent they exist, and examine the impact they will have on the patient. It is also important to understand the dynamics and respond to the challenges inherent in **bilingualism** (the habitual use of two different languages, particularly when speaking), **multiculturalism** (when individuals live and function in two or more cultures simultaneously), and **cultural identity** (the cultural definition or cultural orientation with which an individual self-identifies) of their patients. In addition, consideration should be given to the potential for **culture shock**: the disorientation, uncertainty, and alienation that can occur during the process of adjusting to a new cultural group.

Assessing a patient's cultural beliefs, values, and customs through observation and interview is an essential part of health assessment for culturally competent nursing care. When assessing a patient, a balance is needed between the data related to the specific individuals and their families who are being assessed and the data related to the cultural group to which they have been **enculturated** (the informal process through which the beliefs, values, norms, and practices of a culture are learned by members born into the culture). The nurse, therefore, needs to have experience with a range of individuals and families from any given cultural group in order to determine where in this range the patient being assessed fits. In addition, knowledge of the patient's racial and ethnic group's physical and biological norm differences, as well as the risks to optimal health that are associated with the patient's racial, ethnic, and cultural group are also relevant.

During the health assessment interview, the nurse needs to avoid stereotyping the patient by depending too heavily on an "ideal" or normative racial, ethnic, or cultural characteristic or trait list. Summaries of any group are inherently imprecise by virtue of being normative. No one individual or family within a culture or subculture will display all of the characteristics representative of that culture, and normative lists or summaries do not include all of the diversity that may be part of a given culture. An understanding of basic racial, ethnic, and cultural concepts associated with the conduct of culturally competent health assessments, however, can serve as a *guide* for the nurse.

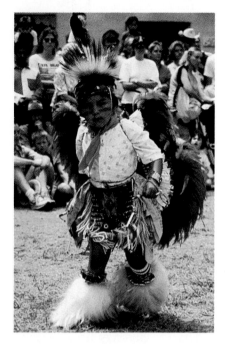

Figure 5-2 Children often adopt the ways of the dominant culture while embracing elements of their parents' culture.   *Photo courtesy of Smithsonian Institution*

BASIC CONCEPTS ASSOCIATED WITH CULTURALLY COMPETENT ASSESSMENTS

Culture

Culture is a learned and socially transmitted orientation and way of life of a group of people. Culture enables members of large groupings of people to find coherence and to survive in the world around them through the development of unique patterns of basic assumptions and shared meanings. The cultural beliefs, values, customs, and norms that result from these assumptions and meanings shape how the group members think, act, and relate to and with others as well as how they perceive aspects of life such as time, space, health, illness, and family, spousal, parental, work, and community-member roles. The beliefs, values, and norms of a cultural group are passed informally from one generation of group members born into the culture to another, exert a powerful force on all group members, and are very difficult to change (refer to Figure 5-2).

Subculture

Subculture refers to membership in a smaller group within a larger culture. These smaller groups possess many of the values, beliefs, and customs of the larger culture but have unique characteristics such as age, education, marital status, preference in life partner, generational placement, occupation, socioeconomic level, health status, or religion. Membership in subcultures is generally involuntary. In addition, membership in subcultures is not usually constrained by obvious physical characteristics such as skin color, body build, or mannerisms.

Numerous subcultures exist within each culture. An individual may be simultaneously a member of several subcultures. For example, a 50-year-old (generational), white (race), overweight (health status), Southern (regional), conservative (political value system), heterosexual (sexual preference), male (special privileges and responsibilities in dominant society), politician (occupation), father of two teenagers (family status), divorced and recently remarried (marital status), Baptist (religious affiliation) of Irish ancestry (genetic) currently living in the Washington, D.C., metropolitan area (lifestyle) is a member of at least 13 subcultures. Each subculture influences to some degree the behavior of its members, as does the primary culture.

It is important to recognize that every individual has a combination of cultural influences, derived from membership in the primary culture as well as multiple subcultures, which creates a **multicultural identity**. This unique multicultural identity makes it critical for the nurse to assess each individual patient in context rather than simply as a normative member of a single culture, subculture, race, ethnic, or minority group.

Racial Groups

Race is defined as the classification of individuals based on shared traits such as skin tone, facial features, and body build that are inherited from biological ancestors and are usually sufficiently obvious to warrant classification as a member of that racial group. Racial characteristics can have an impact on health status and health care, for example, individuals of Asian and American Indian descent have few apocrine glands and therefore perspire little, have mild or no body odor, and dry ear wax. Also, the incidence of skin cancer in darkly pigmented individuals is much lower than in light-skinned individuals, due to a higher level of melanin in the pigmentation. Racial characteristics do not tend to change when acculturation occurs. Nurses need to ask about the patient's self-identified racial group when performing a cultural assessment.

Ethnic Groups

Ethnic group members share a unique national or regional origin and social, cultural, and linguistic heritage. Five ethnic groups are usually recognized in the United States: whites (of European descent such as English, Scottish, Irish, French, Dutch, Polish, Scandinavian, Swiss, Italian, Slavic, and Russian); blacks (of African, Haitian, Jamaican, and Dominican Republic descent); Hispanics (of Spanish-speaking descent such as Cuban, Puerto Rican, Mexican, and Latin and South American); Asian and Pacific Islanders (of Chinese, Japanese, Filipino, Vietnamese, Cambodian, Korean, Hawaiian, Guamanian, East Indian, and Samoan descent); and American Indians (of over 400 American Indian tribes and Eskimo descent) (U.S. Department of Commerce, Bureau of the Census, 1992). Another ethnic group that is increasingly being recognized in the United States is Middle Easterners (of Egyptian, Persian [Iranian], Armenian, Yemeni, and Arab [Palestinian, Lebanonese, Jordanian, Syrian, Saudi Arabian, and Iraqian] descent) (Meleis, Lipson, & Paul, 1992). Table 5-1 specifies ethnic-specific genetic traits and disorders.

It is important to note that although individuals tend to be identified as members of one of these ethnic groups, they may still have significantly different multicultural identities. A person may belong to multiple subcultural groups within the dominant ethnic group as well as have combined hereditary membership in two or more of the racial or ethnic groups.

Ethnic identity, or self-identification with an ethnic group, is subjective and not always obvious. For example, Egyptians tend to identify with their country of origin, but Armenians born in a country such as Iran, and Palestinians born in countries such as Lebanon or Israel, identify with their respective cultures of origin rather than countries of origin (Meleis, Lipson, & Paul, 1992). When conducting a culturally competent assessment, therefore, it is appropriate to determine the patient's self-identified ethnic group as well as place of birth.

Minority Groups

Minority group members are individuals who are considered by themselves or others to be members of a minority because they have a different racial, cultural, ethnic, gender, or sexual orientation, or different socioeconomic level than do members of the dominant cultural group. Minority group members may receive different or unequal treatment and different degrees of acceptance from members of the dominant group. Although members of a minority may not be a true minority worldwide or even within a given region or nation (e.g., women or nurses), it is their membership in a subculture and the difference in the decisional power they have in influencing the dominant cultural environment that leads to their designation and subsequent treatment as a minority.

An example of different treatment based on gender is the tendency of nurses to administer more narcotic analgesics to male patients than to female patients and to white than to Hispanic, black, or Asian American patients (McDonald, 1994). As a nurse, you must continually evaluate your own values and actions to ensure that you provide appropriate care to all patients.

Values, Norms, and Value Orientations

Cultures and subcultures have a fundamental set of principles known as values, which govern the behavior of all members of the group. These values prescribe how each member should think, act, and respond to their internal

---

⊙⊙ THINK ABOUT IT

HIV-Positive Patient

You are working on an orthopedic unit in a city hospital and have just finished admitting a 26-year-old male homosexual social worker who is HIV-positive. The patient sustained multiple lacerations and a compound fracture of his left femur when struck by a speeding car running a red light. As you approach the nurses' station, you overhear the orthopedic intern and a staff nurse making disparaging, homophobic remarks about your new patient.

- What are your thoughts and feelings about working with this patient?
- How would you respond to what you have just overheard?
- How might you help your colleagues increase their cultural sensitivity and ensure the provision of culturally competent care for this patient?
- What research material is available that might support you in your attempt to provide culturally competent care for this patient?

Table 5-1   Ethnic Specific Genetic Traits and Disorders

ETHNIC GROUP	GENETIC TRAIT/DISORDER	ETHNIC GROUP	GENETIC TRAIT/DISORDER
Asian Americans		Karaite Jews	Werdnig-Hoffmann disease
Burmese	Hemoglobin E disease	Libyans (Sephardi Jews)	Cystinuria
Chinese	Adult lactase deficiency Alpha thalassemia Chinese type glucose-6-phosphate dehydrogenase (G-6-PD) deficiency Diabetes mellitus Nasopharyngeal and liver cancer	Lebanese	Dyggus-Melchoir-Clausen syndrome
		Saudi Arabian	Methachromatic leukodystrophy
		Yemenites	Mediterranean type glucose-6-phosphate dehydrogenase (G-6-PD) deficiency Phenylketonuria
Filipino	Diabetes mellitus Thalassemia Glucose-6-phosphate dehydrogenase (G-6-PD) deficiency		
Japanese	Acatalasemia Cleft lip/palate Oguchi's disease	**American Indians**	Chronic liver disease and cirrhosis Diabetes mellitus Tuberculosis Hepatitis B Asthma, infants Nasopharyngeal cancer Trachoma
Korean	Lactase deficiency Osteoporosis Insulin autoimmune syndrome Peptic ulcer disease Hypertension		
		Eskimos	Congenital adrenal hyperplasia Adult lactase deficiency Methemoglobinemia Primary narrow-angle glaucoma Pseudocholinesterase deficiency Haemophilus influenza type b
Papua Melanesian	Burkitt's lymphoma in children		
Polynesians	Clubfoot		
Samoan	Diabetes mellitus		
Thai	Adult lactase deficiency Hemoglobin E disease	Hopi Indians	Tyrosinase-positive albinism
		Navaho Indians	Arthritis Diabetes mellitus Ear anomalies
Vietnamese	Lactase deficiency		
		Zuni Indians	Tyrosinase-positive albinism
Black Americans			
African	Adult lactose deficiency African type glucose-6-phosphate dehydrogenase (G-6-PD) deficiency Beta thalassemia Hemoglobin C disease Hereditary hemoglobin F disease Hypertension Sickle cell anemia Systemic lupus erythematosus Diabetes mellitus Glaucoma	**White Americans**	
		Amish	
		Adams & Allen County, IN	Limb-girdle muscular dystrophy
		Lancaster County, PA	Ellis-van Creveld syndrome
		Mifflin County, OH	Pyruvate kinase deficiency
		Holmes County, PA	Hemophilia B
		Appalachia	Tuberculosis Coronary heart disease Diabetes mellitus
Hispanics	Diabetes mellitus Cleft lip/palate		
Mexican American, Latino, Chicano	Hypertension	Bosnia-Herzegovina (Yugoslavia)	Colon cancer Diabetes mellitus
Costa Rican	Malignant osteoporosis	Danes	Krabbe's disease Phenylketonuria
		East Indians	Lactase deficiency Alpha thalassemia Glucose-6-phosphate dehydrogenase (G-6-PD) deficiency
Middle Eastern			
Armenian	Familial Mediterranean fever Familial paroxysmal polyserositis	English	Cystic fibrosis Hereditary amyloidosis, type III
Habbanite Jews	Metachromatic leukodystrophy		
Iranians	Dubin-Johnson syndrome		
Iraqis	Ichthyosis vulgaris		

continued

Table 5-1 Ethnic Specific Genetic Traits and Disorders *continued*

ETHNIC GROUP	GENETIC TRAIT/DISORDER	ETHNIC GROUP	GENETIC TRAIT/DISORDER
White Americans *continued*		Ashkenazi	Gaucher's disease, adult type Niemann-Pick disease, infantile Tay-Sachs disease, infantile Hypercholesterolemia Polycythemia vera Stomach cancer Myopia
Finns	Congenital nephrosis Diastrophic dwarfism Polycystic liver disease Retinoschisis		
French Canadians (Quebec)	Hypercholesterolemia Osteoarthritis	Sephardi	Ataxia-telangiectasia Cystinuria Familial Mediterranean fever Glycogen storage disease III
Greeks	Tay-Sachs disease	New Zealanders	Asthma
Czechs	Beta thalassemia Familial Mediterranean fever Mediterranean type glucose-6-phosphate dehydrogenase (G-6-PD) deficiency Congenital glaucoma	Norwegians	Cholestasis-lymphedema Krabbe's disease Phenylketonuria
Icelanders	Phenylketonuria	Nova Scotia Acadians	Niemann-Pick disease, type D
Irish	Neural tube defects Phenylketonuria	Polish	Phenylketonuria
Italians	Beta thalassemia Familial Mediterranean fever Mediterranean type glucose-6-phosphate dehydrogenase (G-6-PD) deficiency	Portuguese	Joseph's disease
		Scots	Cystic fibrosis Hereditary amyloidosis, type III Krabbe's disease Phenylketonuria Rett's syndrome Sjögren's syndrome
Jews	Inflammatory bowel disease		

Based on data reported in Giger, J. N., & Davidhizar, R. E. (1995). Transcultural nursing: Assessment and intervention (2nd ed.). Baltimore: Mosby; Wong, D. L. (1995). Whaley and Wong's nursing care of infants and children (5th ed.). Baltimore: Mosby; Geissler, E. (1994). Pocket guide to cultural assessment. Baltimore: Mosby–Year Book, Inc.; and Johnson, K. E., & Rogers, S. (1994).

and external environments. **Cultural values** tend to be acquired subconsciously during the process of enculturation and are a fundamental, often unshakable, unchanging set of principles that serve as the base on which an individual's beliefs, customs, goals, and aspirations are built.

Cultural norms are the often unwritten but generally understood prescriptions for acceptable behavior in designated situations encountered by group members in the course of their daily lives. Every group member is bound by these norms and may be criticized, punished, or ostracized by other group members when the norms are violated.

All cultures have a fundamental set of values and concurrent **value orientations**, i.e., patterned principles that provide order and give direction to individuals' thoughts and behaviors related to the solution of commonly occurring human problems (Kluckholn & Strodtbeck, 1961; Spector, 1996; Giger & Davidhizar, 1995). Five areas about which cultures have their own unique value orientations have major relevance for culturally competent health assessments and care (see Table 5-2). These value orientations are time, human nature, activity, relational, and people-to-nature.

Beliefs

Cultural beliefs consist of the explanatory ideas and knowledge that members of a given culture have about various aspects of their world and are based on cultural values and norms, including commonly held opinions,

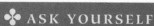

ASK YOURSELF

Fundamental Cultural Values

- What is your time orientation?
- What do you believe about the basic nature of human beings? What do you believe is your basic nature?
- What do you believe is your primary purpose in life?
- What do you believe about the purpose of human relations?
- What do you believe your relation is to nature and the supernatural?

Table 5-2   Basic Cross-Cultural Values, Value Orientations, and Beliefs

VALUE	VALUE ORIENTATION AND BELIEFS
Time What is the time orientation of human beings?	*Past* focus: Reverence for long-standing traditions. *Present* focus: Live in "here and now," perceive time in a linear fashion. *Future* focus: Willing to defer gratification to ensure they can meet a future goal; tend to be disciplined in scheduling and using time.
Human Nature What is the basic nature of human beings?	Human beings are *basically good.* Human beings are *evil but* have a *perfectable* nature. Human beings are a combination of *good and evil* requiring *self-control to perfect* nature; *lapses* occasionally occur and are *accepted.* Human beings are *neutral, neither good nor evil.*
Activity What is the primary purpose of life?	*Being* orientation: Human beings' value resides in their *inherent existence* and spontaneity. *Becoming-in-being* orientation: Human beings' value is inherent but they must engage in *continuous self-development* as integrated wholes. *Doing* orientation: Human beings exist to be *active* and to *achieve.*
Relational What is the purpose of human relations?	*Linear* relationships: Welfare and goals of the *hereditary and extended family* are emphasized. Goals of the family take precedence over the individual's. *Collateral* relationships: Welfare and goals of *social and family group* are emphasized. Group goals take precedence. *Individual* relationships: *Individual* goals and accountability for own behavior emphasized.
People to Nature What is the relationship of human beings to nature?	Human beings *dominate nature* and have control over their environment. Human beings *live in harmony with nature* and must maintain that balance. Human beings are *subjugated to nature* and have no control over their environment.

Compiled from information in: Kluckhorn, K., & Strodtbeck, F. (1961). Variations in value orientations. New York: Row, Peterson; and Giger, J. N., & Davidhizar, R. E. (1995). Transcultural nursing: Assessment and intervention (2nd ed.). Baltimore: Mosby.

knowledge, and attitudes about time, relationships, human nature, purpose in life, and nature (see Figure 5-3). Such beliefs influence the meaning individuals attach to health and illness, by whom and how they prefer to treat illness, and the health behaviors in which they are willing to engage. Because health and illness are culturally determined, what may be considered to be health or illness in one culture may not be in another. In addition, many cultures distinguish between a **"folk illness,"** believed to be caused by disharmony or an imbalance or as punishment, and a **"scientific illness,"** in which the presence of pathology is the defining characteristic. In these cultures, a **folk**

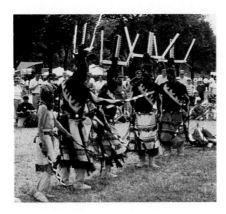

Figure 5-3   Values, customs, and beliefs are shared by members of cultural groups.   *Photo courtesy of Smithsonian Institution.*

practitioner (a healer or other individual who is not part of the scientific health care system but is believed to have special knowledge or power to prevent, treat, or provide resources needed to heal folk illnesses) is consulted for a folk illness because health care practitioners are not believed to be knowledgeable in recognizing or treating such illnesses.

Folk Illnesses

Two major types of folk illnesses are usually delineated: naturalistic and personalistic. **Naturalistic illnesses** are believed to be caused by an imbalance or disequilibrium between essentially impersonal factors. For example, the most common imbalance is between "hot" and "cold" (see Table 5-3). Illnesses and treatments that are classified as either hot or cold are culturally determined and do not have any relationship to the actual temperature of the patient or of the substances used to treat the illness. In general, "hot" illnesses are treated with "cold" substances and vice versa to restore the balance between the two. These beliefs are held by many Hispanic, Arab, and Asian ethnic groups and cultures. Although most cultures who share these beliefs use the hot and cold terminology, among traditional Chinese, these forces are called *yin* (cold) and *yang* (hot).

Understanding the health belief patterns of patients and the meanings attached to symptoms, illnesses, and treatments can be helpful in understanding why patients may refuse to participate in a given treatment regimen or why they insist on a specific treatment. For example, some Hispanic patients may insist on being given penicillin, which is considered to be a *caliente* (hot) treatment, for a viral upper respiratory infection (URI), which is considered to be a *frio* (cold) condition. Explanations about the lack of benefit in treating viral URIs with penicillin and the potential for building a resistance to penicillin when used unnecessarily rarely dissuade those who insist on its use. Substituting another substance such as vitamins, which are also considered to be "hot" treatments, shows an acceptance of their beliefs and "does the least harm."

Personalistic illnesses are believed to occur because an individual has committed some offense and is being punished, or the illness results from acts of aggression (sometimes unintentional) by other individuals. Witchcraft and the "evil eye" are two sources of personalistic illnesses. Witchcraft is believed to be the cause of illness among Haitians, Puerto Ricans, and some black Americans. More often than not, witchcraft is used to punish individuals for an emotional or a physical injury, an illness, or a death they are thought to have caused, or occasionally because they possess something that is coveted by another.

The "evil eye" belief is shared by many Mediterranean (e.g., Italian, Sicilian, and Greek), African, and Spanish-speaking cultures. The "evil eye" is more often than not given unintentionally, for example, by complimenting a child unprotected by an amulet, gold cross, or other protective device or by not touching the child while offering the compliment. It is feared that a child who is complimented for her looks, for example, will lose her good looks (if she was unprotected by a device) or develop symptoms such as severe headache, restlessness, irritability, high fever, diarrhea, weight loss, and sleeplessness if the person complimenting the child was not touching the child at the time.

Self-Care Practices

All cultural groups use a variety of self-care practices that may include the use of "folk medicine" and remedies. Self-care includes practices in which persons engage on their own behalf to aid in health promotion and maintenance, disease or injury prevention or protection, and disease or injury treatment.

Self-care encompasses a wide range of remedies, rituals, and folk medicine. For example, increasing numbers of Americans believe that they can prevent

Table 5-3   Hot and Cold Conditions, Foods, and Treatments

HOT (*Caliente/Yang*) CONDITIONS	COLD (*Frio/Yin*) CONDITIONS
Constipation	Cancer
Diarrhea	Colds
Fever	Depression
Hypertension	Earache
Infections	Infertility
Kidney problems	Headache
Liver problems	Joint pain
Pregnancy	Lactation
Skin rashes, sores	Malaria
Sore throat	Menstruation
Ulcers	Paralysis
	Pneumonia
	Postpartum psychoses
	Rheumatism
	Stomach cramps
	Teething
	Tuberculosis

HOT (*Caliente/Yang*) FOODS	COLD (*Frio/Yin*) FOODS
Aromatic beverages	Avocado
Beans	Barley water
Cereal grains	Bean curds
Cheese	Bland foods
Chili peppers	Bottled whole milk
Chocolate	Cashew nuts
Eggs	Dairy products
Evaporated milk	Fresh vegetables (carrots,
Fried foods	turnips, squash, eggplant)
Goat's milk	Green vegetables
Hard liquor	Honey
Meats (beef, lamb, waterfowl)	Meats (chicken, fish, goat)
Oils	Tropical fruits (banana,
Onions	grapefruit, mango, orange,
Peas	pineapple)
Spicy, hot foods	Raisins
Temperate-zone fruits (apple, grapes,	
pears, peaches)	
Vinegar	
Wine	

HOT (*Caliente/Yang*) MEDICINES AND HERBS	COLD (*Frio/Yin*) MEDICINES AND HERBS
Anise	Bicarbonate of soda
Aspirin	Linden
Castor oil	Milk of magnesia
Cinnamon	Orange flower water
Cod-liver oil	Sage
Garlic	
Ginger root	
Iron preparation	
Penicillin	
Tobacco	
Vitamins	

Compiled from data obtained in: Wilson, H., & Kneisl, C. (1996). Psychiatric Nursing (5th ed.). Reading, MA: Addison-Wesley; Spector, R. (1991). Cultural diversity in health and illness. Norwalk, CT: Appleton & Lange; and Giger, J. N., & Davidhizar, R. E. (1995). Transcultural nursing: Assessment and intervention (2nd ed.). Baltimore: Mosby.

> ❖ ASK YOURSELF
>
> **Self-Care Practices**
>
> - What self-care practices do you use and when do you use them?
> - Where or from whom did you learn the self-care practices you use most often?
> - Which of these self-care practices are based on medical research and which are not?

> ❖ ASK YOURSELF
>
> **Multicultural Identity**
>
> - What are the values and beliefs that most characterize each culture and subculture to which you belong, and with which do you agree?
> - Do any of your values and beliefs that are derived from membership in one culture or subculture conflict with those from any other?
> - If there is any conflict between the values of two or more of the cultures or subcultures with which you identify (e.g., health care professional subculture, religious subculture, socioeconomic subculture, political party subculture), have you resolved these conflicts, and if so, how have you done this and what helped you to reconcile these conflicts?

cardiac problems by taking an aspirin a day, that they can decrease hypertension by eating garlic daily, or that they can prevent their children from getting colds by giving them daily chewable vitamin C tablets with breakfast. Many over-the-counter drugs and preparations for everything from baldness to arthritis are often no more than folk remedies with Fifth Avenue packaging and marketing. When providing nursing care, be sure to ascertain what self-care and folk remedies are used by the patient, and the patient's opinion of their effectiveness.

Values and Beliefs of the Nurse

Nurses, as do patients, tend to assimilate the general values, attitudes, and behaviors of the respective societies in which they have been raised as well as those of their immediate families and cultural groups.

One way to develop self-awareness of your cultural beliefs and values is by composing a list of culture(s) and subcultures of which you are a member. You may belong to a dominant culture by birth or by acculturation and at the same time be a member of a unique combination of subcultures based on age, gender, race, religion, national origin, health status, socioeconomic status, educational level, occupation, political affiliation, and many other factors. The major values and practices of each of these cultures and subcultures can be analyzed to identify who you are, how you perceive the world, and how you behave in relation to others.

Carnevali and Patrick (1993) suggest another strategy that can be used to identify and analyze the cultural values and beliefs that may influence how you think and act when providing patient care. The first step is to state a general value that you hold about patients. Start with a value statement contained in the nursing philosophy for the unit in which you work; the Patient's Bill of Rights, the Code of Nursing, your job description, or a similar document that has patient- or profession-relevant belief and value statements with which you agree.

The value statement selected for analysis might be: "I value the right of all patients to make decisions about their own care based on adequate information provided by health care professionals." After selecting such a value statement, observe your own practice as well as that of other health care professionals, noting occasions when patients were or were not given enough information to make informed choices about their own care. Collect such information until definite patterns begin to emerge that are representative of circumstances that influenced why and when patients were and were not given information and permitted to make their own care decisions.

Then restate the ideal value as it is actually implemented. If circumstances were present that prompted you and other health care professionals to make exceptions in providing patients with information and permitting them to participate in their own care decisions, the working value might be restated as: "I value the right of patients to make decisions about their own care based on adequate information provided by health care professionals *except when . . .*"

1. the patients' cognitive abilities are limited by pathology or their responses to treatment,

2. the patients do not have sufficient energy for making their own care decisions,

3. the health care professionals or the families believe that the patients should not be given particular information about themselves for their own good, and

4. the patients fail to make decisions that the health care professionals or the responsible family members believe are in their best interests.

Assessing the Potential for Harm Associated with a Cultural Belief or Behavior

When assessing one's own cultural values and beliefs and the behaviors that result from these values and beliefs, a nurse is often faced with having to decide when it is appropriate for the nurse's cultural value orientation to take precedence over that of the patient's. In other words, how culturally competent is a nurse to evaluate and decide when a patient's behavior is adaptive, harmful, or neutral? Sprott (1993) has suggested that nurses might make these judgments using Korbin's (1977) work on assessing whether an ethnic group's child-rearing practices constitute harm.

The conditions cited in Korbin's schema have relevance for evaluating the potential physical or psychological harm that health practices may have on a family member as perceived by health professionals or the agents of the family. Using this schema, a practice would not be considered harmful if:

1. The practice is sanctioned by that culture.
2. The practice is within the limits of deviations that are acceptable in that culture.
3. The practice is important for the acceptance of the patient as a member of the culture.
4. The patient on whom the practice will be carried out perceives that it is an appropriate practice in that situation.
5. The intent of the health care provider or agent of the family is consistent with the cultural "rules" that govern the practice.

For many situations, these five conditions can be quite helpful in clarifying the issues associated with evaluating whether an anticipated health practice is harmful or not. For other situations in which the practices of agents of the family, such as folk or traditional practitioners, must be evaluated or when the family requests that the nurse participate in a practice that is in conflict with the nurse's value system, the judgment that must be made is more difficult.

For example, circumcision of young girls (removal of all or part of the clitoris, labia minora, and labia majora) from early childhood through adolescence is widespread in many African countries such as Somalia, Djibouti, Ethiopia, Mali, and northern Sudan, and among Muslim groups in the Middle East, the Philippines, Pakistan, Indonesia, and Malaysia, as well as in some areas of Mexico, Brazil, and Peru (Johnson & Rogers, 1994). Although male circumcision is relatively common in the United States, female circumcision is not a part of the dominant Euro-American culture to which most American nurses have been enculturated.

For the health care professional in the United States who is enculturated into the Euro-American value system and bound by the health care professional oath to "do no harm," surgical removal of female genitalia constitutes a physiological and psychological threat to a child from our dominant culture. But does it pose the same threat to a child who is a member of one of the ethnic groups that practice female circumcision and who is now living in the United States? When the female circumcision procedure on a child from one of these ethnic groups is contemplated in the United States, the primary health care provider to the family may be faced with a cultural conflict: to assist with the procedure by ensuring sterile conditions, pain control, and possible anesthesia versus refusing to have anything to do with it and possibly reporting the parents for child abuse if they go through with the circumcision ritual.

Using Korbin's five criteria, a nurse from the Euro-American culture might conclude that: (1) the practice of female circumcision is sanctioned by the minority cultural group; (2) the practice is within the limits of deviations acceptable to the minority group; (3) the practice is important for the acceptance of the patient as a member of her minority cultural group; (4) the practice of female circumcision may or may not be perceived to be an appropriate

Female Circumcision

- Would you assist with a female circumcision?
- Under what conditions would you participate?
- When would you not participate and why?

practice by the patient (depending on her ability to understand the implications of the practice on her future health status and on how enculturated she is in her minority culture versus how acculturated she is in the dominant culture); (5) the practice is consistent with the cultural "rules" that govern behavior in the minority culture and is not perceived by the minority cultural group as doing physical or psychological harm to the child, but is considered in the dominant Euro-American culture to be physically and psychologically harmful to the child and, thus, a form of child abuse (particularly infibulation).

Although the preceding analysis helps to clarify the issues associated with the cultural conflict of whether or not to assist with female circumcision, going through this process of analysis does not ensure an answer to the question for every nurse. Each nurse must ultimately resolve this and other such cultural and ethical conflicts on an individual patient basis.

Customs and Rituals

Customs and rituals are culturally learned behaviors that are much easier to observe or learn about through interviewing than are the values and beliefs on which the customs and rituals are based. **Customs** are frequent or common practices carried out by tradition and include communication patterns, family and kinship relations, work patterns, dietary and religious practices (see Chapters 6 and 7), and health behaviors and practices (see Table 5-4). **Cultural rituals** are highly structured and prescribed patterns of behavior used by a cultural group to respond to or in anticipation of specific life events such as birth, death, illness, healing, marriage, worship, and other important events.

Communication Patterns

Communication patterns are the means through which members of a cultural group transmit and preserve the values, beliefs, norms, and practices of their culture. Communication practices also reflect, determine, and ultimately mold the culture. Communication patterns include both verbal and nonverbal means of expressing or concealing thoughts and feelings of joy, sorrow, grief, happiness, anger, acceptance, fear, love, and the full range of human experiences.

In some cultures the expression of thoughts and feelings is open and dramatic with frequent touching and sharing of territorial space. In other cultures such open expressions are regarded as unacceptable. For example, among Southeastern Asians it is considered to be positive to avoid confrontation and negative to overtly express annoyance, anger, or hatred. In addition, many new immigrants from East Africa and Southeast Asia may find the immediate, social pleasantness and friendliness of the American health care provider confusing and offensive when they discover that these behaviors do not reflect the depth of a more advanced stage of personal intimacy and friendship that such behaviors signify in their own cultures.

Although the process of communication is universal, the intonation, rhythm, speed, use of silence, facial expressions, eye and head movements, body posture, touch, styles and types of feedback, as well as other "rules" for communication may be culturally unique.

In some cultures, movement of the head may mean the exact opposite of what it means in Western cultures. For example, Bulgarians nod the head to indicate "no" and move the head back and forth to indicate "yes." In other cultures a "yes" answer may be indicated in some other way, such as among Tongans, who raise their eyebrows to answer "yes" to a question. Sometimes a verbal "yes" may actually mean "no." For example, when Tunisians say "yes *N'sha'llah*" (God willing), it reflects the belief that only God has control over the future, and, therefore, can mean "no."

There are many communication variables that are culture specific. Some of these are eye contact, proximity to others, role of social small talk, direct versus nondirect questioning, topic taboos or topics the patient is reluctant to talk about, as well as who makes health decisions for family members in a given culture. For example, African and Mexican Americans value eye contact, but Filipinos do not. Anglo-Americans and German Americans require more personal space than do Hispanic, Japanese, and Arab Americans. Western European and Spanish Americans value social small talk prior to discussing the actual purpose for an interaction, such as an interview about current illness.

The nurse can communicate respect for the patient and the patient's behavior through respectful listening, reflection, restating, and validation of inferences drawn about the meaning of the patient's responses and behavior. Other critical communication techniques include conveying willingness and the time to listen by giving the patient undivided attention and by allowing the patient sufficient time to formulate and give answers to interview questions.

Cultural Meaning of Symptoms

One of the most important techniques when performing a culturally competent health assessment is to make every effort to discover the cultural meaning of the patient's perceptions and to encourage the patient to communicate interpretations of health, illness, and symptoms. When people experience pain or other symptoms associated with sickness or illness, they interpret the symptoms and react to them in ways that fit their cultural norms. When attempting to discover the cultural meaning the patient gives to symptoms, the nurse must be concerned with eliciting statements about symptoms the patient considers to be significant as well as symptoms the patient believes to be an expected part of one's life.

In addition, each culture has its own system for communicating the distress associated with illness. For example, many Mexican Americans value enduring pain stoically and expect this behavior from both children and adults. In contrast, many Italians use expressive reactions to communicate distress, especially from chronic pain, but tend to hide pain from their families and closest friends and are not likely to describe the details of the pain. Persians (Iranians) may report emotional distress as "heart distress," whereas Cambodians often refer to the depression associated with the cumulative trauma of war experiences and the cultural adaptation to the American inner-city environment as "thinking too much."

To discover the cultural meaning that a patient attaches to symptoms, Wenger (1993) proposes that nurses use a bidirectional translation process. This method of ascribing cultural meaning involves collecting the symptom statements of the patient and analyzing them in the context of meanings and patterns of thought that are shared by other members of the patient's culture. As the patient communicates these meanings, link this cultural knowledge to the health care practices and therapeutic regimens that are perceived to be the most culturally congruent and efficacious. Listen to the patient's symptom descriptions, reflect on the meaning the patient seems to attach to the symptoms, restate the inferred meaning, and allow the patient time to determine if the reflected inferred meaning statement accurately reflects the patient's own reality. Then restate and restructure the inferred meaning until the patient validates its accuracy.

Language Barriers

In seeking clarification of the meaning patients from other cultures attach to their illness experiences, it is important to accurately identify and then remove or overcome any language barriers that may exist. A variety of language barriers may exist even among two people for whom English is the first language, particularly if different forms of English are used by the individuals. Language barriers may be due to different connotative meanings for words, the use of clichés, a reliance on jargon specific to one individual's background but not to the other's, the complexity of the sentence structure, the different meanings

NURSING TIP

Overcoming Language Barriers

Special approaches for overcoming language barriers:
- Speak slowly and distinctly in a normal tone.
- Use gestures or pictures to illustrate meaning.
- Avoid clichés, jargon, and value-laden terms.
- Avoid defensive or offensive body language.
- Obtain feedback to confirm accurate understanding.
- Provide reading material written in the appropriate language.
- Use a culturally sensitive interpreter with fluency in health care terminology.
- Speak to the patient, rather than to the interpreter.
- Use the same interpreter for each interaction.

attached to specific types of body language, and the use of value-laden terms. When English is the patient's second language, a serious language barrier may occur (even for those proficient in their second language) if the patient is too anxious or ill to invest limited energy in speaking and understanding English.

Family and Kinship Relations

Family and kinship patterns are usually linear, collateral, or individualist. When the family has a linear pattern, the welfare, continuity, and goals of the hereditary family and extended family are emphasized, and the goals of the group take precedence over those of the individual. The family is usually patriarchal, places a strong emphasis on the enculturation of children, and is respectful of elder members. Asian, Middle Eastern, and upper-class Euro-American families tend to have linear family and kinship patterns.

Among families in which collateral patterns are the norm, the welfare and goals of lateral group members such as siblings or peers, in addition to the nuclear family, are emphasized, and the goals of the individual are subordinate to those of the lateral group. These families tend to hold most of their social activities with their social family groups, are generally open in their expressions of friendship, and value their children highly (refer to Figure 5-4). Although the male is often the head of the family group, women play a major role in decision making, particularly in relation to child-rearing and caring. Examples of collateral family and kinship patterns are found among Hispanic and American Indian families.

In cultures in which individualistic family and kinship patterns are prevalent, the individual family member's goals take precedence, and self-responsibility and accountability for one's own behavior is the norm. Generosity in times of crisis, however, is characteristic. There is less respect for authority figures and less respect and sense of responsibility for the elder family members. Sharing of parental and family responsibilities between the mother and father is common. The middle-class Euro-American family, single-parent family, and gay family typify the individualistic family and kinship pattern (refer to Figure 5-5).

When assessing the family, kinship, and work patterns, it is important to determine the family's actual structure. It may be helpful to draw a diagram, known as an **ecogram**, of the patient and the relationships with family members and significant friends, peers, neighbors, and work associates, noting those with whom the patient has the most frequent contact and their relative importance to the patient. The nature of the relationships may also be important. For example, is the relationship dependent versus independent or interdependent? Is it intimate or friendly versus hostile? Is there shared decision making versus being subject to the decision? Figure 5-7 on page 126 illustrates an ecogram.

Health Beliefs and Health Practices

Understanding culturally based health belief practices can also prevent their misidentification. For example, the Vietnamese American may use *cao gio* (skin rubbing with a coin) to treat diseases they believe to be caused by wind entering the body (e.g., upper respiratory infections). After applying oil or an ointment on the skin over the affected body area (chest, shoulders, upper back), the edge of a coin is moved along the skin until ecchymotic stripes appear, demonstrating that the treatment is successful. *Cao gio* is rarely painful or injurious and more often than not is perceived to be helpful by the recipient. Finding these areas of ecchymosis, however, can lead to a misdiagnosis of abuse if knowledge of this folk practice is lacking. Table 5-4 summarizes cultural characteristics and health care beliefs and practices. Keep in mind that general information is provided and there are variants in any cultural group.

For assistance in conducting a culturally competent health assessment of patients and their families, see Table 5-5 (refer also to Figure 5-6). The assessment should be tailored to those areas having a direct impact on the patient's immediate health status.

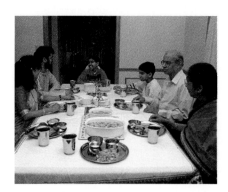

Figure 5-4 Sharing meals together is often an important family function. *Courtesy of Delmar Publishers, Albany, NY*

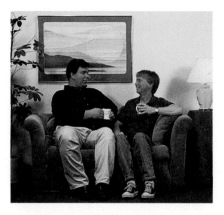

Figure 5-5 Families come in many shapes and configurations.

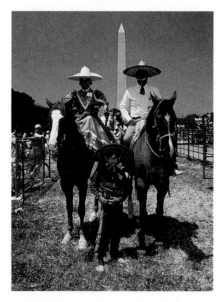

Figure 5-6 Appreciation of family and cultural ties is the first step in delivering culturally sensitive nursing care. *Photo courtesy of Smithsonian Institution*

Table 5-4 Cultural Characteristics and Health Care Beliefs and Practices

CULTURAL GROUP	COMMUNICATIONS STYLES	FAMILY, SOCIAL, AND WORK RELATIONSHIPS	HEALTH VALUES AND BELIEFS	HEALTH CUSTOMS AND PRACTICES
Asian-American				
Chinese	Nonverbal and contextual cues important. Silence after a statement is used by a speaker who wishes the listener to consider the importance of what is said. Self-expression repressed. Value silence. Touching limited. May smile when do not understand. Hesitant to ask questions.	Hierarchical, extended family pattern. Deference to authority figures and elders. Both parents make decisions about children. Value self-reliance and self-restraint. Important to preserve family's honor and save face. Value working hard and giving to society.	Health viewed as gift from parents and ancestors and the result of a balance between the energy forces of *yin* (cold) and *yang* (hot). Illness caused by an imbalance. Blood is the source of life and cannot be regenerated. Lack of blood and chi (innate energy) produces debilitation and long illness. Respect for the body and belief in reincarnation dictates that one must die with the body intact. Believe a good physician can accurately diagnose an illness by simply examining a person using the senses of sight, smell, touch, and listening.	May use medical care system in conjunction with Chinese methods of acupuncture (a *yin* treatment consisting of the insertion of needles to meridians to cure disease or relieve pain) and moxibustion (a *yang* treatment during which heated, pulverized wormwood is applied to appropriate meridians to assist with labor and delivery and other *yin* disorders). Medicinal herbs, e.g., ginsing, are widely used. Fear painful, intrusive diagnostic tests, especially the drawing of blood. May refuse intrusive surgery or autopsy. May be distrustful of physicians who order and use painful or intrusive diagnostic tests. Accept immunizations as valid means of disease prevention. Heavy use of condiments such as monosodium glutamate and soy sauce.
Japanese	Attitude, action, and feeling more important than words. Tend to listen empathically. Touching limited. Direct eye contact considered a lack of respect. Stoic, suppress overt emotion. Value self-control, politeness, and personal restraint.	Close, interdependent, intergenerational relationships. Individual needs subordinate to family's needs. Will endure great hardship to ensure success of next generation. Belonging to right clique or society important to status and success. Obligation to kin and work group. Education highly valued.	Believe illness caused by contact with polluting agents (e.g., blood, skin diseases, corpses), social or family disharmony, or imbalance from poor health habits. Cleanliness highly valued.	Tend to rely on Euro-American medical system for preventive and illness care. Oldest adult child responsible for care of elderly. Care of disabled is a family's responsibility. Take pride in good health of children. Believe in removal of diseased areas. Practice of emotional control may make pain assessment more difficult. When visiting ill, often bring fruit or special Japanese foods.
Vietnamese	Respect and harmony most important values. Disrespectful to question authority figures. Avoid direct eye contact.	Family close, multigenerational, and primary social network. Filial piety of primary importance. Father is family decision maker. Individual needs are subordinate to family's needs.	Believe illness caused by naturalistic (bad food, water), supernaturalistic (punishment for displeasing a deity), metaphysical (imbalance of hot and cold) forces, or from contamination by germs.	Often use both folk and some parts of the scientific health care system such as drugs. Family orally transmits folk medicine information. Health care regarded as family responsibility.

continued

CULTURAL GROUP	COMMUNICATIONS STYLES	FAMILY, SOCIAL, AND WORK RELATIONSHIPS	HEALTH VALUES AND BELIEFS	HEALTH CUSTOMS AND PRACTICES
Vietnamese *continued*	Strong focus on respect through use of titles and terms indicating family and generational relationships. Modesty of speech and action valued. Relaxed concept of time; punctuality less significant than propriety. Use Ya to indicate listening, not understanding. Avoid asking direct questions.	Training of children shared by extended family. Behavior of individual reflects on total family. Education highly valued.		Use medicinal herbs, therapeutic diets, hygienic measures to promote health, prevent illness, and treat illness. All means and resources available to family are tried before seeking outside help. Folk care practices include *cao gio* (rubbing skin with coin) for respiratory illnesses, *bat gil* (skin pinching) for headaches, inhalation of aromatic oils and liniments for respiratory and gastrointestinal illnesses. May consult priest, astrologer, shaman, or fortune-teller for prediction or instruction about health, or use hot and cold foods and substances to restore balance.
Filipinos	Personal dignity and preserving self-esteem highly valued. Nonverbal communication important. Eye contact avoided. Avoid direct expressions of disagreement, particularly with authority figures. Sex, socioeconomic status, and tuberculosis too personal to discuss. Need to engage in "small talk" before discussing more serious matters.	Multigenerational matrifocal family with strong family ties. Avoid behavior that shames family. Defer to elderly. Individual interests subordinate to family's interests. Value interpersonal relationships over current events.	Tend to believe illness is related to natural (unhealthy environment), supernatural (God's will and providence), and metaphysical (imbalance between hot and cold) forces. Tend to be fatalistic in outlook on life.	If accessible, may use both folk and scientific medical systems. Folk practices include flushing (stimulating perspiration, vomiting, bowel evacuation), heating (hot and cold substances to maintain internal body temperature), and protection (use of amulets, good luck pieces, religious medals, pictures, statues). Tend to be stoic; believe pain is God's will and He will give one the strength to bear it.
Black Americans				
African Americans	Many have high level of caution or distrust of majority group. Expressive use of nonverbal behavior and speech. Many use an English dialect: "black English." Very sensitive to lack of congruence between verbal and nonverbal messages. Value direct eye contact.	Strong kinship bonds in extended family. 50% patriarchical; 50% matriarchical families. Large social networks of family and unrelated members. Elderly members respected, particularly maternal grandparents.	Illness is a collective event that disrupts the total family system. Illness believed to be a natural event resulting from conflict or disharmony in one's life, failure to protect oneself from cold air, pollution, food, and water, or sent by God as punishment.	Health is maintained by proper diet, rest, clean environment. Self-care and folk medicine (usually religious in origin) very prevalent. Individuals from more rural backgrounds are more likely to use folk practitioners.

continued

Table 5-4   Cultural Characteristics and Health Care Beliefs and Practices continued

CULTURAL GROUP	COMMUNICATIONS STYLES	FAMILY, SOCIAL, AND WORK RELATIONSHIPS	HEALTH VALUES AND BELIEFS	HEALTH CUSTOMS AND PRACTICES
African Americans *continued*	May "test" health professionals before submitting self to decisions and care of the majority group's health care providers.	Strong sense of peoplehood: come to aid of others in crisis. Black minister a strong influence in community. Women protect health of family. Worth of education is judged by its "usability in living."	Those more assimilated to dominant culture perceive illness to be due to preventable injury or pathology.	Attempt home remedies first; may not seek help from the medical establishment until illness serious; often will elect to retain dignity rather than seek care if values and sensibilities are demeaned. Prayer is common means for prevention and treatment. When ill or hospitalized, visits by family minister are sought, expected, and valued to help cope with illness and suffering.
Haitians	New immigrants and older persons often speak only Haitian Creole. Hand gesturing and tone of voice frequently used to complement speech. Smiling and nodding often do not indicate understanding. Direct eye contact used in formal and casual conversations. Unassertive — will not ask questions if health care provider appears busy or rushed. Touch is perceived as comforting, sympathetic, and reassuring.	Two-class social system: wealthy and poor. Rural and poor families tend to be matriarchical. Children taught unquestioning obedience to adults. Child-rearing shared by parents and older siblings. Tend to be status conscious, thus parents often choose children's mate to increase family status.	Illness believed to be caused by supernatural forces (angry spirits, enemies, or the dead) or natural forces (irregularities of blood volume, flow, viscosity, purity, color or temperature [hot and cold]; gas [gaz]; movement and consistency of mother's milk; hot/cold imbalance in the body; bone displacement). Believe health is a personal responsibility.	Use medical care and folk medicine simultaneously. Health maintained by good dietary and hygienic habits. Adherence to prescribed treatments directly related to perceived severity of illness; resist dietary and activity restrictions. Hot and cold and light and heavy properties of food are used to gain harmony with one's life cycle and bodily states. Natural illnesses are first treated by home remedies. Supernatural illnesses treated by healers: herbalist or leaf doctor (*dokte fèy*), midwife (*fam saj*), or voodoo priest (*boungan*), or priestess (*mambo*). Use amulets and prayer to protect against supernatural illnesses.
Hispanic Americans				
Mexicans	Most bilingual; may use nonstandard English. Introductory embrace common. Tend to revert to native language in times of stress. Consider prolonged eye contact disrespectful but value direct eye contact.	Strong kinship bonds among nuclear and extended families including *compadres* (godparents). Strong need for family group togetherness. Respect wisdom of elders. Children highly desired and valued; accompany family everywhere.	Illness can be prevented by: being good, eating proper foods, and working proper amount of time; also accomplished through prayer; wearing religious medals or amulets, and sleeping with relics at home.	Magico-religious practices common. Usually seek help from older women in family before going to a Jerbero, who specializes in the use of herbs and spices to restore balance/health or *curandero* or *curandera* (holistic healers) with whom they have a uniquely personal relationship and share a common worldview.

continued

CULTURAL GROUP	COMMUNICATIONS STYLES	FAMILY, SOCIAL, AND WORK RELATIONSHIPS	HEALTH VALUES AND BELIEFS	HEALTH CUSTOMS AND PRACTICES
Mexicans *continued*	Appreciate "small talk" before initiating actual conversation topic. Appreciate a nondirective approach with open-ended questions. Hesitant to talk about sex but may do so more freely with nurse of same sex. Father should be present when speaking with a male child.	Entire family contribute to family's financial welfare. Homes frequently decorated with statues, medals, and pictures of saints. Children often reluctant to share communal showers in schools. Relaxed concept of time.	Some believe illness is due to: body imbalance between *caliente* (hot) and *frio* (cold) or "wet" and "dry"; dislocation of parts of the body (*empacho* — ball of food stuck to the stomach wall or *caida de la mollera* — more serious, depression of fontanelle in infant); magic or supernatural (*mal ojo* [evil eye] or punishment from God); strong emotional state (*susto* — soul loss following an extreme fright); or *envidio* (success leads to envy by others resulting in misfortune). More concerned with present than with future and therefore may focus on immediate solutions rather than long-term goals. May view hospital as place to go to die.	Prevent and treat illness with "hot" and "cold" food prescriptions and prohibitions. For severe illness, use scientific medical system but also make promises, visit shrines, use medals and candles, offer prayers — elements of Catholic and Pentecostal rituals and artifacts. Extreme modesty; may avoid seeking medical care and open discussions of sex. Children and adults expected to and do endure pain stoically.
Puerto Ricans	Older, newly moved to the mainland often speak only Spanish; others usually bilingual. May use nonstandard English. Personal and family privacy valued. Consider questions regarding family disrespectful and presumptuous. Tend to have a relaxed sense of time.	Paternalistic, hierarchical family; father is family provider and decision maker. Family of central importance. Families usually large. Parents demand absolute obedience and respect from children. Women in family tend to all ill members and dispense all medicines. Children valued — seen as gift from God.	Many believe illness is caused by imbalance of hot and cold, evil spirits, and forces. Many believe in spirits and spiritualism, having visions, and hearing voices. Accept many idiosyncratic behaviors; often perceive behavioral disturbances as symptoms of illness that need to be treated rather than judged. Suspicious and fearful of hospitals.	Use folk practitioners and medical establishment or both. When ill: first seek advice from women in family; if not sufficient, seek help from a *senoria* (woman especially knowledgeable about causes and treatment of common illnesses); if unable to help, consult an *espiritista*, *curandera*, or *santeria* (if psychiatric problem) who listens nonjudgmentally; often use herbs, lotions, salves, and massage and *caliente* (hot), *fresco* (cool), and *frio* (cold) treatments; if no relief, may go to a medical physician; if not satisfied, may return to any of the preceding.

continued

Table 5-4 Cultural Characteristics and Health Care Beliefs and Practices *continued*

CULTURAL GROUP	COMMUNICATIONS STYLES	FAMILY, SOCIAL, AND WORK RELATIONSHIPS	HEALTH VALUES AND BELIEFS	HEALTH CUSTOMS AND PRACTICES
Cuban Americans	Most new immigrants are bilingual. Expect some social talk before getting to actual reason for discussion.	Strong family and maternal and paternal kinship ties. Mother tends to explain and reason constantly to obtain child's conformity to family norms. Elderly cared for at home. Mother primary health care provider in home and must be included in all health education programs for family members. Children often supported and assisted by parents long after becoming adults. Extensive network of support for family and family members from social institutions such as schools, health clinics, and social clubs. Ambitious and take advantage of any opportunity to be successful in their work.	Believe good health results from prevention and good nutrition. Believe plump babies and young children are most healthy and admirable.	Combine use of medical practitioners with religious and nonreligious folk practitioners. Tend to be eclectic in health-seeking practices and, in some instances, may seek assistance of *santeros* (Afro-Cuban healers) and *espiritista* to complement treatment by medical practitioners. Parents very concerned about eating habits of their children; may spend a considerable part of the family budget on food.
American Indians	Most speak their Indian language and English. Nonverbal communication important. Unwavering eye gaze viewed as insulting. Tend to take time to form an opinion of health professionals. Consider silence essential to understanding and respecting another. A pause following a question signifies that the question is important enough to be given thoughtful consideration.	Strong extended family and kinship structure — usually including relatives from both sides of the family. Believe family members are responsible for one another. Elder members greatly respected and assume leadership roles. Children valued. Children taught respect for traditions and to honor wisdom and those who possess it.	Medicine and religion strongly interwoven. Believe health results from being in harmony with nature and universe. Reject germ theory as cause of illness; believe every sickness and pain is a price to be paid for something that occurred in the past or will happen in the future. May carry objects believed to guard against witchcraft.	Use total immersion in water, sweat lodges, and special rituals in the gathering, preparation, and use of herbs to regain harmony and thus health. Diviner-diagnosticians determine cause of illness, recommend treatment, and refer to a specific medicine man — diagnose but do not have powers or skill to implement medical treatment. Medicine man — traditional healer in whom most faith placed — uses herbs and special chants and rituals to cure illness. Singers effect cures by laying on of hands and by the power of the songs they obtain from supernatural beings.

continued

CULTURAL GROUP	COMMUNICATIONS STYLES	FAMILY, SOCIAL, AND WORK RELATIONSHIPS	HEALTH VALUES AND BELIEFS	HEALTH CUSTOMS AND PRACTICES
American Indians *continued*	Hesitant to discuss personal affairs until trust is developed, which can take some time. Believe it is ethically wrong to speak for another person. Hesitant to talk about sex but may do so more freely with a nurse of the same sex. Sensitive about having their words and behavior written down.			
Middle Eastern	Men and women do not shake hands or touch each other in any manner outside immediate family or marital relationship. Touching and embracing on arrival and on departure are common among same sex. Use silence to show respect for another.	Providing family care and support is an important responsibility. Male-dominated. Eldest male is the decision maker. Male children valued more than females. Adult male must not be alone with any female except wife.	Magico-religious; follow will of Allah — passive role is norm. Various beliefs about the causes of disease coexist: "hot" and "cold" and "evil eye." Physically robust person considered healthier. Emotional distress expressed as "heart disease." Obligation and responsibility to visit the sick, help others when they are ill, especially children and elderly. Expect immediate pain relief from health professionals.	Use magico-religious, folk, self-care, and medical science. Use amulets inscribed with verses of the Koran, turquoise stones, charm of a hand with five fingers to enhance protective powers against evil eye. Male health professionals prohibited from touching or examining a female patient. May refuse to have female health professionals care for males. The dead must be buried with the body intact. May perform female circumcision to ensure Muslim females become "good wives" and are accepted by other women in the family and community.
White Americans Euro-Americans (middle class)	Often separate into male and female groups at social events unless the activity is for couples. Nod to denote understanding or indicate agreement. Tend to maintain a "neutral" facial expression in public. Tolerate hugs and embraces among intimates and close friends.	Nuclear family professed norm. Two primary family goals: encourage and nurture each individual, produce healthy, autonomous children. Power more egalitarian. Socialize primarily with work-related and neighborhood friends. Generosity in time of crisis.	Generally future oriented and believe one's internal and external environments can be controlled. Expect the most modern medical technology to be used when ill. Believe good health is a personal responsibility. Accept the germ theory and perceive illness to be the result of	Engage in self-care practices: strive for balanced diet, rest and activity, and work and leisure. Utilize self-care over-the-counter remedies for minor illnesses. Utilize medical health care system and health professionals for health screening, illness care, and follow-up.

continued

Table 5-4   Cultural Characteristics and Health Care Beliefs and Practices *continued*

CULTURAL GROUP	COMMUNICATIONS STYLES	FAMILY, SOCIAL, AND WORK RELATIONSHIPS	HEALTH VALUES AND BELIEFS	HEALTH CUSTOMS AND PRACTICES
Euro-Americans (middle class) *continued*	Pat on shoulder denotes camaraderie; firm handshake symbolic of goodwill. Good social manners include smiling, speaking pleasantly and warmly to put the other person at ease. Insist on own personal space.	Espouse the Protestant work ethic: work and plan for the future. Competitive and achievement oriented. Value education and knowledge from books as well as from experience.	injury or pathology that can usually be prevented or contained through individual lifestyle and community health efforts.	Intolerant of delays in health care services and of health professionals whose practices they believe are out of date. Read and access other media sources to increase understanding of risk factors, health promotion practices, and treatment techniques. Want to be consulted by health professionals before treatment is initiated but tend to accept health professionals' medical and health care judgments.
Appalachian	Avoid answering questions related to income, children's school attendance, the affairs of others in the household and of neighbors. May consider direct eye contact impolite or aggressive. Uncomfortable with the impersonal and bureaucratic orientation of the American health system. May evaluate health professional on basis of interpersonal skills rather than on professional competence.	Community interdependence. Stay near home for protection. Keep ties with kin. Guard against strangers and outsiders. Kindness to others valued. Do more for others, less for self.	Disability an inevitable part of life and aging. Severity of illness perceived in terms of degree of dependency it necessitates during the period of illness. Believe cold and lack of personal care cause illness. Frugal; always use home remedies first. The hospital is "the place where people die."	Use folk practices "first and last." Rule for primary prevention: "eat right, take fluids, keep the body strong, stay warm when it's cold." Self-care for minor illnesses. Medical care for serious illnesses. Help from kin as needed for primary care. Help from family members and extended family expected and accepted.

Compiled from information in Giger, J. N., & Davidhizar, R. E. (1995). Transcultural nursing: Assessment and intervention (2nd ed.). Baltimore: Mosby; Leininger, M. M. (1994). Transcultural nursing: Concepts, theory, research, and practice (2nd ed.). Columbus, OH: McGraw Hill and Greyden Press; Geissler, E. (1994). A pocket guide to cultural assessment. Baltimore: Mosby; Spector, R. E. (1991). Cultural diversity in health and illness (3rd ed.). Norwalk, CT: Appleton & Lange; and Wong, D. L. (1995). Whaley and Wong's nursing care of infants and children (5th ed.). Baltimore: Mosby.

Table 5-5 Culturally Competent Assessment Guide

1. Ethnic Group Affiliation and Racial Background

   a. How long have you lived here in _____?

   b. Where are you from originally?

   c. What is the primary ethnic group in _____? How closely do you identify with this ethnic group or combination of ethnic groups?

   d. What health problems did you experience or were you exposed to when you lived in each place? What helped you to recover from each of the health problems?

2. Major Beliefs and Values

   a. What are some of the traditions and beliefs that are the most important in your culture? Which ones are related to your health and health practices that you want us to know about? (For example, infant circumcision, hot and cold observance.)

3. Health Beliefs and Practices

   a. What does being healthy mean to you?

   b. What do you do to help you stay healthy? (self-care practices)

   c. What does being ill or sick mean to you?

   d. What do you usually do when you are sick or not feeling well?

   e. Who do you want to be with you when you are sick?

   f. Who in your family is primarily responsible for making health care decisions? Who should be taught how to deal with your specific health problems?

   g. Are there any cultural or ethnic sanctions or restrictions that you want to or must observe (such as exposure of body parts, certain types of medical treatments)?

   h. Whom do you prefer to provide your health and medical care: A nurse, physician, or other health care provider? Do you prefer that they have the same cultural background (or be the same age or gender) as your own?

4. Language Barriers and Communication Styles

   a. In what language are you most comfortable communicating?

   b. Do you need an interpreter when discussing health care information and treatments?

   c. Are there special ways of showing respect or disrespect in your culture?

   d. Are there any cultural preferences or restrictions related to touching, social distance, making eye contact, or other verbal or nonverbal behaviors when communicating?

5. Role of the Family, Spousal Relationship, and Parenting Styles*

   a. With what ethnic group(s) does your family as a whole identify? How does their ethnic identity affect their health status? What ethnic traditions affect their health status?

   b. What is the composition of your family? Who is considered to be a member of your family? (Include an ecogram if needed.)

   c. Which of your relatives live nearby? With what family members and relatives do you interact the most often?

   d. In what ways do your family members believe that the nurse, the physician, or other health care practitioners can help the family members to achieve their goals and dreams for the health and well-being of the family?

*Adapted from Sprott, J. E. (1993). The black box in family assessment: Cultural diversity. In S. L. Feetham, S. B. Meister, J. M. Bell, & C. L. Gilliss (Eds.), The nursing of families: Theory, research, education, practice. Newbury Park, CA: Sage Publications.

CASE STUDY

The case study illustrates the application and objective documentation of the cultural assessment.

A Mexican American Patient Recently Relocated to the Metropolitan Washington, D.C., Area

Maria and Carlos Mendoza have brought their 2½-year-old daughter, Anita, to the pediatric clinic of X-HMO in northern Virginia for follow-up after her hospitalization for a recent episode of severe upper respiratory infection. They are accompanied by Maria's mother, Mrs. Carmen Garcia, who cares for Anita and four of Carlos' nieces and nephews while their parents work. Also present is Ramon Mendoza, Carlos' older brother, who financed the family's move to the area from Laredo, Texas, 9 months ago.

This is the first posthospitalization clinic visit for members of the Mendoza family, who only recently have been covered by an HMO plan under Mr. Mendoza's health insurance at work. Anita was seen briefly 1 week ago, found to be in acute respiratory distress, and immediately admitted to the local hospital. There is a history of repeated URIs since birth for which she has been hospitalized three times in Texas.

The records from the local hospital indicate that health personnel experienced difficulty communicating with the family, who tended to use a blend of Spanish and English and frequently reverted to rapid Spanish when stressed. In addition, when Anita's parents were notified that her lab work was positive for cystic fibrosis (CF) and that CF is an autosomal recessive trait inherited from both parents, Mr. Mendoza refused to believe that any of his genes were defective. He questioned whether Anita was really his child, avoided eye contact with his wife, and refused to discuss the diagnosis further. He left the hospital and did not return until 2 days later when Anita was discharged.

Cultural Assessment

Pt's father answered questions except where noted.

1. Ethnic Group Affiliation and Racial Background

   a. How long have you lived here in *Fairfax, Virginia? 9 mo*

   b. Where are you from originally?
      Laredo, Texas (border town south of San Antonio)

   c. What is the primary ethnic group in *Fairfax*? How closely do you identify with this ethnic group or combination of ethnic groups?
      Ramon (pt's uncle): "We were born in the USA, but we were born Mexican."

   d. What health problems did you experience or were you exposed to when you lived in each place? What helped you to recover from each of these health problems?
      Pt began having repeated URIs shortly after birth. By 6 mo, when prayer did not prevent respiratory problems from getting worse, grandmother encouraged parents to take pt to curandera (folk healer). While being examined by curandera, pt began to experience acute respiratory distress & was rushed to hospital where she was admitted for the 1st X. Family was pleased when pt was treated for pneumonia, a frio (cold) condition, with PCN, a caliente (hot) medicine. With repeated URIs, grandmother urged parents to have pt undergo cure for mal ojo ("evil eye"). A hen's egg was placed in water & put under pt's crib at night, with no improvement. Relatives light a candle at church & offer prayers when pt is ill.

2. Major Beliefs and Values

   a. What are some of the traditions and beliefs that are the most important in your culture? Which ones are related to your health and health practices that you want us to know about?
      "Our family is more important to us than anybody else. We can't make it without our family."
      Mother: "We can't really do anything if it's God's will. I mean, you can be good and try to stay balanced, but if God lets you get sick, there's just nothing you can do but pray."
      Parents want curandera(o) (using hot-cold tx) to treat pt initially; if unsuccessful, then HMO.

3. Health Beliefs and Practices

   a. What does being healthy mean to you?
      Mother: "Health is a reward from God. It is the result of maintaining a balance between forces like hot & cold, wet & dry."

continued

b. What do you do to help you stay healthy?

"Prayer, proper diet & rest, & avoiding getting a chill in wet weather will help achieve the balance between God and people, between hot & cold, wet & dry forces."

c. What does being ill or sick mean to you?

"If your child is ill, it is God's will to teach you a lesson. Your life isn't in balance."

d. What do you usually do when you are sick or not feeling well?

"We seek help from the wisest, eldest women in the family; if unsuccessful, a curandera(o) *is contacted. There are a few* curandera(o) *here."*

e. Who do you want to be with you when you are sick?

Pt wants her mother or grandmother; if pt is left alone when she is sick, her wheezing gets worse.

f. Who in your family is primarily responsible for making health care decisions? Who should be taught how to deal with your specific health problems?

Father makes decisions for his nuclear family after consulting with wife, mother-in-law, & brother (& sometimes his & wife's siblings & other members of his extended family in Texas if he's not certain what to do).

"I must be consulted before any health care decisions are made & must be invited to be involved in any patient teaching or counseling sessions that are conducted. My wife will provide care for Anita."

g. Are there any cultural or ethnic sanctions or restrictions that you want to or must observe?

If anyone compliments pt or any of her family, they must touch them as they give the compliment. Only father will sign papers.

h. By whom do you prefer to have your health and medical care provided: a nurse, physician, or other health care provider? Do you prefer that they have the same cultural background as your own?

Pt prefers women RN & MD who speak Spanish, particularly if doing any tx that causes pain or fear; family member or female RN must be present if a male MD examines pt; object to male RN.

4. Language Barriers and Communication Styles

a. In what language are you most comfortable communicating?

Parents are comfortable speaking English; grandmother prefers Spanish; when grandmother is present, all family members use combination of English & Spanish.

b. Do you need an interpreter when discussing health care information and treatments?

"When Ramon is present, there is no need for an interpreter; he has lived here for 12 yr & works in another hospital as x-ray tech. He can explain any medical information."

Ramon: "It would be best to share new information only if I'm present."

c. Are there special ways of showing respect or disrespect in your culture?

"We would appreciate and respect any health professional who respects how Mexican families function. We discuss everything together and handle everything as a family."

d. Are there any cultural preferences or restrictions related to touching, social distance, making eye contact, or other verbal or nonverbal behaviors when communicating?

"It is important to give explanations to everyone in the family, to take the time to listen & make certain everyone understands; to show an interest in Anita's health, & to touch Anita if you compliment her. We like to engage in "small talk" before "getting down to business." We Mexicans don't come back if you make us stay in the waiting room while only the mother is permitted in the examining room or if you only give us a 5-minute office visit!"

"We don't like to talk about family matters to just anyone outside the family. That's why we like to see the same RN & MD each time we have to bring Anita in. And we don't feel comfortable with Anglo humor."

5. Role of the Family, Spousal Relationship, and Parenting Styles

a. With what ethnic group(s) does your family as a whole identify? How does their ethnic identity affect their health status? What ethnic traditions affect their health status?

See above.

b. What is the composition of your family? Who is considered to be a member of your family? (Refer to Figure 5-7.)

c. Which of your relatives lives nearby? With what family members and relatives do you interact the most often?

continued

All noted preceding live within 2 blocks of one another & interact primarily with one another.

d. In what ways do your family members believe that the nurse, the physician, or other health care practitioners can help the family members to achieve their goals and dreams for the health and well-being of the family?

"Respect our ways . . . remember that I'm responsible for my family."

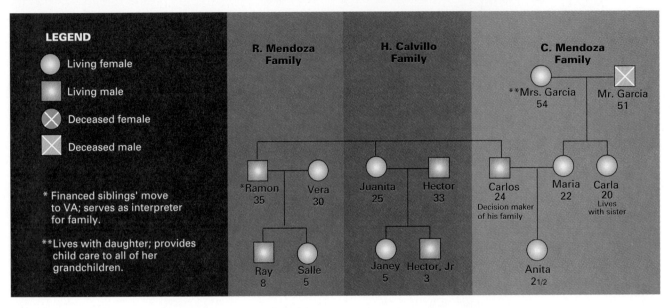

Figure 5-7 Ecogram: Mendoza/Calvillo Collateral Family

REVIEW QUESTIONS AND ACTIVITIES

1. Describe the process for providing culturally competent nursing care.

2. To provide culturally competent nursing care, you must first be able to identify your own cultural values, beliefs, and behaviors. To assist in this process of cultural self-discovery, complete the Culturally Competent Assessment Guide (Table 5-5) as honestly and completely as you can. After doing so, review your responses. What patterns, orientations, and practices do you see emerging that may influence how you interact with individuals from a different culture?

3. You are assessing a patient for increased health risks and genetic traits and disorders prevalent among individuals from the patient's ethnic group. For what health risks and disorders would you assess a Chinese American? An African American? A Jewish American? An American Indian? A Swedish American?

4. Compare your own health-seeking behaviors and health practices identified in number 2 above with those identified in Table 5-3 for the ethnic or cultural group with which you identify. How are they similar? How are they different?

5. For this exercise, you will need a tape recorder and a volunteer (preferably another health care provider student or graduate) who has a cultural or ethnic identity that is different from yours. Record the interaction as you interview the other person using the initial assessment items in the Culturally Competent Assessment Guide (Table 5-5). After completing the interview, listen to the recording together and identify the most significant patterns, orientations, and practices that emerge.

Compare these findings with those identified in Table 5-4 for the ethnic or cultural group with which your volunteer identifies. How are they similar? How are they different? Are there any identified values, beliefs, customs, or norms with which you and the volunteer may be in conflict to any degree? Select one potential conflict area and discuss why you disagree and ways to resolve the conflicting views or practices.

Questions 6–8 refer to the following scenario:

Mrs. Carmen Manjo, a 42-year-old Filipino American, has been admitted to the hospital with the diagnosis of uncontrolled diabetes mellitus. This is Mrs. Manjo's second admission associated with her lack of diabetic control. Although Mrs. Manjo is a second-generation American, her husband (employed as a construction worker) immigrated to the United States as a young adult. Mrs. Manjo has been repeatedly counseled about the lifestyle changes in diet, exercise, and medication she must make to bring her diabetes under control. She has continued to cook using the same recipes and meal plans, however, that she used for the family prior to her diagnosis a year ago. She also is sporadic in testing her blood glucose level and in monitoring and restricting her food intake. When asked what she most consistently does to manage her diabetes, Mrs. Manjo replies, "I leave it up to God."

6. Mrs. Manjo's continuing to cook using the same recipes and meal plans she used prior to her diagnosis a year ago is most likely due to which value orientation held by many Filipinos?
   a. Human beings are basically "good."
   b. Past focus: reverence for long-standing traditions.
   c. Goals of the family take precedence over those of the individual.
   d. Human beings are subjugated to nature and have no control over their environment.

   The correct answer is (c).

7. Ethnic genetic traits and disorders to which Filipinos are most subject are:
   a. Tuberculosis, coronary heart disease, diabetes mellitus
   b. Lactase deficiency, thalassemia, alcohol sensitivity, G-6-PD deficiency
   c. Diabetes mellitus, hypertension, beta thalassemia
   d. Diabetes mellitus, thalassemia, G-6-PD deficiency

   The correct answer is (d).

8. Which of the following communication styles is probably *not* characteristic of Mrs. Manjo?
   a. Considers direct eye contact to be a sign of disrespect
   b. Believes it is ethically wrong to speak for another person
   c. Appreciates "small talk" before initiating actual conversation topic
   d. Hesitant to talk about sex, tuberculosis, or socioeconomic status

   The correct answer is (b).

Spiritual Assessment

1. Identify your personal spiritual beliefs and how they affect your nursing care.
2. Describe how different spiritual beliefs might influence the patient's view of health, growth and development, illness, and death.
3. Conduct a spiritual assessment on a patient.
4. Identify signs and symptoms that indicate the patient is experiencing spiritual distress.
5. Formulate nursing interventions that promote the patient's spiritual well-being.

Spiritual beliefs can determine whether a patient will keep a clinic appointment, follow a diet, take medications, agree to surgery, or execute a living will. Spirituality is an important — and for some patients, perhaps the most essential — ingredient in health care (Guzzetta & Dossey, 1993). It is therefore imperative to **holistic nursing** care, that is, nursing care that addresses all aspects of a patient's health and well-being, to assess and intervene in the physical, mental, and spiritual dimensions of the patient (Andrews, 1989).

SPIRITUALITY AND RELIGION

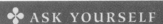

❖ ASK YOURSELF

Know Yourself

Knowing your own spirituality will help you identify and understand your own biases and point of view, which will help you to empathize with patients who make health care decisions based on their spiritual beliefs. Are your own spiritual beliefs more or less important than maintaining your health? If a medical decision forced you to choose between your health and your spiritual and/or religious beliefs, which would you choose? For instance, imagine that your child is bleeding profusely following an accident and requires a blood transfusion. The transfusion is against your religion. How would you decide what to do?

Spirituality is the concern for the meaning and purpose of life. Spirituality integrates values and ultimate concern with oneself, one's relationship with a higher power, and the surrounding environment. Spiritual beliefs help the individual define the self and the self's ultimate purpose in life. For many, health is a concern, but it may not be the primary concern. Factors such as leaving behind a good reputation, passing on morals to the next generation, being in a good relationship with God, and being in harmony with the forces in the universe may be of ultimate concern for the patient and could therefore drive the patient's health care choices.

An example of spirituality is the belief that both animals and human beings can feel pain and joy, and therefore animals must be treated with the same respect shown to humans. A person who has this belief would probably believe the self to be important but only as important as all other beings on the earth. The implication for health care is that this person would likely be a vegetarian and may refuse any treatment (such as a porcine cardiac valve) that resulted from the sacrifice or suffering of an animal.

By contrast, **religion** is an organized system of beliefs usually centered around the worship of a supernatural force or being, which in turn defines the self and the self's purpose in life. Religion exists in group form over time, and is a tradition of shared beliefs. Although many variances may exist among believers within any given religion, there will be common threads uniting the followers. A religious system of beliefs can be highly organized and include **rituals**, which often are solemn, and ceremonial acts that reinforce faith. **Faith** is the assent to the truth of the beliefs and may also refer to the total orientation of the self's entire life to the belief structure. **Dogma** refers to the beliefs of the religion that are so essential to the identity of the religion that to deny them is to deny the religion itself. Religions also include **codes of ethics**, which are codified beliefs and lists of mandatory or prohibited acts that help define the self's relation to the object of worship.

An example of a religion is Judaism. Followers of the Jewish faith worship Yahweh (God) and define humans as the special creations of God who must in turn worship God. Judaism is highly organized. Who God is, why He should be worshipped, and how humans ought to act by virtue of being created by Him is delineated in a system of biblical commentary and teachings by the leaders of the religion. Judaism has different kinds of religious leaders (rabbis, cantors, mohels), codes of ethics (the biblical Ten Commandments is the most well-known example), and rituals (circumcision, bar mitzvah). There are many forms of Judaism, but broadly speaking, implications for health care for a religious Jew could include a special diet (pork-free or kosher) and consultation with a rabbi before any complex bioethical decisions are made.

The relationship between spirituality and religion is illustrated in Figure 6-1. One can be spiritual without being religious. In the example of spirituality given previously, the patient espouses a spiritual belief about the interconnectedness of humans and animals that includes the patient in a harmonious

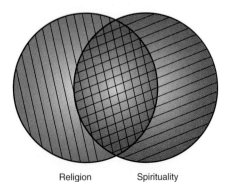

Religion   Spirituality

Figure 6-1   The Relationship Between Religion and Spirituality

belief system with all living beings on the planet. However, there are not necessarily rituals, involvement of a supernatural force that is being worshipped, or an organized system of beliefs that make this spirituality a religion. Nevertheless, this spirituality can have a profound impact on the person's outlook on life and sense of spiritual well-being.

Likewise, one can be religious without being spiritual. For example, a particular Jew may fulfill religious obligations to attend temple and participate in required rituals without believing in or worshipping Yahweh, which is the central tenet of the religion. The religion may have no impact on the Jew's behavior or outlook on life and may not help define what is important to that person.

Finally, one can be both spiritual and religious by participating in a religion and by holding its spiritual core at the center of one's being, actions, and beliefs. For example, a Jew who believes in God and worships God in the manner specified by Judaism, and whose belief in God is manifested in thought, actions, purpose, and identity exhibits the properties of both religion and spirituality.

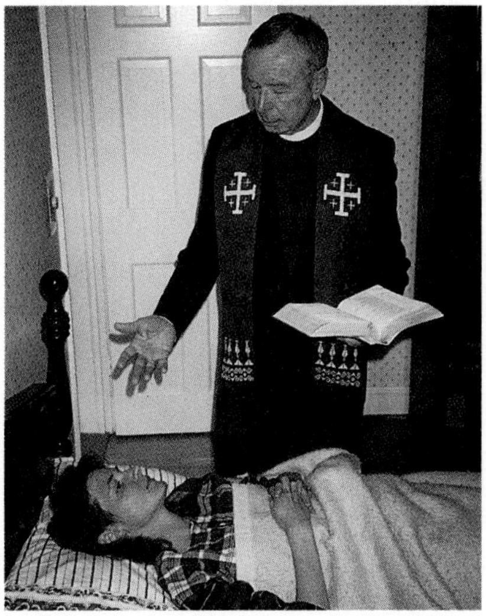

SPIRITUAL THEORY

Almost all religions attempt to explain why human beings suffer from illness and death and how higher powers can affect healing. It is important to realize that religion rarely, if ever, describes disease as resulting from a strictly biological cause with a scientific solution (Sullivan, 1988). Instead, some religious explanations of disease indicate that it was sent directly by the creator or a lesser god, caused by sin or by the poor performance of a ritual act, or resulted from the malevolence of relatives, neighbors, or ancestors. Based on these explanations, the cure for disease is to be found in confessing sin, purification rites, exorcism, or the transmission of power to the patient such as by the laying on of hands (refer to Figure 6-2), plastering, or other rituals. These acts of healing are not performed by physicians and nurses, but by priests, elders, mediums, and other specialists who have access to the higher powers that control disease. It may be more important to the patient to see a neighbor who has had experience with a disease and was successfully able to repel it with certain prayers, for example, than to take a prescribed medication.

Being familiar with various religious and spiritual terms may help you to communicate more effectively with your patients (see Figure 6-3). The concept of **god** may vary from a dispassionate, distant deity to a dynamic, personal, present being. "God" may be called by many names, such as Allah, Yahweh, Jehovah, or Shiva, and one religion, Judaism, considers the name of God to be so sacred that believers are not supposed to pronounce the name at all. **Prayer** is the means by which one communicates with the higher power(s). Prayer may range from silence to the repetition of sounds, words, or prayers or may include chanting, singing, or dancing. Some religions dictate how prayers are to be conducted; for instance, Muslims are required to pray facing in the direction of Mecca, Saudi Arabia. **Monotheistic religions** such as Judaism, Christianity, and Islam believe in only one all-powerful, omnipresent, and omnipotent God (capital *G*) who created the universe. **Polytheistic religions** such as Hinduism recognize many gods (spelled with a lower-case *g*) that may have different levels of power and status. These gods may even compete with each other, but are all ultimately manifestations of the one true higher power behind existence.

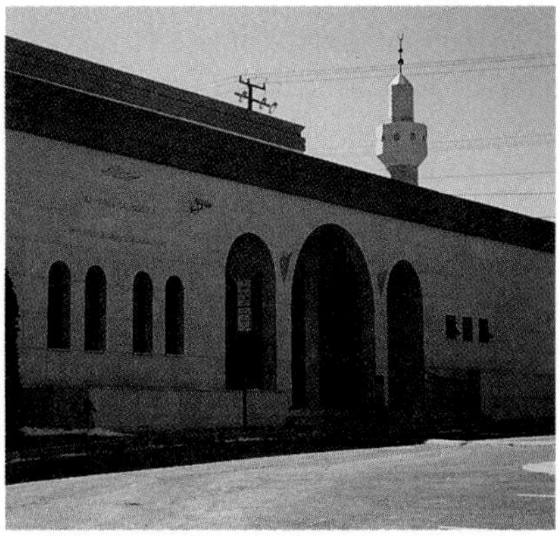

A **sin** exists when someone has gone against the teachings of the belief system. A **heretic** is someone who rejects the official teachings or dogma of a religion or belief system. A **schismatic** is a person who shares the essential beliefs or dogma of a religion but who is separated by political or other disagreements from the group of believers.

A patient may claim to be an **atheist** (*a-theist*, that is, without God), or one who does not believe in God. An **agnostic** (*a-gnosis*, that is, without

Figure 6-2 Rituals such as the laying on of hands may be an integral part of certain expressions of spirituality.

Figure 6-3 Spirituality and religion may be important aspects of your patients' lives.

knowledge) is one who is unsure if God exists. Atheists or agnostics may be very spiritual if they hold certain beliefs to be of utmost importance to their lives, such as attaining great knowledge, living in harmony with humanity, or showing kindnesses to others. A **pagan** is someone who is without religion; the term may also be used to describe someone who does not believe in the one God of the monotheistic religions.

A person may belong to a **cult**, which is the religious devotion to a set of beliefs or to a person. Cults are thought to be fanatical and are societally disapproved, but the difference between a religion and a cult may be in the eyes of the person who makes the definition. A patient may be insulted if his or her religion is referred to as a cult, so you must show sensitivity to all expressions of spirituality.

The concept of the **soul** varies from the essential, spiritual part of a person to the part of the person that continues to exist after physical death. This is a concept central to many religions. **Spirit** can encompass the same concept as soul, or may refer to a disembodied being or supernatural force, or may indicate the Christian trinitarian concept of God, as in the Holy Spirit. **Animism** is the belief that all things in nature have souls. Many American Indian religions contain this concept. Many religions and spiritual belief systems contain the belief in life after death, wherein the soul and/or body of a person continues to live on in some form after physical death. This idea is central to Christianity. **Reincarnation** is the belief that the person after death lives another life on earth in another body. In Hinduism, one seeks, through good deeds, to obtain release from endless reincarnations. Many religions describe a peaceful or joyful place or state one goes to or becomes if the ethics of the religion are followed. Christians, for example, believe in **heaven**, whereas Buddhists believe in **nirvana**, which is the state of perfect blessedness and peace of the soul.

HOLISTIC HEALTH AND SPIRITUALITY

A goal of nursing is to support the patient's spiritual well-being. Spiritual well-being can be defined as the state in which a patient is satisfied with the way in which particular circumstances fit into the belief system. There is evidence that **spiritual well-being** is a positive factor in coping with chronic illness (Soeken, 1987). Holistic nursing is the simultaneous recognition and integration of body-mind-spirit unity in nursing practice (Guzzetta & Dossey, 1993). Patients in a state of spiritual well-being will react in ways consistent with their belief systems to the normal rhythms of life from birth to death. It is important, therefore, to know what the patient's spiritual and religious beliefs are and how different belief systems define acceptable behavior through the life cycle (Andrews, 1989). Table 6-1 illustrates how certain religions view sentinel events, from birth to death.

Spiritual distress is the state in which a patient feels that the belief system, or his or her place within it, is threatened. Commonly, the circumstances in which nurses find themselves providing care — birth, accidents, illness, and the dying process — are the same events that provoke spiritual distress. As Holst (1985) writes, "Hospitals do not create paradoxes and mysteries, they merely focus them. Suffering dispels the illusion that we are infinite without limits. In that regard, suffering can be a great moment of [spiritual] truth for the sufferer" (p. 11).

Any threat to one's own life, any reminder of one's own mortality, can serve to evoke both wonderment about the meaning and purpose of life and disquiet about the answers that spirituality and/or religion provide. Spiritual distress may manifest as anxiety, withdrawal, distractedness, hopelessness, or crying behaviors. Nursing interventions are directed toward resolving spiritual distress, and therefore you need to be astute about assessing the spiritual status of the patient.

❖ ASK YOURSELF

Self-Evaluation of Spirituality

Are you spiritual? Are you religious? Are you both? Are you neither? What is most important in your life? What are your beliefs? Have your beliefs changed from when you were younger? How do you feel about people whose beliefs differ markedly from yours?

☺ THINK ABOUT IT

Meeting Patients' Spiritual Needs

What would you do if a patient requested that you participate in a religious practice that conflicted with your own spiritual, religious, or institutional practices? For example, suppose a Hindu family asked you to help move a dying Hindu patient out of his hospital bed and onto the floor, in accordance with their religious beliefs. Or suppose a Muslim family asked a non-Muslim nurse to whisper "There is no God but Allah, and Mohammed is His Prophet" into the ear of a dying Muslim patient, in accordance with their religious beliefs. What would you do? What would you say? How would you reconcile the institution's policies with the patient's spiritual requests? How would you handle these situations?

Table 6-1 Religions and Health Care

RELIGION	JUDAISM	ISLAM	ROMAN CATHOLIC/ORTHODOX	PROTESTANT
Description	Judaism is an ancient religion dating to about 2000 BCE. It is a monotheistic religion that believes that God (Yahweh) has chosen the Jewish people and made a covenant with them. The covenant is that the Jews will worship God and follow His laws, and in return God will protect and preserve them. Over its long history, Judaism has developed several traditions, among them Orthodox, which believes in a strict interpretation of the Scriptures; Conservative, which allows for some modern interpretation of the Scriptures; and Reform, which is a blending of tradition with modern-day moral demands. Jews are largely concentrated in the Middle East, Europe, and the United States, but can be found worldwide, including Asia, Africa, and South America.	Islam is a monotheistic religion sharing early Judeo-Christian religious roots. It was established when the Prophet Mohammed (d. 632 CE) preached the word of God as revealed to him by an angel. The essence of Mohammed's prophecies is that God (Allah) is the one, true God and is absolutely sovereign. The central tenet of the faith is "There is no God but Allah and Mohammed is His Prophet." Several versions of Islam have developed, among them Sunni, Sufi, and Shiite. Islam has spread beyond its origins in the Middle East to Europe, Asia, Africa, and the Americas.	A monotheistic religion and an off-shoot of Judaism, Christianity dates from the birth of Jesus in 30 BCE. Christians believe that Jesus is the son of God, that Jesus died on the cross to serve as a sacrifice for the sins of humanity, that Jesus was resurrected from the dead, and that God exists in three forms: God (Father), Jesus (Son), and the Holy Spirit. Roman Catholicism is the oldest and largest of the Christian denominations with members worldwide. Orthodoxy was an early offshoot emphasizing mysticism. Centered in Eastern Europe, the Middle East, and Slavic countries. Roman Catholicism and Orthodoxy emphasize the Eucharist (bread and wine representing the body and blood of Jesus) and use a version of the Bible that includes several Old Testament chapters not found in the Hebrew or Protestant Bibles.	Protestants hold the same basic beliefs of Roman Catholics and Orthodox Christians. The Reformation led to the divorce from Roman Catholicism on other doctrinal and theological issues. In brief, the Protestants de-emphasized the Eucharist and the pivotal position of the priest and placed more emphasis on the centrality of the Bible and the individual's relationship with God. Mainline Protestants (Anglicans, Methodists, Presbyterians, Lutherans) retain some sacramentalism and liturgy but emphasize the individual's relationship with God. Fundamental Protestants (Baptist) emphasize the centrality of the Bible and further de-emphasize the Eucharist. Evangelical Protestants (Pentecostal) emphasize the continued presence of the Holy Spirit.
Religious Leaders	Rabbi: a religious authority of the faith. A rabbi renders decisions interpreting the laws that Jews are required to abide by to preserve their covenant with God. Cantor: a trained person who leads prayer services, performs marriages and funerals, and provides the musical part of prayer services. Mohel: A person trained in the ritual and spiritual aspects of the tradition of circumcision.	Imam: a trained Muslim preacher and teacher.	Priests: administer the sacraments, lead the worship, and provide church leadership. Must be male. Bishops: provide church leadership. Monks and Nuns: members of religious orders.	Priests (Anglican): perform the same functions as Roman Catholic priests but may be female. Ministers (Methodist): lead the worship, preach the Bible, provide church leadership; may be male or female. Pastors (Lutheran, Baptist, Pentecostal): Same functions.
Holy Books and Artifacts	Bible: a collection of divinely inspired writings concerning God's interaction with and revelations to the Jewish people. Torah: the first five books of the Bible contained in a scroll.	Koran (Qur'an): the collection of the prophecies of Mohammed. The Koran is central to the faith of Muslims. Shari'a: the body of Islamic law. Hadith: the tradition of Islamic law.	The Bible, which includes several Old Testament chapters not seen in the Hebrew or Protestant Bible. The Bible is central to the Christian faith. Priests dress distinctively in black with a white stiff collar. Nuns may or	The Bible, without the Apocrypha (the old testament chapters used in the Roman Catholic Bible). Protestants may wear crosses, which emphasize the resurrection of Jesus.

continued

Table 6-1   Religions and Health Care   *continued*

RELIGION	JUDAISM	ISLAM	ROMAN CATHOLIC/ORTHODOX	PROTESTANT
Holy Books and Artifacts *continued*	Talmud: the tradition of interpretation of holy law. Observant men may wear yarmulkes, small, round caps for the top of the head. Men may also wear a prayer shawl.	Islamic women may cover their heads and faces with veils.	may not wear habits, distinctive dress with headgear. Monks may or may not wear distinctive robes. Church members may wear crucifixes, depicting Jesus being crucified on the cross, and may carry rosary beads, a string of beads that aids prayer. Roman Catholics and Orthodox may also use religious medals to remind them of the presence and blessings of God and the saints of God.	Priests and ministers may dress distinctively with white collars. Baptist and Pentecostal pastors wear street clothes.
Holy Day of the Week	Friday from sundown until Saturday at sundown.	Friday.	Sunday.	Sunday.
Holy Holidays, Festivals, Observances	Rosh Hashana: Jewish new year; it usually occurs in the fall. Yom Kippur: occurs 10 days after Rosh Hashana; a solemn day of atonement and fasting. Sukkot: the feast of tabernacles, a harvest festival; it occurs 5 days after Yom Kippur. Hanukkah: this lesser feast is a 7-day feast of lights. Passover: usually falls in early spring and recalls the exodus of the Jews from enslavement in Egypt. Shavuot: festival occurring 50 days after Passover and commemorating the giving of the Torah to Moses on Mt. Sinai.	Muslims are expected to pray five times a day from before sunup to after sundown. Prayer should be done in a clean place, and the believer should be clean. A person is considered to be unclean if he or she has recently eliminated body wastes, passed flatus, or is asleep. Proper cleansing for prayer includes washing the hands, face, nostrils, ears, arms to the elbows, and feet to the ankles, and moistening the head. After menstruation, childbirth, or sexual intercourse, a complete bath including washing the hair is required before prayer. Muharam 1 Rasal-Sana: the New Year. Ramadan: the ninth month in the Muslim lunar calendar is a time of fasting, meditation, and spiritual purification. Shawwal 1 "Id ad-Fitr": a 3-day celebration following Ramadan. Dhu-al-Hijjah 1–10: this last month of the Muslim calendar is when the journey to Mecca is made. The journey to Mecca is one of the religious pillars of Islam and Muslims are obligated to go once in their lifetimes if they are able.	There are several days of "obligation" for the Roman Catholic, on which attendance is required in church. Important church observances are Christmas (the birth of Jesus), Good Friday (the crucifixion of Jesus), Easter (the resurrection of Jesus), Pentecost (the sending of the Holy Spirit), and the Assumption (when Mary, the mother of Jesus, went to heaven).	All Protestant churches observe Christmas and Easter, but some denominations eliminate or de-emphasize other observations.

continued

RELIGION	JUDAISM	ISLAM	ROMAN CATHOLIC/ORTHODOX	PROTESTANT
Dietary Restrictions	Dietary rules are complex and are not kept by all Jews. Kosher food denotes food prepared according to strict dietary laws, which prohibit pork and any other meat of an animal with a cloven hoof that chews a cud, as well as shellfish. Any meat to be eaten must be ritually slaughtered according to strict laws. Meat and dairy products must not be taken together.	Pork and products made from pork, such as gelatin and lard, are forbidden. Alcohol and street drugs are also forbidden. Strictly speaking, all meat should be ritually slaughtered according to religious laws, but in practice, even religious Muslims are relaxed about this requirement.	There is a tradition of not eating meat on Fridays during Lent in the Roman Catholic church.	None. Some Protestant denominations (Baptist, Pentecostal) forbid the use of alcohol and smoking.
Periods of Fasting	Fasting is associated with Yom Kippur and also with some minor holidays. Fasting may be set aside on the advice of a physician.	There is fasting from dawn to sundown during the 28-day month of Ramadan. Pregnant women, menstruating women, and the sick are not required to fast, but they must make up the fast at a later time.	Fasting is practiced on Ash Wednesday and Good Friday during Lent.	Fasting is de-emphasized in the Protestant tradition.
Medical Treatment	Jews are encouraged to seek medical care and treatment when needed as part of the religious obligation to take care of oneself. Jews hold medicine and physicians in high esteem. Prayers and visitation are proper for the sick.	Healing the sick is considered the highest service to God after religious requirements. Seeking medical treatment for illness is encouraged, and there is no prohibition for doing so. Privacy should be maintained for women and girls during illness and hospitalization. Female bodies should remain covered; gowns should have long sleeves if possible.	Medical treatment is encouraged, even obligated, as part of the obligation to care for oneself. Anointing of the sick with oil and prayers is appropriate at the time of illness. Anointing may be done many times, not just at the time of death. Prayers and visitation are appropriate for the sick.	Same as Roman Catholicism/Orthodoxy, although some Fundamental and Pentecostal offshoots may emphasize prayer and spiritual healing over medical treatment. Mainline Protestants may practice the anointing of the sick. Prayers and visitation are appropriate for the sick.
Birth Control	Sexual relations are permitted only within marriage. Birth control is allowed within marriage.	Sexual relations are permitted only within marriage. Teachings on birth control are contradictory, but in general, the use of birth control within marriage to control family size or to protect the health of the wife is permitted.	Sexual relations are permitted only within marriage. Procreation is one of the celebrated purposes of marriage. Birth control is forbidden by the Roman Catholic Church. Natural family planning, in which intercourse is timed with the menstrual cycle to prevent conception to limit family size or protect the health of the mother, is permitted.	Sexual relations are permitted only within marriage. Birth control is permitted.
Infertility Treatment	A primary purpose of marriage is the procreation of children, and infertility treatments are permitted. Whether to allow the use of gametes from outside the marriage (that is, donor egg or donor sperm) is under discussion.	Procreation is one of the celebrated purposes of marriage, so medical treatment used to treat infertility is acceptable as long as gametes from within the marriage are used and as long as the couple is still married and both husband and wife are alive. Using gametes from outside the marriage (donor egg, donor sperm) would be considered adultery.	Infertility treatment is permitted as long as gametes from within the marriage are used. Since masturbation is prohibited, collection of sperm is difficult for treatment.	Infertility treatment is permitted. The use of donor egg or donor sperm is not condemned by most Protestant churches.

continued

Table 6-1 Religions and Health Care *continued*

RELIGION	JUDAISM	ISLAM	ROMAN CATHOLIC/ORTHODOX	PROTESTANT
Abortion	Judaism has a high respect for life, including prenatal life. However, the fetus is not considered to be fully human until birth. Jewish law does reluctantly permit abortion under some circumstances, such as to preserve the life or welfare of the mother.	Abortion is forbidden after the fetus is "ensouled." There is some controversy as to whether the ensoulment occurs at 40 or 120 days of pregnancy. The father must give permission for the abortion. Abortion after the time of ensoulment is considered murder.	The fetus is considered human from the time of conception. Abortion is therefore prohibited, except when it is done as the effect of another procedure, the purpose of which is not to cause the death of the fetus (for example, a hysterectomy of a pregnant, cancerous uterus is permitted, but the direct abortion of the same fetus is not).	Most Protestant denominations consider fetal life human, but reluctantly allow for abortion to preserve the health of the mother. Baptists and Pentecostals forbid abortion.
Observances at Birth	Circumcision is performed on all males, traditionally at the age of 8 days. Girls may undergo a naming ceremony.	At the time of birth, the baby's father, or nearest male relative, or the mother whispers the central tenet of the Islamic faith into the baby's ear: "There is no God but Allah, and Mohammed is His Prophet." These are the first words the baby should hear. Some Muslim women may refuse to be attended to by male nurses or physicians. A birth is considered legitimate only if it occurs 6 months after marriage.	Prayers and blessings are customary at the time of birth. If the child is ill at birth, baptism should be performed (baptism is a sacrament that brings the recipient into the church).	Prayers and blessings are customary at the time of birth. If the child is ill at birth, baptism may be performed by most Protestants except Baptists and Pentecostals.
Rites of Initiation	Boys undergo a bar mitzvah at age 13, a celebration of religious adulthood. In the Reform and Conservative traditions, girls may undergo a parallel ceremony called a bat mitzvah.	Males are routinely circumcised at or near birth. Females may also undergo circumcision as young girls. In practice, this female circumcision may be a symbolic nick on the genitals to the actual removal of the clitoris.	Baptism is traditionally performed for children as infants. Children are confirmed at about age 12, when they complete instruction about the church.	Baptism is performed on infants by all Protestant denominations except Baptists and Pentecostals, who perform baptism on children (or adults) when they reach an age to consent to belong to the church.
Withdrawal of Life Support	Active euthanasia and assisted suicide are forbidden because of the position of the sanctity of human life and the prohibition of murder. Hastening death is equivalent to murder. The withdrawal of life support is allowed under the right circumstances, as it is simply the removal of impediments to a natural death.	Active euthanasia and assisted suicide are forbidden because of the sanctity of human life and the prohibition of murder. It is permitted to withdraw life support if the treatment is serving only to prolong the patient's death, or if the patient's condition is medically hopeless.	Suicide and active euthanasia are forbidden because of the principle of the sanctity of life. The withdrawal of life support has been the subject of much controversy in the church, but is permitted if the condition of the patient is hopeless and as long as the purpose of the withdrawal of support is to reduce pain and suffering, and not to kill the patient.	Suicide is forbidden. Some mainline Protestant denominations have expressed some sympathy for assisted suicide and active euthanasia, but in general, suicide and active euthanasia are forbidden, because of the sanctity of life and the prohibition of murder. The withdrawal of life support is appropriate when the patient's condition is hopeless and the treatment is serving only to prolong the patient's death.

continued

RELIGION	JUDAISM	ISLAM	ROMAN CATHOLIC/ORTHODOX	PROTESTANT
Death	Suicide is forbidden. Orthodox Jews may position and wash a dead body. Autopsies are controversial but are permitted if they will serve to provide information that will save other lives in the future. Burial should be done within 24 hr of death, although this may be extended to 48 hr in special circumstances. Cremation is forbidden. There is a 7-day period of mourning called *Shiva* that begins the day of the funeral. Some Jews customarily may not shave during this time and may cover mirrors.	Suicide is forbidden. Relatives and friends are normally present when a person dies. There may be an expectation for the patient to say, or for a person to whisper into the ear of the patient, the central tenet of the Islamic faith, "There is no God but Allah, and Mohammed is His Prophet," so that these are the last words the person hears before death. After death the body is washed. Men wash a man's body, and women wash a woman's body. Autopsies are permitted if they serve to help solve a crime or will provide further medical knowledge. Burial should be commenced without delay. There are detailed teachings regarding funerals and burials. Attending funerals is a meritorious act. Funerals may be held in absentia for an important person.	Prayers are appropriate at the time of death. Burial or cremation is permitted. Autopsies are permitted, especially if they will aid medical knowledge.	Same as Roman Catholicism/Orthodoxy.
Organ Donation	Organ donations and receiving transplanted organs are permitted, since the procedure saves life. One exception is Orthodox Jews, who reject the "brain death" definition of death and agree with the cardiac definition of death only.	Organ donations and receiving transplanted organs are permitted, as are blood transfusions.	Organ donation is permitted.	Organ donation is permitted, though some Baptists or Pentecostals may be against organ donation, believing that they should go to heaven with all their body parts.

RELIGION	CHRISTIAN SCIENCE	JEHOVAH'S WITNESSES	BUDDHISM	HINDUISM
Description	Christian Science is a religious movement founded in the 1860s by American Mary Baker Eddy (1821–1910). Mrs. Eddy experienced a healing after Bible study, and subsequently devoted her life to Bible study and the ministry of healing. Christian Scientists believe that Eddy identified the scientific method and divine laws Jesus used in his healings. The church teaches that Jesus is central to individual salvation, but was not God.	Founded in the 1870s, the beliefs of Jehovah's Witnesses are centered around a unique interpretation of the Bible. They differ from traditional Christianity in their belief that Jesus is God's son but inferior in status to God, and their beliefs concerning the end-time (how and when it will occur and its character) differ as well. Their name for God is Jehovah.	Buddhism is a varied, intellectual and psychological religion that originated with the life of Siddhartha Gautama, the Buddha ("enlightened one") in India in the 4th century BCE. Buddhism centers around the imaged ideal of the Buddha, the transformation of consciousness, and the transformation of karma, or practical destiny. Buddhism holds that ordinary life is unsatisfactory because it is based on ignorance and desire, resulting in the inability to realize that there is no real "self" (Ellwood, 1982). Today, Buddhism has many forms, among them Zen, Bodhisattva, and	Hinduism is an ancient religion that originated in India around 1500 BCE. It is a complex religion that embraces a variety of gods, practices, and spiritual paths. Hinduism is a polytheistic religion that teaches that ultimately there is only one god, or essence of existence — Brahman. Brahman appears in different forms, most notably in the forms of Krishna, Shiva, and Vishnu. Hinduism teaches that although the universe goes through endless cycles, the divine does not change. Humans are expected to follow the cosmic order (dharma) in life and

continued

Table 6-1 Religions and Health Care *continued*

RELIGION	CHRISTIAN SCIENCE	JEHOVAH'S WITNESSES	BUDDHISM	HINDUISM
Description *continued*			Tantric, Theravada and Mahayana are two different approaches to reality within Buddhism. Buddhism has spread into and become enmeshed with cultures throughout the world. Because Buddhism has proved to be so highly adaptable to local culture and religions, it is difficult to isolate one strict Buddhist dharma, or way.	hope to achieve spiritual liberation (moksha). This occurs through selfless acts and good thoughts (karma). The cultural caste system of India was early on incorporated into Hinduism. The castes range from brahmins (priest caste) to untouchables (lowest class). Complex social and religious rules govern these castes (Ellwood, 1995).
Religious Leaders	None. The church is entirely run by lay people. Christian Science practitioner: a person devoted full-time to the ministry of Christian healing. Every practicing Christian Scientist has a practitioner to call in case healing is needed. Christian Science nurse: These nurses are not registered nurses, but undergo 2 to 5 years of training in bedside nursing skills and spirituality. They assist patients with bedside care and prayer while healing is ongoing.	All baptized persons are considered ordained ministers. Jehovah's Witnesses believe that a clergy class and special titles are improper. Elders (all male) lead each congregation and lead worship, provide pastoral care, visit the sick, teach, and preach sermons. Ministerial students are young men who assist elders in the functioning of the Kingdom Hall.	Monks and Nuns: usually celibate, monks and nuns function as teachers and bearers of Buddhist tradition. Buddhist tradition also holds that all followers are leaders.	Priests: offer sacrifices to the gods and idols; control worship. Guru: a teacher of spiritual ways. Sadhu: a "peaceful man," a sort of Hindu holy man, like a monk, but not in a formal order. May wander from village to village. Yogi: a spiritual teacher.
Holy Books and Artifacts	The Bible. *Science and Health with Key to the Scriptures* by M. B. Eddy. This book is central to the Christian Science theology and is used to interpret the Bible.	The *New World Translation* of the Bible, which Jehovah's Witnesses believe to be the most accurate translation of the ancient languages of the Bible. Kingdom Hall is where Jehovah's Witnesses meet and worship.	*The Tibetan Book of the Dead*: intended to be read into the ear of one who is dying or has just died. *The Buddha Dharma*: 100 volumes of the collected words of the Buddha with the commentary of scholars. Statues of the Buddha are common.	*The Vedas*: four ancient (1500 BCE) holy books containing hymns and stories. The hymns are sung to the gods during the presentation of sacrifices. *Upanishads*: a book dating from 500 BCE and including philosophical stories. *Bhagavad Gita*: often called the bible of Hinduism. It details the story of Krishna and explores the themes of destiny and salvation. Cows are sacred in Hinduism, symbolizing mother earth, bounty, and Krishna. Feeding a cow is an act of worship. The Ganges River: in India, it is a symbol of life without end, and most Hindus want to bathe in and/or drink its spiritual waters.

continued

RELIGION	CHRISTIAN SCIENCE	JEHOVAH'S WITNESSES	BUDDHISM	HINDUISM
Holy Books and Artifacts *continued*				Other worship artifacts: statues or dolls depicting various gods are common, as well as sandalwood, flat stones, incense, water, candle or oil lamp, flowers, and food for offerings.
Holy Day of the Week	None. Church is attended on Sunday, but this is not a holy day. Short services that include testimonials about healings occur on Wednesdays.	No one day is any holier than any other. Most services are held in the evenings during the week or on Sunday.	Buddhist tradition teaches that every day is a holy day. Various cultures and traditions within Buddhism may hold different days as special days (such as the first and 15th days of the month).	There is no particular holy day to Hindus. Devotees of particular gods may observe chosen holy days.
Holy Holidays, Festivals, Observances	There is a special Thanksgiving service recognized by all Christian Scientists on the American Thanksgiving Day. Otherwise, Christian Scientists do not observe Christmas, Easter, or other Christian holidays.	Memorial of Jesus' death: celebrated annually at the time of the Last Supper of Jesus. Falls in the spring at the time of Passover. Jehovah's Witnesses do not celebrate Christmas or Easter, because there is no command by Jesus to do so.	Wesak: The birth of the Buddha is celebrated for 1 to 15 days. This festival usually falls in April or May. There can be many other holidays, depending on the form of Buddhism.	Divali: New Year, Festival of Lights. Holi: spring festival dedicated to Krishna. Dasara: 10 days of celebration in honor of Kali. Tarpan: a time of oblation to forefathers. Makar Sankranji/Pongal: a celebration of spring; homage paid to the sun. Shivaratri: a 24-hour celebration and fasting in honor of Lord Siva. Ram Navami: a celebration of Lord Rama's birth. The story of Rama is chanted for 24 hr. Janmashtami: Lord Krishna's birthday. Ganesh Chaturthi: day to honor Lord Ganesh. Navaratri: 9-day festival in praise of Lord Rama.
Dietary Restrictions	None. Most Christian Scientists avoid alcohol, smoking, and caffeine, because these can affect overall well-being.	No food containing blood (such as blood sausages) is allowed, because Jehovah's Witnesses believe it is forbidden to take in blood. Meat should have all blood drained out of it before cooking; meat approved by the American Dietetic Association meets this criterion.	Some Buddhists, but not all, are vegetarians. Different schools of thought in Buddhism have different views on diet. Strict Buddhists may refuse strong spices.	Since the cow is sacred, no beef is eaten, although milk and milk products, particularly yogurt, are staples of a Hindu's diet. Some Hindus are vegetarians, others are not. Nonvegetarians do not eat pork. Roasted meat may be eaten after a sacrificial ceremony. If one has dedicated a specific fruit to God, one is forbidden to eat that fruit for the rest of one's life.

continued

Table 6-1   Religions and Health Care *continued*

RELIGION	CHRISTIAN SCIENCE	JEHOVAH'S WITNESSES	BUDDHISM	HINDUISM
Periods of Fasting	None.	None.	Some Buddhists may fast as a path to spiritual enlightenment, presenting an opportunity to think and reflect. Other Buddhists may not support fasting.	Fasting is associated with spiritual purposes such as spiritual training and special worship services, some holy festivals, and mourning. At such times, Hindus who eat meat may be vegetarians or may fast altogether.
Medical Treatment	There is no prohibition in the Christian Science Church against seeking medical care. However, Christian Scientists believe that illness is caused by a spiritual disruption in the relationship with God. Healing in its most holistic sense is obtained through spiritual guidance. Practicing Christian Scientists avoid hospitals and medical care. There are a few accepted exceptions to this: x-rays and other treatments for broken bones; dental care by a dentist; MD or midwife care during childbirth; and vaccinations and other treatment required by law. In the case of illness, the Christian Scientist would (1) pray and study the Bible and texts, (2) call his or her Christian Science practitioner, (3) seek care from a Christian Science nurse if assistance with activities of daily living is needed, and (4) repeat steps 1 and 2 until the expected healing occurs.	Jehovah's Witnesses do seek medical care for all infirmities. The only limitation on their use of health care services is an important religious belief that the Bible forbids the ingestion of blood. This belief prohibits the use of whole blood, packed RBCs, plasma, WBCs, and platelets. Other preparations in which the amount of blood is very minute, such as albumin, immune globulins, and hemophiliac preparations, are up to the conscience of the individual. Jehovah's Witnesses understand the implications (including possible death) of refusing blood. However, full medical treatment is acceptable as long as no blood is used. They appreciate and seek nonblood treatments for bleeding, such as Hespan, vasopressors, MAST trousers, intraoperative blood salvage, etc. Jehovah's Witnesses are encouraged to carry cards indicating refusal of blood as well as general advance directives.	Medical treatments that may enhance life and the search for enlightenment are approved of. Buddhism has a high regard for the healing nature of the doctor-patient relationship. Doctors and nurses are respected.	Taking care of the body is seen as a good thing. There is no conflict between religion and seeking medical care, as long as a person is not harmed without purpose. The study of medicine has a long and honored tradition in Hindu culture. Traditional Hindu medicine offers homeopathic, herbal, non-Western care for diseases.
Birth Control	Sex is permitted only within marriage. Birth control is acceptable. Christian Scientists prefer barrier methods over medications such as the pill.	Sex is permitted only within marriage. Birth control is a matter of personal choice. Birth control that prevents implantation (such as some forms of the pill) are prohibited.	Birth control is discouraged because it is unnatural.	The traditional Hindu point of view is against birth control because children are seen as a gift, and many children are even a greater blessing.
Infertility Treatment	Infertility, like other physical problems, is believed to have a spiritual cause, therefore healing should be sought through prayer, not through medical treatment.	Infertility treatment is up to the individual conscience. No donor gametes from outside of the marriage are permitted.	Infertility may be seen as Buddha's plan. Infertility treatments may be seen as unnatural. This is controversial.	Infertility treatment is permitted, as long as gametes from outside the marriage (donor egg, sperm) are not used. Donor gametes are seen as being against the marriage.

continued

RELIGION	CHRISTIAN SCIENCE	JEHOVAH'S WITNESSES	BUDDHISM	HINDUISM
Abortion	There is no official church teaching on abortion. Abortion is very uncommon among Christian Scientists, although it is seen as an individual's choice.	Abortion is prohibited if it is done solely to prevent the birth of an unwanted child. However, abortion is permitted if needed to save the life of the mother.	The morality of abortion would depend on the circumstances. Abortion may be supported if the child is suffering in the womb. Nothing is absolute in Buddhism, however, and in general, any form of killing may be seen as adding to bad karma, and thus abortion would be discouraged. Compassion and wisdom must be emphasized.	The traditional Hindu view prohibits abortion, because it is seen as a form of killing that would lead to the accumulation of bad karma. In modern practice, however, some Hindus practice abortion.
Observances at Birth	None. Christian Scientists do not practice baptism.	None.	At an early age — from 1 month to 100 days of age — the parents of a new baby give thanks to the Buddha and dedicate the child to Buddha.	On the 10th to 11th day after birth, a priest performs a naming ceremony for the newborn, invoking the blessings of gods and goddesses.
Rites of Initiation	None. Christian Scientists do not observe birthdays or anniversaries.	Baptism by immersion is done when the child (or adult) can and does give consent to be a Jehovah's Witness, usually at puberty.	It depends on the child. A child may be taken to a temple for a ceremony of further dedication.	Mundan: the first haircut for a boy. Dvija: for boys of the upper three castes, a rite of initiation at age 15. The boy is invested with three strands of the sacred thread, signifying right thought, right speech, right actions.
Withdrawal of Life Support	Most Christian Scientists have advance directives to avoid medical treatment. Critical illness should be dealt with by prayer, not medical treatment. Withdrawal of medical treatment is in accordance with a practicing Christian Scientist's wishes. A Christian Scientist never prays for death to avoid physical misery. Instead, a Christian Scientist prays for healing, even at an advanced age and in the face of critical illness. No illness is seen as hopeless by Christian Science standards.	Life is sacred and the willful taking of life under any circumstances is wrong. Reasonable and humane effort should be made to sustain and prolong life. However, the Scriptures do not require that extraordinary, complicated, distressing, or costly measures be taken to sustain a person if such measures would merely prolong the dying process and/or leave the patient with no quality of life. Any advance directives of patients that specifically define what is to be done are to be respected.	Buddhism values life, but sees death as a natural part of life. Maintenance, comfort care, and withdrawal of life support would be acceptable for those patients who are crossing the threshold of death. But good karma results from saving, prolonging, or improving life. The most weighty sin for a Buddhist is to take the life of another living being (Bhikkhu, 1991).	When the body is beyond repair, Hinduism supports the withdrawal of artificial life support in order to allow for a natural death. The point of life is liberation — moksha — from the endless cycles of life and death through good karma.
Death	Death is not a failure. Spiritual life goes on beyond death. When death occurs, the person's Christian Science practitioner should always be notified. Autopsies are permitted. Cremation and memorial service are the usual practices.	The soul dies with the body, but resurrection will occur for 144,000 at the end-time, and such will be born again as spiritual sons of God. Euthanasia is forbidden. Suicide is not approved of but understood as the product of mental illness. Autopsies are permitted only if legally necessary, so that the body will not be subjected to unnecessary mutilation. Burial and cremation are permitted.	Death is a natural part of life. At death, existence for the Buddhist can take a sudden turn for the better or the worse, depending on the good or evil done in life. Suicide is strongly criticized, except for self-sacrifice. Cremation is common. After death, the body should not be disturbed with movement, talking, or crying.	The atmosphere around the dying person must be peaceful, a spiritual silence, so the last thoughts are of God. Holy water, such as from the Ganges River, is poured into the mouth of the dying person. Hindus prefer to die at home, as close to mother earth as possible, so many prefer to die on the floor or even on the ground. A married woman's nuptial

continued

Table 6-1 Religions and Health Care *continued*

RELIGION	CHRISTIAN SCIENCE	JEHOVAH'S WITNESSES	HINDUISM	BUDDHISM
Death *continued*			thread (necklace) or amulets are removed just before death to allow the soul's free journey to infinity. The family washes the body, and the eldest son arranges for a funeral and cremation within 24 hr of death. The body should lie under a white sheet and be disturbed as little as possible. Embalming or beautifying the body are discouraged. Autopsies are discouraged. Children under 2 are buried, and there are no rituals for infants, because the soul from the last life had not yet lived. The names of gods are chanted at the funeral, and the family fasts and wears white for purity. Suicide and active euthanasia are forbidden, because killing accumulates bad karma.	
Organ Donation	Christian Scientists do not donate or receive organs, because they believe this is not the way to treat the spiritual cause of organ failure.	Organ transplants and organ donations are matters of individual choice. There is no biblical injunction against taking in body tissue or bone as there is against taking in blood.	Traditional Hindu thought is against receiving organ donations because organ donation is not natural. Donating organs involves disturbing the body after death, which is discouraged.	This is controversial. Some Buddhists accept the concepts of brain death and organ donation. If the donation of organs would help others, this may bring good karma and be approved of.

RELIGION	CHURCH OF JESUS CHRIST OF LATTER-DAY SAINTS (MORMONS)	UNITARIAN-UNIVERSALIST ASSOCIATION OF CONGREGATIONS (UUA)	SHINTO	AMERICAN INDIAN RELIGIONS
Description	The Church of Jesus Christ of Latter-Day Saints was founded in the 1800s. Church members believe that messages and a set of texts were divinely revealed to Joseph Smith. The Mormons differ from traditional Christianity in elevating these texts to the level of the Bible, and in believing that the church, as it grew after the resurrection of Christ, was corrupt, and that its authority was replaced by Joseph Smith's followers.	The Unitarians began in Europe in the 1600–1700s. The movement affirms the moral perfection of God but differs from traditional Christianity in that it believes that Jesus was human, and not the son of God (that is, unitarian, not trinitarian). The Universalist movement began in England in the eighteenth century, with the basic belief in a benevolent God and that all humans are inherently good, that is, a rejection of the Doctrine of Original Sin held by mainstream Christianity (the belief that humankind does not need redemption	Shinto is the ancient, traditional religion of Japan. Although it has been influenced by Buddhism, Shintoism has remained a distinct religion. Shintoism is a polytheistic, animistic religion. Shintoism teaches that the Japanese islands were a special, favored creation by the gods. The religion teaches that the sun goddess *Amaterasu* sent her grandson down to Earth to rule the world for her. He spawned the long line of emperors that have ruled Japan for hundreds of years. The emperors thus enjoyed a semidivine status until so-called "State	While there are many hundreds of distinct American Indian (and Canadian American Indian, Australian Indian, etc.) religions (note that all of these religions are not interchangeable) there are nevertheless certain common characteristics that may serve to illustrate the spiritualism of native people. Native religions are usually classed as "primal" religions. These religions arise from people close to nature, who are aware of nature's mysterious powers, and who have a belief in a spiritual world of powers or beings who are greater than humans and who give

continued

RELIGION	CHURCH OF JESUS CHRIST OF LATTER-DAY SAINTS (MORMONS)	UNITARIAN-UNIVERSALIST ASSOCIATION OF CONGREGATIONS (UUA)	SHINTO	AMERICAN INDIAN RELIGIONS
Description *continued*		by Jesus). The Unitarians and Universalists merged in 1961. UUA is a creedless church that has seven principles that all churches have agreed to, such as respecting the worth and dignity of all human beings. Church members live primarily in the United States and Canada, with some churches in Romania and Europe.	"Shinto" was outlawed at the end of World War II. "Folk" Shinto still exists. Shintoism centers around shrines, which have a characteristic gate and are built, often at special sites such as the tops of mountains, to house a kami (god). Numerous kamis exist. There are thousands of shrines in Japan, but fewer than a dozen in the United States.	meaning to events in life. Central to these religions is the belief that all life is sacred, and all things are inter-connected, and the importance of the community is emphasized. Often, the view of humanity is humble. These religions are polytheistic and animistic, involving an original or supreme creator god who is now withdrawn. There are no temples, holy books, or creeds.
Religious Leaders	Bishop: a volunteer lay leader of the church. Bishops are male and usually serve 5-year terms as church leaders. Home teacher: a male church member assigned to look after a member of the church. The home teacher provides practical as well as spiritual help to his assigned church member. Every member of the church has a home teacher, and that teacher is called in case of an illness.	Minister: an ordained male or female church leader who leads worship services.	Priests: priesthood is a hereditary office limited to males who are usually married. Only priests are allowed into the holiest part of the shrine, where the kami is said to exist. Priests lead worship and conduct ceremonies such as marriages.	Most often, a specialist in the religion is involved — a medicine man, a teacher, or an elder who is able to communicate with the spirits or the Great Spirit and convey the wishes of the petitioner or people. Such a person may look after sacred objects, organize ceremonies, interpret omens or dreams, know of techniques or remedies for problems, and function as a healer. Some may specialize in one of these functions. Often, such a leader is identified as a child as having special spiritual gifts and subsequently serves a long apprenticeship. Wisdom is associated with age.
Holy Books and Artifacts	The "standard works" include: The Bible, *The Book of Mormon*, the *Doctrine and Covenants*, and the *Pearl of Great Price*. Endowed church members, that is, members who have been to a Mormon temple, may also wear special underclothing that are considered sacred.	The Bible is not a definitive source for the UUA. Many members consider the Bible flawed.	Kojiki: written 712 CE Nihongi: written 720 CE, mostly in Chinese. Both works are important and honored, but are rarely recited or studied by ordinary believers. Believers may have at home a kami shelf, where daily prayers are said and offerings made. Daruma dolls, actually representations of the Buddha, are popular. Paper strips, broken arrows, and protective charms may be used by a practicing Shinto.	Usually, there are no holy books, and the religious tradition is passed on orally and through experience with rituals and festivals. Religious artifacts may include feathers, gourds, drums, shells, a medicine pouch worn around the neck and with important religious symbols inside, and grasses or other sources for incense.
Holy Day of the Week	Sunday	Sunday	None	None

continued

Table 6-1   Religions and Health Care *continued*

RELIGION	CHURCH OF JESUS CHRIST OF LATTER-DAY SAINTS (MORMONS)	UNITARIAN-UNIVERSALIST ASSOCIATION OF CONGREGATIONS (UUA)	SHINTO	AMERICAN INDIAN RELIGIONS
Holy Holidays, Festivals, Observances	Church members celebrate Christmas and Easter.	UUA members celebrate Christmas and Easter, but the holidays have more cultural than religious significance. Easter is seen as a celebration of spring and new life, rather than as a recognition of the resurrection of Jesus.	New Year's Day is popular, with celebrations lasting for 1 to 3 days. The Meiji shrine in Tokyo often is visited on this day. Spring Day, March 20. Children's Day, May 5. Respect for Old Age Persons Day, September 15. Autumn Day, September 23. Thanksgiving for Work Day, November 23. Japanese Emperor's Birthday, December 23.	Festivals are often associated with changes in seasons and with harvests. Often, believers may dress up as well-known spirits or gods.
Dietary Restrictions	Church members abstain from illicit drugs, alcohol, tobacco, tea, and coffee. The church advises all members to practice moderation in all things including diet, and to eat wholesome food, eat meat sparingly, and get rest and exercise.	None	None	Varies
Periods of Fasting	None	None	Priests may fast on a day before a festival by eating no meat or just rice. Fasting is not usually done by lay people.	Fasting may be a special form of prayer, supervised by the elder.
Medical Treatment	Church members are encouraged to seek medical care when needed and to exercise their best judgment based on competent medical advice. When sick, church members may call on their home teachers or other church members for the laying on of hands, or a blessing for healing. The blessing is done by two male members of the church at the request of the patient.	There is no prohibition against seeking medical care and treatment when necessary. The UUA is a socially active organization that has lobbied for the right to health care for all. When UUA members are ill, members of the congregation's caring committee may visit the person and provide practical and spiritual support.	Shinto followers with illnesses are encouraged to seek medical treatment. Those with illnesses may go to a shrine to ask for prayers for healing.	Illness may be related to a sin or an unhappy spirit or god. A specialist in the religion may be consulted to discern the cause of the illness or seek the ritual that will appease the unhappy spirit.
Birth Control	Sexual relations are permitted only within marriage. Birth control is permitted for family planning but discouraged for family prevention. Surgical sterilization is discouraged unless it is for health reasons. The decision to use birth control is left up to the prayerful	There are no prohibitions against birth control. Sexual relations are permitted between consenting adults in a mutually respectful relationship.	No restrictions.	Usually not practiced. Children are seen as blessings and essential to survival.

continued

RELIGION	CHURCH OF JESUS CHRIST OF LATTER-DAY SAINTS (MORMONS)	UNITARIAN-UNIVERSALIST ASSOCIATION OF CONGREGATIONS (UUA)	SHINTO	AMERICAN INDIAN RELIGIONS
Birth Control *continued*	decision of the husband and wife, based on competent medical advice.			
Infertility Treatment	Infertility treatment is a decision left up to the prayerful decision making of husband and wife, based on competent medical advice. Use of surrogate mothers and donor insemination is discouraged.	There are no prohibitions against seeking treatment for infertility.	No particular teachings. Medical treatment for infertility is allowed without restrictions.	A couple may seek treatment from the tribal elder for infertility, but may be reluctant to seek outside medical assistance.
Abortion	Abortion is permitted in instances of rape and incest, or when the health of the mother is jeopardized, or is left up to the prayerful consideration between husband and wife, based on competent medical advice.	The UUA is in favor of all reproductive rights for women, including the right to an abortion.	No particular teachings. Abortion is not forbidden but not encouraged.	Usually not practiced or tolerated openly.
Observances at Birth	The child is named and blessed in a church service, usually within 6 weeks of birth.	No special observances.	Newborns are commonly taken to a shrine for a blessing and for prayers for good health. Boys are taken on the 31st day of life, girls on the 33rd day of life.	Often, a dedication or thanksgiving ceremony.
Rites of Initiation	Baptisms are done at age 8.	Infants and children can undergo a dedication ceremony in the church.	Children at ages 3, 5, and 7 are blessed with special prayers on Children's Day. At age 20, an adult blessing is received.	Often, a boy reaching puberty or adulthood undergoes an initiation rite that includes some shedding of blood, if only a small amount.
Withdrawal of Life Support	The decision to withdraw life support is left up to the patient or family, based on competent medical advice.	There is no prohibition against withdrawing life support based on competent medical advice. UUA members have been in the forefront of the movement to withdraw life support when the quality of life is poor and suffering is great. However, assisted suicide and active euthanasia remain controversial.	No real teachings about withdrawal of life support.	Life support is seen as unnatural and therefore not necessary.
Death	Burials are arranged by the church, especially if the person was endowed. Cremation is discouraged. The decision for an autopsy is up to the family.	Suicide is seen as a tragedy but not a sin. There are no UUA requirements concerning burial. Autopsies are permitted when necessary.	Upon death, the deceased person becomes a spirit, according to Shinto beliefs. The person's name often is inscribed in wood at the ancestor shrine used by the family. The body is usually, but not always, cremated.	There are usually complex beliefs about death and the treatment and disposal of the body. Often, the spirit of the person is believed to live on after death, and ancestor worship is often involved.
Organ Donation	The decision for organ donation is left up to the family, based on competent medical advice.	There are no UUA restrictions on organ donation.	No particular teachings or restrictions. Organ donation is tolerated.	Organ donation is discouraged because of death and burial practices.

SPIRITUALITY AND THE NURSING PROCESS

The nurse's role in the spiritual care of the patient includes:

1. Conducting a spiritual assessment
2. Formulating nursing diagnoses
3. Planning and implementing nursing interventions designed to address the patient's diagnoses
4. Evaluating the plan of care

Spiritual Assessment

✓ NURSING CHECKLIST
General Approach to Spiritual Assessment

1. Conduct this assessment as part of the history-taking portion of a general patient assessment once trust has been established, rather than as a stand-alone interview.
2. Choose a quiet, private room that will be free from interruptions.
3. Ensure that the room's light is sufficiently bright to observe the patient's verbal and nonverbal reactions.
4. Greet the patient, introduce yourself, and explain that you will be taking a health history.
5. Position yourself at eye level with the patient.
6. Portray an interested, nonjudgmental manner throughout the interview. Respect silence and diversity.

Conducting the Spiritual History

1. The spiritual assessment should obtain the following information:
   a. the nature of the patient's spiritual beliefs
   b. the nature of the patient's spiritual support
   c. how the patient's spiritual beliefs have an impact on the treatment of health and illness
   d. the patient's state of spiritual well-being or spiritual distress.

2. Begin the interview with the physical history of the patient. Move on to the psychological history and end with the spiritual history. Make your transitions as smooth as possible. Keep in mind that the physical history may itself raise spiritual issues. For example, the patient may reveal a requirement for a vegetarian diet, or a history of circumcision at birth, or that a tatoo was imprinted for religious reasons. Use these facts to launch your spiritual assessment of the patient by saying, "Are you a vegetarian for spiritual reasons, or for health reasons, or some other reason?" or, "You mentioned circumcision — was that done for religious reasons?" or, "That's interesting. Can you tell me what that symbol in the tatoo means?"

3. Ask the patient if he or she has an **advance directive** (Living Will or Durable Medical Power of Attorney) stating what should be done if the patient is too ill to self-direct medical care. This is a good topic for opening the door to a discussion about spiritual beliefs, because the patient's answer to the question may involve spirituality. For example, the patient may say, "I don't believe in keeping the body alive when the soul is gone," or, "It's for God to decide when I die, not me." By probing with

❀ NURSING TIP

Required Information

Many states have Required Request laws, which obligate hospital staff to inquire about a patient's interest in organ or tissue donation. Furthermore, since 1992, the Patient Self-Determination Act has required that every hospital in the United States ask each inpatient on admission about the existence of an advance directive. While these questions currently are not required for outpatients, home visits, or clinic visits, it is a good idea to ask all patients about this important information. It is essential to know whether the patient has an advance directive or an organ donor card. Learning the techniques of tactfully approaching this delicate subject will aid you in showing sensitivity to patients and their families.

👁👁 THINK ABOUT IT

Abortion

What would you say if a patient tells you confidentially that she had an abortion, but that the religion to which she belongs doesn't approve of abortion?

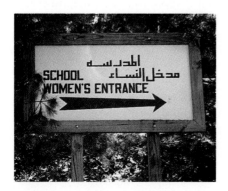

Figure 6-4 Awareness of cultural and religious norms and customs will help you deliver appropriate nursing care.

gentle, interested, open-ended questions into the patient's response, you can delve further into the details of the patient's spiritual beliefs. For example, you can ask, "Can you tell me more about that?" or restate the belief, "So, you believe that God should decide," in an attempt to get the patient to elaborate further. If the patient does not know what an advance directive is, take the opportunity for teaching and try to elicit the same spiritual information.

4. Ask the patient whether he or she has signed an organ donor card or given any thought to donating organs or tissue after death. Again, the patient's answers to these questions will probably involve spiritual beliefs. If the patient states that he or she is an organ donor, note this information and ask what led to this decision and if it has been discussed with the family or significant others. If the patient seems reluctant to discuss the issue, ask, "What do you believe about all this?" Try to get the patient to elaborate by asking open-ended questions such as "Can you tell me more about that?" If the patient does not understand organ donation, use the opportunity to do some teaching. As the issue becomes clear to the patient, you should be able to elicit some information about the patient's spiritual beliefs. Whatever the patient's response, be sure not to imply approval or disapproval of the patient's position on the matter.

5. Ask the patient if there are any spiritual or religious beliefs that will affect the health care received (refer to Figure 6-4). The patient may be unsure of what to expect from medical care, so you may need to probe for the answers you are seeking. What you are looking for is whether the patient needs to be on a special diet, such as a diet without pork, if the patient has specific beliefs about certain forms of treatment, such as a refusal of blood products, or if the patient wants to have a certain religious ritual performed at a certain time, such as baptism of a critically ill infant. It is helpful to know the general requirements for various religions so you know what areas to assess (see Table 6-1). However, it is important to remember that not every member of an organized religion adheres to the formal requirements of that religion. Do not assume that every Muslim will fast during Ramadan, or that every Jehovah's Witness will refuse blood transfusions.

6. While conducting the interview, observe the patient for clues about spiritual beliefs. Is the patient wearing any religious clothing or jewelry, such as a yarmulke, a cross, or a turban? Does the patient have religious reading material, such as a Koran or religious pamphlets? Are other religious artifacts, such as small statues, shawls, or amulets, on display? Comment on these items and use them to ask about the patient's spiritual beliefs. For example, "I see you have several crystals with you. Are you a spiritual person?" or, "This is interesting — what is it? What does it mean?" or, "I see you're reading a book about philosophy. Are you interested in philosophical and spiritual things?"

7. Ask the patient who should be notified in the event that there is a change in condition. After noting this, ask if the patient also wants you to notify a place of worship or a specific religious leader. Ask who will be supportive to the patient, family, and significant others during the illness. The patient may name other relatives, friends, or a religious organization. This is another opportunity to probe gently into the spiritual beliefs of the patient.

8. If the patient's affiliation with a specific religion or faithfulness to a particular spiritual belief has not yet been identified, you might say, "Experiencing an illness or surgery can be very emotionally difficult and stressful. Do you have any particular spiritual beliefs? Do you belong to any particular religion?" This is a gentler approach than asking "What is your religion?" which implies that everyone belongs to some sort of

NURSING TIP

Clues to a Patient's Spirituality

When you are caring for a patient in the home or in an institution such as a hospital, a hospice, or a nursing home, use your access to the patient to observe for clues about the patient's spirituality. Does the patient pray before meals? Do the patient's get-well cards contain religious or spiritual messages? Who visits the patient — family and friends, or also members of the patient's religious or spiritual organization (Andrews, 1989)?

NURSING TIP

Through the Back Door

A patient may resist answering questions about spiritual beliefs even during considerable spiritual distress. One key to assessing the patient's spirituality is to inquire about the spiritual and emotional state of the patient's significant other. Simple questions such as "How is your wife holding up under all this?" or "How are things going at home while you're here in the hospital?" are often helpful in encouraging the patient to discuss spiritual issues. The patient may display considerable worry about the effect the illness is having on significant others, and this in turn is often a reflection of the patient's own concern, spiritual and otherwise, about his or her fate.

religion, and may embarrass or insult a patient who does not. Depending on the patient's response, you can ask gentle, probing questions that will elicit more information. Helpful questions are "Do you go to a temple around here?" or "Do you mean you're an atheist?" or "Do you believe that your religion is a private matter?" Don't be surprised if the patient is reluctant to talk about spirituality and religion. This may be an area more private than the patient's own bowel or sexual habits. If the patient is reluctant to open up, don't push it. As you work with the patient, observe the patient, and develop a trusting relationship, more information will become available to you, and opportunities will arise to discuss this with the patient again.

9. If the patient in your care is experiencing any threat to his or her health and well-being, such as being newly diagnosed with a chronic illness, being admitted to a hospital because of an acute illness, or undergoing an assessment after an accident that was frightening or caused an injury, overtly state the obvious and ask how the patient is thinking spiritually about the change. For example, "You just had a heart attack two days ago and I wonder how you are feeling about that. How does your faith interpret that for you?" or, "You're having surgery first thing in the morning. What's going through your mind?" or, "How do you feel about being told that you have cancer?"

10. Document the answers to these questions in the patient's chart. It is important to record in an easily accessible place whether the patient has an advance directive or is an organ donor. If the patient names a particular religion, you should ask if he or she would like you to call that place of worship or a specific religious leader under certain circumstances, such as if the patient needs to be admitted to a hospital. Chart this information also.

Nursing Diagnosis

There are two North American Nursing Diagnosis Association (NANDA) nursing diagnoses that address the spiritual care of the patient. The first is: *Spiritual distress (distress of the human spirit)*, which is defined as "Disruption in the life principle which pervades a person's entire being and which integrates and transcends one's biological and psychosocial nature" (NANDA, 1996, p. 47). This diagnosis is used for patients with an actual disruption in spiritual well-being.

The second nursing diagnosis concerning spirituality is: *Potential for enhanced spiritual well-being*, which is defined as "the process of an individual's developing/unfolding of mystery through harmonious interconnectedness that springs from inner strengths" (NANDA, 1996, p. 48). This diagnosis is appropriate when you anticipate that spiritual support may be helpful to the patient.

Spiritual support is often helpful during times of change or crisis and during times of spiritual distress, including:

1. Birth, accidents, and death

2. Sudden change in condition

3. The imparting of bad news, such as a grim prognosis

4. Serious discussions concerning difficult plans to be made for patients with complex needs, such as a patient care conference about a patient with terminal cancer focusing on pain control and placement in hospice or home care

5. Withdrawal of life support, or discussions about it, or other discussions about bioethical dilemmas

Planning and Implementation

Once a nursing diagnosis has been made, you can plan and implement nursing interventions for the patient. The following interventions are appropriate for both spiritual nursing diagnoses:

1. Listen actively. It is important for patients to verbalize their feelings — either of spiritual distress or of their appreciation of their spiritual beliefs in times of trial. You should be alert to times when the patient wants to talk and should avoid waving off the patient's concerns with simple platitudes such as "It'll all look better tomorrow." Take the patient's concerns seriously. Allow the patient to talk and encourage the patient to continue talking by appearing interested, nodding, restating, and asking questions that gently probe for more information. Verbalization of doubts and suffering can be therapeutic, and you should resist the temptation to try to convince the patient that the spiritual concerns are not valid.

2. Project an empathetic, warm, interested response to the patient's concerns. Part of the cause of spiritual distress is often the fear that no one really cares about the patient's existence or fate. It is a therapeutic use of self for you to show interest in the patient and the patient's ultimate concerns, and not just physical and technical issues.

3. Show respect for the patient's spiritual beliefs. The patient may fear ridicule if spiritual beliefs are revealed. This fear may be particularly real if the patient has beliefs that are outside the mainstream. For example, Hindus prefer to die on the floor or, even more preferably, on the ground. You will help promote a sense of relief in the patient by respecting the patient's beliefs and by giving him or her permission to exercise his or her spirituality. You can also demonstrate respect for religious beliefs by waiting to speak until a patient finishes praying, providing privacy for a spiritual advisor visiting the patient, or asking the patient what should be done with religious or spiritual artifacts: "This looks special — do you have a particular place you want me to put this?"

4. Provide privacy for the patient for the purpose of religious practices, such as prayer or rituals. This may be as simple as drawing a curtain or leaving the room, or it may involve some negotiation around certain treatments. A meal or a treatment could be timed around a service, for example. A patient may require a private room or a change in roommates in order to practice a religious belief. Rather than forbidding chanting because it bothers the roommate, for example, find a private room, chapel, or even report room for that patient to use, if possible. A room change may also be necessary if a patient's roommate is verbal in expressing disapproval of the patient's spiritual beliefs.

5. Make appropriate referrals to the hospital chaplain and/or the patient's own spiritual or religious leader from the community. Hospital chaplains of any religion generally function as spiritual and religious resource people within a health care institution. Do not fail to take advantage of their expertise just because the patient is Buddhist and the chaplain is Jewish, for example. The chaplain can visit a patient and discuss the patient's spiritual concerns without judging the patient or trying to convert the patient to the chaplain's own religion. The chaplain can also make appropriate referrals and will be in a better position to find Buddhist support for a Buddhist patient, for example.

6. Provide support for the patient's practice of religion. This can be done by simply pointing out that Mass is televised on the hospital's inside channel at 7 A.M., or by spreading out a prayer shawl on the bed at the patient's request, or by suggesting creative solutions to religious prob-

NURSING TIP

Signs of Spiritual Distress

Signs of spiritual distress may be subtle or overt, but you should be alert to their deep meanings and not brush them off as the patient's "having a bad day." Such signs may include:

- Crying, sighing, withdrawn behavior.
- Verbalization of questions about spiritual beliefs, such as "What does it all mean?" or "An experience like this really makes you put things into perspective," or "I just don't understand why this is happening to me."
- Verbalizations about worthlessness or death, such as "I'd be better off dead" or "I guess we've all got to go sometime."
- Verbalizations about God and God's purposes, such as "I guess the gods have it in for me," or "It's payback time," or "I wonder what I did to deserve this," or "When God says it's your time to go, you go no matter what, I guess."
- Explicit requests to the nurse or others for spiritual assistance, such as requests for prayers or the special placement of religious artifacts (Labun, 1988).

NURSING TIP

Arranging for Pastoral Care

Most institutional chaplains have received special training in **pastoral care**, which is the care and response needed when a person is in a spiritual crisis. Chaplains are employed to visit and support patients in spiritual distress. In their practice of pastoral care, these chaplains can be valuable aids for the patient in spiritual distress. However, some patients, when asked, will refuse a visit with a chaplain based on the incorrect belief that they are present only to visit dying patients, practice their own religious rituals, or preach their own dogmas. If your patient's diagnosis is spiritual distress, initiate a chaplaincy referral. The chaplain will provide a satisfying explanation for the visit, such as "I normally visit with all patients before surgery," and the patient will not miss out on a valuable resource for alleviating spiritual distress.

ASK YOURSELF

A Patient Asks for Your Participation

- What would you do if a patient asked you to pray for him?
- What would you do if a patient asked you to pray with him?
- What would you do if a patient asked you to perform a religious ritual (such as a baptism)?

lems. For example, where hospital regulations forbid open flames, suggest a menorah with electric lights instead of candles. The Muslim patient who needs a blanket for prayer purposes may need a bath blanket set aside and labeled for that purpose. A patient with strict dietary restrictions may need some creative nursing interventions to meet nutritional needs, the patient's family may need to be taught how the food should be prepared to meet cholesterol or salt restrictions ordered by the physician, or you may need to enlist the aid of the dietician to get the kitchen to meet religious dietary needs.

7. Coordinate medical care with respect to the patient's beliefs. For example, suggest cutting down on blood sampling for a Jehovah's Witness whose hematocrit is decreasing. Insist on including the patient's religious leader in a patient care conference if that is what the patient wants. Knowing that the patient is a member of a small spiritual group, you could, with the patient's permission, investigate that group as a possible source of volunteers for posthospital care. In your report, pass on spiritual information as part of the care plan, such as "the patient's mother has asked us to pin the St. Christopher medal on her pillow."

8. There are several interventions you should avoid when working with a patient's spirituality, and these are listed in Table 6-2.

Table 6-2   Nursing Actions to Avoid When Intervening in the Patient's Spiritual Condition

You need to know and be comfortable and secure with your own spiritual beliefs before you can help your patients with their spiritual concerns. Avoid these actions because of their detrimental effects on the patient's spirituality:

1. Do not proselytize your own spiritual beliefs. You may share your beliefs, if the issue comes up, but it is never appropriate to try to convert the patient to another set of beliefs. In a worst-case scenario, you may instill fear in the patient that you will not provide care unless the patient espouses your own beliefs. You may also unwittingly undermine the patient's support system at a time when the patient needs support.

2. Do not instruct the patient in religious or spiritual doctrine. Your expertise is nursing, not religion or spirituality. Furthermore, in a time of spiritual distress, a patient needs support, not instruction. Let the religious or spiritual leader take the lead in any instruction that is required, and follow nursing interventions that will enhance spiritual well-being.

3. Do not perform the function of a spiritual advisor for the patient. This is not an area of nursing expertise, and you and the patient may become confused about your role.

4. Do not respond to the patient with clichés. Well-known and overused clichés such as "no sense crying over spilled milk" or "there's always someone else around who's worse off than you" are inappropriate because they tend to diminish the anguish of the patient (Linn, 1986). Clichés about religion are just as inappropriate, because they are patronizing and tend to trivialize both the sufferer's problems and the sufferer's religion. Additionally, most well-known religious clichés are based on Western Judeo-Christian culture and have no bearing on those with other kinds of religions or spiritual beliefs. Some examples of religious clichés to avoid are "God helps those who help themselves," "when God closes a door, He opens a window," and "it was God's will" (Linn, 1986). Respond instead with real, heartfelt words or, in some cases, with silence or with touch, if appropriate.

◎◎ THINK ABOUT IT

Privacy Versus Spirituality

In your role as a registered nurse, you recognize a patient who is being admitted to another unit. You have seen her praying at the Shinto shrine where you worship. The patient is asleep after surgery, and her family is not around. She is listed as being in serious condition. Should you notify your priest that the patient has been admitted? How would you decide?

Evaluation

Evaluate the effect of your nursing interventions by observing the patient. Signs that the patient's spiritual distress has decreased include:

1. Acceptance of spiritual support from the source with which the patient feels most comfortable.
2. Decrease in crying, restlessness, and sleeplessness. There may even be a decrease in complaints of pain or the severity of pain.
3. Decrease in statements of worthlessness and hopelessness.
4. Verbalization of satisfaction with spiritual beliefs and the support and comfort they provide. The patient may talk openly about spiritual beliefs and even offer spiritual insights to other patients, to you, or to other health care professionals. This is a healthy sign that the patient is admitting acceptance of spiritual beliefs.

CASE STUDY

The case study illustrates the application and documentation of the spiritual assessment.

The Spiritual Side of the Withdrawal of Life Support

Mulu is a 20-year-old immigrant from Pakistan who is admitted to the hospital after a motor vehicle accident. She was not wearing a seat belt and sustained severe closed-head injuries. Three days after her admission to the ICU, she has shown no signs of consciousness, has no spontaneous movements, and is ventilator dependent. EEGs done yesterday and today show no electrical brain activity, and during an apnea test done today the patient showed no signs of respiratory attempts. Her physician has declared that the patient is brain dead and wants to meet with the family to discuss organ donation before life support is withdrawn.

❖ HEALTH HISTORY

PATIENT PROFILE

20 yo SBF

History of Present Illness

(From the chart & from interviews with the pt's mother, brothers, & friends): pt admitted s/p MVA. Was in front passenger seat, no seat belt, when car hit a tree at high speed. Driver killed. Pt found in ditch 30 ft away by rescue squad, pulseless & breathless. CPR begun & pt intubated & transported to ER. CAT scan showed expanding subdural hematoma (SDH). Underwent emergency sgy to relieve SDH, but intracranial pressures remained ↑ & CAT scan next day showed brain stem herniation.

Spiritual Assessment

Entire family is Islamic, although their practice of some rituals of the faith, such as regular prayer, have gone by the wayside since their emigration to the United States 8 yr ago. Family does not belong to a mosque, but does keep dietary practices. Family fasts during Ramadan. Pt refused to wear veil in public because of c/o of ridicule from schoolmates. Family does not know if the pt had advance directive or organ donor card. Oldest brother became animated at these questions & asked several questions about what organ donation was, why the hospital wanted to know, & whether the hospital intended to sell his sister's organs. p̄ explanations, the brother's voice lowered but he stated he was unsure if their religion allows for organ donation. Pt has no organ donor card c̄ her driver's license.

continued

Family appears to be in crisis. Waiting room is filled c̄ pt's extended family, family friends, & high school- & college-aged friends. Pt's mother cries continually, rocks back & forth in her chair, moans, & is attended to by other women. Pt's brothers appear angry & upset. One of them says, "She didn't do anything to deserve this!" Another says, "Allah is good! How did He allow this to happen?" The ICU staff has been flooded with phone calls from relatives from out of state & from Pakistan.

REVIEW QUESTIONS AND ACTIVITIES

1. Organize two or more small groups and discuss spiritual beliefs and abortion. Identify whether the group is in agreement about abortion and whether there is bias for or against abortion within the group. What is each group member's spiritual or religious belief that makes that person for or against abortion? Are individuals who belong to religions acting in accordance with the official teachings of their faiths? Is it difficult to discuss those beliefs in the group? How might any bias or an individual's beliefs be unwittingly communicated to a patient or a patient's family? Compare the groups' results. Afterwards, take a secret poll of the members to determine whether any group member felt intimidated about discussing spiritual beliefs and abortion, and whether anyone withheld an unpopular viewpoint during discussion.

2. Form a small group and discuss the case study. Discuss how your own beliefs for or against organ donation might have an impact on your reaction to the family's choice. Imagine that the family makes a decision that is opposite to what you would have chosen. How would you interact with the family after that decision? Would your disapproval be evident? Assign different roles — MD, RN, mother, brother, imam, etc. — to the members of the group and act out how the patient care conference alluded to in the case study might proceed.

3. Interview other nurses of different religious or spiritual backgrounds. Then have them critique your sensitivity, knowledge, and verbal and nonverbal communication.

4. Which of the following religions does not allow blood transfusions?
   a. Roman Catholic
   b. Shinto
   c. Jehovah's Witness
   d. Islam

   The correct answer is (c).

5. Which of the following religions permits the use of donor egg and donor sperm for the treatment of infertility?
   a. Judaism
   b. Roman Catholicism
   c. Islam
   d. None of the above

   The correct answer is (d).

7

Nutritional Assessment

1. Describe the recommended dietary allowances for adequate nutritional intake for all age groups.
2. Identify nutritional differences for different age groups.
3. Perform a thorough nutritional history.
4. Perform necessary anthropometric measurements.
5. Describe the most common pathophysiologies for abnormal findings.
6. Describe laboratory analyses needed and their clinical significance to the nutritional assessment.

Nutrition, or the processes by which the body metabolizes and utilizes nutrients, affects every system in the body, both positively and negatively. We must have food and drink to sustain life, but what type and how much are the questions that must be asked when assessing a person's nutritional health. Health care providers must also understand how the body digests and absorbs nutrients, the importance of meeting daily nutritional requirements, the causes and results of an imbalance of nutrients, and how to assess them. Psychological, social, and cultural issues must also be considered during a nutritional assessment.

The U.S. Public Health Service's *Put Prevention into Practice* (1994) campaign focuses on preventive care for all Americans. This campaign stresses the importance of nutritional counseling for individuals of all ages to promote good health throughout life. The risk of many chronic conditions (coronary artery disease, hypertension, diabetes mellitus) may be reduced by developing proper dietary habits.

DIETARY GUIDELINES

Dietary guidelines are published by various government agencies to educate the general population regarding dietary needs. **Recommended dietary allowances (RDA)** are the recommended amounts of nutrients that should be eaten daily. Recommendations differ based on sex, age, and whether the patient is pregnant or lactating. These are recommendations, not requirements. Requirements are the amounts needed to prevent deficiencies. Recommendations exceed the required amounts in order to ensure that the entire population is considered.

These recommendations must be used as guidelines only and should be modified to fit individual needs. The "Basic Four" food guide, first issued in 1956, divided foods into four groups: milk and dairy, meats, vegetables and fruits, and breads and cereals. The USDA published recommendations in 1992 using the **Food Guide Pyramid**, which expands on the original basic four

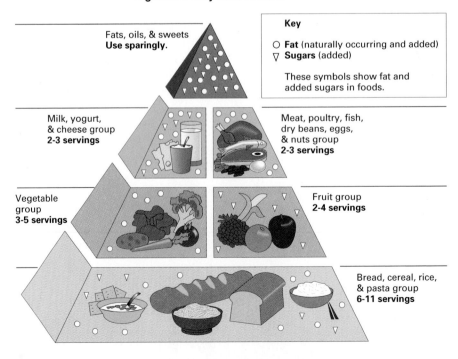

**The Food Guide
Pyramid
A guide to daily food choices**

Fats, oils, & sweets
Use sparingly.

Key

○ **Fat** (naturally occurring and added)
▽ **Sugars** (added)

These symbols show fat and added sugars in foods.

Milk, yogurt,
& cheese group
2-3 servings

Meat, poultry, fish,
dry beans, eggs,
& nuts group
2-3 servings

Vegetable
group
3-5 servings

Fruit group
2-4 servings

Bread, cereal, rice,
& pasta group
6-11 servings

Figure 7-1   Food Guide Pyramid
Courtesy of United States Departments of Agriculture and Health and Human Services (1992). The food guide pyramid: A guide to daily food choices. Washington, DC (leaflet no. 572)

Table 7-1 Daily Food Guide for Specific Age Groups

Food Group	Portion Size	NUMBER OF SERVINGS FOR SPECIFIC AGE GROUPS				
		Child*	Adolescent	Adult	Pregnancy	Lactation
Bread, cereal, rice, and pasta	1 ounce = 1 serving 1 slice bread ½ English muffin 4 saltines ½ cup cooked cereal ½ cup cooked rice ½ cup cooked pasta ½ oz cold cereal	6–11	6–11	6–11	6–11	6–11
Vegetable	½ cup cooked ½ cup raw 1 cup leafy raw vegetables 1 small baked potato 1 ear of corn	3–5	3–5	3–5	3–5	3–5
Fruits	¾ cup juice 1 medium apple, banana, or orange ½ cup fresh, cooked, or canned	2–4	2–4	2–4	2–4	2–4
Milk, yogurt, and cheese	1 cup milk 1 cup yogurt ½ cup evaporated milk 1½ oz natural cheese 2 oz process cheese	2 cups	4 cups	2–3 servings	4 servings	4 servings
Meat, poultry, fish, dry beans, eggs	3 oz meat, poultry, fish ½ cup cooked beans 2 tablespoons peanut butter 1 oz = 1 egg	2–3 oz	4–5 oz	2–3 servings (5–7 oz)	2–3 servings (5–7 oz)	2–3 servings (5–7 oz)
Fats, oils, and sweets	Limit the use of fats to 30% total daily calories. Limit sugars to 6 teaspoons/day for 1,600 calorie diet, 12 teaspoons for 2,200 calorie diet. Avoid alcohol while pregnant or lactating.					

*1–5 year old portion size 1 tablespoon per year of age for all food groups

Adapted from the United States Department of Agriculture and United States Department of Health and Human Services (1990). Nutrition and your health: Dietary guidelines for Americans (3rd ed.). (Home and Garden Bulletin no. 232), Washington, DC.

food groups to include guidelines on proportions and moderation. The Food Guide Pyramid was introduced to provide Americans with guidelines to improve their diets (refer to Figure 7-1). The six different groups represent specific nutrients. Table 7-1 illustrates the number of servings for specific age groups based on the Food Guide Pyramid.

Canada's Food Guide to Healthy Eating combines a food rainbow, which depicts types of food from each group, and a bar representation of the range of servings for each food group for people over age 4. Note that food with the smallest number of daily servings is on the bottom, the shortest arc of the rainbow, and the food with the largest number of daily servings is on the top, the broadest arc of the rainbow (refer to Figure 7-2).

NUTRIENTS

To perform a proper nutritional assessment you must have a clear understanding of the various nutrients needed to provide an adequate diet, the reason they are needed, and the food sources that provide them. **Nutrients** are the substances found in food that are nourishing and useful to the body.

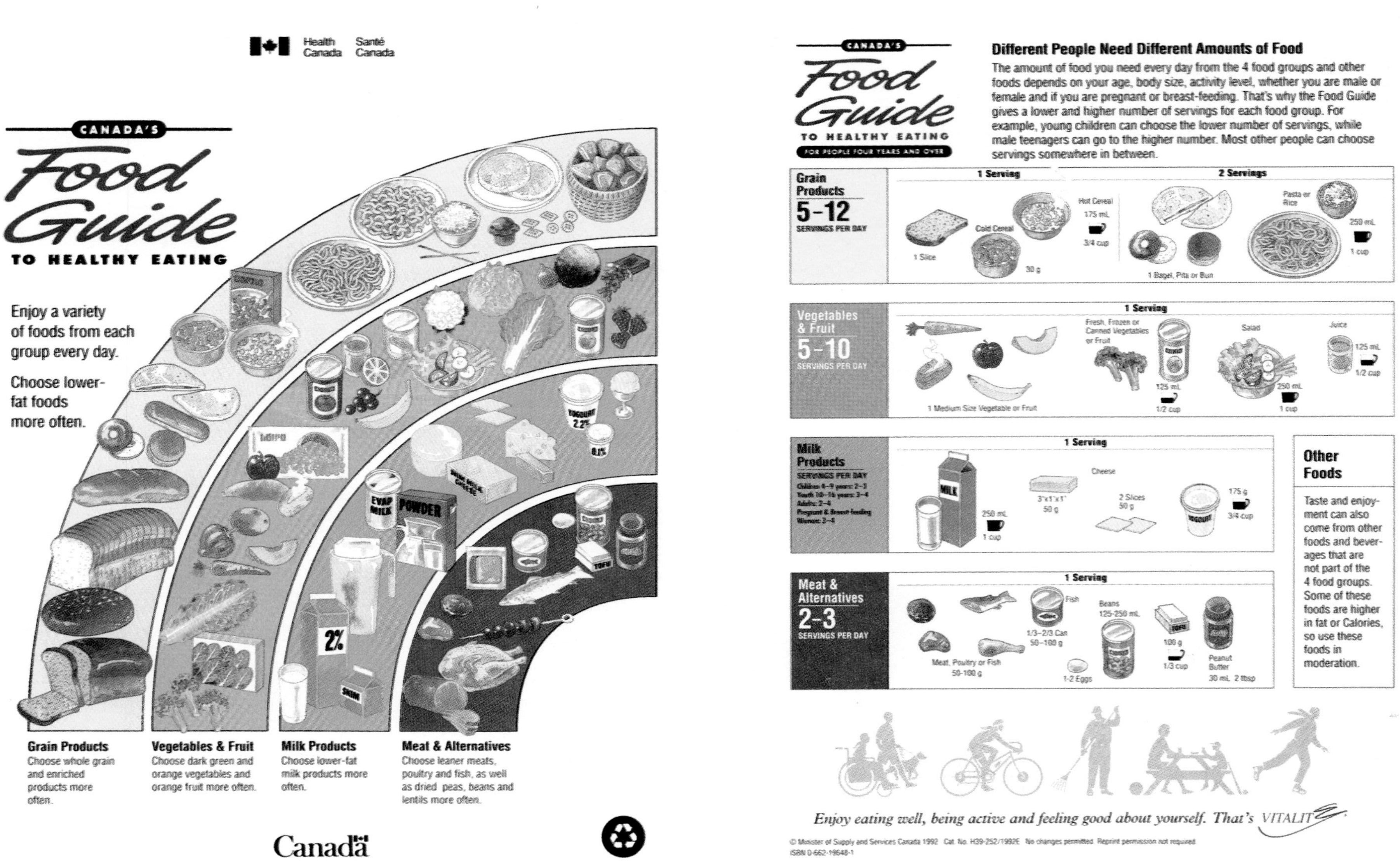

Figure 7-2 Canada's Food Guide to Healthy Eating *Courtesy of Minister of Supply and Services, 1992. Cat. No. H39-252, 1992E*

Carbohydrates, proteins, fats, vitamins, minerals, and water are the nutrients essential for life.

Carbohydrates, proteins, and fats supply the body with energy, which is measured in units called kilocalories (kcal). A **kilocalorie** (also called calorie) is the amount of heat required to raise 1 gram of water 1 degree centigrade. The USDA guidelines for calculating caloric requirements are based on activity level and the ideal body weight (IBW) multiplied by a specific number of calories per pound.

CALORIES/POUND OF IBW		
Activity	**Males**	**Females**
Sedentary	16	14
Moderate	21	18
Heavy	26	22

A 130-pound female who performs a moderate amount of exercise should have a daily intake of 2,340 calories (18 × 130), and a 165-pound male who performs a moderate amount of exercise should have an intake of 3,465 calories (21 × 165). This is compared to a 1,820 calorie intake (14 × 130) for the 130-pound woman and a 2,640 calorie intake (16 × 165) for the 165-pound man who lead sedentary lifestyles.

Carbohydrates

The major source of energy for the various functions of the body is **carbohydrates**. Each gram of carbohydrates contains 4 calories. Adults require 50 to 100 grams of carbohydrates per day to prevent carbohydrate deficiencies (ketosis and protein breakdown of muscles). This constitutes approximately 50%–60% of the daily caloric intake.

Carbohydrates help form adenosine triphosphate (ATP), which is needed to transfer energy within the cells. Carbohydrates supply fiber and assist in the utilization of fat. The primary sources of carbohydrates are bread, potatoes, pasta, corn, rice, dried beans, and fruits. A deficiency of carbohydrates in the diet may produce an electrolyte imbalance, fatigue, and depression. An excess in carbohydrates may produce obesity and tooth decay and may adversely affect those with diabetes mellitus.

Diets high in fiber have been shown to be beneficial in disease prevention. The possible benefits are decreases in the risks of colon cancer, rectal cancer, heart disease (decreases serum cholesterol levels), dental caries, constipation, and diverticulosis; and decreased weight.

Proteins

There are 4 calories in every gram of protein, but foods usually are a combination of protein and fat (meats, milk) or protein and carbohydrates (legumes). Adults require 0.8 g/kg/day of protein, or approximately 10%–20% of the daily caloric intake. **Protein** is required to give the body the nine essential amino acids, which are the amino acids that the body is unable to synthesize. These are needed to form the basis of all cell structures in the body. The major sources of protein are meat, poultry, fish, eggs, cheese, and milk. Legumes (dried beans and peas) are a good source of protein when eaten with corn or wheat (e.g., beans and rice provide a good source of protein). This is helpful information for vegetarians and people whose incomes will not cover the purchase of meat and milk products.

Protein-calorie malnutrition (PCM), or protein-energy malnutrition (PEM), is a major health problem that can occur anywhere but is most often associated

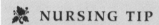

NURSING TIP

High-Fiber Diet

- Eat fresh foods instead of processed foods.
- Eat whole grain flour and breads.
- Eat at least five servings of fruits and vegetables per day.
- Increase water intake; minimum is six to eight glasses per day.
- Obtain fiber from the diet rather than from supplements.

with developing countries. Kwashiorkor and marasmus are two severe forms of PCM.

Kwashiorkor, which means "the disease of the displaced child when the next one is born," is a severe deficiency in good-quality protein. It occurs most often in children ages 1 to 4, usually as a result of being weaned too abruptly from the breast after a sibling is born. In the adult, it can occur with the ingestion of liquid diets that are low in protein, malabsorption diseases, hypermetabolic states, cancer, and AIDS. The physical signs are muscle wasting, edema, scaly, flaky skin, depigmentation of the hair, enlarged liver, and mental apathy.

Marasmus affects primarily 6- to 18-month-old infants and has symptoms similar to kwashiorkor except that sufferers appear more emaciated and do not have edema. Marasmus occurs when there is an inadequate intake of protein and calories or from poor absorption of protein such as with infections, burns, anorexia nervosa, tuberculosis, cancer, AIDS, malabsorption diseases, and chronic liver disease.

Fats

Lipids, or fats, contain 9 calories per gram. The Food Guide Pyramid recommends using fats in the diet sparingly, and the recommendation of many health care experts is to reduce fat to 20%–30% of the total calories consumed. **Fats** supply the essential fatty acids, which form a part of the structure of all cells. They also help to lower the serum cholesterol. Essential fatty acids must be supplied by the diet. Fats influence the texture and taste of food. The food sources of fat are animal fat (butter, shortening, lard) and vegetable fat (vegetable oil, margarine, and nuts). The types of fats consumed in the diet should be evaluated. **Saturated fats** come from both animal sources (butter, lard, fatty meats) and vegetable sources (coconut, palm, and partially hydrogenated oils that occur in some processed foods). Saturated fats have been found to raise the cholesterol level. **Monosaturated fats** (olive and canola oils) lower the "bad" cholesterol (LDL) and do not lower the "good" cholesterol (HDL). **Cholesterol** is a lipid found only in animal products. It is found in muscle, red blood cells, and cell membranes. Cholesterol is transported in the blood by **high-density lipoproteins** (HDL) and **low-density lipoproteins** (LDL). The HDL are useful in carrying cholesterol away from the heart and arteries and toward the liver. The LDL carry the cholesterol toward the heart. There is a strong association between high levels of LDL and coronary artery disease (CAD). High levels of HDL protect against CAD.

Triglycerides account for most of the lipids stored in the body's tissues. In the bloodstream, triglycerides produce energy for the body. An elevated triglyceride level occurs in hyperlipidemia, a risk factor for CAD.

A deficiency of fat in the diet can cause a decrease in weight, lack of satiety, and skin and hair changes. An excess of fat in the diet contributes to obesity and is linked to CAD. There has also been a correlation between high-fat diets and certain cancers (colon, breast, and prostate, in particular).

Vitamins

Vitamins are organic substances needed to maintain the function of the body. They are not supplied by the body in sufficient amounts and must be obtained from dietary sources. Vitamins stored in dietary fat and absorbed in the fat portions of the body's cells are **fat-soluble vitamins**. These are vitamins A, D, E, and K. **Water-soluble vitamins** include C, thiamine (B_1), riboflavin (B_2), niacin, pyridoxine (B_6), folacin (folate), cobalamin (B_{12}), pantothenic acid, and biotin. They are not stored in the body and are excreted in the urine. Various disease conditions occur when a vitamin source is lacking. Table 7-2 discusses the signs and symptoms of vitamin deficiencies and excesses.

Table 7-2 Fat-Soluble Vitamins and Water-Soluble Vitamins

NAME	FOOD SOURCES	FUNCTIONS	DEFICIENCY/TOXICITY

Vitamin A (retinol)	Animal
	  Liver
	  Whole milk
	  Butter
	  Cream
	  Cod liver oil
	Plants
	  Dark-green leafy vegetables
	  Deep-yellow or orange fruit
	  Fortified margarine
		Dim light vision
		Maintenance of mucous
		  membranes
		Growth and development
		  of bones
			Deficiency
			  Night blindness
			  Xerophthalmia
			  Respiratory infections
			  Bone growth ceases
			Toxicity
			  Cessation of menstruation
			  Joint pain
			  Stunted growth
			  Enlargement of liver

Vitamin D (cholecalciferol)	Animal
	  Eggs
	  Liver
	  Fortified milk
	Plants
	  None
		Bone growth	Deficiency
			  Rickets
			  Osteomalacia
			  Poorly developed teeth
			  Muscle spasms
			Toxicity
			  Kidney stones
			  Calcification of soft tissues

Vitamin E (alphatocopherol)	Animal
	  None
	Plant
	  Margarines
	  Salad dressing
		Antioxidant	Deficiency
			  Destruction of RBCs
			Toxicity
			  Hypertension

Vitamin K	Animal
	  Egg yolk
	  Liver
	  Milk
	Plant
	  Green leafy vegetables
	  Cabbage
		Blood clotting	Deficiency
			  Prolonged blood clotting
			Toxicity
			  Hemolytic anemia
			  Jaundice

Thiamine (vitamin B_1)	Animal
	  Pork
	  Beef
	  Liver
	  Eggs
	  Fish
	Plants
	  Whole and enriched grains
	  Legumes
		Coenzyme in oxidation of
		  glucose
			Deficiency
			  Gastrointestinal tract, nervous, and
			  cardiovascular system problems
			Toxicity
			  None

Riboflavin (vitamin B_2)	Animal
	  Milk
	Plants
	  Green vegetables
	  Cereals
	  Enriched bread
		Aids release of energy from
		  food
			Deficiency
			  Cheilosis
			  Glossitis
			  Photophobia
			Toxicity
			  None

Pyridoxine (vitamin B_6)	Animal
	  Pork
	  Milk
	  Eggs
	Plants
	  Whole-grain cereals
	  Legumes
		Synthesis of nonessential
		  amino acids
		Conversion of tryptophan
		  to niacin
		Antibody production
			Deficiency
			  Cheilosis
			  Glossitis
			Toxicity
			  Liver disease

Vitamin B_{12}	Animal
	  Seafood
	  Meat
	  Eggs
	  Milk
	Plants
	  None
		Synthesis of RBCs
		Maintenance of myelin
		  sheaths
			Deficiency
			  Degeneration of myelin sheaths
			  Pernicious anemia
			Toxicity
			  None

Niacin (nicotinic acid)	Animal
	  Milk
	  Eggs
	  Fish
	  Poultry
		Transfers hydrogen atoms
		  for synthesis of ATP
			Deficiency
			  Pellagra
			Toxicity
			  Vasodilation of blood vessels

continued

Table 7-2   Fat-Soluble Vitamins and Water-Soluble Vitamins *continued*

NAME	FOOD SOURCES	FUNCTIONS	DEFICIENCY/TOXICITY

Folacin (folic acid)	Animal
	  None
	Plants
	  Spinach
	  Asparagus
	  Broccoli
	  Kidney beans
		Synthesis of RBCs	Deficiency
			  Glossitis
			  Macrocytic anemia
			Toxicity
			  None

Biotin	Animal
	  Milk
	  Liver
	Plants
	  Legumes
	  Mushrooms
		Coenzyme in carbohydrate
		  and amino acid metabolism
		Niacin synthesis from
		  tryptophan
			Deficiency
			  None
			Toxicity
			  None

Pantothenic acid	Animal
	  Eggs
	  Liver
	  Salmon
	  Yeast
	Plants
	  Mushrooms
	  Cauliflower
	  Peanuts
		Metabolism of carbohydrates,
		  lipids, and proteins
		Synthesis of acetylcholine
			Deficiency
			  None
			Toxicity
			  None

Vitamin C (ascorbic acid)	Fruits
	  All citrus
	Plants
	  Broccoli
	  Tomatoes
	  Brussel sprouts
	  Potatoes
		Prevention of scurvy
		Formation of collagen
		Healing of wounds
		Release of stress hormones
		Absorption of iron
			Deficiency
			  Scurvy
			  Muscle cramps
			  Ulcerated gums
			Toxicity
			  Raised uric acid level
			  Hemolytic anemia
			  Kidney stones
			  Rebound scurvy

RBC = red blood cell; ATP = adenosine triphosphate.

Courtesy of Delmar Publishers, Albany, NY

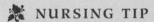 **NURSING TIP**

Preventing Iron-Deficiency Anemia

- Identify those patients at risk.
- Perform a complete nutritional assessment on high-risk patients.
- Encourage patients to eat foods high in iron. These include lean meats, poultry, fish, enriched breads, legumes, leafy green vegetables, dried fruits, and nuts.

Minerals

Minerals are inorganic elements. Minerals regulate body processes and build body tissue. These processes are fluid balance, acid-base balance, nerve cell transmission, vitamin, enzyme, and hormonal activity, and muscle contractions. Minerals are divided into two classifications. **Macrominerals** are needed by the body in large amounts (>100 mg/day), and are sometimes called the major minerals (refer to Table 7-3). **Microminerals**, or trace minerals, are needed in smaller amounts by the body (<15 mg/day) (refer to Table 7-4).

The most common nutrient deficiency in the world is lack of iron. This is particularly prevalent among infants, adolescents, and pregnant and menstruating women. It can result in iron-deficiency anemia.

Water

Water is essential to life; we cannot survive more than a few days without it. Water accounts for 50% to 60% of the body's weight. The daily amount needed depends on the size of the person, the climate, and the amount of activity. The average adult needs 5 to 6 cups of water a day; athletes and those living

NAME	FOOD SOURCES	FUNCTIONS	DEFICIENCY/TOXICITY
Table 7-3 **Major Minerals**			
Calcium (Ca)	Milk exchanges Milk, cheese Meat exchanges Sardines Salmon Vegetable exchanges Green vegetables	Development of bones and teeth Permeability of cell membranes Transmission of nerve impulses Blood clotting	Deficiency Osteoporosis Osteomalacia Rickets
Phosphorus (P)	Milk exchanges Milk, cheese Meat exchanges Lean meat	Development of bones and teeth Transfer of energy Component of phospholipids Buffer system	(Same as calcium)
Potassium (K)	Fruit exchanges Oranges, bananas Dried fruits	Contraction of muscles Maintaining water balance Transmission of nerve impulses Carbohydrate and protein metabolism	Deficiency Hypokalemia Toxicity Hyperkalemia
Sodium (Na)	Table salt Meat exchanges Beef, eggs Milk exchanges Milk, cheese	Maintaining fluid balance in blood Transmission of nerve impulses	Toxicity Increase in blood pressure
Chlorine (Cl)	Table salt Meat exchanges	Gastric acidity Regulation of osmotic pressure Activation of salivary amylase	Deficiency Imbalance in gastric acidity Imbalance in blood pH
Magnesium (Mg)	Vegetable exchanges Green vegetables Bread exchanges Whole grains	Synthesis of ATP Transmission of nerve impulses Activation of metabolic enzymes Relaxation of skeletal muscles	
Sulfur (S)	Meat exchanges Eggs, poultry, fish	Maintaining protein structure Formation of high-energy compounds	

Courtesy of Delmar Publishers, Albany, NY

in hot, dry climates require more. Thirst may not always be an adequate indicator of water intake needs, especially in infants or very ill individuals who may have a poor thirst mechanism. Those who engage in intense physical activity may have a decreased thirst sensation as well (see Figure 7-3).

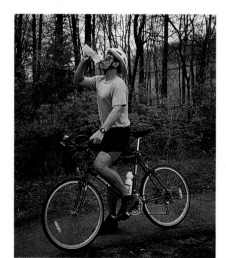

Figure 7-3 Preventing dehydration is an important element of proper nutrition.

⬡ NURSING ALERT

Signs and Symptoms of Dehydration

- Health history reveals inadequate intake of fluids.
- Decrease in urine output.
- Urine specific gravity >1.035.
- Weight loss (% body weight): 3%–5% for mild, 6%–9% for moderate, and 10%–15% for severe dehydration.
- Eyes appear sunken; tongue has increased furrows and fissures.
- Oral mucous membranes are dry.
- Decreased skin turgor.
- Venous filling and emptying times are delayed (>3–5 seconds).
- Sunken fontanels in infants.
- Changes in neurological status may occur with moderate to severe dehydration.

Table 7-4   Trace Minerals

NAME	FOOD SOURCES	FUNCTIONS	DEFICIENCY/TOXICITY
Iron (Fe)	Meat exchanges Meat, fish, poultry Dried fruits, beans Fortified cereals	Transports oxygen and carbon dioxide	Iron-deficiency anemia

Iodine (I)	Meat exchanges
	    Seafood
	Iodized salt
		Regulates basal metabolic rate	Deficiency
			    Goiter
			    Cretinism

Zinc (Zn)	Meat exchanges Eggs, oysters Milk exchange	Formation of collagen Component of insulin Component of many vital enzymes	
Selenium (Se)	Meat exchanges Liver, seafood	Antioxidant	
Copper (Cu)	Meat exchanges Oysters, liver	Oxidation of glucose	
Manganese (Mn)	Meat exchanges Nuts, peas, beans	Component of metabolic enzymes	
Fluoride (F)	Drinking water, seafoods	Reduces dental caries	Toxicity Mottled-looking teeth
Chromium (Cr)	Meat exchanges Eggs, meats	Binds insulin to cell membranes	

Molybdenum (Mo)	Meat exchanges
	    Liver, legumes
	Bread exchanges
	    Whole grains
		Metabolism of nucleic acids to uric acid	

Courtesy of Delmar Publishers, Albany, NY

NUTRITION THROUGH THE LIFE CYCLE

Assessment of the patient's developmental needs must always be included with a nutritional assessment. Nutritional needs change throughout the life cycle and are affected by both physical and developmental changes. A clear understanding of those changes, how they affect the patient, and what anticipatory guidance is indicated are needed to conduct a nutritional assessment. **Anticipatory guidance** covers health promotion, informs at-risk individuals of physical, cognitive, psychological, and social changes that occur, and explains their nutritional needs.

Children

Recommended daily requirements for children change with each age group. An understanding of development with regard to physical, cognitive, and psychosocial changes is needed to properly assess the nutritional needs of children. This includes educating the caregiver about these changes before they occur. Families can then have more realistic expectations and understand what is within the normal range and what should be cause for concern.

Infants

Infants grow more during the first 6 to 12 months of life than at any other time. This is also the time when there are great neurological changes, which indicates a need for proper nutrients for growth and development. The American Academy of Pediatrics recommends the use of breast milk for infants instead of formula feeding for the first 6 to 12 months (AAP, 1982). If this is not possible, even a few weeks is beneficial, except in cases where the mother is HIV-positive because HIV infection can be transmitted via breast milk. Be prepared to support the caregiver's feeding decision, and discuss schedules, habits, and warning signs of problems or inadequate intake.

Infants are born with several reflexes that should be assessed when evaluating their nutritional status — sucking, rooting, and swallowing. Infants are able to feel hunger and express the need to eat by crying. Between 4 and 6 months, infants can feed themselves a cracker. When infants are 8 to 12 months old, they may drink from a cup by themselves. The use of a developmental assessment tool helps you monitor the infant's ability to achieve these milestones (refer to the DDST II, Chapter 23). Assessing the infant's physical development (such as head control and the ability to sit) is also helpful to determine readiness for solid food. Foods should be introduced one at a time to observe for possible allergic reactions. The recommended order of new foods starts with the least allergenic as outlined in the nursing tip.

NURSING TIP

Infant Feeding Guidelines

Birth to 6 months: breast milk or infant formula only. Increases gradually to 28–32 oz per day by the third to fourth month of life.

4 to 6 months: iron-fortified cereals. Rice cereal is the least allergenic and is usually introduced first. Wheat cereals are usually not added until after 6 months of age. Help the infant adjust to spoon-feeding. Offer only one new food every 3 to 4 days to observe for signs of allergic reactions. Do not use mixed foods that may have other ingredients added.

5 to 8 months: fruits and vegetables. Encourage parents to read the labels of all foods to determine what has been added. Fruit juices that are noncitrus may be introduced. It is helpful to use a cup. This prevents the infant from associating sweet fruit juices with a bottle and also limits the amount they ingest. Do not add sugar or seasoning to foods. Introduce egg yolks, then gradually introduce meats last. Egg whites may be given when all other foods have been introduced.

9 to 10 months: finger foods may be introduced. Small bite-size pieces that are cooked, mashed, and soft will allow the child independence and will provide increased texture that requires chewing. Gradually increase foods with texture as the child's chewing skills improve and teeth emerge.

✓ NURSING CHECKLIST
Nutritional Assessment of Infants

- If the infant is breastfed, how often and for how long?
- How much formula does the infant take at each feeding, and how often does the infant eat? (Estimate how much is consumed in 24 hours.)
- How is the formula prepared? (It is important to make sure the formula is prepared correctly; this also helps establish how much the infant is eating.) How is the prepared formula stored?
- How does the infant react to eating? Does the infant appear satisfied?
- Does the infant appear to have any distress or problems while eating? Are there any problems with constipation or diarrhea, and how is it treated? Have any allergies been discovered?
- Is the infant taking any supplemental food?
- Is the infant ever put in bed with a bottle? If the answer is yes, instruct the caregivers about infant bottle caries and the importance of not propping the bottle or placing it in the bed (see Figure 7-4). (If the caregivers do not want to comply, try to get them to put only water in the bottle.)

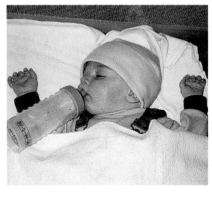

Figure 7-4 Allowing infants to sleep with a bottle contributes to dental caries.

Toddlers

Toddlers have their own unique nutritional needs. Growth and development play a very important role in the toddler's diet and in providing appropriate assessment and anticipatory guidance to the caregivers. As children experience increased independence and control over their bodies, some of this independence is demonstrated in their eating patterns. There is an increased problem with food refusal or the desire for only certain foods (this can change from day to day). This is a normal response to the developmental stage and should not be a problem unless it is excessive. Toddlers may say "no" even to food they desire to demonstrate that they are in charge.

Instruct parents to offer foods that the toddler can self-feed in small portions and offer only one new food at a time. A serving size should be about 1 to 2 tablespoons of food for each year of age. Toddlers are very good at imitating and often exhibit food dislikes that are shown at home (particularly if there is an older sibling). Encourage routine mealtimes that are enjoyed together to provide the toddler with role models for developing good eating habits.

Preschoolers

Preschoolers continue to have food dislikes and become picky eaters. They verbalize their likes and dislikes and show their independence by being in conflict with their caregivers. Giving choices, serving small amounts of foods children can eat easily (finger foods), and providing a routine and enjoyable eating environment helps to foster good eating habits by decreasing conflicts.

Preschoolers often have smaller appetites compared to toddlers. This may be caused by drinking too many beverages (milk, juice, Kool-Aid), and a slower increase in growth. They often are resistant to new foods and may eat only one food at a time. Encourage the caregivers to offer other foods. Discuss the need to provide healthy snacks and prevent the preschooler from eating foods that are too high in sugar. The preschooler benefits by helping to prepare food, setting the table, and making some decisions. Providing them with acceptable options is an easy way to ensure an appropriate diet.

School-Age Children

School-aged children tend to have erratic growth patterns that are reflected in their equally erratic eating patterns. They also tend to continue having strong likes and dislikes. Encourage families to maintain a balanced diet and to limit highly sweetened snacks and foods. Caregivers should be advised to teach children proper nutrition and should be encouraged to show children how to read nutrition and ingredient labels. Advise caregivers and children that pubescent chubbiness is a normal part of growth that often precedes a rapid increase in height.

Adolescents

Adolescence is a period of rapid growth and change. Adolescents' nutritional needs fluctuate accordingly. Adolescents are concerned with body image and often compare their bodies to those of their peers in an attempt to fit into an identity that is acceptable to them. A poor body image can lead to eating disorders such as anorexia nervosa, bulimia nervosa, and obesity. Although anorexia nervosa and bulimia nervosa can occur at any age, they are frequently seen in adolescents. There are several important elements to look at when assessing for anorexia nervosa or bulimia nervosa (refer to Table 7-5 and Figure 7-5).

Level of physical activity must also be taken into account for a nutritional evaluation. An understanding of the different sports and their requirements

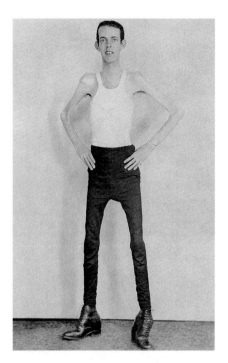

Figure 7-5 Anorexia Nervosa
Copyright © Zee, 1995

Table 7-5 Diagnostic Criteria for Eating Disorders

ANOREXIA NERVOSA

A. Refusal to maintain body weight at or above a minimally normal weight for age and height (e.g., weight loss leading to maintenance of body weight less than 85% of that expected; or failure to make expected weight gain during period of growth, leading to body weight less than 85% of that expected).

B. Intense fear of gaining weight or becoming fat, even though underweight.

C. Disturbance in the way in which one's body weight or shape is experienced, undue influence of body weight or shape on self-evaluation, or denial of the seriousness of the current low body weight.

D. In postmenarcheal females, amenorrhea, i.e., the absence of at lease three consecutive menstrual cycles. (A woman is considered to have amenorrhea if her periods occur only following hormone, e.g., estrogen, administration.)

Specify type:

Restricting Type: during the current episode of Anorexia Nervosa, the person has not regularly engaged in binge-eating or purging behavior (i.e., self-induced vomiting or the misuse of laxatives, diuretics, or enemas)

Binge-Eating/Purging Type: during the current episode of Anorexia Nervosa, the person has regularly engaged in binge-eating or purging behavior (i.e., self-induced vomiting or the misuse of laxatives, diuretics, or enemas)

BULIMIA NERVOSA

A. Recurrent episodes of binge eating. An episode of binge eating is characterized by both of the following:
   (1) eating, in a discrete period of time (e.g., within any 2-hour period), an amount of food that is definitely larger than most people would eat during a similar period of time and under similar circumstances
   (2) a sense of lack of control over eating during the episode (e.g., a feeling that one cannot stop eating or control what or how much one is eating)

B. Recurrent inappropriate compensatory behavior in order to prevent weight gain, such as self-induced vomiting; misuse of laxatives, diuretics, enemas, or other medications; fasting; or excessive exercise.

C. The binge eating and inappropriate compensatory behaviors both occur, on average, at least twice a week for 3 months.

D. Self-evaluation is unduly influenced by body shape and weight.

E. The disturbance does not occur exclusively during episodes of Anorexia Nervosa.

Specify type:

Purging Type: during the current episode of Bulimia Nervosa, the person has regularly engaged in self-induced vomiting or the misuse of laxatives, diuretics, or enemas.

Nonpurging Type: during the current episode of Bulimia Nervosa, the person has used other inappropriate compensatory behaviors, such as fasting or excessive exercise, but has not regularly engaged in self-induced vomiting or the misuse of laxatives, diuretics, or enemas.

EATING DISORDER NOT OTHERWISE SPECIFIED

The Eating Disorder Not Otherwise Specified category is for disorders of eating that do not meet the criteria for any specific Eating Disorder. Examples include

1. For females, all of the criteria for Anorexia Nervosa are met except that the individual has regular menses.

2. All of the criteria for Anorexia Nervosa are met except that, despite significant weight loss, the individual's current weight is in the normal range.

3. All of the criteria for Bulimia Nervosa are met except that the binge eating and inappropriate compensatory mechanisms occur at a frequency of less than twice a week or for a duration of less than 3 months.

4. The regular use of inappropriate compensatory behavior by an individual of normal body weight after eating small amounts of food (e.g., self-induced vomiting after the consumption of two cookies).

5. Repeatedly chewing and spitting out, but not swallowing, large amounts of food.

6. Binge-eating disorder: recurrent episodes of binge eating in the absence of the regular use of inappropriate compensatory behaviors characteristic of Bulimia Nervosa.

Reprinted with permission. American Psychiatric Association. Diagnostic and statistical manual of mental disorders (4th ed.). Washington, DC: American Psychiatric Association.

🌸 NURSING TIP

Preventing Eating Disorders

- Encourage healthy dietary habits and adequate exercise.
- Emphasize a healthy lifestyle over physical appearance and weight loss.
- Encourage increased self-esteem and stress a positive self-worth.
- Avoid pressuring children to achieve perfection or perform beyond their abilities.
- Recognize signs and symptoms of eating disorders, and seek professional help when suspected.

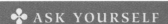

Figure 7-6 Adolescent athletes are at risk for anabolic steroid abuse.

may help you screen for potential problems. In some sports (e.g., football), players are encouraged to be large and heavy; this puts them at a risk for possible anabolic steroid use (see Figure 7-6). Toxic effects of steroid use include possible cancer of the liver, short stature, behavioral changes, endocrine problems (acne, impotence, testicular atrophy), and hypertension. In sports where decreased weight is desirable (e.g., wrestling, gymnastics), athletes may try many methods to "make weight." Instruction about proper nutrition to help reduce body fat without compromising health is needed when working with all athletes.

✓ **NURSING CHECKLIST**
Nutritional Assessment of Adolescents

- Are you involved in any sports? If so, are there any requirements regarding weight or food?
- Are you on any specific diet or meal plan?
- Do you skip any meals?
- Do you feel content with your weight? If not, how much do you feel you should weigh? What do you do to control your weight?
- How often do you weigh yourself?
- Have you ever induced vomiting, used laxatives, diuretics, or diet pills to help with weight control?
- Do you eat snacks? What type of snacks? What are your between-meal eating habits?
- Do you exercise regularly? How often and what kind of exercise?

❧ **ASK YOURSELF**

Obese Patient

An obese patient is concerned about her appearance.
- What are your biases about obesity?
- How would you react to this patient?
- What resources and information would you provide to assist your patient?

Young and Middle-Aged Adults

Growth and caloric needs usually stabilize in young and middle-aged adults. Eating habits may be altered by changes in activity levels and by the effects of work and life stressors.

Obesity is a weight greater than 120% of the ideal body weight (IBW). Obesity occurs when calories consumed are greater than calories expended. This can occur when there is an increase in food consumption, a decrease in activity level, or both. Obesity can occur at any age but is frequently seen in young and middle-aged adults (see Figure 7-7). Many factors affect whether a person is prone to obesity: genetic, physiological, psychological, and environmental factors. Obesity places a person at risk for hyperlipidemia, CAD, hypertension, diabetes mellitus, and chronic disorders.

Patients who are overweight or obese frequently experience yo-yo dieting, or weight cycling. In weight cycling, patients diet for some period of time, achieve their goal weights, and cease dieting. The majority of people return to their usual eating habits and regain the lost weight, and may add a few more pounds as well. Because many weight reduction programs neither address behavior modification for eating nor include an exercise regimen, most diets fail. The use of fad diets (i.e., diets that promise results without effectively altering lifestyle) and fad exercise regimens (e.g., use of vibrating machine to lose fat, use of sauna to decrease weight) may be deleterious to a person's health. Some fad programs are relatively safe if followed for a short period of time with adequate professional supervision.

Osteoporosis is a disease that reduces bone mass. It is more common in women, especially after menopause, and is often not detected until the person falls and fractures a bone. The risk factors for osteoporosis include: family history, estrogen deficiency, sedentary lifestyle, smoking, alcohol abuse, and long-standing calcium deficiency.

Non–insulin-dependent diabetes mellitus, or type II diabetes, is a disease usually diagnosed after age 40. It is associated with family history and obesity.

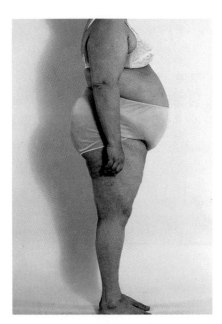

Figure 7-7 Obese Adult *Courtesy of the Armed Forces Institute of Pathology*

It is often undiagnosed until there are complications, because often the person has few or mild symptoms.

Coronary artery disease is one of the leading causes of death in the United States. The primary cause is **atherosclerosis**, which is the development of plaques along the coronary arteries. The risk factors include family history, diabetes mellitus, cerebrovascular or peripheral vascular disease, smoking, high blood pressure, and high cholesterol levels.

Pregnant and Lactating Women

It is important to assess and counsel the pregnant woman regarding nutrition to promote a healthy pregnancy. Proper nutrition for the mother from the time of conception is required for the development of a healthy infant. The infant is at risk of being small for gestational age if the woman does not gain adequate weight, and the woman is at risk for gestational diabetes and hypertension if the weight gain is excessive. Target weight gain is dependent on the woman's weight at conception. The woman at IBW should gain 24 to 28 pounds. If she is more than 20% above IBW, she should gain 15 to 20 pounds, and 30 to 35 pounds if she is 10% under IBW. Assessment includes a general knowledge of physical changes and their relationships to nutrition. Some of the common complaints experienced during pregnancy (e.g., heartburn, constipation, nausea, and vomiting) can be alleviated by dietary changes such as small frequent meals, increased fluid intake, and a well-balanced diet.

Iron supplements are given routinely during pregnancy because diet alone is not adequate in meeting the requirements. Prenatal vitamins are usually prescribed for all pregnant women. There is evidence that folic acid helps to reduce the risk of neural tube defects, especially when the folic acid supplement is instituted 3 months prior to pregnancy. The U.S. Public Health Service recommends that all women of childbearing age consume 0.4 mg of folic acid per day. An additional 300 calories per day is recommended during pregnancy and an additional 500 calories per day during lactation. The Food Guide Pyramid does not specify any differences other than an increase in milk consumption, which increases both protein and caloric intake. Fluid intake is important and pregnant women are encouraged to drink 6 to 8 glasses of fluid daily (in the form of water, fruit juices, and milk). Lactating women need additional fluid intake and may need 2 to 3 quarts of fluid daily.

Pica, or cravings for substances other than food, is a phenomenon documented primarily in pregnant women. It is the practice of eating dirt, clay, starch, or even ice cubes, and may lead to nutritional difficulties, including an increased risk of anemia. Research is being conducted to ascertain the degree of health problems caused by pica, particularly in pregnant women.

✓ **NURSING CHECKLIST**
Nutritional Assessment of Pregnant Women

- What was your prepregnancy weight? (Take IBW from Table 7-9, page 174 to determine targeted pregnancy weight gain.)
- What is your activity level and are there any changes since you became pregnant?
- Do you take any supplemental vitamins?
- Do you have a history of problems during previous pregnancies? What were they? How were they resolved?
- How often do you use caffeine, artificial sweeteners, alcohol, cigarettes, or drugs (legal or illegal)?
- Do you experience constipation, nausea, vomiting, or heartburn?
- Do you have any food cravings?
- Do you have cravings for substances other than food?

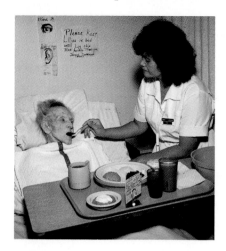

Figure 7-8 Older adults may have health problems that affect their ability to self-feed. *Courtesy of Delmar Publishers, Albany, NY*

Older Adults

Good eating habits and nutrition established early in life will benefit adults as they age, whereas poor eating habits may contribute to disease processes (e.g., hypertension, diabetes mellitus, CAD, and obesity). Caloric needs decrease as a person ages due to the reduction in basal metabolic rate. The Food Guide Pyramid may be used to assess and teach proper proportions, but modifications to the Food Guide Pyramid are needed to decrease portion size in conjunction with reduced activity and decreased caloric requirements. Planning with the patient to include modifications that are acceptable and providing education and support help to ensure compliance.

Possible problems that may be noted when assessing the elderly are difficulty chewing (oral problems), difficulty swallowing (possible stroke or Parkinson's disease), decreased appetite, decreased ability to feed self (see Figure 7-8), and decreased taste and smell. There is also a decreased emptying time of the esophagus, making the older adult more susceptible to aspiration. The older adult should eat in a sitting position to avoid aspiration. Constipation, due to a decrease in gastrointestinal motility, is a common problem that can be alleviated through adequate fluid intake and foods high in fiber. It is significant to note that one-third of hospitalized older adults as well as those in long-term care facilities experience protein calorie malnutrition (Jensen, 1996).

 NURSING TIP

Psychosocial Implications of Food

The psychosocial implications of food and eating cannot be stressed enough. Food elicits certain memories and feelings of when we were younger (e.g., the smell of mom's pie baking or the taste of Aunt Edna's cookies). It is also important to take into account other aspects of the nutritional history. If an older adult lives alone, there may be a problem obtaining food or preparing it; loneliness at mealtimes may also be a factor.

 NURSING CHECKLIST
Nutritional Assessment of Older Adults

- Do you have any physical limitations?
- Do you have any difficulty swallowing? (History of cerebrovascular accident, neuromuscular disorders?)
- Do you have any dental problems?
- Who buys and prepares the food?
- Do you eat alone or with someone?

CULTURAL DIFFERENCES

It is not possible to have knowledge of all cultural differences, but an open and understanding attitude and acceptance of various religious and cultural beliefs is imperative. Certain foods may have special meanings and memories for individual patients or may be traditional among many with the same cultural backgrounds (e.g., turkey for Thanksgiving). There may also be regional considerations, food preferences, and religious beliefs that restrict certain foods. An understanding of the food practices for various cultural groups is needed to provide appropriate nutritional assessment and education (see Figure 7-9). This is also helpful to establish rapport and individualize the

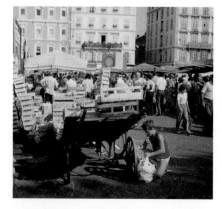

Figure 7-9 Cultural influences often affect food purchases.

nutritional plan. Be sure to inquire about various cultural and religious influences on dietary practices during the nutritional assessment; refer to Chapters 5 and 6 for a more in-depth discussion.

◎◎ THINK ABOUT IT

Culturally Based Nutritional Practices

- Your Islamic patient has been fasting during the ninth month of the Muhammadan year. He is diabetic and continues to become hypoglycemic. What would be your plan of care? How would you help him balance his religious and nutritional needs?
- LoAn is a pregnant Vietnamese female who is HIV-positive. She incorporates the observance of yin and yang into her daily rituals. LoAn confides that she is looking forward to breastfeeding her child. You realize that pregnancy is a "yang" condition and lactation is a "yin" condition, which is in line with LoAn's beliefs. What information would you discuss with LoAn, knowing that a female who is HIV-positive is advised against breastfeeding?

❖ HEALTH HISTORY

The nutritional history or subjective information gathered is one of the most significant aspects of the nutritional assessment. It gives an understanding of the patient's dietary habits and practices. Information about nutrition is gathered throughout the entire health history.

The nutritional health history provides insight into the link between a patient's lifestyle and nutritional information and pathology.

PATIENT PROFILE — *Diseases that are age- and sex-specific for nutrition are listed.*

Age — Anorexia nervosa (adolescents)
Bulimia nervosa (adolescents)

Sex

Female — Over 90% of patients with anorexia nervosa are female.

CHIEF COMPLAINT — *Common chief complaints for nutrition are defined and information on the characteristics of each sign and symptom is provided.*

Weight Gain — Number of pounds gained above usual weight

Associated Manifestations — Use of medications (corticosteroids), pregnancy, sedentary lifestyle, high-calorie, high-fat diet

Setting — Stress, depression, and negative body image

Weight Loss — Number of pounds lost below usual weight

Associated Manifestations — Nausea, vomiting, diarrhea, use of laxatives or diuretics, medication side effects, malabsorption diseases, diseases increasing demand of nutrients

Setting — Stress, depression, and negative body image

continued

PAST HEALTH HISTORY	*The various components of the past health history are linked with nutrition pathology and nutrition-related information.*
Medical	
Nutrition-Specific	Obesity, malnutrition, malabsorption, anorexia nervosa, bulimia nervosa, dysphagia, weight cycling, increased cholesterol level
Non–Nutrition-Specific	Diabetes mellitus, coronary artery disease, cerebrovascular accident, hypertension, cancer, diverticulosis, muscular dystrophy, multiple sclerosis, Parkinson's disease
Surgical	Gastric reduction (bypass or stapling), jaw wiring to reduce intake of food in morbid obesity, any surgical procedure that would alter food intake from postsurgical complications, nausea, or normal recovery
Medications	Review all medications for actual or potential side effects that may affect appetite or growth (antibiotics may cause gastrointestinal disturbances, Ritalin may cause anorexia, and long-term steroid use may affect linear growth).
Communicable Diseases	Children with AIDS: failure to thrive; adults with AIDS: wasting syndrome
Allergies	Gastrointestinal disturbances may occur with medication, food, and environmental allergies; infants may manifest allergies as dietary disturbances (milk intolerance)
Injuries and Accidents	Affect eating or the ability to self-feed, such as facial or mouth trauma; need for nasogastric tube feeding, gastrostomy
Disabilities and Handicaps	Affect ability to cut, handle, chew, or swallow food
Childhood Illnesses	Anorexia nervosa, bulimia nervosa, obesity, or malabsorption diseases (celiac disease, cystic fibrosis, hypoproteinemia)
FAMILY HEALTH HISTORY	*Nutritional diseases that are familial are listed.*
	Food intolerances, eating disorders, obesity, as well as any medical conditions that may contribute to nutritional problems (e.g., diabetes mellitus)
SOCIAL HISTORY	*The components of the social history are linked to nutritional factors and pathologies.*
Alcohol Use	Alcohol has very little nutrient value and abuse may lead to nutritional deficiencies. These include an inadequate intake of food, decreased sense of taste and smell, altered metabolism of nutrients (decreases storage and increases excretion of nutrients), and decreased absorption through intestinal mucosa. There is also an increased excretion of calcium with alcohol consumption that increases the risk of osteoporosis. In a pregnant woman, chronic alcohol consumption can lead to a low-birth-weight baby.
Tobacco Use	Smoking is associated with decreased estrogen levels in women, which increases their risk of osteoporosis. Tobacco is also an appetite suppressant that may stimulate weight gain when the person quits smoking. Tobacco may also alter the senses of taste and smell.

continued

Drug Use	Drug abuse alters nutrition due to the patient's increased dependence on the substance and decreased intake of proper nutrients. Many drugs alter food intake by causing anorexia (amphetamines) and decreasing sense of smell and taste (cocaine).
Travel History	Recent travel may cause problems with gastrointestinal disturbances. It may also temporarily change the normal dietary habits of the patient.
Hobbies and Leisure Activities	Food-related hobbies or food activities (gourmet cooking), or the amount of physical activity
Education	Education level may not necessarily translate into an adequate knowledge of nutritional needs.
Economic Status	Resources for purchase of adequate food
Religion	Refer to Chapter 6 for religious restrictions on diet.
Ethnic Background	Refer to Chapter 5 for ethnic considerations regarding diet.
HEALTH MAINTENANCE ACTIVITIES	*This information provides a bridge between health maintenance activities and nutritional function.*
Sleep	Stress increases when a patient is sleep deprived, which may contribute to nutritional problems.
Diet	The first question regarding nutrition should always be: "Do you have any concerns about your diet or eating?" Following the nutritional screening guidelines outlined in Table 7-6 is useful as an initial indicator of nutritional status. Refer to Table 7-7 for guidelines for a comprehensive assessment when nutritional problems are suspected.
Exercise	Patients with anorexia nervosa may exercise to excess.
Stress Management	Increasing or decreasing food consumption
Health Check-Ups	Cholesterol level results, last weight, height, and any other measurements

EQUIPMENT

- Wall-mounted unit (stadiometer), rod attached to the scale that has a right-angle headboard
- Tape measure
- Scale (preferably a balance-beam scale or electronic scale)
- Skinfold calipers (ideally one with a spring-loaded lever)

NUTRITIONAL ASSESSMENT

Table 7-7 illustrates a comprehensive nutritional assessment. It includes physical assessment, anthropometric measurements, laboratory data, and diagnostic data.

Table 7-6   Nutritional Screening

HISTORY

In the last 6–12 months:

- Have you experienced any change in weight?
- Has your appetite or dietary habits changed?
- Do you have any difficulty in feeding self, eating, chewing, or swallowing?
- Have you experienced any nausea, vomiting, or diarrhea?
- What are your food likes and dislikes?
- How do you prepare and store your food?
- Do you eat alone or with a family or group?
- Do you take any vitamins or supplements (liquid diets)?
- Do you follow a particular diet?
- Do you have any especially strong cravings?

Review 24-hour diet history:

Time	Food Eaten	Amount	Method of Preparation	Where Eaten

ASSESSMENT

Appearance of Patient

Height _____ feet & inches/cm

Weight _____ lb/kg

- Do you have any familial risk factors, such as obesity, high cholesterol, diabetes mellitus, hypertension, coronary artery disease, cerebrovascular disease, or cancer?
- What nutritional concerns would you like to discuss?

Table 7-7   Comprehensive Nutritional Assessment

Add information from nutritional screening (refer to Table 7-6)

PHYSICAL ASSESSMENT: REFER TO TABLE 7-8

ANTHROPOMETRIC MEASUREMENTS:

Height: _____ feet & inches/cm

Weight: _____ lb/kg

$$\% \text{ Ideal Body Weight} = \frac{\text{Current Weight}}{\text{IBW}^*} \times 100 = \text{_____}$$

*IBW obtained from Table 7-9

$$\% \text{ Usual Body Weight} = \frac{\text{Current Weight}}{\text{Usual Body Weight}} \times 100 = \text{_____}$$

$$\% \text{ Weight Change} = \frac{\text{Usual Weight} - \text{Current Weight}}{\text{Usual Weight}} \times 100 = \text{_____}$$

Triceps Skinfold (TSF) _____ mm

Mid-Arm Circumference (MAC) _____ cm

Mid-Arm Muscle Circumference (MAMC)

MAMC (cm) = MAC (cm) − [3.14 × TSF* (cm)] = _____

*The TSF is measured in mm. You will need to convert the TSF from mm to cm in order to calculate MAMC.

LABORATORY DATA

Hematocrit (HCT): _____ %

Hemoglobin (HGB): _____ g/dl

Cholesterol: _____ mg/dl   HDL: _____ mg/dl   LDL: _____ mg/dl

Triglycerides: _____ mg/dl

TIBC: _____ µg/dl

Transferrin (0.8 × TIBC) − 43 = _____ mg/dl

Iron: _____ µg/dl

Total Lymphocyte Count: _____ cells/mm³

Antigen Skin Testing: _____

Albumin: _____ g/dl

Glucose: _____ mg/dl

$$\% \text{CHI} = \frac{\text{Actual 24-hr Creatinine Excretion}}{\text{Ideal 24-hr Creatinine Excretion}} \times 100 = \text{_____}$$

$$\text{Nitrogen Balance} = \frac{\text{Grams Protein Eaten}}{6.25} - (\text{UUN}^* + 4) = \text{_____} \text{ g}$$

*UUN = 24-hr urine urea nitrogen (in g)

DIAGNOSTIC DATA

X-rays _____

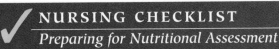

Preparing for Nutritional Assessment

1. Explain all procedures to patients and/or family members.
2. Ask patient to remove shoes prior to height measurement.
3. Have older children or adults remove heavy clothing (an adult may wear a hospital gown).
4. Between patients, place clean paper on scale.
5. Explain and review results with patient and/or family.

NURSING TIP

Interpreting Anthropometric Measurements

It is important to interpret anthropometric, laboratory, and diagnostic data collectively. One abnormal result does not provide sufficient evidence to diagnose malnutrition. Deficiencies and toxicities usually occur in more than one assessment area. Monitor the results of the nutritional assessment and observe trends that occur.

PHYSICAL ASSESSMENT

Certain physical signs may indicate poor nutrition. Refer to Table 7-8 for a list of signs and symptoms of poor nutritional status.

Anthropometric Measurements

Anthropometric measurements are the various measurements of the human body, including height, weight, and body proportions. They measure growth patterns in children and changes in nutritional status in adults.

Table 7-8 Physical Signs and Symptoms of Poor Nutritional Status

	SUBJECTIVE	OBJECTIVE
1. General appearance	Fatigue, poor sleep, change in weight, frequent infections	Dull affect, apathetic, increased weight, decreased weight
2. Skin	Pruritus, swelling, delayed wound healing	Dry, rough, scaling, flaky, edema, lesions, decreased turgor, changes in color (pallor, jaundice), petechiae, ecchymoses, xanthomas (slightly elevated yellow nodules)
3. Nails	Brittle	Dry, splinter hemorrhages, spoon-shaped, pale
4. Hair	Easily falls out, brittle	Less shiny, dry, changes in color pigment
5. Eyes	Vision changes, night blindness, eye discharge	Hardening and scaling of cornea, conjunctiva pale or red
6. Mouth	Mouth sores	Lips: cracked, dry, swollen, fissures around corners
		Gums: recessed, swollen, bleeding, spongy
		Tongue: smooth, beefy red, magenta, pale, fissures, sores, increased or decreased in size, increased or decreased papillae
		Teeth: missing, caries
7. Head and neck	Headaches, decreased hearing	Xanthelasma, irritation and crusting of nares, swollen cheeks (parotid gland enlargement), goiter
8. Heart and peripheral vasculature	Palpitations, swelling	Cardiac enlargement, changes in blood pressure, tachycardia, heart murmur, edema
9. Abdomen	Tender, changes in appetite, nausea, changes in bowel habits	Edema, hepatosplenomegaly
10. Musculoskeletal system	Weakness, pain, cramping, frequent fractures	Muscle tone is decreased, flabby muscles, bowing of lower extremities
11. Neurological system	Irritable, changes in mood, numbness, paresthesia	Slurred speech, unsteady gait, tremors, decreased deep tendon reflexes, loss of position and vibratory sense, paresthesia, decreased coordination
12. Female genitalia	Changes in menstrual pattern	None

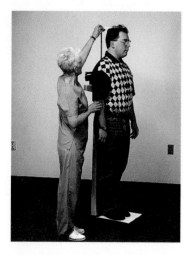

Figure 7-10 Measuring Patient Height

Table 7-9	Adult Growth Chart*	
	METROPOLITAN 1983 WEIGHTS	
HEIGHT	**FOR AGES 25–59†**	
	Men	Women
ft-in	*lb*	*lb*
4-10	—	100–131
4-11	—	101–134
5-0	—	103–137
5-1	123–145	105–140
5-2	125–148	108–144
5-3	127–151	111–148
5-4	129–155	114–152
5-5	131–159	117–156
5-6	133–163	120–160
5-7	135–167	123–164
5-8	137–171	126–167
5-9	139–175	129–170
5-10	141–179	132–173
5-11	144–183	135–176
6-0	147–187	—
6-1	150–192	—
6-2	153–197	—
6-3	157–202	—
6-4	—	—

*Values in this table are for height without shoes and weight without clothes. To convert inches to centimeters, multiply by 2.54; to convert pounds to kilograms, multiply by 0.455

†The weight range is the lower weight for small frame and the upper weight for large frame.

Reproduced courtesy of Metropolitan Life Insurance Company

E	**Examination**
N	**Normal Findings**
A	**Abnormal Findings**
P	**Pathophysiology**

Measurements are easily obtained and can assist in an objective assessment that can be compared over time. Standardized charts should be used to compare the specific measurements with expected norms.

Height

A standing height is obtained for patients 3 years and older (see Figure 7-10).

E   **1.** Have the patient stand erect with back and heels against the wall or measuring device.
     2. Place the headboard at a right angle to the wall and along the crown of the patient's head.
     3. Record height to the nearest one-eighth inch or 1 mm.

N   *Compare to standardized growth charts. Bear in mind that patients will reflect familial growth patterns (refer to Table 7-9).*

A   Insufficient growth is abnormal.

P   Chronic malnutrition may result in a decrease in height because the body does not have the nutrients necessary for proper growth.

A   Excessive growth is abnormal.

P   Hormone abnormalities may cause excessive growth, as in acromegaly, giantism, and precocious puberty.

P   Genetic and metabolic syndromes that affect growth are Marfan's syndrome and Klinefelter's syndrome.

🌿 NURSING TIP

Measuring Height of the Bedridden Patient

When a patient is bedridden or immobile, measure recumbent length with a rod or yardstick.

Weight

E   **1.** Have patient stand on scale, facing weights (see Figure 7-11).
     2. Slide weight until balanced.
     3. Read and record to the nearest 100 g or one-quarter lb (10 g or one-half oz for infants).
     4. Calculate percentage of ideal body weight.
     5. Calculate the percentage of usual body weight.
     6. Calculate the percentage of weight change.

N   *Compare to standardized growth charts (refer to Table 7-9).*

A   Obesity is abnormal. Mild obesity occurs when the patient is 20%–40% above the IBW; moderate obesity occurs when the patient is 40%–100% above the IBW; and morbid obesity occurs when a patient is more than 100% above the IBW.

P   Obesity occurs when there is excess body fat because of increased food intake, decreased activity level, or both.

P   Some medications may contribute to weight gain (e.g., steroids).

P   Some disease processes may contribute to weight gain, such as hypothyroidism (decreased metabolic rate).

P   Genetics may influence weight gain.

A   A weight under 90% of IBW is termed undernutrition. A weight between 80% and 90% of the IBW is mild undernutrition, between 70% and 80% is moderate undernutrition, and below 70% is severe undernutrition.

P   Decreased food intake may occur with HIV, dental problems, depression, medications, alcoholism, anorexia nervosa, and poverty.

P   Inadequate nutrition may occur with impaired absorption, as present in malabsorption diseases (e.g., celiac disease), AIDS, and small bowel disease.

P   There may be a loss of nutrients with diarrhea, vomiting, and diabetes mellitus.

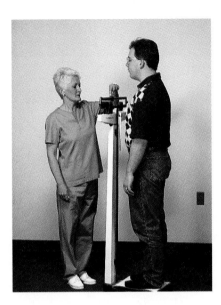

Figure 7-11 Measuring Patient Weight

P Increased demand for nutrients may be present in malignancies, fever, and hyperthyroidism. This increased demand may account for the weight loss that occurs early in cancer even when calories are not decreased. If this continues, the patient exhibits signs of extreme malnutrition and wasting, which is called **cachexia**.

Skinfold Thickness

Skinfold thickness (refer to Figure 7-12) is used to determine body fat stores and nutritional status. It is a more reliable indicator of body fat than is weight, because more than half of the body's total fat is located in the subcutaneous tissue. The most common measurement site is the **triceps skinfold** (TSF). Measurements can also be performed in subscapular and suprailiac skinfolds.

E
1. Place the patient in a sitting or standing position.
2. Take the measurements on the nondominant arm, with the patient in a relaxed position.
3. Make a mark on the posterior portion of the upper arm midway between the acromion process and the olecranon process.
4. Using your nondominant hand, grasp the skin and pull it free from the muscle.
5. Apply the caliper with your dominant hand and align the markers.
6. Note the measurement to the nearest 0.5 mm.
7. Release the skin and repeat two or three times.
8. Average the findings to determine the TSF.

N *Refer to Table 7-10. Normal measurements fall between the 5th and 95th percentiles.*

A/P Refer to page 176.

Mid-Arm and Mid-Arm Muscle Circumferences

The **mid-arm circumference (MAC)** provides information on skeletal muscle mass. This measurement alone is not of great significance but it is used to calculate the **mid-arm muscle circumference (MAMC)**.

E
1. Instruct patient to flex the arm.
2. Measure the circumference of the upper arm (MAC) midway between the acromion process and the olecranon process.
3. Calculate MAMC (refer to Table 7-7).

E	**Examination**
N	**Normal Findings**
A	**Abnormal Findings**
P	**Pathophysiology**

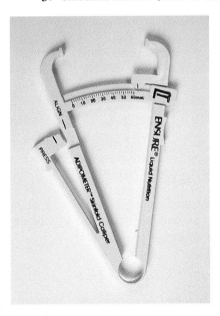

A. Skinfold Caliper

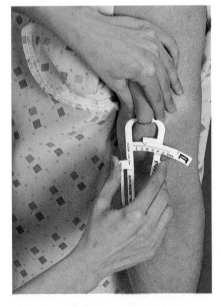

B. Measuring Triceps Skinfold

Figure 7-12 Skinfold Thickness

Table 7-10 Triceps Skinfold Percentiles†

TRICEPS SKINFOLD PERCENTILES (MM²)

Age (yr)	Males n	5	10	25	50	75	90	95	Females n	5	10	25	50	75	90	95
1–1.9	228	6	7	8	10	12	14	16	204	6	7	8	10	12	14	16
2–2.9	223	6	7	8	10	12	14	15	208	6	8	9	10	12	15	16
3–3.9	220	6	7	8	10	11	14	15	208	7	8	9	11	12	14	15
4–4.9	230	6	6	8	9	11	12	14	208	7	8	8	10	12	14	16
5–5.9	214	6	6	8	9	11	14	15	219	6	7	8	10	12	15	18
6–6.9	117	5	6	7	8	10	13	16	118	6	6	8	10	12	14	16
7–7.9	122	5	6	7	9	12	15	17	126	6	7	9	11	13	16	18
8–8.9	117	5	6	7	8	10	13	16	118	6	8	9	12	15	18	24
9–9.9	121	6	6	7	10	13	17	18	125	8	8	10	13	16	20	22
10–10.9	146	6	6	8	10	14	18	21	152	7	8	10	12	17	23	27
11–11.9	122	6	6	8	11	16	20	24	117	7	8	10	13	18	24	28
12–12.9	153	6	6	8	11	14	22	28	129	8	9	11	14	18	23	27
13–13.9	134	5	5	7	10	14	22	26	151	8	8	12	15	21	26	30
14–14.9	131	4	5	7	9	14	21	24	141	9	10	13	16	21	26	28
15–15.9	128	4	5	6	8	11	18	24	117	8	10	12	17	21	25	32
16–16.9	131	4	5	6	8	12	16	22	142	10	12	15	18	22	26	31
17–17.9	133	5	5	6	8	12	16	19	114	10	12	13	19	24	30	37
18–18.9	91	4	5	6	9	13	20	24	109	10	12	15	18	22	26	30
19–24.9	531	4	5	7	10	15	20	22	1,060	10	11	14	18	24	30	34
25–34.9	971	5	6	8	12	16	20	24	1,987	10	12	16	21	27	34	37
35–44.9	806	5	6	8	12	16	20	23	1,614	12	14	18	23	29	35	38
45–54.9	898	6	6	8	12	15	20	25	1,047	12	16	20	25	30	36	40
55–64.9	734	5	6	8	11	14	19	22	809	12	16	20	25	31	36	38
65–74.9	1,503	4	6	8	11	15	19	22	1,670	12	14	18	24	29	34	36

†The Lange caliper was used in these studies.

Reprinted with permission from Frisancho, A.R. (1981). American Journal of Clinical Nutrition, 34, 2540, American Society for Clinical Nutrition.

🌹 NURSING TIP

Differentiating Marasmus and Kwashiorkor

Marasmus
- Decreased TSF, MAC
- Decreased weight
- Visceral proteins (albumin) within normal limits or decreased
- Immune function within normal limits

Kwashiorkor
- TSF, MAC within normal limits
- Weight possibly within normal limits
- Decreased visceral proteins
- Decreased immune function

E	Examination
N	Normal Findings
A	Abnormal Findings
P	Pathophysiology

N Refer to Table 7-11. Normal measurements fall between the 5th and 95th percentiles.

A Results less than the 5th percentile on the standard charts are abnormal.

P Possible malnutrition is present when the protein stores are diminished in the muscle. This is seen in disease processes such as AIDS, cancer, and chronic illnesses.

A Results greater than the 95th percentile on the standard charts are abnormal.

P Obesity is suggested.

P If edema is present on the assessed body parts, the measurement may not be a reliable indicator of nutritional status.

Laboratory Data

Laboratory analysis is used for screening for potential nutritional problems and to assist with diagnosis when problems are suspected after a thorough history and a physical are conducted.

Hematocrit and Hemoglobin

Hematocrit determines the percentage of red cells to volume of whole blood. It reflects the body's iron supply. **Hemoglobin** is the iron component of the blood that transports oxygen. Both values are obtained from a venous blood sample.

Table 7-11 MAC and MAMC Percentiles†

Age (yr)	ARM CIRCUMFERENCE (mm)						ARM MUSCLE CIRCUMFERENCE (mm)					
	5th	50th	95th	5th	50th	95th	5th	50th	95th	5th	50th	95th
	Males			Females			Males			Females		
1–1.9	142	159	183	138	156	177	110	127	147	105	124	143
2–2.9	141	162	185	142	160	184	111	130	150	111	126	147
3–3.9	150	167	190	143	167	189	117	137	153	113	132	152
4–4.9	149	171	192	149	169	191	123	141	159	115	136	157
5–5.9	153	175	204	153	175	211	128	147	169	125	142	165
6–6.9	155	179	228	156	176	211	131	151	177	130	145	171
7–7.9	162	187	230	164	183	231	137	160	190	129	151	176
8–8.9	162	190	245	168	195	261	140	162	187	138	160	194
9–9.9	175	200	257	178	211	260	151	170	202	147	167	198
10–10.9	181	210	274	174	210	265	156	180	221	148	170	197
11–11.9	186	223	280	185	224	303	159	183	230	150	181	223
12–12.9	193	232	303	194	237	294	167	195	241	162	191	220
13–13.9	194	247	301	202	243	338	172	211	245	169	198	240
14–14.9	220	253	322	214	252	322	189	223	264	174	201	247
15–15.9	222	264	320	208	254	322	199	237	272	175	202	244
16–16.9	244	278	343	218	258	334	213	249	296	170	202	249
17–17.9	246	285	347	220	264	350	224	258	312	175	205	257
18–18.9	245	297	379	222	258	325	226	264	324	174	202	245
19–24.9	262	308	372	221	265	345	238	273	321	179	207	249
25–34.9	271	319	375	233	277	368	243	279	326	183	212	264
35–44.9	278	326	374	241	290	378	247	286	327	186	218	272
45–54.9	267	322	376	242	299	384	239	281	326	187	220	274
55–64.9	258	317	369	243	303	385	236	278	320	187	225	280
65–74.9	248	307	355	240	299	373	223	268	306	185	225	279

†The Lange caliper was used in these studies.

Reprinted with permission from Frisancho, A.R. (1981). American Journal of Clinical Nutrition, 34, 2540, American Society for Clinical Nutrition.

Table 7-12 Normal Values for Hematocrit and Hemoglobin

Age	NORMAL VALUES	
	Hematocrit (%)	Hemoglobin g/dl
1 mo	33–55	10.7–17.1
12 mo	33–41	11.3–14.1
1–2 yr	32–40	11.0–14.0
12–14 yr		
Female	34–44	11.5–15.0
Male	35–45	12.0–16.0
18–44 yr		
Female	35–45	12.0–15.0
Male	39–49	13.0–17.0
45–64 yr		
Female	35–47	12.0–16.0
Male	39–50	13.0–17.0
65–74 yr		
Female	35–47	12.0–16.0
Male	37–51	13.0–17.0

N *Hemoglobin and hematocrit results should fall within expected values as shown in Table 7-12. Increased hematocrit and hemoglobin may normally occur with people living in high altitudes due to the decrease in partial pressure of oxygen in those areas.*

A Decreased hematocrit and hemoglobin are abnormal.

P Moderate to severe anemia may indicate leukemia, cirrhosis, hyperthyroidism, hemorrhage, hemodilution, or hemolytic reactions.

A Increased hematocrit and hemoglobin are abnormal.

P Severe dehydration may result from hemoconcentration.

Cholesterol and Triglycerides

Cholesterol and triglyceride levels are both obtained from a venous blood sample.

N *Normal levels of cholesterol are:*

Desirable range: Adults: 140–220 mg/dl
Children: 70–175 mg/dl

High-density lipoproteins (HDL): Women: 38–85 mg/dl
Men: 35–70 mg/dl
Children: 30–65 mg/dl

Low-density lipoproteins (LDL): <130 mg/dl: within the desirable range
130–159 mg/dl: borderline high risk
>160 mg/dl: high risk

Triglycerides: Women: 35–135 mg/dl
Men: 40–150 mg/dl
Children: 30–138 mg/dl

A Elevated cholesterol, LDL, and triglycerides above desirable range are abnormal. HDL less than 35 mg/dl is abnormal in adults.

P Elevated cholesterol and/or triglycerides can be due to increased fat intake, genetics, and some medications (e.g., cyclosporin).

Transferrin, Total Iron-Binding Capacity (TIBC), and Iron

Transferrin is a protein that regulates iron absorption. Transferrin can be measured by the **total iron-binding capacity (TIBC)** (the amount of iron with which it can bind). **Serum iron** is the amount of transferrin-bound iron. These data are obtained from a venous blood sample.

N *Normal adult levels are:*
Transferrin: 170–250 mg/dl
TIBC: 240–450 μg/dl
Serum iron (women): 65–165 μg/dl
Serum iron (men): 75–175 μg/dl

A An increase in transferrin is abnormal.

P Increased levels of transferrin are found in inadequate dietary iron, iron-deficiency anemia, hepatitis, and oral contraceptive use.

A Decreased levels of transferrin are abnormal.

P Decreased levels of transferrin are found in pernicious anemia, sickle cell anemia, anemia associated with infection or chronic diseases, cancer, and malnutrition.

A Increases in serum iron levels are abnormal.

P Increases in serum iron levels are found in hemolytic anemias and lead poisoning.

A Decreases in serum iron levels are abnormal.

P Decreases in serum iron levels are found in iron deficiency, chronic diseases, third-trimester pregnancy, and severe physiological stress.

Total Lymphocyte Count

Total lymphocyte count (TLC) is measured in the complete blood count with differential and measures immune function and visceral protein status. When the white blood cell count is abnormally elevated or decreased, such as in bacterial infections or AIDS, respectively, the TLC is not always a reliable indicator of nutritional status.

N *Normal adult levels are 1500–1800 cells/mm³.*

A A decrease in the total lymphocyte count of less than 1500 indicates moderate protein deficiency, while less than 900 indicates severe protein deficiency.

P Protein deficiency occurs when the body is malnourished, such as when a patient is immunocompromised.

Antigen Skin Testing

Antigen skin testing is another test of immune function. Intradermal injections of various antigens can be used. Antigens commonly used are PPD tuberculin skin tests, mumps virus, *Candida albicans*, streptokinase, *Streptococcus*, and tetanus toxoid. Results are read at 24 and 48 hours postinjection.

N *A negative skin reaction after being tested with various antigens is normal. These are antigens to which most people have been exposed and have developed an antibody response.*

A A positive reaction to antigens placed intradermally is abnormal, which is indicated by a red area 5 mm or more around the test site 24 hours or more after the injection. A negative reaction to only one of the antigens tested or a delayed positive reaction may occur with malnutrition.

P Poor antibody response occurs in patients who are immunocompromised. They have a decreased ability to fight infection and build antibodies. Protein malnutrition has been shown to decrease immune function. This diminished reaction to antigens is called **anergy**. Antigen skin testing is often called anergy panels.

Albumin

Albumin is formed in the liver. It transports nutrients, blood, and hormones, and helps maintain osmotic pressure. Albumin must have functioning liver cells and an adequate amount of amino acids to be synthesized. It is an indicator of visceral protein status. Because albumin has a long half-life (about 20 days), it is not an indicator that detects subtle or early changes in nutritional status. It is measured from a venous blood sample.

N *The normal range for serum albumin is 3.5 to 5.0 g/dl.*

A Less than 3.5 g/dl is abnormal.

P Decreased levels of albumin may indicate malnutrition because of a decrease in visceral protein stores, or a decrease in the amount of protein stored in organs. The decrease may not be seen until the protein deficiency reaches a chronic stage.

P Decreased levels of albumin are also found in massive hemorrhage, burns, and kidney disease.

Glucose

Serum glucose tests the body's ability to metabolize glucose. It is best assessed after a fasting period and from a venous blood sample.

N *The normal glucose levels are:*

Adult:	*Fasting serum:*	*70–110 mg/dl*
	Nonfasting:	*85–125 mg/dl*
Child:		*60–100 mg/dl*

A An increase in glucose level is abnormal.

P **Hyperglycemia** occurs in diabetes mellitus, impaired glucose tolerance, vitamin B_1 deficiency, and convulsive states. This indicates that glucose is not being transported into the cells by insulin.

A A decrease in serum glucose level is abnormal.

P **Hypoglycemia** occurs in pancreatic disorders, liver disease, and insulin overdose. This occurs when there is too much insulin and not enough glucose in the blood.

Creatinine Height Index (CHI)

Creatinine is a substance normally excreted in the urine; it is dependent on the amount of skeletal muscle mass and it measures the amount of protein reserves. Urine creatinine is tested after collecting a 24-hour urine sample. An ideal urine creatinine level by height table is used to establish the denominator in the equation used to calculate CHI.

N *Normal CHI values are greater than 90%.*

A CHI between 80% and 90% indicates mild protein deficiency.
CHI between 70% and 80% indicates moderate protein deficiency.
CHI of less than 70% indicates severe protein deficiency.

P Protein malnutrition may be indicated by the loss of lean body mass as can occur in severe trauma, prolonged fever, and stress.

Nitrogen Balance

Nitrogen is usually taken into the body in the form of food protein sources. It is one of the compounds of amino acids. Nitrogen is incorporated into protein and excreted in urine and feces. This balance of intake of nitrogen to output of nitrogen is compared, usually with a 24-hour urine sample.

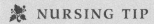

NURSING TIP

Accurate Urine Tests

Urine samples for CHI and nitrogen balance require the observance of strict collection procedures. Check your institution's procedure manual to ensure accuracy of the 24-hour samples.

E	**Examination**
N	**Normal Findings**
A	**Abnormal Findings**
P	**Pathophysiology**

N *A zero balance is normal. A positive balance indicates tissue formation, found in growing children and in pregnant women.*

A A negative nitrogen balance is abnormal and indicates a catabolic state (the body excretes more nitrogen than is consumed).

P More nitrogen is excreted than taken in, which means there is destruction or wasting of tissue. This can occur in malnutrition and in catabolic states (burns, severe stress, trauma, surgery).

Diagnostic Data

E Examination
N Normal Findings
A Abnormal Findings
P Pathophysiology

Radiographic studies are used to determine bone formation and to assess development. Rickets and scurvy are both examples of long-term nutritional deficiencies that have radiographic manifestations. Rickets is a deficiency of vitamin D, and scurvy is a deficiency of vitamin C; both are characterized by softening and deformities of the bones. Osteoporosis, which can be linked to nutrition, can show up on x-rays as a decrease in bone density.

CASE STUDY

The case study illustrates the application and objective documentation of the nutritional assessment.

The Patient with Anorexia Nervosa

Karen came to the student health clinic at the university she attends because she has not had a menstrual period for 6 months. She was encouraged to come by her parents, but she feels this is not necessary. There are no previous records except her school admission history and physical, which was completed 2 years ago. There is no information on that history except her immunization status.

❖ HEALTH HISTORY

PATIENT PROFILE	21 yo SWF
CHIEF COMPLAINT	"I haven't had a period for 6 mo."
HISTORY OF PRESENT ILLNESS	Pt states she is here only b/c her parents insisted. Uses enemas or suppositories q 4–5 d; Ø menses × 6 mo.; previously q 28 d, 1–2 d in duration. Pt states she is very healthy & has no other hl problems x̄ frequent constipation.
PAST HEALTH HISTORY	
Medical	Seen 3 yr PTA for problem c̄ "wt loss" but she says "there are no problems now."
Surgical	Tonsillectomy 12 yo; Ø complications
Medications	Laxatives, enemas q 4–5 d for constipation
Communicable Diseases	Denies
Allergies	No known medication or food allergies Has seasonal allergic rx during spring when pollen count is ↑; tx c̄ seldane
Injuries and Accidents	Denies
Disabilities or Handicaps	Denies

Blood Transfusions	Denies
Childhood Illnesses	Overwt in early adolescence; family was very concerned & made her follow a strict diet; would not say how many lb overwt; was not addressed as a problem by her pediatrician.
Immunizations	Last dT & MMR: 15 yo

FAMILY HEALTH HISTORY

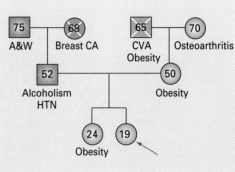

LEGEND

- ⬤ Living female
- ⬛ Living male
- ⊗ Deceased female
- ⊠ Deceased male
- ╱ Points to patient

A&W = Alive & well
CA = Cancer
CVA = Cerebrovascular accident
HTN = Hypertension

Denies family hx of food intolerances.

SOCIAL HISTORY	
Alcohol Use	Denies
Tobacco Use	Denies
Drug Use	Denies
Sexual Practice	Heterosexual: Ø sexual intercourse × 2 yr
Travel History	No recent travels
Work Environment	Not currently employed (student)
Home Environment	Living in dorm (suite of 4 rooms adjoining a living area); shares room c̄ roommate; has a small hot plate & refrigerator
Hobbies and Leisure Activities	Likes to cook gourmet meals
Stress	Occurs when she feels she doesn't have enough time to exercise
Education	Junior at university majoring in geology
Economic Status	Full college scholarship
Military Status	None
Religion	No organized religious affiliation
Ethnic Background	Denies any specific ethnic background

continued

Roles/Relationships	Has no boyfriend at present, & dates infrequently; has several friends but not one close friend; describes her relationship c̄ her parents as "strained," refuses to elaborate.
Characteristic Patterns of Daily Living	Pt feels school causes a very hectic lifestyle & has a hard time getting into a routine. Gets up at 6 AM to exercise ā 8 AM class. Keeps routine even on weekends and holidays; p̄ class all day, has quick meal in her room before studying either in her room or library; occasionally goes to a movie c̄ roommates. Bedtime between MN to 2 AM.

HEALTH MAINTENANCE ACTIVITIES

Sleep	Erratic sleep & rest schedule due to school work; averages 4 hr, feels this is enough.
Diet	Very knowledgeable about nutrition & writes down everything she eats to maintain her diet. Likes to prepare her own meals & refuses to eat in the university cafeteria b/c food is "too fatty." Likes to prepare gourmet meals for roommates; does her own shopping & rarely eats out at restaurants.

24-hour diet recall:

Food	Amount	Prepared	Comments
Dry toast	1 slice		Eaten while walking
Coffee	1 cup	Black	
Salad	Small bowl	No dressing	Eaten in dorm by self
Diet soda	1 can		

Didn't eat dinner b/c "was too busy."
Feels her wt is fine but she would like to lose a couple of more lb to be perfect.

Exercise	1½–2 hr qd; stationary bike & step aerobics.
Stress Management	Feels she handles stress very well. Exercise helps to keep her in control. Feels she organizes her work well & this ↓ stress from her studies.
Use of Safety Devices	Always wears safety belt.
Health Check-Ups	Last seen 2 yr ago for school physical.

NUTRITIONAL ASSESSMENT

Physical Assessment

	Subjective	Objective
1. General appearance	Feels she needs to lose wt	Very thin in appearance; slightly flat affect
2. Skin	Pruritus × 2 mo	Pale & dry
3. Nails	Break easily	Pale
4. Hair	None	Dry, ↓ shine
5. Eyes	No d/c	Conjunctiva pink
6. Mouth	Denies sores	Dried, cracked lips, small fissures along corners of mouth

continued

	Subjective	Objective
7. Head and neck	Occasional H/A	Gross hearing intact, clear nasal d/c, nares patent c̄ mild erythema
8. Heart and peripheral vasculature	Palpitations when exercising	HR: 100, rhythm regular, Ø murmur
9. Abdomen	Frequent constipation	Flat, firm, s̄ masses, Ø organomegaly
10. Musculoskeletal system	Leg cramps c̄ exercising	Muscles weak & flabby
11. Neurological system	None	Steady gait, alert, irritable during interview, ↓ sensation lower extremities, reflexes WNL
12. Genitalia	LMP 6 mo ago, see hx	

Anthropometric Measurements

Height: 66 inches
Weight: 100 lbs
%IBW: $\dfrac{100}{120} \times 100 = 83\%$
TSF: 14 mm
MAC: 23 cm
MAMC: 23 cm − (3.14 × 0.14) = 22.6

Laboratory Data

Hct: 33%
Hgb: 11 g/dl
TIBC: 220 µg/dl
Transferrin: (0.8 × 220) − 43 = 133 mg/dl
TLC: 1.5–3.0 k/mm³
Further laboratory tests not available in school health clinic.

✓ NURSING CHECKLIST
Nutritional Assessment

Physical Assessment (Refer to Table 7-8)
Anthropometric Measurements
- Height
- Weight
- Skinfold Thickness
- Mid-Arm and Mid-Arm Muscle Circumference

Laboratory Data
- Hematocrit/Hemoglobin
- Cholesterol and Triglycerides
- Transferrin, Total Iron-Binding Capacity, and Iron
- Total Lymphocyte Count
- Antigen Skin Testing
- Albumin
- Glucose
- Creatinine Height Index
- Nitrogen Balance

Diagnostic Data

REVIEW QUESTIONS
AND ACTIVITIES

1. Name the food group divisions of the Food Guide Pyramid. In what order do they occur? Use the Food Guide Pyramid to evaluate what you ate yesterday.

2. Which is the "good" cholesterol that helps decrease the risk of coronary artery disease?
   a. LDL
   b. HDL
   c. Triglycerides
   d. None of the above
   The correct answer is (b).

3. Identify five macrominerals and microminerals, their functions, and the results of mineral deficiency or toxicity.

4. Why is it important not to put an infant to bed with a bottle?

5. What is the significance of anthropometric measurements?

6. Plan a 24-hour menu for an adolescent female.

7. Several high-risk factors may indicate the need for further nutritional assessment. Name at least four high-risk health problems.

Questions 8–10 refer to the following situation:

Tattiana is a 42-year-old, slightly overweight (HT 65 in, WT 159 lb) woman being seen in your clinic for the first time. She is being seen for a routine check-up. She leads a sedentary lifestyle and lives alone with her dog.

8. What are some specific diseases for which Tattiana may be at risk and that should be addressed when discussing nutrition?
   a. Osteoporosis
   b. Coronary artery disease
   c. Diabetes mellitus
   d. All of the above
   The correct answer is (d).

9. What specific changes in lifestyle may be beneficial for Tattiana?
   a. Taking up new, challenging sports
   b. Losing weight quickly
   c. Increasing walks with the dog
   d. Decreasing calcium intake
   The correct answer is (c).

10. Tattiana tells you that her weight was consistently the same for 3 years until 6 months ago when she lost 11 lb. What is her % weight change?
    a. 94%
    b. 107%
    c. 6.5%
    d. 6.9%
    The correct answer is (c).

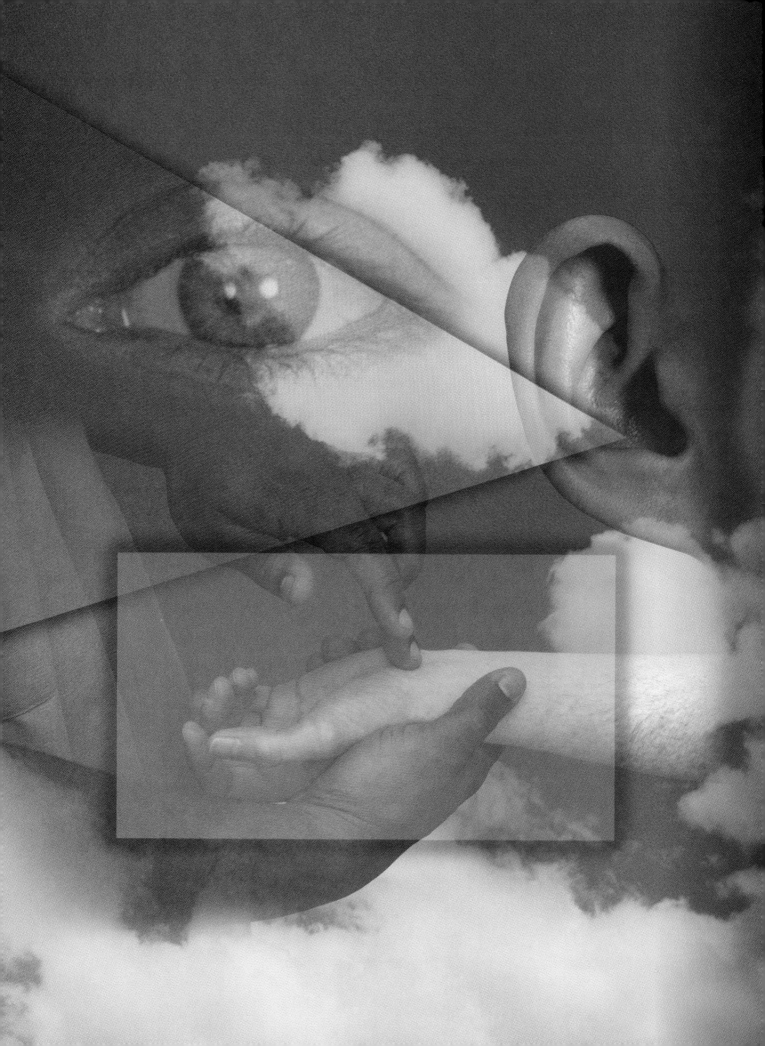

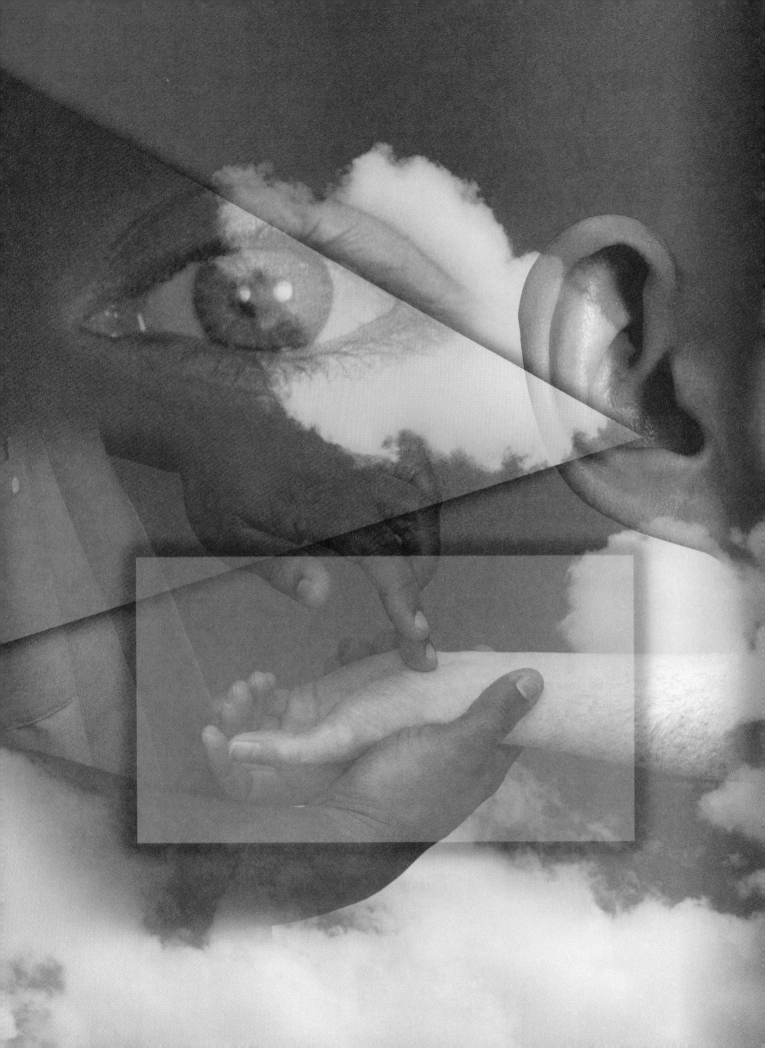

Physical Assessment

UNIT III

There are a great many observations, of such importance both physiologically and practically, which might be made by nurses, if they were educated to observation, and indeed, can only be made by nurses.

Florence Nightingale

Physical Assessment Techniques

1. Describe how to maintain standard precautions during the physical assessment.
2. Describe how to perform inspection, palpation, percussion, and auscultation, and which areas of the body are assessed with each technique.
3. Establish an environment suitable for conducting a physical assessment.
4. Demonstrate inspection, palpation, percussion, and auscultation in the clinical setting.

Inspection, palpation, percussion, and auscultation are the techniques used by the nurse to assess the patient during a physical examination. This chapter introduces the assessment techniques and equipment used to conduct physical examinations.

ASPECTS OF PHYSICAL ASSESSMENT

Physical assessment of a patient serves many purposes:

1. Validation of the complaints that brought the patient to seek health care.
2. Screening of general well-being. The findings will serve as baseline information for future assessments.
3. Monitoring of current health problems.
4. Formulation of diagnoses and treatments.

The need for physical assessment depends on, among other factors, the patient's health status, concept of health care, and accessibility to health care. For example, a brittle diabetic with arthritis and glaucoma who has access to health care is likely to enter the health care delivery system more often than a healthy college student.

Role of the Nurse

The professional nurse plays a vital role in the physical assessment of patients. Educational preparation and clinical experience in part determine the extent to which the nurse participates in the assessment process. For example, a nurse in primary care may perform physical assessments of patients for all of the reasons mentioned previously, while a critical care nurse may conduct patient assessments only to monitor and treat current health problems. In either case, nurses are expected to be familiar with and comfortable using physical assessment skills. Today's nurses are sophisticated professionals who require information in order to make clinical decisions. The physical assessment findings provide this information.

Standard Precautions

The transmission of hepatitis, human immunodeficiency virus (HIV), and other infectious diseases is a primary concern for you and for the patient. **Standard precautions**, formerly known as universal precautions, were developed by the Centers for Disease Control and Prevention (CDC) to protect health care professionals and patients. The primary goal of standard precautions is to prevent the exchange of blood and body fluids. Standard precautions should be practiced with every patient throughout the entire encounter. Figure 8-1 illustrates the standard precautions recommended by the CDC.

❖ ASK YOURSELF

Self-Evaluation of Standard Precaution Practices

Think back to the last day that you worked in the clinical setting.

- Did you consistently use standard precautions?
- If not, what was the occasion when you did not use standard precautions? What factors influenced this decision? What are the short-term ramifications of this decision? Long-term consequences?

⚡ NURSING ALERT

Latex Allergies

In accordance with standard precautions, nurses frequently use gloves when dealing with patients' body fluids. Be alert to the possibility that you, as well as your patients, may have latex allergies. Reactions range from eczematous contact dermatitis to anaphylactic shock. Ask patients if they have any known allergy to latex products prior to touching patients while wearing latex gloves.

STANDARD PRECAUTIONS

FOR INFECTION CONTROL

Wash Hands (Plain soap)
Wash after touching **blood**, **body fluids**, **secretions**, **excretions**, and **contaminated items**.
Wash immediately **after gloves are removed** and **between patient contacts**.
Avoid transfer of microorganisms to other patients or environments.

Wear Gloves
Wear when touching **blood**, **body fluids**, **secretions**, **excretions**, and **contaminated items**.
Put on **clean** gloves just **before touching mucous membranes** and **nonintact skin**.
Change gloves between tasks and procedures on the same patient after contact with material that may contain high concentrations of microorganisms. Remove gloves promptly after use, before touching noncontaminated items and environmental surfaces, and before going to another patient, and wash hands immediately to avoid transfer of microorganisms to other patients or environments.

Wear Mask and Eye Protection or Face Shield
Protect mucous membranes of the eyes, nose and mouth during procedures and patient–care activities that are likely to generate **splashes** or **sprays** of **blood**, **body fluids**, **secretions**, or **excretions**.

Wear Gown
Protect skin and prevent soiling of clothing during procedures that are likely to generate **splashes** or **sprays** of **blood**, **body fluids**, **secretions**, or **excretions**. Remove a soiled gown as promptly as possible and wash hands to avoid transfer of microorganisms to other patients or environments.

Patient-Care Equipment
Handle used patient–care equipment soiled with **blood**, **body fluids**, **secretions**, or **excretions** in a manner that prevents skin and mucous membrane exposures, contamination of clothing, and transfer of microorganisms to other patients and environments. Ensure that reusable equipment is not used for the care of another patient until it has been appropriately cleaned and reprocessed and single use items are properly discarded.

Environmental Control
Follow hospital procedures for routine care, cleaning, and disinfection of environmental surfaces, beds, bedrails, bedside equipment and other frequently touched surfaces.

Linen
Handle, transport, and process used linen soiled with **blood**, **body fluids**, **secretions**, or **excretions** in a manner that prevents exposures and contamination of clothing, and avoids transfer of microorganisms to other patients and environments.

Occupational Health and Bloodborne Pathogens
Prevent injuries when using needles, scalpels, and other sharp instruments or devices; when handling sharp instruments after procedures; when cleaning used instruments; and when disposing of used needles.

Never recap used needles using both hands or any other technique that involves directing the point of a needle toward any part of the body; rather, use either a one-handed "scoop" technique or a mechanical device designed for holding the needle sheath.

Do not remove used needles from disposable syringes by hand, and do not bend, break, or otherwise manipulate used needles by hand. Place used disposable syringes and needles, scalpel blades, and other sharp items in puncture–resistant sharps containers located as close as practical to the area in which the items were used, and place reusable syringes and needles in a puncture–resistant container for transport to the reprocessing area.

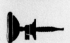

Use **resuscitation devices** as an alternative to mouth–to–mouth resuscitation.

Patient Placement
Use a **private room** for a patient who contaminates the environment or who does not (or cannot be expected to) assist in maintaining appropriate hygiene or environmental control. Consult Infection Control if a private room is not available.

The information on this sign is abbreviated from the HICPAC Recommendations for Isolation Precautions in Hospitals.

Form No. **SPR**   BREVIS CORP., 3310 S 2700 E, SLC, UT 84109   © 1996 Brevis Corp.

Figure 8-1   Standard Precautions   *Courtesy of BREVIS Corporation*

In addition, you need to exercise infection control practices. The most important infection control practice is handwashing. You must begin every physical assessment with a thorough handwash. Some nurses perform this in the assessment area with the patient present. It is a nonthreatening way to start the physical assessment and allows the patient time to ask questions concerning the process.

Legal Issues

In today's litigious society, you must be ever vigilant when engaging in nursing practice. Documentation issues have previously been addressed. Equally important is how you execute the nursing assessment. Establishing a trusting and caring relationship is the primary element in avoiding malpractice claims. While performing each step in the physical assessment process, you need to inform the patient of what to expect, where to expect it, and how it will feel. Protests by the patient need to be addressed prior to continuing the examination. Otherwise, the patient may claim insufficient informed consent, sexual abuse, or physical harassment.

All assessments and procedures, including any injury that was caused during the physical assessment, must be completely documented. The institutional policy regarding patient injury in the workplace must be followed.

ASSESSMENT TECHNIQUES

Physical assessment findings, or objective data, are obtained through the use of four specific diagnostic techniques: inspection, palpation, percussion, and auscultation. Usually, these assessment techniques are performed in this order when body systems are assessed. An exception is in the assessment of the abdomen, when auscultation is performed prior to percussion and palpation, as the latter two can alter bowel sounds. These four techniques validate information provided by a patient in the health history, or they can verify a suspected physical diagnosis.

Usually, the easiest assessment skills to master are inspection and basic auscultation. Percussion and palpation may take more time and practice to perfect.

Inspection

"A conscientious nurse is not necessarily an observing nurse; and life or death may lie with the good observer." This statement by Florence Nightingale provides inspiration and direction for inspection, which is usually the first assessment technique used during the assessment process. Inspection is an ongoing process that you use throughout the entire patient interaction. **Inspection** is the use of one's senses of vision and smell to consciously observe the patient.

Vision

Use of sight can reveal many facts about a patient. Visual inspection of a patient's respiratory status, for example, might reveal a rate of 38 breaths per minute and blue nailbeds. In this case, the patient is tachypneic and possibly hypoxic and would need a more thorough respiratory assessment. The process of visual inspection necessitates full exposure of the body part being inspected, adequate overhead lighting, and when necessary, **tangential lighting** (light that is shone at a right angle on the patient to accentuate shadows and highlight subtle findings).

Smell

The nurse's olfactory sense provides vital information about a patient's health status. The patient may have a fruity breath odor characteristic of diabetic ketoacidosis. The classic odor that is emitted by a *Pseudomonas* infection is another well-recognized smell to the trained nurse.

Palpation

The second assessment technique is **palpation**, which is the act of touching a patient in a therapeutic manner to elicit specific information. Prior to palpating a patient, some basic principles need to be observed. You should have short fingernails to avoid hurting the patient as well as yourself. Also, you should warm your hands prior to placing them on the patient; cold hands can make a patient's muscles tense, which can distort assessment findings. Encourage the patient to continue to breathe normally throughout the palpation. If pain is experienced during the palpation, discontinue the palpation immediately. Most significantly, inform the patient where, when, and how the touch will occur, especially when the patient cannot see what you are doing. In this way, the patient is aware of what to expect in the assessment process.

Your hands are the tools used to perform the palpation process. Different sections of the hands are best used for assessing certain areas of the body. The dorsum of the hand is most sensitive to temperature changes in the body. Thus, it is more accurate to place the dorsum of the hand on a patient's forehead to assess the body temperature than it is to use the palmar surface of the hand. The palmar surface of the fingers at the metacarpophalangeal joints, the ball of the hand, and the ulnar surface of the hand best discriminate vibrations, such as a cardiac thrill and fremitus. The finger pads are the portion of the hand used most frequently in palpation. The finger pads are useful in assessing fine tactile discrimination, skin moisture, and texture; the presence of masses, pulsations, edema, and crepitation; and the shape, size, position, mobility, and consistency of organs (refer to Figure 8-2).

There are two distinct types of palpation: light and deep palpation. Each of these techniques is briefly described here and will be covered in greater detail in chapters describing body systems where palpation is specifically used.

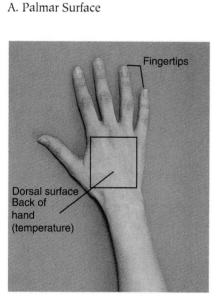

Finger pads assess:
Fine tactile discrimination
Moisture, Texture
Masses, Pulsations, Edema, Crepitation, Organ size, shape, position, mobility and consistency

A. Palmar Surface

B. Dorsal Surface

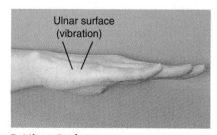

C. Ulnar Surface

Figure 8-2 Parts of the Hand Used in Palpation

> ## ❀ NURSING TIP
>
> ### Order of Assessment Procedures
>
> A good rule of thumb to follow when sequencing assessment procedures is to progress from the least intrusive to the most intrusive. That is, assessments that may cause discomfort should be performed last whenever possible in order to prevent patient anxiety, fear, and muscle guarding, which could affect the assessment process. For example, palpation of a tender area in the abdomen should be performed last. In the pediatric patient, the assessment of the ears and throat is usually performed last because these are the most uncomfortable for the child and may cause crying.

Light Palpation

Light palpation is done more frequently than deep palpation and is always performed before deep palpation. As the name implies, **light palpation** is superficial, delicate, and gentle. In light palpation, the finger pads are used to gain information on the patient's skin surface to a depth of approximately 1 centimeter (cm) below the surface. Light palpation reveals information on skin texture and moisture; overt, large, or superficial masses; and fluid, muscle guarding, and superficial tenderness. To perform light palpation:

1. Keeping the fingers of your dominant hand together, place the finger pads lightly on the skin over the area that is to be palpated. The hand and forearm will be on a plane parallel to the area being assessed.

2. Depress the skin 1 cm in light, gentle, circular motions.

3. Keeping the finger pads on the skin, let the depressed body surface rebound to its natural position.

4. Using a systematic approach, move the fingers to an adjacent area and repeat the process.

5. Continue to move the finger pads until the entire area being examined has been palpated.

6. If the patient has complained of tenderness in any area, palpate this area last. Refer to Figure 8-3, which shows how light palpation is performed.

Deep Palpation

Deep palpation can reveal information about the position of organs and masses, as well as their size, shape, mobility, and consistency. Deep palpation uses the hands to explore the body's internal structures to a depth of 4 to 5 cm or more (see Figure 8-4). This technique is most often performed for the abdominal and male and female reproductive assessments. Variations in this technique are single-handed and bimanual palpation and are discussed in Chapter 16.

Percussion

Percussion is the technique of striking one object against another to cause vibrations that produce sound. The density of underlying structures produces characteristic sounds. These sounds are diagnostic of normal and abnormal findings. The presence of air, fluid, and solids can be confirmed, as can organ size, shape, and position. Any part of the body can be percussed, but only limited information can be obtained in specific areas such as the heart. The thorax and abdomen are the most frequently percussed locations.

Percussion sound can be analyzed according to its intensity, duration, pitch (frequency), quality, and location. **Intensity** refers to the relative loudness or softness of the sound. It is also called the amplitude. **Duration** of percussed sound describes the time period over which a sound is heard when elicited. Frequency describes the concept of **pitch**. Frequency is caused by the sound's vibrations, or the highness or lowness of a sound. Frequency is measured in

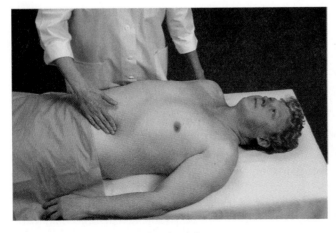

Figure 8-3 Technique of Light Palpation

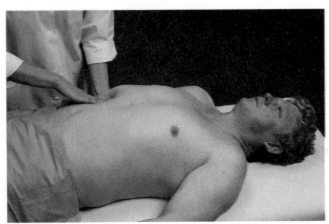

Figure 8-4 Technique of Deep Palpation

cycles per second (cps) or hertz (Hz). More rapidly occurring vibrations have a pitch that is higher than that of slower vibrations. Figure 8-5 illustrates this concept. The **quality** of a sound is its timbre, or how one perceives it musically. Location of sound refers to the area where the sound is produced and heard.

The process of percussion can produce five distinct sounds in the body: **flatness**, **dullness**, **resonance**, **hyperresonance**, and **tympany**. Specific parts of the body elicit distinct percussable sounds. Therefore, when an unexpected sound is heard in a particular part of the body, the cause must be further investigated.

Table 8-1 illustrates each of the five percussion sounds in relation to its respective intensity, duration, pitch, quality, location, and relative density. In addition, examples are provided of normal and abnormal locations of percussed sounds.

Sound waves are better conducted through a solid medium than through an air-filled medium because of the increased concentration of molecules. The basic premises underlying the sounds that are percussed are:

1. The more solid a structure, the higher its pitch, the softer its intensity, and the shorter its duration.

2. The more air-filled a structure, the lower its pitch, the louder its intensity, and the longer its duration.

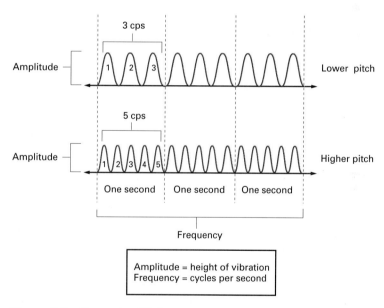

Figure 8-5   Percussion Pitch

Table 8-1	Characteristics of Percussion Sounds						
SOUND	INTENSITY	DURATION	PITCH	QUALITY	NORMAL LOCATION	ABNORMAL LOCATION	DENSITY
Flatness	Soft	Short	High	Flat	Muscle (thigh) or bone	Lungs (severe pneumonia)	Most dense
Dullness	Moderate	Moderate	High	Thud	Organs (liver)	Lungs (atelectasis)	
Resonance	Loud	Moderate-long	Low	Hollow	Normal lungs	No abnormal location	
Hyperresonance	Very loud	Long	Very low	Boom	No normal location	Lungs (emphysema)	
Tympany	Loud	Long	High	Drum	Gastric air bubble	Lungs (large pneumothorax)	Least dense

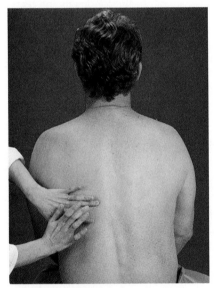

Figure 8-6 Technique of Immediate Percussion

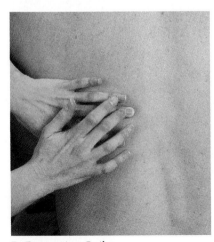

A. Position of Hands for Posterior Thorax Percussion

B. Percussion Strike

Figure 8-7 Technique of Mediate Percussion

There are four types of percussion techniques: immediate, mediate, direct fist percussion, and indirect fist percussion. It is important to keep in mind that the sounds produced from percussion are generated from body tissue up to 5 cm below the surface of the skin. If the abdomen is to be percussed, the patient should have the opportunity to void before the assessment.

Immediate Percussion

Immediate, or **direct**, **percussion** is the striking of an area of the body directly. To perform immediate percussion:

1. Spread the index or middle finger of the dominant hand slightly apart from the rest of the fingers.
2. Make a light tapping motion with the finger pad of the index finger against the body part being percussed.

Percussion of the sinuses (Figure 8-6) illustrates the use of immediate percussion in the physical assessment.

Mediate Percussion

Mediate percussion is also referred to as **indirect percussion**. This is a skill that takes time and practice to develop and to use effectively. Most sounds are produced using mediate percussion. Follow these steps to perform mediate percussion (Figure 8-7):

1. Place the nondominant hand lightly on the surface to be percussed.
2. Extend the middle finger of this hand, known as the **pleximeter**, and press its distal phalanx and distal interphalangeal joint firmly on the location where percussion is to begin. The pleximeter will remain stationary while percussion is performed in this location.
3. Spread the other fingers of the nondominant hand apart and raise them slightly off the surface. This prevents interference and, thus, dampening of vibrations during the actual percussion.
4. Flex the middle finger of the dominant hand, called the **plexor**. The fingernail of the plexor finger should be very short to prevent undue discomfort and injury to the nurse. The other fingers on this hand should be fanned.
5. Flex the wrist of the dominant hand and place the hand directly over the pleximeter finger of the nondominant hand.
6. With a sharp, crisp, rapid movement from the wrist of the dominant hand, strike the pleximeter with the plexor. At this point, the plexor should be perpendicular to the pleximeter. The blow to the pleximeter should be between the distal interphalangeal joint and the fingernail. Use the finger pad rather than the fingertip of the plexor to deliver the blow. Concentrate on the movement to create the striking action from the dominant wrist only.
7. As soon as the plexor strikes the pleximeter, withdraw the plexor to avoid dampening the resulting vibrations. Do not move the pleximeter finger.
8. Note the sound produced from the percussion.
9. Repeat the percussion process one or two times in this location to confirm the sound.
10. Move the pleximeter to a second location, preferably the contralateral location from where the previous percussion was performed. Repeat the percussion process in this manner until the entire body surface area being assessed has been percussed.

Recognizing Percussion Sound

When using mediate and immediate percussion, the change from resonance to dullness is more easily recognized by the human ear than is the change from dullness to resonance. It is often helpful to close your eyes and concentrate on the sound in order to distinguish if a change in sounds occurs. This concept has implications for patterns of percussion in areas of the body where known locations have distinct percussable sounds. For example, the techniques of diaphragmatic excursion and liver border percussion can proceed in a more defined pattern because percussion can be performed from an area of resonance to an area of dullness. Another helpful hint is to validate the change in sounds by percussing back and forth between the two areas where a change is noted to confirm this change.

As stated earlier, the percussion technique can take considerable time to develop and perfect. Practicing the technique in the home environment can be a helpful learning experience; refer to the accompanying Nursing Tip.

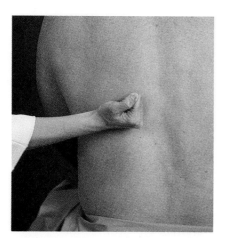

Figure 8-8 Technique of Direct Fist Percussion: Kidneys

Direct Fist Percussion

Direct fist percussion is used to assess the presence of tenderness in internal organs, such as the liver or the kidneys. To perform direct fist percussion (see Figure 8-8):

1. Explain this technique thoroughly so the patient does not think you are hitting him or her.
2. Draw the dominant hand up into a fist.
3. With the ulnar aspect of the closed fist, directly hit the area where the organ is located. The strike should be of moderate force, and it may take some practice to achieve the right intensity.

The presence of pain in conjunction with direct fist percussion indicates inflammation of that organ or a strike of too high an intensity.

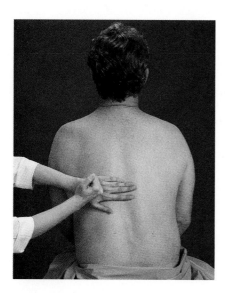

Figure 8-9 Technique of Indirect Fist Percussion: Kidneys

Indirect Fist Percussion

The purpose of **indirect fist percussion** is the same as direct fist percussion. In fact, the indirect method is preferred over the direct method. It is performed in the following manner (see Figure 8-9):

1. Place the palmar side of the nondominant hand on the skin's surface over the organ to be examined. Place the fingers adjacent to one another and in straight alignment with the palm.
2. Draw up the dominant hand into a closed fist.
3. With the ulnar aspect of the closed fist, use moderate intensity to hit the outstretched nondominant hand on the dorsum.

The nondominant hand absorbs some of the force of the striking hand. The resulting intensity should be of sufficient force to produce pain in the patient if organ inflammation is present.

Auscultation

Auscultation is the act of active listening to body organs to gather information on a patient's clinical status. Auscultation includes listening to sounds that are voluntarily and involuntarily produced by the body. An exasperated sigh illustrates a voluntary sound, and heart sounds illustrate involuntary sounds. A quiet environment is necessary for auscultation. Auscultated sounds should be analyzed in relation to their relative intensity, pitch, duration, quality, and location. There are two types of auscultation: direct and indirect.

Direct Auscultation

Direct, or **immediate**, **auscultation** is the process of listening with the unaided ear. This can include listening to the patient from some distance away or placing the ear directly on the patient's skin surface.

Indirect Auscultation

Indirect, or **mediate**, **auscultation** describes the process of listening with some amplification or mechanical device. The nurse most often performs mediate auscultation with an acoustic stethoscope, which does not amplify the body sounds, but instead blocks out environmental sounds. Amplification of body sounds can also be achieved with the use of a Doppler ultrasonic stethoscope. This text describes the use of an acoustic stethoscope.

Figure 8-10 illustrates the acoustic stethoscope. The earpieces come in various sizes. Choose an earpiece that fits snugly in the ear canal without causing pain. The earpieces block out noises in the environment. The earpieces and binaurals should be angled toward the nose. This angle permits the natural direction of the ear canal to be accessed. In this manner, sounds will be directed toward the adult tympanic membrane. The rubber or plastic tubing should be no more than 35 cm (13½ in.). Stethoscopes with longer tubing will diminish the body sounds that are auscultated.

The acoustic stethoscope has two listening heads: the bell and the diaphragm. The diaphragm is flat and the bell is a concave cup. The diaphragm transmits high-pitched sounds and the bell transmits low-pitched sounds. Breath sounds and normal heart sounds are examples of high-pitched sounds. Bruits and some heart murmurs are examples of low-pitched sounds.

Prior to auscultating, remove dangling necklaces or bracelets that can move during the examination and cause false noises. Warm the headpieces of the stethoscope in your hands prior to use, because shivering and movement can obscure assessment findings. To use the diaphragm, place it firmly against the skin surface to be auscultated. If the patient has a large quantity of hair in this area, it may be necessary to wet the hair to prevent it from interfering with the sound that is being auscultated. Otherwise, a grating sound may be heard. To use the bell, place it lightly on the skin surface that is to be auscultated. The bell will stretch the skin and act like a diaphragm and transmit high-pitched sounds if it is pressed too firmly on the skin. In both instances, auscultation requires a great deal of concentration. It may be helpful to close your eyes during the auscultation process to help you concentrate on the sound and block out the environment. Remember, auscultation is a skill that requires practice and patience. Don't expect to become an expert overnight!

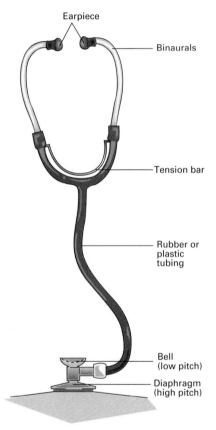

Figure 8-10 Acoustic Stethoscope

Earpiece

Binaurals

Tension bar

Rubber or plastic tubing

Bell (low pitch)

Diaphragm (high pitch)

🌺 NURSING TIP

Headpiece Mnemonic

The word "bellow" can be used to remember which frequency is transmitted by the headpiece of the stethoscope. The "bell" transmits "low" sounds.

EQUIPMENT

The physical assessment will proceed in an efficient manner if you have gathered all of the necessary equipment beforehand. The equipment needed to perform a complete physical examination of the adult patient includes:

- Pen and paper
- Marking pen
- Tape measure
- Clean gloves
- Penlight or flashlight
- Scale (You may need to walk the patient to a central location if a scale cannot be brought to the patient's room.)
- Thermometer
- Sphygmomanometer
- Gooseneck lamp
- Tongue depressor
- Stethoscope
- Otoscope
- Nasal speculum
- Ophthalmoscope
- Transilluminator
- Visual acuity charts
- Tuning fork
- Reflex hammer
- Sterile needle
- Cotton balls
- Odors for cranial nerve assessment (coffee, lemon, flowers, etc.)
- Small objects for neurological assessment (paper clip, watch, pen, etc.)
- Lubricant
- Various sizes of vaginal speculums
- Cervical brush
- Cotton-tip applicator
- Cervical spatula
- Slide and fixative
- Guaiac material
- Specimen cup
- Goniometer

The use of these items is discussed in the chapters describing the assessments for which they are used. Figure 8-11 illustrates some of the equipment used in the physical assessment.

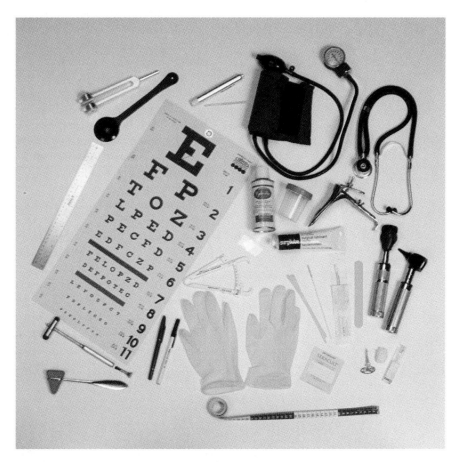

Figure 8-11 Equipment Used in Physical Assessment

✓ NURSING CHECKLIST
Preparing for a Physical Assessment

- Always dress in a clean, professional manner; make sure your name pin or workplace identification is visible.
- Remove all bracelets, necklaces, or earrings that can interfere with the physical assessment.
- Be sure that your fingernails are short and your hands are warm for maximum patient comfort.
- Be sure your hair will not fall forward and obstruct your vision or touch the patient.
- Arrange for a well-lit, warm, and private room.
- Assemble and arrange all the necessary equipment.
- Introduce yourself to the patient: "My name is Mary Gill. I am a nurse and I will be performing a physical assessment on you."
- Clarify with the patient how he or she wishes to be addressed: Miss Jones, José, Dr. Casy, Rev. Grimes, etc.
- Explain what you plan to do and how long it will take; allow the patient to ask questions.
- Instruct the patient to undress; the underpants can be left on until the end of the assessment; provide a gown and drape for the patient and explain how to use them.
- Allow the patient to undress privately; inform the patient when you will return to start the assessment.
- Have the patient void prior to the assessment.
- Wash your hands in front of the patient to show your concern for cleanliness.
- Observe standard precautions as indicated.
- Ensure that the patient is accessible from both sides of the examining bed or table.
- If a bed is used, raise the height so that you do not have to bend over to perform the assessment.
- Position the patient as dictated by the body system being assessed; refer to Figure 8-12 for positioning and draping techniques.
- Enlist the patient's cooperation by explaining what you are about to do, where it will be done, and how it may feel.
- Warm all instruments prior to their use (use your hands or warm water).
- Explain to the patient why you may be spending a long time performing one particular skill: "Listening to the heart requires concentration and time."
- If the patient complains of fatigue, continue the assessment later (if possible).
- Avoid making crude or negative remarks; be cognizant of your facial expression when dealing with malodorous and dirty patients or with disturbing findings (infected wounds, disfigurement, etc.).
- Conduct the assessment in a systematic fashion every time. (This decreases the likelihood of forgetting to perform a particular assessment.)
- Thank the patient when the physical assessment is concluded; inform the patient what will happen next.
- Document assessment findings.

Position   **System Assessed**

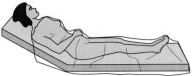

A. Semi-Fowler's 45° angle

Skin; head and neck; eyes, ears, nose, mouth, and throat; thorax and lungs; heart and peripheral vasculature; neurological; patients who cannot tolerate sitting up at a 90° angle

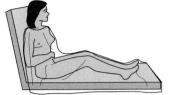

B. High Fowler's 90° angle

Same as Semi-Fowler's

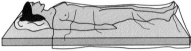

C. Horizontal recumbent

Breasts; heart and peripheral vasculature; abdomen; musculoskeletal

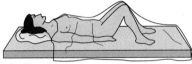

D. Dorsal recumbent

Female genitalia; patients who cannot tolerate knee flexion

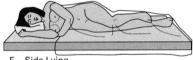

E. Side Lying

Skin; thorax and lungs; bedridden patients who cannot sit up

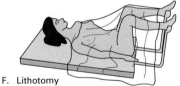

F. Lithotomy

Female genitalia

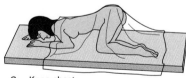

G. Knee-chest

Rectum and prostate

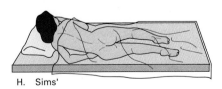

H. Sims'

Rectum and female genitalia

Figure 8-12 Positioning and Draping Techniques

NURSING TIP

Golden Rules for Physical Assessment

- Stand on the right side of the patient; establishing a dominant side for assessment will decrease your movement around the patient.
- Perform the assessment in a head-to-toe approach.
- Always compare the right- and left-hand sides of the body for symmetry.
- Proceed from the least invasive to the most invasive procedures for each body system.
- Always perform the physical assessment using a systematic approach; if it is performed the same way each time, you are less likely to forget some part of the assessment.

✓ NURSING CHECKLIST
Physical Assessment Techniques

Inspection
- Vision
- Smell

Palpation
- Light Palpation
- Deep Palpation

Percussion
- Immediate, or Direct, Percussion
- Mediate, or Indirect, Percussion
- Direct Fist Percussion
- Indirect Fist Percussion

Auscultation
- Immediate, or Direct, Auscultation
- Mediate, or Indirect, Auscultation

REVIEW QUESTIONS AND ACTIVITIES

1. Perform the "percussion at home" drills described in the Nursing Tip on page 197. Practice percussion of various body parts on a colleague.

2. Match the following percussion sounds with their characteristics:
   a. Tympany _____ loud, low pitched, hollow
   b. Hyperresonance _____ soft, high pitched, flat
   c. Resonance _____ loud, high pitched, drumlike
   d. Dullness _____ moderate intensity, high pitched, thudlike
   e. Flatness _____ very loud, very low pitched, boomlike

3. Match the following auscultation sounds with the stethoscope headpiece that is used to assess them:
   a. Diaphragm _____ breath sounds
   b. Bell _____ bowel sounds
   _____ bruit

4. Mrs. Q. visits the clinic for treatment of a leg ulcer that is actively draining. Mrs. Q. is well known to the clinic staff because she is being treated for pulmonary tuberculosis. Describe the standard precautions you would use when examining her.

Questions 5 and 6 refer to the following situation:

Pei C. is a 21-year-old female admitted to the emergency room complaining of abdominal pain.

5. In what order would you conduct the physical assessment of the abdomen?
   a. Inspection, palpation, percussion, auscultation
   b. Inspection, auscultation, percussion, palpation
   c. Auscultation, percussion, palpation, inspection
   d. Palpation, percussion, inspection, auscultation
   The correct answer is (b).

6. What position best facilitates this assessment?
   a. Semi-Fowler's
   b. Side lying
   c. Horizontal recumbent
   d. Dorsal recumbent
   The correct answer is (c).

9

General Assessment and Vital Signs

Acomplete physical assessment is initiated by collecting general data through making observations of the patient and by obtaining the patient's **vital signs**. Initial observations can provide data about the patient's general state of health. Vital signs include the patient's respirations, pulse, temperature, and blood pressure (BP). These measurements provide information about the patient's basic physiological status.

GENERAL ASSESSMENT

Initial observations include collecting information about the patient's physical presence, psychological presence, and signs and symptoms of distress.

Physical Presence

Observe the patient's:
E 1. Stated age versus apparent age
    2. Body fat
    3. Stature
    4. Motor activity
    5. Body and breath odors

Stated Age Versus Apparent Age

N *The patient's stated chronological age should be congruent with the apparent age.*

A It is abnormal for a patient to appear significantly older or younger than the stated chronological age.

P Endocrine deficiencies of growth hormone associated with dwarfism can manifest in a younger-than-chronological-age appearance in younger life and premature aging later in life.

P Genetic syndromes (e.g., Turner's) manifest in an "old-person" facial appearance.

Body Fat

N *Body fat is normally evenly distributed. Body fat composition is difficult to estimate accurately without the use of immersion tanks or calipers. Research has indicated, however, that it is body fat content, not body weight, that is most closely linked to pathology. For example, a person can be within normal limits on height and weight charts but have a high proportion of body fat to lean body mass.*

A Obesity occurs when there are large amounts of body fat distributed evenly over the body. This poses a serious health risk to the patient and warrants a comprehensive nutritional assessment (refer to Chapter 7).

P Excess caloric intake and/or decreased energy expenditure are the most common causes of obesity.

P Some disease processes, such as hypothyroidism, which slows the basic metabolic rate, may result in obesity.

A Cushing's syndrome manifests in a rounded moonlike face, truncal obesity, fat pads on the neck, and relatively thin limbs.

P Excessive production of cortisol resulting from an anterior pituitary tumor or large doses of prolonged steroid therapy produces Cushing's syndrome.

A A thin or frail appearance occurs when there are limited body fat stores. Severely limited fat stores can be a life-threatening condition.

NURSING TIP

Environmental Cues

In addition to observing the patient, look around the room for clues about the patient's health status. For example, eye drops, nasal spray or an inhaler, and used handkerchiefs may all provide information about the patient's health.

EQUIPMENT

- Stethoscope
- Watch with a second hand
- Thermometer (gloves & lubricant if using a rectal thermometer)
- Sphygmomanometer

E **Examination**
N **Normal Findings**
A **Abnormal Findings**
P **Pathophysiology**

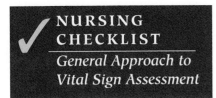

NURSING CHECKLIST
General Approach to Vital Sign Assessment

- Gather equipment.
- Explain procedure to patient.
- Select equipment according to patient's age, size, and developmental level, and site selected for assessment. Specific decision-making criteria are discussed under each section.
- Warm stethoscope headpiece before touching the patient with it.
- Assess vital signs and record findings.

☺☺ THINK ABOUT IT

Assessing the Patient with Severe Odors

A patient has a strong breath or body odor. You need to complete a physical exam. How would you handle this situation? What questions would you pose to discover the cause of the odors, while maintaining respect for the patient's dignity?

E Examination
N Normal Findings
A Abnormal Findings
P Pathophysiology

P Energy expenditures that exceed caloric intake will result in inadequate fat stores. This may be caused by several conditions, including:
- Anorexia nervosa, which results in inadequate intake of calories from food and/or overexpenditure of energy by means of exercise.
- Hyperkinetic states in which body metabolic needs are greater than the ability to ingest calories. Adolescent growth spurts result in tall, thin teens because the increased metabolic demands for growing tissue exceed the calories they can consume.
- Many chronic disease processes may be due to hyperkinetic states or a result of malabsorption diseases.

Stature

N *Limbs and trunk should appear proportional to body height; posture should be erect.*
A A slumped or humpbacked appearance is abnormal.
P In older women, osteoporosis and loss of bone density in the spine may cause a slumped or humpbacked appearance.
P Patients experiencing depression may also present with a slumped posture.
A Long limbs relative to trunk length are abnormal.
P Marfan's syndrome, an inherited disease, can result in the development of long limbs, a tall, thin appearance, and poorly developed muscles due to a defect in the elastic fibers of connective tissues.

Motor Activity

N *Normal walking gait as well as other body movements should be smooth and effortless. All body parts should have controlled, purposeful movement.*
A An unsteady gait or movements that are slow, absent, or require great effort are abnormal. Tremors or movements that seem uncontrollable by the patient are also abnormal.
P Arthritis can result in slow and difficult movement because joint movement is painful.
P Neurological disturbances can result in tics, paralysis, or ataxia, and can cause difficulty with the smoothness of movement.

Body and Breath Odors

N *Normally, there is no apparent odor from patients. It is normal for some people to have bad breath related to the types of foods ingested or due to individual digestive processes.*
A Severe body or breath odor is abnormal.
P Poor hygiene can cause body odors due to perspiration and bacteria left on the skin.
P An alcohol smell on the breath can result from alcohol ingestion or from ketoacidosis in a diabetic patient.
P Bad breath can result from poor oral hygiene or from oral or pulmonary infections such as tonsillitis, sinusitis, or pneumonia.
P Severe vaginal infections can result in an offensive body odor.

Psychological Presence

Observe the patient's:
E 1. Dress, grooming, and personal hygiene
2. Mood and manner
3. Speech
4. Facial expressions

Dress, Grooming, and Personal Hygiene

N *Normally, patients should appear clean and neatly dressed. Clothing choice should be appropriate for the weather. Norms and standards for dress and cleanliness may vary among cultures.*

A A disheveled, unkempt appearance or clothing that is inappropriate for the weather (such as a wool coat in hot weather) is abnormal.

P Psychological or psychiatric disorders such as depression (characterized in part by lethargy, mood swings, anhedonia [or lack of pleasure in activities], fatigue, etc.), psychotic disorders (characterized by a distortion in thinking), and dementia (processes that alter perceptions of reality) may be reflected in inappropriate appearance (hair, makeup) or through inappropriate clothing selection.

P Poor self-esteem or a homeless lifestyle may be reflected by general neglect of personal hygiene, grooming, and dress.

P An unshaven, unclean appearance may reflect abuse or neglect of the patient by the patient's caretaker.

Mood and Manner

N *Generally, a patient should be cooperative and pleasant.*

A An uncooperative, hostile, or tearful adult, or an adult who seems unusually elated or who has a flat affect needs further assessment.

P Psychiatric conditions such as depression, manic disorders, paranoid disorders, and psychotic disorders produce a distortion in reality (distorted thinking and perceptions), resulting in abnormal behaviors. Dementia or confusion in the elderly can also result in disturbances of mood and manner. See Chapter 18 for a more complete discussion.

Speech

N *The patient should respond to questions and commands easily. Speech should be clear and understandable. Pitch, rate, and volume should vary normally.*

A Speech that is slow, slurred, mumbled, very loud, or rapid is abnormal.

P Hyperthyroidism, a syndrome that results when tissues are exposed to excessive amounts of thyroid hormone, can cause rapid speech. These hormones are stimulatory in nature and result in hypermetabolism and hyperactivity.

P Alcohol ingestion can cause slow, mumbled, or slurred speech because alcohol affects the central nervous system, causing transient brain dysfunction.

P Hearing difficulties may be associated with loud speech because individuals with decreased ability to hear may not be able to hear themselves at normal conversational decibels.

P Strokes can result in speech aphasia if the speech center in the brain is affected.

Facial Expression

N *The patient should appear awake and alert. Facial expressions should be appropriate for what is happening in the environment. Facial expression should change naturally.*

A Unchanging or flat facial expression, inappropriate facial expression, tremors, or tics are abnormal.

P Apathy or depression may cause lack of facial expression due to feelings of lethargy or sadness.

P Dementia may cause inappropriate facial expression because the patient's perception of reality is distorted.

E	Examination
N	Normal Findings
A	Abnormal Findings
P	Pathophysiology

P Bell's palsy, a condition resulting in paralysis of the muscles in the face, may cause the mouth to droop and the affected side of the face to appear flaccid.

Distress

Observe for:

E 1. Labored breathing, wheezing or cough, labored speech
   2. Painful facial expression, sweating, or physical protection of painful area
   3. Signs of emotional distress or anxiety that may include but are not limited to tearfulness, nervous tics or laughter, avoidance of eye contact, cold, clammy hands, excessive nail biting, inability to pay attention, autonomic responses such as diaphoresis, or changes in breathing patterns

N *Breathing should be effortless, without cough or wheezing. Speech should not leave a patient breathless. Face should be relaxed and the patient should be willing to move all body parts freely. The patient should not perspire excessively or show signs of emotional distress such as nail biting or avoidance of eye contact.*

A The presence of shortness of breath with labored speech, wheezing, or cough is abnormal.

P Pulmonary disease may be present. See Chapter 14 for additional information.

A Pain as evidenced by facial grimacing, sweating, or protection of a body part is an abnormal finding.

P Tissue damage results in pain and needs further investigation into the character, location, intensity, and occurrence of the pain as well as factors associated with increased and decreased pain.

A Excessive nail biting, avoidance of eye contact, nervous laughter, tearfulness, or lack of interest may be indicators of emotional distress or emotional pain.

P Nervous habits are often displayed when a person is in an uncomfortable or new situation. A tearful or sad affect can result from emotional pain related to situations the patient may be experiencing or has experienced. Often, there is an attempt made to disguise emotional distress.

VITAL SIGNS

Respiration

Respiration is the act of breathing. Breathing supplies oxygen to the body and occurs in response to changes in the concentration of oxygen (O_2), carbon dioxide (CO_2), and hydrogen (H^+) in the arterial blood. Inhalation, or inspiration, occurs when air is taken into the lungs. Exhalation, or expiration, refers to the airflow out of the lungs.

Inspiration occurs when the diaphragm and the intercostal muscles contract. This can be observed by the movement of the abdomen outward and the movement of the chest upward and outward, resulting in the lungs filling with air. Expiration occurs when the external intercostal muscles and the diaphragm relax. The abdomen and the chest return to a resting position.

Respiratory rate is measured in breaths per minute. One respiratory cycle consists of one inhalation and one expiration. Respiratory rate varies with age, exercise, stress or anxiety, medications, and altitude. A complete discussion of respiratory assessment is found in Chapter 14.

To assess respiratory rate:

E 1. Stand in front of or to the side of the patient.
   2. Discretely observe the patient's breathing (rise and fall of the chest).

☙ NURSING TIP

Assessing Vital Signs

Vital signs should be assessed at the beginning of each visit. If the patient is hospitalized, vital signs should be assessed as often as prescribed or as often as the patient's condition requires.

E Examination
N Normal Findings
A Abnormal Findings
P Pathophysiology

Table 9-1 Respiratory Rate		
AGE	RESTING RESPIRATORY RATE (Breaths/Minute)	AVERAGE
Newborn	30–50	40
1 Year	20–40	30
3 Years	20–30	25
6 Years	16–22	19
10 Years	16–20	18
14 Years	14–20	17
Adult	16–20	18

🌸 NURSING TIP

Respiration Assessment

Most frequently, respirations can be measured while measuring radial or apical pulse. If respirations are shallow and the patient is supine, put the patient's arm across the chest while taking a radial pulse and feel the chest rise while observing for respirations.

E   **Examination**
N   **Normal Findings**
A   **Abnormal Findings**
P   **Pathophysiology**

These observations are best done with the patient unaware of what you are doing. If the patient is aware that you are counting respirations, the breathing pattern may be altered.

3. Count the number of respiratory cycles that occur in 1 minute.

N   *Table 9-1 lists the normal respiratory rates for different ages. Normal respiratory rates decrease with age and may vary with excitement, anxiety, or fever.*

A   **Tachypnea** is a respiratory rate greater than 20 breaths per minute in an adult.

P   Hypoxia and metabolic acidosis are common causes of tachypnea. The increased respiratory rate is a compensatory mechanism to provide the body with more oxygen in hypoxic states and eliminate excess hydrogen ions when the body is in an acidotic state.

P   Stress and anxiety cause the release of catecholamines, which can elevate the respiratory rate.

A   **Bradypnea** is a respiratory rate less than 12 breaths per minute in an adult at rest.

P   Head injury resulting in increased intracranial pressure in the respiratory center of the brain can cause bradypnea.

P   Medications or chemicals such as narcotics, barbiturates, or alcohol depress the respiratory center of the brain and can cause bradypnea.

P   A lower metabolic rate that occurs during normal sleep can result in bradypnea.

A   **Apnea** is the absence of breathing for 10 or more seconds.

P   Many causes of apnea are unknown.

P   Traumatic brain injury may lead to apnea from injury of the brain stem. Death ensues in the absence of respirations and pulse.

Pulse

As the heart contracts, blood is ejected from the left ventricle (stroke volume) into the aorta. A pressure wave is created as the blood is carried to the peripheral vasculature. This palpable pressure is the **pulse**. Pulse assessment can determine heart rate, rhythm, and the estimated volume of blood being pumped by the heart.

Rate

Pulse rate is the number of pulse beats counted in 1 minute. Several factors influence heart rate or pulse rate. These include:

- The SA node, which fires automatically at a rate of 60 to 100 times per minute and is the primary controller of pulse rate and heart rate.
- Parasympathetic or vagal stimulation of the autonomic nervous system, which can result in decreased heart rate.
- Sympathetic stimulation of the autonomic nervous system, which results in increased heart rate.
- Baroreceptor sensors, which can detect changes in blood pressure and influence heart rate. Elevated blood pressure can decrease heart rate, whereas decreased blood pressure can increase heart rate.

Other factors influencing heart rate include:

- Age: heart rate generally decreases with age.
- Gender: the average female's pulse is higher than a male's pulse.
- Activity: heart rate increases with activity. Athletes will have a lower resting heart rate than the average person because of their increased cardiac strength and efficiency.
- Emotional status: heart rate increases with anxiety.
- Pain: heart rate increases.
- Environmental factors: temperature and noise level can alter heart rate.

- Stimulants: caffeinated beverages and tobacco elevate heart rate.
- Medications: drugs such as digoxin decrease heart rate, and drugs such as amphetamines increase heart rate.

Table 9-2   Scales for Measuring Pulse Volume

3-POINT SCALE

Scale	Description of Pulse
0	Absent
1+	Thready/weak
2+	Normal
3+	Bounding

4-POINT SCALE

Scale	Description of Pulse
0	Absent
1+	Thready/weak
2+	Normal
3+	Increased
4+	Bounding

Rhythm

Pulse rhythm refers to the pattern of pulses and the intervals between pulses. Pulses can be regular or irregular.

Volume

Pulse volume (also called pulse strength or amplitude) reflects the stroke volume and the **peripheral vasculature resistance** (afterload). It can range from absent to bounding. Table 9-2 displays the two most commonly used scales: a 3-point and a 4-point scale. When reporting pulse volume, 2+/4+ indicates a normal pulse (2+) on a 4-point scale, whereas 2+/3+ indicates a normal pulse (2+) on a 3-point scale.

Site

Peripheral pulses can be palpated where the large arteries are close to the skin surface. There are nine common sites for assessment of pulse as indicated in Figure 9-1. When routine vital signs are assessed, the pulse is generally measured at one of two sites: radial or apical.

The radial pulse can be palpated where the radial artery runs along the radial bone on the thumb side of the inner wrist. The apical pulse can be palpated and auscultated at the apex of the heart. In an adult, the apex is on the left side of the chest, to the left of the sternum, between the fourth and sixth intercostal spaces. Measuring the apical pulse is indicated for patients with irregular pulses or known cardiac or pulmonary disease. The assessment of apical pulse can be accomplished through palpation but is most commonly accomplished through auscultation.

Radial Pulse

To palpate the radial pulse:

E 1. Place the pad of your first, second, or third finger on the site of the radial pulse.
   2. Press your fingers gently against the artery with enough pressure so that you can feel the pulse. Pressing too hard will obliterate the pulse.
   3. Count the pulse rate using the secondhand of a watch. If the pulse is regular, count for 30 seconds and multiply by 2 to obtain the pulse rate per minute. If the pulse is irregular, count for 60 seconds.
   4. Identify the pulse rhythm as you palpate (regular or irregular).
   5. Identify the pulse volume as you palpate (using scales from Table 9-2).

N/A/P   Refer to section on Rate, page 210.

Apical Pulse

To assess the apical pulse:

E 1. Place the diaphragm of the stethoscope on the apical pulse site.
   2. Count the pulse rate for 30 seconds if regular, 60 seconds if irregular.
   3. Identify the pulse rhythm and volume.
   4. Identify a **pulse deficit** (apical pulse rate greater than the radial pulse rate) by listening to the apical pulse and palpating the radial pulse simultaneously.

N/A/P   Refer to section on Rate, page 210.

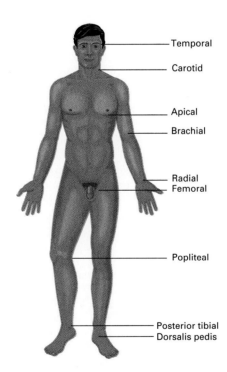

Temporal
Carotid
Apical
Brachial
Radial
Femoral
Popliteal
Posterior tibial
Dorsalis pedis

Figure 9-1   Pulse Sites

E	Examination
N	Normal Findings
A	Abnormal Findings
P	Pathophysiology

Table 9-3 Pulse Rate: Normal Range According to Age		
AGE	**RESTING PULSE RATE (Beats/Minute)**	**AVERAGE**
Newborn	100–170	140
1 year	80–170	120
3 years	80–130	110
6 years	70–115	100
10 years	70–110	90
14 years	60–110	85–90
Adult	60–100	72

Rate

N *Normal pulse rates vary with age. Table 9-3 depicts ranges for normal pulse rates by age. The heart rate normally increases during periods of exertion.*

A **Tachycardia** refers to a pulse rate faster than 100 beats per minute in an adult.

P Psychophysiological stressors such as trauma, blood volume losses, anemias, infection, fear, fever, pain, hyperthyroidism, shock, and anxiety can increase pulse rate because of increased metabolic demands placed on the body.

P Some tachycardia may not have clinical significance; however, in patients with myocardial disease, tachycardia can be a sign of decreased cardiac output, congestive heart failure, myocardial ischemia, or dysrhythmias.

A **Bradycardia** refers to slow pulse rates. Pulse rates that fall below 60 in adults are considered to be bradycardic.

P Athletes commonly have resting heart rates below 60 because of the increased strength and efficiency of the cardiac muscle.

P Medications such as cardiotonics (digoxin) and beta blockers decrease the heart rate.

P Bradycardia usually occurs with excessive vagal stimulation or decreased sympathetic tone. Conditions that may cause bradycardia are eye surgery, increased intracranial pressure, myocardial infarction, hypothyroidism, and prolonged vomiting.

A **Asystole** refers to the absence of a pulse. Feel or auscultate for a pulse for 5 to 10 seconds to establish asystole.

P Cardiac arrest resulting from biological or clinical death can result in asystole.

P Pulseless electrical activity (electromechanical dissociation) caused by, for example, hypovolemia, pneumothorax, cardiac tamponade, or acidosis results in the absence of a pulse despite the presence of electrical activity in the heart muscle.

A A pulse deficit occurs when the apical pulse rate is greater than the radial pulse rate.

P Dysrhythmias (such as atrial fibrillation, premature ventricular contractions, second degree heart block, and third degree heart block) or heart failure can cause pulse deficits because some heart contractions are too weak to produce a pulse pressure to the peripheral site. Severe vascular disease can also cause pulse deficits.

Rhythm

N *Normal pulse rhythm is regular with equal intervals between each beat.*

A **Dysrhythmias**, or **arrhythmias**, refer to pulse rhythms that are not regular. They may consist of irregular beats that are random or irregular beats that present in a regular pattern.

P Cardiac dysrhythmias that are atrial and ventricular in origin cause abnormal rhythms, such as atrial fibrillation and premature ventricular contractions.

Volume

N *The pulse volume is normally the same with each beat. A normal pulse volume can be felt with a moderate amount of pressure of the fingers and obliterated with greater pressure.*

A Small, weak pulses are referred to as weak or thready pulses or pulses easily obliterated with light pressure.

P Decreased cardiac stroke volume caused by heart failure, hypovolemic shock, and cardiogenic shock can result in weak pulses.

E	**Examination**
N	**Normal Findings**
A	**Abnormal Findings**
P	**Pathophysiology**

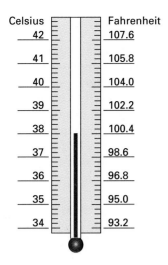

Celsius | Fahrenheit
42 — 107.6
41 — 105.8
40 — 104.0
39 — 102.2
38 — 100.4
37 — 98.6
36 — 96.8
35 — 95.0
34 — 93.2

To convert:
(9/5 x temperature in Celsius) + 32° = temperature in Fahrenheit

5/9 x (temperature in Fahrenheit – 32°) = temperature in Celsius

Figure 9-2 Correlation between Celsius and Fahrenheit Scales

P A low pulse amplitude occurs in states of increased peripheral vascular resistance, such as in aortic stenosis and constrictive pericarditis.

P Weak pulses occur in conditions when ventricular filling time is decreased, such as in dysrhythmias.

A Bounding pulses are full, forceful pulses that are difficult to obliterate with pressure.

P Hyperkinetic states such as exercise, fever, anemia, anxiety, and hyperthyroidism can cause bounding pulses.

P Early stages of septic shock are characterized by bounding pulses because of decreased peripheral vascular resistance.

Temperature
Temperature Scales

Both the Celsius and the Fahrenheit scales are commonly used to measure **temperature**, which is the degree of core body heat. Patients are most often familiar with the Fahrenheit scale, whereas institutions often use the Celsius scale. Therefore, it is important that you know temperature scale correlations. Figure 9-2 summarizes these correlations and the conversion formula.

Measurement Routes

There are four basic routes by which temperature can be measured: oral, rectal, axillary, and tympanic. Each method has advantages and disadvantages. The advantages and disadvantages of each route are summarized in Table 9-4.

Table 9-4 Advantages and Disadvantages of Four Routes for Body Temperature Measurement			
ROUTE	**NORMAL RANGE**	**ADVANTAGES**	**DISADVANTAGES**
Oral			
Average 37.0°C or 98.6°F	36.0°–38.0°C 96.8°–100.4°F	Convenient; accessible	**Safety:** Glass thermometers with mercury can be bitten and broken, causing patient injury. Patients need to be alert and cooperative and cognitively capable of following instructions for safe use.
			Physical abilities: Patients need to be able to breathe through the nose, and be without oral pathology or recent oral surgery; route not applicable for comatose or confused patients.
			Accuracy: Oxygen therapy by mask, as well as ingestion of hot or cold drinks immediately before oral temperature measurement, affects accuracy of the reading.
Rectal			
Average 0.7°C or 0.4°F higher than oral	36.7°C–38.7°C 100.8°F–104.0°F	Considered most accurate	**Safety:** Contraindicated following rectal surgery. Risk of rectal perforation in children less than 2 years of age. Risk of stimulating valsalva maneuver in cardiac patients.
			Physical Aspects: Invasive and uncomfortable.
Axillary			
Average 0.6°C or 1°F lower than oral	35.4°C–37.4°C 95.8°F–99.4°F	Safe; noninvasive	**Accuracy:** Glass thermometer must be left in place for 5 minutes to obtain accurate measurement. Placement and position of thermometer tip affect reading.
Tympanic			
Calibrated to oral or rectal scales	See oral or rectal	Convenient; fast; safe; noninvasive. Does not require contact with any mucous membrane.	**Accuracy:** Research is inconclusive as to accuracy of readings and correlations with other body temperature measurements. Technique affects reading. Tympanic membrane is thought to reflect the core temperature.

Variables Affecting Body Temperature

Core body temperature is established by the temperature of blood perfusing the area of the hypothalamus (the body's temperature control center), which triggers the body's physiological response to temperature. An ideal thermometer would accurately measure central brain stem temperature at the hypothalamus. Invasive procedures that provide temperatures of the arterial blood, esophagus, or bladder are reliable indicators of core temperature, but are impractical. More practical methods for measurement of body temperature are less reliable and can result in variations in body temperature readings. In addition, there are physiological variables that affect body temperature. These include:

- **Circadian rhythm** patterns: Normal body temperature (as well as pulse and blood pressure) fluctuates with a patient's activity level and the time of day. Core body temperature is lower during sleep than during waking activities, being the lowest in the early morning just before awakening from sleep and the highest in the afternoon or early evening. A 0.5°C to 1.0°C, or a 1°F to 2°F, fluctuation in body temperature throughout the day is considered within the normal range.
- Hormones: In women, increased production of progesterone at the time of ovulation raises the basal body temperature about 0.35°C, or 0.5°F.
- Age: Infants and young children are affected by the environmental temperature to a much greater extent than adults because their thermoregulation mechanisms are not fully developed. The elderly are more sensitive to extremes of environmental temperature due to a decrease in thermoregulatory controls.
- Exercise: Body temperature rises due to increased metabolic activity.
- Stress: Stimulation of the sympathetic nervous system increases the production of epinephrine, resulting in increased metabolic activity and higher body temperature.
- Environmental extremes of hot or cold.

Measurement

Oral Method

E 1. Place the thermometer at the base of the tongue and to the right or left of the frenulum, and instruct the patient to close the lips around the thermometer.
2. Leave the thermometer in the mouth for the time recommended by your agency or institution (usually 3 to 10 minutes).
3. Read the thermometer and record the temperature.

Rectal Method

E 1. Position patient with the buttocks exposed. Adults may be more comfortable lying on the side (with the knees slightly flexed), facing away from you, or prone.
2. Put on clean gloves.
3. Lubricate the tip of the thermometer with lubricant such as K-Y® Jelly.
4. Ask the patient to take a deep breath; insert the thermometer into the anus 0.5 to 1.5 inches, depending on the patient's age.
5. Do not force the insertion of the thermometer or insert into feces.
6. Hold thermometer in place for 3 to 5 minutes or the time recommended by your institution.

Axillary Method

E 1. Place the thermometer into the middle of the axilla and fold the patient's arm across the chest to keep the thermometer in place.
2. Leave the thermometer in place 5 to 10 minutes, depending on your institution's protocol.

✿ NURSING TIP

Using Oral and Rectal Thermometers

Do not use the same thermometer to take rectal and oral temperatures, because doing so may result in the transfer of pathogens.

E   Examination
N   Normal Findings
A   Abnormal Findings
P   Pathophysiology

Electronic Thermometer

E   **1.** Remove electronic thermometer from the charging unit.
         2. Attach a disposable cover to the probe.
         3. Using a method described (oral, rectal, or axillary), measure the temperature.
         4. Listen for the sound or look for the symbol that indicates maximum body temperature has been reached.
         5. Observe and record the reading.
         6. Remove and discard the probe cover.
         7. Return the electronic thermometer to the charging unit.

Tympanic Thermometer

E   **1.** Attach the probe cover to the nose of the thermometer.
         2. Gently place the probe of the thermometer over the entrance to the ear canal. If the patient is under 3 years old, pull the pinna down, aiming the probe toward the opposite eye. If the patient is over 3 years old, grasp the pinna and pull gently up and back, aiming the probe toward the opposite ear. Make sure there is a tight seal.
         3. Press the start button on the thermometer handle.
         4. Wait for the beep, remove the probe from the ear, and read the temperature.
         5. Discard the probe cover.
         6. Return the tympanic thermometer to the charger unit.

N   *Normal body temperatures are described in Table 9-4.*

A   **Hyperthermia**, pyrexia, or fever are conditions in which body temperatures exceed 38.5°C, or 101.5°F. Clinical signs of hyperthermia include increased respiratory rate and pulse, shivering, pallor, and thirst.

P   There can be many causes of hyperthermia (including infection), which results from an increased basal metabolic rate.

A   **Hypothermia** occurs when the body temperature is below 34°C, or 93.2°F. Clinical signs of hypothermia include decreased body temperature and initial shivering that ceases as drowsiness and coma ensue. Hypotension, decreased urinary output, lack of muscle coordination, and disorientation also occur as hypothermia progresses.

P   Hypothermia can be caused by prolonged exposure to cold such as immersion in cold water or administration of large volumes of unwarmed blood products.

P   Hypothermia can be induced to decrease the tissues' need for oxygen, such as during cardiac surgery.

Blood Pressure

Blood pressure measures (in millimeters of mercury [mm Hg]) the force exerted by the flow of blood pumped into the large arteries. Arterial blood pressure is determined by blood flow and the resistance to blood flow as indicated in the following formula:

$$MAP = CO \times TPR$$

mean arterial pressure (MAP) = cardiac output (CO) × total peripheral resistance (TPR)

Changes in blood pressure can be used to monitor changes in cardiac output. Ineffective pumping, decreased circulating volume, as well as changes in the characteristics of the blood vessels can affect blood pressure. There is a diurnal variation in blood pressure as characterized by a high point in the early evening and a low point during the early deep stage of sleep.

Korotkoff Sounds

Korotkoff sounds are generated when the flow of blood through the artery is altered by inflating the blood pressure cuff that is wrapped around the

E	**Examination**
N	**Normal Findings**
A	**Abnormal Findings**
P	**Pathophysiology**

ම THINK ABOUT IT

Assessing Vital Signs in Reluctant Patients

You are the rural health nurse substituting for a sick colleague. Today you are visiting 3-year-old Amalia, who has been followed for many months since her congenital heart repair. Her mother tells you that Amalia feels hot and that she has been unable to find a thermometer to take Amalia's temperature. You prepare to assess Amalia's rectal temperature when she tells you that she doesn't want you to touch her. She will only let Nurse Fauntleroy take care of her. How would you handle this situation? What would you say? What would you do?

extremity. Korotkoff sounds can be heard by listening over a pulse site that is distal to the blood pressure cuff. As the air is released from the bladder of the cuff, the pressure on the artery changes from that which completely occludes blood flow to that which allows free flow. As the pressure against the artery wall decreases, five distinct sounds occur. These are:

Phase I: The first audible sound heard as the cuff pressure is released. Sounds like clear tapping and correlates to systolic pressure (the force needed to pump the blood out of the heart).

Phase II: Sounds like swishing or a murmur. Created as the blood flows through blood vessels narrowed by the inflation of the blood pressure cuff.

Phase III: Sounds like clear intense tapping. Created as blood flows through the artery but cuff pressure is still great enough to occlude flow during diastole.

Phase IV: Sounds are muffled and are heard when cuff pressure is low enough to allow some blood flow during diastole. The change from the tap of Phase III to the muffled sound of Phase IV is referred to as the first diastolic reading.

Phase V: No sounds are heard. Occurs when cuff pressure is released enough to allow normal blood flow. This is referred to as the second diastolic reading.

Measuring Blood Pressure

Systolic pressure represents the pressure exerted on the arterial wall during **systole**, when the ventricles are contracting. Diastolic pressure represents the pressure in the arteries when the ventricles are relaxed and filling. Blood pressure is recorded as a fraction with the top number representing the systole and the bottom number(s) representing the **diastole**. If first and second diastolic sounds are recorded, the first diastolic sound is written over the second. For example, 120/90/80 indicates that 120 mm Hg is the systolic pressure, 90 mm Hg is the first diastolic sound, and 80 mm Hg is the second diastolic sound. An explanation of the blood pressure sounds is found in the section entitled *Korotkoff Sounds*. **Pulse pressure** is the difference between diastole and systole.

Measurement Sites

There are several potential sites for blood pressure measurement. The preferred site is the upper arm pulse site, where the brachial artery runs across the antecubital fossa. The thigh, where the popliteal artery runs behind the knee joint, can also be used. A site should not be used if there is pain or injury around or near the site; for instance, a postmastectomy patient should have blood pressure assessed on the unaffected side. Surgical incisions, intravenous, central venous, or arterial lines, or areas with poor perfusion should be avoided for blood pressure measurement. Patients with arteriovenous (AV) fistulas or AV shunts should not have blood pressure measured in those extremities.

Equipment

Blood pressure is measured indirectly with a stethoscope or Doppler and a **sphygmomanometer**, which consists of the blood pressure cuff, connecting tubes and air pump, and manometer. Blood pressure cuffs come in several sizes. The size of the cuff from top to bottom should be two-thirds the circumference of the limb being assessed. The cuff should completely encircle the limb.

A manometer is attached to the cuff via a second tube. There are two types of manometers: aneroid and mercury. The **aneroid manometer** is a calibrated dial with a needle that points to numbers representing the air pressure

E	Examination
N	Normal Findings
A	Abnormal Findings
P	Pathophysiology

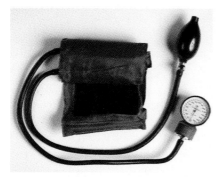

A. Aneroid Sphygmomanometer

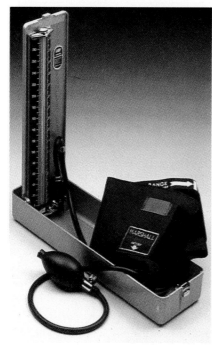

B. Mercury Sphygmomanometer
Courtesy of Omron Marshall Products, Inc.

Figure 9-3 Sphygmomanometers

◎◎ THINK ABOUT IT

Inability to Auscultate
Korotkoff Sounds

You are taking Ms. Qualm's blood pressure and are unable to hear the Korotkoff sounds. What would you do?

E   Examination
N   Normal Findings
A   Abnormal Findings
P   Pathophysiology

---

within the cuff. The **mercury manometer** uses a calibrated column of mercury to provide the blood pressure readings. An eye-level view of the meniscus of mercury (crescent-shaped top surface of the mercury column) is important in obtaining accurate readings. Figure 9-3 displays two types of sphygmomanometers.

Doppler or ultrasound stethoscopes can also be used to obtain blood pressure readings. They are especially useful when blood pressure sounds are difficult to hear such as with infants or very obese patients.

E   1. Select appropriate size cuff.
   2. Position the patient. The patient may be sitting, standing, or supine. At first encounter, all three positions are recommended.
   3. Position the arm or leg to be used so that the extremity is at a level equal to or lower than the heart to prevent a false reading.
   4. Apply deflated blood pressure (BP) cuff:
      a. Upper arm: wrap the BP cuff snugly around the bare upper arm. The bottom of the BP cuff should be slightly above the antecubital fossa. The center of the bladder should be directly above the brachial artery.
      b. Leg: wrap the BP cuff around the bare thigh, with the bottom of the BP cuff slightly above the knee. The popliteal artery below the cuff is used for BP measurement.
   5. Establish a baseline systolic blood pressure (palpating the blood pressure), if needed:
      a. Palpate the artery with the finger pads of your nondominant hand distal to the BP cuff.
      b. Inflate the BP cuff and note when the artery pulsation is no longer palpable.
      c. Release the air from the BP cuff and wait 1 to 2 minutes.
   6. Palpate the pulse distal to the BP cuff.
   7. Place the bell of the stethoscope over the blood pressure site (diaphragm may be used if sounds are hard to hear):
      a. If a Doppler ultrasonic stethoscope is to be used, apply conducting gel to the site where the pulse was palpated.
      b. Place Doppler transducer over the site.
   8. Inflate the BP cuff to approximately 20 mm Hg above the established baseline blood pressure or 20 mm Hg above where the Korotkoff sounds disappear.
   9. Slowly open the valve and release the pressure at a rate of 2 to 3 mm Hg per second.
  10. Listen for the Korotkoff sounds:
      a. Onset of Korotkoff sounds correlates to systolic pressure.
      b. Muffling or disappearance of sounds correlates to diastolic pressures.
  11. Deflate BP cuff completely.
  12. Record blood pressure reading(s). The extremity used and position of patient may be important data to record along with the blood pressure reading.

N   *Normal blood pressure varies with age. As a person ages, blood pressure generally increases. Table 9-5 presents general ranges for normal blood pressure at different ages. Normally, **baroreceptors** (receptors that are located in the walls of most of the great arteries and sense hypotension and initiate reflex vasoconstriction and tachycardia to bring the blood pressure back to normal) help a patient to maintain normal blood pressure when changing from a supine to a sitting or a standing position. Pulse pressure is normally 30 to 40 mm Hg. Table 9-6 lists errors in blood pressure measurement.*

A   **Hypertension**, or high blood pressure, is usually confirmed when an adult patient has blood pressure readings remaining consistently above 140 mm Hg systolic and 90 mm Hg diastolic on two consecutive visits.

NURSING ALERT

Automatic Blood Pressure Cuffs

Your patient may be receiving a drug such as heparin, aspirin, or thrombolytic therapy that makes him or her susceptible to bleeding complications (see Figure 9-4). If you are using an automatic blood pressure cuff on your patient, take these precautions to prevent any bleeding complications that may occur in the arm that is being used for non-invasive blood pressure monitoring:

1. Adjust the maximal inflation pressure on the automatic blood pressure machine to your patient's last systolic blood pressure. Otherwise, the blood pressure cuff could inflate as high as to a systolic blood pressure of 200 mm Hg.
2. Once your patient's blood pressure is stable, increase the intervals between measurements. If you do not, the blood pressure cuff could inflate as often as every minute. Also, you can switch the mode to manual from automatic so that you avoid unnecessary inflations of the blood pressure cuff.
3. Place the blood pressure cuff on the arm opposite any intravenous infusions. If this is not possible, then try the thigh as a site for blood pressure measurement.
4. Whenever permissible, rotate the cuff site and remember to remove it at least every shift to assess the patient's skin.

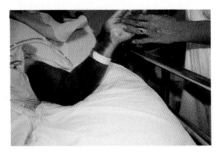

Figure 9-4 Proper placement and monitoring of an automatic blood pressure cuff will reduce the risk of injury or trauma to the patient.

Table 9-5 Blood Pressure: Normal Range According to Age

AGE	SYSTOLIC (mm Hg)	DIASTOLIC (mm Hg)	AVERAGE
Newborn	65–95	30–60	80/46
Infant	65–115	42–80	90/61
3 years	76–122	46–84	99/65
6 years	85–115	48–64	100/56
10 years	93–125	46–68	109/58
14 years	99–137	51–71	118/61
Adult	100–140	60–90	120/80
Elderly	100–160	60–90	130/80

Table 9-6 Errors in Blood Pressure Measurement

IF READING SHOWS:	SUSPECT:
Inaccurately high blood pressure	Blood pressure cuff is too short or too narrow (e.g., using a regular blood pressure cuff on an obese arm), or the brachial artery may be positioned below the heart.
High diastolic blood pressure	Unrecognized auscultatory gap (a silent interval between systolic and diastolic pressures that may occur in hypertensive patients or because you deflated the blood pressure cuff too rapidly); immediate reinflation of the blood pressure cuff for multiple blood pressure readings (resultant venous congestion makes the Korotkoff sounds less audible); if the patient supports his or her own arm, then sustained muscular contraction can raise the diastolic blood pressure by 10%.
Inaccurately low blood pressure	Blood pressure cuff is too long or too wide; the brachial artery is above the heart.
Low systolic blood pressure	Unrecognized auscultatory gap (a rapid deflation of the cuff or immediate reinflation of the cuff for multiple readings can result in venous congestion, thus making the Korotkoff sounds less audible and the pressure appear lower).

Table 9-7 Hypertension Classification*

INITIAL SCREENING BLOOD PRESSURE (mm Hg)**

Systolic	Diastolic	Follow-up Recommended***
<130	<85	Recheck in 2 years
130–139	85–89	Recheck in 1 year****
140–159	90–99	Confirm within 2 months
160–179	100–109	Evaluate or refer to source of care within 1 month
180–209	110–119	Evaluate or refer to source of care within 1 week
≥210	≥120	Evaluate or refer to source of care immediately

   * *Recommendations are for adults age 18 and older.*
  ** *If the systolic and diastolic categories are different, follow recommendation for the shorter time follow-up.*
 *** *The scheduling of follow-up should be modified by reliable information about past blood pressure measurements, other cardiovascular risk factors, or target-organ disease.*
**** *Consider providing advice about lifestyle modifications.*

(From Fifth Report of the Joint National Committee on Detection, Evaluation, and Treatment of High Blood Pressure)

Refer to Table 9-7 for recommendations on the detection, evaluation, and treatment of hypertension.

P The cause of hypertension in 90% of patients who have it is unknown. It is thought that the mechanisms that maintain the therapeutic fluid volume in the body (e.g., the heart, kidneys, nervous system, renin-angiotensin-aldosterone system) may be abnormal. The other 10% of the population who have high blood pressure have secondary hypertension. All of the following pathophysiologies of hypertension are secondary in nature.

P Arteriosclerosis reduces arterial compliance. Elastic and muscular tissues of arteries are replaced with fibrous tissue as part of the normal aging process, making the vessels less able to contract and relax in response to systolic and diastolic pressures.

P Processes decreasing the size of arterial lumen cause hypertension. Hypercholesterolemia results in deposits of plaque along the inner walls of the vessels, reducing the size of the lumen and increasing blood pressure.

P Processes increasing cardiac output will increase blood pressure. Exercise increases O_2 demands on the body, and the body's response is to increase cardiac output.

P Processes that increase the viscosity of the blood, such as sickle cell crisis, cause greater friction between molecules of the blood and, thus, higher blood pressure.

P High blood pressure may result from diseases affecting other regulatory blood pressure processes. For example, kidney disease, which affects the production of antidiuretic hormone, a hormone that helps control body fluid balance, can cause hypertension. An adrenal gland tumor, or pheochromocytoma, can increase blood pressure because of epinephrine and norepinephrine secretion.

P Overloads of fluids from poor renal function or indiscriminant intravenous fluid administration (particularly in children) can result in hypertension.

P Stress can increase blood pressure. Stimulation of the sympathetic nervous system increases cardiac output and vasoconstriction, thus increasing blood pressure.

A Blood pressure falling below normal range is considered to be **hypotension**, or low blood pressure, which results in inadequate tissue perfusion and oxygenation. If the standing systolic blood pressure is more than 30 mm Hg below the supine systolic pressure, it may indicate that the person has orthostatic hypotension. Slow response by baroreceptors when an individual transitions from a lying to a standing position can result in transitory orthostatic hypotension. When this occurs, the individual may feel dizzy and is at risk for falls.

P Processes drastically reducing circulatory blood volume, such as hypovolemic shock, cause hypotension.

P Medications such as nitroglycerin or antihypertensives lower blood pressure.

P Anaphylactic shock, resulting from massive histamine release, and circulatory collapse cause severe hypotension.

A A difference of greater than 10 to 15 mm Hg between the blood pressure in both arms is abnormal.

P This can be caused by coarctation of the aorta, aortic aneurysm, atherosclerotic obstruction, and subclavian steal syndrome, because these conditions all result in an increased pressure proximal to the narrowing and a decreased pressure distal to the narrowing of the aorta or whatever is causing the obstruction.

A A systolic blood pressure that is greater in the arms than in the legs is abnormal.

P This is caused by constriction or obstruction of the aorta, which can result from an increase in stroke volume ejection velocity, increased cardiac output, peripheral vasodilation, and decreased distensibility of the aorta or major arteries.

E	**Examination**
N	**Normal Findings**
A	**Abnormal Findings**
P	**Pathophysiology**

Using Clinical Judgment When Taking Vital Signs

Mr. Goldstein is a 75-year-old hospitalized for pneumonia. He is wearing a 40% oxygen face mask. Mr. Goldstein has a history of confusion and combative behavior, particularly at night. His IV had to be replaced last night because, in his confusion and agitation, he pulled it out. You are working the night shift and it is 2:00 A.M. Mr. Goldstein is sleeping comfortably. He has vital signs ordered every 4 hours. His signs were last taken at 10:00 P.M. and were as follows:

Respirations: 14
Pulse: 90
Blood pressure: 132/88 (left arm)
Temperature: 37.1°C (rectal)

• What are the major issues related to taking Mr Goldstein's vital signs right now?
• What are the possible actions you could take, and what are the potential consequences of each?

E   Examination
N   Normal Findings
A   Abnormal Findings
P   Pathophysiology

A A decreased pulse pressure is abnormal.
P A decreased pulse pressure can result from a decreased stroke volume (cardiac tamponade, shock, and tachycardia) or increased peripheral resistance (aortic stenosis, coarctation of the aorta, mitral stenosis or mitral regurgitation, and cardiac tamponade).
A An increased pulse pressure is abnormal.
P An increased pulse pressure can result from increased stroke volume (aortic regurgitation) or increased peripheral vasodilatation (fever, anemia, heat, exercise, hyperthyroidism, and arteriovenous fistula).

✓ **NURSING CHECKLIST**
General Assessment and Vital Signs

General Assessment
• Physical Presence
  – Stated Age Versus Apparent Age
  – Body Fat
  – Stature
  – Motor Activity
  – Body and Breath Odors
• Psychological Presence
  – Dress, Grooming, and Personal Hygiene
  – Mood and Manner
  – Speech
  – Facial Expression
• Distress

Vital Signs
• Respiration
• Pulse
• Temperature
• Blood Pressure

REVIEW QUESTIONS AND ACTIVITIES

1. Body temperature can be assessed through oral, rectal, axillary, and tympanic routes. Which site would be most appropriate for assessing the following patients' temperatures? Why?
   a. An adult with oral thrush
   b. A patient with cystic fibrosis receiving 2 liters of O_2 via face mask
   c. An adult postsubmersion hypothermia

2. Pulse can be assessed at several sites. Which sites would you chose for pulse assessment for the following patients? Why?
   a. An adult with bilateral wrist injury
   b. An adult with known cardiovascular disease
   c. An unconscious adult following a car accident

3. There are several considerations for selecting the site for measuring blood pressure. Decide which sites would be most appropriate in the following instances. Why?

a. Patient who has an IV infusing in the right arm and an AV fistula for dialysis in the left arm

b. Patient who complains of being dizzy every morning when getting out of bed

c. Patient who is obese and whose blood pressure is difficult to hear

d. Patient who has an IV in left forearm and cast on right arm

e. Elderly patient with extreme dehydration

4. Using a volunteer or yourself, measure and compare body temperature using oral, rectal, axillary, and tympanic routes.

5. Measure and record your early morning and late afternoon temperatures using the same route at each time for several days. Compare the temperatures. Measure and compare your temperature before and after your regular exercise. What factors may have influenced the temperatures?

6. Obtain obese-, adult-, and child-sized blood pressure cuffs. Ask a small adult to volunteer to have blood pressure measured in the arm with each of the cuffs. Compare the readings. Now use the guidelines to select the proper-sized cuff. Which cuff produced an erroneously high reading? An erroneously low reading? Which cuff would you select to measure the pressure if you had to use the leg as a site?

Questions 7 and 8 refer to the following situation:

You are making a home visit to Ms. Margaret Dix, a 78-year-old female discharged yesterday post hip fracture. You notice as you walk in that the house is dimly lit by one lamp in the hall and that Ms. Dix is wearing a beautiful mink fur coat. There is a smell of kerosene in the house. She walks using her walker with a slow, shuffling gait and a slightly hunched-over posture. Her body appears frail and thin. Her hair is matted and she apologizes for the way she looks. As she brings her hand to her hair, you notice a slight tremor. Her speech flows naturally, she smiles, and she seems to respond appropriately to your verbal communication. As you glance around the room, you notice an inhaler at her bedside and a large-print *Guideposts* magazine. She muses about what a cold spring it has been. You agree and recall that last night it dropped down into the low 30°s.

You collect her vital signs. They are as follows:
- Respiratory rate: 18
- Pulse: 96 regular, and 2+/4+
- Temperature: 36.8°C by mouth
- BP: 135/100 (right arm)

7. Based on this set of vital signs, you conclude that Ms. Dix is:
a. Tachypneic
b. Hypothermic
c. Tachycardic
d. Hypertensive

The correct answer is (d).

8. You wonder why Ms. Dix is wearing her beautiful full-length mink coat. Some possible explanations that need further investigation are:
a. She lives on a fixed income and has limited amounts of kerosene. To save kerosene, she turns the heater off at night and as much as possible during the warmer parts of the day.
b. She has difficulty with thermoregulation and is easily chilled.
c. She is suffering from a psychiatric disorder or dementia.
d. All of the above.

The correct answer is (d).

9. Becky Engquist is a 37-year-old triathlete and avid snow skier who lives in Williamsburg, Virginia. During her annual physical, her vital signs were recorded as follows:
   - Respirations: 12
   - Pulse: 51
   - Blood pressure: 110/82/60 (right arm)
   - Temperature: 37.2°C oral

   a. Why is she bradycardic?
   b. Each winter she takes a ski trip to the mountains outside Denver, Colorado. Why does she feel breathless and tachypneic and have an increased heart rate at this higher altitude?

10

Skin, Hair, and Nails

COMPETENCIES

1. Describe the anatomy and physiology of the integumentary system.
2. Explain the process of describing and classifying skin lesions.
3. Identify common skin lesions and discuss possible etiologies.
4. Identify pathophysiological changes to hair and nails and discuss possible etiologies.
5. State the warning signs of carcinoma in pigmented lesions.
6. Describe methods used to assess integumentary changes in both light- and dark-skinned patients.

The skin, also known as the **integumentary system**, or cutaneous tissue, is the largest organ system of the body. It shelters most of the other organ systems, and if assessed carefully, it can provide a noninvasive window to observe the body's level of functioning.

This chapter will provide a review of the skin and its appendages, hair, and nails. Techniques for assessment of the integumentary system will be addressed as will be an approach to evaluating skin lesions.

ANATOMY AND PHYSIOLOGY

Skin

The surface area of the skin covers approximately 20 square feet in the average adult, with a thickness varying from 0.2 mm to 1.5 mm, depending on the region of the body and the patient's age. Morphologically speaking, the skin is composed of three main layers: the epidermis, the dermis, and the subcutaneous tissue, or hypodermis (Figure 10-1).

Epidermis

The **epidermis** is a multilayered outer covering consisting of four layers throughout the body, except for the palms of the hands and soles of the feet, where there are five layers (Figure 10-2). The deepest layer of the epidermis is the **stratum germinativum**, or basal cell layer. It is composed of columnar-shaped cells that rest on a basement membrane. These columnar cells undergo continuous mitosis to produce new cells that replace cells that are lost from the top layer of the epidermis. This layer provides the skin with tone and also creates pigment-producing melanocytes, which filter ultraviolet light. The **stratum spinosum** overlays the stratum germinativum. The stratum spinosum consists of layers of polyhedral-shaped cells. Intercellular bridges

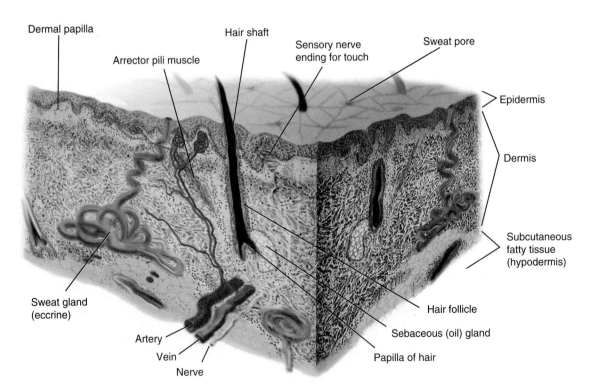

Figure 10-1   Structures of the Skin

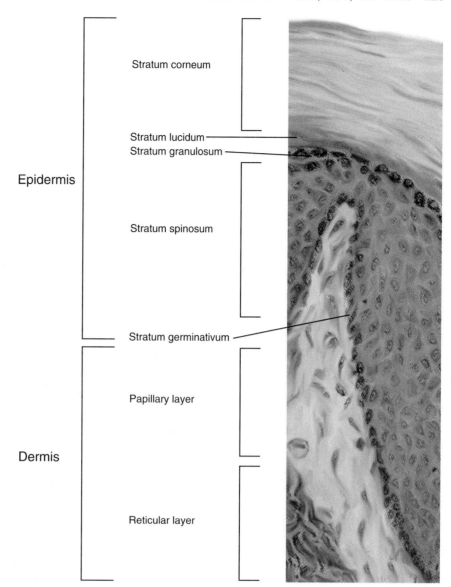

Figure 10-2   Epidermal and Dermal Layers

provide for the irregular shape. Skin cell death occurs in the **stratum granulosum**, which overlays the stratum spinosum. The stratum granulosum is composed of cells with shriveled nuclei and strands of keratin.

The additional layer, which is found exclusively on the palmar and plantar surfaces, is the **stratum lucidum**. It contains a thin layer of translucent **eleidin** that aids in the formation of keratin. Finally, the **stratum corneum**, also known as the horny layer, completes the epidermis. The stratum corneum is composed of enucleated dead epithelial cells. These cells contain keratin, which provides a waterproof barrier. This layer is in a continual state of **desquamation** (shedding), as new skin cells are pushed up from the lower layers; a complete turnover of cells occurs every 3 to 4 weeks.

The epidermis, with the exception of the palmar and plantar surfaces, is normally smooth. All epidermal surfaces are devoid of blood vessels. Despite the absence of vessels, blood pigments, such as oxyhemoglobin and reduced hemoglobin in the corium or dermis, are responsible for the vascular color transmitted to the skin's surface. Other factors that affect the skin's color are various pigments such as melanin and carotene. Epidermal thickness and the ability of the skin to reflect light, known as the Tyndall effect, also influence integumentary color.

Dermis

The **dermis**, or corium, is the second layer of the skin. It is approximately 20 times thicker than the epidermis in certain areas of the body and can be divided into two layers: the papillary layer and the reticular layer (see Figure 10-2). The **papillary layer**, or upper layer, is composed primarily of loose connective tissue, small elastic fibers, and an extensive network of capillaries that serve to nourish the epidermis. The **reticular layer**, the lower layer of the dermis, is formed by a dense bed of vascular connective tissue that also includes nerves and lymphatic tissue. This layer also provides structural support for the skin. In the deeper portions of the reticular layer, collagen fibers in combination with elastic fibers are surrounded in a gelatinous matrix. Intermeshed with the connective tissue are hair follicles, sweat glands, sebaceous glands, and adipose tissue.

The fibrous connective tissue in the dermis gives the skin its strength and elasticity. The fibrous tissues provide structural support for the epidermis and form dermal "ridges" to which the epidermis conforms and anchors, creating "epidermal ridges" known as fingerprints. These ridges develop during the first trimester of fetal development and although they enlarge with growth, their pattern remains the same throughout life and enhances with age.

In general, the dermis is thicker over the dorsal and lateral surfaces such as the palmar and plantar surfaces. It is much thinner over the ventral and medial surfaces, and is especially thin in areas such as the eyelids, scrotum, and penis.

Subcutaneous Tissue

Beneath the dermis is the **subcutaneous tissue**, or superficial fascia. It is composed of loose areolar connective tissue or adipose tissue, depending on its location in the body. The subcutaneous layers attach the skin to the underlying bones. These layers act as a temperature insulator and help regulate body heat; they also encompass fat stores for energy use and contain an extensive venous plexus layer, which acts as a reservoir for the blood that warms the surface of the skin.

Distributed around the dermal blood vessels and the subcutaneous tissue are the skin's mast cells. These cells number from 7,000 to 20,000 per cubic centimeter of skin. **Mast cells** are the body's major source of tissue histamine and trigger the body's reaction to allergens.

Glands of the Skin

There are two main groups of glands in the skin: the sebaceous glands and the sweat glands.

Sebaceous Glands The **sebaceous glands** are sebum-producing glands that are found almost everywhere in the dermis except for the palmar and plantar surfaces. They are also part of the apparatus that contains the hair follicle and the **arrector pili muscle**, which causes contraction of the skin and hair, resulting in "goose bumps." The ducts of the sebaceous glands open into the upper part of the hair follicle and are responsible for producing **sebum**, an oily secretion that is thought to retard evaporation and water loss from the epidermal cells. Sebaceous glands are most prevalent in the scalp, forehead, nose, and chin.

Sweat Glands The two main types of **sweat glands** are **apocrine glands**, which are associated with hair follicles, and **eccrine glands**, which are not associated with hair follicles. The secretory apparatus of both types of sweat glands is located in the subcutaneous tissue. Eccrine glands open directly onto the skin's surface and are widely distributed throughout the body. Apocrine glands are found primarily in the axillae, genital and rectal areas, nipples, and navel. These glands become functional during puberty, and secretion occurs during emotional stress or sexual stimulation. After puberty, apocrine glands are responsible for the characteristic body odor when sweat mixes with the natural bacterial flora normally present on the skin surface.

Hair

With few exceptions (the palmar and plantar surfaces, lips, nipples, and the glans penis), hair is distributed over the entire body surface. Its abundance and texture are dependent on an individual's age, sex, race, and heredity. **Vellus**, or fine, faint hair, covers most of the body. In general, **terminal hair** is the coarser, darker hair of the scalp, eyebrows, and eyelashes. In the axillary and pubic areas, terminal hair becomes increasingly evident in both males and females with the onset of puberty. Males will also tend to develop coarser, thicker chest and facial hair.

Specialized epidermal cells are located in depressions at the base of each hair follicle and are responsible for the formation of each individual hair shaft. The cells are nourished by blood vessels in the dermis so that they grow and divide, pushing the older cells toward the surface of the skin.

Most hair shafts are composed of three layers: the cuticle, or outer layer; the cortex, or middle layer; and the medulla, or innermost layer. Hair color is determined by the **melanocytes** produced in the cells at the base of each follicle; an abundance of pigment produces darker hair color and smaller amounts produce a lighter color.

Nails

Nails are composed of keratinized, or horny, layers of cells that arise from undifferentiated epithelial tissue called the **matrix**. The **nail plate**, tissue that covers the distal portion of the digits and provides protection, is approximately 0.5–0.75 mm thick. The nails consists of the **nail root**, which lies posteriorly to the cuticle and is attached to the matrix; the **nail bed**, which is the vascular bed located beneath the nail plate; and the **periungual tissues**, which surround the nail plate and the free edge of the nail (Figure 10-3). At

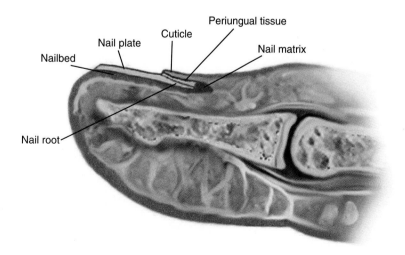

Figure 10-3   Structures of the Nail

the proximal end of each nail is a white, crescent-shaped area known as the **lunula**. This structure is obscured by the cuticle in some individuals.

The normally translucent nail plate is given a pinkish cast by the underlying vascular bed in light-skinned individuals and a brownish cast in dark-skinned individuals. In many disease processes, the color of the nailbed may vary. For instance, a decrease in oxygen content of the blood will cause the nailbeds to appear **cyanotic**, or blue.

The nail plate is formed continuously as the plate is pushed forward by new growth from the germinative layer of the matrix. Normal growth for an adult is 0.1 mm to 1.0 mm per day, but growth varies with age, season, nutrition, climate, health status, and activity.

Function of Skin

The skin has many functions, but perhaps the most important one is its ability to serve as a protective barrier against invasion from environmental hazards and pathogens. It provides boundaries for materials that might enter the body, such as toxic chemicals, and provides boundaries for fluids and mobile tissues, such as blood, within the body. An intact integument is also responsible for the protection of underlying organs, which would otherwise be vulnerable to injury because of exposure.

Temperature regulation is carried out by the skin through the production of perspiration. During states of increased body temperature, large quantities of sweat are produced by the eccrine glands. As perspiration reaches the skin's surface, rapid evaporation takes place and the body's temperature begins to decrease. The skin's vascular system also plays a role in heat control. When vasodilation occurs, much of the heat can be lost through radiation and conduction. Conversely, vasoconstriction helps to maintain body heat.

The skin contains receptors for pain, touch, pressure, and temperature. These receptors originate in the dermis and terminate as either free nerve endings throughout the skin's surface or as special touch receptors that are encapsulated and found predominantly in the fingertips and lips. Each hair found on the body also contains a basal nerve fiber that acts as a tactile receptor. Sensory signals that help determine precise locations on the skin are transmitted along rapid sensory pathways, and less distinct signals such as pressure or poorly localized touch are sent via slower sensory pathways.

The skin acts as an organ of excretion for substances such as water, salts, and nitrogenous wastes. The skin produces cells for wound repair and is the site for the production of vitamin D. It is also an indicator of nonverbal language and emotions via blushing and facial expressions.

Function of Hair

Hair provides warmth, protection, and sensation to the underlying systems. Terminal hair of the scalp and face provides warmth, shields against ultraviolet light, and filters dust and particulate matter. Vellus hair enhances tactile sensation and sensory perception. In many cultures, hair is a status symbol of beauty and wealth.

Function of Nails

Nails provide protection to the distal surface of the digits and can be used for self-protection. In many cultures, nail length in both men and women is a qualifier of social and economic status.

❖   HEALTH HISTORY

The skin, hair, and nails health history provides insight into the link between a patient's life/lifestyle and skin, hair, and nails information and pathology.

PATIENT PROFILE	*Diseases that are age-, sex-, and race-specific for the skin, hair, and nails are listed.*
Age	
Skin	Fungal infections, diseases of sebaceous glands, such as acne vulgaris (13–26) Lupus erythematosus, psoriasis, hyperpigmented macular lesions, skin tags (acrochordon), dermatophyte infections (25–60) Basal cell carcinoma (older adults)
Hair	Male pattern alopecia (adolescence to young adulthood) Thinning, graying, loss of hair in axillary and pubic areas, excessive facial hair (middle to old age)
Sex	
Skin	Male: Skin pathology is consistently more prevalent among males than females; dermatophyte infections; skin tumors; fungal infections and increased incidence of tumors related to occupational hazards and hygiene; Kaposi's sarcoma associated with immunodeficiency conditions
Hair	Female: Female pattern alopecia, increased facial hair with aging Male: Alopecia, increased coarse nose and ear hair with aging
Race	
Dark Skinned	Keloid formation, dermatosis papulosa nigra, hyper- and hypopigmentation, traumatic marginal alopecia, seborrheic dermatitis, pseudofolliculitis barbae, acne keloidalis, granuloma inguinale, Mongolian spots, albinism, hypopigmented sarcoidosis, granulomatosis skin lesions
Light Skinned	Squamous and basal cell carcinoma, actinic keratosis, psoriasis
CHIEF COMPLAINT	*Common chief complaints for the skin, hair, and nails are defined, and information on the characteristics of each sign/symptom is provided.*
Pruritus	Cutaneous itching that may have a multitude of etiologies
Location	Generalized or localized
Quality	Superficial or deep sensation of itching, intensity of itching, interference with sleep habits

continued

Associated Manifestations	Rashes, lesions, edema, angioedema, anaphylaxis, excoriation or ulcers as the result of scratching, **lichenification** (thickening of the skin), systemic disease
Aggravating Factors	Exposure to chemicals, sunlight, plants, food, animals, stress, climate, parasites, xerosis, drug reaction, systemic disease processes, contact dermatitis, types of clothing (frequently wool)
Alleviating Factors	Dietary changes, medications, antihistamines, biofeedback, cool baths, types of clothing (frequently cotton), increased skin hydration, ultraviolet band light therapy
Setting	Work, home, school, or recreational environment
Timing	Pre- or postprandial, nocturnal, seasonal, during periods of stress, associated with menstrual cycle
Rash	A cutaneous eruption that may be localized or generalized.
Lesion	A circumscribed pathological change in the tissues
Location	Location of, where did it start and spread, distribution over the body, percent of body involved, following dermatomes
Quantity	"Grouping or arrangement": discrete, grouped, confluent, linear, annular, polycyclic, generalized, zosteriform
Quality	"Morphology": macule, patch, papule, plaque, nodule, cyst, wheal, vesicle, pustule, bullae, tumor, lichenification, crust, erosion, fissure, ulcer, or atrophy
Associated Manifestations	Edema, angioedema, anaphylaxis, excoriation or ulcers as the result of scratching, lichenification, systemic disease, allergies, fever, induration
Aggravating Factors	Exposure to chemicals, sunlight, plants, food, animals, stress, climate, parasites, xerosis, drug reaction, systemic disease processes, contact dermatitis, radiation, types of clothing (frequently wool)
Alleviating Factors	Dietary changes, medications, antihistamines, biofeedback, cool baths, types of clothing (frequently cotton), increased skin hydration, ultraviolet band light therapy, surgery
Setting	Work, home, school, or recreational environment
Timing	When did it start, pre- or postprandial, nocturnal, seasonal, during periods of stress, associated with menstrual cycle
PAST HEALTH HISTORY	*The various components of the past health history are linked to skin, hair, and nails pathology and skin-, hair-, and nails-related information.*
Medical	
Skin Specific	Allergies, eczema, melanoma, albinism, vitiligo, psoriasis, skin cancer, athlete's foot

continued

Nonskin Specific	Renal disease, diabetes mellitus, lupus erythematosus, peripheral vascular disease, idiopathic thrombocytopenia purpura (ITP), Rocky Mountain spotted fever, liver disease, hepatitis, collagen diseases, cardiac dysfunction, sexually transmitted diseases, Lyme disease, arthritis, lymphoma, thyroid disease, pregnancy, Addison's disease, pernicious anemia, HIV, cytomegalovirus, Epstein-Barr virus, measles, mumps, rubella, coxsackievirus, adenovirus, typhoid, drug hypersensitivities, varicella, herpes zoster, herpes simplex, Kawasaki disease, toxic shock syndrome, carcinoma, asthma, tuberculosis
Hair Specific	Allergies, alopecia, lice, bacterial or fungal infections of the scalp, brittle hair, rapid hair loss, trichotillomania, trauma, congenital anomalies
Nonhair Specific	Renal disease, diabetes mellitus, cardiac dysfunction, peripheral vascular disease, thyroid disease, pregnancy, Addison's disease, HIV, anemia, malnutrition, stress, chemotherapy, radiation therapy
Nail Specific	Allergies, psoriasis, bacterial or fungal infections, trauma, brittle nails, nail biting, congenital anomalies
Non-Nail Specific	Iron deficiency, anemia, chronic infection, malnutrition, Raynaud's disease, hypoxia, acute infections, syphilis
Surgical	Keloid and scar formation, plastic surgery for birthmarks, skin grafts, reconstructive surgery, tattoos, excision biopsy
Medications	Reaction manifested in skin changes after use of prescription or over-the-counter drugs
Communicable Diseases	Chickenpox, roseola, measles, scabies, bacterial or fungal infections, HIV, etc. Sexually transmitted diseases: syphilis, gonorrhea, chancroid, genital warts (refer to Chapters 19 and 20 for further information)
Allergies	Medication, insect stings, foods, soaps, laundry detergent, chemicals, fibers (wool), metals (gold), animal dander, pollens, grasses, cosmetics, first manifestation of allergic reaction
Injuries/Accidents	Chemical inhalation, trauma, burns, toxin contamination
Disabilities/Handicaps	Poor eyesight can lead to poor hygiene, frequent skin trauma, prevents early detection and treatment of skin diseases
Blood Transfusions	Skin eruptions, pruritus
Childhood Illnesses	Refer to section on communicable diseases
FAMILY HEALTH HISTORY	*Skin, hair, and nail diseases that are familial in nature are listed.*
Skin Specific	Allergies, eczema, melanoma, albinism, vitiligo, psoriasis
Hair Specific	Allergies, alopecia, brittle hair, hair loss

continued

Nail Specific	Allergies, brittle nails
SOCIAL HISTORY	*The components of the social history are linked to skin, hair, and nail factors/pathology.*
Alcohol Use	Hepatotoxicity and subsequent skin manifestations that accompany liver failure, such as jaundice and pruritus; skin bruising and trauma from falls and ataxia; telangiectasia (spider veins) of the nose, neck, and upper chest
Tobacco Use	Yellow discoloration of fingertips on smoking hand, leathery facial appearance
Drug Use	Skin manifestations from intravenous drug use, such as injection sites or tracks; these are especially prevalent in the forearms, behind the knees, toe webs, finger webs, and under the nails
Sexual Practice	Various sexually transmitted diseases may manifest in the genital region; these are discussed in Chapters 19 and 20
Travel History	Central and South America: fungal infections, contact dermatitis, tropical eczema, leishmaniasis Insect bites: insects indigenous to certain climates, such as the tsetse fly in Africa and the deer tick in wooded areas of the northern and southeastern United States High altitude areas: light-sensitive eruptions and winter eczema Southeastern United States, Mississippi, and Ohio River valleys, and South America: blastomycosis most likely caused by infected soil
Work Environment	Chemical: contact dermatitis and burns Sunlight: skin eruptions, increased incidence of basal or squamous cell carcinoma, burns, wrinkles, senile freckles, lightened hair, excessive exposure to ultraviolet radiation Excessive exposure to water: drying and cracking of skin, pruritus, soft nails, damaged hair shafts Insect bites: rashes, urticaria, edema, angioedema, pruritus Operating heavy or sharp equipment: trauma, laceration Excessive exposure to wind and cold temperatures: aging, drying, and cracking of skin Pollution: contact dermatitis Tar and pitch: act as both photosensitizers and carcinogens
Home Environment	Chemicals used in cleaning can cause contact dermatitis; excessive exposure to water can cause dry, cracked skin, soft nails and damaged hair shafts; excessive heat in the home can dry skin and cause pruritus; infected kittens and puppies may lead to tinea capitis
Hobbies/Leisure Activities	Gardening with exposure to chemicals, sunlight, and insect bites; outdoor summer sports or activities increase sun and insect-bite exposure; outdoor winter activities increase frostbite and exposure; excessive exposure to chlorine and salt water damages hair; excessive use of tanning salons may lead to skin carcinoma

continued

Stress	Skin eruptions such as eczema, urticaria, acne, and psoriasis may have a psychological component in some cases; body image disorder as a result of skin disease and hair loss
Economic Status	People of lower socioeconomic status may develop skin eruptions associated with poor hygiene because of insufficient resources, infestations associated with overcrowding, and infections associated with malnutrition
Ethnic Background	
Scandinavian and Northern European	Psoriasis
Mexican American	Lupus erythematosus
Hawaiian and Brazilian	Leprosy is endemic in these populations
Central and South American	Fungal infections, contact dermatitis, tropical ulcers, and eczema related to increased heat and humidity; light-sensitivity eruptions and winter eczema related to high altitude
HEALTH MAINTENANCE ACTIVITIES	*This information provides a bridge between the health maintenance activities and the skin, hair, and nails function.*
Sleep	Sleep disturbances caused by symptoms such as itching or burning
Diet	Allergies to food can cause skin eruptions such as urticaria; diets high in fat and cholesterol may be connected to the development of xanthelasmatous lesions; vitamin deficiencies result in skin, hair, and nail changes; refer to Chapter 7 for further information
Exercise	Increased risk for cutaneous trauma associated with contact sports
Use of Safety Devices	Sunblock with appropriate sun protection factor (SPF) to prevent ultraviolet exposure; lotions and creams to prevent drying and cracking of skin; apply products to hydrated skin; protective gloves when handling harsh irritating chemicals
Health Check-Ups	Moles and birthmarks assessed for changes in size, shape, or color; skin lesions from sun exposure assessed

❖ ASK YOURSELF

Dealing with a Chemical-Dependent Patient

What would you do if during an assessment of a patient you found signs of IV drug use? Would you confront the patient regarding substance use and practices? How would you feel about providing care to this patient? Should drug users receive the same care and treatment as other individuals? Should they receive Medicaid if their addictions are disabling?

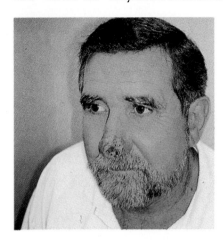

Figure 10-4A Blastomycosis
*Courtesy of Dr. Mark Dougherty,
Lexington, KY*

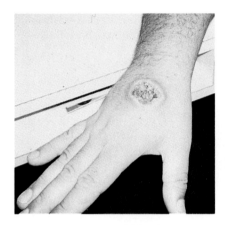

Figure 10-4B Leishmaniasis
*Courtesy of Dr. Mark Dougherty,
Lexington, KY*

 NURSING TIP

***Reducing Exposure to
Integumentary Irritants***

- In the workplace, always follow Occupational Health and Safety Administration (OSHA) and employer's safety guidelines.
- Follow the directions on the labels of all products; pay special attention to warning labels.
- If using a personal care product for the first time, perform a patch test to evaluate for sensitivity.
- Use rubber gloves when handling toxins or caustic substances.
- Contact poison control center for treatment guidelines if exposed to toxic or caustic substances.

 NURSING TIP

Eliciting the Travel History

Figure 10-4A depicts a patient with blastomycosis, and Figure 10-4B shows a patient with leishmaniasis. Both conditions are most frequently seen in individuals who live in regions associated with these disorders, although travelers to these areas are also susceptible to the diseases. These photographs graphically demonstrate the importance of inquiring about a patient's home and work environments and travel history.

 ASK YOURSELF

Skin, Hair, and Nails Risk Assessment

1. Identify the health maintenance activities that you use to protect your skin, hair, and nails.
2. Are there any safety devices or techniques that you should use but do not? If yes, what are your reasons? Is the rationale based on scientific evidence?

✓ NURSING CHECKLIST
Specific Health History Questions Regarding the Skin, Hair, and Nails

Skin Care Habits
- Do you use lotions, perfumes, cologne, cosmetics, soaps, oils, shaving cream, after-shave lotion, electric or standard razor?
- What type of home remedies do you use for skin lesions and rashes?
- How often do you bathe or shower?
- Do you use a tanning bed or salon?
- What type of sun protection do you use?
- Have you ever had a reaction to jewelry that you wore?
- Do you wear hats, visors, gloves, long sleeves or pants, sunscreen?
- How much time do you spend in the sun?

Hair Care Habits
- Do you use shampoo, conditioner, hair spray, setting products?
- Do you color, dye, bleach, frost, or use relaxants on your hair?
- What products do you use?
- Do you wear a wig or hairpiece?
- Do you have graying hair or hair loss?
- Do you use a hair dryer, heated curlers, or curling iron?
- Do you tightly braid your hair?

Nail Care Habits
- Do you get manicures or pedicures?
- What type of nail care do you practice (trimming, clipping, use of polish, nail tips, acrylics)?
- Do you bite your nails?
- Do you suffer from nail splitting or discoloration?

NURSING ALERT

Manicures and Pedicures

Recently, there has been an increased incidence of hepatitis B infections related to manicures and pedicures obtained in commercial salons. Advise your patients to verify that the facilities in which they obtain these type of cosmetic treatments sterilize the equipment between clients. Also advise patients to bring their own equipment to be used during the manicures or pedicures.

NURSING CHECKLIST

General Approach to Skin, Hair, and Nails Assessment

1. Ensure that the room is well lit. Daylight is the best source of light, especially when determining skin color. However, if daylight is unavailable, overhead fluorescent lights should be added.
2. Use a hand-held magnifying glass to aid in inspection when simple visual inspection is not adequate.
3. Explain to the patient each step of the assessment process prior to initiating the assessment.
4. Ensure patient privacy by providing drapes.
5. Ensure the comfort of the patient by keeping the room at an appropriate temperature.
6. Warm hands by washing them in warm water prior to the assessment.
7. Gather equipment on a table prior to initiating the assessment.
8. Ask the patient to undress completely and put on a patient gown, leaving the back untied.
9. Perform assessment in a cephalocaudal fashion.

EQUIPMENT

- Magnifying glass
- Good source of natural light
- Penlight
- Clean gloves
- Microscope slide
- Small centimeter ruler

For Special Techniques

- Wood's lamp
- #15 scalpel blade
- Microscope slide with cover slips
- Mineral oil
- 10% potassium hydroxide (KOH)
- Lighter or alcohol burner
- Microscope

E	Examination
N	Normal Findings
A	Abnormal Findings
P	Pathophysiology

ASSESSMENT OF THE SKIN, HAIR, AND NAILS

Inspection of the Skin

In each area, observe for: color, bleeding, ecchymosis, vascularity, lesions, moisture, temperature, texture, turgor, and edema.

E
1. Facing the patient, inspect the color of the skin of the face, eyelids, ears, nose, lips, and mucous membranes.
2. Inspect the anterior and lateral aspects of the neck, then behind the ears.
3. Inspect arms and dorsal and palmar surfaces of the hands. Pay special attention to the webs between the fingers.
4. Have the patient move to a supine position, with arms placed over the head.
5. Lower gown to uncover chest and breasts.
6. Inspect intramammary folds and ridges. Pendulous breasts may need to be raised to complete this inspection.
7. Assess axillae and cover chest and breasts with gown.
8. Raise gown to uncover abdomen and anterior aspect of the lower extremities; place a sheet over the genital area.
9. Inspect abdomen, anterior aspect of the lower extremities, dorsal and plantar surfaces of the feet, and toe webs.
10. Don gloves and uncover genital area.
11. Inspect inguinal folds and genitalia.
12. Remove gloves.
13. Have the patient turn to a side-lying position on the examination table so the patient's back is facing you.
14. Inspect back and posterior neck and scalp. Specifically look for nevi or other lesions.

15. Inspect posterior aspect of the lower extremities.

16. Don clean gloves and raise the gluteal cleft and inspect the gluteal folds and perianal area; then remove and discard the gloves.

17. Cover the patient and assist back to a sitting position.

NURSING TIP

Targeting Integumentary Assessment

Assessment of the skin, hair, and nails is usually incorporated into the cephalocaudal patient assessment. If the patient presents with a skin, hair, or nail complaint, or if pathology of the skin, hair, or nails is found on examination, a thorough assessment is warranted.

Color

E Assess for coloration.

N *Normally, the skin is a uniform whitish pink or brown color, depending on the patient's race. Exposure to sunlight results in increased pigmentation of sun-exposed areas. Dark-skinned persons may normally have a freckling of the gums, tongue borders, and lining of the cheeks; the gingiva may appear blue or variegated in color.*

A The appearance of cyanotic (dusky blue) fingers, lips, or mucous membranes is abnormal in both light- and dark-skinned individuals. In light-skinned individuals, the skin has a bluish tint. The earlobes, lower eyelids, lips, oral mucosa, nailbeds, and palmar and plantar surfaces may be especially cyanotic. Dark-skinned individuals have an ashen-gray to pale tint, and the lips and tongue are good indicators of cyanosis.

P Cyanosis occurs when there is greater than 5 g/dl of deoxygenated hemoglobin in the blood. In order for cyanosis to be an accurate indicator of arterial blood oxygen (PaO_2), two conditions must be met. The patient must have normal hemoglobin and hematocrit as well as normal perfusion. For example, a patient with **polycythemia** (elevated number of red blood cells) can be cyanotic but have adequate oxygenation. The problem lies in the fact that the patient has too many red blood cells rather than too little oxygen. Conversely, a patient with **anemia** (reduced number of red blood cells) can be hypoxemic but not cyanotic. In this case, the patient has too little hemoglobin. Central cyanosis is secondary to marked heart and lung disease; peripheral cyanosis can be secondary to systemic disease or vasoconstriction stimulated by cold or anxiety.

A The appearance of **jaundice** (yellow-green to orange cast or coloration) of skin, sclera, mucous membranes, fingernails, and palmar or plantar surfaces in the light-skinned individual is abnormal (see Figure 10-5A). Jaundice in dark-skinned individuals may appear as yellow staining in the sclera, hard palate, and palmar or plantar surfaces.

P Jaundice is caused by an increased serum bilirubin level of greater than 2 mg/dl associated with liver disease or hemolytic disease. Severe burns and sepsis also can produce jaundice.

A Orange-yellow coloration of palmar and plantar surfaces and forehead but no involvement of the mucous membranes is abnormal.

P **Carotenemia**, elevated levels of serum carotene, results from the excessive ingestion of carotene-rich foods such as carrots.

A A grayish cast to the skin is abnormal.

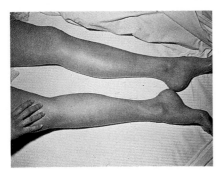

A. Jaundice *Courtesy of the Centers for Disease Control and Prevention (CDC)*

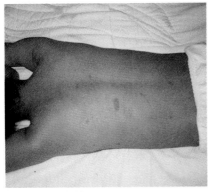

B. Café au Lait Spots

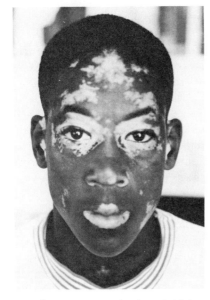

C. Vitiligo *Courtesy of Delmar Publishers, Albany, NY*

Figure 10-5 Skin Coloration Abnormalities

E	**Examination**
N	**Normal Findings**
A	**Abnormal Findings**
P	**Pathophysiology**

P A grayish cast is seen in renal patients and is associated with chronic anemia along with retained urochrome pigments. Slight jaundice may also be found in the renal patient.

A A combination of pallor and ecchymosis with a jaundiced appearance is abnormal.

P Uremia secondary to renal failure results in serum urochrome pigment retention.

A Sustained bright red or pink coloration in light-skinned individuals is abnormal. Dark-skinned individuals may have no underlying change in coloration. Palpation may be used to ascertain signs of warmth, swelling, or induration.

P Hyperemia occurs because of dilated superficial blood vessels, increased blood flow, febrile states, local inflammatory condition, or excessive alcohol intake.

A A bright red to ruddy sustained appearance that is evident on the integument, mucous membranes, and palmar or plantar surfaces is abnormal in both light- and dark-skinned individuals.

P Polycythemia, as noted earlier, is an increased number of red blood cells and results in this ruddy appearance.

A A dusky rubor of the extremities when in a dependent position, which can be associated with tissue necrosis, is abnormal.

P Venous stasis results from venule engorgement and diminished blood flow, which occurs in congestive heart failure and atherosclerosis.

A A pale cast to the skin that may be most evident in the face, mucous membranes, lips, and nailbeds is abnormal in light-skinned individuals. A yellow-brown to ashen-gray cast to the skin along with pale or gray lips, mucous membranes, and nailbeds is abnormal in dark-skinned individuals.

P Pallor is due to decreased visibility of the normal oxyhemoglobin. This can occur when the patient has decreased blood flow in the superficial vessels, as in shock or syncope, or when there is a decreased amount of serum oxyhemoglobin, as in anemia. Localized pallor may be secondary to arterial insufficiency.

A A brown cast to the skin can be generalized or discrete.

P A brown coloration occurs when there is a deposition of melanin that can be caused by genetic predisposition, pregnancy, Addison's disease (deficiency in cortisol leads to enhanced melanin production), café au lait spots (see Figure 10-5B), and sunlight.

A A white cast to the skin as evidenced by generalized whiteness including of the hair and eyebrows is abnormal.

P This lack of coloration is caused by **albinism**, a congenital inability to form melanin.

A **Vitiligo** is a condition marked by patchy symmetrical areas of white on the skin and is abnormal (see Figure 10-5C).

P This condition can be caused by an acquired loss of melanin. Trauma can also lead to hypopigmentation, especially in dark-skinned individuals.

Bleeding, Ecchymosis, and Vascularity

E Inspect the skin for evidence of bleeding, ecchymosis, or increased vascularity.

N *Normally, there are no areas of increased vascularity, ecchymosis, or bleeding.*

A Bleeding from the mucous membranes, previous venipuncture sites, or lesions should be considered abnormal.

P Spontaneous bleeding can be indicative of clotting disorders, trauma, or use of antithrombolytic agents such as coumadin or heparin.

E Examination
N Normal Findings
A Abnormal Findings
P Pathophysiology

A **Petechiae** are red-purple discolorations of less than 0.5 cm in diameter (see Figure 10-6A). Petechiae do not blanch. In dark-skinned individuals, evaluate for petechiae in the mucous membranes and axillae.

P Petechiae can indicate an increased bleeding tendency or embolism; causes include intravascular defects or infections.

A **Purpura** is a condition characterized by the presence of confluent petechiae or confluent ecchymosis over any part of the body (see Figure 10-6B).

P Purpura or peliosis is characterized by hemorrhage into the skin and can be caused by decreased platelet formation. Lesions vary based on the type of purpura; pigmentation changes may become permanent.

A **Ecchymosis** is a red-purple discoloration of varying size, also called a black-and-blue mark (see Figure 10-6C). In dark-skinned patients, these red-purple discolorations are deeper in color.

P Ecchymosis is caused by extravasation of blood into the skin as a result of trauma and can also occur with heparin or coumadin use or liver dysfunction.

A **Spider angiomas** are bright red and star shaped. There is often a central pulsation noted with pressure and this results in blanching in the extensions. Most often, these lesions are noted on the face, neck and chest.

P Causes of spider angiomas include pregnancy, liver disease, and hormone therapy. They are normal in a small percentage of the population and are more prevalent in women.

A **Venous stars** are linear or irregularly shaped blue vascular patterns that do not blanch with pressure (see Figure 10-6D). These are often noted on the legs near veins or on the anterior chest.

P Venous stars are caused by increased venous pressure in the superficial veins.

A **Cherry angiomas** are bright-red circumcised areas that may darken with age (see Figure 10-6E). They can be flat or raised and may show partial blanching with pressure. Most often, they are found on the trunk.

P These vascularities are of unknown etiology and are pathologically insignificant except for cosmetic appearance.

A A bright-red, raised area that has well-defined borders and does not blanch with pressure is abnormal (see Figure 10-6F).

P Strawberry hemangiomas, or strawberry marks, are congenital malformations of closely packed immature capillaries. This condition is also known as nevus vascularis.

A A burgundy, red, or purple macular vascular patch that is located along the course of a peripheral nerve is abnormal (see Figure 10-6G).

P This is a port-wine stain, or nevus flammeus. The port-wine stain is composed of mature but thin-walled capillaries. The lesion is usually present at birth and is frequently located on the face. A port-wine stain can be indicative of underlying disorders.

A In light-skinned individuals, a purple to black discoloration is abnormal (see Figure 10-6H). In dark-skinned individuals, very dark to black discoloration is abnormal.

P These findings can indicate different stages of necrosis, or tissue death. Conditions that starve the affected body part of oxygen, whether in acute or chronic situations, can cause necrosis. Diabetes mellitus, disseminated intravascular coagulation, acute hypovolemia, and severe electric charge are some of the conditions that can cause necrosis.

A Dark-brown or blackened areas of skin that are edematous and painful are abnormal (see Figure 10-6I). These areas may drain a thin liquid that has a sweet, foul odor. Crepitus may be palpated in the affected areas.

P Gas gangrene, or clostridial myonecrosis, is a gram-positive infection that affects skeletal muscles that have decreased oxygenation. The clostridia organisms are endogenous to the gastrointestinal tract and are also found

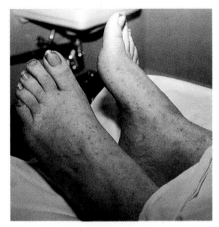

A. Petechiae   *Courtesy of Dr. Mark Dougherty, Lexington, KY*

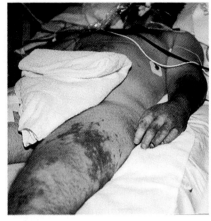

B. Purpura   *Courtesy of Dr. Mark Dougherty, Lexington, KY*

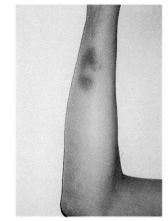

C. Ecchymosis

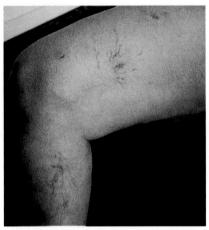

D. Venous Star

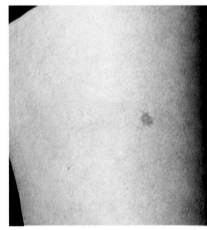

E. Cherry Angioma

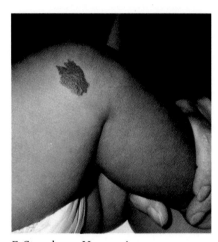

F. Strawberry Hemangioma

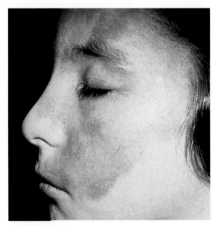

G. Nevus Flammeus   *Courtesy of Robert A. Silverman, M.D., Clinical Associate Professor, Department of Pediatrics, Georgetown University*

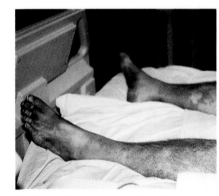

H. Necrosis   *Courtesy of Dr. Mark Dougherty, Lexington, KY*

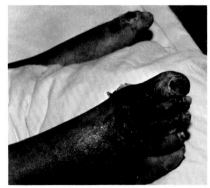

I. Gas Gangrene   *Courtesy of Delmar Publishers, Albany, NY*

Figure 10-6   Bleeding, Ecchymosis, and Vascular Abnormalities of the Skin

in the soil. Patients who experience circulatory compromise, such as in diabetes mellitus, arterial insufficiency, trauma, and constricting casts, are at risk for developing gas gangrene. Patients who have contaminated wounds and decreased vascularity to the affected area are also at risk for developing gas gangrene.

Lesions

E   1. Inspect the skin for lesions, noting the anatomic location. Lesions can be localized, regionalized, or generalized. They can involve exposed areas or skin folds (see Table 10-1).
2. Note the grouping or arrangement of the lesions: discrete, grouped, confluent, linear, annular, polycyclic, generalized, or zosteriform (see Figure 10-7).
3. Inspect the lesions for elevation (flat or raised).
4. Using a ruler, measure the lesions.
5. Describe the color of the lesions.
6. Note any exudate for color or odor.
7. Note the morphology of the skin lesions. Skin lesions can be primary, originating from previously normal skin, or secondary, originating from primary lesions. For specific descriptions of primary lesion morphology, refer to Figure 10-8. For specific descriptions of secondary lesion morphology, refer to Figure 10-9.

N   *No skin lesions should be present except for freckles, birthmarks, or moles (**nevi**), which may be flat or elevated.*

Table 10-1   Anatomic Locations of Various Skin Lesions

LESION	LOCATION
Basal cell carcinoma	Medial and lateral canthi and nasolabial fold
Rosacea	Face
Acne vulgaris	Face, back, shoulders, chest
Furuncle	Nose, neck, face, axillae, and buttocks
Lesions resulting from light exposure (squamous cell carcinoma, solar lentigo, solar keratosis)	Forehead, cheeks, tops of the ears, neck, dorsal surface of hands and forearms, and lateral arms
Seborrheic keratosis, spider angioma	Face, trunk and upper extremities
Impetigo, verruca vulgaris (warts)	Arms, legs, buttocks, face, hands, fingers, and knees
Herpes zoster	Along the cutaneous spinal nerve tracks, almost always unilateral
Kaposi's sarcoma	Widespread: trunk, head, tip of nose, periorbital, penis, legs, palms, and soles
Erythema nodosum	Lower legs
Stasis dermatitis	Sock area
Cutaneous moniliasis	Moist folds behind the ears, under the breasts, in the axilla, umbilicus, along the inguinal and pudendal regions, and in the gluteal and perineal areas
Adult atopic eczema	Mainly flexor surfaces of the body
Psoriasis	Mainly scalp, elbows, and extensor surfaces of the body (rarely on the face and skin folds)
Contact dermatitis	Affects surfaces in contact with irritating agents
Pediculosis pubis	Pubic and axillary areas

E   **Examination**
N   **Normal Findings**
A   **Abnormal Findings**
P   **Pathophysiology**

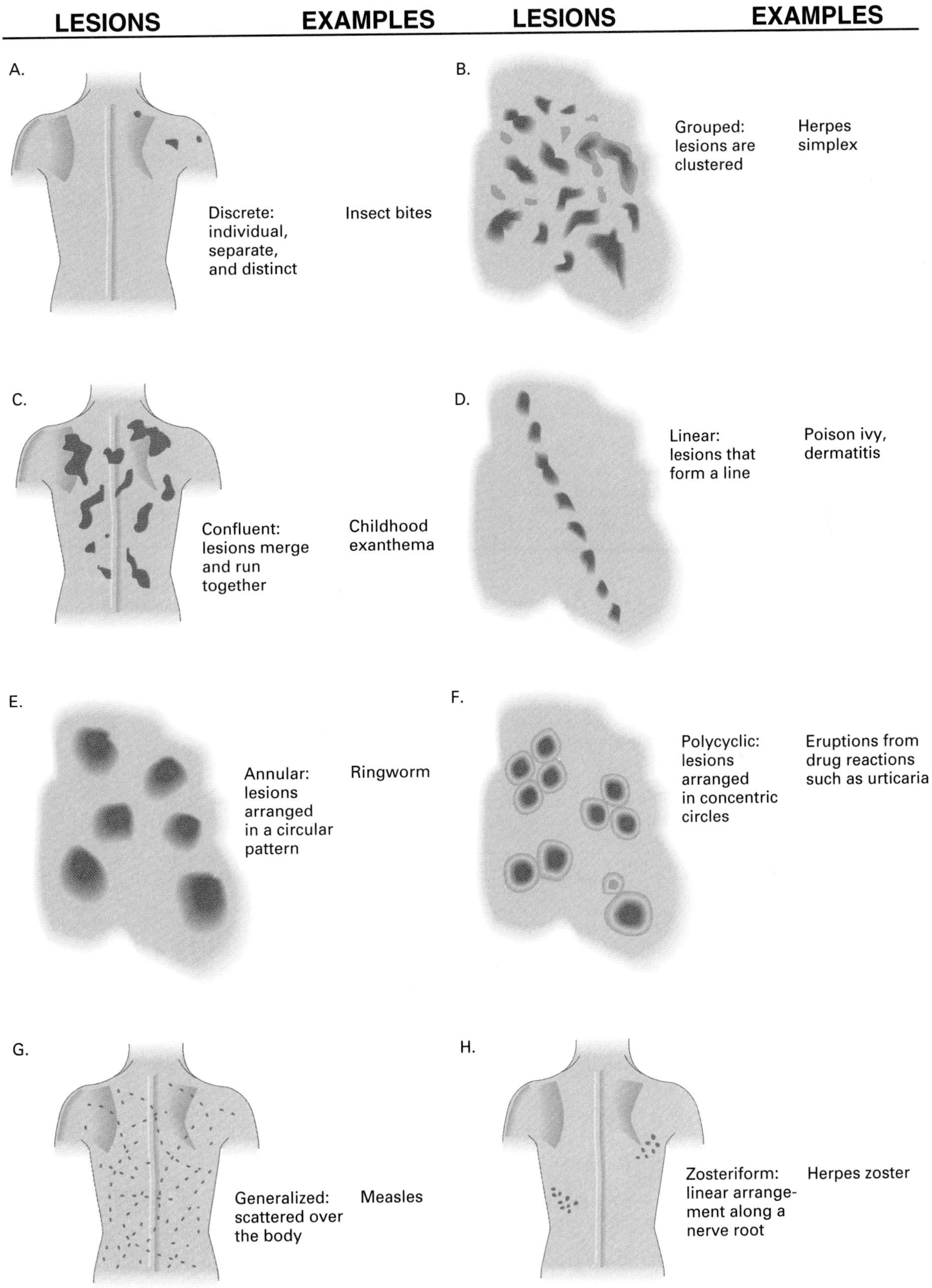

LESIONS	EXAMPLES	LESIONS	EXAMPLES

A.

Discrete: individual, separate, and distinct

Insect bites

B.

Grouped: lesions are clustered

Herpes simplex

C.

Confluent: lesions merge and run together

Childhood exanthema

D.

Linear: lesions that form a line

Poison ivy, dermatitis

E.

Annular: lesions arranged in a circular pattern

Ringworm

F.

Polycyclic: lesions arranged in concentric circles

Eruptions from drug reactions such as urticaria

G.

Generalized: scattered over the body

Measles

H.

Zosteriform: linear arrangement along a nerve root

Herpes zoster

Figure 10-7 Arrangement of Lesions

NONPALPABLE

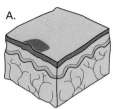

A.

Macule:
Localized changes in skin color of less than 1 cm in diameter
Example:
Freckle

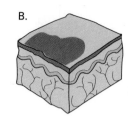

B.

Patch:
Localized changes in skin color of greater than 1 cm in diameter
Example:
Vitiligo, stage 1 of pressure ulcer

PALPABLE

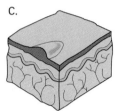

C.

Papule:
Solid, elevated lesion less than 0.5 cm in diameter
Example:
Warts, elevated nevi

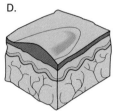

D.

Plaque:
Solid, elevated lesion greater than 0.5 cm in diameter
Example:
Psoriasis

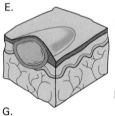

E.

Nodules:
Solid and elevated; however, they extend deeper than papules into the dermis or subcutaneous tissues, 0.5-2.0 cm
Example:
Lipoma, erythema nodosum, cyst

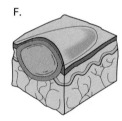

F.

Tumor:
The same as a nodule only greater than 2 cm

Example:
Carcinoma (such as advanced breast carcinoma); **not** basal cell or squamous cell of the skin

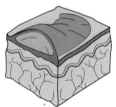

G.

Wheal:
Localized edema in the epidermis causing irregular elevation that may be red or pale
Example:
Insect bite or a hive

FLUID-FILLED CAVITIES WITHIN THE SKIN

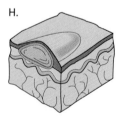

H.

Vesicle:
Accumulation of fluid between the upper layers of the skin; elevated mass containing serous fluid; less than 0.5 cm
Example:
Herpes simplex, herpes zoster, chickenpox

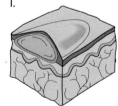

I.

Bullae:
Same as a vesicle only greater than 0.5 cm
Example:
Contact dermatitis, large second-degree burns, bulbous impetigo, pemphigus

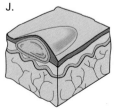

J.

Pustule:
Vesicles or bullae that become filled with pus, usually described as less than 0.5 cm in diameter
Example:
Acne, impetigo, furuncles, carbuncles, folliculitis

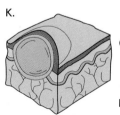

K.

Cyst:
Encapsulated fluid-filled or a semi-solid mass in the subcutaneous tissue or dermis
Example:
Sebaceous cyst, epidermoid cyst

Figure 10-8 Morphology of Primary Lesions

ABOVE THE SKIN SURFACE

A.
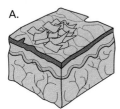
Scales:
    Flaking of the skin's surface
Example:
    Dandruff or psoriasis, xerosis

B.
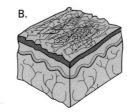
Lichenification:
    Layers of skin become
    thickened and rough as a
    result of rubbing over a
    prolonged period of time
Example:
    Chronic contact dermatitis

C.
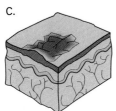
Crust:
    Dried serum, blood, or pus
    on the surface of the skin
Example:
    Impetigo

D.
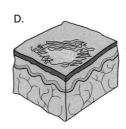
Atrophy:
    Thinning of the skin surface
    and loss of markings
Example:
    Striae, aged skin

BELOW THE SKIN SURFACE

E.
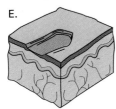
Erosion:
    Loss of epidermis
Example:
    Ruptured chickenpox vesicle

F.
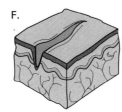
Fissure:
    Linear crack in the epidermis
    that can extend into the dermis
Example:
    Chapped hands or lips,
    athlete's foot

G.
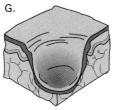
Ulcer:
    A depressed lesion of
    the epidermis and upper
    papillary layer of the dermis
Example:
    Stage 2 pressure ulcer

H.
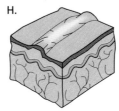
Scar:
    Fibrous tissue that replaces
    dermal tissue after injury
Example:
    Surgical incision

I.
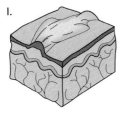
Keloid:
    Enlarging of a scar past
    wound edges due to excess
    collagen formation (more
    prevalent in dark-skinned
    persons)
Example:
    Burn scar

J.
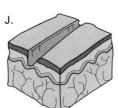
Excoriation:
    Loss of epidermal layers
    exposing the dermis
Example:
    Abrasion

Figure 10-9   Morphology of Secondary Lesions

🌺 NURSING TIP

Wound Evaluation

If a wound is present, remove the dressing and assess the wound for location, color, drainage, odor, size, and depth. Measure the borders of the wound with a centimeter ruler and draw a picture in your notes if necessary to depict necrotic areas, drains, etc.

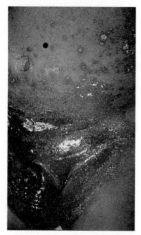

A. Moniliasis   *Courtesy of the Centers for Disease Control and Prevention (CDC)*

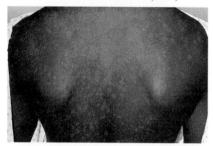

B. Tinea Versicolor   *Courtesy of Robert A. Silverman, M.D., Clinical Associate Professor, Department of Pediatrics, Georgetown University*

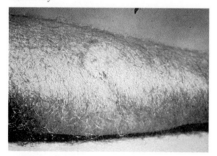

C. Tinea Corpis   *Courtesy of the Centers for Disease Control and Prevention (CDC)*

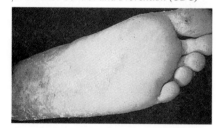

D. Tinea Pedis   *Courtesy of the Centers for Disease Control and Prevention (CDC)*

Figure 10-10   Common Skin Lesions

E	Examination
N	Normal Findings
A	Abnormal Findings
P	Pathophysiology

A Intertriginous exudative patches that are well demarcated, pruritic, and erythematous are abnormal.

P Moniliasis, also known as candidiasis, is a yeast infection that may invade numerous areas of the body but normally occurs in the axillae, inframammary areas, groin, and gluteal regions (see Figure 10-10A).

A Scaly macular patches of white, reddish brown, or tan hyperpigmentation, or hypopigmentation of the skin is abnormal (see Figure 10-10B).

P These occur in tinea versicolor, which is caused by superficial fungal infections. The lesions usually occur on the trunk and proximal extremities.

A A pink to red papulosquamous annular lesion with raised borders that expands peripherally and has a clearing center is abnormal.

P Tinea corpis is caused by a *Trichophyton*, a dermatophyte (fungal) infection (see Figure 10-10C).

A Toe web lesions that are macerated and have scaling borders are abnormal.

P Tinea pedis (athlete's foot) is very common and often erupts in the third and fourth interdigital spaces; with time, the lesions will spread over the plantar surface. Tinea pedis is caused by *Trichophyton mentagrophytes* (see Figure 10-10D).

A A slightly erythematous, rose- or fawn-colored oval patch that may have slightly raised borders is abnormal (see Figure 10-10E).

P A herald patch is normally found on the trunk and is indicative of pityriasis rosea. This condition is often seen in young adults and may resemble ringworm. The herald patch is normally followed in 5 to 10 days by a generalized eruption of similar lesions. The etiology is thought to be viral.

A Vesicles or bullae that measure 1 to 2 cm and become pustular and rupture easily, discharging straw-colored fluid are abnormal. The purulent drainage becomes thick as it dries, producing light-brown or golden-yellow crusts (see Figure 10-10F).

P Impetigo is usually caused by group A streptococcus or *Staphylococcus aureus* and is highly contagious. It is typically found in preschoolers in the late summer and can be associated with poor hygiene, crowding, contact sports, and minor skin trauma that is untreated.

A Red, shiny, indurated (with a peau d'orange appearance), and warm edematous lesions are abnormal. These lesions may be elevated, have defined margins, and may be painful. Vesicles and bullae may also be present (see Figure 10-10G).

P Erysipelas is a type of superficial cellulitis that is usually found in older adults and in young children. Erysipelas can originate in cuts or incisions infected by group A streptococcus either from the patient's respiratory tract or the respiratory tract of someone who was in close contact with the patient.

A A diffuse red area that is warm, edematous, painful, and indurated is abnormal (see Figure 10-10H).

P These findings suggest cellulitis, an acute bacterial infection (usually staphylococcal or streptococcal) of the skin and subcutaneous tissues. Cellulitis can result from trauma to the skin, .foreign bodies in the skin, and underlying infection. The patient shown in Figure 10-10H developed periorbital cellulitis from ethmoid sinusitis.

A A flat or raised lesion with a black interior is abnormal (see Figure 10-10I).

P A comedo, or blackhead, is usually seen on the face, chest, shoulders, or back. Comedones are due to increased keratinization in the hair follicle from an unknown etiology. They are associated with acne.

A Comedones accompanied by pustules (with yellow or white centers), red papules, nodules, and cysts are abnormal (see Figure 10-10J).

P Acne vulgaris usually occurs in the middle to late teen years and is caused by an inflammation of the sebaceous follicles. Acne vulgaris is associated with hormonal changes. It can be located on the face, chest, shoulders, and back. Lesions that appear punched out may be present from scarring of previously active acne lesions (see Figure 10-10K).

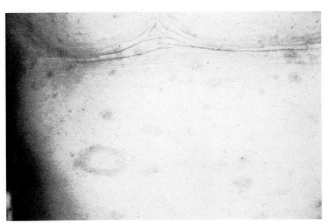

E. Pityriasis Rosea   *Courtesy of the Centers for Disease Control and Prevention (CDC)*

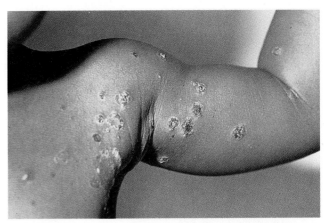

F. Impetigo   *Courtesy of Robert A. Silverman, M.D., Clinical Associate Professor, Department of Pediatrics, Georgetown University*

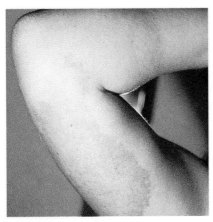

G. Erysipelas   *Courtesy of Robert A. Silverman, M.D., Clinical Associate Professor, Department of Pediatrics, Georgetown University*

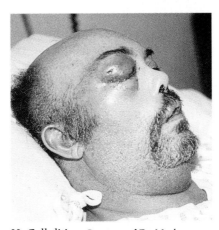

H. Cellulitis   *Courtesy of Dr. Mark Dougherty, Lexington, KY*

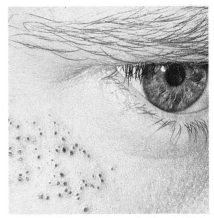

I. Comedones   *From Plewig, G., Kligman, A. B., eds: Acne Vulgaris ©1975 by Springer-Verlag, Berlin, Heidelberg. Used with permission.*

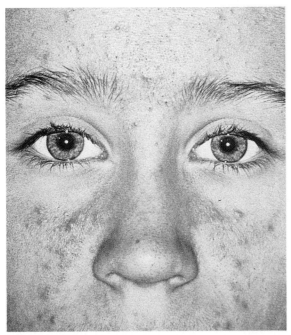

J. Acne Vulgaris   *From Plewig, G., Kligman, A. B., eds: Acne Vulgaris ©1975 by Springer-Verlag, Berlin, Heidelberg. Used with permission.*

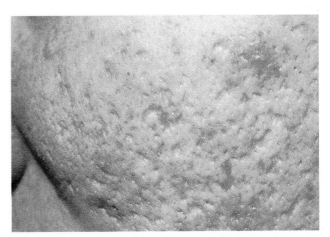

K. Facial Scarring from Acne Vulgaris   *From Plewig, G., Kligman, A. B., eds: Acne Vulgaris ©1975 by Springer-Verlag, Berlin, Heidelberg. Used with permission.*

Figure 10-10   Common Skin Lesions   *continued*

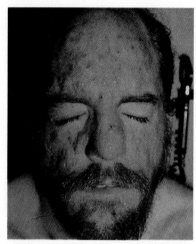

L. Acne Rosacea *Courtesy of Timothy Berger, M.D., San Francisco, CA*

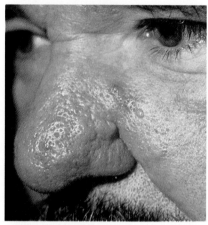

M. Rosacea Rhinophyma *Courtesy of Robert A. Silverman, M.D., Clinical Associate Professor, Department of Pediatrics, Georgetown University*

Figure 10-10 Common Skin Lesions *continued*

E **Examination**
N **Normal Findings**
A **Abnormal Findings**
P **Pathophysiology**

A Redness, with dilatation of the blood vessels on the cheeks, and acne are abnormal.

P Acne rosacea is a chronic inflammation seen primarily in middle-aged and older adults. The cause is unknown, although it is aggravated by alcohol, spicy food, hot liquids, sunlight, extremes in temperature, and stress (see Figure 10-10L).

A Rosacea that is red or purple on the lower nose and is accompanied by thickening of the affected skin and enlargement of the follicular orifices is abnormal (see Figure 10-10M).

P This is rosacea rhinophyma. The pathophysiology is the same as for rosacea.

A Reddish salmon-colored macular lesions are abnormal.

A Elevated purple to brown lesions (in light-skinned patients) and bluish lesions (in dark-skinned patients) that are spongy, painful, and pruritic are abnormal (see Figure 10-10N).

P Both of these abnormal findings are typical lesions of Kaposi's sarcoma. The reddish-salmon lesions are early findings, and the purplish or bluish lesions are more advanced lesions. Kaposi's sarcoma is a neoplastic disorder that is thought to have a genetic, hormonal, and viral etiology. It is frequently found in homosexual males infected with the AIDS virus, immunocompromised patients, and older adults.

A Pruritic silvery scales of the epidermis that have clearly demarcated borders and underlying erythema are abnormal. These lesions are circular and are found primarily on the elbows, knees, and behind the ears (see Figure 10-10O).

P The etiology of psoriasis is unknown, but it has a genetic component and may be aggravated by cold weather, trauma, and infection.

A A chronic superficial inflammation of the face, scalp, buttocks, or extremities that evolves into pruritic, red, weeping, crusted lesions is abnormal (see Figure 10-10P).

P Eczema, also known as atopic dermatitis, is a multifaceted disease process that is often associated with asthma and allergic rhinitis. The etiology is unknown and a family history of related disorders is usually noted.

A It is abnormal to have edema and erythema as well as red, pruritic vesicles that may discharge an exudate that leads to crusting (see Figure 10-10Q).

P This describes allergic contact dermatitis. In Figure 10-10Q, the allergen is poison oak. The patient must come in direct contact with the irritant to develop the dermatitis.

A Red, pruritic papules or vesicles with S-shaped or straight-line burrows are abnormal (see Figure 10-10R). These lesions can be intensely pruritic.

P Scabies is caused by the *Sarcoptes scabiei* mite, and may be visible as a small, dark area within the vesicle. It is highly contagious and can sometimes be spread through infected clothing or bedding.

A Red papules, vesicles, open sores, and crusting on the face, in the mouth, or on the genitalia are abnormal (see Figure 10-10S).

P Herpes simplex virus I is usually responsible for these lesions, which are more common on the face and in the mouth. After the initial exposure, the patient can often predict an outbreak because of the presence of burning, itching, or soreness at the eruption site.

A Red macular and papular lesions that are intensely pruritic are abnormal (see Figure 10-10T).

P Varicella, or chickenpox, usually starts on the trunk and proceeds to the extremities. Papules progress to thin-walled vesicles, pustules, and crusts. The patient may exhibit all of the different lesions simultaneously. Varicella is caused by the varicella-zoster virus, which is highly contagious, especially in children.

A Red, extremely painful vesicles with paresthesia that are closely grouped in a dermatomal pattern are abnormal (see Figure 10-10U).

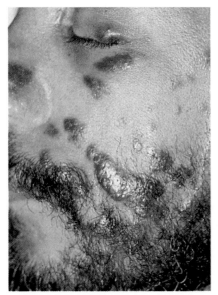

N. Kaposi's Sarcoma   *Courtesy of Robert A. Silverman, M.D., Clinical Associate Professor, Department of Pediatrics, Georgetown University*

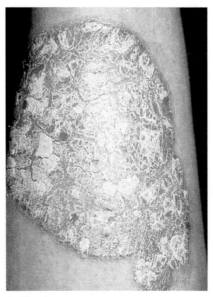

O. Psoriasis   *Courtesy of Robert A. Silverman, M.D., Clinical Associate Professor, Department of Pediatrics, Georgetown University*

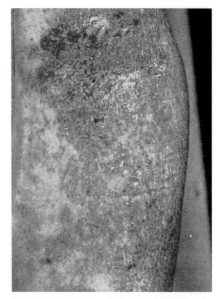

P. Eczema   *Courtesy of the Centers for Disease Control and Prevention (CDC)*

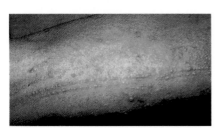

Q. Allergic Contact Dermatitis from Poison Oak; Note Linear Pattern to Lesions.   *Courtesy of the Centers for Disease Control and Prevention (CDC)*

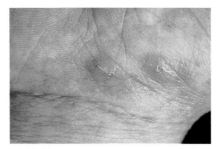

R. Scabies   *Courtesy of Robert A. Silverman, M.D., Clinical Associate Professor, Department of Pediatrics, Georgetown University*

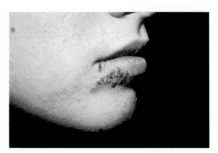

S. Herpes Simplex Virus I   *Courtesy of Robert A. Silverman, M.D., Clinical Associate Professor, Department of Pediatrics, Georgetown University*

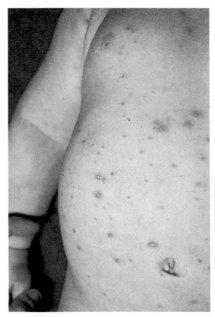

T. Varicella   *Courtesy of Robert A. Silverman, M.D., Clinical Associate Professor, Department of Pediatrics, Georgetown University*

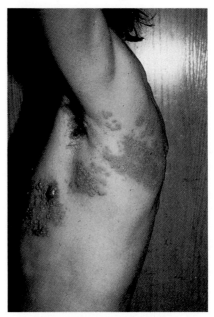

U. Herpes Zoster   *Courtesy of Robert A. Silverman, M.D., Clinical Associate Professor, Department of Pediatrics, Georgetown University*

Figure 10-10   Common Skin Lesions
continued

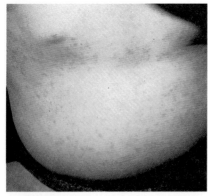

V. Roseola   *Courtesy of Robert A. Silverman, M.D., Clinical Associate Professor, Department of Pediatrics, Georgetown University*

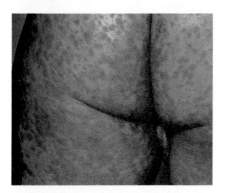

W. Rubeola   *Courtesy of the Centers for Disease Control and Prevention (CDC)*

Figure 10-10   Common Skin Lesions *continued*

E   Examination
N   Normal Findings
A   Abnormal Findings
P   Pathophysiology

P   Herpes zoster, or shingles, is caused by a reactivation of the varicella-zoster virus. The virus remains dormant after the initial varicella inoculation. It frequently occurs in elderly individuals. The lesions are similar to those of varicella, but they tend to develop more slowly.

A   Discrete pink macules or papular lesions with clear halos are abnormal. These lesions usually start on the trunk and progress to the face, neck, and extremities and are accompanied by a high fever (see Figure 10-10V).

P   Roseola, or exanthem subitum, is most likely viral in origin.

A   A maculopapular rash that is brownish pink and starts around the ears, face, and neck then progresses over the truck and limbs is abnormal (see Figure 10-10W).

P   Rubeola (measles) is a viral infection that is highly contagious, and is characterized by high fever, cough, rash, and Koplik's spots (see Figure 10-10X) on the buccal or labial mucosa.

A   Rubella (German measles) displays a fine, pinkish, macular rash that becomes confluent and pinpoint after the second day (see Figure 10-10Y).

P   Rubella is an RNA virus in nature and spreads from the face and neck to the trunk.

A   A diffuse, pinkish red flush of the skin that is confluent over the entire body surface is abnormal (see Figure 10-10Z).

P   Scarlet fever is caused by streptococcal bacteria (usually group A) and is associated with a strawberry tongue, circumoral pallor, fever, and chills.

A   A blotchy, maculopapular rash that may be reticular is abnormal (see Figure 10-10AA).

P   Erythema infectiosum (fifth disease) usually starts on the cheeks and spreads to the arms and trunk. Its cause is human parovirus B19.

A   A maculopapular rash with erythemic borders that appears first on the wrists, ankles, palms, soles, and forearms and is associated with a high fever is abnormal (see Figure 10-10BB)

P   Rocky Mountain spotted fever is associated with a history of tick bites. This febrile disease is caused by *Rickettsia rickettsii* and is transmitted by several types of ticks.

A   Pruritic, red wheals (urticarial rash) that vary in size from very small to large and are sometimes accompanied by maculopapular eruptions, vesicles, and bullae are abnormal (see Figure 10-10CC).

P   These findings occur in exanthematous drug eruption. The patient may exhibit these dermatological findings when experiencing an allergic reaction to medications.

A   Lesions that are brownish tan, red, white, blue, pink, purple, or gray and that have irregular borders and notching are abnormal. These lesions can be flat or elevated.

P   Malignant melanoma is a cancerous lesion that is associated with repeated sun exposure. Those individuals with light skin and blue eyes are particularly at risk for malignant melanoma. These neoplastic lesions can also be related to precancerous lesions such as nevi. Figure 10-10DD depicts lentigo malignant melanoma.

A   Perifollicular papules are abnormal (see Figure 10-10EE).

P   Pseudofollicultis barbae, or ingrown hair, is caused by hair tips that penetrate into the skin rather than exiting through the follicular orifice. It usually occurs in the beard area, particularly in African American men, because their hair may be curly and leave the skin at a sharp angle.

A   Pustules at the opening of the hair follicle are abnormal (see Figure 10-10FF).

P   Folliculitis is an inflammation of the hair follicle. Figure 10-10FF depicts a staphylococcal folliculitis; however, the causative agent may be fungal and therefore tinea barbae (see Figure 10-10GG).

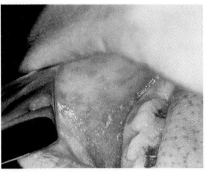

X. Koplik's Spots in Rubeola *Courtesy of the Centers for Disease Control and Prevention (CDC)*

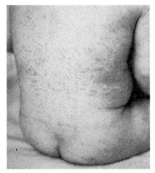

Y. Rubella *Courtesy of the Centers for Disease Control and Prevention (CDC)*

Z. Scarlet Fever *Courtesy of the Centers for Disease Control and Prevention (CDC)*

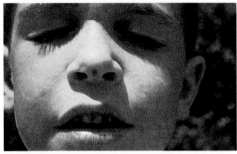

AA. Erythema Infectiosum *Courtesy of the Centers for Disease Control and Prevention (CDC)*

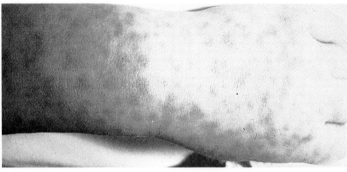

BB. Rocky Mountain Spotted Fever *Courtesy of the Centers for Disease Control and Prevention (CDC)*

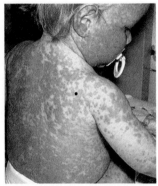

CC. Exanthematous Drug Eruption
Courtesy of Robert A. Silverman, M.D., Clinical Associate Professor, Department of Pediatrics, Georgetown University

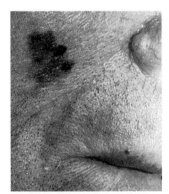

DD. Lentigo Malignant Melanoma
Courtesy of Robert A. Silverman, M.D., Clinical Associate Professor, Department of Pediatrics, Georgetown University

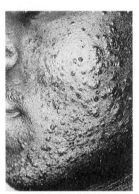

EE. Pseudofolliculitis Barbae *From Plewig, G., Kligman, A. B., eds: Acne Vulgaris ©1975 by Springer-Verlag, Berlin, Heidelberg. Used with permission.*

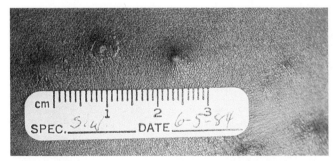

FF. Folliculitis *Courtesy of Robert A. Silverman, M.D., Clinical Associate Professor, Department of Pediatrics, Georgetown University*

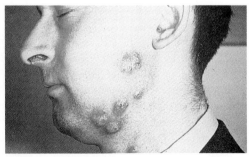

GG. Tinea Barbae *Courtesy of the Centers for Disease Control and Prevention (CDC)*

Figure 10-10 Common Skin Lesions *continued*

NURSING TIP

Self-Inspection of Moles

Instruct the patient to check moles once a month for the danger signs listed in the Nursing Alert. If the mole is on posterior surfaces, the patient should ask a significant other to assess moles for changes, or use a mirror. If a change is noted, the mole should be evaluated.

⚙ NURSING ALERT

Danger Signs in Potentially Cancerous Lesions

1. Rapid change in size
2. Change in coloration
3. Irregular border or butterfly-shaped border
4. Elevation in a previously flat mole
5. Multiple colorations in a lesion
6. Change in surface characteristics, such as oozing
7. Change in sensation, such as pain, itching, or tenderness
8. Change in surrounding skin, such as inflammation or induration
9. Bleeding or ulcerative appearance in a mole

Patient referral is required for any of the above-mentioned abnormal findings because of the risk of basal cell or squamous cell carcinoma.

⚙ NURSING ALERT

Stages of Pressure Ulcers

Uniform standards for staging pressure ulcers are used for patients with pressure sores on any portion of the body.

Stage 1 In light-skinned patients, area is reddened, but the skin is not broken; in dark-skinned patients, the pigmentation is enhanced (see Figure 10-11A).

Stage 2 Epidermal and dermal layers have sustained injury (see Figure 10-11B).

Stage 3 Subcutaneous tissues have sustained injury (see Figure 10-11C).

Stage 4 Muscle tissue and perhaps bone have sustained injury (see Figure 10-11D).

NURSING TIP

Wound Healing

Wound healing includes **reepithelialization**, which is the migration of epithelial cells inward from the wound edges and from any surrounding hair follicles or eccrine glands. Scab formation may prohibit reepithelialization because of diminished moisture. **Granulation tissue** is a combination of inflammatory cells, new vessels, and white blood cells that form a matrix at the base of the wound. The granulation tissue provides a foundation on which reepithelialization occurs. Scar formation may take several months. New scars are thick, darkened, and vascular in appearance. Over time, the scar tissue flattens and becomes less vascular; however, old scars remain slightly darker or discolored compared to the surrounding tissue.

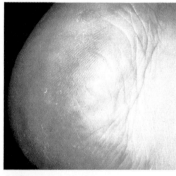

A. Stage 1

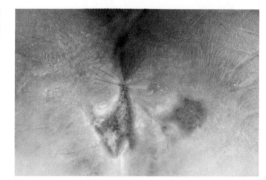

B. Stage 2

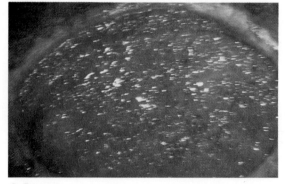

C. Stage 3

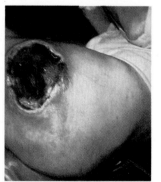

D. Stage 4

Figure 10-11   Pressure Ulcers   *Courtesy of Emory University Hospital, Atlanta, Georgia*

❧ NURSING TIP

Decrease Sun Exposure

Advise your patients to decrease their exposure to the sun by applying sunscreens with SPF 15 or greater, limiting exposure to the sun during the hours of 10 AM to 2 PM, wearing long-sleeved shirts and trousers, wearing hats that shade the face, head, and neck, and avoiding tanning salons.

❧ NURSING TIP

Identifying Burns

A burn patient frequently has varying degrees of injury on the body. Parts of the body may have first-degree burns, and other parts may have second-, third-, or fourth-degree burns. The following descriptions and photographs will assist you in identifying burn injuries:

First-Degree Burn (see Figure 10-12A): the epidermis is injured or destroyed; there may be some damage to the dermis; hair follicles and sweat glands are intact; the skin is red and dry; painful.

Second-Degree Burn (see Figure 10-12B): the epidermis and upper layers of the dermis are destroyed; the deeper dermis is injured; hair follicles, sweat glands, and nerve endings are intact; the skin is red and blistery with exudate; painful.

Third-Degree Burn (see Figure 10-12C): the epidermis and dermis are destroyed; subcutaneous tissue may be injured; hair follicles, sweat glands, and nerve endings are destroyed; the skin is white, red, black, tan, or brown with a leathery-looking appearance; painless because nerve endings are destroyed.

Fourth-Degree Burn (see Figure 10-12D): the epidermis and dermis are destroyed; subcutaneous tissue, muscle, and bone may be injured; hair follicles, sweat glands, and nerve endings are destroyed; the skin is white, red, black, tan, or brown with exposed and damaged subcutaneous tissue, muscle, or bone; painless.

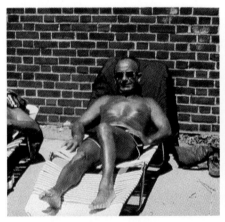

A. First-Degree Burn

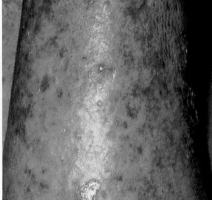

B. Second-Degree Burn

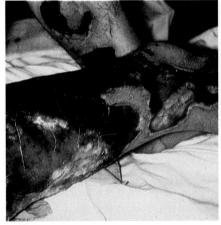

C. Third-Degree Burn

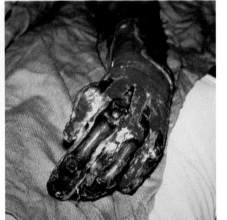

D. Fourth-Degree Burn

Figure 10-12   Types of Burns   *Courtesy of the Phoenix Society for Burn Survivors, Inc.*

Palpation of the Skin

Moisture

E Palpate all nonmucous membrane skin surfaces for moisture using the dorsal surfaces of the hands and fingers.

N *Normally, the skin is dry with a minimum of perspiration. Moisture on the skin will vary from one body area to another with perspiration normally present on the hands, axilla, face, and in between the skin folds. Moisture also varies with changes in environment, muscular activity, body temperature, stress, and activity levels. Body temperature is regulated by the skin's production of perspiration, which evaporates to cool the body.*

A Excessive dryness of the skin, **xerosis**, as evidenced by flaking of the stratum corneum and associated pruritus is abnormal.

P Hypothyroidism and exposure to extreme cold and dry climates can lead to xerosis.

A Diaphoresis is the profuse production of perspiration.

P Causes include hyperthyroidism, increased metabolic rate, sepsis, anxiety, or pain.

Temperature

E Palpate all nonmucosal skin surfaces for temperature using the dorsal surfaces of the hands and fingers.

N *Skin surface temperature should be warm and equal bilaterally. Hands and feet may be slightly cooler than the rest of the body.*

A **Hypothermia** is a cooling of the skin and may be generalized or localized.

P Generalized hypothermia is indicative of shock or some other type of central circulatory dysfunction. Localized hypothermia is indicative of arterial insufficiency in the affected area.

A Generalized **hyperthermia** is the excessive warming of the skin and may be generalized or localized.

P Generalized hyperthermia may be indicative of a febrile state, hyperthyroidism, or increased metabolic function caused by exercise. Localized hyperthermia may be caused by infection, trauma, sunburn, or windburn.

Texture

E
1. Evaluate the texture of the skin using the finger pads.
2. Evaluate surfaces such as the abdomen and medial surfaces of the arms first.
3. Compare these areas to areas that are covered with hair.

N *Skin should normally feel smooth, even, and firm except where there is significant hair growth. A certain amount of roughness can be normal.*

A Roughness can occur on exposed areas such as the elbows, the soles of the feet, and the palms of the hands.

P Roughness can be due to wool clothing, cold weather, or the use of soap. In addition, generalized roughness can be associated with systemic diseases such as scleroderma, hypothyroidism, and amyloidosis. Localized thickening and roughness can be a result of chronic pruritus (lichenification) due to scratching, which causes a thickening of the epidermis.

A Areas of hyperkeratosis and increased roughness that are found in the lower extremities are abnormal.

P This type of texture change may be indicative of peripheral vascular disease, which causes abated circulation and diminished nourishment of cutaneous layers.

A The skin can feel very soft and silklike.

P Generalized softness can result from hyperthyroidism secondary to elevated metabolism.

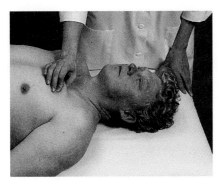

Figure 10-13   Assessment of Skin Turgor

🌺 **NURSING TIP**

Enhancement Techniques

Magnification: Use of a magnifying glass may be beneficial in the evaluation of lesions and discolorations for morphology.

Wood's Lamp: Also known as an ultraviolet light, it is valuable in the diagnosis of certain skin and hair diseases. Dermatophytosis and erythrasma are easily diagnosed by the fluorescent changes that occur under ultraviolet exposure. Dermatophytosis in the hair shaft will appear green to yellow, and erythrasma will appear coral red.

Diascopy: Consists of pressing a microscope slide over a skin lesion. Diascopy is useful in determining if a red lesion's coloration is due to erythema, which will blanch, or extravasation of blood, which will not blanch. Diascopy can also be useful in the detection of the glassy, yellow-brown appearance of papules found in tuberculosis of the skin, lymphoma, and sarcoidosis.

Turgor

Palpate the skin **turgor**, or elasticity, which reflects the skin's state of hydration.

E   1. Pinch a small section of the patient's skin between your thumb and forefinger. The anterior chest, under the clavicle, and the abdomen are optimal areas to assess.
　　2. Slowly release the skin.
　　3. Observe the speed with which the skin returns to its original contour when released (see Figure 10-13).

N   *When the skin is released, it should return to its original contour rapidly.*

A   Decreased skin turgor is present when the skin is released and it remains pinched, and then slowly returns to its original contour.

P   **Dehydration**, or lack of fluid in the tissues, is the main cause of decreased skin turgor. The aging process and scleroderma can also decrease the turgor of the skin.

A   Increased turgor or tension causes the skin to return to its original contour too quickly.

P   Increased turgor can be indicative of connective tissue disease caused by an increase of granulation tissue.

Edema

Palpate the skin for **edema**, or accumulation of fluid in the intercellular spaces.

E   1. Firmly imprint your thumb against a dependent portion of the body, such as the arms, hands, legs, feet, ankle, or sacrum.
　　2. Release pressure.
　　3. Observe for an indentation on the skin.
　　4. Rate the degree of edema. Pitting edema is rated on a 4-point scale:
　　　　+0" no pitting
　　　　+1, 0"–¼" pitting (mild)
　　　　+2, ¼"–½" pitting (moderate)
　　　　+3, ½"–1" pitting (severe)
　　　　+4, greater than 1" pitting (severe)
　　5. Check for symmetry and measure circumference of affected extremities.

N   *Edema is not normally present.*

A   Edema is present if the skin feels puffy and tight. It can be localized in one area or generalized throughout the body. There are many different types of edema (refer to Table 10-2).

P   Localized edema may be due to dependency (see Figure 10-14); however, generalized or bilateral edema is caused by increased hydrostatic pressure, decreased capillary osmotic pressure, increased capillary permeability, or obstruction to lymph flow. This occurs in congestive heart failure or kidney failure.

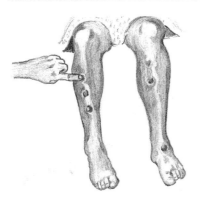

Figure 10-14   Pitting Edema

⚡ **NURSING ALERT**

Evaluation of Edema

If the edema is severe enough, it can prohibit the evaluation of pathological conditions that are manifested by coloration changes. Plus two (+2) edema warrants referral if it is newly onset. Severe edema (+3–+4) warrants immediate evaluation.

Table 10-2	Types of Edema
TYPE	DESCRIPTION
Pitting	Edema that is present when an indentation remains on the skin after applying pressure
Nonpitting	Edema that is firm with discoloration or thickening of the skin; results when serum proteins coagulate in tissue spaces
Angioedema	Recurring episodes of noninflammatory swelling of skin, brain, viscera, and mucous membranes; onset may be rapid with resolution requiring hours to days
Dependent	Localized increase of extracellular fluid volume in a dependent limb or area
Inflammatory	Swelling due to an extracellular fluid effusion into the tissue surrounding an area of inflammation
Noninflammatory	Swelling or effusion due to mechanical or other causes not related to congestion or inflammation

🌺 NURSING TIP

Hair Inspection

Ask patients to remove hair bands and hair pieces or to unbraid hair prior to the inspection process. If this is not possible, inspect the exposed areas as completely as possible.

E   **Examination**
N   **Normal Findings**
A   **Abnormal Findings**
P   **Pathophysiology**

Inspection of the Hair
Color

E   Inspect scalp hair, eyebrows, eyelashes, and body hair for color.
N   *Hair varies from dark black to pale blonde based on the amount of melanin present. As melanin production diminishes, hair turns gray. Hair color may also be chemically changed.*
A   Patches of gray hair that are isolated or occur in conjunction with a scar are abnormal.
P   Patches of gray hair not associated with aging can be indicative of nerve damage.

Distribution

E   Evaluate the distribution of hair on the body, eyebrows, face, and scalp.
N   *The body is covered in vellus hair. Terminal hair is found in the eyebrows, eyelashes, and scalp, and in the axilla and pubic areas after puberty. Males may experience a certain degree of normal balding and may also develop terminal facial and chest hair. Indians and Asians may have a light distribution of hair.*
A   The absence of pubic hair, unless purposefully removed, is abnormal in the adult.
P   Diminished or absent pubic hair may be indicative of endocrine disorders such as anterior pituitary adenomas.
A   Male or female pattern baldness (**alopecia**) may be abnormal in some individuals if associated with pathology. Alopecia areata is a circumscribed bald area (see Figure 10-15A).
P   Androgenetic alopecia is a common, progressive hair loss that is caused by a combination of genetic predisposition and androgenetic effects on the hair follicle; however, alopecia may be secondary to chemotherapy and radiation, infection, stress, drug reactions, lupus, and traction. A pathological etiology of alopecia should be ruled out.
A   Total scalp baldness, or alopecia totalis, is abnormal.
P   Autoimmune diseases, emotional crisis, stress, or heredity can cause alopecia totalis.
A   Hair loss in linear formations in conjunction with hair style is abnormal.

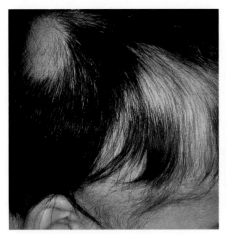

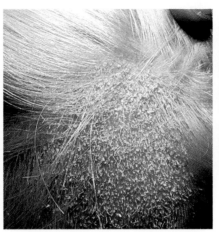

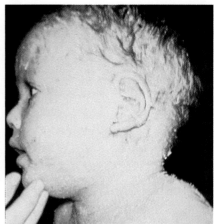

A. Alopecia Areata *Courtesy of Robert A. Silverman, M.D., Clinical Associate Professor, Department of Pediatrics, Georgetown University*

B. Tinea Capitis *Courtesy of Robert A. Silverman, M.D., Clinical Associate Professor, Department of Pediatrics, Georgetown University*

C. Seborrheic Dermatitis *Courtesy of the Centers for Disease Control and Prevention (CDC)*

Figure 10-15 Abnormalities of the Hair and Scalp

❖ ASK YOURSELF

Caring for Patients with Infestations

When providing care to a patient who has an infestation, would you follow your institution's guidelines and thoroughly wash your hands? Would you keep the cuffs of your clothing away from the patient to keep from contaminating yourself and the patient? Would you wear gloves when appropriate? (Standard precautions help protect you and the patient.) Would you style your hair to prevent it from falling forward and touching the patient? How would you feel after taking care of the patient? Would you run home, wash all your clothing, and shower?

P Traction alopecia can be caused by the use of curlers and wearing the hair in a tightly pulled ponytail where traction is continually applied. This is common among individuals who wear cornrows.

A Excess facial and body hair is abnormal.

P **Hirsutism** is manifested by excessive body hair. It is indicative of endocrine disorders such as hypersecretion of adrenocortical androgens. In women, this disorder is manifested as excess facial and chest hair.

P Hirsutism can also result as a side effect of medications such as cyclosporin.

A Areas of broken-off hairs in irregular patterns with scaliness but no infection are abnormal.

P Trichotillomania is the manipulation of the hair by twisting and pulling, leading to reduced hair mass. This can be an unconscious action or a sign of emotional problems.

A Broken-off hairs with scaliness and follicular inflammation is abnormal (see Figure 10-15B). The area may be painful and purulent with boggy nodules.

P Tinea capitis (ringworm) is a fungal infection, frequently caused by dermatophytic trichomycosis.

A The scalp is covered with yellow-brown scales and crusts. The scalp may be oily. Edema may be present (see Figure 10-15C).

P Seborrheic dermatitis is caused by increased production of sebum by the scalp.

Lesions

E 1. Don gloves and lift the scalp hair by segments.
    2. Evaluate the scalp for lesions or signs of infestation.

N *The scalp should be pale white to pink in light-skinned individuals and light brown in dark-skinned individuals. There should be no signs of infestation or lesions. **Seborrhea**, commonly known as dandruff, may be present.*

A Abnormal manifestations include head lice.

P Head lice (pediculosis capitis) may be distinguished from dandruff in that dandruff can be easily removed from the scalp or hair whereas nits (see Figure 10-16), which are the lice larvae, are attached to the hair shaft and are difficult to remove. Both seborrhea and head lice may cause itching.

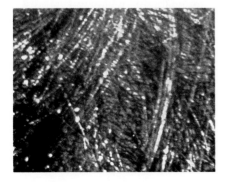

Figure 10-16 Head Lice *Courtesy of Reed and Carnrick Pharmaceuticals*

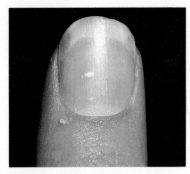

A. Leukonychia *Courtesy of Delmar Publishers, Albany, NY*

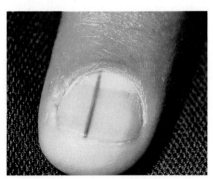

B. Leukonychia Totalis *Courtesy of Robert A. Silverman, M.D., Clinical Associate Professor, Department of Pediatrics, Georgetown University*

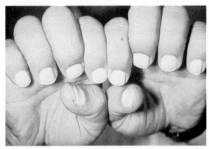

C. Longitudinal Melanochyia *Courtesy of Robert A. Silverman, M.D., Clinical Associate Professor, Department of Pediatrics, Georgetown University*

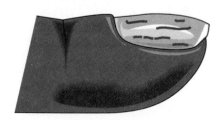

D. Splinter Hemorrhages

Figure 10-17 Abnormal Color Changes of the Nailbed

E	Examination
N	Normal Findings
A	Abnormal Findings
P	Pathophysiology

Palpation of the Hair

Texture

E **1.** Palpate the hair between your fingertips.
   2. Note the condition of the hair from the scalp to the end of the hair.

N *Hair may feel thin, straight, coarse, thick, or curly. It should be shiny and resilient when traction is applied and should not come out in clumps in your hands.*

A Brittle hair that easily breaks off when pulled or hair that is listless and dull is abnormal.

P Brittle, dull hair or hair that is broken off can be indicative of malnutrition, hyperthyroidism, use of chemicals such as permanents, or infections secondary to damage of the hair follicle.

Inspection of the Nails

Color

E **1.** Inspect the fingernails and toenails, noting the color of the nails.
   2. Check capillary refill by depressing the nail until blanching occurs.
   3. Release the nail and evaluate the time required for the nail to return to its previous color.
   4. Perform a capillary refill check on all four extremities.

N *Normally, the nails have a pink cast in light-skinned individuals and are brown in dark-skinned individuals. Capillary refill is an indicator of peripheral circulation. Normal capillary refill may vary with age, but color should return to normal within 2 to 3 seconds.*

A White striations or dots in the nailbed are abnormal (see Figure 10-17A).

P Leukonychia (Mees bands) may result from trauma, infections, vascular diseases, psoriasis, and arsenic poisoning.

A An entire nail plate that is white is abnormal (see Figure 10-17B).

P Leukonychia totalis may result from hypercalcemia, hypochromic anemia, leprosy, hepatic cirrhosis, and arsenic poisoning.

A A brown color in the nail plate is abnormal (see Figure 10-17C).

P Melanochyia may result from Addison's disease and malaria.

A Bluish nails are abnormal.

P Bluish nails may result from cyanosis, venous stasis, and sulfuric acid poisoning.

A Red or brown linear streaks in the nailbed are abnormal (see Figure 10-17D).

P Splinter hemorrhages can result from subacute bacterial endocarditis, mitral stenosis, trichinosis, cirrhosis, and nonspecific causes.

A It is abnormal if the proximal end of the nailbed is white and the distal portion is pink.

P Lindsey's nails (half and half nails) can result from chronic renal failure and hypoalbuminemia.

Shape and Configuration

E **1.** Assess the fingernails and toenails for shape, configuration, and consistency.
   2. View the profile of the middle finger and evaluate the angle of the nail base.

N *The nail surface should be smooth and slightly rounded or flat. Curved nails are a normal variant. Nail thickness should be uniform throughout, with no splintering or brittle edges. The angle of the nail base should be approximately 160° (see Figure 10-18).*

Normal nail angle

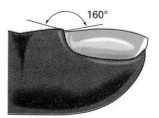

160°

Curved nail
variant
of normal

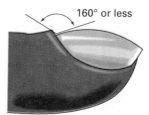

160° or less

Early clubbing

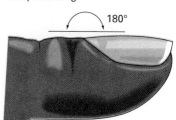

180°

Figure 10-18   Nail Angles

A   Thin nail plates with cuplike depressions and concave, or spoon-shaped, nails are abnormal (Figure 10-19A).

P   Koilonychia can result from iron deficiency anemia, chronic infections, malnutrition, or Raynaud's disease.

A   An angle of the nail base greater than 160° (see Figure 10-19B), along with sponginess of the nailbed is abnormal.

P   Clubbing can result from long-standing hypoxia and lung cancer.

A   A transverse furrow in the nail plate is abnormal (see Figure 10-19C).

P   Beau's line is caused by an arrest of nail growth at the matrix. It can be associated with an acute phase of an infectious disease, malnutrition, and anemia.

A   Separation of the nail from the nailbed is abnormal (see Figure 10-19D).

P   Onycholysis can result from hypo- and hyperthyroidism, repeated trauma, Raynaud's disease, syphilis, eczema, and acrocyanosis.

A   Painful, red swelling of the nail fold is abnormal (see Figure 10-19E).

P   Paronychia can be caused by *Candida albicans*, bacteria, and repeated exposure of the nails to moisture.

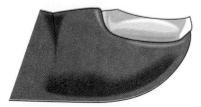

A. Koilonychia

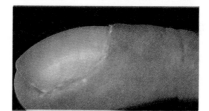

B. Clubbing   *Courtesy of Robert A. Silverman, M.D., Clinical Associate Professor, Department of Pediatrics, Georgetown University*

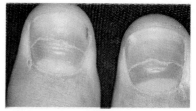

C. Beau's Line   *Courtesy of Robert A. Silverman, M.D., Clinical Associate Professor, Department of Pediatrics, Georgetown University*

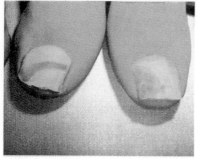

D. Onycholysis, with Hyperkeratosis (Thickening of the Nail Plate)
Courtesy of Judith A. Mysliborski, MD, Albany, NY

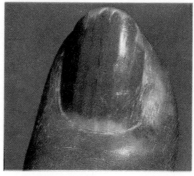

E. Paronychia   *Courtesy of Delmar Publishers, Albany, NY*

Figure 10-19   Abnormalities of the Shape and Configuration of the Nail

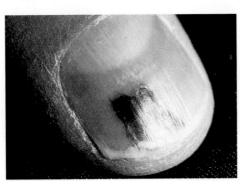

F. Subungal Hematoma   *Courtesy of Robert A. Silverman, M.D., Clinical Associate Professor, Department of Pediatrics, Georgetown University*

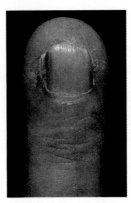

G. Onychocryptosis   *Courtesy of Delmar Publishers, Albany, NY*

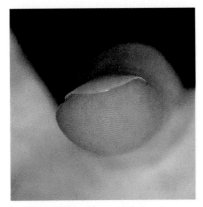

H. Eggshell Nails   *Courtesy of Delmar Publishers, Albany, NY*

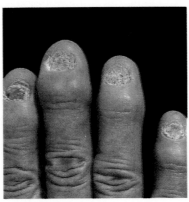

I. Onychatrophia   *Courtesy of Delmar Publishers, Albany, NY*

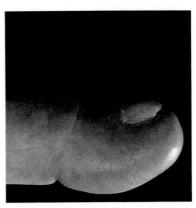

J. Onychauxis   *Courtesy of Delmar Publishers, Albany, NY*

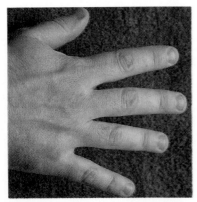

K. Onychophagy   *Courtesy of Delmar Publishers, Albany, NY*

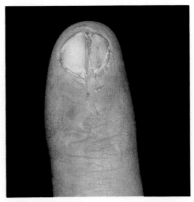

L. Onychorrhexis   *Courtesy of Delmar Publishers, Albany, NY*

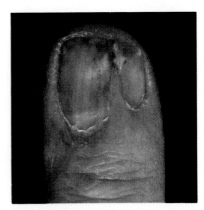

M. Pterygium   *Courtesy of Delmar Publishers, Albany, NY*

Figure 10-19   Abnormalities of the Shape and Configuration of the Nail   *continued*

A Numerous horizontal depression ridges or a depression down the middle of the nail is abnormal.

P Habit tic deformity is caused by continuous picking of the cuticle and nail by a finger of the same hand. Trauma ensues to the nail base and nail matrix.

A Purpura or ecchymosis under the nail plate is abnormal (see Figure 10-19F).

P Subungal hematoma is caused by trauma to the digit and nail, leading to hemorrhage into the matrix and nailbed.

A The distal portion of the nail plate is embedded in periungual tissues (see Figure 10-19G). The periungual tissues may become inflamed.

P Onychocryptosis (ingrown nail) is caused by growth of the distal nail plate into periungual tissues, resulting in trauma to the tissues.

A Nails that become white, thin, and curved under the free edge are abnormal (see Figure 10-19H).

P Eggshell nails may be caused by systemic diseases, medications, dietary deficiencies, nervous disorders, or sleeping with the hand fisted.

A Nails that atrophy, shrink, and fall off are abnormal (see Figure 10-19I).

P Onychatrophia may result from injury to the nail matrix and from systemic diseases.

A Nails that hypertrophy (become abnormally thick and overgrown) are abnormal (see Figure 10-19J).

P Onychauxis is caused by systemic infection, electrolyte imbalance, and hereditary predisposition.

A Nails deformed in shape are abnormal (see Figure 10-19K).

P Onychophagy results from excessive biting of the nails.

A A nail that is split or brittle with lengthwise ridges is abnormal (see Figure 10-19L).

P Onychorrhexis may result from trauma to the nail, toxic exposure to solvents, or harsh nail filing.

A It is abnormal for the cuticle to overgrow the nail and become attached to the nail (see Figure 10-19M). The cuticle growth may persist to the free edge.

P Pterygium can occur in Raynaud's disease.

Palpation of the Nails

Texture

E **1.** Palpate the nail base between your thumb and index finger.
　　2. Note the consistency.

N *The nail base should be firm on palpation.*

A A spongy nail base is an early indication of clubbing.

P Clubbing is the result of chronic bronchitis, emphysema, or heart disease. See Chapters 14 and 15 for further information.

✳ SPECIAL TECHNIQUES

Skin Scraping for Scabies

1. Place a drop of mineral oil on a sterile #15 scalpel blade.
2. Scrape the suspected papule or known scabies burrow vigorously in order to excavate the top of the papule or burrow. Flecks of blood will mix with the oil.
3. Place some of the oil and skin scrapings onto a microscope slide and cover with a cover slip.
4. Examine the slide for mites, ova, or feces.

continued

E	**Examination**
N	**Normal Findings**
A	**Abnormal Findings**
P	**Pathophysiology**

Skin Scraping for Mycelia

1. Scrape the roof of suspected vesicle or scales or take a sample of hair follicle.
2. Place a drop of 10% KOH on the sample to clear it of other organisms.
3. Warm it gently over a lighter or alcohol burner.
4. Examine the slide under a microscope for mycelia.

GERONTOLOGICAL VARIATIONS

The most visible signs of aging are manifested in the skin and hair. These changes include wrinkles, sagging skin folds, graying hair, and hair loss. Also, skin disorders are more likely to occur as a person ages. Light-skinned individuals appear to manifest the changes of aging more rapidly than do dark-skinned individuals, and these changes are accelerated by sun exposure.

With aging, the epidermis thins and elastic fibers that provide support to the dermis degenerate and lead to sagging skin folds. The number of sweat and sebaceous glands diminishes as does the vascularity of the skin, which affects thermoregulation. There is increased incidence of hypothermia due to decreased vasodilation and vasoconstriction of the dermal arterioles, and loss of subcutaneous fat.

In elderly individuals, diminished inflammatory response and diminished perception of pain increase the risk of adverse effects from noxious stimuli. The elderly are at a greater risk for frostbite and burns because of diminished pain perception. Their injuries are more serious because of the thinning epidermis and prolonged wound healing. Reepithelialization takes approximately twice as long in patients over the age of 75 than in those who are 25 years of age.

Wrinkling is the change most associated with aging. Wrinkles are most prominent on the face and neck because these areas have the greatest sun exposure. Other factors leading to wrinkling are loss of subcutaneous fat and diminished elasticity of the skin.

Another obvious, early skin change associated with aging is hyperpigmentation. Senile **lentigo**, or liver spots (see Figure 10-20A), are the result of the inability of the melanocytes to produce even pigmentation of the skin. Larger areas of hyperpigmentation are lentigines. These are generally seen on the backs of the hands and wrists of light-skinned individuals and are related to the degree of sun exposure.

Senile pruritus is the most common skin affliction in elderly individuals. Pruritus is due to a decrease in water content of the skin and atrophy of the sweat glands. Dryness and itching are exacerbated during the winter months when humidity is low, indoor temperatures are high, and drying winds are present. The condition is aggravated by frequent bathing in hot water, which robs the skin of moisture. Generalized itching is also associated with systemic diseases such as diabetes mellitus, atherosclerosis, and liver disease. Thus, prolonged itching should receive medical attention.

Keratosis, lesions on the epidermis and characterized by overgrowth of the horny layer, is prevalent among the elderly population. Actinic keratosis, also known as solar keratosis, occurs in those areas where sun exposure has been greatest (neck, ears, bald scalp, hands, forearms). Actinic keratosis is premalignant; seborrheic keratosis is usually not premalignant. However, if either is the precursor of skin cancer, the cancer is usually basal cell carcinoma (see Figure 10-20B). The lesions of seborrheic keratosis are found on the trunk, face, and scalp and are covered with greasy, velvety textured scales.

Although cancer of the skin is common among the elderly population, it is not usually life threatening. Basal cell carcinoma most often affects Caucasian males. Factors associated with this type of cancer include prolonged exposure to sunlight, poor tanning ability, and previous therapy with x-rays for facial acne. Squamous cell carcinoma (see Figure 10-20C) is much less common than basal cell carcinoma. It is almost twice as prevalent in males as in

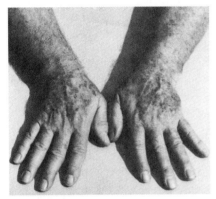

A. Senile Lentigo *Courtesy of Delmar Publishers, Albany, NY*

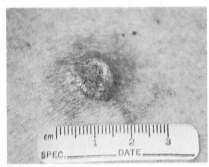

B. Basal Cell Carcinoma *Courtesy of Robert A. Silverman, M.D., Clinical Associate Professor, Department of Pediatrics, Georgetown University*

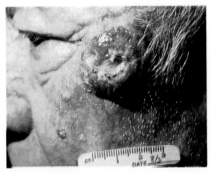

C. Squamous Cell Carcinoma *Courtesy of Robert A. Silverman, M.D., Clinical Associate Professor, Department of Pediatrics, Georgetown University*

Figure 10-20 Skin Changes in the Elderly

females; however, the incidence on the legs of females is higher. Risk factors include the ingestion of arsenic, prolonged exposure to sunlight, and exposure to gamma radiation and x-rays.

The number and thickness of terminal hairs generally diminish, and there is a conversion of vellus hair to terminal hair in areas such as the rims of the ears and nose in men, and on the upper lip and chin in women. Decreased melanin production decreases the melanocytes at the hair follicle and thus leads to graying.

The nails in elderly persons may thicken and yellow. There may be an overcurvature of the toenails if tight shoes were worn for most of the individual's life.

While most changes seen in aging are part of the normal aging process, many can also indicate underlying systemic or localized disease. Therefore, it is prudent not to generalize changes seen in elderly patients as routine.

🍂 NURSING TIP

Safety Tips to Help the Elderly Patient Avoid Integumentary Damage

1. Assist elderly patients in identifying hazards in the home that could cause trauma (e.g., loose rugs, sharp table edges, glass items in the bathroom, stoves, electric appliances, etc.). Assist them in finding avenues to decrease the risk of trauma.

2. Remind elderly patients that sensation to temperature diminishes with age and that they may therefore wish to check their bath water with a thermometer (should not be warmer than 105°F).

3. Advise elderly patients to wear multiple layers of clothing in cooler temperatures, and gloves and socks to protect the distal extremities from hypothermia and frostbite.

4. Remind elderly patients to keep electric blankets and heating pads on a medium setting to prevent burns.

5. Advise elderly patients to apply emollient lotions to decrease xerosis and pruritus but to avoid lotions with a high alcohol content, which can cause further drying of the skin.

6. Warn elderly patients that their skin will tear more easily and be prone to shearing because their epidermal layers are thinner and that because the integumentary system is slower to recover from trauma, healing from such injuries will take longer.

CASE STUDY

The case study illustrates the application and objective documentation of the skin, hair, and nails assessment.

The Patient with Scabies

Bob is a 15-year-old white male. Two nights ago, he was awakened by generalized intractable pruritus on his wrists, hands, and fingers. He reported to the school nurse this morning after a teacher noticed his discomfort and saw the condition of his hands. The school nurse referred him to the primary care clinic; his mother brought him to the clinic.

❖ HEALTH HISTORY

PATIENT PROFILE	15 yo SWM
CHIEF COMPLAINT	"The itching is so bad on my hands, I can't stop scratching."

continued

HISTORY OF PRESENT ILLNESS	Woke up in middle of night 2 d PTA c̄ intractable itching of wrists & hands; noticed small lesions on wrists & webs of fingers; unable to sleep; many lesions scratched to bleeding; denies lesions or itching of head, pubic area, buttocks, or axillae; not aware of any friends or family members having any infestations or lesions; itching temporarily relieved by warm water soaks; sx seem worse at night

PAST HEALTH HISTORY

Medical	Denies any medical problems
Surgical	Tonsillectomy at 4 yo, no complications
Medications	Occasional acetaminophen for H/A
Communicable Diseases	Denies
Allergies	Denies allergy to medication, food, animals, or environmental conditions
Injuries/Accidents	Fell skateboarding at 12 yo & lacerated scalp requiring 6 stitches, no complications
Disabilities/Handicaps	Denies
Blood Transfusions	Denies
Childhood Illnesses	Chickenpox at 4 yo, no complications, denies any other illness
Immunizations	"Up to date"; school nurse sent immunization records c̄ the patient

FAMILY HEALTH HISTORY

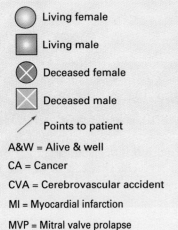

LEGEND

Living female

Living male

Deceased female

Deceased male

Points to patient

A&W = Alive & well

CA = Cancer

CVA = Cerebrovascular accident

MI = Myocardial infarction

MVP = Mitral valve prolapse

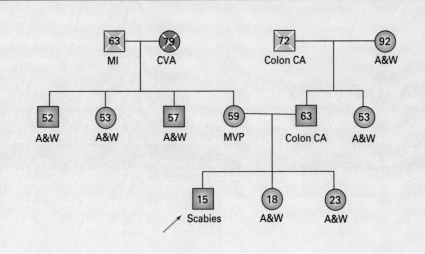

Denies family hx of skin dz or infestations.

continued

SOCIAL HISTORY

Alcohol Use	Denies
Tobacco Use	Denies
Drug Use	Denies use of inhalants, & other drugs
Sexual Practice	States he is not sexually active
Travel History	At summer camp last month; somewhat crowded when sleeping in tents & rented sleeping bags
Home Environment	Lives at home c̄ parents & 2 sisters in 3-bedroom home
Hobbies/Leisure Activities	Plays basketball & swims
Stress	Appearance of hands & wrists; starting to date & is concerned that girls will be afraid to come near him if they find out he is infested c̄ scabies
Education	Currently enrolled in the 10th grade in public school
Economic Status	Middle class
Religion	Protestant
Ethnic Background	Denies any affiliation
Roles/Relationships	Son, brother, denies problem c̄ parents or siblings
Characteristic Patterns of Daily Living	Wakes 7 AM, breakfast c̄ sister, & goes to school; school from 8 AM to 3 PM; plays basketball c̄ friends until 6 PM; dinner c̄ family, does homework until 10 PM; watches TV until MN, goes to bed

HEALTH MAINTENANCE ACTIVITIES

Sleep	6–8 hr per night
Diet	Reports a balanced diet
Exercise	See Hobbies/Leisure Activities
Stress Management	Talking to friends & playing basketball
Use of Safety Devices	Wears seat belt, does not wear helmet when riding bike, does not use sunscreen
Health Check-Ups	Annual physical in order to participate in sports

continued

PHYSICAL ASSESSMENT

Inspection of the Skin

Color
Skin of wrists & hands pink c̄ areas of erythema

Bleeding, Ecchymosis, Vascularity
No ecchymosis, frank bleeding, or vascular Δ

Lesions
Lesions noted over ant & post aspects of wrists, prevalent in finger webs & scattered on dorsal & palmar surfaces bilaterally. Primary lesions: numerous threadlike burrows that look like gray to skin-colored ridges; linear in appearance; minute vesicles & papules at distal aspects of burrows; burrows between 0.5 cm & 1.0 cm; numerous vesicles; Ø nodules present. Secondary lesions: small urticarial papules c̄ plaques & small amt crusting noted. Ø other pigmented lesions. Ø other similar lesions found on rest of body.

Palpation of the Skin

Moisture
Dorsal surfaces of hands dry & flaking bilaterally; sl sweaty palmar surface

Temperature
Hands & fingers warm bilaterally

Texture
Skin surface rough over dorsal & palmar surfaces of hands as well as ant & post aspects of wrists 2° to lesions

Turgor
Skin returns to original contour immediately

Edema
Ø edema on affected surfaces

Inspection of the Hair

Color
Vellus hair on hands & wrists light brown & s̄ gray

Distribution
Body hair distribution appropriate for teenaged male

Lesions
Ø lesions on scalp

Palpation of the Hair

Texture
Vellus hair of wrists & hands smooth & soft; Ø terminal hair growth noted in these areas

Inspection of the Nails

Color
Pink c̄ capillary refill of 1 second

Shape and Configuration
Smooth & flat, Ø splintering or brittle edges; nail angle 160°

Palpation of the Nails

Texture
Firm

Laboratory Data
Skin Scraping for Scabies: ⊕ microscopic evaluation from 2 distinct lesions of mites & ova

⊚⊚ THINK ABOUT IT

Dealing with Pediculosis

As the school nurse in an elementary school, you are asked to conduct an assessment of each first grade student's hair for lice. You discover that seven children are infested with lice. You call the affected children's parents to pick up their children. One father screams at you on the phone, "My child is OK. You must be mistaken. Every few weeks you tell me that my daughter has lice. It's not my problem!"

- What is your response to this parent?
- What are your responsibilities for the well-being of the entire school?
- Plan an educational program to be disseminated to each class.

✓ NURSING CHECKLIST
Skin, Hair, and Nails Assessment

Inspection of the Skin
- Color
- Bleeding, Ecchymosis, and Vascularity
- Lesions

Palpation of the Skin
- Moisture
- Temperature
- Texture
- Turgor
- Edema

Inspection of the Hair
- Color
- Distribution
- Lesions

Palpation of the Hair
- Texture

Inspection of the Nails
- Color
- Shape and Configuration

Palpation of the Nails
- Texture

Special Techniques
- Skin Scraping for Scabies
- Skin Scraping for Mycelia

REVIEW QUESTIONS AND ACTIVITIES

1. Describe anticipated normal findings of inspection and palpation of the skin, hair, and nails. Assess your own integumentary system and appendages for normal variations.

2. It is helpful to practice positioning, assessment techniques, and handling the equipment prior to working with a patient. You will need an examination table, drapes, penlight, magnifying glass, microscope slide, and a volunteer. Practice positioning and draping the patient as well as assessing the integumentary system. Practice diascopy procedures.

3. Illustrate the differences between a primary lesion and a secondary lesion and provide examples of dermatological conditions that illustrate each lesion.

4. Develop a teaching plan that would assist patients in recognizing the warning signs of skin cancer.

5. Discuss the normal changes associated with aging that you would expect to find in a geriatric patient.

6. You are caring for a 21-year-old Latina who has come to your clinic complaining of a rash on her scalp, arms, and trunk for the past 48 hours. She is in her last semester of college and started student teaching 2 weeks ago. Three types of lesions are noted: macules, papules, and vesicles. Vesicles are noted mostly on the trunk, and macules and papules are noted on the arms and scalp. She states the lesions changed from macules to vesicles over a 24-hour period. Vesicles on the trunk also appear to be crusting. She has a temperature of 100°F and is complaining of pruritus. Based on your assessment, you conclude that this patient may be experiencing:
   a. Scabies
   b. Insect bites
   c. Varicella
   d. Herpes simplex

The correct answer is (c).

7. Macules, papules, and vesicles are all examples of which type of lesions?
   a. Secondary lesions
   b. Primary lesions
   c. Primary and secondary lesions
   d. None of the above

The correct answer is (b).

Head and Neck

COMPETENCIES

1. Identify the anatomic structures of the head and neck.
2. Locate the lymph nodes of the head and neck.
3. Describe the system-specific health history for the head and neck.
4. Demonstrate the physical assessment of the head and neck.
5. Describe normal findings in the physical assessment of the head and neck.
6. List common abnormalities found in physical assessment of the head and neck.
7. Explain pathophysiology of common abnormalities found in physical assessment of the head and neck.

Assessment of the head and neck is the gateway to a wide range of critical clues about the function of various body systems. As you assess the head and neck, you will learn about the skin, endocrine function, musculoskeletal integrity, and neurological function.

ANATOMY AND PHYSIOLOGY

Skull

The skull is a complex bony structure that rests on the superior end of the vertebral column (refer to Figure 11-1). The skull protects the brain from direct injury and provides a surface for the attachment of the muscles that assist with mastication and produce facial expressions.

Cranial bones of the skull are connected by immovable joints called **sutures**. The most prominent sutures are the coronal suture, the sagittal suture, and the lambdoidal suture. The junction of the coronal and sagittal sutures is called the **bregma**.

Face

The face of every individual has its own unique characteristics influenced by factors such as race, state of health, emotions, and environment. Facial structures are symmetrical so that eyes, eyebrows, nose, mouth, nasolabial folds, and palpebral fissures look the same on both sides.

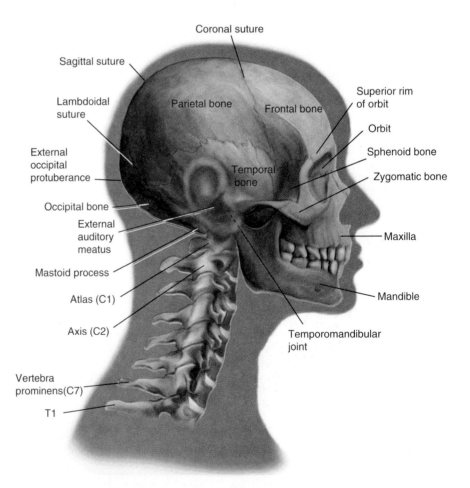

Figure 11-1 Bones of the Face and Skull (Lateral View)

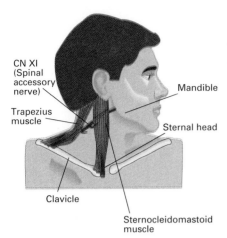

CN XI (Spinal accessory nerve)

Trapezius muscle

Mandible

Sternal head

Clavicle

Sternocleidomastoid muscle

Figure 11-2   Major Cervical Muscles

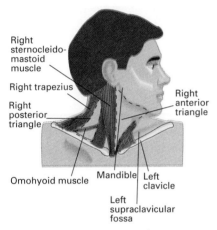

Right sternocleido-mastoid muscle

Right trapezius

Right posterior triangle

Right anterior triangle

Omohyoid muscle

Mandible

Left clavicle

Left supraclavicular fossa

Figure 11-3   Anterior and Posterior Cervical Triangles

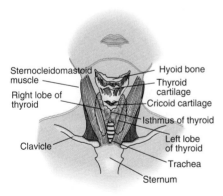

Sternocleidomastoid muscle

Right lobe of thyroid

Clavicle

Hyoid bone

Thyroid cartilage

Cricoid cartilage

Isthmus of thyroid

Left lobe of thyroid

Trachea

Sternum

Figure 11-4   Structures of the Thyroid Gland

Neck

The neck is made up of seven flexible cervical vertebrae that support the head while allowing it maximum mobility. The first cervical vertebra, the **atlas**, articulates with the occipital condyles to support and balance the head. The second vertebra, the **axis**, has an odontoid process that extends into the ring of the atlas, allowing it to pivot as the head is turned from side to side. The seventh cervical vertebra has a long spinous process called the **vertebra prominens**, which serves as a useful landmark during physical assessment of the neck, back, and thorax.

The major muscles of the neck are the sternocleidomastoids and the trapezii (see Figure 11-2). The sternocleidomastoid muscles extend from the upper portion of the sternum and the clavicle to the mastoid process and allow the head to bend laterally, rotate, flex, and extend. They also divide each side of the neck into two triangles: the anterior cervical and the posterior cervical, which serve as assessment landmarks. The **anterior triangle** is formed by the mandible, the trachea, and the sternocleidomastoid muscles and contains the anterior cervical lymph nodes, the trachea, and the thyroid gland. The **posterior triangle**, the area between the sternocleidomastoid and the trapezius muscles with the clavicle at the base, contains the posterior cervical lymph nodes (see Figure 11-3).

The trapezii extend from the occipital bone down the neck to insert at the outer third of the clavicles, at the acromion process of the scapula, and along the spinal column to the level of T12. They allow the shoulders and scapula to move up and down and rotate the scapula medially.

Thyroid

The thyroid gland, the largest endocrine gland in the body, secretes thyroxine (T_4) and triiodothyronine (T_3), which regulate the rate of cellular metabolism. The gland, a flattened, butterfly-shaped structure with two lateral lobes connected by the **isthmus**, weighs about 25 to 30 grams and is slightly larger in females (refer to Figure 11-4).

Lymphatics

An extensive system of lymphatic vessels drains the head and neck and is an important part of the immune system (refer to Figure 11-5). Lymphatic tissue in the nodes is responsible for the filtering and sequestration of pathogens and other harmful substances. When nodes are enlarged or tender, it is important to assess for infection or other causes in the area they drain.

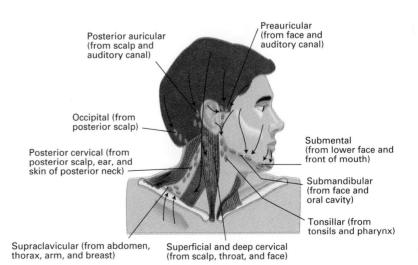

Posterior auricular (from scalp and auditory canal)

Preauricular (from face and auditory canal)

Occipital (from posterior scalp)

Posterior cervical (from posterior scalp, ear, and skin of posterior neck)

Submental (from lower face and front of mouth)

Submandibular (from face and oral cavity)

Tonsillar (from tonsils and pharynx)

Supraclavicular (from abdomen, thorax, arm, and breast)

Superficial and deep cervical (from scalp, throat, and face)

Figure 11-5   Lymph Nodes of the Head and Neck; Drainage Patterns

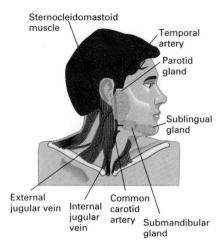

Sternocleidomastoid muscle
Temporal artery
Parotid gland
Sublingual gland
External jugular vein
Internal jugular vein
Common carotid artery
Submandibular gland

Figure 11-6 Major Veins and Arteries of the Neck

Blood Supply

The blood supply to the head and neck is quite extensive, with similar arterial and venous patterns. Major vessels carrying blood to the head and neck include internal and external carotids, internal and external jugulars, and the subclavian veins and arteries (see Figure 11-6).

> ❀ **NURSING TIP**
>
> **Cranial Nerve Assessment**
>
> The twelve cranial nerves that innervate the head and neck are assessed during this portion of the examination. Refer to Chapters 12 and 18.

❖ HEALTH HISTORY

The head and neck health history provides insight into the link between a patient's life/lifestyle and head and neck information and pathology.

PATIENT PROFILE *Diseases that are age- and sex-specific for the head and neck are listed.*

Age Lymphadenopathies related to Hodgkin's disease (11–29)
Cervical spine trauma (young adults)
Hyperthyroidism (reproductive years in young women)
Temporal arteritis (elderly)
Decreased mobility of the cervical spine related to an inflammatory or degenerative process (elderly)

Sex

Female Hypo- or hyperthyroidism, thyroid cancer
Degenerative cervical bone disease

Male Lymphadenopathy related to Hodgkin's disease
Trauma-related cervical spine injury

CHIEF COMPLAINT *Common chief complaints for the head and neck are defined, and information on the characteristics of each sign/symptom is provided.*

Stiff Neck Painful movement of the neck that restricts range of motion

Quality Limited range of motion, either passive or active

Associated Manifestations Headache, neck tenderness, swelling, fever, numbness and tingling in arms or hands

Aggravating Factors Position (sitting, standing, lying down), mobility, stress, weather

Alleviating Factors Immobility or rest, certain position, analgesics, heat

Setting Work, driving

continued

Timing	With all movements, with rotating movements only, with flexion and extension only, with weather changes; after falls, motor vehicle or other accidents
Hoarseness	Husky or harsh quality of the voice
Quality	Audible, inaudible
Associated Manifestations	Fever, sore throat, malaise
Aggravating Factors	Inhalation of chemicals or noxious fumes, smoking, overuse of voice, alcohol use, recent upper respiratory infections, recent head and neck surgery, intubation, neck trauma
Alleviating Factors	Medications, adequate hydration, voice rest
Setting	Public speaking, singing, yelling, normal speech
Timing	Continuous, intermittent
Neck Mass	Discrete area of swelling found in the neck
Quality	Mobile, nonmobile, smooth, irregular, tender, nontender
Associated Manifestations	Shortness of breath, hoarseness, weight loss, fever and chills, dysphagia, ear pain
Aggravating Factors	Eating, talking, movement, tight clothing around the neck, swallowing
Alleviating Factors	Avoidance of tight clothing, analgesic medications, decreased dietary intake
Timing	Long-standing, recent
Headache	Pain felt within the head, behind the eyes, or at the nape of the neck (see Table 11-1)
Location	Temporal, frontal, occipital, behind the eyes, neck and upper shoulders
Quality	Neck pain: aching, sore, dull, sharp; head pain: throbbing, sharp, dull, aching
Associated Manifestations	Neck pain: fever, headache, swelling, tenderness; head pain: nausea and vomiting, aura, diplopia, blurred vision, irritability, sneezing, rhinorrhea, weakness
Aggravating Factors	Neck pain: stress, trauma, aging, position, mobility, weather changes; head pain: stress, fatigue, foods, noxious odors, caffeine intake, coughing, alcohol intake, smoke, hunger, season, weather, menstrual periods
Alleviating Factors	Medications such as analgesics, anti-inflammatory agents, ergotamine, or sumatriptan; position change; rest; sleep; shaking head; food intake
Setting	Work, outdoors
Timing	Neck pain: with movement, at rest, weather changes; head pain: constant, intermittent, in the morning, at the end of the day, premenstrual, seasonal

continued

PAST HEALTH HISTORY	*The various components of the past health history are linked to head and neck pathology and head- and neck-related information.*
Medical	
Head and Neck Specific	Hypo- or hyperthyroidism, sinus infections, migraine headache, cancer, closed head injury or skull fracture
Nonhead and Neck Specific	Pheochromocytoma
Surgical	Thyroidectomy, facial reconstruction, cosmetic surgery, neurosurgery, other surgery related to the head or neck
Medications	Antibiotics, steroids, anticonvulsants, chemotherapy, thyroxine, propranolol, analgesics, oral contraceptives
Communicable Diseases	Meningitis, encephalitis
Injuries/Accidents	Obstruction caused by foreign bodies, trauma to the head or neck, chemical splashes to the face, noxious fumes, sports injuries, motor vehicle accidents
Disabilities/Handicaps	Tracheostomy, paralysis
FAMILY HEALTH HISTORY	*Head and neck diseases that are familial are listed.*
	Thyroid disease, headaches
SOCIAL HISTORY	*The components of the social history are linked to head and neck factors/pathology.*
Alcohol Use	Predisposes to accidents and head injury
Work Environment	Risk of head injury, exposure to toxins or chemicals
Home Environment	Risk of falls and head injury due to loose throw rugs or absence of handrails
Stress	Demands of employment, home, school
HEALTH MAINTENANCE ACTIVITIES	*This information provides a bridge between the health maintenance activities and head and neck function.*
Sleep	May be increased due to head injury
Diet	Recent weight gain or loss
Use of Safety Devices	Protective headgear for sports and work

NURSING TIP

Assessing Patients with Headaches

Patients who complain of headaches should always have blood pressure measured to rule out hypertension as a potential etiology of their headaches.

 THINK ABOUT IT

Preventing Head and Neck Injury

Ivan is a 20-year-old bicycle courier for a large business in the downtown area. He presents to the clinic with a swollen ankle that he sustained after running a red light and colliding with a car. You note that Ivan has extensive bruises on his face. You inquire about his use of a helmet. He replies, "I'm careful. I don't need it." How would you respond to this comment? What teaching strategies might you use?

EQUIPMENT:

- Stethoscope
- Cup of water

Table 11-1 Causes of Headaches

MUSCLE CONTRACTION
Tension headache

VASCULAR CAUSES
Migraine headache
Cluster headache

SYSTEMIC CAUSES
Infection
Post-lumbar puncture
Hypertension
Carbon monoxide inhalation
Exertion

INTRACRANIAL CAUSES
Masses such as tumors
Hemorrhage
Intracranial infection

FACIAL OR CERVICAL CAUSES
Sinusitis
Temporomandibular joint dysfunction
Dental lesions
Temporal arteritis
Trigeminal neuralgia
Narrow angle glaucoma

Adapted from: Johnson, C. J. (1995). Headaches and facial pain. In R. L. Barker, J. R. Burton, and P. D. Zieve (Eds.), Principles of Ambulatory Medicine (4th ed., pp. 1162–1197). Baltimore: Williams & Wilkins.

 NURSING TIP

Nonpharmaceutical Headache Remedies

The patient may benefit from instructions on methods to reduce or alleviate headaches by nonchemical means. Some suggestions include: relaxation techniques, a quiet environment, a dark room, lying down, walking, soothing music, muscle stretching, warm or cool compresses to the head, herbal tea, and a neck or temple massage. Encourage the patient to experiment with these techniques to determine what is effective, and to use the effective method when headaches occur.

✓ **NURSING CHECKLIST**
General Approach to Head and Neck Assessment

1. Greet the patient and explain the assessment techniques that you will be using.
2. Ensure that the environment is at a warm, comfortable room temperature to provide the patient comfort.
3. Use a quiet room that will be free from interruptions.
4. Ensure that the light in the room provides sufficient brightness to allow adequate observation of the patient.
5. Place the patient in an upright sitting position on the examination table, or
5A. Gain access to the head of the supine, bedridden patient by removing nonessential equipment or bedding (for patients who cannot tolerate the sitting position).
6. Ask the patient to remove wig or headpiece.
7. Visualize the underlying anatomic structures during the assessment process to permit an accurate description of the location of any pathology.
8. Always compare the right and left sides of the head, neck, and face to one another.
9. Use the same systematic approach every time the assessment is performed.

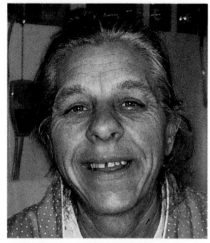

A. Hydrocephalus *Courtesy of Armed Forces Institute of Pathology*

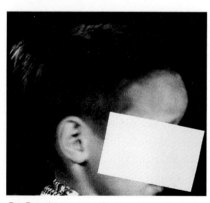

B. Acromegaly (Note wide nose, spaced teeth, and large lips.) *Courtesy of Matthew C. Leinung, M.D., Albany Medical College, Albany, NY*

C. Craniosynostosis *Courtesy of Armed Forces Institute of Pathology*

Figure 11-7   Abnormal Head Shapes

E	Examination
N	Normal Findings
A	Abnormal Findings
P	Pathophysiology

ASSESSMENT OF THE HEAD AND NECK

Inspection of the Shape of the Head

E   **1.** Have the patient sit in a comfortable position.
    2. Face the patient, with your head at the same level as the patient's head.
    3. Inspect the head for shape and symmetry.

N   *The head should be normocephalic and symmetrical.*

A   **Hydrocephalus** is an enlargement of the head without enlargement of the facial structures (see Figure 11-7A).

P   Hydrocephalus is caused by an abnormal accumulation of cerebrospinal fluid within the skull.

A   **Acromegaly** is an abnormal enlargement of the skull and bony facial structures.

P   Acromegaly is caused by excessive secretion of growth hormone from the pituitary gland (see Figure 11-7B).

A   **Craniosynostosis** is characterized by abnormal shape of the skull or bone growth at right angles to suture lines, exophthalmos, and drooping eyelids (see Figure 11-7C).

P   Craniosynostosis is caused by the premature closure of one or more sutures of the skull before brain growth is complete.

Palpation of the Head

E   **1.** Place the finger pads on the scalp and palpate all of its surface, beginning in the frontal area and continuing over the parietal, temporal, and occipital areas.
    2. Assess for contour, masses, depressions, tenderness.

N   *The normal skull is smooth, nontender, and without masses or depressions.*

A   Masses in the cranial bones that feel hard or soft are abnormal.

P   These types of masses may be carcinomatous metastasis from other regions of the body or may result from lymphomas, multiple myeloma, or leukemia.

A   Palpation elicits localized edema over the bony frontal portion of the skull.

P   Osteomyelitis of the skull may develop following acute or chronic sinusitis if the infection extends out from the sinuses into the surrounding bone.

A   Firm palpation reveals a softening of the outer bone layer.

P   **Craniotabes** is a softening of the skull caused by hydrocephalus or demineralization of the bone due to rickets, hypervitaminosis A, or syphilis.

> ✿ **NURSING TIP**
>
> **Assessment of Temporal Arteries**
>
> Inspection and palpation of the temporal arteries are normally done while palpating the head in order to maintain efficiency of effort. Refer to Chapter 15 for a description of the technique.

Inspection and Palpation of the Scalp

E   **1.** Part the hair repeatedly all over the scalp and inspect the scalp for lesions or masses.
    2. Place the finger pads on the scalp and palpate for lesions or masses.

N   *The scalp should be shiny, intact, and without lesions or masses.*

A   A laceration or a laceration with bleeding is abnormal.

P   Direct trauma can cause lacerations to the scalp.

Gaping Lacerations

Gaping lacerations of the scalp require emergency treatment under aseptic conditions because of their access to the brain and potential to threaten the patient's life.

Hematomas

Hematomas may be life-threatening conditions and require immediate referral to a physician.

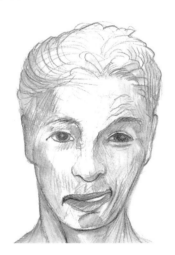

Figure 11-8 Bell's Palsy

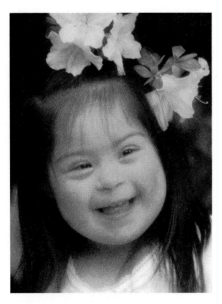

Figure 11-9 Down Syndrome
© Marijane Scott, Marijane's Designer Portraits, Down Right Beautiful 1996 Calendar

A A gaping laceration with profuse bleeding is abnormal.

P If the laceration on the scalp is gaping, it indicates a deep wound that may indicate a compound skull fracture as a result of some type of trauma.

A Palpation reveals a localized, easily movable accumulation of blood in the subcutaneous tissue.

P Hematomas can result from direct trauma to the skull.

A Palpation may reveal either single or multiple masses that are easily movable. They are round, firm, nontender, and arise from either the skin or the subcutaneous tissue.

P These are sebaceous cysts that form as a result of a retention of secretions from sebaceous glands.

A Nonmobile, fatty masses with smooth, circular edges may be palpated deeper in the scalp.

P These masses are benign fatty tumors known as **lipomas**.

Inspection of the Face

Facial Piercing

How would you react to the patient who has pierced lips, cheeks, or nose? What would be appropriate verbal and nonverbal responses? Are there any cultural or religious implications?

Symmetry

E 1. Have the patient sit in a comfortable position facing you.
2. Observe the patient's face for expression, shape, and symmetry of the following structures: eyebrows, eyes, nose, mouth, ears.

N *The facial features should be symmetrical. Both palpebral fissures should be equal and the nasolabial fold should present bilaterally. It is important to remember that slight variations in symmetry are common. Slanted eyes with inner epicanthal folds are normal findings in patients of Asian descent.*

A Structures are absent or deformed. There is a definite asymmetry of expression, the palpebral fissures, the nasolabial folds, and the corners of the mouth.

P Asymmetry of the palpebral fissures, nasolabial folds, the mouth, and facial expression may indicate damage to the nerves innervating facial muscles, as in stroke or **Bell's palsy** (see Figure 11-8).

Shape

E 1. Face the patient.
2. Observe the patient's face for changes in shape, swelling, abnormal features, or unusual movement.

N *The shape of the face can be oval, round, or slightly square. There should be no edema, disproportionate structures, or involuntary movements.*

A Inspection of the face may reveal slanted eyes with inner epicanthal folds; a short, flat nose; and a thick, protruding tongue.

P These findings are likely to indicate the presence of **Down syndrome**, a chromosomal aberration (see Figure 11-9).

A An abnormally wide distance between the eyes is **hypertelorism**.

P Hypertelorism is a congenital anomaly.

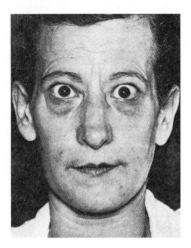

Figure 11-10 Graves' Disease
From DeGroot, The Thyroid and Its Diseases, *4th ed., ©1975. Reprinted by permission of John Wiley & Sons, Inc.*

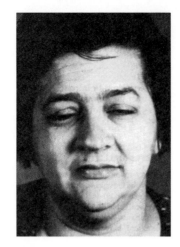

Figure 11-11 Myxedema *Courtesy of Delmar Publishers, Albany, NY*

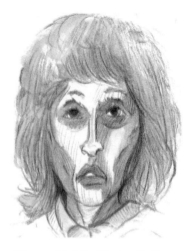

Figure 11-12 Cachectic Face

A The face is thin with sharply defined features and prominent eyes in Graves' disease (see Figure 11-10).

P Graves' disease is an autoimmune disorder associated with increased circulating levels of T_3 and T_4.

A The patient's face is round and swollen with characteristic periorbital edema and dry, dull skin (see Figure 11-11).

P This condition is known as myxedema and is associated with hypothyroidism.

A The eyes are sunken and cheeks are hollow in cachexia (see Figure 11-12).

P Cachexia is a profound state of wasting of the vital tissues associated with cancer, malnutrition, and dehydration.

A The patient's face is immobile and expressionless with a staring gaze and raised eyebrows in Parkinson's disease (see Figure 11-13).

P Parkinson's disease is the degeneration of basal ganglia, resulting from a deficiency of the neurotransmitter dopamine.

A The face of Caucasians shows a dusky blue discoloration beneath the eyes along with creases in the lower eyelids and mouth breathing (see Figure 11-14).

P The patient with chronic allergies develops this characteristic allergic facies.

A The patient's face has a rounded, "moonface" along with red cheeks and excess hair on the jaw and upper lip (see Figure 11-15).

P This is the facies of Cushing's syndrome, which is caused by increased production of adrenocorticotropic hormone (ACTH) or steroid ingestion.

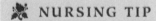

NURSING TIP

Color of Facial Skin

In order to proceed in an organized manner, it is appropriate to evaluate the color of facial skin during inspection. Please refer to Chapter 10 for assessment of skin.

E Examination
N Normal Findings
A Abnormal Findings
P Pathophysiology

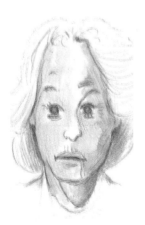

Figure 11-13 Parkinson's Disease

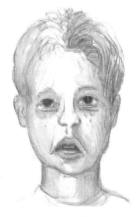

Figure 11-14 Allergic Facies

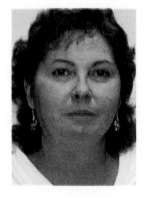

Figure 11-15 Cushing's Syndrome
Courtesy of Matthew C. Leinung, M.D., Albany Medical College, Albany, NY

☸ NURSING TIP

Assessment of the Cranial Nerves

The integrity of cranial nerves V and VII is usually evaluated during assessment of the face. For a description of the technique, see Chapter 18.

◎◎ THINK ABOUT IT

Sensitivity to Patients with Severe Facial Burns

During your first day working in the burn unit, you are assigned to care for a patient who has multiple second-degree burns to his face and upper extremities. As you meet him for the first time, he says, "I look horrible; you won't be able to stand to look at me." How would you respond verbally and nonverbally to his comment and his disfigurement?

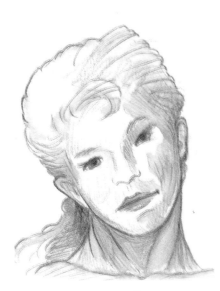

Figure 11-16   Torticollis

E	**Examination**
N	**Normal Findings**
A	**Abnormal Findings**
P	**Pathophysiology**

Palpation and Auscultation of the Mandible

E   1. Use the fingertips of both index and middle fingers to locate the temporomandibular joint anterior to the tragus of the ear on both sides.
  2. Hold the fingertips firmly in place over the joints and ask the patient to open and close the mouth.
  3. As the patient opens and closes the mouth, observe the relative smoothness of the movement and whether or not the patient notices any discomfort.
  4. Remove the hands.
  5. Hold the bell of the stethoscope over the joint.
  6. Listen for any sound while the patient opens and closes the mouth.

N   *The patient should experience no discomfort with movement. The temporomandibular joint should articulate smoothly and without clicking or crepitus.*

A   The patient complains of tenderness when the mouth is opened and closed. Palpation or auscultation reveals clicking or crepitus.

P   Tenderness in the joint may be from the inflammation of migratory arthritis.

A   Crepitus is present from the articulation of irregular bone surfaces found in osteoarthritis.

P   Clicking may follow a "snapping" sound if there is displaced cartilage.

A   The mouth remains in an open and fixed position.

P   Following a wide yawn or trauma to the chin, the temporomandibular joint is dislocated and will not function. This condition requires reduction.

Inspection and Palpation of the Neck

Inspection of the Neck

E   1. Have the patient sit facing you, with the head held in a central position.
  2. Inspect for symmetry of the sternocleidomastoid muscles anteriorly, and the trapezii posteriorly.
  3. Have the patient touch the chin to the chest, to each side, and to each shoulder.
  4. Assess for limitation of motion.
  5. Note the presence of a stoma or tracheostomy.

N   *The muscles of the neck are symmetrical with the head in a central position. The patient is able to move the head through a full range of motion without complaint of discomfort or noticeable limitation. The patient may be breathing through a stoma or tracheostomy.*

A   The patient complains of pain with flexion or rotation of the head.

P   Pain with flexion can be associated with the pain and muscle spasm caused by meningeal irritation of meningitis (see Chapter 18). Generalized discomfort may be related to trauma, spasm, or inflammation of muscles or diseases of the vertebrae.

A   There is a slight or prominent lateral deviation of the patient's neck (see Figure 11-16). The sternocleidomastoid muscles, and to a lesser extent the trapezius and scalene muscles, may also be prominent on the affected side. The muscles frequently hypertrophy as the result of powerful contractions.

P   This condition is called **torticollis**. Causes can be:
  1. Congenital: resulting from a hematoma or partial rupture at birth of the sternocleidomastoid, causing a shortening of the muscle.
  2. Ocular: a head posture assumed to correct for ocular muscle palsy and resulting diplopia.

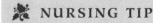

NURSING TIP

Evaluation of Cranial Nerve XI

When inspecting and palpating the neck, it is prudent to evaluate cranial nerve XI. Refer to Chapter 18 for a description of the technique.

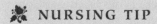

NURSING TIP

Assessment of the Trachea

It is appropriate to assess the trachea at this point in the examination. Refer to Chapter 14 for a description of the technique.

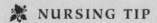

NURSING TIP

Assessment of the Carotid Arteries and Jugular Veins

It is important to assess the carotid arteries and jugular veins at this point in the examination. Refer to Chapter 15 for a description of the technique.

E	Examination
N	Normal Findings
A	Abnormal Findings
P	Pathophysiology

3. Acute spasm: commonly associated with the inflammation of viral myositis or trauma such as sleeping with the head in an unusual position.
4. Other: phenothiazine therapy, hysteria, and Parkinson's disease as the result of increased cholinergic activity in the brain.

A Range of motion of the neck is reduced.

P Degenerative changes of osteoarthritis may result in decreased ability for full range of motion. This condition is usually painless unless nerve root irritation has occurred. Crepitus, or a crunching sound on hyperextension of the neck, may also be observed.

Palpation of the Neck

E 1. Stand in front of the patient.
2. With the finger pads, palpate the sternocleidomastoids.
3. Note the presence of masses or tenderness.
4. Stand behind the patient.
5. With the finger pads, palpate the trapezius.
6. Note the presence of masses or tenderness.

N *The muscles should be symmetrical without palpable masses or spasm.*

A A mass is palpated in the musculature.

P A mass may be a tumor, either primary or metastatic.

A A spasm may be felt in the muscles.

P Muscle spasm may be due to varied causes such as infections, trauma, chronic inflammatory processes, or neoplasms.

Inspection of the Thyroid Gland

E 1. Secure strong, tangential lighting.
2. Face the patient.
3. Ask the patient to look straight ahead with the head slightly extended.
4. Have the patient drink a sip of water and swallow twice.
5. As the patient swallows, observe the front of the neck in the area of the thyroid and the isthmus for masses and symmetrical movement.

N *Thyroid tissue moves up with swallowing but often the movement is so small it is not visible on inspection. In males, the thyroid cartilage, or "Adam's apple," is more prominent than in females.*

A A mass or enlargement of the thyroid that moves upward with swallowing is not normal.

P Many **goiters** (enlarged thyroid glands) or thyroid nodules are visible and may indicate a variety of thyroid diseases.

Palpation of the Thyroid Gland

Palpation of the thyroid gland may be done using both anterior and posterior approaches (see Figure 11-17).

Posterior Approach

E 1. Have the patient sit comfortably. Stand behind the patient.
2. Have the patient lower the chin slightly in order to relax the neck muscles.
3. Place the thumbs on the back of the patients's neck and bring the other fingers around the neck anteriorly with their tips resting on the lower portion of the neck over the trachea.
4. Move the finger pads over the tracheal rings.

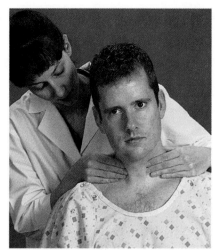

A. Posterior Approach

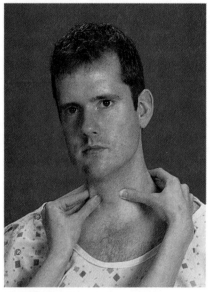

B. Anterior Approach

Figure 11-17 Examination of the Thyroid Gland

E **Examination**
N **Normal Findings**
A **Abnormal Findings**
P **Pathophysiology**

5. Instruct the patient to swallow. Palpate the isthmus for nodules or enlargement.
6. Have the patient incline the head slightly forward.
7. Press the fingers of the left hand against the left side of the thyroid cartilage to stabilize it while placing the fingers of the right hand gently against the right side.
8. Instruct the patient to swallow sips of water.
9. Note consistency, nodularity, or tenderness as the gland moves upward.
10. Repeat on the other side.

N/A/P Refer to Anterior Approach.

Anterior Approach

E 1. Stand in front of the patient.
  2. Ask the patient to flex the head slightly forward.
  3. Place the right thumb on the thyroid cartilage and displace the cartilage to the patient's right.
  4. Grasp the elevated and displaced right lobe of the thyroid gland with the thumb and index and middle fingers of the left hand.
  5. Palpate the surface of the gland for consistency, nodularity, and tenderness.
  6. Have the patient swallow, and palpate the surface again.
  7. Repeat the procedure on the opposite side.

N *No enlargement, masses, or tenderness should be noted on palpation.*

A Palpation reveals the gland to be smooth, soft, and slightly enlarged but less than twice the size of a normal thyroid gland.

P This is referred to as physiological hyperplasia and can be seen premenstrually, during pregnancy, or from puberty to young adulthood in the female. Symmetrical enlargement may also be noted in patients who live in areas of iodine deficiency. These are referred to as nontoxic diffuse goiters or endemic goiters.

A Palpation reveals the gland to be two to three times larger than normal size.

P This is diffuse toxic hyperplasia of the thyroid, or Graves' disease, an autoimmune disorder that is the most common type of hyperthyroidism.

A Asymmetrical enlargement of the thyroid and the presence of two or more nodules are found.

P These are thyroid adenomas (benign epithelial tumors) that usually occur after the age of 30. A nontoxic diffuse goiter may become nodular as the patient ages.

A Palpation reveals a solitary nodule in the thyroid tissue.

P A solitary nodule is suggestive of carcinoma.

A Lateral deviation of the trachea is noted on palpation, but you are unable to identify a specific goiter.

P This may be a retrosternal goiter. This type of goiter sometimes occurs in a patient with a short neck or a goiter with many adenomatous nodules.

A Tenderness of the thyroid is found on palpation.

P Tenderness of an enlarged, firm thyroid suggests thyroiditis.

Auscultation of the Thyroid Gland

If the thyroid is enlarged, auscultation should be done.

E 1. Stand in front of the patient.
  2. Place the bell of the stethoscope over the right thyroid lobe.
  3. Auscultate for bruits.
  4. Repeat on the left thyroid lobe.

N *Auscultation should not reveal bruits.*

A Auscultation reveals the presence of a bruit over an enlarged thyroid gland.

P Bruits occur with increased turbulence in a vessel and are due to the increased vascularization of a thyroid gland that is enlarged due to diffuse toxic goiter.

Inspection of the Lymph Nodes

E 1. Stand in front of the patient.
2. Expose the area of the head and neck to be assessed.
3. Inspect the nodal areas of the head and neck for any enlargement or inflammation.

N *Lymph nodes should not be visible or inflamed.*

A Enlargement and inflammation is present in specific nodes.

P Lymph nodes can be enlarged and inflamed when there is a localized or generalized infection in the body. This attempt to prevent the spread of infection occurs as a part of the body's immune response to infection.

Palpation of the Lymph Nodes

E 1. Have the patient sit comfortably.
2. Face the patient and conduct the assessment of both sides of the neck simultaneously.
3. Move the pads and tips of the middle three fingers in small circles of palpation using gentle pressure.
4. Follow a systematic, routine sequence beginning with the preauricular, postauricular, occipital, submental, and submandibular nodes. Moving down to the neck, evaluate the anterior cervical chain, the posterior cervical chain, the tonsillar nodes, and the supraclavicular nodes (see Figure 11-18).
5. Note size, shape, delimitation (discrete or matted together), mobility, consistency, and tenderness.

N *Lymph nodes should not be palpable in the healthy adult patient; however, small, discrete, movable nodes are sometimes present but are of no significance.*

A Palpable lymph nodes are abnormal.

P Palpable lymph nodes are frequently seen in acute bacterial infections such as streptococcal pharyngitis. The anterior cervical nodes are usually affected and may be warm, firm, tender, and mobile.

P An enlarged postauricular node is sometimes found in patients with ear infections.

P Enlarged, hard, tender nodes are seen in lymphadenitis (inflammation of the lymph nodes). The affected node is the site of the inflammation.

P Enlarged nodes, particularly of the anterior and posterior cervical chains, may be found in infectious mononucleosis. These nodes are usually tender.

P An enlarged node in the left supraclavicular area (Virchow's node) may point to malignancy in the abdominal or thoracic regions.

P Nontender, firm or hard nodes that are nonmobile may indicate a malignancy in the head and neck area, or metastasis from the region that the lymph node drains.

P Patients with malignant lymphomas may also present with nodes that are firm, hard, or rubbery; nontender; and fixed. In Hodgkin's disease, the cervical nodes are frequently the first to be palpable.

P Palpable lymph nodes can result from a variety of other pathological processes, including blood dyscrasias, AIDS, tuberculosis, surgical procedures that traumatize the nodes, blood transfusions, or chronic illness.

E   **Examination**
N   **Normal Findings**
A   **Abnormal Findings**
P   **Pathophysiology**

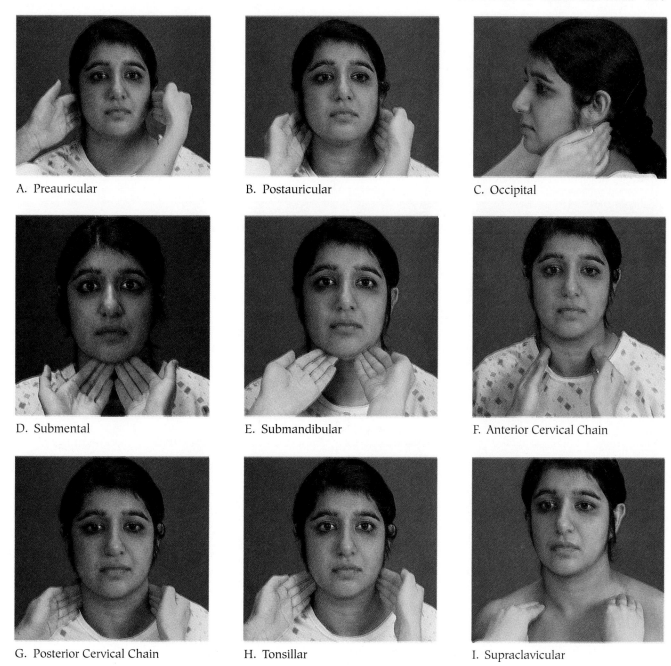

A. Preauricular

B. Postauricular

C. Occipital

D. Submental

E. Submandibular

F. Anterior Cervical Chain

G. Posterior Cervical Chain

H. Tonsillar

I. Supraclavicular

Figure 11-18 Palpation of Lymph Nodes

GERONTOLOGICAL VARIATIONS

Loss of subcutaneous fat and musculoskeletal changes due to the aging process affect the appearance and function of the head and neck. Facial symmetry may be altered because of the presence of dentures or loss of teeth. Neck veins may be more prominent due to loss of fat.

The head, neck, and lower jaw may be thrust forward, especially with a kyphotic posture. A "buffalo hump" may appear as an accumulation of fat over the posterior cervical vertebrae. Range of motion of the head may be limited, painful, or possible only with a jerking or "cogwheel" motion. Dizziness accompanying movement of the head may create safety problems. All of these changes may affect the elderly patient's ability to maintain normal activities of daily living.

✪ NURSING ALERT

Patient Safety During Assessment

Maintain safety for elderly patients by allowing them to remain seated during the head and neck assessment. Doing so will prevent dangerous falls if dizziness and instability occur.

CASE STUDY

The case study illustrates the application and objective documentation of the head and neck assessment.

The Patient with Thyromegaly

Bob is a 38-year-old high school physical education teacher. For the past week he has been aware of a tenderness and fullness in his neck. At first he thought he was coming down with a cold, but his symptoms haven't changed and he has no fever. Because the problem hasn't gone away, he made an appointment with his nurse practitioner to find out what is wrong.

❖ HEALTH HISTORY

PATIENT PROFILE	38 yo SWM
CHIEF COMPLAINT	"My neck has been sore for a week."
HISTORY OF PRESENT ILLNESS	Pt in usual state of good health until 1 wk PTA when he noticed soreness & swelling in lower front of neck; pt dismissed as a "cold"; mild discomfort at all times but aggravated by mvt & buttoned shirt collars. Pain doesn't disturb sleep or interfere $\bar{c}$ eating. Pt concerned that he might have "cancer in his lymph glands." More tired recently, gained 4 lb due to lack of energy, c/o mild constipation. Denies unusual stress, irritability, frequent infections, fever, thirst, urination, hunger, heat or cold intolerance, hx of DM.
PAST HEALTH HISTORY	
Medical	Denies past problems
Surgical	Uncomplicated appendectomy at City General Hospital 12 yo; uncomplicated removal of wisdom teeth 20 yo in local oral surgeon's office
Medications	Occasional acetaminophen for H/A
Communicable Diseases	Chickenpox 7 yo. Denies other childhood dz or STD
Allergies	Mild pollen allergy in spring (no meds required)
Injuries/Accidents	fx Ⓡ ring finger playing basketball 15 yo $\bar{s}$ sequelae
Disabilities/Handicaps	Denies
Blood Transfusions	Denies
Childhood Illnesses	See communicable dz
Immunizations	"Usual" childhood immunizations; tetanus booster 1 yr ago; flu shot q yr
FAMILY HEALTH HISTORY	

continued

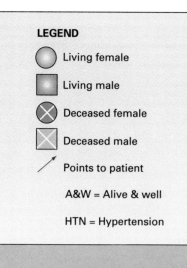

LEGEND

- (circle) Living female
- (square) Living male
- (circle with X) Deceased female
- (square with X) Deceased male
- (arrow) Points to patient
- A&W = Alive & well
- HTN = Hypertension

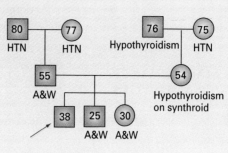

Denies family hx of H/A.

SOCIAL HISTORY

Alcohol Use	Drinks 6 pack of beer on weekends
Tobacco Use	Has never smoked cigarettes
Drug Use	Denies
Sexual Practice	Monogamous relationship c̄ fiancee
Travel History	Camping in mountains last month
Work Environment	Spends most of day in gym, locker rooms, outdoors at school, or classroom
Home Environment	Lives c̄ fiancee in rented apt
Hobbies/Leisure Activities	Enjoys playing & watching sports, especially tennis; enjoys music & scuba diving
Stress	Denies
Education	Masters degree in education
Economic Status	Middle class, comfortable c̄ income
Military Service	None
Religion	Nonpracticing Methodist
Ethnic Background	Polish ancestry
Roles/Relationships	"Very close" to parents & siblings. Helps parents c̄ yard work & other "heavy" household chores. Engaged to be married in 6 mo.
Characteristic Patterns of Daily Living	Workday: gets up at 6:30 AM, eats breakfast, drives to school & arrives at 8:15 AM; lunch in school cafeteria at noon; classes until 2:15, when he supervises sports team practices then runs on school track or at a fitness club; dinner at 7 or 7:30 & goes to bed around 11 PM. Weekends: sleeps till 8 or 8:30 AM; runs before breakfast then does assorted

continued

"weekend chores" at apt or parents' home; sometimes watches sports on TV during weekend afternoons or has social gatherings c̄ friends or family; weekend meals & bedtimes vary c̄ social schedule.

HEALTH MAINTENANCE ACTIVITIES

Sleep	7–8 hrs most nights
Diet	Low-fat diet
Exercise	Active in many sports especially tennis, runs several miles on treadmill at fitness club or school track 4–5 × per wk
Stress Management	Running, tennis, music
Use of Safety Devices	Wears seat belt
Health Check-Ups	Had insurance physical last yr

PHYSICAL ASSESSMENT

Inspection of the Shape of the Head	Normocephalic
Palpation of the Head	Skull smooth, s̄ tenderness, masses, or depressions
Inspection and Palpation of the Scalp	Scalp shiny & intact, no lesions or masses
Inspection of the Face	
Symmetry	Symmetrical s̄ involuntary movements or swelling
Shape	Oval, s̄ edema
Palpation and Auscultation of the Mandible	TMJ articulate smoothly s̄ clicking or crepitus
Inspection of the Neck	s̄ masses or spasm & c̄ full ROM
Palpation of the Neck	Supple & symmetrical s̄ masses or spasm
Inspection of the Thyroid Gland	Symmetrically enlarged & rises c̄ swallowing
Palpation of the Thyroid Gland	Both lobes of thyroid are enlarged Ⓡ > Ⓛ & sl tender to palpation, s̄ nodules
Auscultation of the Thyroid Gland	No bruits
Inspection of the Lymph Nodes	No enlargement

continued

Palpation of the Lymph Nodes	Not palpable		
LABORATORY DATA		Pt's Values	Normal Range
	T_4 (Thyroxine)	4.0 μg/dl	5–12 μg/dl
	T_3 Uptake	24%	25%–35%
	TSH	17.7 μIU/ml	<8 μIU/ml
	HCT	43%	Males: 39%–51%

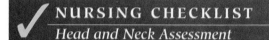

NURSING CHECKLIST
Head and Neck Assessment

Inspection of the Shape of the Head
Palpation of the Head
Inspection and Palpation of the Scalp
Inspection of the Face
  • Symmetry
  • Shape
Palpation and Auscultation of the Mandible
Inspection and Palpation of the Neck
  • Inspection of the Neck
  • Palpation of the Neck
Inspection of the Thyroid Gland
Palpation of the Thyroid Gland
  • Posterior Approach
  • Anterior Approach
Auscultation of the Thyroid Gland
Inspection of the Lymph Nodes
Palpation of the Lymph Nodes

REVIEW QUESTIONS AND ACTIVITIES

1. It is helpful to visualize the location of anatomic landmarks when describing findings of the head and neck assessment. Ask a classmate to assist you with this activity. Using a washable marker, identify the muscles of the neck and mark the outlines of the anterior and posterior triangles. Next, mark the locations of the lymph nodes to be assessed. Finally, mark the locations of the thyroid and cricoid cartilages and the two lobes and isthmus of the thyroid gland.

2. Describe the facial appearance of the patient with hypothyroidism (myxedema).

3. Describe characteristics to be assessed when an enlarged lymph node is noted.

4. Describe two techniques for palpation of the thyroid gland.

5. Describe the assessment of the temporomandibular joint.

Questions 6–8 refer to the following situation:

You are asked to assess Robert Dawson, a 40-year-old African American who is complaining of a headache.

6. What vital sign should always be measured for patients who experience headaches?
   a. Temperature
   b. Respirations
   c. Visual acuity
   d. Blood pressure

   The correct answer is (d).

7. During your palpation of the patient's mandible, he complains of tenderness when he opens and closes his mouth, and you note a clicking sound. Name the possible cause of this patient's headache.
   a. Dental abscess
   b. Swollen lymph nodes
   c. Temporomandibular joint dysfunction
   d. Vascular spasm

   The correct answer is (c).

8. When palpating Mr. Dawson's lymph nodes, which of the following sequences is correct?
   a. Supraclavicular, tonsillar, posterior cervical chain, submental, anterior cervical chain, preauricular, postauricular, occipital, submandibular
   b. Postauricular, preauricular, anterior cervical chain, posterior cervical chain, occipital, submandibular, tonsillar, supraclavicular, submental
   c. Preauricular, postauricular, occipital, submental, submandibular, tonsillar, supraclavicular, anterior cervical chain, posterior cervical chain
   d. Preauricular, postauricular, occipital, submental, submandibular, anterior cervical chain, posterior cervical chain, tonsillar, supraclavicular.

   The correct answer is (d).

Eyes, Ears, Nose, Mouth, and Throat

1. Identify the structures of the eyes, ears, nose, mouth, and throat.
2. Discuss the system-specific history for the eyes, ears, nose, mouth, and throat.
3. Describe normal findings in the physical assessment of the eyes, ears, nose, mouth, and throat.
4. Describe common abnormalities found in the physical assessment of the eyes, ears, nose, mouth, and throat.
5. Explain the pathophysiology of common abnormalities of the eyes, ears, nose, mouth, and throat.
6. Perform the physical assessment of the eyes, ears, nose, mouth, and throat.

Physical assessment of the eyes, ears, nose, sinuses, mouth, and throat provides a wealth of information about the integrity of many body systems and serves as the foundation for assessment of the neurological, respiratory, endocrine, gastrointestinal, musculoskeletal, and cardiovascular systems.

ANATOMY AND PHYSIOLOGY

Eye
External Structures

The external structures of the eyes comprise the eyelids or palpebra, the conjunctiva, the lacrimal glands, and the extraocular muscles. The eyelids consist of smooth muscle covered with a very thin layer of skin; they admit light to the eye while protecting and maintaining lubrication of the eye. The interior surface of the lid muscle is covered with a pink mucous membrane called the **palpebral conjunctiva**. Contiguous with the palpebral conjunctiva is the **bulbar conjunctiva**. The bulbar conjunctiva folds back over the anterior surface of the eyeball and merges with the cornea at the **limbus**, the junction of the sclera and the cornea (see Figure 12-1). The conjunctiva contains blood vessels and pain receptors that respond quickly to outside insult. Eyelashes are evenly spaced along lid margins and curve outward to protect the eye by filtering particles of dirt and dust from the external environment. Eyebrows are symmetrical and evenly distributed above the eyelids.

The opening between the eyelids is called the **palpebral fissure**. Upper and lower eyelids meet at the inner **canthus** on the nasal side and at the outer canthus on the temporal side. Embedded just beneath the lid margins are the meibomian glands, which secrete a lubricating substance onto the surface of the eye. The **tarsal plates** are connective tissue that give shape to the upper lids.

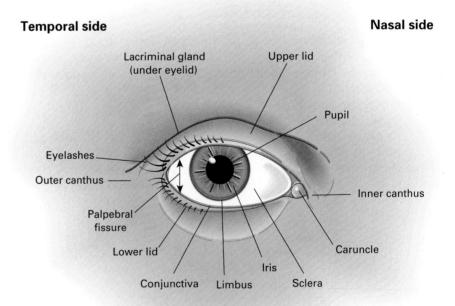

RIGHT EYE

Figure 12-1   External View of the Eye

Lacrimal Apparatus The **lacrimal apparatus** is made up of the lacrimal gland and ducts. The lacrimal glands, located above and on the temporal side of each eye, are responsible for the production of tears, which lubricate the eye. Tears drain through the inferior and superior **puncta** at the inner canthus through the nasolacrimal duct and the lacrimal sac to the inferior turbinate in the nose. The **caruncle**, which contains sebaceous glands, is the round, red structure in the inner canthus.

Extraocular Muscles Six extraocular muscles extend from the scleral surface of each eye and attach to the bony orbit. These voluntary muscles work in concert to move the eyes with great precision in several directions to provide a single image to the brain. These muscles are the superior, inferior, medial, and lateral recti, and the superior and inferior obliques.

Internal Structures

The globes of the eyes are spherical structures that are encased in the protective bony orbits of the face along with the lacrimal gland and extrinsic muscles of the eye. Only a small portion of the anterior surface of the eye is exposed. The eye itself is approximately one inch in diameter and has three layers: a tough, outer, fibrous tunic (sclera); a middle, vascular tunic; and the innermost layer, which contains the retina (refer to Figure 12-2).

Outer Layer The outer tunic consists of the transparent cornea on the outer portion, which is continuous with the **sclera**, an opaque material that appears white and covers the structures inside the eye. The **cornea** is a nonvascular, transparent surface that covers the iris and is continuous with the conjunctival epithelium. The sclera protects the eye and is a surface for the attachment of the extraocular muscles. The posterior portion of the sclera contains an opening for the entrance of the optic nerve and various blood vessels.

Middle Layer The pigmented, middle, vascular tunic, or uveal layer, is composed of the **choroid**, the ciliary body, and the iris. The choroid is a vascular tissue that lines the inner surface of the eye just beneath the retina. It provides nutrition to the retinal pigment epithelium and helps absorb excess light.

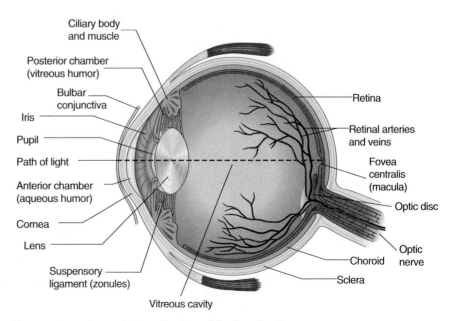

Figure 12-2 Lateral Cross Section of the Interior Eye

The **ciliary body** is an anterior extension of the uveal tract; it siphons serum from the systemic blood flow to produce the aqueous humor needed to nourish the corneal endothelium. Zonules are small strands of tissue extending from the ciliary body to the crystalline **lens**. Zonules hold the lens in place and allow it to change shape in order to refract light from various focusing distances. The **iris**, the most anterior portion of the uveal tract, provides a distinctive color for the eye. The **pupil**, an opening in the center of the iris, regulates the amount of light entering the eye. The pupil reacts to light and closeness of objects by stimulation of the sympathetic nervous system, which dilates it, and parasympathetic nervous system, which constricts it.

The central cavity of the eye posterior to the lens is filled with a clear, gelatinous material called **vitreous humor**, which helps maintain the shape of the eye and the position of the internal structures.

Visual images pass through the structures and aqueous humor of the **anterior chamber**, the space anterior to the pupil and iris, and the vitreous humor of the **posterior chamber**, the space immediately posterior to the iris, to the fundus of the eye, where the retina is located.

Inner Layer   The innermost layer of the eyeball, or the **retina**, is an extension of the optic nerve, which lines the inside of the globe and receives light impulses to be transmitted to the occipital lobe of the brain. Paired retinal arteries and veins branch from the optic disc toward the periphery, growing smaller as they extend outward. Generally, retinal arteries are smaller and lighter red than veins and often have a silver-looking "arterial light reflex." Normal arterial-to-venous width is a ratio of 2:3 or 4:5.

The **optic disc** is a round or oval area with distinct margins located on the nasal side of the retina. Retinal fibers join at the optic disc to form the optic nerve. Nerve fibers from the temporal visual fields cross at the optic chiasm.

The **physiologic cup** is a pale, central area in the optic disc occupying one-third to one-fourth of the disc. In the temporal area of the retina, the tiny, darker **macula**, with the **fovea centralis** at its center, contains a high concentration of **cones** necessary for color vision, reading ability, and other tasks requiring fine visual discrimination. The fovea is the area of sharpest vision. Other portions of the retina contain a high concentration of **rods**, which provide dark and light discrimination and peripheral vision.

Visual Pathway

Objects in the field of vision reflect light that is received by sensory neurons in the retina; these images are received upside down and reversed. From there they pass along nerve fibers through the optic disc and the optic nerve. Fibers from the left half of each eye pass through the optic chiasm to the right side of the brain, and fibers from the right side of each eye pass to the left side of the visual cortex of the occipital lobe of the brain (see Figure 12-3).

Ear

The ear has three sections: the external, the middle, and the inner ears.

External Ear

The external ear, which is also called the **auricle** or pinna, extends through the auditory canal to the tympanic membrane. The auricle receives sound waves and funnels them through the auditory canal to produce vibrations on the tympanic membrane. The auricle is composed of cartilage (see Figure 12-4).

The external auditory canal is an S-shaped tube approximately 2.5 cm in length, with the outer third made up of cartilage and the remainder of bone

LEFT VISUAL FIELD   **RIGHT VISUAL FIELD**

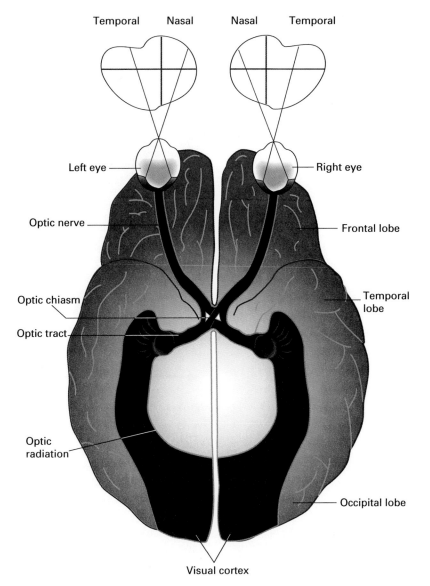

Figure 12-3 Visual Pathway

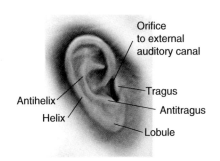

Figure 12-4 External Ear

covered by a thin layer of skin (see Figure 12-5). The canal is lined with tiny hairs and modified sweat glands that secrete a thick, waxlike substance called **cerumen**, which can vary in consistency from dry and flaky to wet and waxy. Cerumen ranges from a pale, honey color in light-skinned individuals to dark-brown or black in dark-skinned people.

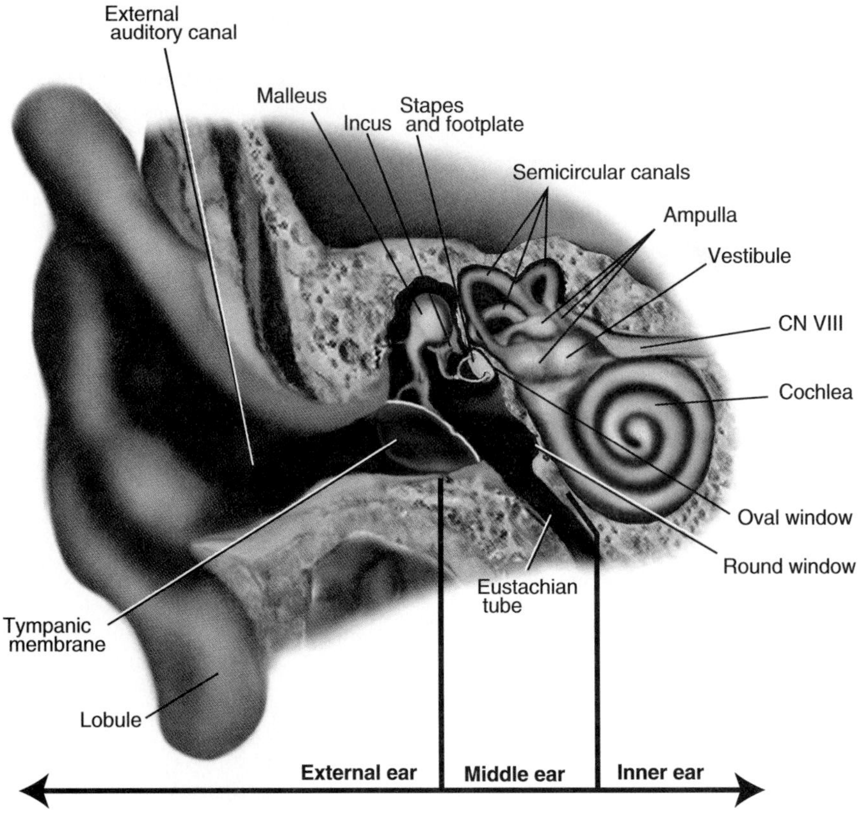

External auditory canal

Malleus

Stapes and footplate

Incus

Semicircular canals

Ampulla

Vestibule

CN VIII

Cochlea

Oval window

Round window

Eustachian tube

Tympanic membrane

Lobule

External ear | Middle ear | Inner ear

Figure 12-5 Cross Section of the Ear

Middle Ear

The middle ear is composed of the tympanic membrane, the ossicles, and the tympanic cavity. The cavity is an air-filled compartment that separates the external ear from the internal ear. The tympanic membrane, which is circular or oval and is about an inch in diameter, sits in an oblique position in the external canal so that it leans slightly forward. The rim of the tympanic membrane is called the annulus, the superior portion is the pars flaccida, and the tighter, largest area of the drum is the pars tensa (refer to Figure 12-6).

The **ossicles** are three tiny bones — the malleus (hammer), the incus (anvil), and the stapes (stirrup) — that play a crucial role in the transmission of sound. The long handle, or manubrium, of the malleus extends downward from the short process and meets the tympanic membrane at the umbo. The stapes is held against the wall of the tympanic membrane at the oval window by tiny ligaments. The head of the malleus articulates with the incus, which in turn articulates with the stapes; they work as a unit when the tympanic membrane begins to vibrate. Vibrations set up in the tympanic membrane by sound waves reaching it through the external auditory canal are transmitted to the inner ear by rapid movement of the ossicles.

The tensor tympani and the stapedius are two tiny muscles involved in movement of the ossicles. The tensor tympani maintains the tension of the tympanic membrane and pulls the malleus inward when it contracts. The stapedius works in opposition by pulling the stapes outward. This coordinated movement is an important mechanism in reducing the intensity of loud sounds that might otherwise result in serious damage to hearing receptors in the inner ear.

The middle ear is connected to the nasopharynx by the auditory or **eustachian tube**, which serves as a channel through which air pressure within the cavity can be equalized with air pressure outside to maintain normal hearing. Equalization of pressure is aided by yawning or swallowing, which causes the opening of valvelike flaps that cover the openings of the eustachian tubes.

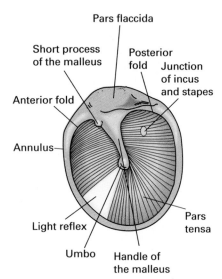

Pars flaccida

Short process of the malleus

Posterior fold

Junction of incus and stapes

Anterior fold

Annulus

Light reflex

Umbo

Handle of the malleus

Pars tensa

Figure 12-6 Landmarks of the Tympanic Membrane

Inner Ear

The inner ear is a complex, closed, fluid-filled system of interconnecting tubes called the **labyrinth**, which is essential for hearing and equilibrium. The labyrinth has bony and membranous portions. The bony labyrinth is composed of the cochlea, the semicircular canals, and the vestibule. The **vestibule** is located between the cochlea and the **semicircular canals** and is important in both hearing and balance. The three semicircular canals located at right angles to each other provide balance and equilibrium for the body. The **cochlea** is a snail-shaped structure made up of three compartments. The first two compartments contain perilymph, and the third contains endolymph. As sound waves travel through the ear, they cause the perilymph and the endolymph to vibrate, stimulating the thousands of hearing-receptor cells of the organ of Corti. Nearby nerve fibers transmit impulses along the cochlear branch of the vestibulocochlear nerve to the brain, allowing us to hear.

Nose

The nose consists of the external or outer nose and the nasal fossae, or internal nose (see Figure 12-7). The outer nose is made up of bone and cartilage and is divided internally into two nasal fossae by the nasal septum. Anterior openings into the nasal fossae are nostrils, or nares. Each fossa has a vestibule just inside the nostril. Superior, middle, and inferior meatuses or grooves are located on the lateral walls of the nostrils just below the corresponding conchae, or **turbinates**. The nasal turbinates are covered by mucous membranes and greatly increase the surface area of mucous membrane in the nose because of their shape.

Air enters the anterior nare, passes through the vestibule, and enters the fossa. The vestibule contains nasal hairs and sebaceous glands. The fossae have both olfactory and respiratory functions. To protect the lungs from noxious agents, these structures of the nose clean, filter, humidify, and control the temperature of inspired air. The mucous covering in the nose and sinuses traps fine dust particles, and lysosomes kill most of the bacteria. The tiny hairs of the nose (cilia) transport the mucus and the particles to the pharynx to be swallowed.

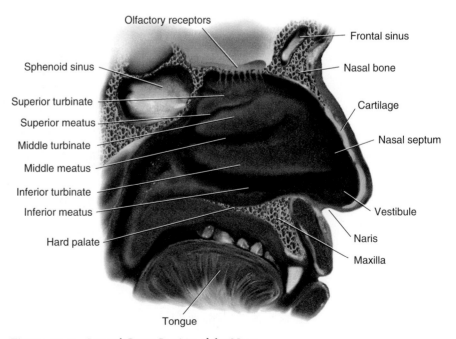

Figure 12-7 Lateral Cross Section of the Nose

The nasal mucosa is capable of adding large amounts of water to inspired air through evaporation from its surface. The rich vascular supply to the turbinates radiates heat to the incoming air as it passes through.

Olfactory receptor cells are located in the upper parts of the nasal cavity, the superior nasal conchae, and on parts of the nasal septum and are covered by hairlike cilia that project into the cavity. The chemical component of odors binds with the receptors, causing nerve impulses to be transmitted to the olfactory cortex, located in the base of the frontal lobe.

Sinuses

Air-filled cavities lined with mucous membranes are present in some of the cranial bones and are referred to as **paranasal sinuses** (see Figure 12-8). These air-filled sinuses lighten the weight of the skull and add resonance to the quality of the voice. The frontal, maxillary, ethmoid, and sphenoid paranasal sinuses open into the nose. Only the frontal and maxillary sinuses can be assessed in the physical examination.

Mouth and Throat

The lips are sensory structures found at the opening of the mouth (see Figure 12-9). The cheeks form the lateral walls of the mouth and are lined with buccal mucosa. The posterior pharyngeal wall is at the back of the mouth.

The roof of the mouth consists of the hard palate anteriorly and the soft palate posteriorly. The **linear raphe** is a linear ridge in the middle of the hard palate that is formed by two palatine bones and part of the superior maxillary bone. The mucous membrane on either side of the linear raphe is thick, pale, and corrugated, while the posterior mucous membrane is thin, a deeper pink, and smooth.

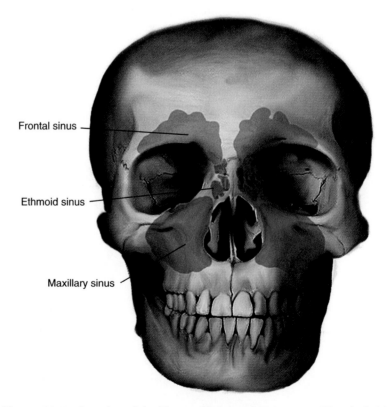

Frontal sinus

Ethmoid sinus

Maxillary sinus

Figure 12-8 Location of the Sinuses (Sphenoid Sinuses are Directly Behind Ethmoid Sinuses)

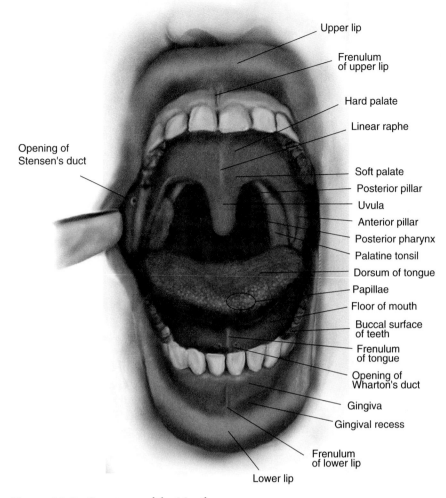

Upper lip

Frenulum
of upper lip

Hard palate

Linear raphe

Opening of
Stensen's duct

Soft palate

Posterior pillar

Uvula

Anterior pillar

Posterior pharynx

Palatine tonsil

Dorsum of tongue

Papillae

Floor of mouth

Buccal surface
of teeth

Frenulum
of tongue

Opening of
Wharton's duct

Gingiva

Gingival recess

Frenulum
of lower lip

Lower lip

Figure 12-9 Structures of the Mouth

Situated in the floor of the mouth, the tongue is a muscular organ connected to the hyoid bone posteriorly and to the floor of the mouth anteriorly by the **frenulum**. The tongue assists with mastication, swallowing, speech, and mechanical cleansing of the teeth.

The mucous membrane covering the upper surface of the tongue has numerous projections called **papillae**, which assist in handling food and contain taste buds. Four qualities of taste are found in taste buds distributed over the surface of the tongue: bitter is located at the base, sour along the sides, and salty and sweet near the tip. The **sulcus terminalis** is the midline depression that separates the anterior two-thirds of the tongue from the posterior one-third.

Two of the three pairs of salivary glands open into the mouth on the ventral surface of the tongue. Submaxillary glands secrete fluid through **Wharton's ducts**, located on both sides of the frenulum. Sublingual glands open into the floor of the mouth posteriorly to Wharton's ducts. The larger parotid glands are located in the cheeks and secrete their amylase-rich fluid through **Stensen's ducts**, located just opposite the upper second molars.

These salivary glands produce 1,000 to 1,500 cc of saliva per day to assist with digestion of food and maintenance of oral hygiene. Saliva prevents dental caries and bacterial damage of healthy oral tissue by washing away bacteria and destroying it with antibodies and proteolytic enzymes.

Gums, or gingivae, appear pink or coral in light-skinned individuals and brown with a darker melanotic line along the edges in dark-skinned individuals. Gums hold the teeth in place.

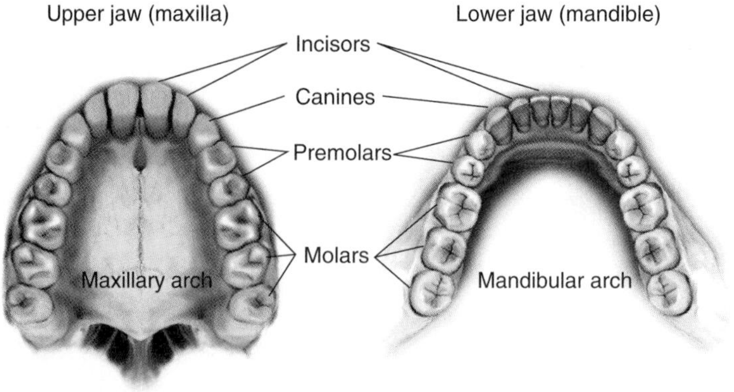

Upper jaw (maxilla)   Lower jaw (mandible)

Incisors

Canines

Premolars

Molars

Maxillary arch   Mandibular arch

Figure 12-10   Permanent Teeth

Adults have 32 permanent teeth: four incisors, two canines, four premolars, and six molars in each half of the mouth (see Figure 12-10). The three parts of the tooth are the top, or the crown, the root, which is embedded in the gum, and the neck, which connects the root and the crown. The teeth are well designed for chewing. Incisors provide strong cutting action, and molars provide strong grinding action.

The soft palate is suspended from the posterior border of the hard palate and extends downward as folds called palatine arches or pillars, forming an incomplete septum between the mouth and the nasopharynx. The **uvula** is a fingerlike projection of tissue that hangs down from the center of the soft palate. Two palatine tonsils containing primarily lymphoid tissue are connected to the palatine arches; they vary greatly in size from one individual to another. Lymphoid tissue in the tonsils plays a role in the control of infection.

❖ HEALTH HISTORY

The eyes, ears, nose, mouth, and throat health history provides insight into the link between a patient's life/lifestyle and eyes, ears, nose, mouth, and throat information and pathology.

PATIENT PROFILE   *Diseases that are age-, sex-, and race-specific for the eyes, ears, nose, mouth, and throat are listed.*

Age

Eyes   Cataract (congenital, elderly)
Presbyopia (middle age)
Hypertensive retinopathy (middle age to elderly)
Glaucoma (middle age to elderly)
Macular degeneration (elderly)
Entropion, ectropion (elderly)
Dry eyes (elderly)

Ears   Hearing loss related to sensorineural degeneration or otosclerosis (elderly)
Excessive or impacted cerumen (elderly)

continued

Mouth and Throat	Orthodonture (middle age) Tooth loss and gum disease (elderly) Thrush related to immunosuppression (elderly) Decrease in ability to taste (elderly)
Sex	
Eyes	Female: Dry eyes, thyroid-related ophthalmopathy
Ears	Female: Calcifications of the ossicles
Nose	Male: Rhinophyma, deviated septum related to trauma
Mouth and Throat	Male: Singer's nodule on the larynx (over 30), cancer of the larynx, leukoplakia of the tongue, gums, and buccal mucosa
Race	
Eyes	Melanoma of the eye (Caucasians), glaucoma (African Americans)
CHIEF COMPLAINT	*Common chief complaints for the eyes, ears, nose, mouth, and throat are defined, and information on the characteristics of each sign/symptom is provided.*
Eyes	
Changes in Visual Acuity	Change in ability to see clearly
Location	One eye or both eyes
Quality	Dimming of vision, blurred vision, diplopia, visual field loss, legal blindness
Associated Manifestations	Headache, rhinorrhea, sneezing, vertigo, "floaters" (spots of different sizes that float across the visual field and caused by changes in the vitreous humor), "flashes" of light, aura, nausea and vomiting, generalized muscle weakness, eye pain or pressure, infection (herpes or cytomegalovirus)
Aggravating Factors	Allergens, stress, lack of sleep, decreased lighting, darkness (night), refractive changes, systemic diseases
Alleviating Factors	Improved lighting, medication, corrective glasses, rest or sleep
Setting	Work environment, increased reading, computer work, night driving
Timing	With aging, at night, after trauma, with or after a headache, seasonal, sudden onset, gradual onset
Pain	Discomfort in the eye
Quality	Aching, sharp, throbbing, burning

continued

Associated Manifestations	Drainage, conjunctival injection, decreased vision, herpes simplex or zoster lesions, increased tearing, headache
Aggravating Factors	Foreign body in the eye, sunlight or very bright light, contact lenses, trauma, allergens
Alleviating Factors	Closing of eye or eyes, removal of contacts, medications, sunglasses, avoiding allergens
Setting	Work environment (increased reading or computer work), recreational area, outdoors
Timing	Sudden onset, gradual onset, with reading
Drainage	Discharge of liquid from the eye
Quality	Type, color
Associated Manifestations	Crusting on the lids, pain, itching, redness of the eye or the lids, headache
Aggravating Factors	Allergens, eye makeup, chlorine, poor hygiene, upper respiratory infection
Alleviating Factors	Medications, hypoallergenic or no eye makeup, avoiding allergens, good handwashing
Setting	Outdoors, swimming pool
Timing	In the morning, continuous, intermittent, seasonal
Itching	Irritation that causes the patient to scratch
Quality	Mild, severe
Associated Manifestations	Rhinitis, sneezing, drainage, burning sensation in the eye, "gritty" sensation in the eye, conjunctivitis, headache
Aggravating Factors	Allergens, contact lenses, eye makeup
Alleviating Factors	Medications, cold compresses to the eyes, removal of contacts, avoiding allergens and eye makeup
Setting	Indoors, outdoors
Timing	Seasonal, intermittent, continuous
Dryness	Reduced amount of lubricating secretions in the eye
Associated Manifestations	With systemic disease, redness of the eye, reduced tearing, itching
Aggravating Factors	Decreased humidity, wind, reading
Alleviating Factors	Artificial tears, humidified air

continued

Setting	Outdoors, indoors with decreased humidity
Timing	With aging, during the winter (decreased humidity), post menopause
Ear	
Change in or Loss of Hearing	Reduction in the perception of sound
Location	Unilateral, bilateral
Quality	Loud sounds heard, soft sounds heard
Quantity	Partial or complete
Associated Manifestations	Tinnitus, vertigo, drainage, swelling, fever, ear pain
Aggravating Factors	Loud noises, excessive or impacted cerumen, swimming
Alleviating Factors	Hearing aid, removal of excessive cerumen, turning up volume when possible, cupping the ear, facing the speaker
Setting	Work (jobs with loud background noise)
Timing	Constant, intermittent, after drug therapy, onset sudden, gradual, or slow
Discharge	Drainage of liquid from the ear
Location	Unilateral or bilateral
Quality	Painful or nontender, watery, bloody or purulent, foul odor
Associated Manifestations	Hearing loss, headache, fever, vertigo, upper respiratory infection
Aggravating Factors	Upright or supine position
Alleviating Factors	Upright or supine position
Timing	Following trauma, continuous, intermittent
Pain	Discomfort in the ear
Location	Unilateral or bilateral
Quality	Aching, dull, sharp
Associated Manifestations	Drainage, tinnitus, dysphagia, sore throat, vertigo, diminished hearing
Aggravating Factors	Tooth infection, upper respiratory infection, perforated tympanic membrane, insect bites in the ear, upright or supine position, objects in ear
Alleviating Factors	Analgesics, upright or supine position, avoiding swimming, avoiding pressure changes, removal of objects
Setting	Outdoors, high altitudes, noisy environments

continued

Timing	Continuous, intermittent, after swimming, following trauma to the head or ear, following loud noises, after pressure changes
Tinnitus	"Ringing" in the ears
Location	Unilateral or bilateral
Quality	Pulsatile, buzzing, high-pitched ringing
Associated Manifestations	Vertigo, drainage, pain, nausea, fullness or pressure in the ears, hearing loss, upper respiratory infection, allergies, middle ear infection, inner ear lesions, eustachian tube inflammation
Aggravating Factors	Medications, fluid in the middle ear, perforation of the tympanic membrane, position, pressure on the neck, excessive cerumen
Alleviating Factors	Discontinuing medications, position change, avoiding allergens
Setting	Work (high noise levels), outdoors
Timing	Long-standing, recent, constant, intermittent, following drug therapy, after exposure to loud noises
Nose	
Pain	Discomfort in the nose
Quality	Aching, throbbing, sharp
Associated Manifestations	Fever, chills, visual changes, swelling, sneezing, nasal discharge
Aggravating Factors	Exposure to allergens, decreased humidity indoors, cocaine use
Alleviating Factors	Use of medications (decongestant or antihistamine), removal of allergens, humidification of the environment, discontinuation of cocaine
Setting	Outdoors, dry heat, low humidity
Timing	Seasonal, in the morning
Drainage	Excessive discharge of nasal secretions
Quality	Unilateral or bilateral, amount, viscosity, color, odor
Associated Manifestations	Fever, sneezing, pain, mouth breathing, swelling, skin irritation around drainage site, itchy eyes
Aggravating Factors	Allergens, infections
Alleviating Factors	Medication, hydration, avoiding allergens
Setting	Outdoors, indoor
Timing	In the morning, seasonal, after trauma
Blockage or Congestion	Reduced ability to move air through the nose secondary to obstruction

continued

Quality	Complete, partial
Associated Manifestations	Mouth breathing, snoring, pain, disfigurement, sneezing, itchy eyes, sinus infection
Aggravating Factors	Infection, allergens, medications, objects in nose
Alleviating Factors	Mouth breathing, medications, avoidance of allergens, removal of objects
Setting	Outdoors, indoors
Timing	Following drug therapy, trauma after oral intake, after nasal surgery

Mouth and Throat

Halitosis	Unpleasant odor of the breath
Quality	Ammonia, acetone, newly mown grass or old wine odor, foul
Associated Manifestations	Gum disease, caries, systemic disease, sinusitis, pharyngitis
Aggravating factors	Poor oral hygiene, poor nutrition, poor diabetic control, alcohol intake, decreased hydration, inadequate renal function
Alleviating Factors	Good oral hygiene, control of systemic diseases, breath mints, good nutrition, adequate dental care, treatment of infection
Timing	Associated with systemic disease or acute infectious process
Pain	Discomfort in the mouth or throat
Quality	Dull, sharp, aching, burning
Associated Manifestations	Bleeding, exudate, lesions, fever
Aggravating Factors	Hot, cold, or spicy stimulation; eating; chemotherapy; dehydration; smoking; alcohol
Alleviating Factors	Medications, hydration, avoiding hot, cold, or spicy stimuli, avoiding smoking and alcohol
Setting	During meals
Timing	Continuous, intermittent, with eating, with brushing of teeth, with swallowing, with coughing
Lesions	Disruptions in the mucosa of the mouth or tongue
Quality	Tender, nontender
Associated Manifestations	Malnutrition, odor, pain, swelling, fever, stress
Aggravating Factors	Eating, drinking, spices, smoking, hot or cold stimuli, alcohol, dehydration
Alleviating Factors	Medications, avoiding eating, hydration, proper nutrition, avoiding smoking and alcohol
Timing	Associated with systemic disease, intermittent, continuous

continued

Swelling	Edema of the pharynx
Quality	Mild, moderate, severe
Associated Manifestations	Dysphagia, urticaria, wheezing, pruritus, rhinorrhea, difficulty breathing, lesions, chills, sweats, fever, sneezing, itchy eyes
Aggravating Factors	Exposure to allergens, heat
Alleviating Factors	Medications, avoiding allergens, ice, saltwater gargles
Setting	Outdoors
Timing	Following drug therapy, after eating, after an insect bite, after trauma, during or after an infectious process
PAST HEALTH HISTORY	*The various components of the past health history are linked to eyes, ears, nose, mouth, and throat pathology and eyes-, ears-, nose-, mouth-, and throat-related information.*
Medical	
Eye Specific	Glaucoma, cataracts, conjunctivitis, trachoma
Ear Specific	Acute otitis media, acute otitis externa, serous otitis media
Nose Specific	Polyps, septal deviation, sinus infection, allergic rhinitis
Mouth and Throat Specific	Tonsillitis, caries, herpes simplex virus, *Candida* infections, strep throat, frequent upper respiratory infections, tonsillar abscess
Non-Eye, Ear, Nose, Mouth, and Throat Specific	Diabetes mellitus, renal disease, atherosclerotic disease, hypertension, inflammatory processes, infections (viral or bacterial), immunosuppressive disease, dental pathology, blood dyscrasias, sexually transmitted diseases, anaphylaxis, nutritional disturbances
Surgical	Cataract extraction, lens implant, repair of detached retina, neurosurgery, enucleation of eye, optic nerve decompression, tonsillectomy, adenoidectomy, tumor removal, cosmetic surgery of head or neck, repair of septal deviation, oral surgery, tympanostomy tube placement
Medications	Antibiotics, antihistamines, decongestants, steroids, chemotherapy, immunosuppressive drugs
Allergies	Pollen: sneezing, nasal congestion, watery or itchy eyes, cough Insect stings: swelling of the throat, around the eyes Animal dander: sneezing, nasal congestion, watery or itchy eyes, cough
Injuries/Accidents	Foreign bodies; trauma to the eyes, ears, nose, mouth, throat; noxious fumes; sports injuries to the face; motor vehicle accidents

continued

Disabilities/Handicaps	Legal blindness, deafness, speech disorders
Childhood Illnesses	Frequent tonsillitis, frequent ear infections, rubella and visual sequelae (blindness)
FAMILY HEALTH HISTORY	*Eyes, ears, nose, mouth, and throat diseases that are familial are listed.*
	Hearing loss, neonatal blindness secondary to cataracts from mother contracting rubella in pregnancy
SOCIAL HISTORY	*The components of the social history are linked to eyes, ears, nose, mouth, and throat factors/pathology.*
Alcohol Use	Predisposes the patient to cancer of the oral cavity as well as decreased nutrition leading to cheilosis
Tobacco Use	Snuff or chewing tobacco predisposes the patient to mouth, lip, or throat cancer
Drug Use	Snorting cocaine may cause perforation of the nasal septum
Sexual Practice	Herpes simplex viruses I and II and gonorrhea can be contracted from oral sex
Work Environment	Exposure to toxins, chemicals, infections, excess noise, allergens
Home Environment	Exposure to loud music may cause hearing loss
Hobbies/Leisure Activities	Hunting without proper ear protection may cause hearing loss
Stress	Relationship to frequent upper respiratory infections, decreased vision or hearing
Ethnic Background	Trachoma: Middle Easterners, American Indians Nasopharyngeal cancer: Chinese Rhinoscleroma: individuals from Mediterranean countries, Southeast Asians, Indonesians, South Americans
HEALTH MAINTENANCE ACTIVITIES	*This information provides a bridge between the health maintenance activities and eyes, ears, nose, mouth, and throat functions.*
Sleep	Deprivation may be associated with frequent upper respiratory infections
Diet	Deficiencies may affect integrity of nasal and oral mucosa
Use of Safety Devices	Use of mouth guard for sports participants; goggles or face shields for sports, job, or home projects; ear protection when around loud noise to prevent damage to hearing
Health Check-Ups	Eye examination, hearing check, dental examination

EQUIPMENT

- Ophthalmoscope
- Otoscope with earpieces of different sizes and pneumatic attachment
- Nasal speculum
- Penlight
- Tuning fork, 512 Hz
- Tongue blade
- Watch
- Gauze square
- Clean gloves
- Snellen chart, Snellen E chart, Rosenbaum near-vision pocket screening card
- Vision occluder
- Transilluminator
- Cotton-tipped applicator

NURSING CHECKLIST
General Approach to Eyes, Ears, Nose, Mouth, and Throat Assessment

1. Greet the patient and explain the assessment techniques that you will be using.
2. Use a quiet room that will be free from interruptions.
3. Ensure that the light in the room provides sufficient brightness to allow adequate observation of the patient.
4. Place the patient in an upright sitting position on the examination table, or
4A. For patients who cannot tolerate the sitting position, gain access to the patient's head so that it can be rotated from side to side for assessment.
5. Visualize the underlying structures during the assessment process to allow adequate description of findings.
6. Always compare right and left eyes and ears, as well as right and left sides of the nose, sinuses, mouth, and throat.
7. Use a systematic approach that is followed consistently each time the assessment is performed.

 NURSING TIP

Prosthetic Eyes

Observe the patient to determine whether or not a prosthetic eye is worn. If so, determine the reason for the loss of the natural eye. A prosthetic eye may be needed following eye trauma or extensive disease of the eye. Ask the patient if he or she has any difficulties with the eye prosthesis.

ASSESSMENT OF THE EYE

Assessment of the eyes should be carried out in an orderly fashion, moving from the extraocular structures to the intraocular structures. The eye assessment usually includes testing of associated cranial nerves and can be performed in the following order:

1. Determination of visual acuity
2. Determination of visual fields
3. Assessment of the external eye and lacrimal apparatus
4. Evaluation of extraocular muscle function
5. Assessment of the anterior segment structures
6. Assessment of the posterior segment structures

Visual Acuity

The assessment of visual acuity (cranial nerve II) is a simple, noninvasive procedure that is carried out with the use of a Snellen chart and an occluder to cover the patient's eye. The **Snellen chart** contains letters of various sizes with standardized numbers at the end of each line of letters (see Figure 12-11A). The numbers indicate the degree of visual acuity when the patient is able to read that line of letters at a distance of 20 feet. For instance, a patient who has a visual acuity of 20/70 can read at 20 feet what a patient with 20/20 vision is able to read at 70 feet.

It is sometimes difficult to have a space of 20 feet available for the placement of the chart, but the distance can be simulated with the use of mirrors. For all vision screening, the chart should be illuminated with a diffuse light source to prevent spot lighting or glare.

Distance Vision

E 1. Ask the patient to stand or sit facing the Snellen chart at a distance of 20 feet (see Figure 12-11B).

E	**Examination**
N	**Normal Findings**
A	**Abnormal Findings**
P	**Pathophysiology**

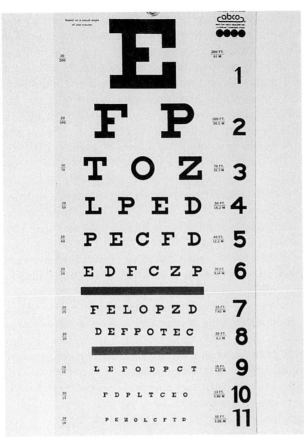

A. Snellen Vision Chart

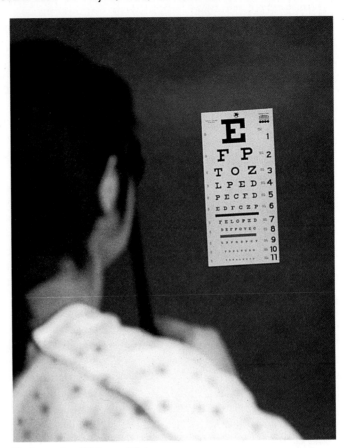

B. Assessing Distance Vision

Figure 12-11 Visual Acuity

> ### 🌺 NURSING TIP
>
> ***Use of the Snellen E Chart***
>
> When testing visual acuity of illiterate or preschool (ages 3 to 6) patients, use the Snellen E chart, which shows the letter "E" facing in different directions, rather than the standard Snellen alphabet chart. Ask the patient to identify the direction to which the "E" or "legs" of the E point.

2. If the patient normally wears glasses, ask that they be removed. Contact lenses may be left in the eyes.
3. Instruct the patient to cover the left eye with the occluder and to read as many lines on the chart as possible.
4. Note the number at the end of the last line the patient was able to read.
5. If the patient is unable to read the letters at the top of the chart, move the patient closer to the chart. Note the distance at which the patient is able to read the top line.
6. Repeat the test, occluding the right eye.
7. If the patient normally wears glasses, the test should be repeated with the patient wearing the glasses, and it should be so noted (corrected or uncorrected).

E Examination
N Normal Findings
A Abnormal Findings
P Pathophysiology

N *The patient who has a visual acuity of 20/20 is considered to have normal visual acuity.*

A The patient is unable to read the chart with an uncorrected visual acuity of 20/30 in one eye, vision in both eyes is different by two lines or more, or acuity is absent.

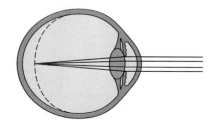

A. Normal eye
Light rays focus on the retina

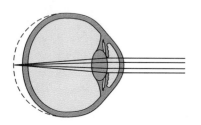

B. Myopia (nearsightedness)
Light rays focus in front
of the retina

C. Hyperopia (farsightedness)
Light rays focus behind
the retina

Figure 12-12 Eye Refraction

NURSING TIP

Blindness versus Legal Blindness

Be sure to describe visual loss correctly. For example, many more people are legally blind than totally blind, i.e., they have no light perception. The definition of legal blindness can vary from state to state, but a commonly used parameter is corrected vision that is 20/200 or worse, or peripheral vision that is less than 20°.

E   Examination
N   Normal Findings
A   Abnormal Findings
P   Pathophysiology

P   The patient may have a refractive error related to a difference in the refractive power of the cornea. Figure 12-12A illustrates how light rays focus on the retina in a normal eye. In **myopia** (nearsightedness), the axial length of the globe is longer than normal, resulting in the image not being focused directly on the retina; this condition can be changed with corrective lenses (see Figure 12-12B). If the patient is amblyopic, no corrective lenses will improve vision. **Amblyopia** is the permanent loss of visual acuity resulting from strabismus that has not been corrected in early childhood, or certain medical conditions (alcoholism, uremia, diabetes mellitus).

P   The patient may have corneal opacities that are congenital, from lesions that have scarred the cornea (e.g., herpes simplex), from trauma, or from degeneration and dystrophies.

P   Visual acuity can be decreased because of opacities of the lens caused by senile or traumatic cataracts.

P   Systemic autoimmune diseases such as inflammatory bowel disease, arthritis, or other collagen vascular diseases can be associated with inflammation of the iris (iritis), which will affect visual acuity. Iritis can also be idiopathic.

P   Inflammation of the retina caused by toxoplasmosis or by the presence of blood in the vitreous humor following hemorrhage can be responsible for decreased visual acuity.

P   Systemic diseases such as hypertension or diabetes mellitus and trauma may damage the choroid and retina, causing decreased visual acuity.

P   Visual acuity can be impaired by pathology affecting the optic nerve, such as multiple sclerosis, tumors or abscesses of the nerve itself, optic atrophy, papilledema resulting from increased intracranial pressure, optic neuritis, or neovascularization of the optic nerve with resultant bleeding and related to diabetes mellitus.

Near Vision

E   1. Use a pocket Snellen chart, Rosenbaum card, or any printed material written at an appropriate reading level.
   2. If the pocket vision card is available, have the patient sit comfortably and hold the card 14 inches from the face without moving it.
   3. Ask the patient to read the smallest line possible. If other printed material is used, you will be able to gain only a general understanding of the patient's near vision.

N   *Until the patient is in the late 30s to the late 40s, reading is generally possible at a distance of 14 inches.*

A   A patient in this age range who cannot read at 14 inches is considered presbyopic. Younger persons may have difficulty seeing up close because they have **hyperopia**, or farsightedness (see Figure 12-12C).

P   The normal aging process causes the lens to harden (nuclear sclerosis), decreasing its ability to change shape and therefore focus on near objects.

Color Vision

E   For routine testing of color vision, test the patient's ability to identify primary colors found on the Snellen chart or in the examining room. For more specific testing, ask the patient to view Ishihara plates and identify the numerals on them.

N   *The patient who is able to identify all six screening Ishihara plates correctly has normal color vision.*

A   The color vision defect is designated as red/green, blue/yellow, or complete when the patient sees only shades of gray.

P   Defects in color vision can result from diseases of the optic nerve, macular degeneration, pathology of the fovea centralis, nutritional deficiency, or heredity.

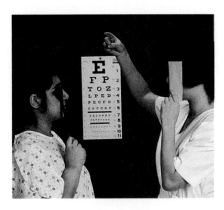

Figure 12-13 Testing Visual Fields by Confrontation

🌺 NURSING TIP

Visual Field Assessment

Although this test can detect gross hemianopsia (blindness in one-half of the visual fields in one or both eyes), quadrantanopsia (blindness in one-fourth of the visual fields of one or both eyes), or large scotomas (areas of depressed vision within the visual field), more precise evaluation can be accomplished only by an ophthalmologist.

Visual Fields

The confrontation technique is used to test visual fields of each eye (CN II). The visual field of each eye is divided into quadrants, and a stimulus is presented in each quadrant.

E
1. Sit or stand approximately 2 to 3 feet opposite the patient, with your eyes at the same level as the patient's (see Figure 12-13).
2. Have the patient cover the right eye with the right hand or an occluder.
3. Cover your left eye in the same manner.
4. Have the patient look at your uncovered eye with his or her uncovered eye.
5. Hold your free hand at arm's length equidistant from you and the patient and move it or a held object such as a pen into your and the patient's field of vision from nasal, temporal, superior, inferior, and oblique angles.
6. Ask the patient to say "now" when your hand is seen moving into the field of vision. Use your own visual fields as the control for comparison to the patient's.
7. Repeat the procedure for the other eye.

N *The patient is able to see the stimulus at about 90° temporally, 60° nasally, 50° superiorly, and 70° inferiorly.*

A If the patient is unable to identify movement that you perceive, a defect in the visual field is presumed. The portion of the visual field loss should be noted (see Figure 12-14).

P Defects in the patient's visual field can be associated with tumors or strokes or neurological diseases such as glaucoma or retinal detachment.

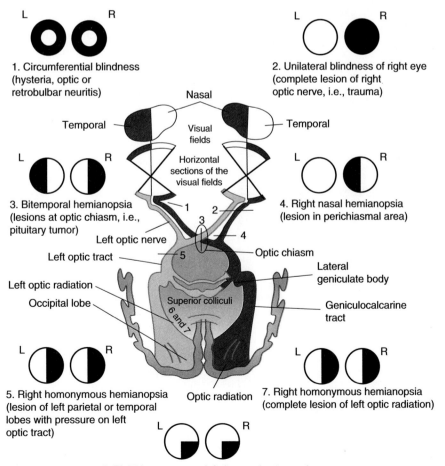

1. Circumferential blindness (hysteria, optic or retrobulbar neuritis)

2. Unilateral blindness of right eye (complete lesion of right optic nerve, i.e., trauma)

3. Bitemporal hemianopsia (lesions at optic chiasm, i.e., pituitary tumor)

4. Right nasal hemianopsia (lesion in perichiasmal area)

5. Right homonymous hemianopsia (lesion of left parietal or temporal lobes with pressure on left optic tract)

6. Right homonymous inferior quadrantanopsia (partial lesion of left optic radiations)

7. Right homonymous hemianopsia (complete lesion of left optic radiation)

Labels within figure: Nasal, Temporal, Visual fields, Horizontal sections of the visual fields, Left optic nerve, Left optic tract, Left optic radiation, Occipital lobe, Superior colliculi, Optic radiation, Optic chiasm, Lateral geniculate body, Geniculocalcarine tract

Figure 12-14 Visual Field Defects

External Eye and Lacrimal Apparatus

The assessment of the external eye includes the eyelids and the lacrimal apparatus. Pathology of the eyelids is among the most common eye complaints of patients seeing a health care provider.

Eyelids

E
1. Ask the patient to sit facing you.
2. Observe the patient's eyelids for drooping, infection, tumors, or other abnormalities.
3. Note the distribution of the eyelashes and eyebrows.
4. Instruct the patient to focus on an object or a finger held about 10 to 12 inches away and slightly above eye level.
5. Move the object or finger slowly downward and observe for a white space of sclera between the upper lid and the limbus.
6. Observe the blinking of the eyes.
7. Ask the patient to elevate the eyelids.

N *The eyelids should appear symmetrical with no drooping, infections, or tumors of the lids. Eyelids of Asians normally slant upward. When the eyes are focused in a normal frontal gaze, the lids should cover the upper portion of the iris. The patient can raise both eyelids symmetrically (CN III). Slight **ptosis**, or drooping of the lid, can be normal. When the eye is closed, no portion of the cornea should be exposed. Normal lid margins are smooth with the lashes evenly distributed and sweeping upward from the upper lids and downward from the lower lids. Eyebrows are present bilaterally and are symmetrical and without lesions or scaling.*

A The patient has either unilateral or bilateral, constant or intermittent ptosis of the lid (see Figure 12-15). If part of the pupil is occluded, there may be wrinkling of the forehead above the affected eye in an attempt to compensate by using the frontalis muscle to lift the lid.

P Ptosis can be either congenital or acquired. In congenital ptosis there is failure of the levator muscle to develop. This condition may be associated with pathology of the superior rectus muscle as well. If the ptosis is acquired, it is related to one of three factors:
  1. Mechanical: heavy lids from lesions, adipose tissue, swelling, or edema
  2. Myogenic: muscular diseases such as myasthenia gravis or multiple sclerosis
  3. Neurogenic: paralysis from damage or interruption of the neural pathways.

A An area of white sclera appears between the upper lid and the limbus, widening as the object is moved downward.

P This condition is called lid lag and may indicate the presence of thyrotoxicosis or increased circulating levels of free thyroxine or triiodothyronine.

A The patient is unable to bring about complete lid closure. This is generally a unilateral condition.

P This condition is referred to as **lagophthalmos** and can be associated with Bell's palsy, stroke, trauma, or **ectropion** (everted eyelid).

A During inspection of the lids, a disparity of the palpebral fissure is noted with apparent lid retraction, indicating a protrusion of the globe. This condition may be unilateral or bilateral (see Figure 12-16).

P This abnormality is **exophthalmos** (or proptosis) and can be present unilaterally in orbital tumors, thyroid disease, trauma, or inflammation. Bilateral exophthalmos is related to thyroid disease.

A There is apparent disparity in the size of the globe, manifested by a narrowing of the palpebral fissure.

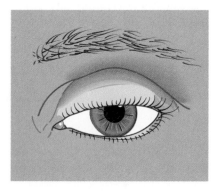

Figure 12-15 Ptosis

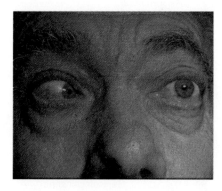

Figure 12-16 Exophthalmos
© Phototake/CNRI/PNI

E	Examination
N	Normal Findings
A	Abnormal Findings
P	Pathophysiology

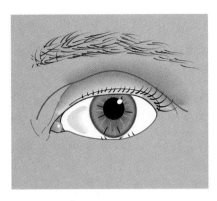

Figure 12-17   Entropion

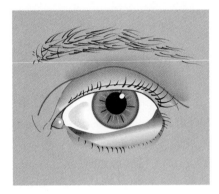

Figure 12-18   Ectropion

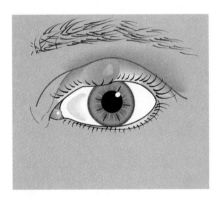

Figure 12-19   Hordeolum

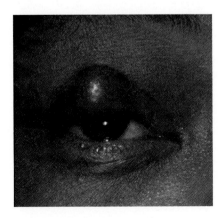

Figure 12-20   Chalazion
© *Phototake/Margaret Cubberly/PNI*

P **Enophthalmos** is a backward displacement of the globe in the orbit, generally caused by orbital blowout fracture due to trauma. When this occurs, the orbital contents herniate through the fracture site.

A The turning inward, or inversion, of the lower lid is referred to as **entropion** and can cause severe discomfort to the patient as the eyelashes abrade the cornea (trichiasis) (see Figure 12-17). If left untreated, it can cause inflammation, corneal scarring, and eventual ulceration.

P Entropion is caused by spasms or advancing age (senile). In senile entropion, there is a loss of muscle tone, which causes the lid to fold inward.

A The turning outward, or eversion, of the lower lid is referred to as ectropion and may be unilateral or bilateral (see Figure 12-18). With ectropion, the lower lids appear to be sagging outward.

P The normal aging process can cause the muscles to lose their tone and relax, or they may be affected by Bell's palsy.

A The patient exhibits excessive blinking that may or may not be accompanied by increased tearing and pain.

P The causes of excessive blinking are:
   1. Voluntary: irritation to the cornea or the conjunctiva, or stress and anxiety (usually disappears when stimulus is removed)
   2. Involuntary: tonic spasms of the orbicularis oculi muscle, called blepharospasm; often seen in elderly individuals as well as in patients with CN VII lesions, irritation of the eye, fatigue, and stress.

A The lids are black and blue, bluish, yellow, or red, depending on race and skin color.

P Color changes in the lids can result from the following:
   1. Redness: generalized redness is nonspecific; however, redness in the nasal half of the lid may indicate frontal sinusitis. Redness adjacent to the lower lid can indicate disease of the lacrimal sac or nasolacrimal duct, such as dacryocystitis; and redness in the temporal portion of the lid can result from dacryoadenitis, an inflammation of the lacrimal gland.
   2. Bluish: cyanosis can result from orbital vein thrombosis, orbital tumors, or aneurysms in the orbit.
   3. Black and blue: ecchymosis is caused by bleeding into the surrounding tissues following trauma (black eye).

A Swelling or edema is noted in the eyelid.

P Swelling or edema may be noted in nonocular conditions such as inflammation associated with allergies, systemic diseases, medications that contribute to swelling from fluid overload, trichinosis, early myxedema, thyrotoxicosis, or contact dermatitis.

A There is an acute localized inflammation, tenderness, and redness, with the patient complaining of pain in the infected area (refer to Figure 12-19). This is called a **hordeolum**.

P *Staphylococcus* is generally the infecting organism that causes a hordeolum. There are two types of hordeolum:
   1. Internal: affects the meibomian glands, is usually large, and can point either to the skin or to the conjunctival side of the lid.
   2. External: often called a "sty," an infection of a sebaceous gland that usually points to the skin side of the lid.
Infections of the glands of the eyelid can be caused by improper removal of makeup, dry eyes, or seborrhea. There may be some connection between a hordeolum and increased handling of the lids in activities such as inserting and removing contact lenses.

A There is a chronic inflammation of the meibomian gland in either the upper or the lower lid. It generally forms over several weeks and, in many cases, points toward the conjunctival side of the lid (see Figure 12-20). There is no redness or tenderness.

P This inflammation is referred to as a **chalazion** and its cause is unknown.

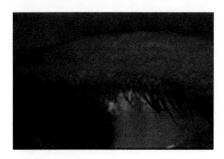

Figure 12-21 Blepharitis
© *Phototake/Barts Medical Library/PNI*
Credit Phototake

A The lids are inflamed bilaterally and are red rimmed, with scales clinging to both the upper and the lower lids. The patient complains of itching and burning along the lid margins (refer to Figure 12-21). There may also be some loss of the eyelashes.

P This is chronic marginal **blepharitis**, which may be either staphylococcal or seborrheic. Often a patient has both types simultaneously. If the patient has seborrheic infections elsewhere (scalp or eyebrows), it is more likely that the blepharitis is of the seborrheic type.

A Raised, yellow, nonpainful plaques are present on upper and lower lids near the inner canthus.

P These lesions are **xanthelasma**, a form of xanthoma frequently associated with hypercholesterolemia.

✿ ASK YOURSELF

The Patient with Suspected Physical Abuse

How would you react to a patient who has swollen and discolored eyelids that you believe to be the result of physical abuse? What would be an appropriate verbal response? What resources are available in your community or institution to support and assist victims of physical abuse?

Lacrimal Apparatus

Inspection

E 1. Have the patient sit facing you.
  2. Identify the area of the lacrimal gland. Note any swelling or enlargement of the gland or elevation of the eyelid. Note any enlargement, swelling, redness, increased tearing, or exudate in the area of the lacrimal sac at the inner canthus.
  3. Compare to the other eye in order to determine whether there is unilateral or bilateral involvement.

N *There should be no enlargement, swelling, or redness, no large amount of exudate, and minimal tearing.*

A There is inflammation and swelling in the upper lateral aspect of one or both eyes and the patient complains of pain in the affected area.

P Acute inflammation of the lacrimal gland is called **dacryoadenitis** and does not occur commonly. Dacryoadenitis may result from trauma or may be found in association with measles, mumps, and mononucleosis.

A There is inflammation and painful swelling beside the nose and near the inner canthus and possibly extending to the eyelid.

P **Dacryocystitis** is caused by inflammatory or neoplastic obstruction of the lacrimal duct.

Palpation

E 1. To assess the lacrimal sac for obstruction, don gloves.
  2. Gently press the index finger near the inner canthus, just inside the rim of the bony orbit of the eye.
  3. Note any discharge from the punctum.

N *There should not be excessive tearing or discharge from the punctum.*

A Mucopurulent discharge is noted.

P Obstruction anywhere along the system from the lacrimal sac to the point at which the ducts empty below the inferior nasal turbinate can cause mucopurulent discharge.

A There is an overflowing of tears from the eye.

P This condition is epiphora, which is caused by obstruction of the lacrimal duct.

E	**Examination**
N	**Normal Findings**
A	**Abnormal Findings**
P	**Pathophysiology**

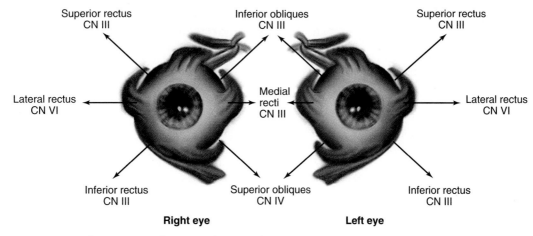

Superior rectus
CN III

Inferior obliques
CN III

Superior rectus
CN III

Lateral rectus
CN VI

Medial recti
CN III

Lateral rectus
CN VI

Inferior rectus
CN III

Superior obliques
CN IV

Inferior rectus
CN III

Right eye   **Left eye**

Figure 12-22 Direction of Movement of Extraocular Muscles

> ### 🌸 NURSING TIP
>
> ***Extraocular Muscles***
>
> One method of remembering names of extraocular muscles and associated cranial nerves is: LR (lateral rectus) VI; SO (superior oblique) IV; all others (superior, inferior, and medial rectus and inferior oblique) are III.

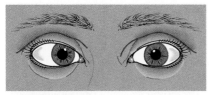

A. Right esotropia

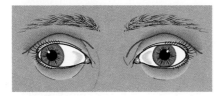

B. Right exotropia

Figure 12-23 Asymmetrical Corneal Light Reflex

E	**Examination**
N	**Normal Findings**
A	**Abnormal Findings**
P	**Pathophysiology**

Extraocular Muscle Function

Six extraocular muscles control the movement of each eye in relation to three axes: vertical, horizontal, and oblique (see Figure 12-22). Assessing extraocular function is carried out by observing corneal light reflex or alignment, using the cover/uncover test, and by testing the six cardinal fields of gaze (cranial nerves III, IV, and VI).

Corneal Light Reflex (Hirschberg Test)

E 1. Instruct the patient to look straight ahead.
  2. Focus a penlight on the corneas from a distance of 12 to 15 inches away at the midline.
  3. Observe the location of reflected light on the cornea.

N *The reflected light (light reflex) should be seen symmetrically in the center of each cornea.*

A There is a discrepancy in the placement of one of the light reflections.

P Asymmetrical corneal light reflexes indicate an extraocular muscle imbalance that may be related to a variety of causes, depending on the patient's age and medical condition: neurological, such as myasthenia gravis, multiple sclerosis, stroke, neuropathies of diabetes mellitus; uncorrected childhood strabismus (misalignment); trauma; or hypertension. The condition of one eye constantly being deviated is called **strabismus**, or tropia: **esotropia** is an inward turning of the eye; **exotropia** is an outward turning of the eye (see Figure 12-23).

Cover/Uncover Test

E 1. Ask the patient to look straight ahead and to focus on an object in the distance.
  2. Place an occluder over the left eye for several seconds and observe for movement in the uncovered right eye.
  3. As the occluder is removed, observe the covered eye for movement.
  4. Repeat the procedure with the same eye, having the patient focus on an object held close to the eye.
  5. Repeat on the other side.

N *If the eyes are in alignment, there will be no movement of either eye.*

A If the uncovered eye shifts position as the other eye is covered, or if the covered eye shifts position as it is uncovered, a **phoria**, or latent misalignment of an eye, exists.

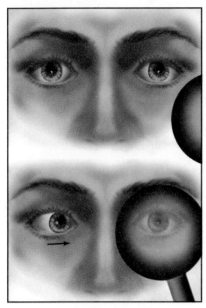

Right uncovered eye is weaker.
(Right Esophoria)

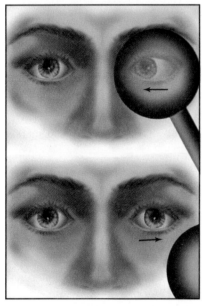

Left covered eye is weaker.
(Left Exophoria)

Figure 12-24 Cover/Uncover Test

E	Examination
N	Normal Findings
A	Abnormal Findings
P	Pathophysiology

P This condition is a mild weakness elicited by the cover/uncover test and has two forms: **esophoria**, nasal or inward drift, and **exophoria**, a temporal or outward drift (see Figure 12-24).

Cardinal Fields of Gaze (Extraocular Muscle Movements)

E 1. Place the patient in a sitting position facing you.
  2. Place the nondominant hand just under the patient's chin or on top of the head as a reminder to hold the head still.
  3. Ask the patient to follow an object (finger, pencil, or penlight) with the eyes.
  4. Move the object through the six fields of gaze (see Figure 12-25) in a smooth and steady manner, pausing at each extreme position to detect any **nystagmus**, or involuntary movement, and returning to the center after each field is tested.
  5. Note the patient's ability to move the eyes in each direction.
  6. Move the object forward to about 5 inches in front of the patient's nose at the midline.
  7. Observe for convergence of gaze.

N *Both eyes should move smoothly and symmetrically in each of the six fields of gaze and converge on the held object as it moves toward the nose. A few beats of nystagmus with extreme lateral gaze can be normal.*

A There is a lack of symmetrical eye movement in a particular direction.

P Inability to move the eye in a given direction indicates a weakness in the muscle responsible for moving the eye in that direction.

A Abnormal eye movements consist of failure of an eye to move outward (CN VI), inability of the eye to move downward when deviated inward (CN IV), or other defects in movement (CN III).

P Traumatic ophthalmoplegia may be caused by fracture of the orbit near the foramen magnum, causing damage to the extraocular muscles or CN II, III, IV, and VI. Basilar skull fractures that involve the cavernous sinus may also cause extraocular muscle palsy.

P Vitamin deficiency, especially thiamine (which may occur in chronic alcoholism), may cause extraocular muscle palsy and nystagmus. Usually CN VI is affected.

P Herpes zoster, syphilis, scarlet fever, whooping cough, or botulism are infections that may affect CN III, IV, and VI, causing extraocular muscle palsy.

A Ophthalmoplegia is paralysis of one or more of the optic muscles.

P Increased intracranial pressure may cause strangulation of CN VI. CN VI palsy occurs late after the onset of increased intracranial pressure.

P Parasellar meningiomas or tumors in the sphenoid sinus may impinge on the wall of the cavernous sinus and involve one or more cranial nerves (CN III, IV, and VI).

A Vertical gaze is a paralysis of upward gaze and it is abnormal.

P Destruction at the area of the midbrain-diencephalic junction or the medial longitudinal fasciculus, or tumors of the pineal gland that press on the brain stem at the superior colliculus can cause a vertical gaze deviation.

A Paralysis of horizontal gaze is abnormal.

P Damage to the motor areas of the cerebral cortex causes the loss of the ability of both eyes to look to the contralateral side, so the eyes tend to deviate toward the side of the lesion.

A With internuclear ophthalmoplegia, the eyes are unable to look medially, but convergence may be maintained because the pathway for convergence is different from that for conjugate gaze.

P The medial rectus muscle is involved, so the eyes are unable to look medially. Internuclear ophthalmoplegia may be caused by demyelinization due to multiple sclerosis.

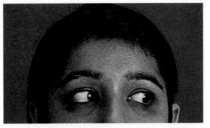

A. Eyes Midline

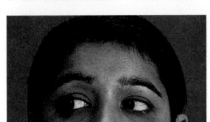

B. Left Lateral Gaze

C. Left Lateral Inferior Gaze

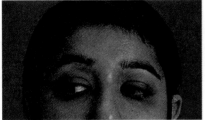

D. Right Lateral Inferior Gaze

E. Right Lateral Gaze

F. Right Lateral Superior Gaze

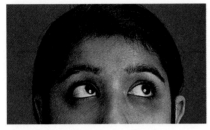

G. Left Lateral Superior Gaze

Figure 12-25 Cardinal Fields of Gaze

A If one eye deviates down and the other eye deviates up, it is called skew deviation.

P Cerebellar disease or a lesion in the pons on the same side as the eye that is deviated down may cause skew deviation.

A There is a rhythmic, beating, involuntary oscillation of the eyes as the object is held at points away from the midline. Movement is usually lateral, vertical, or rotary. Nystagmus can be jerky, with fast and slow components, or rhythmic, similar to the pendulum of a clock.

P Nystagmus may be caused by a lesion in the brain stem, cerebellum, vestibular system, or along the visual pathways in the cerebral hemispheres.

Anterior Segment Structures

Conjunctiva

To assess the bulbar conjunctiva:

E 1. Separate the lid margins with the fingers.
2. Have the patient look up, down, and to the right and left.
3. Inspect the surface of the bulbar conjunctiva for color, redness, swelling, exudate, or foreign bodies. Note whether **injection** or redness is around the cornea, foreign bodies, or toward the periphery.
4. With the thumb, gently pull the lower lid toward the cheek and inspect the surface of the bulbar conjunctiva for color, inflammation, edema, lesions, or foreign bodies.

N *The bulbar conjunctiva is transparent with small blood vessels visible in it. It should appear white except for a few small blood vessels, which are normal. No swelling, injection, exudate, foreign bodies, or lesions are noted.*

A/P Refer to palpebral conjunctiva.

The palpebral conjunctiva is examined only when there is a concern about its condition. To examine the palpebral conjunctiva of the upper lid:

E 1. Explain the procedure to the patient to alleviate the fear of pain or damage to the eye.
2. Don gloves. Have the patient look down to relax the levator muscle (see Figure 12-26A).
3. Gently pull the eyelashes downward and place a sterile, cotton-tipped applicator about 1 cm above the lid margin.
4. Gently exert downward pressure on the applicator while pulling the eyelashes upward to evert the lid (see Figure 12-26B).

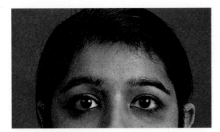

A. Patient Position

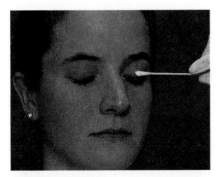

B. Everting the Eyelid

Figure 12-26 Assessing Palpebral Conjunctiva

5. Inspect the palpebral conjunctiva for injection, swelling or **chemosis**, exudate, and foreign bodies.

6. Return the lid to its normal position by instructing the patient to look up and then pulling the eyelid outward and removing the cotton-tipped applicator. Ask the patient to blink.

N *The palpebral conjunctiva should appear pink and moist. It is without swelling, lesions, injection, exudate, or foreign bodies.*

A Bilateral injected conjunctiva with purulent, sticky discharge and lid edema are noted.

P These findings usually indicate the presence of bacterial conjunctivitis.

A Unilateral injection with moderate pain and without purulent discharge is noted but the patient complains of increased lacrimation.

P These symptoms indicate that the conjunctivitis is viral. Viral conjunctivitis is most commonly due to adenovirus, which may become epidemic. Herpes simplex may also be a viral cause of conjunctivitis. A preauricular node is often felt on palpation.

A Mild inflammation and injection and follicles of palpebral conjunctiva are present with scant discharge. The patient reports an itching and burning sensation as well as increased lacrimation.

P This is allergic conjunctivitis and is often associated with hay fever.

A A yellow nodule is noted on the nasal side of the bulbar conjunctiva adjacent to the cornea. It may be on the temporal side as well. This lesion is painless unless it becomes inflamed.

P This lesion is called a **pinguecula**. It is a nodular degeneration of the conjunctiva and is thought to be a result of increased exposure to ultraviolet light.

A A unilateral or bilateral triangle-shaped encroachment onto the conjunctiva is abnormal (see Figure 12-27). This lesion always occurs nasally and remains painless unless it becomes ulcerated. If the lesion covers the cornea, loss of vision may occur.

P This lesion is called a **pterygium** and is also caused by excessive ultraviolet light exposure.

A The patient exhibits a sudden onset of a painless, bright-red appearance on the bulbar conjunctiva.

P This is a subconjunctival hemorrhage and may result from the pressure exerted during coughing, sneezing, or a Valsalva maneuver. It can also be attributed to anticoagulant medications or uncontrolled hypertension.

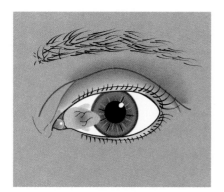

Figure 12-27 Pterygium

Sclera

E While assessing the conjunctiva, inspect the sclera for color, exudates, lesions, and foreign bodies.

N *In light-skinned individuals, the sclera should be white with some small, superficial vessels and without exudate, lesions, or foreign bodies. In dark-skinned individuals, the sclera may have tiny brown patches of melanin or a grayish blue or "muddy" color.*

A The color of the sclera is uniformly yellow.

P This condition is known as jaundice or scleral icterus and is due to coloring of the sclera with bilirubin, which infiltrates all tissues of the body. This is an early manifestation of systemic conditions such as hepatitis, sickle cell disease, gallstones, and physiological jaundice of the newborn.

A The sclera is blue.

P This finding is a distinctive feature of osteogenesis imperfecta and is due to the thinning of the sclera, which allows the choroid to show through.

Cornea

E **1.** Stand in front of the patient.
2. Shine a penlight directly on the cornea.

E **Examination**
N **Normal Findings**
A **Abnormal Findings**
P **Pathophysiology**

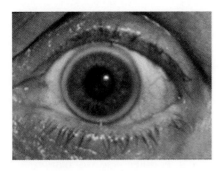

Figure 12-28 Arcus Senilis
© Phototake/Barts Medical Library/PNI

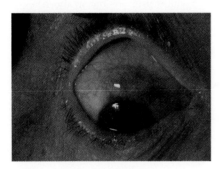

Figure 12-29 Glaucoma
© Phototake/Barts Medical Library/PNI

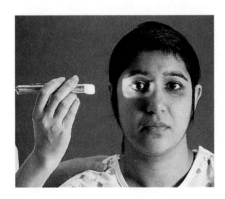

Figure 12-30 Examining the Anterior Chamber

3. Move the light laterally and view the cornea from that angle, noting color, discharge, and lesions.

N *The corneal surface should be moist and shiny, with no discharge, cloudiness, opacities, or irregularities.*

A A grayish, well-circumscribed ulcerated area on the cornea is abnormal.

P The most common cause of this is a corneal ulceration resulting from a bacterial invasion.

A A treelike configuration on the corneal surface is identified. The patient complains of mild discomfort, photophobia, and in some cases blurred vision (depending on the location of the lesions).

P This type of ulceration is caused by the herpes simplex virus. The patient usually has a history of having had a cold sore somewhere on the face.

A There is a hazy gray ring about 2 mm in width just inside the limbus (see Figure 12-28).

P This common finding is **arcus senilis**, a bilateral, benign degeneration of the peripheral cornea. It can be found at any age but is most common in older individuals. If found in a young person, it may be associated with hypercholesterolemia.

A A steamy or cloudy cornea is abnormal (see Figure 12-29). The patient also has ocular pain.

P Glaucoma is caused by increased intraocular pressure. Refer to anterior chamber assessment.

Anterior Chamber

The anterior chamber is that compartment of the eye found between the cornea and the iris. The space between the flat plane of the iris and the periphery of the cornea must be adequate to allow drainage of aqueous fluid out of the eye. If this angle is too narrow, drainage is inadequate, the pressure of the aqueous fluid in the anterior chamber increases, and **glaucoma** develops. If intraocular fluid pressure remains high, optic nerve damage and visual field loss occur.

To differentiate a normal from a narrowed angle:

E **1.** Face the patient and shine a light obliquely through the anterior chamber from the lateral side toward the nasal side (see Figure 12-30).

2. Observe the distribution of light in the anterior chamber (see Figure 12-31).

3. Repeat the procedure with the other eye.

N *In a normal eye, the entire iris will be illuminated.*

E	**Examination**
N	**Normal Findings**
A	**Abnormal Findings**
P	**Pathophysiology**

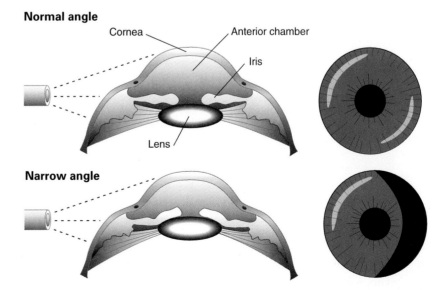

Normal angle

Cornea — Anterior chamber — Iris — Lens

Narrow angle

Figure 12-31 Evaluating the Anterior Chamber

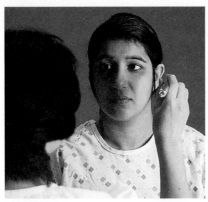

A. Starting Position with Penlight to Side of Pupil

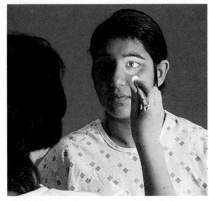

B. Move Penlight Directly in Front of Pupil

Figure 12-32 Pupil Assessment

A   The eye has a narrow angle, with the decreased space between the iris and the cornea appearing as a crescent-shaped shadow on the far portion of the iris.

P   The narrow angle is an anatomic variant that can predispose an individual to the development of angle closure glaucoma. As aging progresses, the lens thickens, which may cause even further narrowing of the angle.

Iris

E   With the penlight, inspect the iris for color, nodules, and vascularity.

N   *Normally, the color is evenly distributed over the iris, although there can be a mosaic variant. It is normally smooth and without apparent vascularity.*

A   There is a heavily pigmented, slightly elevated area visible in the iris.

P   This lesion can be a benign iris nevus or a malignant melanoma. An iris nevus is much more common than melanoma.

A   The inferior portion of the iris is obscured by blood.

P   This is a **hyphema** and is caused by bleeding from vessels in the iris as a result of direct trauma to the globe. It can also occur as a result of eye surgery.

A   An absent wedge portion of the iris is abnormal.

P   The shape of the iris changes after surgical removal of a cataract; the pupil may also have an irregular shape.

Pupil

E   1. Stand in front of the patient in a darkened room.
2. Note the shape and size of the pupils in millimeters.
3. Move a penlight from the side to the front of one eye without allowing the light to shine on the other eye (see Figure 12-32).
4. Observe the pupillary reaction in that eye. This is the direct light reflex. Note the size of the pupil receiving light stimulus and the speed of pupillary response to light.
5. Repeat in the other eye.
6. Move the penlight in front of one eye and observe the other eye for pupillary constriction. This is the consensual light reflex.
7. Repeat the procedure on the other eye.
8. Instruct the patient to shift the gaze to a distant object for 30 seconds.
9. Instruct the patient to then look at your finger or an object held in your hand about 10 cm from the patient.
10. Note the reaction and size of the pupils. **Accommodation** occurs when pupils constrict and converge to focus on objects at close range.

N   *The pupils should be deep black, round, and of equal diameter, ranging from 2 to 6 mm. Pupils should constrict briskly to direct and consensual light and to accommodation (CN III). Small differences in pupil size (**anisocoria**) may be normal in some people.*

A   The pupil that constricts to less than 2 mm in diameter is termed miotic. The pupil that dilates to more than 6 mm in diameter is termed mydriatic.

P   Abnormal pupillary size can be caused by medications such as sympathomimetics or parasympathomimetics, iritis, or disorders such as CN III paralysis, which can occur as a result of a carotid artery aneurysm. These abnormalities may also be due to nerve damage or trauma (see Table 12-1 for further pathologies).

A   The pupil has an irregular shape.

P   This is a common finding associated with the surgical removal of cataracts and iridectomy.

🌿 NURSING TIP

Assessment of the Pupils

The beginning examiner should focus the beam of light a total of four times, twice in each eye, to assess direct light reflex and to assess consensual light reflex. This will ensure accuracy of examination.

E   Examination

N   Normal Findings

A   Abnormal Findings

P   Pathophysiology

Table 12-1   Pupil Abnormalities

A.

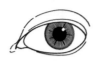

A: The size of pupils is unequal but both pupils react to light and accommodation.
P: Inequality of pupillary size is called **anisocoria** and may be congenital or due to inflammation of ocular tissue or disturbances of neurophthalmic pathways.

B.

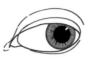

A: A fixed and dilated pupil is observed on one side. The abnormal pupil does not react to direct or consensual light stimulation and does not accommodate. Ptosis and lateral downward deviation may also be noted.
P: This abnormality is caused by **oculomotor nerve damage** due to head trauma and increased intracranial pressure. Atropine-like agents applied topically may cause an even more widely fixed and dilated pupil.

C.

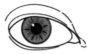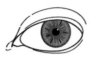

A: A unilateral, small, regularly shaped pupil is observed. Both pupils react directly and consensually and accommodate. Ptosis and diminished or absent sweating on the affected side may also be noted.
P: This finding is **Horner's syndrome,** which is caused by a lesion of the sympathetic nerve pathway.

D.

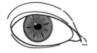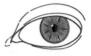

A: Pupils are bilaterally small and irregularly shaped. They react to accommodation but sluggishly or not at all to light.
P: These abnormalities are **Argyll Robertson** pupils and are usually caused by central lesions of neurosyphilis. Other causes include encephalitis, drugs, diabetes, brain tumors, and alcoholism.

E.

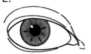

A: A unilateral, large, regularly shaped pupil is noted. The affected pupil's reaction to light and accommodation is sluggish or absent. The patient may report blurred vision because of the slow accommodation. You may observe diminished ankle and knee deep-tendon reflexes.
P: This abnormality, a tonic or **Adie's** pupil, is due to impaired sympathetic nerve supply.

F.

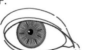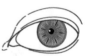

A: Both pupils are **small, fixed,** regularly shaped, and do not react to light or accommodation.
P: This abnormality may be caused by opiate ingestion, topical application of miotic drops, or lesions in the brain.

A: Pupils are small, equal, and reactive.
P: Diencephalic injury or metabolic coma may cause these findings.

G.

A: Both pupils are **dilated** and **fixed,** and do not react to light or accomodation.
P: Severe head trauma, brain stem infarction, cardiopulmonary arrest (after **4** to **6** min).

H.   Blind eye

Light

A: Light shone into a blind eye (amaurotic pupil) will cause no reaction (direct or consensual) in either pupil. If light is shone in the other eye, and CN III is intact, both pupils should constrict.
P: Due to a lesion in the retina or the optic nerve, the light stimulus shown in the amaurotic pupil is unable to pass along the sensory pathway; therefore, the oculomotor response in both eyes is absent.

A When the direct light reflex is defective, the pupil dilates in response to light, but consensual reaction is appropriate. This is called a Marcus Gunn pupil.

P Optic nerve damage in the optic chiasm, such as in trauma, results in destruction of the afferent pathways of the pupillary light reflex (deafferentated pupil).

A The hippus phenomenon occurs after the pupil has been stimulated by direct light. Light causes the pupil to constrict, but then the pupil appears to rhythmically vacillate in size from a larger to a smaller diameter.

P Hippus may be caused by a lesion in the midbrain.

A The presence of midposition, round, regular, and fixed (5 to 6 mm) pupils that may show hippus is abnormal.

P These signs usually indicate midbrain damage that interrupts the light reflex but may leave accommodation intact.

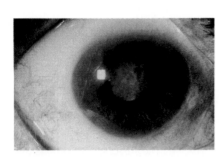

Figure 12-33 Cataract *Courtesy of the National Eye Institute*

Lens

E 1. Stand in front of the patient.

2. Shine a penlight directly on the pupil. The lens is behind the pupil.

3. Note the color.

N *The lens is transparent in color.*

A One or more of the pupils are not deep black.

P In an adult, a pearly gray appearance of one or both pupils may indicate an opacity (cloudiness) in the lens (**cataract**) (refer to Figure 12-33).

P A senile cataract is the most common type. Progressively blurred distance vision is the main symptom, although near vision may be improved because of greater convexity of the lens.

P A unilateral cataract may occur soon after eye injury caused by a foreign body. Along with the lens opacity, there may be intraocular hemorrhage or aqueous or vitreous humor leaking from the globe. The patient reports an immediate blurring of vision.

P Bilateral cataracts found in infants or young children are congenital cataracts. These cataracts are probably genetically determined, although maternal rubella in the first trimester can also be responsible.

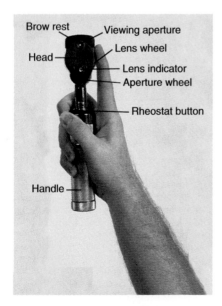

Brow rest — Viewing aperture
Head — Lens wheel
— Lens indicator
— Aperture wheel
— Rheostat button
Handle —

Figure 12-34 Ophthalmoscope

Posterior Segment Structures

The funduscopic assessment (CN II) requires the use of a direct ophthalmoscope to assess the structures in the posterior segment of the eye (see Figure 12-34). The ophthalmoscope consists of two parts: the head and the handle. To activate the light source in the head, depress the rheostat button and move it as far as possible. Move the aperture wheel to produce the largest beam of light that can be visualized by focusing the beam of light on the palm of the hand. The larger beam is preferred when assessing an average-sized pupil, and the smaller beam makes assessment of a smaller pupil easier. The diopter wheel allows you to choose lenses of varying power for different parts of the assessment. These lenses are marked with red and black numbers, signifying different focal lengths. The 0 lens sits between the red- and black-numbered lenses and has no correction. In some ophthalmoscopes, there is no color designation (red or black) and the lens power is signified by + or − signs in front of the numbers. A + sign is equivalent to black and focuses closer to the ophthalmoscope; a − sign is equivalent to red and focuses further from the instrument. These lenses compensate for the refractive error of both the patient and the nurse.

Retinal Structures

In a darkened room, ask the patient to remove eyeglasses; contact lenses may be left in place.

E 1. Instruct the patient to look at a distant object across the room. This will help to dilate the eyes.
   2. Set the ophthalmoscope on the 0 lens and hold it in front of your right eye.
   3. From a distance of 8 to 12 inches from the patient and about 15° to the lateral side, shine the light into the patient's right pupil, eliciting a light reflection from the retina; this is called the red reflex (see Figure 12-35A).
   4. While maintaining the red reflex in view, move closer to the patient and move the diopter wheel from 0 to the + or black numbers in order to focus on the anterior ocular structures.
   5. For optimum visualization, keep the ophthalmoscope within an inch of the patient's eye (see Figure 12-35B).
   6. At this point, move the diopter wheel from the + or black numbers, through 0, and into the − or red numbers in order to focus on structures progressively more posterior.
   7. Focus on the optic disc at the nasal side of the retina by following any retinal vessels centrally (see Figure 12-36).
   8. You may need to reverse direction along the vessel if the disc does not appear.
   9. Observe the retina for color and lesions, the retinal vessels for configuration and characteristics of their crossing, and the optic disc for color, shape, size, margins, and comparison of cup-to-disc ratio.
   10. Describe the size, position, and location of any abnormality. Use the diameter of the disc (DD) as a guide to describe the distance of the abnormality from the optic disc. Use the optic disc as a clock face as a reference point to describe the location of the abnormality. Describe the size of the abnormality in relation to the size of the optic disc.
   11. Repeat on the left eye.

N *Refer to Table 12-2. The red reflex is present. The optic disc is pinkish orange in color, with a yellow-white excavated center known as the physiologic cup (see Figure 12-36). The ratio of the cup diameter to that of the entire disc is 1:3. The border of the disc may range from a sharp, round demarcation from the surrounding retina to a more blended border but should be on the same plane as the retina. In general, there are four main vascular branches emanating from the disc, each branch consisting of an arteriole and a venule. The venules are approximately four times the size of the accompanying arterioles and are darker in color. Light often produces a glistening "light reflex" from the arteriolar vessel. Normal arterial-to-venous width is a ratio of 2:3 or 4:5.*

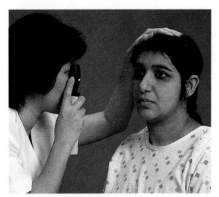

A. Eliciting the Red Reflex

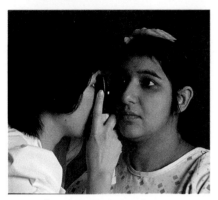

B. Funduscopic Examination

Figure 12-35 Examining Retinal Structures

Table 12-2 Retinal Color Variations	
FINDINGS	**CHARACTERISTICS**
Fair-skinned individual	• Retina appears a lighter red-orange color • Tessellated appearance of the fundi (pigment does not obscure the choroid vessels)
Dark-skinned individual	• Fundi appear darker in color; grayish purple to brownish (from increased pigment in the choroid and retina) • No tessellated appearance • Choroidal vessels usually obscured
Aging individual	• Vessels are straighter and narrower • Choroidal vessels are easily visualized • Retinal pigment epithelium atrophies and causes the retinal color to become paler

E **Examination**
N **Normal Findings**
A **Abnormal Findings**
P **Pathophysiology**

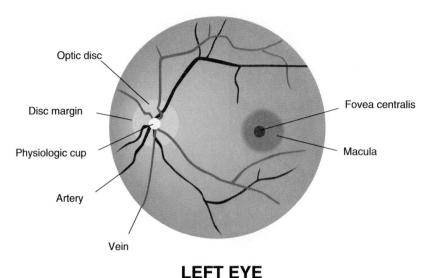

LEFT EYE

Figure 12-36 Optic Disc

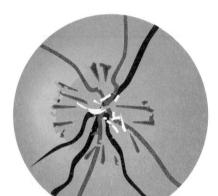

A. Papilledema

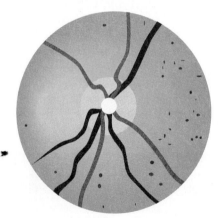

B. Deep Retinal Hemorrhages

Figure 12-37 Retinal Structure Abnormalities

E	**Examination**
N	**Normal Findings**
A	**Abnormal Findings**
P	**Pathophysiology**

A The optic disc is pale.

P Pallor is due to optic atrophy caused by increased intracranial pressure or from congenital syphilis; an intracranial space-occupying lesion, e.g., meningioma; or end-stage glaucoma.

A The physiologic cup exceeds the normal 1:3 ratio. The disc appears elevated above the plane of the surrounding retina.

P Disc edema and loss of vision are caused by the papillitis resulting from optic neuritis. The disc is hyperemic, the margins are blurred, and the disc surface is elevated.

P Disc edema and an elevated disc without loss of vision are found in papilledema (see Figure 12-37A), which is caused by increased intracranial pressure obstructing return blood flow from the eye. This is also called a "choked disc."

A Superficial retinal hemorrhages are flame-shaped hemorrhages found in the fundi or they may appear as red hemorrhages with white centers called Roth's spots. These hemorrhages form a pattern related to the nerve fibers that radiate from the optic disc.

P These hemorrhages may be due to severe hypertension, occlusion of the central retinal vein, and papilledema. Roth's spots are sometimes associated with infective endocarditis.

A Deep retinal hemorrhages appear as small red dots or irregular spots in the deep layer of the retina (see Figure 12-37B).

P Deep retinal hemorrhages can be associated with diabetes mellitus.

A Diffuse preretinal hemorrhages occur in the small space between the vitreous and the retina.

P Preretinal hemorrhages may occur in conjunction with a sudden increase in intracranial pressure.

A Microaneurysms are tiny red dots that can be seen in peripheral and macular areas of the retina.

P These dots are small vessels that dilate in diabetic retinopathy.

A Neovascularization is the formation of new vessels that are very narrow and disorderly in appearance and may extend into the vitreous (see Figure 12-37C). These vessels may bleed, resulting in a loss of vision.

P Neovascularization occurs in proliferative diabetic retinopathy.

A Fluffy white areas that appear on the retina and are patchy in shape are abnormal (see Figure 12-37D).

P Cotton wool spots represent microscopic infarcts of the nerve fiber layer and are due to diabetic or hypertensive retinopathy.

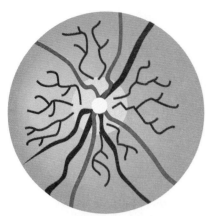

C. Neovascularization

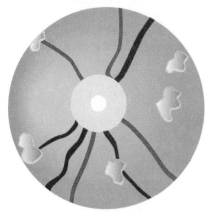

D. Cotton Wool Spots

Figure 12-37 Retinal Structure Abnormalities *continued*

 NURSING TIP

The Patient with Decreased Hearing

Observe the patient for signs of hearing difficulty and deafness during the health history and physical exam. Turning the head to facilitate hearing, lip reading, speaking in a loud voice, or asking you to write words are signs of hearing difficulty. If the patient is wearing a hearing aid, ask if it is turned on, when the batteries were last changed, and if the device causes any irritation of the ear canal.

A Drusen are small white dots in the fundus that are arranged in an irregular pattern. They may also occur on the optic disc, and may become shiny with calcification.

P Drusen are findings of the normal aging process. They may cause loss of vision if they occur in the macular region.

A Hard exudates are yellow with distinct borders, and are small unless they coalesce. They are arranged in round, linear, or star-shaped patterns.

P Hard exudates are associated with diabetes mellitus or hypertension.

A A cleft defect of the choroid and retina is abnormal. The size ranges from medium to large.

P **Coloboma** is a congenital abnormality.

A The red-orange retinal reflex is absent in the area of a retinal detachment. The area appears pearly gray and is elevated and wrinkled.

P A detached retina may be associated with severe myopia, cataract surgery, or diabetic retinopathy, or it may be caused by trauma.

A Fibrous white bands that obscure the retinal vessels are abnormal. Neovascularization may also be present.

P These findings occur in proliferative diabetic retinopathy.

Macula

When the retinal structures and the optic disc have been assessed:

E 1. Move the ophthalmoscope approximately two disc diameters temporally to view the macula or ask the patient to look at the light. The red-free filter lens of the ophthalmoscope may also be helpful in assessing the macula. Because the macula is not clearly demarcated and because it is very light sensitive, you may have difficulty assessing it. The patient tends to turn away when the light strikes the fovea, making it difficult to assess details of the macular area.

2. Note the fovea centralis and observe for color, shape, and lesions.

3. Repeat with the other eye.

N *The macula is a darker, avascular area with a pinpoint reflective center known as the fovea centralis.*

A The retina is pale with the macular region appearing as a cherry-red spot.

P This finding is central retinal artery occlusion, an indication of Tay-Sachs disease.

A Sharply defined, small red spots are found in and around the macula.

P These microaneurysms are pathognomonic of diabetes mellitus.

A Macular borders are blurred, with a few spots of pigment near the macula; a hole may appear to be present in the center of the region, or a hemorrhage may have occurred.

P This finding is characteristic of age-related macular degeneration. Hemorrhages, patches of retina atrophy, and pigmented areas may also be associated with this condition.

ASSESSMENT OF THE EAR

Physical assessment of the ear consists of three parts:

1. Auditory screening (CN VIII)

2. Inspection and palpation of the external ear

3. Otoscopic assessment

Auditory Screening

Voice-Whisper Test

E 1. Instruct the patient to occlude one ear with a finger.

2. Stand 2 feet behind the patient's other ear and whisper a two-syllable word or phrase that is evenly accented.

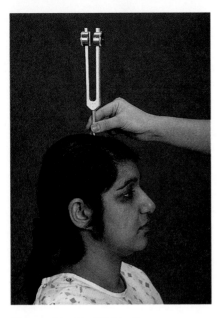

Figure 12-38   Weber Test

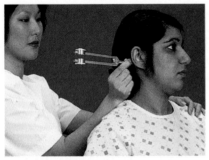

A. Assessing Bone Conduction

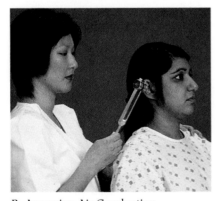

B. Assessing Air Conduction

Figure 12-39   Rinne Test

E	**Examination**
N	**Normal Findings**
A	**Abnormal Findings**
P	**Pathophysiology**

3. Ask the patient to repeat the word or phrase.

4. Repeat the test with the other ear.

N *The patient should be able to repeat words whispered from a distance of 2 feet.*

A The patient is unable to repeat the words correctly or states that he or she was unable to hear anything.

P This indicates a hearing loss in the high-frequency range that may be caused by excessive exposure to loud noises.

Tuning Fork Tests

Weber and **Rinne** tests help to determine whether the type of hearing loss the patient is experiencing is conductive or sensorineural. In order to understand how these tests are evaluated, it is important to know the difference between air and bone conduction. Air conduction refers to the transmission of sound through the ear canal, tympanic membrane, and ossicular chain to the cochlea and auditory nerve. Bone conduction refers to the transmission of sound through the bones of the skull to the cochlea and auditory nerve.

Weber Test

E **1.** Hold the handle of a 512-Hz (vibrates 512 cycles per second to create a specific frequency) tuning fork and strike the tines on the ulnar border of the palm to activate it.

  2. Place the stem of the fork firmly against the middle of the patient's forehead, on the top of the head at the midline, or on the front teeth (see Figure 12-38).

  3. Ask the patient if the sound is heard centrally or toward one side.

N *The patient should perceive the sound equally in both ears or "in the middle." No lateralization of sound is known as a "negative" Weber test.*

A The sound lateralizes to the affected ear.

P This occurs with unilateral conductive hearing loss because the sound is being conducted directly through the bone to the ear. Conductive hearing loss occurs when there are external or middle ear disorders such as impacted cerumen, perforation of the tympanic membrane, serum or pus in the middle ear, or a fusion of the ossicles.

A The sound lateralizes to the unaffected ear.

P This occurs with sensorineural loss related to nerve damage in the impaired ear. Sensorineural hearing loss occurs when there is a disorder in the inner ear, the auditory nerve, or the brain; disorders include congenital defects, effects of ototoxic drugs, and repeated or prolonged exposure to loud noise.

Rinne Test

E **1.** Stand behind or to the side of the patient and strike the tuning fork.

  2. Place the stem of the tuning fork against the patient's right mastoid process to test bone conduction (see Figure 12-39A).

  3. Instruct the patient to indicate if the sound is heard.

  4. Ask the patient to tell you when the sound stops.

  5. When the patient says that the sound has stopped, move the tuning fork, with the tines facing forward, in front of the right auditory meatus, and ask the patient if the sound is still heard. Note the length of time the patient hears the sound (testing air conduction) (see Figure 12-39B).

  6. Repeat the test on the left ear.

N *Air conduction is heard twice as long as bone conduction when the patient hears the sound through the external auditory canal (air) after it is no longer heard at the mastoid process (bone).*

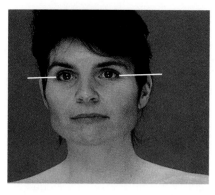

Figure 12-40 Normal Ear Alignment

E	Examination
N	Normal Findings
A	Abnormal Findings
P	Pathophysiology

A The patient reports hearing the sound longer through bone conduction; that is, bone conduction is equal to or greater than air conduction.

P This occurs when there is a conductive hearing loss resulting from disease, obstruction, or damage to the outer or middle ear.

External Ear

Inspection

E 1. Inspect the ears and note their position, color, size, and shape.
2. Note any deformities, nodules, inflammation, or lesions.
3. Note color, consistency, and amount of cerumen.

N *The ear should match the flesh color of the rest of the patient's skin and should be positioned centrally and in proportion to the head. The top of the ear should cross an imaginary line drawn from the outer canthus of the eye to the occiput (see Figure 12-40). Cerumen should be moist and not obscure the tympanic membrane. There should be no foreign bodies, redness, drainage, deformities, nodules, or lesions.*

A The ears are pale, red, or cyanotic.

P Vasomotor disorders, fevers, hypoxemia, and cold weather can account for various color changes.

A The ears are abnormally large or small or unusually shaped.

P These abnormalities can be congenitally determined or the result of trauma.

A Purulent drainage is abnormal.

P Purulent drainage usually indicates an infection.

A Clear or bloody drainage is present.

P Clear or bloody drainage may be due to cerebrospinal fluid leaking as a result of head trauma or surgery.

A Nodules are present on the external ear.

P Tophi are uric acid nodules and may indicate the presence of gout. Many other nodules are benign fibromas.

A Lymph nodes anterior to the tragus or overlying the mastoid are abnormal.

P Lymph nodes may be enlarged due to a malignancy or an infection such as external otitis.

A Sebaceous cysts are abnormal.

P Sebaceous cysts or retention cysts form as a result of the blockage of the ducts to the sebaceous gland.

Palpation

E 1. Palpate the auricle between the thumb and the index finger, noting any tenderness or lesions.
2. Using the tips of the index and middle fingers, palpate the mastoid tip, noting any tenderness.
3. Using the tips of the index and middle fingers, press inward on the tragus, noting any tenderness.
4. Hold the auricle between the thumb and the index finger and gently pull up and down, noting any tenderness.

N *The patient should not complain of pain or tenderness during palpation.*

A Auricular pain or tenderness is noted.

P Auricular pain is a common finding in external ear infection and is called acute otitis externa.

A There is tenderness over the mastoid process.

P Mastoid tenderness is associated with middle ear inflammation or mastoiditis.

A The tragus is edematous or sensitive.

P This finding may indicate inflammation of the external or middle ear.

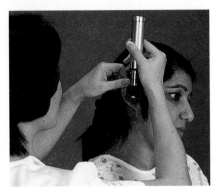

Figure 12-41 Position for Otoscopic Examination

Otoscopic Assessment

E
1. Ask the patient to tip the head away from the ear being assessed.
2. Select the largest speculum that will comfortably fit the patient.
3. Hold the otoscope securely in the dominant hand, with the head held downward and the handle held like a pencil between the thumb and the forefinger.
4. Rest the back of the dominant hand on the right side of the patient's head (see Figure 12-41).
5. Use the ulnar aspect of the free hand to pull the right ear in a manner that will straighten the canal. In adults and in children over 3 years old, pull the ear up and back. See Chapter 23 for the assessment of children.
6. If hair obstructs visualization, moisten the speculum with water or a water-soluble lubricant.
7. If wax obstructs visualization, it should be removed only by a skilled practitioner, either by curettement (if the cerumen is soft or the tympanic membrane is ruptured) or by irrigation (if the cerumen is dry and hard and the tympanic membrane is intact).
8. Slowly insert the speculum into the canal, looking at the canal as the speculum passes.
9. Assess the canal for inflammation, exudates, lesions, and foreign bodies.
10. Continue to insert the speculum into the canal, following the path of the canal until the tympanic membrane is visualized.
11. If the tympanic membrane is not visible, gently pull the tragus slightly farther in order to straighten the canal to allow adequate visualization.
12. Identify the color, light reflex, umbo, the short process, and the long handle of the malleus. Note the presence of perforations, lesions, bulging or retraction of the tympanic membrane, dilatation of blood vessels, bubbles, or fluid.
13. Ask the patient to close the mouth, pinch the nose closed, and blow gently while you observe for movement of the tympanic membrane. A pneumatic attachment may be used to create this movement if one is available.
14. Gently withdraw the speculum and repeat the process with the left ear.

N *The ear canal should have no redness, swelling, tenderness, lesions, drainage, foreign bodies, or scaly surface areas. Cerumen varies in amount, consistency, and color. The tympanic membrane should be pearly gray with clearly defined landmarks and a distinct cone-shaped light reflex extending from the umbo toward the anteroinferior aspect of the membrane. This light reflex is seen at 5 o'clock in the right ear and at 7 o'clock in the left ear. Blood vessels should be visible only on the periphery, and the membrane should not bulge, be retracted, or have any evidence of fluid behind it. The tympanic membrane should move when the patient blows against resistance.*

A There is redness, swelling, narrowing, and pain of the external ear. Drainage may be present.

P Acute otitis externa is caused by infectious organisms or allergic reactions. Predisposing factors include excessive moisture in the ear related to swimming, trauma from cleansing the ears with a sharp instrument, or allergies to substances such as hairspray.

A Hard, dry, and very dark yellow-brown cerumen is abnormal.

P Old cerumen is harder and drier, and may become impacted if not removed.

A The tympanic membrane is red, with decreased mobility and possible bulging (see Figure 12-42A).

P This is acute **otitis media**, or an inflammation of the middle ear. Pain and fever may accompany the ear infection.

E	**Examination**
N	**Normal Findings**
A	**Abnormal Findings**
P	**Pathophysiology**

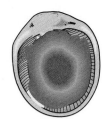

A. Acute Otitis Media

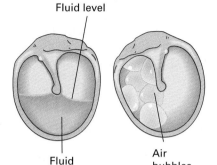

Fluid level

Fluid

Air bubbles

B. Serous Otitis Media

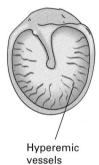

Hyperemic vessels

C. Acute Purulent Otitis Media: Early Stage

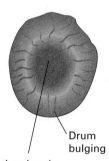

Drum bulging

Landmarks obscured

D. Acute Purulent Otitis Media: Late Stage

Figure 12-42 Abnormalities Found in Otoscopic Examination

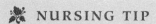

NURSING TIP

Assessing Patency of the Nose

The sense of smell (CN I) is evaluated during testing of cranial nerves. Refer to Chapter 18.

A Amber-yellow fluid on the tympanic membrane is abnormal. It may be accompanied by a fluid line or bubbles behind the membrane. Bulging may be present and mobility of the eardrum may be decreased (refer to Figure 12-42B).

P Serous otitis media can be caused by allergies, infections, and a blocked eustachian tube.

A Light reflex is absent, the eardrum is red with hyperemic blood vessels, and bulging is noted (see Figure 12-42C).

P These findings occur in the early stage of acute purulent otitis media.

A Along with a bulging eardrum and decreased mobility, the landmarks are diffuse, displaced, or absent.

P The late stage of acute purulent otitis media causes landmarks to become progressively obscured (see Figure 12-42D).

A Retraction of the tympanic membrane is noted and the landmarks are exaggerated. Mobility of the tympanic membrane may be decreased.

P Retraction of the tympanic membrane can occur when the intratympanic membrane pressures are reduced, as in eustachian tube blockage caused by serous otitis media or allergies.

A The tympanic membrane appears to have a darkened area or a hole.

P A perforated eardrum is caused by untreated ear infection secondary to increasing pressure. Trauma to the ear canal can also cause a perforation.

A The tympanic membrane is pearly gray and has dark patches.

P These patches are usually old perforations in the tympanic membrane.

A The tympanic membrane is pearly gray and has dense white plaques.

P These plaques represent calcific deposits of scarring of the tympanic membrane from frequent past episodes of otitis media.

NURSING TIP

Cleaning the Ears

Advise patients who have frequent cerumen impactions to use three drops of a hydrogen peroxide/water solution (1:1) once or twice a week to prevent further problems. Instruct patients **not** to use cotton-tipped applicators to clean the ears. Cotton-tipped applicators are likely to make the problem worse by packing the cerumen more tightly into the ear canal. They may also cause traumatic injury to the ear canal or tympanic membrane.

ASSESSMENT OF THE NOSE

External Inspection

E Inspect the nose, noting any trauma, bleeding, lesions, masses, swelling, and asymmetry.

N *The shape of the external nose can vary greatly among individuals. Normally, it is located symmetrically in the midline of the face and is without swelling, bleeding, lesions, or masses.*

A The nose is misshapen, broken, or swollen.

P The shape of the nose is determined by genetics; however, changes can occur because of trauma or cosmetic surgery.

Patency

E 1. Have the patient occlude one nostril with a finger.
2. Ask the patient to breathe in and out through the nose as you observe and listen for air movement in and out of the nostril.
3. Repeat on the other side.

N *Each nostril is patent.*

A You observe or the patient states that air cannot be moved through the nostril(s).

P Occlusion of the nostrils can occur with a deviated septum, foreign body, upper respiratory infection, allergies, or nasal polyps.

Internal Inspection

E
1. Position the patient with the head in an extended position.
2. Place the nondominant hand firmly on top of the patient's head.
3. Using the thumb of the same hand, lift the tip of the patient's nose.
4. Gently insert a nasal speculum or an otoscope with a short, wide nasal speculum (see Figure 12-43). If using a nasal speculum, use a penlight to view the nostrils.
5. Assess each nostril separately.
6. Inspect the mucous membranes for color and discharge.
7. Inspect the middle and inferior turbinates and the middle meatus for color, swelling, drainage, lesions, and polyps.
8. Observe the nasal septum for deviation, perforation, lesions, and bleeding.

N *The nasal mucosa should be pink or dull red without swelling or polyps. The septum is at the midline and without perforation, lesions, or bleeding. A small amount of clear, watery discharge is normal.*

A The nasal mucosa is red and swollen with copious clear, watery discharge. This is called rhinitis, an inflammation of the nasal mucosa (see Figure 12-44).

P These findings indicate the occurrence of the common cold (coryza) when there is an acute onset of symptoms. Discharge may become purulent if a secondary bacterial infection develops.

A Nasal mucosa is pale and edematous with clear, watery discharge.

P These findings usually indicate the presence of allergies or hay fever.

A Following trauma to the head, there is a clear, watery nasal discharge with normal-appearing mucosa. This discharge tests positive for glucose.

P These findings indicate the presence of cerebrospinal fluid. This may occur following head injury or complications of nose or sinus surgery or dental work. Immediate referral is warranted.

A Nasal mucosa is red and swollen with purulent nasal discharge. These findings are usually worse on one side but may be found bilaterally.

P These are common findings in bacterial sinusitis, a secondary infection associated with the common cold.

A There is unilateral purulent discharge; however, the patient does not experience other symptoms of an upper respiratory infection. Nasal mucosa on the unaffected side appears normal.

P Unilateral purulent discharge without other findings of an upper respiratory infection indicates the development of a local infection. A common cause of localized infection is the presence of a foreign body.

A Nasal mucosa is inflamed and friable with possible septal perforation. There is no infection present.

P These findings may indicate nasal inhalation of cocaine or amphetamines or the overuse of nasal spray.

ASSESSMENT OF THE SINUSES

Inspection

E Observe the patient's face for any swelling around the nose and eyes.

N *There is no evidence of swelling around the nose and eyes.*

A Swelling is noted above or below the eyes.

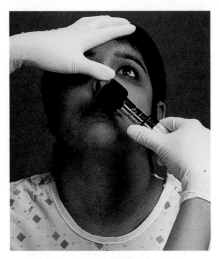

A. Use of Otoscope with Nasal Speculum

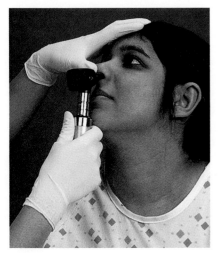

B. Lateral View of Internal Nose Assessment

Figure 12-43   Internal Inspection of Nose

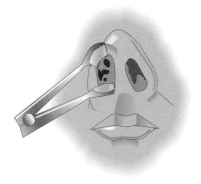

Figure 12-44   Rhinitis

E   Examination
N   Normal Findings
A   Abnormal Findings
P   Pathophysiology

P Acute sinusitis may result in swelling of the face around the eyes due to inflammation and accumulation of purulent material in the paranasal sinuses.

◎◎ THINK ABOUT IT

Septal Perforation from Cocaine Use

How do you feel about the use of illegal drugs? Would you treat the patient differently because of your views about street drug use? What would be an appropriate verbal response to the patient whom you believe to be using cocaine?

Palpation and Percussion

To palpate and percuss the frontal sinuses:

E 1. Stand facing the patient.
   2. Gently press the thumbs under the bony ridge of the upper orbits (see Figure 12-45A). Avoid applying pressure on the globes themselves.
   3. Observe for the presence of pain.
   4. Percuss the areas using the middle or index finger of the dominant hand (immediate percussion).
   5. Note the sound.

N/A/P Refer to maxillary sinuses.

To palpate and percuss the maxillary sinuses:

E 1. Stand in front of the patient.
   2. Apply gentle pressure in the area under the infraorbital ridge using the thumb or middle finger (see Figure 12-45B).
   3. Observe for the presence of pain.
   4. Percuss the area using the dominant middle or index finger.
   5. Note the sound.

N *The patient should experience no discomfort during palpation or percussion. The sinuses should be air filled and therefore resonant to percussion.*

A The patient complains of pain or tenderness at the site of palpation or percussion.

P Sinusitis can be due to viral, bacterial, or allergic processes that cause inflammation of the mucous membranes and obstruction of the drainage pathways.

A Percussion of the sinuses elicits a dull sound.

P Dullness can be caused by fluid or cells present in the sinus cavity from an infectious or allergic process, or congenital absence of a sinus.

A An extremely bright glow is abnormal.

P This phenomenon may be present in an elderly patient with decreased subcutaneous fat.

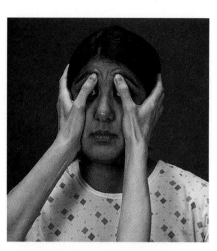

A. Palpation of Frontal Sinuses

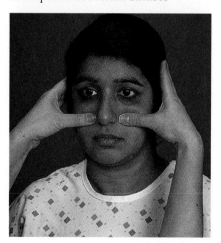

B. Palpation of Maxillary Sinuses

Figure 12-45 Palpation of Sinuses

✳ SPECIAL TECHNIQUE

Transillumination of the Sinuses

If palpation and percussion of the sinuses suggest sinusitis, transillumination of the frontal and maxillary sinuses should be performed.

To evaluate the frontal sinuses:

E 1. Place the patient in a sitting position facing you in a dark room.
   2. Place a strong light source such as a transilluminator, penlight, or tip of an otoscope with the speculum under the bony ridge of the upper orbits (see Figure 12-46A).
   3. Observe the red glow over the sinuses and compare the symmetry of the two sides.

N/A/P Refer to maxillary sinuses.

continued

E	Examination
N	Normal Findings
A	Abnormal Findings
P	Pathophysiology

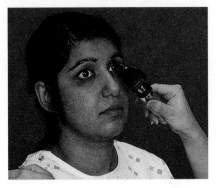
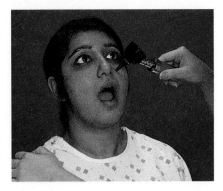

A. Frontal Sinus   B. Maxillary Sinus

Figure 12-46   Transillumination of Sinuses

To evaluate the maxillary sinuses:

E   **1.** Place the patient in a sitting position facing you in a dark room.

      2. Place the light source firmly under each eye and just above the infra-orbital ridge (see Figure 12-46B).

      3. Ask the patient to open the mouth; observe the red glow on the hard palate.

      4. Compare the two sides.

N   *The glow on each side is equal, indicating air-filled frontal and maxillary sinuses.*

A   Absence of glow is abnormal.

P   Absence of glow suggests sinus congestion or the congenital absence of a sinus.

❧ NURSING TIP

Percussing the Sinuses

Before percussing the sinuses, explain to the patient that you are assessing for infection and warn him or her that some minor discomfort may be experienced during the procedure.

ASSESSMENT OF THE MOUTH AND THROAT

Assessment of the Mouth

Breath

E   **1.** Stand facing the patient and about 12 inches away.

      2. Smell the breath.

N   *Breath should smell fresh.*

A   The breath smells foul.

P   The foul smell of halitosis can be a symptom of tooth decay, poor oral hygiene, or diseases of the gums, tonsils, or sinuses.

A   The breath smells of acetone.

P   Acetone or "fruity" breath is common in patients who are malnourished or who have diabetic ketoacidosis.

A   The breath smells musty.

P   Fetor hepaticas is the musty smell of the breath of a patient in liver failure and is caused by the breakdown of nitrogen compounds.

A   The breath smells of ammonia.

P   The smell of ammonia can be detected in a patient in end-stage renal failure (uremia) because of the inability to eliminate urea.

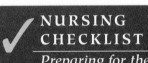

✓ NURSING CHECKLIST

Preparing for the Assessment of the Mouth and Throat

1. Physical assessment of the oral cavity should include the following:
- Breath, lips, tongue, buccal mucosa, gums and teeth, hard and soft palates, throat (oropharynx), and temporomandibular joint (see Chapters 11 and 17).

2. If the patient is wearing dentures or removable orthodontia, ask that they be removed before the examination begins.

3. Use gloves and a good light source such as a penlight for optimum visualization of the oral cavity and pharynx.

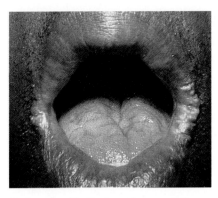

A. Angular Cheilosis *Courtesy of Dr. Joseph Konzelman, School of Dentistry, Medical College of Georgia*

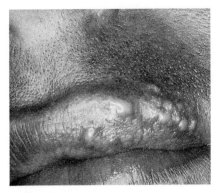

B. Fever Blister (Herpes Simplex Virus I) *Courtesy of Dr. Joseph Konzelman, School of Dentistry, Medical College of Georgia*

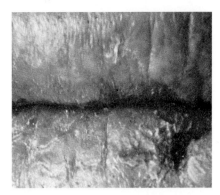

C. Squamous Cell Carcinoma *Courtesy of Dr. Joseph Konzelman, School of Dentistry, Medical College of Georgia*

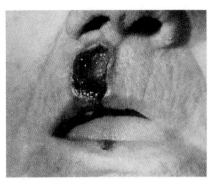

D. Basal Cell Carcinoma *Courtesy of Delmar Publishers, Albany, NY*

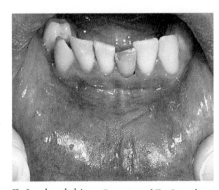

E. Leukoplakia *Courtesy of Dr. Joseph Konzelman, School of Dentistry, Medical College of Georgia*

Figure 12-47 Lip Abnormalities

E	**Examination**
N	**Normal Findings**
A	**Abnormal Findings**
P	**Pathophysiology**

Lips

Inspection

E 1. Observe the lips for color, moisture, swelling, lesions, or other signs of inflammation.
2. Instruct the patient to open the mouth.
3. Use a tongue blade to inspect the membranes that connect the upper and lower lips to the gums for color, inflammation, lesions, and hydration.

N *The lips and membranes should be pink and moist with no evidence of lesions or inflammation.*

A The lips are pale or cyanotic.

P Refer to Chapter 15.

A The lips are dry and cracked.

P Chapping or superficial cracking of the lips may be due to exposure to wind, sun, or a dry environment, dehydration of the patient, or persistent licking of the lips.

A Swelling of the lips is noted.

P Allergic reactions to medications, foods, or other allergens can result in swelling of the lips.

A The skin at the outer corners of the mouth is atrophic, irritated, and cracked (see Figure 12-47A).

P Angular cheilosis may be due to increased accumulation of saliva in the corners of the mouth or constant drooling from the mouth. This occurs in nutritional deficiencies (such as riboflavin), poorly fitting dentures, and deficiencies of the immune system. *Candida* infections may also be present.

A Vesicles on erythematous bases with serous fluid are found on the lips, gums, or hard palate, either singly or in clusters. They later rupture, crust over, and become painful (refer to Figure 12-47B).

P These are herpes simplex lesions, which are commonly called cold sores or fever blisters. This common viral infection may be precipitated by febrile illness, sunlight, stress, or allergies.

A A round, painless lesion with central ulceration is noted. This lesion may become crusted.

P This is a chancre, the primary lesion of syphilis.

A A plaque, wart, nodule, or ulcer is noted, usually on the lower lip.

P This may be squamous cell carcinoma, the most common form of oral cancer, which is more frequent in males (see Figure 12-47C).

P Basal cell carcinoma lesions can have pearly borders, crusting, and central ulcerations (see Figure 12-47D).

A Persistent, painless, white, painted-looking patches are noted on the lips (see Figure 12-47E). They are associated with heavy smoking and the use of chewing tobacco.

P   These patches are called leukoplakia and are considered premalignant lesions. They often occur at sites of chronic irritation from dentures, tobacco, or excessive alcohol intake.

Palpation

E   1. Don clean gloves.
2. Gently pull down the patient's lower lip with the thumb and index finger of one hand and pull up the patient's upper lip with the thumb and index finger of the other hand.
3. Note the tone of the lips as they are manipulated.
4. If lesions are present, palpate them for consistency and tenderness.

N   *Lips should not be flaccid and lesions should not be present.*

A/P   See inspection of the lips for pathologies.

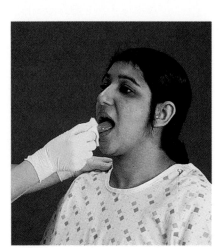

Figure 12-48   Tongue Assessment

Tongue

E   1. Ask the patient to stick out the tongue (CN XII assesses tongue movement).
2. Observe the dorsal surface for color, hydration, texture, symmetry, fasciculations, atrophy, position in the mouth, and the presence of lesions.
3. Ask the patient to move the tongue from side to side and up and down.
4. With the patient's tongue back in the mouth, ask the patient to press it against the cheek. Provide resistance with your finger pads held on the outside of the cheek. Note the strength of the tongue and compare bilaterally.
5. Ask the patient to touch the tip of the tongue to the roof of the mouth. You may also grasp the tip of the tongue with a gauze square held between the thumb and the index finger of the gloved hand (see Figure 12-48).
6. Inspect the ventral surface of the tongue, the frenulum, and Wharton's ducts for color, hydration, lesions, inflammation, and vasculature.
7. With the gauze square, pull the tongue to the left and inspect and palpate the tongue using the finger pads.
8. Repeat with the tongue held to the right side.

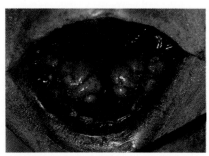

A. Mandibular Tori

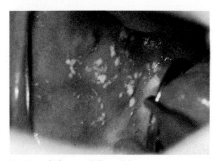

B. Candidiasis (Thrush)

Figure 12-49   Tongue Conditions
All photos in this series courtesy of Dr. Joseph Konzelman, School of Dentistry, Medical College of Georgia

N   *The tongue is in the midline of the mouth. The dorsum of the tongue should be pink, moist, rough (from the taste buds), and without lesions. The tongue is symmetrical and moves freely. The strength of the tongue is symmetrical and strong. The ventral surface of the tongue has prominent blood vessels and should be moist and without lesions. Wharton's ducts are patent and without inflammation or lesions. The lateral aspects of the tongue should be pink, smooth, and lesion free. Some patients may have mandibular tori (Figure 12-49A), which are bony nodules on the inside of the mandible.*

A   The tongue is enlarged.

P   An enlarged tongue may be associated with myxedema, acromegaly, Down syndrome, or amyloidosis. Transient enlargement may be associated with glossitis, stomatitis, cellulitis of the neck, angioneurotic edema, hematoma, or abscess.

A   The tongue is red and smooth with absent papillae.

P   This indicates glossitis caused by a vitamin B$_{12}$, iron, or niacin deficiency. It may also be a side effect of chemotherapy.

A   There is a thick, white, curdlike coating on the tongue that leaves a raw, red surface when it is scraped off (see Figure 12-49B).

P   This is candidiasis, or thrush, which may also be red in the absence of the coating. Thrush can result from changes in the normal oral flora due to chemotherapy, radiation therapy, disorders of the immune system such as AIDS, antibiotic therapy, or excessive use of alcohol, tobacco, or cocaine.

E	Examination
N	Normal Findings
A	Abnormal Findings
P	Pathophysiology

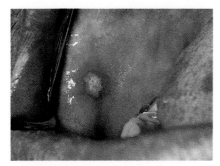

C. Aphthous Ulcer (Canker Sore)

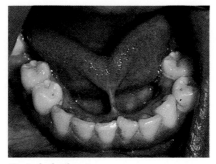

D. Ankyloglossia

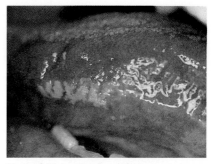

E. Oral Hairy Leukoplakia

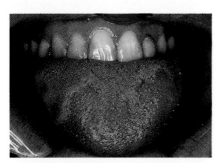

F. Geographic Tongue

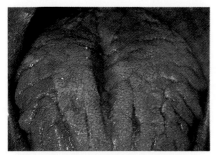

G. Fissured Tongue (Scrotal Tongue)

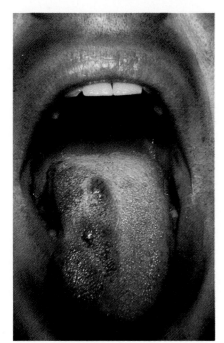

H. Hemangioma

Figure 12-49 Tongue Conditions
continued

A Thin, pearly white lesions that coalesce and become thick and palpable are noted on the sides of the tongue. These white lesions are firmly attached to the underlying tissue and will not scrape off.

P This is leukoplakia. Refer to pages 327–328.

A A painful, small, round, white, ulcerated lesion with erythematous borders is abnormal (refer to Figure 12-49C).

P This is an aphthous ulcer (canker sore), which can be associated with stress, extreme fatigue, food allergies, and oral trauma.

A A short lingual frenulum is observed (see Figure 12-49D).

P Ankyloglossia is a congenital abnormality.

A The tongue has a hairy appearance and is yellow, black, or brown (see Figure 12-49E).

P This is known as oral hairy leukoplakia, or hairy tongue, a benign condition that can result from antibiotic therapy. The hairy appearance is caused by elongated papillae.

A Lesions are noted on the ventral surface of the tongue.

P The ventral surface of the tongue is an area where malignancies are likely to develop, especially in patients who drink alcohol and smoke or use smokeless tobacco.

A Indurations, or ulcerations, are present on the lateral surfaces of the tongue.

P Most lingual cancers are located in this area and are associated with use of alcohol and tobacco.

A Patches of red denuded areas on the lingual surface of the tongue, frequently at the papillae, surrounded by ridges of pale-yellow epithelium are abnormal (see Figure 12-49F).

P This harmless condition, known as geographic tongue, has no known cause. Its name is derived from the patterns of regular and irregular surfaces on the tongue that resemble a map.

A Numerous furrows or grooves are observed, often radiating horizontally from the midline of the dorsal surface of the tongue (see Figure 12-49G).

P This is a harmless and often inherited condition known as fissured or scrotal tongue. It is different from syphilitic glossitis, which is characterized by longitudinal furrows.

A Engorged blood vessels of the tongue are abnormal (see Figure 12-49H).

P A hemangioma of the tongue is a benign overgrowth of vascular tissue.

A Deviation of the tongue toward one side, atrophy, and asymmetrical shape of the tongue are abnormal.

P Unilateral paralysis of the tongue muscles will cause the tongue to deviate toward the affected side because the muscles on the paralyzed side are unable to oppose the strong muscles of the unaffected side. The patient is unable to push the tongue toward the nonparalyzed side. Lesions of the hypoglossal nucleus or nerve fiber cause these unilateral symptoms.

A Atrophy of the tongue and the inability to protrude the tongue are abnormal.

P Bilateral paralysis of the tongue muscles will prevent the patient from protruding the tongue. Syringobulbia or trauma to CN XII may cause hypoglossal nerve paralysis.

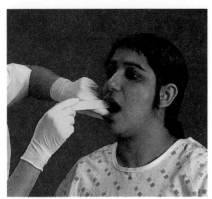

Figure 12-50   Assessment of Buccal Mucosa

Buccal Mucosa

E   1. Ask the patient to open the mouth as wide as possible.
   2. Use a tongue depressor and a penlight to assess the inner cheeks and the openings of Stensen's ducts (see Figure 12-50).
   3. Observe for color, inflammation, hydration, and lesions.

N   *The color of the oral mucosa on the inside of the cheek may vary according to race. African Americans have a bluish hue; Caucasians have pink mucosa. Frecklelike macules may appear on the inside of the buccal mucosa. The buccal mucosa should be moist, smooth, and free of lesions.*

A   Painless, white, painted-looking patches are noted.

P   Leukoplakia may be found in the buccal mucosa. Refer to pages 327–328 for information.

A   Small, round, white ulcers, each surrounded by a halo of reddened mucosa are found on the mucosa.

P   These are aphthous ulcers. Refer to page 329.

A   The mucosa is pale.

P   Pallor is caused by vasoconstriction that may occur when the sympathetic nervous system is stimulated, such as in shock.

A   The mucosa is cyanotic.

P   Cyanosis can indicate systemic hypoxemia. Refer to Chapters 10 and 15.

A   The mucosa is erythematous.

P   Erythema can be associated with stomatitis.

A   There is excessive dryness of the mucosa.

P   This is xerostomia, which occurs when salivary gland activity is decreased or when the patient is hypovolemic.

A   Excessive moisture is noted in the mouth.

P   This condition may be noted in the early stages of inflammation or when the patient is hypervolemic.

A   Flat-topped papules with thin, bluish white spider-web lines resembling leukoplakia are noted on the mucosa or tongue.

P   These are the lesions of lichen planus, which is an inflammatory and pruritic disease of the skin and mucous membranes. It is usually a benign disease and the cause is unknown.

Gums

E   1. Instruct the patient to open the mouth.
   2. Observe dentures or orthodontics for fit.
   3. Remove any dentures or removable orthodontia.
   4. Shine the penlight in the mouth.
   5. Use the tongue depressor to move the tongue to visualize the gums.
   6. Observe for redness, swelling, bleeding, retraction from the teeth, or discoloration.

N   *In light-skinned individuals, the gums have a pale-red stippled surface. Patchy brown pigmentation may be present in dark-skinned patients. The gum margins should be well defined with no pockets existing between the gums and the teeth and no swelling or bleeding.*

A   The gingiva are red, tender, and swollen and bleed easily (see Figure 12-51).

P   This describes gingivitis, which may be caused by poor dental hygiene, improperly fitted dentures, and scurvy. Gingivitis can also occur with stomatitis that occurs in mouth infections and upper respiratory tract infections.

A   Gingival borders are red and there is infection of the pockets formed between receding gums and teeth. Purulent drainage may be present.

P   This is periodontitis, which is an inflammation of the periodontium due to chronic gingivitis. This condition is caused by infrequent brushing of the teeth and poor oral hygiene.

A   Blue lines are noted approximately 1 mm from the gingival margin.

P   These are lead bismuth lines caused by chronic exposure to lead or bismuth.

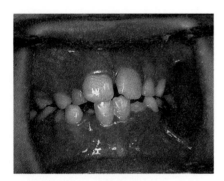

Figure 12-51   Gingivitis with Herpes Simplex Virus II and Stomatitis
Courtesy of Dr. Joseph Konzelman, School of Dentistry, Medical College of Georgia

E	**Examination**
N	**Normal Findings**
A	**Abnormal Findings**
P	**Pathophysiology**

A The gums are brownish.

P This occurs in association with Addison's disease.

A A grayish membrane is noted over an inflamed and ulcerated area of the mucosa.

P This condition is Vincent's stomatitis, or trench mouth, a bacterial infection of the gums that may extend into pharyngeal structures and bones.

A A nontender, immobile tumor lighter than the gums is noted on the gum.

P This lesion is epulis, a fibrous tumor of the gums.

A The gums are retracted from the teeth, sometimes exposing the roots of the teeth.

P This recession of the gums often occurs in older individuals due to poor oral hygiene.

A Hypertrophy of gum tissue is abnormal.

P This is called gingival hyperplasia and is usually painless; it occurs in pregnancy or with the use of some medications such as phenytoin.

Teeth

E
1. Instruct the patient to open the mouth.
2. Count the upper and lower teeth.
3. Observe the teeth for discoloration, loose or missing teeth, caries, malocclusion, and malformation.

N *The adult normally has 32 teeth, which should be white with smooth edges, in proper alignment, and without caries.*

A Teeth are absent.

P This problem may be due to loss or failure of development. The patient's nutritional status may be seriously impaired when the teeth are insufficient.

A There are white or black patches on the surface of a tooth. These patches may become eroded as damage progresses.

P These are dental caries, or cavities, resulting from poor oral hygiene.

A The teeth are worn at an angle.

P Biting surfaces of the teeth may become worn down by repetitive biting on hard substances or objects or grinding of teeth, called bruxism, especially at night.

A A tooth is dark in color and the patient reports insensitivity to cold.

P This is usually a dead tooth, which results in a darkening of the enamel.

Palate

E
1. Ask the patient to tilt the head back and open the mouth as wide as possible.
2. Shine the penlight in the patient's mouth.
3. Observe both the hard and the soft palates.
4. Note their shape and color, and the presence of any lesions or malformations.

N *The hard and soft palates are concave and pink. The hard palate has many ridges; the soft palate is smooth. No lesions or malformations are noted.*

A The palates are red, swollen, tender, or with lesions.

P These findings are symptoms of infection.

A There is a bony ridge in the midline of the hard palate.

P This is a benign condition called torus palatinus, which develops in adulthood.

A A fibrous, encapsulated tissue growth on the palate is abnormal (see Figure 12-52).

P A fibroma may be idiopathic or neoplastic in origin. Chronic trauma can also lead to fibroma formation.

A A lesion that has become eroded is noted on the palate.

P This may be a cancerous lesion in the epithelium of the hard palate.

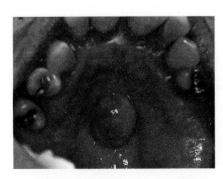

Figure 12-52 Fibroma *Courtesy of Dr. Joseph Konzelman, School of Dentistry, Medical College of Georgia*

E Examination
N Normal Findings
A Abnormal Findings
P Pathophysiology

A The palate is highly arched.
P This finding is associated with Turner's syndrome and Marfan's syndrome.
A There is a hole in the hard palate.
P Palatine perforation is related to syphilis or radiation therapy.

Inspection of the Throat

E 1. Ask the patient to tilt the head back and to open the mouth widely. The patient can either stick out the tongue or leave it resting on the floor of the mouth.
  2. With the right hand, place the tongue blade on the middle third of the tongue.
  3. With the left hand, shine a light at the back of the patient's throat.
  4. Ask the patient to say "ah."
  5. Observe the position, size, color, and general appearance of the tonsils and uvula.
  6. Touch the posterior third of the tongue with the tongue blade.
  7. Note movement of the palate and the presence of the gag reflex.
  8. Assess the color of the oropharynx. Note the presence of swelling, exudate, or lesions.

N *When the patient says "ah," the soft palate and the uvula should rise symmetrically (CN IX and X). The uvula is midline. The throat is normally pink and vascular and without swelling, exudate, or lesions. Normal tonsillar size is evaluated as 1+ to 2+. (Refer to Figure 12-53 for grading scale.) This indicates that both tonsils are behind the pillars. The patient's gag reflex should be present but is congenitally absent in some patients (CN IX and X).*

A The posterior pharynx is red with white patches. The tonsils are large and red with white patches, and the uvula is red and swollen.
P Viral pharyngitis and tonsillitis are common illnesses with these findings.
A Tonsils, pillars, and uvula are very red and swollen, with patches of white or yellow exudate on the tonsils. The posterior pharynx is bright red (see Figure 12-54). The patient reports soreness of the throat with swallowing.

🌸 **NURSING TIP**

Eliciting the Gag Reflex

Before eliciting the gag reflex, be sure to warn the patient about what to expect during your assessment. It may not be necessary to elicit the gag reflex if the palate and uvula rise symmetrically with phonation.

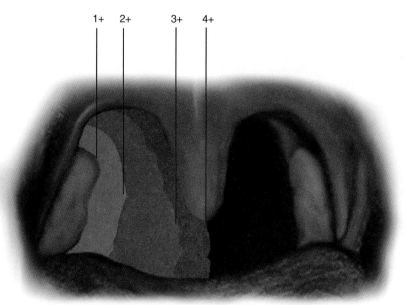

Figure 12-53 Grading of Tonsils
1+ tonsils are visible
2+ tonsils are between the pillars and the uvula
3+ tonsils are touching uvula
4+ one or both tonsils extend to the midline of the oropharynx

E Examination
N Normal Findings
A Abnormal Findings
P Pathophysiology

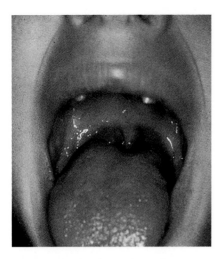

Figure 12-54 Streptococcal Pharyngitis *Courtesy of the Centers for Disease Control and Prevention (CDC)*

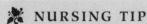

NURSING TIP

Diminished Sense of Taste

If a patient is experiencing some loss of taste, you can suggest adding seasonings to the diet, such as garlic, pepper, and curry. Heavy use of salt should be avoided. You can also suggest preparing aromatic foods that first stimulate the olfactory sense to enhance appetite.

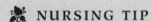

NURSING TIP

Night Driving

Many older persons find that driving at night is not safe because of their decreased night-time vision. Being unable to drive at night results in major changes in the ability to participate in activities such as shopping and social events.

E Examination
N Normal Findings
A Abnormal Findings
P Pathophysiology

P These findings are typical of streptococcal pharyngitis and tonsillitis and are usually associated with significant lymphadenopathy. However, diagnosis requires throat culture or rapid strep test.
A There is a grayish membrane covering the tonsils, uvula, and soft palate.
P These findings are typical of diphtheria, acute tonsillitis, or infectious mononucleosis.
A The patient speaks with a hoarse voice and the oropharynx is red.
P Causes of hoarseness are varied and may include overuse of the voice, inflammation due to viral or bacterial infection, lesions of the larynx, foreign bodies, and pressure on the larynx from masses or an enlarged thyroid gland.

GERONTOLOGICAL VARIATIONS

Visual and hearing impairments are among the most prevalent chronic conditions in the older patient. Sight and hearing facilitate communication; taste, smell, and temperature perception provide information to enable the patient to function safely in the environment. Prevention of sensory impairment and resulting handicaps are challenges for patients and health care providers.

During the aging process, the eye undergoes significant changes. First, by the age of 42, the lens cortex becomes more dense, compromising its ability to change shape and focus. This condition, **presbyopia**, is responsible for farsightedness and the need for bifocals. Next, there is a tendency for the lens to yellow and become cloudy. This change impairs a person's ability to discern various colors, especially blues and greens. In addition, pupils become smaller so that the amount of light reaching the retina is reduced. As a consequence, elderly individuals need more light to see and their eyes take longer to accommodate to darkness and glare. Finally, a decrease in tear production predisposes the individual to corneal irritation and conjunctivitis.

Cataracts, age-related macular degeneration, and glaucoma are the most common visual problems among elderly persons. Cataracts involve opacity and yellowing of the lens, which results in dimmed and blurred vision. Cataracts can be surgically removed.

Age-related macular degeneration is loss of central vision. Individuals experiencing this change require the use of magnification to compensate for visual loss. Systemic diseases that aggravate macular degeneration include diabetes mellitus and hypertension.

Glaucoma may cause total blindness if not treated. Increased intraocular pressure and inability of aqueous humor to flow out into collecting channels places pressure on the optic nerve. Early detection of glaucoma is critical; screening is recommended for all adults over age 40.

Inspection of the eyelids of the older individual often reveals slightly drooping upper and lower lids. The globe appears to be deeper in the socket, and the lacrimal gland may be visible because of lost subcutaneous fat around the eye.

Hearing loss, **presbycusis**, is also a common problem among elderly individuals. Conductive hearing loss occurs in the outer or middle ear and usually makes things sound softer. However, the more common age-related hearing loss is sensorineural, which involves the inner ear. Otoscopic assessment may reveal more pronounced landmarks if atrophic or sclerotic changes have occurred.

Taste may not diminish with age but may become less reliable. As one ages, the ability to taste sweetness remains, and the ability to taste bitterness declines. Sense of smell also diminishes slightly with age.

Common alterations in the mouths of elderly individuals are precancerous and cancerous lesions, untreated caries, periodontal disease, tooth loss resulting from oral disease, oral alterations related to systemic disease, side effects from medications, and orofacial pain. The increased incidence of chronic systemic disease, depression, and physical limitations in elderly individuals contribute to development of these problems.

A loss of teeth may affect closure of the mouth. The amount of saliva is reduced, and the mucosa is shinier, thinner, and less vascular. Gums are likely to be more pale, and the teeth appear larger as the gums recede with the resorption of supporting bone.

CASE STUDY

The case study illustrates the application and objective documentation of the eyes, ears, nose, mouth, and throat assessment.

The Patient with Bacterial Pharyngitis

Bridget is a 21-year-old college student who has a severe sore throat. She came to the student health clinic so that she can get well in time to study for exams.

❖ HEALTH HISTORY

PATIENT PROFILE	21 yo SBF
CHIEF COMPLAINT	"I feel awful today; my throat is sore & my head aches."
HISTORY OF PRESENT ILLNESS	Pt in usual state of good hl until this AM when awakened c̄ severe sore throat, malaise, H/A. Took 2 acetaminophen; swallowing made pain worse. C/o tender, swollen glands in neck. Thinks she has fever but doesn't have a thermometer; felt very cold during the PM & this AM. Has not eaten anything for 18 hr b/c "It hurts too much & besides, I'm not hungry." Denies exposures to others who are ill; denies ear, abdominal, muscle, or joint pain, nasal congestion, cough, or recent illness.
PAST HEALTH HISTORY	
Medical	Denies any major illnesses
Surgical	Denies
Medications	Takes 3 ibuprofen (200 mg tabs) × 1–2 d q month for menstrual cramps
Communicable Diseases	Chickenpox age 6 s̄ sequelae
Allergies	Denies allergies to medication, food, environmental conditions, pets
Injuries/Accidents	Denies
Disabilities/Handicaps	Denies
Blood Transfusions	Denies
Childhood Illnesses	See above
Immunizations	Up to date; tetanus booster at age 18; has not had hepatitis B immunization

continued

FAMILY HEALTH HISTORY

LEGEND

- ⬤ Living female
- ⬛ Living male
- ⊗ Deceased female
- ⊠ Deceased male
- ╱ Points to patient

A&W = Alive & well
BP = Blood Pressure
NIDDM = Non-insulin-dependent diabetes mellitus
PVD = Peripheral vascular disease

```
   78        83           73         73
   PVD     ↑ BP          NIDDM      A&W
         Cataracts

        45              46
       A&W             A&W

           21      18
                  A&W
```

Denies family hx of hearing loss.

SOCIAL HISTORY

Alcohol Use	Wkend use at college parties; usually 3–4 beers
Tobacco Use	Denies
Drug Use	Denies
Sexual Practice	Never involved in sexual relationship
Travel History	Spent last summer studying in France
Work Environment	Spends most days in classrooms or library
Home Environment	Lives c̄ 40 women students in sorority house
Hobbies/Leisure Activities	Swimming, tennis, reading, music
Stress	School, conflicts c̄ parents
Education	College senior majoring in French
Economic Status	Upper middle class; father is MD
Military Service	None
Religion	Attends Episcopal church regularly
Ethnic Background	Both parents are African American
Roles/Relationships	Has many close friends at school & started dating a new boyfriend; participates in sorority community service literacy project; sees parents q 3–4 wk either at home or at school & usually talks on phone c̄ mother 1 ×/wk.
Characteristic Patterns of Daily Living	Wakes at 8 AM, eats bagel & walks to 9 AM class; in classes till noon; eats lunch at cafeteria c̄ boyfriend; reads or exercises to 4 PM; returns to sorority house & talks c̄ friends; has dinner at house; studies in library c̄ boyfriend until MN; boyfriend walks her home; goes to bed about 2 AM.

continued

HEALTH MAINTENANCE ACTIVITIES

Sleep	5–6 hr during wk; 8–10 on wkends
Diet	Watches fats & sweets
Exercise	Swims 3–4 ×/wk for 1 hr
Stress Management	Swimming, music
Use of Safety Devices	Wears seat belt; doesn't walk alone at night on campus
Health Check-Ups	Routine gyn exam 2 mo ago

PHYSICAL ASSESSMENT

This assessment is more in-depth than a physical examination would typically be for this type of patient. The complete assessment is included to illustrate documentation methods.

Eyes

Visual Acuity

Distance vision: 20/30 OD, 20/20 OS
Near vision: reads newspaper s̄ errors
Color vision: identifies colors in room correctly

Visual Fields

Intact

External Eye and Lacrimal Apparatus

Eyelids: s̄ inflammation, Ø ptosis or lid lag
Lacrimal apparatus
    Inspection: s̄ enlargement, swelling, redness, tearing, Ø exudate
    Palpation: s̄ d/c

Extraocular Muscle Function

Corneal light reflex: symmetric s̄ strabismus
Cover/uncover test: s̄ deviation
Cardinal fields of gaze: intact s̄ nystagmus

Anterior Segment Structures

Conjunctiva: sl injected s̄ lesions, foreign bodies, purulent d/c, or
    excessive tearing
Sclera: white s̄ redness or lesions
Cornea: moist & shiny, clear, s̄ d/c or opacities
Anterior chamber: clear, entire iris illuminated
Iris: brown & intact
Pupils: PERRLA (pupils equal [5 mm], round, & react to light &
    accommodation)
Lens: clear, s̄ opacities

Posterior Segment Structures

Retinal structures: red reflex present bilaterally, discs flat c̄ sharp margins,
    vessels are in A/V ratio of 2:3; s̄ nicking; background uniformly
    brownish s̄ hemorrhages or exudates
Macula: c̄ even color

continued

Ears

Auditory Screening

Voice-whisper test: intact
Tuning fork tests
    Weber: midline $\bar{s}$ lateralization
    Rinne: air conduction > bone conduction (AC>BC) & = bilaterally

External Ear

Inspection: $\bar{s}$ redness, drainage, nodules, lesions; EAC clear $\bar{s}$ inflammation
    & $\bar{c}$ small amt light brown cerumen
Palpation: $\bar{s}$ tenderness

Otoscopic Assessment

TMs shiny gray & mobile $\bar{c}$ visible landmarks, $\bar{s}$ bulging or perforation

Nose

External Inspection

Midline $\bar{s}$ swelling, bleeding, lesions, or masses

Patency

Nares patent

Internal Inspection

Septum midline $\bar{s}$ perforations or polyps; mucosa pink & moist $\bar{s}$ swelling
    or purulent d/c

Sinuses

Inspection

Ø swelling of frontal/maxillary sinuses

Palpation and Percussion

Nontender

Mouth and Throat

Mouth

Breath

Foul smelling

Lips

Inspection: pink & dry $\bar{s}$ lesions, masses, or tenderness
Palpation: $\bar{s}$ lesions

Tongue

Midline, pink, well papillated & $\bar{s}$ fasciculations, lesions, swelling, or
    bleeding

Buccal Mucosa

Bluish hue, moist $\bar{s}$ lesions

Gums

Pink & moist, $\bar{s}$ swelling or bleeding

Teeth

All present in proper alignment $\bar{s}$ caries

Palate

Intact, rises $\bar{c}$ phonation

Throat

Red & swollen $\bar{c}$ 2⊕–3⊕ tonsils & $\bar{c}$ white exudates; uvula midline;
    Ø gag reflex

LABORATORY DATA

Rapid Strep Test: Positive (normal value is negative)

NURSING CHECKLIST
Eyes, Ears, Nose, Mouth, and Throat Assessment

Eyes
- Visual Acuity
  - Distance Vision
  - Near Vision
  - Color Vision
- Visual Fields
- External Eye and Lacrimal Apparatus
  - Eyelids
  - Lacrimal Apparatus
    - Inspection
    - Palpation
- Extraocular Muscle Function
  - Corneal Light Reflex
  - Cover/Uncover Test
  - Cardinal Fields of Gaze
- Anterior Segment Structures
  - Conjunctiva
  - Sclera
  - Cornea
  - Anterior Chamber
  - Iris
  - Pupil
  - Lens
- Posterior Segment Structures
  - Retinal Structures
  - Macula

Ears
- Auditory Screening
  - Voice-Whisper Test
  - Tuning Fork Tests
    - Weber Test
    - Rinne Test
- External Ear
  - Inspection
  - Palpation
- Otoscopic Assessment

Nose
- External Inspection
- Patency
- Internal Inspection

Sinuses
- Inspection
- Palpation and Percussion

continued

Mouth and Throat
- Mouth
  - Breath
  - Lips
    Inspection
    Palpation
  - Tongue
  - Buccal Mucosa
  - Gums
  - Teeth
  - Palate
- Throat

Special Techniques
- Transillumination of the Sinuses

REVIEW QUESTIONS AND ACTIVITIES

1. Name and describe the three layers of the eye.

2. Compare and contrast physical assessment findings for bacterial and viral conjunctivitis.

3. Describe the technique for funduscopic examination.

4. Describe the testing of visual fields by confrontation.

5. List and describe four common abnormalities found in examination of the retina.

6. List and describe four common abnormalities found in examination of the ear.

7. Compare and contrast physical assessment findings for allergic and bacterial rhinitis.

Questions 8 and 9 refer to the following situation:
    While making rounds of your patients in a local nursing home, you are asked to assess an 84-year-old woman who is complaining that her left ear is "stopped up." You suspect that she has a cerumen impaction.

8. What physical findings would you expect with a cerumen impaction?
   a. The tympanic membrane is red and bulging.
   b. The tympanic membrane is not visible because a large area of dark brown, waxy substance is blocking your line of vision.
   c. The external ear canal is pink and without swelling.
   d. Gross hearing by watch tick test is intact.

   The correct answer is (b).

9. While performing the assessment, you also note that this woman is unable to completely close her eyelids. This is called:
   a. Lagophthalmos
   b. Exophthalmos
   c. Enophthalmos
   d. Entropion

   The correct answer is (a).

13

Breasts and Regional Nodes

COMPETENCIES

1. Describe the anatomy and physiology of the breasts and regional lymphatics, including age-related variations.
2. Demonstrate assessment techniques for the evaluation of the breasts and regional lymphatics.
3. Distinguish common variations and abnormal changes of the breasts.
4. Discuss methods of teaching breast self-examination to patients.
5. Identify risk factors for breast cancer.

The breasts hold significant symbolism in our society. In women, they are an external symbol of sexuality, femininity, and nurturance. In men, they symbolize strength, fitness, and masculinity. Breast disease and its devastating effects have come to the forefront of public debate in recent years. Breast cancer incidence rates have increased significantly over the past 50 years; however, survival rates remain constant despite increased research dollars and public attention.

Long-term survival rates have a direct correlation to early detection of breast cancer. Nurses can have a major impact on women's health by teaching women breast self-examination techniques and by supporting women in achieving healthier lifestyles that are believed to diminish breast cancer risk.

This chapter will focus primarily on the female breast because it is a more complicated structure than the male gland and because of the higher incidence of breast disease in women.

ANATOMY AND PHYSIOLOGY

Breasts

The female **breasts** are a pair of mammary glands located on the anterior chest wall, extending vertically from the second to the sixth rib and laterally from the sternal border to the axilla. Anatomically, the breast may be divided into four quadrants: the upper inner quadrant, the lower inner quadrant, the upper outer quadrant, and the lower outer quadrant (see Figure 13-1). The upper outer quadrant, which extends into the axilla, is known as the **tail of Spence**. The breasts are supported by a bed of muscles: the pectoralis major and minor, latissimus dorsi, serratus anterior, rectus abdominus, and external oblique muscles, which extend vertically from the deep fascia (see Figure 13-2). **Cooper's ligaments**, which extend vertically from the deep fascia

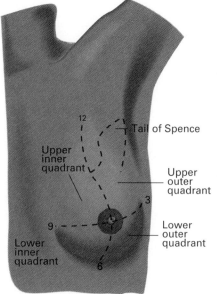

Figure 13-1   Quadrants of the Left Breast

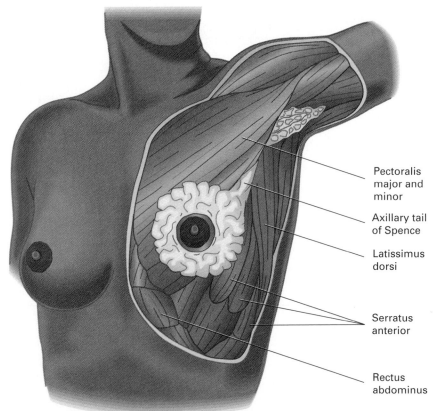

Pectoralis major and minor

Axillary tail of Spence

Latissimus dorsi

Serratus anterior

Rectus abdominus

Figure 13-2   Muscles Supporting the Breast

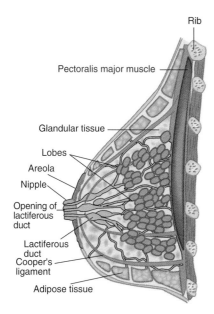

Figure 13-3 Cross Section of the Left Breast

through the breast to the inner layer of the skin, provide support for the breast tissue (refer to Figure 13-3).

In the center of each breast is the **nipple**, a round, hairless pigmented protrusion of erectile tissue approximately 0.5 to 1.5 cm in diameter. The nipple becomes more erect during sexual excitement, pregnancy, lactation, cold temperatures, and certain phases of the menstrual cycle. There are 12 to 20 minute openings on the surface of the nipple. These are openings of the **lactiferous ducts** through which milk and colostrum are excreted.

The **milk line**, or **ectodermal galactic band**, shown in Figure 13-4, develops from the axilla to the groin during the fifth week of fetal development. Most of the band atrophies except in the thoracic area, where it forms a mammary ridge. Incomplete atrophy of the galactic band results in the development of extra nipples or breast tissue known as **supernumerary nipples**. The additional nipples or mammary tissue develop along the milk lines and are a normal variant in a small percentage of adult women.

Surrounding the nipple is the **areola**, a pigmented area approximately 2.5 to 10 cm in diameter. The size and pigmentation vary from woman to woman. Several sebaceous glands (**Montgomery's tubercles**) are present on the surface of the areola. These glands lubricate the nipple, helping to keep it supple during lactation. Hair follicles punctuate the border of the areola.

The breast is composed of glandular, connective (Cooper's ligaments), and adipose tissue. The glandular tissue is arranged radially in the form of 12 to 20 **lobes**. This disbursement is similar to a bicycle wheel; each lobe represents a spoke of the wheel and extends from a central point (the nipple) to the outermost border (see Figure 13-5). Each lobe is composed of 20 to 40 **lobules** that contain milk producing glands called **alveoli** or **acini**. The lobules are arranged in grapelike bunches and are clustered around several ducts. These ducts gradually form one main lactiferous (excretory) duct per lobe. Each lactiferous duct widens to form a sinus that acts as a reservoir for milk during lactation. The duct opens onto the surface of the nipple. The lobes are lodged in tissue composed of subcutaneous and **retromammary adipose tissue**, and it is this tissue that composes the bulk of the breast.

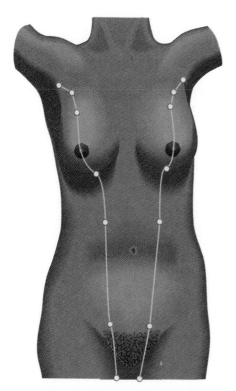

Figure 13-4 Ectodermal Galactic Bands

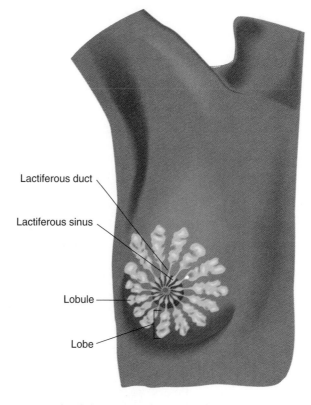

Figure 13-5 Glandular Tissue of the Right Breast

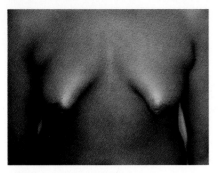

Figure 13-6 Gynecomastia *Courtesy of Steven M. Lynch, M.D.*

The function of the female breast is to produce milk for the nourishment and protection of neonates and infants. In many cultures, breasts provide sensual pleasure during sexual foreplay and breastfeeding. The breasts also provide some protection to the anterior thoracic chest wall.

The male breast is composed of a well-developed areola and a small nipple that has immature tissue underneath. **Gynecomastia**, the enlargement of male breast tissue (see Figure 13-6), may occur normally in adolescent and in elderly males. The condition is normally unilateral and temporary.

Table 13-1   Sexual Maturity Rating for Female Breast Development

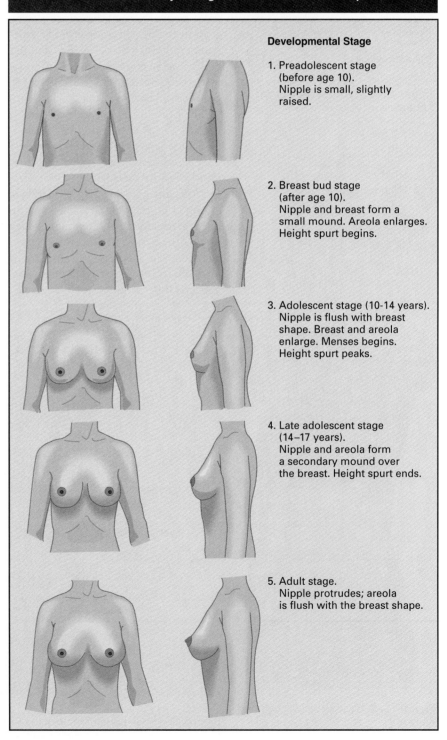

Developmental Stage

1. Preadolescent stage (before age 10). Nipple is small, slightly raised.

2. Breast bud stage (after age 10). Nipple and breast form a small mound. Areola enlarges. Height spurt begins.

3. Adolescent stage (10-14 years). Nipple is flush with breast shape. Breast and areola enlarge. Menses begins. Height spurt peaks.

4. Late adolescent stage (14–17 years). Nipple and areola form a secondary mound over the breast. Height spurt ends.

5. Adult stage. Nipple protrudes; areola is flush with the breast shape.

Regional Nodes

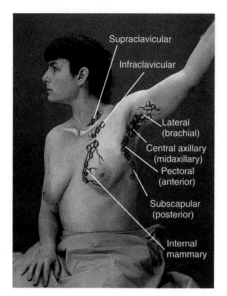

Figure 13-7 Regional Lymphatics and Drainage Patterns of the Left Breast

The **lymphatic drainage** (the yellow alkaline drainage composed primarily of lymphocytes) of the breast is via a complex network of lymph vessels and nodes. It is estimated that a majority of the lymph from the breast flows to the axillary nodes. The **axillary nodes** are composed of four groups: central axillary nodes (midaxillary), pectoral nodes (anterior), subscapular nodes (posterior), and lateral nodes (brachial). The central axillary nodes receive lymph from the three other nodal groups. The lymph is then channeled from the central axillary nodes to the infraclavicular and supraclavicular nodes. The remainder of the lymph flows into the internal mammary chain or directly to the infraclavicular chain via the Rotter's nodes, deep into the chest or abdominal cavity, or to the other breast. The pattern of lymph drainage is illustrated in Figure 13-7.

The axillary nodes are easily accessible by palpation because of their superficial location. The internal mammary nodes are very deep in the chest wall and are inaccessible by palpation.

Adolescent Development

Female breast development usually begins at 10 to 11 years of age and is stimulated by estrogen release during puberty. Enhanced fat deposition increases the size of the breasts, while the ductal system, lobes, and lobules increase in number and in size. Asymmetry in breast development is not abnormal. Tanner's sexual maturity ratings describe the pattern of adolescent breast development (refer to Table 13-1).

❖ HEALTH HISTORY

The breasts and regional nodes health history provides insight into the link between a patient's life/lifestyle and breast information and pathology.

PATIENT PROFILE	*Diseases that are age-, sex-, and race-specific for the breasts and regional nodes are listed.*
Age	Early menarche increases the risk of breast cancer (puberty) Gynecomastia (adolescent and elderly males) Fibroadenoma (15–20), Cystic hyperplasia (benign breast disease) (30–55) Mastitis and plugged milk ducts (childbearing years) Increasing risk of breast cancer (first pregnancy after 30, or nulliparous) Paget's disease (postmenopausal) Incidence of breast cancer increases (50 or older)
Sex	
Female	99% of all breast disease is in women 182,000 new cases of breast cancer in women in 1994, one in every eight or nine women in the United States will develop breast cancer (American Cancer Society, 1994)
Male	1,000 new cases of breast cancer in men in 1994 (American Cancer Society, 1994) Gynecomastia (adolescent and elderly men)
Race	African American cancer death rate is higher than that of Caucasian women in the United States

continued

CHIEF COMPLAINT	*Common chief complaints for the breasts and regional nodes are defined and information on the characteristics of each sign/symptom is provided.*
Breast Mass	Presence of a lump in the breast
Location	Anywhere in the breast or axilla; usually in the upper outer quadrant, unilateral or bilateral
Quality	Size, size in relationship to menstrual cycle, shape, consistency, mobility, delineation of borders
Quantity	Number of masses
Associated Manifestations	Tenderness, presence of dimpling, nipple retraction, nipple discharge, tender palpable lymph nodes
Aggravating Factors	Methylxanthines, recent injury to breast
Alleviating Factors	Aspiration, biopsy, surgery, radiation, chemotherapy
Timing	Incidence rises with age, in relation to menses and ovulation
Breast Tenderness	Sensation of discomfort in the breast
Location	Pinpoint, discrete, generalized, unilateral or bilateral
Quality	Rate pain on a scale of 1 to 10; pain sensation: sharp, dull, pulling
Associated Manifestations	Mass, dimpling, nipple retraction, breast swelling, premenstrual syndrome symptoms (see Chapter 19), induration, discharge, palpable nodes, fever, breastfeeding
Aggravating Factors	Recent injury to breast, palpation, vigorous exercise, oral contraceptives, chlorpromazine, or alpha-methyldopa
Alleviating Factors	Warm compresses, analgesics, massage, support bras, aspiration, biopsy, surgery, breastfeeding, cessation of aggravating medications
Timing	In relation to menses or ovulation, pregnancy, lactation, activity
Discharge	Abnormal substance expressed from the breast
Location	From the nipple or sebaceous gland, unilateral or bilateral
Quality	Color, odor, consistency
Associated Manifestations	Redness, swelling, induration (hardening), mass, dimpling, nipple retraction, breast swelling, palpable nodes, lactation, headaches, history of pituitary disorders, fever
Aggravating Factors	Trauma to breast, breastfeeding, pituitary tumor, hyperthyroidism, chlorpromazine, alpha-methyldopa, digitalis, diuretics, oral contraceptives, papillomas, carcinomas of the ducts
Alleviating Factors	Breastfeeding, biopsy, surgery, cessation of medications
Timing	In relation to pregnancy, menses, lactation, ovulation

continued

PAST HEALTH HISTORY	*The various components of the past health history are linked to breasts and regional nodes pathology and related information.*
Medical	
Breast Specific	Benign breast disease, cysts, fibroadenomas, intraductal papillomas, mammary duct ectasia, mastitis, areas of greater density, breast cancer, masses, breast abscess, Paget's disease
Nonbreast Specific	Thyroid disorders, pituitary tumor, chest radiation, cancer of ovary or endometrium, obesity
Surgical	Breast biopsy, lumpectomy, quadrantectomy, partial mastectomy, radical mastectomy, breast reduction or augmentation
Medications	Oral contraceptives, chlorpromazine, alpha-methlydopa, diuretics, digitalis, steroids, tricyclics may precipitate nipple discharge; use of estrogen-based oral contraceptives has been linked with increased incidences of breast cancer (Love & Lindsey, 1995)
Allergies	Localized rashes of breast contact dermatitis
Injuries/Accidents	May cause hematoma or edema; lumps may result from previous trauma to soft tissue
Disabilities/Handicaps	Grossly pendulous breasts can cause back pain and respiratory distress in compromised patients
Childhood Illnesses	Chicken pox scarring of cutaneous tissue
FAMILY HEALTH HISTORY	*Breasts and regional nodes diseases that are familial are listed.*
	8% to 20% of breast cancers are thought to have a familial link via a primary relative, e.g., mother, sister, grandmother. The link is stronger if the family history includes bilateral breast cancer. Benign breast disease
SOCIAL HISTORY	*The components of the social history are linked to breasts and regional nodes factors/pathology.*
Alcohol Use	Loose association between alcohol intake of more than three glasses per day and increased incidence of breast cancer
Tobacco Use	No association between smoking and breast cancer
Work Environment	Radiation exposure
Home Environment	Increased incidence of breast cancer noted in urban dwellers
Economic Status	Increased incidence of breast cancer in women of upper socioeconomic status (Love & Lindsey, 1995)
Ethnic Background	Incidence of breast cancer among American and European women is higher than that of Japanese and Middle Eastern women
HEALTH MAINTENANCE ACTIVITIES	*This information provides a bridge between the health maintenance activities and breasts and regional nodes function.*

continued

Diet	Strong correlation between high-fat diet and incidence of breast cancer; increased incidence of benign breast disease with caffeine use
Exercise	Strong correlation between obesity and incidence of breast cancer
Use of Safety Devices	Use of restraining devices in motor vehicles to prevent chest trauma
Health Check-Ups	Monthly breast self-examination Clinical physical examination every 3 years for women aged 20–40 Clinical physical examination every year for women over age 40 Baseline screening mammogram at age 40 Mammogram every 1–2 years for women aged 40–49 Annual mammograms after age 50

EQUIPMENT

- Towel
- Drape
- Centimeter ruler
- Teaching aid for breast self-examination

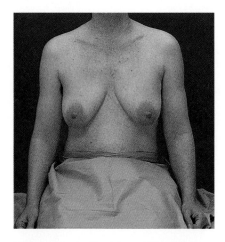

Figure 13-8   Position of Patient for Breast Inspection: Arms at Side

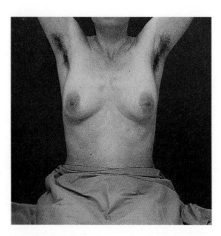

Figure 13-9   Position of Patient for Breast Inspection: Arms Overhead

ASSESSMENT OF THE FEMALE BREASTS AND REGIONAL NODES

Physical assessment produces feelings of fear, anxiety, embarrassment, and loss of control in many women. These feelings may be reduced by the sensitivity of the nurse before, during, and after assessment of the breasts. Assessment of the female breasts and regional nodes includes inspection and palpation.

Inspection of the Breasts

E   **1.** Position the patient uncovered to the waist, seated at the edge of the examination table, and facing you.
  2. Instruct the patient to let her arms relax by her sides as shown in Figure 13-8.
  3. Inspect the breasts, axillae, areolar areas, and nipples for color, vascularity, thickening, edema, size, symmetry, contour, lesions or masses, and exudates.
  4. Repeat the above inspection sequence with the patient's arms raised over her head (see Figure 13-9). This will accentuate any retraction (tissue drawn back) if present.
  5. Repeat inspection sequence with patient pressing hands into hips, which will contract the pectoral muscles (see Figure 13-10). Once again, if retraction is present, it will be more pronounced with this maneuver.
  6. Have the patient lean forward to allow the breasts to hang freely away from the chest wall as shown in Figure 13-11, and repeat the inspection sequence. Provide support to the patient as necessary.

Color

E   Inspect the breasts, areolar areas, nipples, and axillae for coloration.
N   *Normally, the breasts and axillae are flesh colored and the areolar areas and nipples are darker in pigmentation. This pigmentation is normally enhanced during pregnancy. Moles and nevi are normal variants, and terminal hair may be present on the areolar areas.*
A   Reddened areas of the breasts, nipples, or axillae are abnormal findings.
P   Redness may be an indication of inflammation, an infection such as mastitis, or inflammatory carcinoma.
A   Striae (see Figure 13-12) are streaks over the breasts or axillae and are abnormal. In light-skinned individuals, new striae are red and become silver to white in coloration with age. In dark-skinned individuals, new

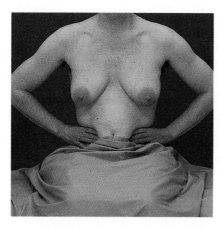

Figure 13-10 Position of Patient for Breast Inspection: Hands Pressed Against Hips

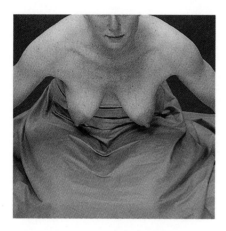

Figure 13-11 Position of Patient for Breast Inspection: Leaning Forward

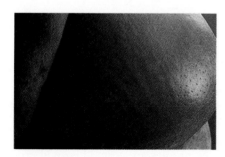

Figure 13-12 Striae Secondary to Inflammatory Breast Cancer. Also note peau d'orange. *Courtesy of Dr. S. Eva Singletary, University of Texas, M.D. Anderson Cancer Center*

E	Examination
N	Normal Findings
A	Abnormal Findings
P	Pathophysiology

striae are a ruddy, dark-brown color, and older striae become lighter than the skin color.

P Striae are caused by rapid stretching of the skin, which damages the elastic fibers found in the dermis. Though normal in pregnancy, striae are often observed with obesity.

✓ NURSING CHECKLIST
General Approach to Breast Assessment

Prior to the assessment:

1. When possible, instruct the patient to neither use creams, lotions, or powders, nor shave her underarms 24 to 48 hours before the scheduled assessment. Application of toiletry products may mask or alter the nature of the surface integument of the breasts, and shaving the underarms may cause folliculitis, which may result in pain upon palpation.

2. Encourage the patient to express any anxieties and concerns about the physical assessment. Acknowledge anxieties and validate concerns. Many women avoid having their breasts assessed because they fear abnormal findings. Assure the patient that she has taken a positive step in her own health care by having her breasts assessed.

3. Inform the patient that the assessment should not be painful but may be uncomfortable at times. This is especially true if the patient is currently experiencing menses or ovulation.

4. Adopt a nonjudgmental and supportive attitude.

5. Be aware of the impact of culture on breast assessment and breast self-examination. In Asian cultures, breast self-examination may be considered a form of masturbation. In some Middle Eastern cultures, baring the breasts to a male is taboo, even if the male is a health care provider.

6. Instruct the patient to remove any jewelry that might interfere with the assessment.

7. Ensure that the room is warm enough to prevent chilling, and provide additional draping material as necessary.

8. Warm your hands with warm water or by rubbing them together prior to the assessment.

9. Ensure that privacy will be maintained during the assessment. Provide screens, closed doors, and door sign stating that an assessment is in progress.

During the assessment:

1. Inform the patient of what you are going to do before you do it.

2. Use this time to educate the patient about her body.

3. Offer the patient the opportunity to ask questions about her body and sexuality.

4. Keep areas not being assessed appropriately draped.

5. Always compare right and left breasts.

6. Wear gloves if the patient has any discharge from the breast.

After the assessment:

1. Assess whether the patient needs assistance in dressing.

2. After the patient is dressed, discuss the experience with her, invite questions and comments, listen carefully, and provide her with information regarding the assessment.

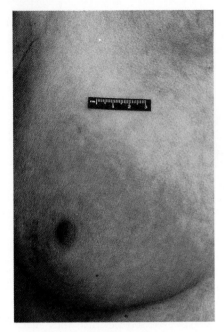

Figure 13-13 Erythema with Abnormal Vascular Pattern Secondary to Inflammatory Breast Cancer *Courtesy of Dr. S. Eva Singletary, University of Texas, M.D. Anderson Cancer Center*

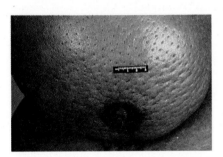

Figure 13-14 Peau d'orange *Courtesy of Dr. S. Eva Singletary, University of Texas, M.D. Anderson Cancer Center*

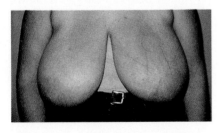

Figure 13-15 Massive Hypertrophy of Breasts *Courtesy of Steven M. Lynch, M.D.*

E	Examination
N	Normal Findings
A	Abnormal Findings
P	Pathophysiology

Vascularity

E Observe the entire surface of each breast for superficial vascular patterns.

N *Normal superficial vascular patterns are diffuse and symmetrical.*

A Abnormal patterns of vascularity are focal or unilateral.

P Focal or unilateral superficial vascular patterns (see Figure 13-13) occur as the result of an increased blood supply and may indicate tumor formation, which requires increased vascularization and an increased blood supply.

Thickening/Edema

E Observe the breasts, axillae, and nipples for thickening or edema.

N *Normally, thickening or edema is not found in the breasts, axillae, and nipples.*

A Thickening or edema of the breast tissue or nipple may present itself as enlarged skin pores that give the appearance of an orange rind (**peau d'orange**). It may be more prevalent in the dependent or inferior portions of the breast (see Figure 13-14).

P This peau d'orange appearance may be indicative of obstructed lymphatic drainage due to a tumor.

Size and Symmetry

E Observe the breasts, axillae, areolar areas, and nipples for size and symmetry.

N *Normally, there is some difference in the size of the breasts and areolar areas, with the breast on the side of the dominant arm being larger. Bilateral hypertrophy of the breasts may be normal for some patients (see Figure 13-15). Nipple inversion, which is present from puberty, is a normal variant and is of no clinical consequence except for difficulty in breastfeeding. Nipples should point upward and laterally, or they may point outward and downward (see Figure 13-16A). Supernumerary nipples are a variant of normal and have no pathological significance in either males or females.*

A Significant differences in the size or symmetry of the breasts, axillae, areolar areas, or nipples are abnormal (see Figure 13-17).

P Significant enlargement of one breast, axilla, or areola may be indicative of tumor formation.

A Recent inversion, flattening, or depression of a nipple is abnormal.

P A sudden onset of nipple inversion, flattening, or depression is indicative of nipple retraction, which is suggestive of an underlying cancer (see Figure 13-18).

A Asymmetry in the directions in which the nipples are pointed is an abnormal finding (see Figure 13-16B).

P Asymmetrical nipple direction is suggestive of an underlying invasive process that is contorting nipple tissue. Often the direction of nipple deviation is toward the underlying process.

A Nipples that have been inverted since puberty and become broader or thicker are abnormal.

P Additional broadening or thickening of a previously inverted nipple may be indicative of tumor formation.

A Lack of breast tissue unilaterally is abnormal.

P Unilateral reduction of breast tissue or structures may result from trauma, mastectomy, or breast reduction.

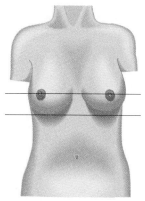
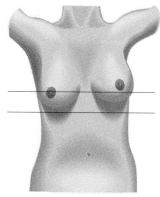

A. Symmetrical without Deviation

B. Asymmetrical with Deviation

Figure 13-16 Deviation of Nipples

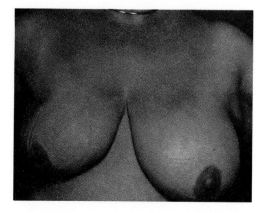

Figure 13-17 Asymmetry of Breasts Due to Cancer *Courtesy of Dr. S. Eva Singletary, University of Texas, M.D. Anderson Cancer Center*

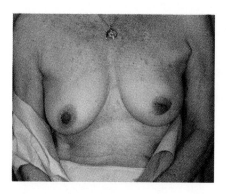

Figure 13-18 Nipple Retraction of Left Breast *Courtesy of Steven M. Lynch, M.D.*

Contour

E **1.** Assess the breasts for contour.
    2. Compare the breasts to each other.
N *The breast is normally convex, without flattening, retractions, or dimpling.*
A Dimpling, retractions, flattening (see Figure 13-19), or other changes in breast contour are abnormal.
P Changes in contour are highly suggestive of cancer. The invasive process that causes the contour changes is the result of fibrotic shortening and disablement of the Cooper's ligament. Fat necrosis and mammary duct ectasia may also cause retraction, dimpling, and puckering.

Lesions/Masses

E Inspect the breasts, axillae, areolar areas, and nipples for lesions or masses.
N *Normally, the breasts, axillae, areolar areas, and nipples are free of masses, tumors, and primary or secondary lesions.*
A Breast masses, tumors, nodules, or cysts of any kind are abnormal.
P See Table 13-2 for common pathologies of breast masses.
A A scaly, eczema-like erosion of the nipple, or persistent dermatitis of the areola and nipple, is abnormal.
P Persistent eczematous dermatitis of the areola and nipple region is suggestive of **Paget's disease**, a malignant neoplasm, which is usually unilateral in its involvement.

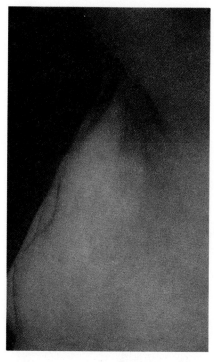

Figure 13-19 Dimpling of Left Breast Tissue *Courtesy of Dr. S. Eva Singletary, University of Texas, M.D. Anderson Cancer Center*

☾☽ THINK ABOUT IT

Oral Contraceptives and Cancer Risk

There have been recent studies indicating a correlation between estrogen-based oral contraceptive use and breast cancer, with a two- to fourfold increased risk noted for some populations. During the breast assessment, the patient asks you about the association between oral contraceptives and increased breast cancer risk because she is considering switching from oral contraceptives to another method of birth control. How would you respond?

Table 13-2 Characteristics of Common Breast Masses

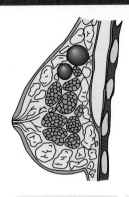 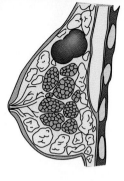 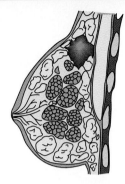

	Gross Cyst	Fibroadenoma	Carcinoma
Age	30-60; diminishes after menopause	puberty to menopause 50 years	most common after
Shape	round	round, lobular, or ovoid	irregular, stellate, or crab-like
Consistency	soft to firm	usually firm	firm to hard
Discreteness	well defined	well defined	not clearly defined
Number	single or grouped	most often single	usually single
Mobility	mobile	very mobile	may be mobile or fixed to skin, underlying tissue or chest wall
Tenderness	tender	nontender	usually nontender
Erythema	no erythema	no erythema	may be present
Retraction/ dimpling	not present	not present	often present

Discharge

E Observe for spontaneous discharge from the nipples or other areas of the breast.

N *In the nonpregnant, nonlactating female, there should be no discharge. During pregnancy and up through the first week after birth, there may be a yellow discharge known as* **colostrum**. *During lactation, there is a white discharge of breast milk.*

A The presence of a nipple discharge in the nonpregnant, nonlactating woman is abnormal.

P Nipple discharge may be caused by the use of tranquilizers, oral contraceptives, manual stimulation, or infection. It may also be indicative of malignant or benign breast disease.

Palpation

Palpation is performed in a sequential manner:

1. Supraclavicular and infraclavicular lymph node areas.
2. Breasts, with the patient in sitting position
   a. Arms at side
   b. Arms raised over head.
3. Axillary lymph node regions.
4. Breasts, with the patient in supine position.

⊘ NURSING ALERT

Examining Nipple Discharge

If a patient is found to have abnormal nipple discharge:

1. Don gloves before proceeding with the assessment.
2. Note the following: color, consistency, amount of discharge, unilateral or bilateral, spontaneous or provoked.
3. With a sterile, cotton-tipped swab, obtain a sample of the discharge so that a culture and sensitivity as well as a gram stain can be obtained.
4. Follow your institution's guidelines for sample preparation.

E	**Examination**
N	**Normal Findings**
A	**Abnormal Findings**
P	**Pathophysiology**

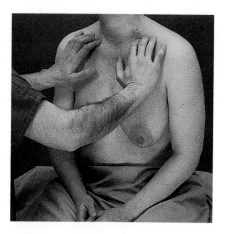

Figure 13-20 Palpation of Supraclavicular Nodes

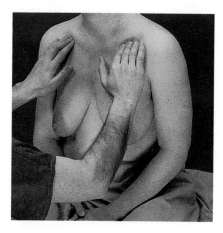

Figure 13-21 Palpation of Infraclavicular Nodes

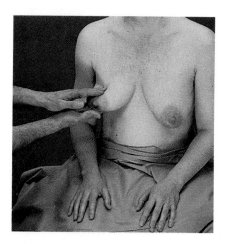

Figure 13-22 Bimanual Palpation of the Breasts While Patient Is Sitting

E	**Examination**
N	**Normal Findings**
A	**Abnormal Findings**
P	**Pathophysiology**

Supraclavicular and Infraclavicular Lymph Nodes

E 1. Have patient seated and uncovered to the waist.
2. Encourage the patient to relax the muscles of the head and neck because this pulls the clavicles down and allows a thorough exploration of the supraclavicular area.
3. Flex the patient's head to relax the sternocleidomastoid muscle.
4. Standing in front of the patient, in a bilateral and simultaneous motion, place the finger pads over the patient's clavicles, lateral to the tendinous portion of the sternocleidomastoid muscles.
5. Using a rotary motion of the palmar surfaces of the fingers, probe deeply into the scalene triangles in order to palpate the supraclavicular lymph nodes (see Figure 13-20).
6. Palpate the infraclavicular nodes using the same rotary motion of the palmar surfaces of the fingers (see Figure 13-21).

N *Palpable lymph nodes less than 1 cm in diameter are usually considered normal and clinically insignificant provided that there are no additional enlarged lymph nodes found in other regions such as the axilla. Palpation should not elicit pain.*

A Fixed, firm, immobile, irregular lymph nodes more than 1 cm in diameter are considered abnormal.

P These nodes are considered suspicious for metastasis from a variety of sources or primary lymphoma.

A Enlarged, painful, or tender nodes that are matted together are abnormal.

P Tender, enlarged nodes may indicate systemic infection or carcinoma.

Breasts: Patient in Sitting Position

E 1. Place the patient in a sitting position with arms at sides.
2. Stand to the patient's right side, facing the patient.
3. Using the palmar surfaces of the fingers of the dominant hand, begin the palpation at the outer quadrant of the patient's right breast.
4. Use the other hand to support the inferior aspect of the breast.
5. In small-breasted patients, the dominant hand can palpate the tissue against the chest wall, but if the breasts are pendulous, use a bimanual technique of palpation as shown in Figure 13-22.
6. Palpate in a downward fashion, sweeping from the outer quadrants to the sternal boarder of each breast.
7. Repeat this sequence on the other breast.
8. Repeat the entire assessment with the patient's arms raised over her head to enhance any potential retraction.

N *The consistency of the breasts is widely variable, depending on age, time in menstrual cycle, and proportion of adipose tissue. The breasts may have a nodular or granular consistency that may be enhanced prior to the onset of menses. The inferior aspect of the breast will be somewhat firmer due to a transverse inframammary ridge. Palpation should not elicit significant tenderness, although the breasts and especially the nipples may become full and slightly tender premenstrually. Breasts that feel fluid filled or firm throughout with accompanying inferior suture-line scars are indicative of breast augmentation.*

A The presence of any lump, mass, thickening, or unilateral granulation that is noticeably different from the rest of the breast tissue should be considered suspicious and abnormal.

P For a description of breast masses and their pathologies, refer to Table 13-2.

A Significant breast tenderness is abnormal and may indicate mammary duct ectasia.

P This is a benign condition in which lactiferous ducts become inflamed.

❧ NURSING TIP

The Patient with a Known Breast Mass

If the patient has a known mass or irregularity in one breast, begin palpation on the unaffected breast. The unaffected breast should indicate the patient's normal physiological state.

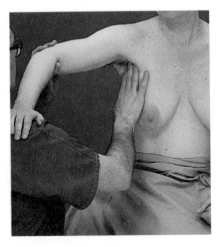

Figure 13-23 Palpation of Axillary Nodes

E	**Examination**
N	**Normal Findings**
A	**Abnormal Findings**
P	**Pathophysiology**

Axillary Lymph Node Region

E 1. Stand at the patient's right side, facing the patient.
   2. Tell the patient to take a deep breath and relax the shoulders and arms (this relaxes the areas to be palpated).
   3. Using your left hand, adduct the patient's right arm so that it is close to the chest wall. This maneuver relaxes the muscles.
   4. Support the patient's right arm with your left hand.
   5. Using the palmar surfaces of the finger pads of your right hand, place your fingers into the apex of the axilla. Your fingers will be positioned behind the pectoral muscles.
   6. Gently roll the tissue against the chest wall and axillary muscles as you work downward.
   7. Locate and palpate the four axillary lymph node groups:
      a. Posterior axillary group (subscapular) at the anterior edge of the latissimus dorsi muscle.
      b. Central axillary group (midaxillary) at the thoracic wall of the axilla.
      c. Anterior axillary group (pectoral) behind the lateral edge of the pectoralis major muscle.
      d. Lateral axillary group (brachial) on the inner aspect of the upper part of the humerus, close to the axillary vein.
   8. Repeat this method of palpation with the patient's arm abducted, i.e., instruct the patient to remain in the same position and lift the upper arm and elbow away from the body. Support the patient's abducted arm on your left shoulder, as shown in Figure 13-23.
   9. Palpate the patient's left axilla using the same technique.

N *Palpable lymph nodes less than 1 cm in diameter are usually considered normal and clinically insignificant provided that there are no additional enlarged lymph nodes found in other regions. Palpation should not elicit pain.*

A Fixed, firm, immobile, irregular lymph nodes more than 1 cm in diameter, are considered abnormal.

P These nodes are considered suggestive of metastasis from a variety of sources or primary lymphoma.

A Enlarged, painful, or tender nodes that are matted together are abnormal.

P Tender, enlarged nodes may be indicative of a systemic infection or carcinoma.

Breasts: Patient in Supine Position

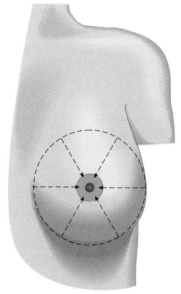

A. Wedge

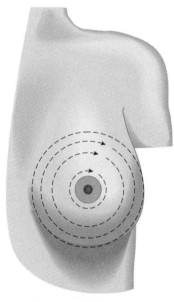

B. Concentric Circles

Figure 13-24   Palpation Methods

E   1. Keep the patient uncovered to the waist.

2. Instruct the patient to assume a supine position. This position spreads the breast tissue thinly and evenly over the chest wall. Palpation is more accurate when there is the least amount of breast tissue between the skin and the chest wall.

3. If the breasts are large, place a small towel or folded sheet under the patient's right shoulder. This helps to flatten the breast more.

4. Stand at the right side of the patient. Palpation can be performed with the patient's arms at her sides or with her right arm above her head.

5. Using the palmar surfaces of the fingers, palpate the right breast by compressing the mammary tissues gently against the chest wall. Palpation may be performed from the periphery to the nipple, in either concentric circles or in wedge sections (see Figure 13-24 and Figure 13-25A).

6. Palpation must include the tail of Spence, periphery, and areola (see Figure 13-25B).

7. Finally, don gloves and compress the nipple to express any discharge, as shown in Figure 13-25C. If discharge is noted, palpate the breast along the wedge radii to determine from which lobe the discharge is originating.

8. Repeat procedure on opposite breast.

N   *See previous section on normal breast tissue findings upon palpation. The nipple should be elastic and return readily to its previous shape. No discharge should be expressed in the nonpregnant, nonlactating patient.*

Refer to Table 13-2 for a description of breast masses. Table 13-3 offers a list of breast mass characteristics that are used to evaluate abnormal findings.

A   Loss of nipple elasticity or nipple thickening is abnormal.

P   Loss of elasticity in the nipple may indicate tumor formation.

A   Milky-white discharge in a nonpregnant, nonlactating patient may be non-puerperal galactorrhea.

P   Nonpuerperal galactorrhea is either hormonally induced from lesions of the anterior pituitary gland or drug induced.

A   Nonmilky discharge from the nipple is abnormal.

P   Nonmilky discharge may be indicative of benign or malignant breast disease such as intraductal papilloma.

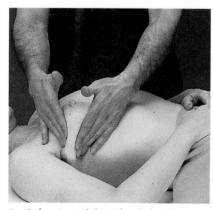

A. Palpation of the Glandular Tissue

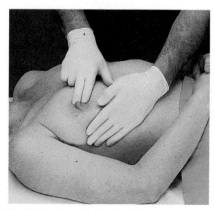

B. Palpation of the Areola

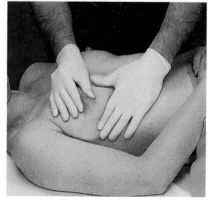

C. Compression of the Nipple

Figure 13-25   Palpation of the Breasts While Patient is Supine

Table 13-3 Evaluation of Breast Mass Characteristics

If a mass is noted during palpation, the following information should be obtained regarding the mass. Always note if one or both breasts are involved.

LOCATION

Identify the quadrant involved or visualize the breast with the face of a clock superimposed upon it. The nipple represents the center of the clock. Note where the mass lies in relation to the nipple, e.g., 3 cm from the nipple in the 3 o'clock position.

SIZE

Determine size in centimeters in all three planes (height, width, and depth).

SHAPE

Masses may be round, ovoid, matted, or irregular.

NUMBER

Note if lesions are singular or multiple. Note if one or both breasts are involved.

CONSISTENCY

Masses may be firm, hard, soft, fluid, or cystic.

DEFINITION

Note if the mass borders are discrete or irregular.

MOBILITY

Determine if the mass is fixed or freely movable in relation to the chest wall.

TENDERNESS

Note if palpation elicits pain.

ERYTHEMA

Note any redness over involved area.

DIMPLING OR RETRACTION

Observe for dimpling or retraction as the patient raises arms overhead and presses her hands into her hips.

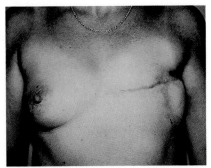

A. Modified Radical

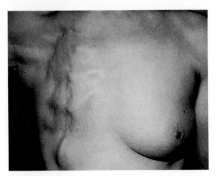

B. Radical

Figure 13-26 Mastectomy Patients
Photos courtesy of Steven M. Lynch, M.D.

🌹 **NURSING TIP**

The Mastectomy Patient

There are four types of **mastectomy** (excision of the breast) procedures. In a simple mastectomy, only the breast is removed. In a modified radical procedure, the breast and lymph nodes from the axilla are removed (see Figure 13-26A). In a radical mastectomy, the breast, lymph nodes from the axilla, and pectoral muscles are removed (see Figure 13-26B). This procedure is rarely performed. In a subcutaneous mastectomy, the skin and nipple are left intact, but the underlying breast tissue and lymph nodes are removed. The patient who has undergone a simple, modified radical, or radical mastectomy literally has had the breast amputated from the chest wall.

Reconstruction techniques include synthetic implants, tissue expansion techniques (in which a temporary device is placed in a subpectoralis-subserratus position between the anterior chest wall and skin and is then inflated with saline over a period of weeks), and latissimus dorsi myocutaneous flap breast reconstruction. A myocutaneous flap reconstruction involves transferring skin from the back or the abdomen to the anterior chest wall.

Assessment of the mastectomy patient will be guided by the type of mastectomy and the presence or absence of reconstructive surgery. Follow the standard assessment procedures and modify your technique to suit the amount of breast tissue and the presence, if any, of a nipple. Always begin the assessment on the unaffected breast. Mastectomy patients should continue to perform monthly breast self-examinations to determine if masses have returned to the excised area. Annual clinical evaluations and mammography are also recommended.

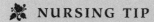

✿ NURSING TIP

Breast Augmentation and Reduction

Breast augmentation, or **augmentation mammoplasty**, is the second most popular surgical procedure among women in the United States. There are three types of synthetic implants: the gel-filled implant, the saline inflatable implant, and the polyurethane-covered implant filled with silicone. When assessing a patient, ask if the breasts have been augmented and what type of implant was used.

Incision sites can be found in the axillae, circumareolar areas, and inframammary creases. Potential complications from augmentation include hematoma; infection; scarring; loss of nipple sensation or skin sensation; pain from engorgement; asymmetry; malpositioning; and breakage of the implant, which can lead to **granulomatous reaction** in the breasts in which small, nodular, inflammatory lesions develop, and a capsular membrane forms over the breasts. The augmented breast will feel firmer upon palpation and remain more erect when the patient is supine.

Breast reduction is usually performed on women who complain of back, neck, or shoulder pain caused by breast hypertrophy. Two types of procedures may be performed to reduce the breasts: free nipple graft and dermal pedicles. The type of procedure can be ascertained from the postoperative scarring. A free nipple graft leaves scars around the nipple and at the inferior mammary fold. A dermal pedicles procedure leaves "keyhole" scars over the breasts.

Potential complications from these breast reduction procedures include hematoma, infection, nipple or skin necrosis, fat necrosis, and asymmetry. Palpation results will depend on the type of procedure performed and the amount of scar tissue formed.

For both breast augmentation and breast reduction, a baseline mammogram should be performed to provide a reference for future mammography. Otherwise, the guidelines for breast self-examination, clinical assessment, and mammography are the same as for women who have not undergone breast surgeries.

Inspection and Palpation of the Male Breasts

Assessment of the male breasts is completed in essentially the same manner as that of the female breast. Modify your technique for a smaller breast with less tissue bulk. Having the patient lean forward is usually not necessary unless gynecomastia is present. Males should perform breast self-examinations every month and have clinical examinations of the breast every 1 to 3 years because 1% of all breast cancer is found in men.

DIAGNOSTIC TECHNIQUES

Etiologic determination of breast or lymphatic masses can be accurately assessed only via a combination of the diagnostic techniques listed below.

1. Mammography: roentgenographic examination of the breasts by means of x-rays, ultrasound, or nuclear magnetic resonance.

2. Ultrasonography: the location, measurement, and delineation of deep structures by measuring the reflection of ultrasonic waves.

❖ ASK YOURSELF

The Patient with a New Breast Mass

What nursing care would you offer to a patient who has a newly diagnosed breast mass? How would you answer her questions about cancer, death, or cure rates? Would you just refer her to a physician to answer her questions? How could you provide positive support, education, and information while working within the framework of nursing practice? Ask yourself how you would want to be treated.

3. Needle aspiration: the withdrawal of fluid or tissue from a cavity via a hollow needle with an aspirator tube attached to one end.

4. Biopsy: the process of removing tissue from a suspicious area for examination. Methods include needle biopsy, punch biopsy, and excisional biopsy.

5. Thermography: measuring the regional temperature of a body part or organ. Malignant lesions are often warmer than nonmalignant areas and are called "hot spots."

 NURSING ALERT

Breast Mass

Any new breast mass or change in a previously benign breast mass must be referred for evaluation.

GERONTOLOGICAL VARIATIONS

The adipose tissue of the breast atrophies with age and is replaced by connective tissue. The glandular tissue gradually decreases and the breasts feel granular instead of lobular. The breasts become smaller, pendulous, and wrinkled. The nipples become smaller and flatter. Ductal tissue becomes more palpable, especially around the nipple, and may become firm and stringy. In addition, the musculature around the breast tends to atrophy, which contributes to the overall "droopiness" of the breasts.

There is increased incidence of breast cancer after the age of 50. In women, it is the second major cause of cancer death, exceeded only by lung cancer.

❀ NURSING TIP

Breast Self-Examination (BSE)

Teaching BSE can be quick and simple.

1. BSE should be performed once a month, 8 days following menses or on any given fixed date. Advise the patient to avoid the time when her breasts might be tender due to menstruation or ovulation. Encourage her to put the BSE on her calendar and include her significant other in the process.

2. **B** (bed): Show the patient how to palpate her breast while supine in bed using the palmar surfaces of her fingers. She should start by placing her right arm over her head and palpating the right breast with the left hand, moving in concentric circles from the periphery inward, including the periphery, tail of Spence, and areola (see Figure 13-27A). Finally, instruct her to squeeze the nipple to examine for discharge. Using the reverse procedure, she should examine the other breast.

3. **S** (standing): Instruct the patient to repeat the above palpation method while standing, as shown in Figures 13-27B and 13-27C.

4. **E** (examination before a mirror): The patient should stand in front of a mirror with her arms at her sides (see Figure 13-27D), then with her arms raised over her head (see Figure 13-27E), and finally with her hands pressed into her hips (see Figure 13-27F). She should examine her breasts for symmetry, retractions, dimpling, inverted nipples, or nipple deviation.

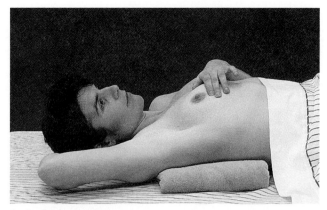

A. In Bed

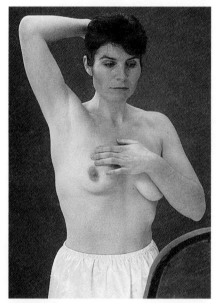

B. Standing

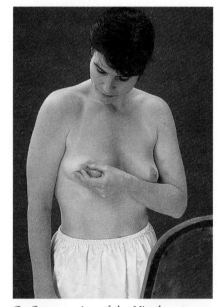

C. Compression of the Nipple

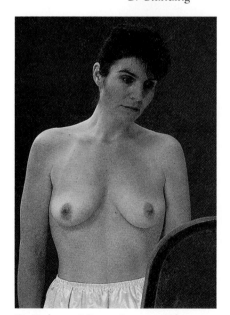

D. Before a Mirror: Arms at Side

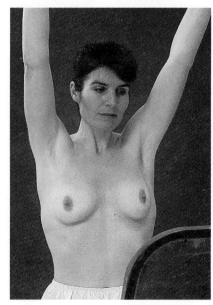

E. Before a Mirror: Arms Overhead

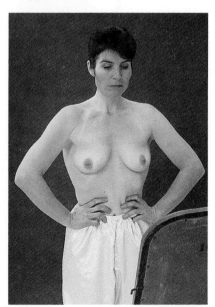

F. Before a Mirror: Hands Pressed into Hips

Figure 13-27 Breast Self-Examination

CASE STUDY

The case study illustrates the application and objective documentation of the breasts and regional nodes assessment.

The Patient with Fibroadenoma of the Left Breast

Ms. Chen came to the family practice clinic after discovering a lump in her left breast while she was showering yesterday.

❖ HEALTH HISTORY

PATIENT PROFILE	31 yo MF (Asian).
CHIEF COMPLAINT	"I felt a lump in my left breast while showering yesterday."
HISTORY OF PRESENT ILLNESS	Ms. Chen palpated a new lump in Ⓛ breast yesterday. States lump "feels like a marble." Denies previous lumps. Denies tenderness, dimpling, nipple retraction, nipple d/c, or painful lymph nodes. Denies recent injury to breasts. LMP was 10 d ago, denies presence of masses during menses or ovulation. "I'm scared that I may have breast cancer" & "worried that my husband might not find me attractive anymore."
PAST HEALTH HISTORY	
Medical	Denies hx of benign breast disease, cysts, fibroadenomas, mastitis, breast cancer, endometrial or ovarian cancer. Denies thyroid disease, pituitary disorders, or exposure to chest radiation. Onset of menarche age 12.
Surgical	Tonsillectomy at age 5, no sequelae; laparoscopy age 18 for dysmenorrhea; no additional tx
Medications	Denies use of oral contraceptives; occasional ASA for H/A & menstrual pain
Communicable Diseases	Denies
Allergies	No known food or drug allergies
Injuries/Accidents	Broken coccyx bone when thrown from a horse at age 28; denies chest trauma; no complications
Disabilities/Handicaps	Denies
Blood Transfusions	Denies
Childhood Illnesses	Chicken pox age 5; mumps age 6
Immunizations	States "all immunizations are current"

continued

FAMILY HEALTH HISTORY

LEGEND

 Living female

 Living male

 Deceased female

Deceased male

Points to patient

A&W = Alive & well

CA = Cancer

CABG = Coronary artery bypass graft

CVA = Cerebrovascular accident

MI = Myocardial infarction

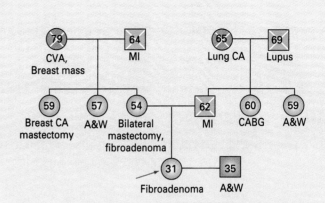

Maternal aunt being treated for breast CA; dx age 45; Ⓛ radical mastectomy performed; pt's mother had modified bilateral mastectomy for fibroadenomas that became painful; pt's maternal grandmother developed mass in Ⓡ breast shortly ā death; mass never evaluated.

SOCIAL HISTORY

Alcohol Use	1–2 scotches/wk
Tobacco Use	Denies
Drug Use	Denies
Sexual Practice	Heterosexual, monogamous relationship
Travel History	Travels to Europe 4×/yr
Work Environment	Urban high rise, denies exposure to toxic substances
Home Environment	Restored home in upscale residential district
Hobbies/Leisure Activities	Walking & reading
Stress	Job is stressful
Education	JD
Economic Status	Upper socioeconomic status
Military Service	Denies
Religion	Presbyterian
Ethnic Background	Chinese
Roles/Relationships	Wife, daughter, employee; denies relationship problems
Characteristic Patterns of Daily Living	Wakens 6:00 AM, breakfast c̄ husband, at work by 8:00 AM. Works through lunch & eats at her desk. Arrives home between 7:00 & 8:00 PM. Shares cooking duties for dinner, in bed by 10:00 PM.

continued

HEALTH MAINTENANCE ACTIVITIES

Sleep	7–8 hr/night
Diet	Eats "a great deal of fast foods"
Exercise	Walks 1–2 miles/wk
Stress Management	Walking & talking to husband
Use of Safety Devices	Wears seat belt
Health Check-Ups	Doesn't perform monthly BSE & never had mammogram; doesn't know how to perform BSE

PHYSICAL ASSESSMENT

Inspection

Color	Breasts & axillae flesh-colored $\bar{c}$ striae bilaterally over breasts & axilla; areolar areas & nipples dark in pigmentation
Vascularity	No enhanced vascular patterns
Thickening/Edema	No thickening or edema
Size and Symmetry	Breasts large & pendulous; Ⓡ breast & areola > Ⓛ; no nipple inversion; both nipples facing downward & outward bilaterally
Contour	Breasts convex in shape & symmetrical $\bar{s}$ dimpling, retraction, or flattening
Lesions/Masses	No fissures or erosion; no supernumerary nipples; no obvious lesions or masses
Discharge	No nipple d/c

Palpation

Supraclavicular and Infraclavicular Lymph Nodes	< 1 cm & discrete $\bar{s}$ tenderness
Breasts: Patient in Sitting Position	No nodes or masses palpable; breast tissue granular & uniform throughout bilaterally
Axillary Lymph Node Region	Discrete, < 1 cm $\bar{s}$ tenderness
Breasts: Patient in Supine Position	Single mass in Ⓛ breast in upper outer quadrant (2 o'clock radii), 7 cm from nipple, 1 cm × 1 cm × 0.5 cm, ovoid in shape, solid consistency, $\bar{c}$ discrete borders, mobile, nontender to palpation, nonerythemic, no dimpling or retraction; ∅ d/c from nipples

DIAGNOSTIC DATA

Mammography	Fibrotic changes noted in Ⓛ breast
Ultrasound	Confirmed fibroadenoma in Ⓛ breast upper outer quadrant (2 o'clock radii)
Thermography	Negative for hot spots

✓ **NURSING CHECKLIST**
Breasts and Regional Nodes Assessment

Inspection
- Color
- Vascularity
- Thickening/Edema
- Size and Symmetry
- Contour
- Lesions/Masses
- Discharge

Palpation
- Supraclavicular and Infraclavicular Lymph Nodes
- Breasts: Patient in Sitting Position
- Axillary Lymph Node Region
- Breasts: Patient in Supine Position

REVIEW QUESTIONS AND ACTIVITIES

1. Perform a breast self-examination. As you perform this assessment, identify the components of the breasts and regional lymphatics. What normal variants are present?

2. Explain the method of palpation for the breasts and regional lymphatics. How does your palpation style change with breast size?

3. Describe anticipated changes in female breast development as noted in Tanner's sexual maturity ratings scale for girls.

4. Describe age-related variants that you would expect to find in the breast and lymphatic assessment of a 65-year-old female.

5. Develop a teaching plan for teaching the identification and reduction of breast cancer risk factors.

Questions 6 and 7 refer to the following situation:
A 55-year-old African American female comes to your clinic complaining of a lump in her left breast. She states that she found the lump while showering 3 days ago. Upon palpation, a single, irregular, firm mass measuring 2 cm × 1.5 cm was noted in the left upper outer quadrant. The borders are not discrete, and the mass is mobile. She denies pain on palpation and no erythema is present, but dimpling is present when the muscles of the chest wall are contracted. No nipple retraction or discharge is noted.

6. Based on your initial assessment, you conclude that this patient may be experiencing:
   a. Fibroadenoma
   b. Carcinoma
   c. Gross cysts
   d. Peau d'orange

   The correct answer is (b).

7. The patient states that she has always been healthy and she denies that she would be at risk for breast cancer. Which answer would not be a risk factor for breast cancer?
   a. Obesity
   b. Smoking
   c. Unopposed estrogen therapy
   d. Primary relative with breast cancer

The correct answer is (b).

Thorax and Lungs

COMPETENCIES

1. Identify the anatomic landmarks of the thorax.
2. Describe the characteristics of the most common respiratory chief complaints.
3. Perform inspection, palpation, percussion, and auscultation on a healthy adult and on a patient with pulmonary pathology.
4. Explain the pathophysiology for abnormal findings.
5. Document respiratory assessment findings.
6. Describe the pathological changes that occur in the lungs with the aging process.

The respiratory system extends from the nose to the alveoli (see Figure 14-1). The normal air pathway is nose, pharynx, larynx, trachea, mainstem bronchus, right and left main bronchi, lobar/secondary bronchi, tertiary/segmental bronchi, terminal bronchioles, respiratory bronchioles, alveolar ducts, alveolar sacs, and alveoli.

The respiratory system is divided into the upper and lower tracts. The upper respiratory tract comprises the nose, pharynx, larynx, and the upper trachea. The nose and pharynx are discussed in Chapter 12. The lower respiratory tract is composed of the lower trachea to the lungs. This chapter deals only with those components of the respiratory system that are located in the thorax.

ANATOMY

Thorax

The thorax is a cone-shaped structure (narrower at the top and wider at the bottom) that consists of bones, cartilage, and muscles. Of these, the bones are the supportive structure of the thorax. On the anterior thorax, these bones are the 12 pairs of ribs and the sternum. Posteriorly, there are the 12 thoracic vertebrae and the spinal column.

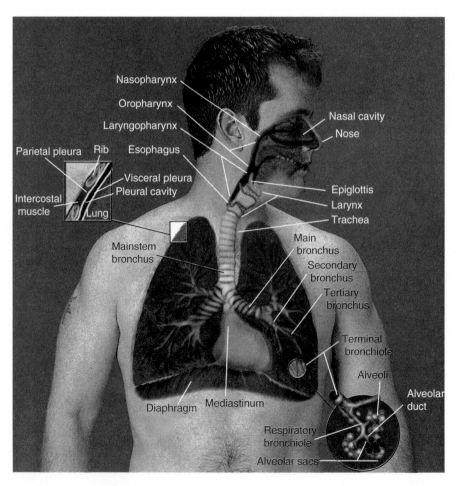

Figure 14-1 The Respiratory Tract

Sternum

The sternum, or breastbone, is a flat, narrow bone approximately 15 cm long. It is located at the median line of the anterior chest wall and is divided into three sections: the **manubrium** (the upper bone of the sternum that articulates with the clavicles and the first pair of ribs), the body, and the **xiphoid process** (a cartilaginous process at the base of the sternum that does not articulate with the ribs).

Ribs

The first seven pairs of ribs are articulated to the sternum via the costal cartilages and are called the **vertebrosternal** or **true ribs**. The **false ribs**, or rib pairs 8–10, articulate with the costal cartilages just above them. The remaining two pairs of ribs (11 and 12) are termed **floating ribs** and do not articulate at their anterior ends. The 10th rib is the lowest rib that can be palpated anteriorly. The 11th rib is palpated on the lateral thorax, and the 12th rib is palpated on the posterior thorax. All ribs articulate posteriorly to the vertebral column. When a rib is palpated, the costal cartilage cannot be distinguished from the rib itself (see Figure 14-2).

Intercostal Spaces

Each area between the ribs is called an **intercostal space** (ICS). There are 11 ICSs.

 NURSING TIP

Identifying Thoracic Landmarks

- Sternum
- Clavicles
- **Suprasternal notch:** With the finger pad of the index finger, feel in the midsternal line above the manubrium; the depression is the suprasternal notch.
- **Angle of Louis** (or **manubriosternal junction** or **sternal angle**): With the finger pads, feel for the suprasternal notch and move your finger pads down the sternum until they reach a horizontal ridge (the junction of the manubrium and the body of the sternum); this is the angle of Louis (or sternal angle); the second rib articulates with this landmark and serves as a convenient reference point for counting the ribs and ICSs (the first rib is difficult to palpate).
- **Costal angle:** Place your right finger pads on the bottom of the patient's anterior left rib cage (10th rib); place your left finger pads on the bottom of the anterior right rib cage (10th rib); move both hands horizontally towards the sternum until they meet in the midsternal line; the angle formed by the intersection of the ribs creates the costal angle.
- **Vertebra prominens:** Flex the neck forward; palpate the posterior spinous processes; if two processes are palpable, the superior process is C7 (vertebra prominens) and the inferior is T1; this landmark is useful in counting ribs to the level of T4; beyond T4 the spinous processes project obliquely and no longer correspond to the rib of the same number as the vertebral process.
- Inferior angle of scapula: Locate the inferior border of the scapula; this level corresponds to the seventh rib or seventh ICS.
- Spine

 NURSING TIP

Counting Anterior Intercostal Spaces

Use the angle of Louis as a landmark for identifying the rib number. Count the ribs in the midclavicular line. Each ICS is named for the number of the rib directly above it. For example, the space between the third and fourth ribs would be called the third ICS.

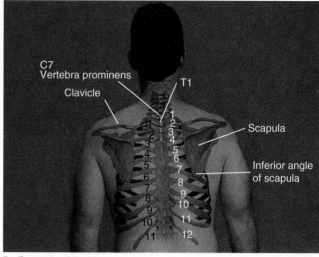

A. Anterior View

B. Posterior View

Figure 14-2 Thorax: (Rib number is shown on the patient's right; intercostal space number is shown on the patient's left.)

Lungs

The lungs are cone-shaped organs that fill the lateral chamber of the thoracic cavity. The lower outer surface of each lung is concave where it meets the convex diaphragm. Likewise, the medial aspect is concave to allow room for the heart, with the left lung having a more pronounced concavity (cardiac notch). The lungs lie against the ribs anteriorly and posteriorly.

The right lung is broader than the left lung because of the position of the heart. Inferiorly, the right lung is about 2.5 cm shorter than the left lung because of the upward displacement of the diaphragm by the liver. The right lung consists of three lobes (upper, middle, and lower) while the left lung has two lobes (upper and lower). In the lung, the **apex** denotes the top of the lung while the **base** refers to the bottom of the lung. Anteriorly, the apices of the lung extend 2.5–4 cm superior to the inner third of the clavicles, and posteriorly, the apices lie near the T1 process. On deep inspiration posteriorly, the lower lung border extends to the level of T12, and to T10 on deep expiration. The anterior inferior border of the lungs is at the sixth rib at the **midclavicular line** (MCL: vertical line drawn from the midpoint of the clavicle) and at the eighth rib at the **midaxillary line** (MAL: vertical line drawn from

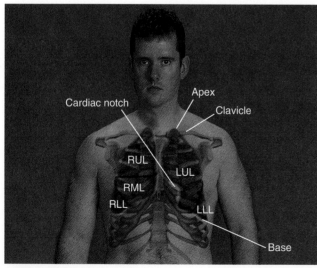

A. Anterior View

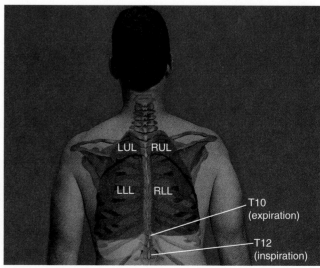

B. Posterior View

Figure 14-3 Lungs: RUL = Right Upper Lobe, RML = Right Middle Lobe, RLL = Right Lower Lobe, LUL = Left Upper Lobe, LLL = Left Lower Lobe

the apex of the axillae and lying midway between the anterior and the posterior axillary lines) (see Figure 14-3).

The lobes of the right and left lungs are divided by grooves called **fissures**. It is important to know the locations of the fissures to describe clinical findings. Figure 14-4 illustrates the right oblique (or diagonal) fissure, the right horizontal fissure, and the left oblique (or diagonal) fissure.

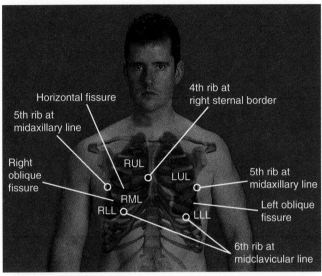

A. Anterior View

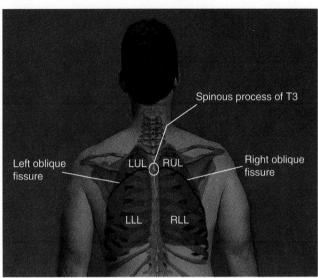

B. Posterior View

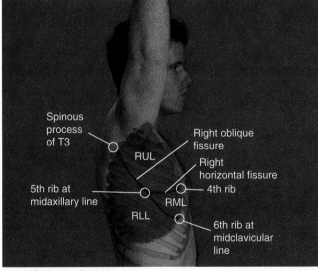

C. Right Lateral View

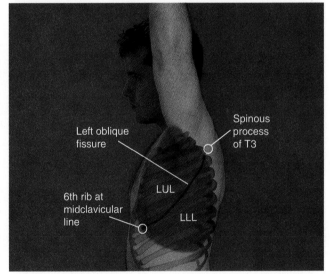

D. Left Lateral View

Figure 14-4 Lung Fissures

🌺 NURSING TIP

Thoracic Anatomic Topography

Additional landmarks that are useful when describing assessment findings are:

- **Anterior axillary line:** vertical line drawn from the origin of the anterior axillary fold and along the anterolateral aspect of the thorax.
- **Midspinal (vertebral) line:** vertical line drawn from the midpoint of the spinous process.
- **Midsternal line:** vertical line drawn from the midpoint of the sternum.
- **Posterior axillary line:** vertical line drawn from the posterior axillary fold.
- **Scapular line:** vertical line drawn from the inferior angle of the scapula.

When assessing the thorax, it is helpful to envision it as a rectangular box, with the four sides being the anterior, posterior, right lateral, and left lateral thoraxes. Figure 14-5 illustrates the imaginary thoracic lines on each of the four sides. These landmarks are helpful in discussing clinical findings.

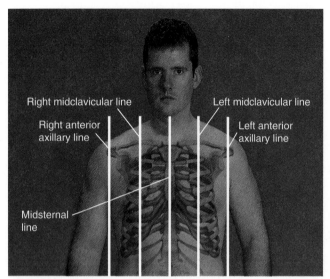

A. Anterior View

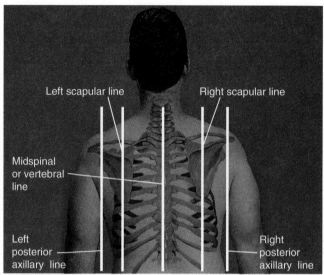

B. Posterior View

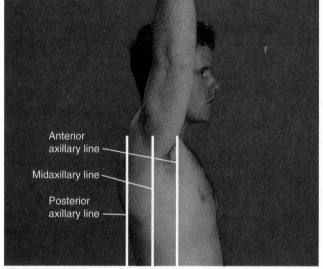

C. Right Lateral View

D. Left Lateral View

Figure 14-5 Imaginary Thoracic Lines

Pleura

Each lung is encased in a serous sac, or **pleura**. The **parietal pleura** lines the chest wall and the superior surface of the diaphragm. The **visceral pleura** lines the external surface of the lungs. Usually, a small amount of fluid is found in the space between these two pleura; this fluid prevents the pleura from rubbing against each other and acts as a cushioning agent for the lungs.

Mediastinum

The **mediastinum**, or **interpleural space**, is the area between the right and left lungs. It extends from the sternum to the spinal column and contains the heart, great vessels, trachea, esophagus, and lymph vessels. The only respira-

🌹 NURSING TIP

Lung Cancer Trends

Lung cancer is currently an equal opportunity disease. It is the primary cause of cancer deaths among men, and now surpasses breast cancer as the number one cause of cancer deaths among women.

tory structures in the mediastinum are the trachea and the pulmonary vasculature. The trachea is a fibromuscular hollow tube located in the anterior thorax in the median plane. It is 11 to 13 cm in length and 2 to 3 cm in width. The trachea lies anterior to the esophagus.

Bronchi

The trachea bifurcates into the left and right mainstem bronchi at the level of the fourth or fifth vertebral process posteriorly and the sternal angle anteriorly. The right mainstem bronchus is wider, shorter, and more vertical than the left. This anatomic difference is critical because it makes the right mainstem bronchus more susceptible to aspiration and endotracheal intubation. The mainstem bronchi further divide into lobar or secondary bronchi. Each lobar bronchus supplies a lobe of the lung. The bronchi transport gases as well as trap foreign particles in their mucus. Cilia aid in sweeping the foreign particles upward in the respiratory tract for possible elimination. Culmination of the tracheobronchial tree is in the alveoli.

Alveoli

The **alveoli** are the smallest functional units of the respiratory system. It is here that gas exchange occurs. It is estimated that approximately 300 million alveoli are present in each lung. This aerating surface is about equal to 100 times the body surface area of an adult. Each alveolus has its own blood supply and lymphatic drainage. Branches of the pulmonary artery carry blood to the capillaries surrounding the alveoli to be oxygenated. Branches of the pulmonary vein transport oxygenated blood from the alveoli to the heart.

Diaphragm

The diaphragm, which is innervated by the phrenic nerve, is a dome-shaped muscle that forms the inferior border of the thorax. Anteriorly, its right edge is located at the fifth rib–fifth ICS at the MCL. The left dome of the diaphragm is the sixth rib–sixth ICS at the MCL. The presence of the liver below the right dome of the diaphragm accounts for the elevated border. On expiration posteriorly, the diaphragm is located at the level of the 10th vertebral process, and at T12 on inspiration. Laterally, the diaphragm is found at the eighth rib at the midaxillary line. The diaphragm is the principal muscle of respiration. Contraction of the diaphragm leads to an increase in volume in the thoracic cavity.

External Intercostal Muscles

The external intercostal muscles are located in the ICS. During inspiration, the external intercostal muscles elevate the ribs, thus increasing the size of the thoracic cavity. The internal intercostal muscles draw adjacent ribs together, thereby decreasing the size of the thoracic cavity during expiration.

Accessory Muscles

Accessory respiratory muscles are used to accommodate increased oxygen demand. Exercise and some diseases lead to the use of accessory muscles. The accessory muscles are the scalene, sternocleidomastoid, trapezius, and abdominal rectus.

🌿 NURSING TIP

Preventing Aspiration

- Never drink alcohol to excess.
- Place the at-risk patient (intoxicated, unconscious) in a side-lying or upright position.
- Turn the head of a vomiting patient to the side.
- Patients receiving intermittent tube feedings should be placed in an upright position for 30 minutes after feeding; patients receiving continuous tube feedings should be maintained in an upright position at all times.
- Delay tube feeding if the gastric residual is significant (amount varies per patient and per amount of usual feeding).
- Suction oropharynx of patients with tracheostomies prior to deflation of their cuffs.

♣ ASK YOURSELF

Tobacco Use

- Do you smoke?
- How do you feel about others who smoke?
- How do you feel about patients who have pathology related to tobacco use?
- Do you treat these patients any differently from nonsmoking patients? If so, what interventions can you implement to deal with this bias?

PHYSIOLOGY

Ventilation

The primary function of the respiratory system is to deliver oxygen to the lungs and to remove carbon dioxide from the lungs. The breathing process includes inspiratory and expiratory phases. During inspiration, the pressure inside the lungs becomes subatmospheric when the diaphragm and external intercostal muscles contract. The diaphragm lowers and the ribs elevate, thus increasing the intrapulmonic volume. As a result of the negative intra-alveolar pressure, atmospheric air is pulled into the respiratory tract until intra-alveolar pressure equals atmospheric pressure. The lungs increase in size with the air.

Expiration is a passive process and occurs more rapidly than inspiration. During expiration, the diaphragm and external intercostal muscles relax, decreasing the volume of the thoracic cavity. The diaphragm rises. The intra-pulmonic volume decreases and the intrapulmonic pressure increases above the atmospheric pressure. The lungs possess elastic recoil capabilities that allow air to be expelled until intrapulmonic pressure equals atmospheric pressure.

External Respiration

External respiration is the process by which gases are exchanged between the lungs and the pulmonary vasculature. Oxygen diffuses from the alveoli into the blood, and carbon dioxide diffuses from the blood to the alveoli. Diffusion is a passive process in which gases move across a membrane from an area of higher concentration to an area of lower concentration. In the lungs, the membrane is the alveolar-capillary network.

Internal Respiration

Internal respiration is the process by which gases are exchanged between the pulmonary vasculature and the body's tissues. Oxygen from the lungs diffuses from the blood into body tissue. Carbon dioxide diffuses from the tissue into the blood. This blood is then carried back to the right side of the heart for reoxygenation.

Control of Breathing

Control of breathing is influenced by neural and chemical factors. The pons and medulla are the central nervous system structures primarily responsible for involuntary respiration. The stimulus for breathing is an increased carbon dioxide level, a decreased oxygen level, or an increased blood pH level.

❖ HEALTH HISTORY

The thorax and lungs health history provides insight into the link between a patient's life/lifestyle and thorax and lungs information and pathology.

PATIENT PROFILE

Diseases that are age-, sex-, and race-specific for the thorax and lungs are listed.

continued

Age	Bronchiectasis (birth–20) Cystic fibrosis (birth–30) Pneumothorax (20–40) Sarcoidosis (30–40) Chronic bronchitis (>35) Pneumonia (>60) Emphysema (50–60) Lung cancer (>50) Intrinsic asthma (>50) Idiopathic pulmonary fibrosis (60–70)
Sex	
Female	Sarcoidosis
Male	Mesothelioma, idiopathic pulmonary fibrosis, pneumothorax
Race	
African American	Sarcoidosis
Caucasian	Cystic fibrosis
CHIEF COMPLAINT	*Common chief complaints for the thorax and lungs are defined and information on the characteristics of each sign/symptom is provided.*
Dyspnea	Subjective feeling of shortness of breath (SOB)
Quantity	The number of steps that can be climbed before SOB occurs; distance that can be walked
Associated Manifestations	Palpitations, leg pain, faintness, anxiety, fatigue, cough, sputum, wheezing, diaphoresis, cyanosis, pain, fever
Aggravating Factors	Smoking, exercise
Alleviating Factors	Pillow orthopnea, side-lying position, tripod position, fresh air, medications (e.g., bronchodilators), supplemental oxygen
Timing	Night time (paroxysmal nocturnal dyspnea)
Cough	Stimulation of afferent vagal endings, which helps to clean the airway of extraneous material by producing a sudden, forceful, and noisy expulsion of air from the lungs
Quality	Dry, hacking, barking, congested, harsh, brassy, high pitched, whooping
Associated Manifestations	SOB, wheezing, sputum, pleuritic pain, chest pain, fever, hemoptysis
Aggravating Factors	Position of patient, exposure to noxious stimuli, exercise
Alleviating Factors	Medications (e.g., dextromethorphan), humidity, cool air, cool liquids
Setting	Temperature and humidity of environment, exertion
Timing	Winter, early morning, bedtime, middle of the night, after eating, prior to fainting, continuous

continued

Sputum	Substance produced by the respiratory tract that can be expectorated or swallowed; it is composed of mucus, blood, purulent material, microorganisms, cellular debris, and, occasionally, foreign objects
Quality	Color: white or clear, purulent, blood tinged, yellow or green, mucoid, rust, black, pink Consistency: thick, thin, moderate; frothy — separates into layers Odor: malodorous
Quantity	Normal daily sputum production is 60–90 ml (normally this is not expectorated); small, moderate, copious
Associated Manifestations	Cough
Aggravating Factors	Exposure to allergens, smoking
Alleviating Factors	Medications (e.g., guaifenesin), liquids
Setting	Sleep, exposure to allergen
Timing	Early morning
Chest Pain	Pain can have a pulmonary, cardiac, gastrointestinal, or musculoskeletal etiology. Chapter 15 differentiates the types of chest pain.
PAST HEALTH HISTORY	*The various components of the past health history are linked to thorax and lung pathology and thorax- and lung-related information.*
Medical	
Respiratory Specific	Asthma, bronchitis, croup, frequent coryza, cystic fibrosis, emphysema, epiglottitis, pleurisy, pneumonia, pneumothorax, pulmonary edema, pulmonary embolus, lung cancer, strep throat
Nonrespiratory Specific	Lupus, drug-induced respiratory pathology, rheumatoid arthritis, congenital musculoskeletal chest defects, severe scoliosis, multiple sclerosis, amyotrophic lateral sclerosis
Surgical	Lobectomy, pneumonectomy, tracheostomy, wedge resection
Medications	Antibiotics, bronchodilators, cough expectorant, cough suppressant, oxygen
Communicable Diseases	Coryza: sneezing, coughing Tuberculosis (TB): pulmonary fibrosis and calcification Flu: pneumonia AIDS: pneumocystis carinii pneumonia Hanta virus: bilateral pulmonary infiltrates, respiratory failure
Allergies	Asthma is the predominant manifestation of allergies in the respiratory patient. Hypersensitivity to drugs, food, pets, dust, cigarette smoke, perfume, or pollen should be closely scrutinized. In addition, any common signs of allergies, such as cough, sneeze, and sinusitis, should be closely evaluated.
Injuries/Accidents	Chest trauma, near drowning

continued

Disabilities/Handicaps	Oxygen dependent, phrenic pacer dependent, ventilator dependent
Childhood Illnesses	Pertussis and measles: bronchiectasis
FAMILY HEALTH HISTORY	*Thorax and lung diseases that are familial are listed.*
	Allergies, alpha$_1$-antitrypsin deficiency, asthma, bronchiectasis, cancer, cystic fibrosis, emphysema, sarcoidosis, TB
SOCIAL HISTORY	*The components of the social history are linked to thorax and lung factors/pathology.*
Alcohol Use	Decreases efficiency of lung defense mechanisms, predisposes to aspiration pneumonia, patients with carbon dioxide retention are more sensitive to alcohol's depressant effect
Tobacco Use	Cigarette smoking is the primary risk factor for chronic bronchitis, emphysema, and lung cancer, as well as other disorders.
Drug Use	Heroin: pulmonary edema Barbiturates or narcotic overdose: respiratory depression Cocaine: tachypnea
Travel History	TB (Haiti, Southeast Asia): poor sanitation and rural conditions San Joaquin Valley fever or coccidioidomycosis (Southwest United States and Mexico): agent is in dirt and dusty winds Pneumonic plague (India): carried by nuclei droplets
Work Environment	Repeated exposure to materials in the workplace can create respiratory complications that range from minor problems to life-threatening events. Numerous categories of respiratory diseases have been identified from repeated exposure to toxic substances. These diseases are listed along with the industries and agents related to them. Silicosis: glass making, tunneling, stonecutting, mineral mining, insulation work, quarrying, cement work, ceramics, foundry work, semiconductor manufacturing Asbestosis: mining, shipbuilding, construction Coal worker's pneumoconiosis: coal mining Pneumoconioses: tin and aluminum production, welding, insecticide manufacturing, rubber industry, fertilizer industry, ceramics, cosmetic industry Occupational asthma: electroplating, grain working, woodworking, photography, printing, baking, painting Chronic bronchitis: coal mining, welding, firefighting Byssinosis: cotton mill dust, flax Extrinsic allergic alveolitis (hypersensitivity pneumonia): animal hair, contamination of air conditioning or heating systems, moldy hay, moldy grains, moldy dust, sugarcane Toxic gases and fumes: welding, cigarette smoke, auto exhaust, chemical industries, firefighting, hair spray Pulmonary neoplasms: radon gas, mustard gas, printing ink, asbestos Pneumonitis: furniture polish, gasoline, or kerosene ingestion; mineral oil, olive oil, and milk aspiration
Home Environment	Air pollution, cigarette smoke, wood-burning stoves, gas stoves and heaters, kerosene heaters, radon gas, pet hair and dander

continued

Hobbies/Leisure Activities	Birds (bird breeder's lung), mushroom growers (mushroom grower's lung), scuba diving (lung rupture, oxygen toxicity, decompression sickness), high-altitude activities (skiing, climbing: pulmonary edema and pulmonary embolus)
Stress	Asthma can be exacerbated by stress.
Economic Status	Poor sanitation and densely populated areas are ideal conditions for the spread of TB
HEALTH MAINTENANCE ACTIVITIES	*This information provides a bridge between the health maintenance activities and thorax and lung function.*
Sleep	Sleep apnea syndrome: absence of inspiratory muscle activation; upper airway occlusion Chronic obstructive pulmonary disease (COPD) or neuromuscular disease: nocturnal oxygen desaturation caused by hypoventilation without apnea
Diet	Obesity: chronic hypoventilation, obstructive apnea (Pickwickian syndrome)
Exercise	Regular exercise improves pulmonary function
Use of Safety Devices	Mask worn when exposed to toxic substances, other occupational precautions as mandated by OSHA; knowledge of Heimlich maneuver
Health Check-Ups	Respiratory rate, lung auscultation, chest x-ray, sputum culture and sensitivity, pulmonary function test, purified protein derivative (tuberculin) (PPD), flu vaccine

 NURSING TIP

Reducing Exposure to Respiratory Hazards in the Workplace

- Always wear a mask if exposed to substances that cause respiratory disease.
- Avoid respiratory irritants when possible.
- Maintain proper ventilation of the environment to ensure minimal breathing of dangerous substances.
- Follow Occupational Safety and Hazard Administration (OSHA) and employer's safety guidelines.

 NURSING CHECKLIST
Maintaining Respiratory Health

- Never smoke around infants and children.
- Don't smoke; never smoke in bed; encourage those living with you to stop smoking.
- If you must live with a smoker, ask that smoking be confined to one well-ventilated room, or preferably outside.
- Clean house frequently to keep the dust level and mold growth minimal, if causes of allergies or aggravating factors for other respiratory ailment.
- Change filters on furnace, heaters, exhaust systems, and range hoods as frequently as the manufacturer specifies.
- Have chimney(s) cleaned at the beginning of each season and more frequently if used heavily.
- Have home inspected for radon and take remedial steps as needed.
- Check smoke detectors on a monthly basis.
- If oxygen is used in the home, use and store away from heat; avoid contact with open flames and cigarettes.

NURSING TIP

The Heimlich Maneuver

You can teach the patient the Heimlich maneuver during the health history when appropriate. This technique is easily demonstrated on yourself and on the patient. Consider teaching the patient this life-saving technique at every opportunity.

 NURSING TIP

Flu Vaccine

A flu vaccine is usually recommended for people over age 60 and for younger adults with chronic illness. Encourage the patient to obtain a flu shot as recommended by the public health department.

✓ **NURSING CHECKLIST**
General Approach to Thorax and Lung Assessment

1. Greet the patient and explain the assessment techniques that you will be using.
2. Ensure that the examination room is at a warm, comfortable room temperature to prevent patient chilling and shivering.
3. Use a quiet room that will be free from interruptions.
4. Ensure that the light in the room provides sufficient brightness to adequately observe the patient.
5. Instruct the patient to remove all street clothes from the waist up and to don an examination gown.
6. Place the patient in an upright sitting position on the examination table, or
6A. For patients who cannot tolerate the sitting position, rotate the supine, bedridden patient from side to side to gain access to the thorax.
7. Expose the entire area being assessed. Provide a drape that women can use to cover their breasts (if desired) when the posterior thorax is assessed.
8. When palpating, percussing, or auscultating the anterior thorax of female or obese patients, ask them to displace the breast tissue. Assessing directly over breast tissue is not an accurate indicator of underlying structures.
9. Visualize the underlying respiratory structures during the assessment process in order to accurately describe the location of any pathology.
10. Always compare the right and the left sides of the anterior thorax and the posterior thorax to one another, as well as the right lateral thorax and the left lateral thorax.
11. Use a systematic approach every time the assessment is performed. Proceed from the lung apices to the bases, right to left to lateral.

ASSESSMENT OF THE THORAX AND LUNGS

EQUIPMENT

- Stethoscope
- Centimeter ruler or tape measure
- Washable marker
- Watch with second hand

E	**Examination**
N	**Normal Findings**
A	**Abnormal Findings**
P	**Pathophysiology**

Inspection

Shape of Thorax

E 1. Stand in front of the patient.
2. Estimate visually the transverse diameter of the thorax.
3. Move to either side of the patient.
4. Estimate visually the width of the anteroposterior (AP) diameter of the thorax.
5. Compare the estimates of these two visualizations.

N *In the normal adult, the ratio of the AP diameter to the transverse diameter is approximately 1:2 to 5:7. In other words, the normal adult is wider from side to side than from front to back. The normal thorax is slightly elliptical in shape. A barrel chest is normal in infants and sometimes in the older adult. See Chapter 23 for a discussion of the pediatric patient. Figure 14-6 illustrates the normal and abnormal configurations of the thorax.*

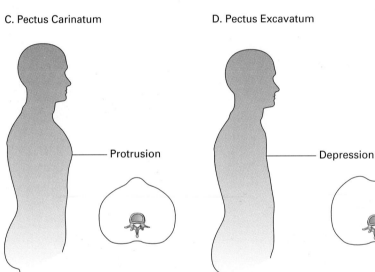

A. Normal Adult   B. Barrel Chest

2x
1:2 ratio   x
                                   1:1 ratio

C. Pectus Carinatum   D. Pectus Excavatum

Protrusion   Depression

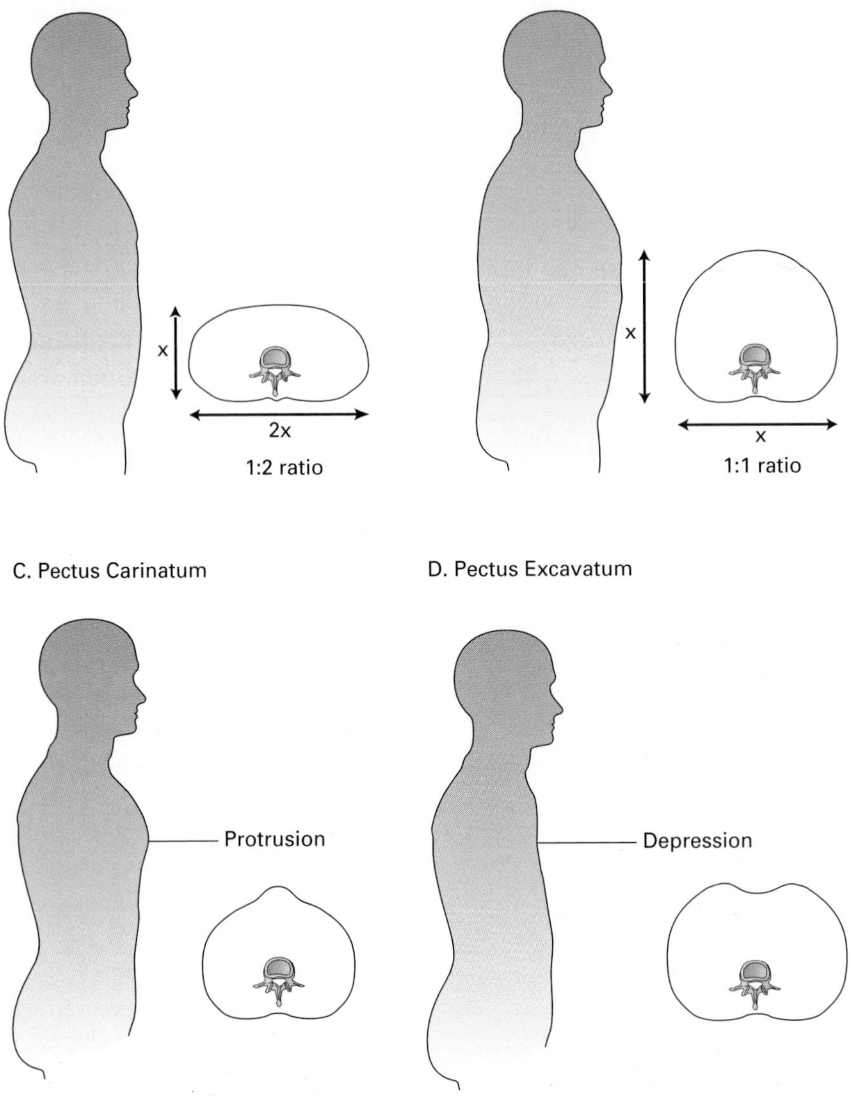

Figure 14-6   Chest Configurations

A   In **barrel chest**, the ratio of the AP diameter to the transverse diameter is approximately 1:1. The patient's chest is circular or barrel shaped in appearance.

P   The patient with COPD has a barrel chest due to air trapping in the alveoli and subsequent lung hyperinflation. Lung volume thus increases and the diaphragm flattens over time. The ribs are forced upward and outward. Collectively these changes result in the barrel-chest appearance.

A   **Pectus carinatum**, or pigeon chest, is a marked protrusion of the sternum. This increases the AP diameter of the thorax.

P   Pectus carinatum can result from a congenital anomaly. A patient with severe pectus carinatum will exhibit respiratory difficulty.

P   Rickets results from a vitamin D deficiency. In this condition, the bones become demineralized and weak. The loss of bone strength allows the intercostal muscles to pull the ribs and sternum forward, resulting in pectus carinatum.

A   **Pectus excavatum**, or funnel chest, is a depression in the lower body of the sternum. This indentation can impede the heart and cause myocardial disturbances. The AP diameter of the chest decreases.

P   Pectus excavatum can result from a congenital anomaly. Respiratory insufficiency can ensue from the compression of the lungs in marked pectus excavatum.

E	**Examination**
N	**Normal Findings**
A	**Abnormal Findings**
P	**Pathophysiology**

A **Kyphosis**, or humpback, is an excessive convexity of the thoracic vertebrae. Gibbus kyphosis is an extreme deformity of the spine.

P The majority of kyphosis cases are idiopathic. Respiratory compromise is manifested only in severe cases.

A **Scoliosis** is a lateral curvature of the thorax or lumbar vertebrae. See page 538 for further discussion.

P The majority of the cases of scoliosis are idiopathic, although scoliosis can also result from neuromuscular diseases, connective tissue diseases, and osteoporosis. Marked scoliosis can interfere with normal respiratory function. The total lung capacity and vital capacity decline in proportion to the severity of the scoliosis.

Symmetry of Chest Wall

E 1. Stand in front of the patient.
2. Inspect the right and the left anterior thoraxes.
3. Note the shoulder height. Observe any differences between the two sides of the chest wall, such as the presence of masses.
4. Move behind the patient.
5. Inspect the right and the left posterior thoraxes, comparing right and left sides.
6. Note the position of the scapula.

N *The shoulders should be at the same height. Likewise, the scapula should be the same height bilaterally. There should be no masses.*

A Having one shoulder or scapula higher than the other is abnormal. The presence of a visible mass is abnormal.

P The presence of scoliosis can lead to a shoulder or a scapula that is higher than its corresponding part. Marked scoliosis impairs lung function.

P A visible chest mass is always abnormal. Likely etiologies are mediastinal tumors or cysts. If large enough, they can compress lung tissue and impair normal lung function.

Presence of Superficial Veins

E 1. Stand in front of the patient.
2. Inspect the anterior thorax for the presence of dilated superficial veins.

N *In the normal adult, dilated superficial veins are not seen.*

A The presence of dilated superficial veins on the anterior chest wall is an abnormal finding.

P Dilated veins on the anterior thorax may be indicative of superior vena cava obstruction. Due to the obstruction, the superficial veins and collateral vessels become engorged with blood and dilate. Venous return to the heart is diminished, compromising oxygenation. A patient may present with dyspnea.

Costal Angle

E 1. Stand in front of the patient.
2. In a patient whose thoracic skeleton is easily viewed, visually locate the **costal margins** (medial borders created by the articulation of the false ribs).
3. Estimate the angle formed by the costal margins during exhalation and at rest. This is the costal angle.
4. In a heavy or obese patient, place your fingertips on the lower anterior borders of the thoracic skeleton.
5. Gently move your fingertips medially to the xiphoid process.
6. As your hands approach the midline, feel the ribs as they meet at the apex of the costal margins. Visualize the line that is created by your fingers as they move up the floating ribs towards the sternum. This is the costal angle (see Figure 14-7A). Approximate this angle.

NURSING TIP

Assessing Oxygenation in the Thorax Assessment

When the chest is exposed, remember to examine the color of the thoracic skin as well as the patient's nailbeds and lips. These areas provide information on oxygenation status. Refer to Chapters 10 and 12.

NURSING TIP

Assessing Nailbed Clubbing and Capillary Refill

The presence of nailbed clubbing provides information on long-term oxygen status, and capillary refill indicates present oxygenation. Note these findings when assessing respiratory function. Assessment techniques for both are described in Chapter 10.

E	**Examination**
N	**Normal Findings**
A	**Abnormal Findings**
P	**Pathophysiology**

N *The costal angle is less than 90° during exhalation and at rest. The costal angle widens slightly during inhalation due to the expansion of the thorax.*

A A costal angle greater than 90° is abnormal.

P Processes where hyperinflation of the lungs (emphysema) or dilation of the bronchi (bronchiectasis) occurs also result in a costal margin angle greater than 90°. The diaphragm flattens out and the ribs are forced upward and outward, leading to the change in the costal margin angle.

Angle of the Ribs

E 1. Stand in front of the patient.
2. In a patient whose thoracic skeleton is easily viewed, visually locate the midsternal area.
3. Estimate the angle at which the ribs articulate with the sternum.
4. In a heavy or obese patient, place your fingertips on the midsternal area.
5. Move your fingertips along a rib laterally to the anterior axillary line. Visualize the line that is created by your hand as it traces the rib. Approximate this angle. Refer to Figure 14-7B.

N *The ribs articulate at a 45° angle with the sternum.*

A An angle greater than 45° is considered abnormal. Patients with particular respiratory pathology may have ribs that are nearly horizontal and perpendicular to the sternum.

P Conditions characterized by an increased AP diameter, such as emphysema, bronchiectasis, and cystic fibrosis, result in an angle greater than 45° because the lungs are forced out due to hyperinflation or dilation of the bronchi.

E **Examination**
N **Normal Findings**
A **Abnormal Findings**
P **Pathophysiology**

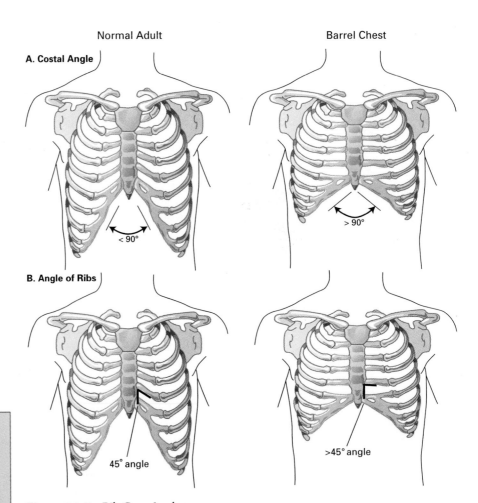

Figure 14-7 Rib Cage Angles

Intercostal Spaces

E 1. Stand in front of the patient.
2. Inspect the ICS throughout the respiratory cycle.
3. Note any bulging of the ICS and any retractions.

N *There should be an absence of retractions and of bulging of the ICS.*

A The presence of bulging of the ICS or of retractions is abnormal. Bulging of the ICS tends to occur during expiration, and retractions occur during inspiration.

P Conditions that obstruct the free inflow of air may lead to retractions. These include emphysema, asthma, tracheal or laryngeal obstruction, and the presence of a foreign body or tumor that compresses the respiratory tract.

P Abnormal bulging of the ICS occurs when there is an obstruction to the free exhalation of air, such as in emphysema, asthma, an enlarged heart, aortic aneurysm, massive pleural effusion, tension pneumothorax, and tumors.

Muscles of Respiration

E 1. Stand in front of the patient.
2. Observe the patient's breathing for a few respiratory cycles, paying close attention to the anterior thorax and the neck.
3. Note all of the muscles that are being used by the patient.

N *No accessory muscles are used in normal breathing.*

A The use of the accessory muscles is a pathological finding.

P Any condition that creates a state of hypoxemia or hypermetabolism may lead to the use of accessory muscles. Accessory muscles are attempting to create an extra respiratory effort to inhale needed oxygen. Patients experiencing hypermetabolic states such as exercise, fever, and infection, or hypoxic events such as COPD, pneumonia, pneumothorax, pulmonary edema, and pulmonary embolus usually present with accessory muscle use.

Respirations

The inspection of the respiration process includes seven components: rate, pattern, depth, symmetry, audibility, patient position, and mode.

Rate

E 1. Stand in front of the patient or to the right side.
2. Observe the patient's breathing without stating what you are doing, because the patient may change the respiratory rate (increase or decrease it) if aware that you are watching the chest rising and falling. This assessment can be conducted simultaneously with the pulse rate assessment.
3. Count the number of respiratory cycles that the patient has for one full minute. A respiratory cycle consists of one inhaled and one exhaled breath.

N *In the resting adult, the normal respiratory rate is 12 to 20 breaths per minute. This type of breathing is termed **eupnea**, or normal breathing.*

A A respiratory rate greater than 20 breaths per minute is termed **tachypnea**.

P Tachypnea is frequently present in hypermetabolic and hypoxic states. By increasing the respiratory rate, the body is trying to supply additional oxygen to meet the body's demands. Tachypnea occurs in many disease states, such as pneumonia, bronchitis, asthma, and pneumothorax.

P Tachypnea is often a sign of stress. In stressful situations, the body releases catecholamines that elevate the respiratory rate to supply sufficient oxygen.

A A respiratory rate lower than 12 breaths per minute is termed **bradypnea**.

P Injury to the brain may cause bradypnea because of excessive intracranial pressure applied to the respiratory center in the medulla oblongata.

NURSING ALERT

Respiratory Rate Emergencies

Extreme tachypnea (greater than 30 breaths per minute in an adult), bradypnea, and apnea are emergency conditions. Assess the patient for additional information and contact the physician immediately.

E	**Examination**
N	**Normal Findings**
A	**Abnormal Findings**
P	**Pathophysiology**

P In drug overdoses (barbiturates, alcohol, and opiates) bradypnea is a sign of the drug's depressant effect on the respiratory center.

P Bradypnea occurs in sleep because of the lowered metabolic state of the body. The respiratory rate also slows in non-REM sleep due to changes in the response of the respiratory center to chemical signals.

A **Apnea** is the lack of respirations for 10 or more seconds.

P Traumatic brain injury may lead to apnea because of herniation of the brain stem.

Pattern (see Figure 14-8)

E **1.** Stand in front of the patient.

    2. While counting the respiratory rate, note the rhythm or pattern of the breathing for regularity or irregularity.

N *Normal respirations are regular and even in rhythm.*

A **Cheyne-Stokes respirations** occur in crescendo and decrescendo patterns interspersed between periods of apnea that can last 15 to 30 seconds. This can be a normal finding in elderly patients and in young children. Cheyne-Stokes respiration is an example of a regularly irregular respiratory pattern, that is, the respirations predictably or regularly become irregular.

P Central cerebral or high brain-stem lesions that occur in brain injury produce Cheyne-Stokes respirations.

P Cheyne-Stokes respirations can also appear in sleep due to alterations in the respiratory center's ability to accurately perceive chemical and mechanical stimuli.

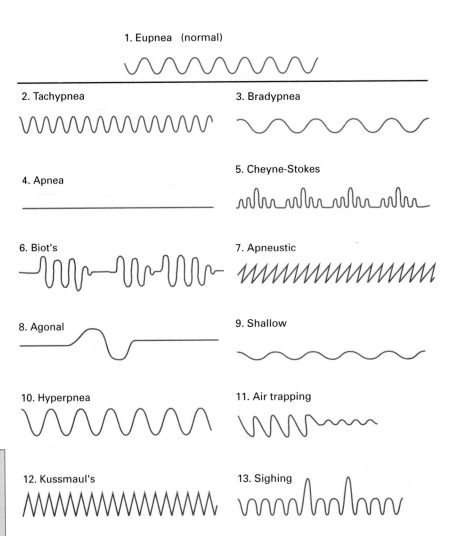

1. Eupnea (normal)

2. Tachypnea

3. Bradypnea

4. Apnea

5. Cheyne-Stokes

6. Biot's

7. Apneustic

8. Agonal

9. Shallow

10. Hyperpnea

11. Air trapping

12. Kussmaul's

13. Sighing

E	Examination
N	Normal Findings
A	Abnormal Findings
P	Pathophysiology

Figure 14-8 Respiratory Patterns

A **Biot's respirations**, or **ataxic breathing** is an example of an irregularly irregular respiratory pattern. In an irregularly irregular rhythm, there is no identifiable pattern to the respiratory cycle. There is an absence of a crescendo and decrescendo pattern. Deep and shallow breaths occur at random intervals interspersed with short and long pauses. Periods of apnea can be long and frequent.

P Biot's breathing indicates damage to the medulla.

A **Apneustic respirations** are characterized by a prolonged gasping during inspiration followed by a very short, inefficient expiration. These pauses can last 30 to 60 seconds.

P Injury to the upper portion of the pons can lead to apneustic breathing.

A **Agonal respirations** are irregularly irregular respirations. They are of varying depths and patterns.

P Impending death, where there is little or no oxygen supplying the brain, or compression of the respiratory center may lead to agonal breaths.

Depth

E 1. Stand in front of the patient.
2. Observe the relative depth with which the patient draws a breath during inspiration.

N *The normal depth of inspiration is nonexaggerated and effortless.*

A In hypoventilation, or shallow respirations, the chest wall is moved minimally during inspiration and expiration. A small tidal volume is being inspired.

P Obese patients frequently have small tidal volumes due to the sheer weight of the chest wall and the effort it takes to move it with each breath.

P The patient in pain or with a recent abdominal or thoracic incision has shallow respirations due to the discomfort of moving the rib cage, the integument, and the respiratory muscles with each breath.

P Shallow respirations are also seen in conditions where lung pathology exists and breathing is painful: pulmonary embolus, pneumonia, pneumothorax.

A **Hyperpnea** is a breath that is greater in volume than the resting tidal volume. The respiratory rate is normal and the pattern is even in hyperpnea.

P In the warm-up and cool-down periods of exercise, hyperpnea is present. The deep breath is drawn to meet the increased metabolic needs of the body.

P Patients in highly emotional states exhibit hyperpnea as the body attempts to meet the increased oxygen demand.

P Patients who are thrust into high-altitude regions will become hyperpneic due to the decreased partial pressure of oxygen. Deep breaths and slight tachypnea represent an attempt to supply the oxygen needs of the body.

A **Air Trapping** is an abnormal respiratory pattern with rapid, shallow respirations and forced expirations.

P Patients with COPD have difficulty with exhaling. When these patients exercise or experience increased heart rate, they have insufficient time to fully exhale. As a result, air is trapped in the lungs, and, over time, the chest overexpands. Likewise, an asthmatic patient experiencing an acute attack has difficulty exhaling due to increased mucus and bronchial constriction. Air trapping ensues.

A **Kussmaul's respirations** are characterized by extreme increased depth and rate of respirations. These respirations are regular and the inspiratory and expiratory processes are both active.

P Diabetic ketoacidosis and metabolic acidosis may result in Kussmaul's respirations. The body is lowering its $paCO_2$ level, thereby raising the pH and correcting the acidosis.

A **Sighing** is characterized by normal respirations interrupted by a deep inspiration and followed by a deep expiration. It may be accompanied by an audible sigh. Sighing is pathological if it occurs frequently.

P Excessive sighing can occur in central nervous system lesions.

E **Examination**
N **Normal Findings**
A **Abnormal Findings**
P **Pathophysiology**

Symmetry

E   **1.** Stand in front of the patient.
    2. Observe the symmetry with which the chest rises and falls during the respiratory cycle.

N   *The healthy adult's thorax rises and falls in unison in the respiratory cycle. There is no paradoxical movement.*

A   Unilateral expansion of either side of the thorax is abnormal.

P   Conditions where the lung is absent or collapsed (pneumonectomy, pneumothorax) are characterized by unilateral thoracic expansion secondary to the lack of active alveolar expansion on inspiration.

P   Absence of expansion is evident on the affected lung side in a patient with pulmonary fibrosis due to the thickening of the lung and decreased elasticity.

P   Acute pleurisy and massive atelectasis are pathologies where pain and collapsed alveoli, respectively, interfere with the respiratory process and prevent adequate bilateral and equal chest symmetry.

A   Paradoxical, or seemingly contradictory, chest wall movement is always abnormal. In paradoxical chest wall movement, the normal part of the thorax will rise during inspiration while the affected area will fall. Conversely, during expiration the normal part of the thorax will fall while the affected area will rise.

P   Broken ribs from trauma to the chest wall or flail chest interferes with the normal rib cage dynamics during the respiratory process and may lead to paradoxical chest wall movement.

A   Hoover's sign is the paradoxical inward movement of the lower ICS during inspiration. This occurs when the diaphragm is flat instead of its normal dome shape. Muscle fibers are horizontal, and diaphragmatic contraction pulls the rib cage inward rather than down.

P   Broken ribs from trauma to the chest wall or flail chest interferes with the normal rib cage dynamics during the respiratory process and may lead to the presence of Hoover's sign.

Audibility

E   **1.** Stand in front of the patient.
    2. Listen for the audibility of the respirations.

N   *A patient's respirations are normally heard by the unaided ear a few centimeters from the patient's nose or mouth.*

A   It is abnormal to hear audible breathing when standing a few feet from the patient. Upper airway sounds may also be heard. These should not be confused with pulmonary sounds. Refer to Chapter 12 for a discussion of upper airway sounds.

P   Any condition where air hunger exists has the potential to create audible and noisy breathing. The body is attempting to meet its oxygen demands. Examples of these states are exercise, COPD, pneumonia, and pneumothorax.

Patient Position

E   **1.** Ask the patient to sit upright for the respiratory assessment.
    2. View the patient either before or after the assessment and note the assumed position for breathing. Ask if the assumed position is required for respiratory comfort.
    3. Note if the patient can breathe normally when in a supine position.
    4. Note if pillows are used to prop the patient upright to facilitate breathing.

N   *The healthy adult breathes comfortably in a supine, prone, or upright position.*

E	**Examination**
N	**Normal Findings**
A	**Abnormal Findings**
P	**Pathophysiology**

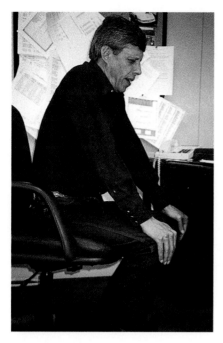

Figure 14-9 Tripod Position

A **Orthopnea** is difficulty breathing in positions other than upright.
P COPD, congestive heart failure, and pulmonary edema exemplify conditions where orthopnea may be present. The upright position maximizes the use of the respiratory muscles in patients who might otherwise be unable to breathe in a supine position, secondary to fluid in the lungs. Patients with COPD may assume the tripod position to breathe easier and make breathing look natural (see Figure 14-9). The tripod position allows for easier use of accessory muscles.

Mode of Breathing

E **1.** Stand in front of the patient.
  2. Note whether the patient is using the nose, the mouth, or both to breathe.
  3. Note for which part of the respiratory cycle each is used.
N *Normal findings vary among individuals but, generally, most patients inhale and exhale through the nose.*
A Continuous mouth breathing is usually abnormal.
P Any type of nasal or sinus blockage obstructs the normal breathing passageway and leads to mouth breathing.
A Pursed-lip breathing is performed by patients who need to prolong the expiration phase of the respiratory cycle. It appears that the patient is trying to blow out a candle or is preparing for a kiss.
P Pursed-lip breathing is performed by patients with COPD. It is the patient's innate mechanism to apply positive-pressure breathing to prevent total alveolar collapse with every breath. Less energy is expended with each breath because the alveoli do not completely collapse after expiration.

Sputum

E **1.** Ask the patient to expectorate a sputum sample.
  2. If the patient is unable to expectorate, ask the patient for a recent sputum sample from a handkerchief or tissue.
  3. Note the color, odor, amount, and consistency of the sputum.
N *A small amount of sputum is normal in every individual. The color is light yellow or clear. Normal sputum is odorless. Depending on the hydration status of the patient, the sputum can be thick or thin.*
A Colors of sputum that are abnormal are mucoid, yellow or green, rust or blood tinged, black, and pink (and frothy).
P Table 14-1 lists the pathologies that are associated with different colors of sputum.
A Foul-smelling sputum is always abnormal.
P Anaerobic infections produce foul-smelling sputum.
A A large amount of sputum can be pathological.
P Chronic bronchitis produces a large amount of sputum as a result of the irritation to the respiratory tract.
P Patients with pneumonia expectorate large quantities of sputum. The sputum is produced in reaction to the infectious process.
P An excessive amount of sputum is found in pulmonary edema, from the fluid that has leaked from pulmonary capillary membranes into large airways.
A Very thick sputum can be abnormal.
P Water is a normal component of the sputum. Therefore, when a patient is dehydrated, the sputum will be thicker because the mucus, blood, purulent material, and cellular debris form the bulk of the sputum.
A Sputum that has a thin consistency can be abnormal.
P In overhydration, the extra fluid tends to dilute the remaining components of the sputum. In pulmonary edema, the sputum is thin, pink, and frothy.

🌸 NURSING TIP

Assisting the Patient in Expectoration

- Increase fluid intake.
- Humidify environment.
- Splint painful areas with a pillow during coughing.
- Teach patient effective coughing technique.
- Use postural drainage and chest physiotherapy prior to cough, when indicated.

E Examination
N Normal Findings
A Abnormal Findings
P Pathophysiology

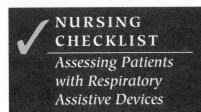

NURSING CHECKLIST
Assessing Patients with Respiratory Assistive Devices

- Oxygen
  - Mode of delivery (e.g., nasal cannula, face mask)
  - Percentage of oxygen that is being delivered (e.g., 25%, 40%)
  - Flow rate of the oxygen (e.g., 2 liters per minute, 4 liters per minute)
  - Humidification provided and oxygen warmed
- Incentive Spirometer
  - Frequency of use
  - Volume achieved (e.g., 1,000 cc, 1,500 cc)
  - Number of times patient reaches goal with each use
- Endotracheal Tube
  - Size of endotracheal tube
  - Nasal or oral insertion
  - Tube secured to the patient
  - Length of the endotracheal tube as it exits the nose or the mouth (e.g., 24 cm at the lips or 27 cm at the tip of the left nare)
  - Cuff inflated or deflated
- Tracheostomy Tube
  - Size of tracheostomy tube
  - Cuff present; if yes, cuff inflated or deflated
  - Tracheostomy ties secure the tube
- Mechanical Ventilation
  - Type of ventilator (e.g., Servo, Bear, Emerson)
  - FiO$_2$ setting
  - Mode used (e.g., assist, intermittent mandatory ventilation)
  - Amount of positive end-expiratory pressure
  - Rate and tidal volume
  - Peak inspiratory pressure
  - Temperature of the humidification
  - Alarms set

Table 14-1 Pathologies Associated with Different Colors of Sputum

SPUTUM COLOR	PATHOLOGY
Mucoid	Tracheobronchitis, asthma
Yellow or green	Bacterial infection
Rust or blood tinged	Pneumonia, pulmonary infarction, tuberculosis
Black	Black lung disease
Pink	Pulmonary edema

Palpation

General Palpation

General palpation assesses the thorax for pulsations, masses, thoracic tenderness, and crepitus.

To perform anterior palpation:

E
1. Stand in front of the patient.
2. Place the finger pads of the dominant hand on the apex of the right lung (above the clavicle).
3. Using light palpation, assess the integument of the thorax in that area.
4. Move the finger pads down to the clavicle and palpate.
5. Proceed with the palpation, moving down to each rib and ICS of the right anterior thorax. Palpate any area(s) of tenderness last.
6. Repeat the procedure on the left anterior thorax.

To perform posterior palpation:

E
1. Stand behind the patient.
2. Place the finger pads of the dominant hand on the apex of the right lung (approximately at the level of T1).
3. Using light palpation, assess the integument of the thorax in that area.
4. Move the finger pads down to the first thoracic vertebra and palpate.
5. Proceed with the palpation, moving down to each thoracic vertebra and ICS of the right posterior thorax.
6. Repeat the procedure on the left posterior thorax.

To perform lateral palpation:

E
1. Stand to the patient's right side.
2. Have the patient lift the arms overhead.
3. Place the finger pads of the dominant hand beneath the right axillary fold.
4. Using light palpation, assess the integument of the thorax in that area.
5. Move the finger pads down to the first rib beneath the axillary fold.
6. Proceed with the palpation, moving down to each rib and ICS of the right lateral thorax.
7. Move to the patient's left side.
8. Repeat steps 2–6 for the left lateral thorax.

Pulsations

N *No pulsations should be present.*
A The presence of pulsations on the thorax is abnormal.
P A thoracic aortic aneurysm that is large may be seen pulsating on the anterior chest wall.

Masses

N *No masses should be present.*
A The presence of a thoracic mass is abnormal.
P The presence of a thoracic tumor or cyst should be closely evaluated and malignancy ruled out.

❀ NURSING TIP

Assessing the Thoracic Skin

When palpating the thorax, remember to assess temperature, turgor, moisture, and edema. The expected findings and abnormalities of the temperature, turgor, moisture, and edema assessments are discussed in Chapter 10.

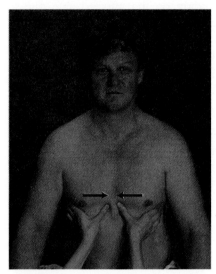

A. Anterior

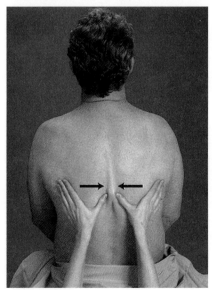

B. Posterior

Figure 14-10 Thoracic Expansion

E	Examination
N	Normal Findings
A	Abnormal Findings
P	Pathophysiology

✵ SPECIAL TECHNIQUE

Locating the Site of a Fractured Rib

To locate the site of a fractured rib:
E 1. Tell the patient what you are going to do and that some pain may be involved.
   2. Place the patient in a supine or upright position. In the latter position, support the patient's back with one hand.
   3. Place your hand over the middle of the sternum and depress lightly.
   4. Quickly remove your hand from the sternum.

Outcome: The patient will complain of pain at the fracture site. Have the patient point to the site of pain. This technique is not effective for the 11th and 12th pairs of ribs because of their anatomic nature and location.

Thoracic Tenderness

N *No thoracic tenderness should be present.*
A Fractured ribs may cause thoracic tenderness.
P Blunt chest trauma can affect any component of the respiratory tract, as well as the heart and great vessels. The region involved, the type of injury, and the impact of the injury dictate the amount of internal damage.

Crepitus

N *Crepitus should be absent.*
A The presence of **crepitus**, also referred to as subcutaneous emphysema, is always an abnormal finding. Fine beads of air escape the lung and are trapped in the subcutaneous tissue. As this area is palpated, a crackling sound may be heard. This air is slowly absorbed by the body. Crepitus is usually felt earliest in the clavicular region, but it can easily be found in the neck, face, and torso. It can also be described as feeling similar to bubble packing material that can be palpated and popped.
P Any condition that interrupts the integrity of the pleura and the lungs has the potential to lead to crepitus. Pathologies where crepitus is frequently found are pneumothorax, chest trauma, thoracic surgery, mediastinal emphysema, alveolar rupture, and tearing of pleural adhesions.

Thoracic Expansion

Thoracic expansion assesses the extent of chest expansion and the symmetry of chest wall expansion. Anterior and posterior thoracic expansions can be assessed (see Figure 14-10).

To perform anterior thoracic expansion:
E 1. Stand directly in front of the patient. Place the thumbs of both hands on the costal margins and pointing towards the xiphoid process. Gather a small fold of skin between the thumbs to assist with the visualization of the results of this technique.
   2. Lay your outstretched palms on the anterolateral thorax.
   3. Instruct the patient to take a deep breath.
   4. Observe the movement of the thumbs, both in direction and in distance.
   5. Ask the patient to exhale.
   6. Observe the movement of the thumbs as they return to the midline.

To perform posterior thoracic expansion:
E 1. Stand directly behind the patient. Place the thumbs of both hands at the level of the 10th spinal vertebra, equidistant from the spinal column and approximately 1 to 3 inches apart. Gather a small amount of skin between the thumbs as directed for anterior expansion.
   2. Place your outstretched palms on the posterolateral thorax.
   3. Instruct the patient to take a deep breath.

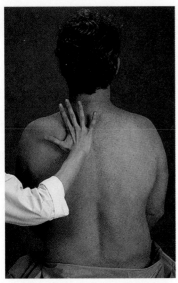

A. Using Palmar Base of Fingers

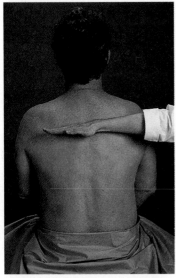

B. Using Ulnar Aspect of Hand

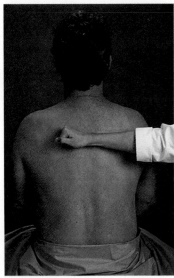

C. Using Ulnar Aspect of Closed Fist

Figure 14-11 Tactile Fremitus

4. Observe the movement of the thumbs, both in direction and in distance.
5. Ask the patient to exhale.
6. Observe the movement of the thumbs as they return to the midline.

N *The thumbs separate an equal amount from the spinal column or xiphoid process (distance) and remain in the same plane of the 10th spinous vertebra or costal margin (direction). The normal distance for the thumbs to separate during thoracic expansion is 3 to 5 cm.*

A Unilateral decreased thoracic expansion is abnormal.

P Unilateral decreased thoracic expansion on the affected or pathological side occurs in pneumothorax, pneumonia, atelectasis, lower lobe lobectomy, pleural effusion, and bronchiectasis. In these conditions, the alveoli are not either present or fully expanding on the affected side due to pathology inside or external to the lung.

A Bilateral decreased thoracic expansion is an abnormal finding.

P Bilateral disease external or internal to the lungs must be present in order for bilateral decreased thoracic expansion to be present. Hypoventilation, emphysema, pulmonary fibrosis, and pleurisy exemplify diseases where the alveoli do not fully expand.

A Displacement of thumbs from the 10th spinal vertebra region (thumbs will not meet in the midline when the patient exhales) is abnormal.

P In scoliosis, the spine is laterally deviated to a particular side. Thus, when the patient takes a deep breath, there can be a slight or marked expansion of the lungs in an unequal fashion due to the compression of the lungs by the spine.

Tactile Fremitus

Tactile or vocal fremitus is the palpable vibration of the chest wall that is produced by the spoken word. This technique is useful in assessing the underlying lung tissue and pleura. The anterior, posterior, and lateral chest walls are assessed. Three different aspects of the hand can be used to perform this skill: the palmar bases of the fingers, the ulnar aspect of the hand, and the ulnar aspect of a closed fist (see Figure 14-11). The beginning nurse may wish to experiment with each technique and decide which is the most comfortable. It is recommended that the ulnar aspect of the hand be used initially because this exposes the least amount of surface area, and, therefore, more discrete areas can be assessed.

To perform tactile fremitus:

E 1. Firmly place the ulnar aspect of an open hand (or palmar bases of the fingers or ulnar aspect of a closed fist) on the patient's right anterior apex (remember that this is above the clavicle).
2. Instruct the patient to say the words "99" or "1, 2, 3" with the same intensity every time you place your hand on the thorax.
3. Feel any vibration on the ulnar aspect of the hand as the patient phonates. If no fremitus is palpated, you may need to have the patient speak more deeply and loudly.
4. Move your hand to the same location on the left anterior thorax.
5. Repeat steps 2 and 3.
6. Compare the vibrations palpated on the right and left apices.
7. Move the hand down 2 to 3 inches and repeat the process on the right and then on the left. Ensure that your hand is in the ICS in order to avoid the bony structures. Minimal or no fremitus will be felt over the ribs because they lie on top of the lungs.
8. Continue this process down the anterior thorax to the base of the lungs.
9. Repeat this procedure for the lateral chest wall and compare symmetry. Either do the entire right then the entire left thorax, or alternate right and left at each ICS.

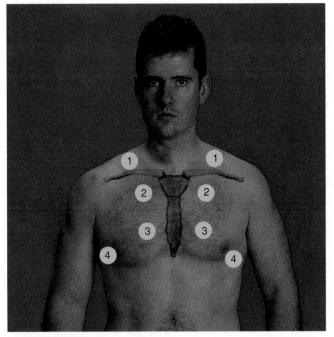

A. Anterior Thorax

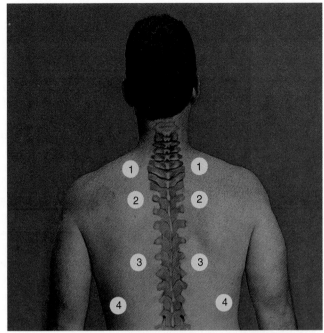

B. Posterior Thorax

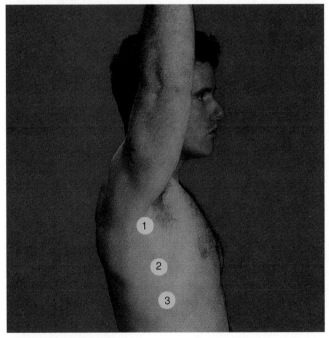

C. Right Lateral Thorax

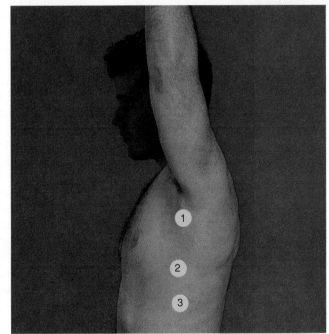

D. Left Lateral Thorax

Figure 14-12   Pattern for Tactile Fremitus

E   Examination
N   Normal Findings
A   Abnormal Findings
P   Pathophysiology

10. Repeat this procedure for the posterior chest wall. Figure 14-12 illustrates the progression of the assessment.

N   *Normal fremitus is felt as a buzzing on the ulnar aspect of the hand. The fremitus will be more pronounced near the major bronchi (second ICS anteriorly, and T1 and T2 posteriorly) and the trachea, and will be less palpable in the periphery of the lung. The diaphragm is approximately at the level of T10–T12 posteriorly and it is slightly higher on the right because of the presence of the liver.*

A   Increased tactile fremitus is abnormal.

P   Diseases that involve consolidation, such as pneumonia, atelectasis, and bronchitis, also involve increased tactile fremitus in the affected area.

A compressed lung will also exhibit increased tactile fremitus because solids conduct sound better than does air.

A Decreased or absent tactile fremitus is a pathological finding.

P Because porous materials conduct vibrations less effectively than do fluids and solids, decreased tactile fremitus will be present in pneumothorax, emphysema, and asthma.

P In a pleural effusion, the exudate is external to the alveoli and therefore acts as a blockade to the transmission of sound waves. This results in decreased tactile fremitus.

P A patient with a large chest wall or the obese patient will have decreased tactile fremitus because the sound waves are dampened as they pass through a greater distance.

A A high diaphragm level is abnormal.

P The diaphragm level is abnormally high in a patient with a lower lobe lobectomy. Tactile fremitus will be present above the surgical site.

A There are three additional findings that can be revealed during tactile fremitus: pleural friction fremitus, tussive fremitus, and rhonchal fremitus.

P **Pleural friction fremitus** is a palpable grating sensation that feels more pronounced on inspiration when there is an inflammatory process between the visceral and the parietal pleuras.

P **Tussive fremitus** is the palpable vibration produced by coughing.

P **Rhonchal fremitus** is the coarse palpable vibration produced by the passage of air through thick exudate in large bronchi or the trachea. This can clear with coughing.

Tracheal Position

To assess the position of the trachea:

E 1. Place the finger pad of the index finger on the patient's trachea in the suprasternal notch (see Figure 14-13).
    2. Move the finger pad laterally to the right and gently move the trachea in the space created by the border of the inner aspect of the sternocleidomastoid muscle and the clavicle.
    3. Move the finger pad laterally to the left and repeat the procedure.

Another method by which the trachea can be palpated is:

E 1. Gently place the finger pad of the index finger in the midline of the suprasternal notch.
    2. Palpate for the position of the trachea.

N *The trachea is midline in the suprasternal notch.*

A Tracheal deviation to the affected side is abnormal.

P The normal midline position of the trachea is maintained by the counterbalancing forces of the air in the alveoli in the right and left lungs. In atelectasis and pneumonia, alveoli are closed to some degree or filled with exudate. Fewer aerating alveoli are present and therefore the trachea is slightly pushed by the healthy lung to the affected side, which contains less air.

P The mechanical pulling force of ventilator tubing that is attached to an endotracheal tube or tracheostomy for a prolonged period of time can cause tracheal deviation toward the side of the pulling.

A Tracheal deviation to the unaffected side is abnormal.

P A tension pneumothorax, pleural effusion, and a tumor may each generate sufficient pressure to force the trachea toward the unaffected side.

P An enlarged thyroid may also deviate the trachea via its space-occupying capacity.

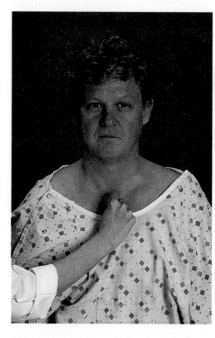

Figure 14-13 Assessing Tracheal Position

⚡ NURSING ALERT

Tension Pneumothorax

A tension pneumothorax constitutes a medical emergency. Contact the physician immediately and prepare for emergency interventions.

E Examination
N Normal Findings
A Abnormal Findings
P Pathophysiology

Percussion

Indirect or mediate percussion is used to further assess the underlying structures of the thorax. Remember that percussion reverberates a sound that is

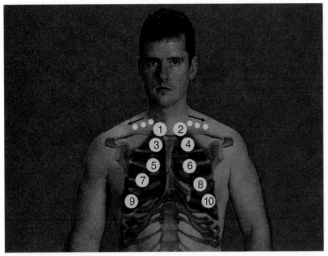

A. Anterior Thorax

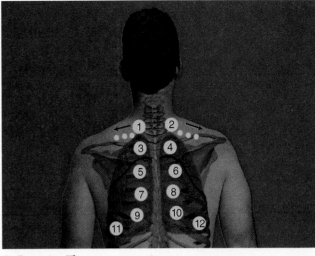

B. Posterior Thorax

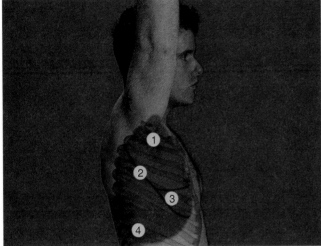

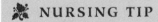

C. Right Lateral Thorax

D. Left Lateral Thorax

Figure 14-14   Percussion Patterns

generated from structures approximately 5 cm below the chest wall. Deep pathological conditions will not be revealed during the percussion process.

General Percussion

Figure 14-14 demonstrates the percussion pattern for the anterior, posterior, right lateral, and left lateral thoraxes.

To perform anterior thoracic percussion:

E   **1.** Place the patient in an upright sitting position with the shoulders back.
   2. Percuss two or three strikes along the right lung apex.
   3. Repeat this process at the left lung apex.
   4. Note the sound produced from each percussion strike and compare the sounds from each. If different sounds are produced or if the sound is not resonant, then pathology is suggested.
   5. Move down approximately 5 cm, or every other ICS, and percuss in that area.
   6. Percuss in the same position on the contralateral side.
   7. Continue to move down until the entire lung has been percussed.

To perform posterior thoracic percussion:

E   **1.** Place the patient in an upright sitting position with a slight forward tilt. Have the patient bend the head down and fold the arms in front at the

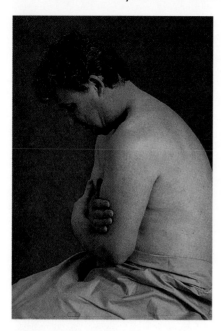

Figure 14-15 Patient Position for Posterior Percussion

waist. These actions move the scapula laterally and maximize the lung area that can be percussed (see Figure 14-15).

2. Percuss the right lung apex located along the top of the shoulder. Approximately three percussion strikes should be struck along this area.

3. Repeat the process on the left lung apex.

4. Note the sound produced from each percussion strike and compare the sounds from each. If different sounds are produced or if the sound is not resonant, then pathology is suggested.

5. Move down approximately 5 cm, or every other ICS, and percuss in that area.

6. Percuss in the same position on the contralateral side.

7. Continue to move down the thorax until the entire posterior lung field has been percussed.

To perform lateral thoracic percussion:

E 1. Place the patient in an upright sitting position, with hands and arms raised directly overhead. This position allows for the greatest exposure of the thorax.

2. Either percuss the entire right lateral thorax and then the entire left lateral thorax, or alternate right and left sides. Start to percuss in the ICS directly below the axilla.

3. Note the sound produced from that strike.

4. Percuss approximately 5 cm below the original location, or about every other ICS.

5. Percuss down to the base of the lung.

N *Normal lung tissue produces a resonant sound. The diaphragm and the cardiac silhouette emit dull sounds. Rib sounds are flat. Hyperresonance is normal in thin adults and in patients with decreased musculature.*

A The presence of hyperresonance in the majority of adults is abnormal.

P Hyperresonance is percussed in air-filled spaces. It can be elicited in pneumothorax, emphysema, asthma, and an emphysematous bulla.

A The healthy human lung never produces a dull sound.

P Dullness is found in solid or fluid-filled structures. Pneumonia, atelectasis, pulmonary edema, pleural effusion, pulmonary fibrosis, hemothorax, empyema, and tumors are dull to percussion.

Diaphragmatic Excursion

Diaphragmatic excursion provides information on the patient's depth of ventilation. This is accomplished by measuring the distance the diaphragm moves during inspiration and expiration.

To perform diaphragmatic excursion:

E 1. Position the patient for posterior thoracic percussion.

2. With the patient breathing normally, percuss the right lung from the apex (resonance in healthy adults) to below the diaphragm (dull). Note the level at which the percussion note changes quality, to orient your assessment to the patient's percussion sounds. If full posterior thoracic percussion has already been performed, then this step can be eliminated.

3. Instruct the patient to inhale as deeply as possible and hold that breath.

4. With the patient holding the breath, percuss the right lung in the scapular line from below the scapula to the location where resonance changes to dullness.

5. Mark this location and tell the patient to exhale and breathe normally.

6. When the patient has recovered, instruct the patient to inhale as deeply as possible, exhale fully, and hold this exhaled breath.

7. Repercuss the right lung below the scapula in the scapular line in a caudal direction. Mark the spot where resonance changes to dullness.

☾☾ THINK ABOUT IT

Diaphragmatic Excursion Technique

You are performing diaphragmatic excursion on a patient. Midway through performing this assessment, the patient states, "Are you sure you know what you are doing? You keep tapping me and I keep breathing over and over." How would you respond to the patient? Would you alter your assessment any after this comment? Why?

E	**Examination**
N	**Normal Findings**
A	**Abnormal Findings**
P	**Pathophysiology**

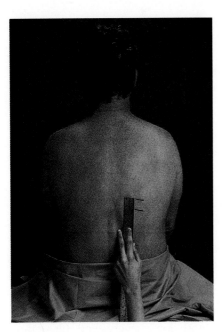

Figure 14-16 Diaphragmatic Excursion

8. Measure the distance between the two marks.

9. Repeat steps 1–8 for the left posterior thorax. Figure 14-16 illustrates diaphragmatic excursion.

N *The measured distance for diaphragmatic excursion is normally 3 to 5 cm. The level of the diaphragm on inspiration is T12, and T10 on expiration. The right side of the diaphragm is usually slightly higher than the left.*

A A diaphragmatic excursion that is less than 3 cm is abnormal.

P Conditions involving hypoventilation, where the patient is unable to inhale deeply or hold that breath, can lead to a reduction in the diaphragmatic excursion. Pain, obesity, lung congestion, emphysema, asthma, and pleurisy are examples.

A A high diaphragm level suggests lung pathology.

P Surgical intervention can elevate the diaphragm. If a lower lobe lobectomy is performed, the diaphragm will move upwards to partially fill the empty space. Likewise, after a pneumonectomy the paralyzed diaphragm will move upwards, leading to a high diaphragm level.

P Space-occupying states such as ascites and pregnancy will lead to an elevated diaphragm due to the upward displacement of the lungs and diaphragm.

P If atelectasis or a pleural effusion is present in a lower lobe, then the diaphragm will seem abnormally high, because these conditions are dull to percussion as is the diaphragm. The border between the diaphragm and the dull lung will thus be indistinguishable.

Auscultation

The aim of respiratory auscultation is to identify the presence of normal breath sounds, abnormal lung sounds, adventitious (or added) lung sounds, and adventitious pleural sounds. The anterior, posterior, and lateral aspects of the chest are auscultated. An acoustic stethoscope is required for this assessment. The diaphragm, which transmits high-pitched sounds, is the headpiece used in this process.

General Auscultation

To perform anterior thoracic auscultation:

E **1.** Place the patient in an upright sitting position with the shoulders back.

2. Instruct the patient to breathe only through the mouth. Mouth breathing, when compared to nasal breathing, decreases air turbulence, which can interfere with the interpretation of breath sounds. Have the patient inhale and exhale deeply and slowly every time the stethoscope is felt or when instructed to do so.

3. Place the stethoscope on the apex of the right lung and listen for one complete respiratory cycle (one inhalation and one exhalation). If the patient has coarse or dense chest hair, dampen the hair to prevent distortion of the auscultation findings by a crackling sound.

4. Note the sound that is auscultated.

5. Repeat on the left apex.

6. Note the breath sound auscultated in each area and compare one side to the other.

7. Continue to move the stethoscope down approximately 5 cm, or every other ICS, comparing contralateral sides. Remember to visualize the anatomic topography of the chest during auscultation.

To perform posterior thoracic auscultation:

E **1.** Place the patient as shown in Figure 14-15, in an upright sitting position with a slight forward tilt, head bent down, and arms folded in front at the waist. These actions move the scapula laterally and maximize the lung area that can be auscultated.

E **Examination**
N **Normal Findings**
A **Abnormal Findings**
P **Pathophysiology**

E Examination
N Normal Findings
A Abnormal Findings
P Pathophysiology

2. Place the stethoscope firmly on the patient's right lung apex. Ask the patient to inhale and exhale deeply and slowly every time the stethoscope is felt on the back.
3. Repeat this process on the left lung apex.
4. Move the stethoscope down approximately 5 cm, or every other ICS, and auscultate in that area.
5. Auscultate in the same position on the contralateral side.
6. Continue to move inferiorly with the auscultation until the entire posterior lung has been assessed. Refer to Figure 14-14 from the percussion section for the recommended stethoscope location for each auscultation.

To perform lateral thoracic auscultation:

E
1. Place the patient in an upright sitting position with the hands and arms directly overhead.
2. Auscultate the entire right thorax first, then the entire left thorax, or auscultate the right and left lateral thoraxes by comparing side to side. The stethoscope should initially be placed in the ICS directly below the axilla.
3. Instruct the patient to breathe only through the mouth. Have the patient inhale and exhale deeply and slowly every time the stethoscope is felt on the lateral thorax.
4. Note the sound that is auscultated and continue to move the stethoscope inferiorly approximately every 5 cm, or every other ICS, until the entire thorax has been auscultated.

Breath Sounds

N *Air rushing through the respiratory tract during inspiration and expiration generates different breath sounds in the normal patient. There are three distinct types of normal breath sounds:*
1. *Bronchial (or tubular)*
2. *Bronchovesicular*
3. *Vesicular*

Each breath sound is unique in its pitch, intensity, quality, relative duration in the inspiratory and expiratory phases of respiration, and location. Table 14-2 depicts this information. It is abnormal to auscultate these breath sounds in locations other than where they are usually found. For example, a patient with emphysema may have bronchial breath sounds in the peripheral lung parenchyma, where vesicular sounds are expected to be found. Also keep in mind that heart sounds may obscure some of the breath sounds during the anterior chest auscultation.

Table 14-2   Characteristics of Normal Breath Sounds

BREATH SOUND	PITCH	INTENSITY	QUALITY	RELATIVE DURATION OF INSPIRATORY AND EXPIRATORY PHASES	LOCATION
Bronchial	High	Loud	Blowing/hollow	I < E	Trachea
Bronchovesicular	Moderate	Moderate	Combination of bronchial and vesicular	I = E	Between scapula, first and second ICS lateral to the sternum
Vesicular	Low	Soft	Gentle rustling/breezy	I > E	Peripheral lung

Breath sounds that are not normal can be classified as either abnormal or adventitious breath sounds. Abnormal breath sounds are characterized by decreased or absent breath sounds. **Adventitious breath sounds** are super-imposed sounds on the normal bronchial, bronchovesicular, and vesicular breath sounds. There are six adventitious breath sounds:

1. Fine crackle
2. Coarse crackle
3. Sonorous wheeze
4. Sibilant wheeze
5. Pleural friction rub
6. Stridor

Table 14-3 depicts general characteristics of adventitious breath sounds.

A Decreased breath sounds are abnormal.

P Decreased breath sounds may be noted when auscultating a large chest because of the distance between the lungs, where the sounds are generated, and the chest wall.

P An emphysematous patient may have decreased breath sounds due to the inability to inhale and exhale deeply.

P Conditions such as bronchial obstruction and atelectasis may lead to decreased breath sounds because a foreign object or sputum occludes some portion of the respiratory tract, thus blocking the passage of air.

A Absent breath sounds are always a pathological finding.

P A pleural effusion, tumor, pulmonary fibrosis, empyema, hemothorax, and hydrothorax lead to absent breath sounds. These states occupy or displace normal aerating lung space internally or externally to the lungs.

P A patient with a large pneumothorax can present with absent breath sounds due to the collapse of the lung.

P Absent breath sounds occur when the lung has been removed (pneumonectomy).

P Blocked passageways in the respiratory tract explain the etiology for absent breath sounds in pulmonary edema, massive atelectasis, and complete airway obstruction.

🌹 NURSING TIP

Upper Airway Sounds

If the patient has secretions in the oropharynx (upper airway), whether from allergies, infection, coryza, etc., the patient's respirations may be loud and gurgling. It may sound as if the patient is having difficulty breathing. Ask the patient to clear the throat, then reassess the breath sounds.

Voice Sounds

The assessment of **voice sounds** will reveal whether the lungs are filled with air, with fluid, or are solid. This auscultation need be performed only if an abnormality is detected during the general auscultation, percussion, or palpation. There are three techniques by which voice sounds can be assessed:

1. Bronchophony
2. Egophony
3. Whispered pectoriloquy

Only one of these assessments needs to be performed because they all are variations of the same physical principle and they all provide the same information. The voice sound findings will parallel those obtained during tactile fremitus. Thus, voice sounds will be heard loudest over the trachea and softest in the lung's periphery.

Table 14-3 Characteristics of Adventitious Breath Sounds

BREATH SOUND	RESPIRATORY PHASE	TIMING	DESCRIPTION	CLEAR WITH COUGH	ETIOLOGY	CONDITIONS
Fine crackle	Predominantly inspiration	Discontinuous	Dry, high-pitched crackling, popping, short duration; roll hair near ears between your fingers to simulate this sound	Possibly	Air passing through moisture in small airways that suddenly reinflate	COPD, congestive heart failure (CHF), pneumonia, pulmonary fibrosis, atelectasis
Coarse crackle	Predominantly inspiration	Discontinuous	Moist, low-pitched crackling, gurgling; long duration	Possibly	Air passing through moisture in large airways that suddenly reinflate	Pneumonia, pulmonary edema, bronchitis, atelectasis
Sonorous wheeze	Predominantly expiration	Continuous	Low pitched; snoring	Possibly	Narrowing of large airways or obstruction of bronchus	Asthma, bronchitis, airway edema, tumor, bronchiolar spasm, foreign body obstruction
Sibilant wheeze	Predominantly expiration	Continuous	High pitched; musical	Possibly	Narrowing of large airways or obstruction of bronchus	Asthma, chronic bronchitis, emphysema, tumor, foreign body obstruction
Pleural friction rub	Inspiration and expiration	Continuous	Creaking, grating	Never	Inflamed parietal and visceral pleura; can occasionally be felt on thoracic wall as two pieces of dry leather rubbing against each other	Pleurisy, tuberculosis, pulmonary infarction, pneumonia, lung abscess
Stridor	Predominantly inspiration	Continuous	Crowing	Never	Partial obstruction of the larynx, trachea	Croup, foreign body obstruction, large airway tumor

To perform **bronchophony**:

E 1. Position the patient for posterior, lateral, or anterior chest auscultation. The area to be auscultated will be that in which an abnormality was found during percussion or palpation or in which adventitious breath sounds were heard.

2. Place the stethoscope in the appropriate location on the patient.

3. Instruct the patient to say the words "99" or "1, 2, 3" every time the stethoscope is placed on the chest or when told to do so.

4. Auscultate the transmission of the patient's spoken word.

To perform **egophony**:

E 1. Repeat steps 1 and 2 from the bronchophony procedure.

2. Instruct the patient to say the sound "ee" every time the stethoscope is placed on the chest or when told to do so.

3. Auscultate the transmission of the patient's spoken word.

To perform **whispered pectoriloquy**:

E 1. Repeat steps 1 and 2 from the bronchophony procedure.

2. Instruct the patient to whisper the words "99" or "1, 2, 3" every time the stethoscope is placed on the chest or when told to do so.

3. Auscultate the transmission of the patient's spoken word.

N *The normal finding when performing tests for bronchophony, egophony, and whispered pectoriloquy is an unclear transmission or muffled sounds.*

A Positive (or present) voice sounds are:

Bronchophony: clear transmission of "99" or "1, 2, 3" with increased intensity.

Egophony: transformation of "ee" to "ay" with increased intensity; the voice has a nasal or bleating quality.

Whispered pectoriloquy: clear transmission of "99" or "1, 2, 3." with increased intensity.

P Any type of consolidation process, such as pneumonia, will produce positive voice sounds. Remember the principle that sound is transmitted reasonably well by a fluid medium.

A Voice sounds are absent or even more decreased than in the normal lung in conditions where the lung is more air filled than usual.

P Air conducts sound poorly. Therefore, air-filled lungs (emphysema, asthma, pneumothorax) will produce absent voice sounds.

Table 14-4 compares physical assessment findings in selected respiratory states.

✸ SPECIAL TECHNIQUE

Forced Expiratory Time

Forced expiratory time is a gross measurement of the forced expiratory volume (FEV).

To perform this assessment:

E 1. Place your stethoscope over the patient's trachea.

2. Instruct the patient to inhale as deeply as possible and then exhale forcefully through the mouth (as if blowing out a candle).

3. Time the exhalation phase.

N *Normal exhalation occurs in less than 4 seconds.*

A The forced expiratory time is abnormal if it is greater than 4 seconds.

P Patients with COPD have a prolonged forced expiratory time and FEV because of the air trapping in the lungs. A complete exhalation is difficult to achieve.

E	Examination
N	Normal Findings
A	Abnormal Findings
P	Pathophysiology

Table 14-4 Comparison of Physical Assessment Findings in Selected Respiratory Conditions

INSPECTION

Condition	Shape of Thorax	Skin Color: Lips and Nails	Clubbing, Angle of Ribs
Healthy adult	1:2 to 5:7	Pink in light-skinned individuals; darker than normal in dark-skinned individuals	No clubbing, rib angle 45°
Atelectasis (obstructed bronchus)	1:2 to 5:7	Pale or cyanotic	No clubbing, rib angle 45°
Atelectasis (patent bronchus)	1:2 to 5:7	Pale or cyanotic	No clubbing, rib angle 45°
Bronchitis	1:2 to 5:7	Possibly pale	No clubbing, rib angle 45°
Consolidation (pneumonia)	1:2 to 5:7	Pale or cyanotic	No clubbing, rib angle 45°
Emphysema	1:1 (barrel chest)	Pale	Clubbing, rib angle >45°
Pleural effusion	1:2 to 5:7	Pale or cyanotic	No clubbing, rib angle 45°
Pneumothorax	1:2 to 5:7	Pale or cyanotic	No clubbing, rib angle 45°
Pulmonary edema	1:2 to 5:7	Pale or cyanotic	No clubbing, rib angle 45°
Asthma	If chronic, may have barrel chest	Pale or cyanotic in acute attack	No clubbing, rib angle 45°
Bronchiectasis	1:1	Pale or cyanotic if severe	Clubbing possible, rib angle >45°
Congestive heart failure	1:2 to 5:7	Pale or cyanotic	Clubbing possible, rib angle 45°

Condition	Capillary Refill	Retractions or Bulging of ICS	Respiratory Rate
Healthy adult	Brisk	Absent	12–20/min eupnea
Atelectasis (obstructed bronchus)	Sluggish	Absent	>20/min tachypnea
Atelectasis (patent bronchus)	Sluggish to moderate	Absent	>20/min tachypnea
Bronchitis	Sluggish to moderate	Absent	>20/min tachypnea
Consolidation (pneumonia)	Sluggish	Absent	>20/min tachypnea
Emphysema	Sluggish	Both present	>20/min tachypnea
Pleural effusion	Sluggish	Bulging	>20/min tachypnea
Pneumothorax	Sluggish	Bulging	>20/min tachypnea
Pulmonary edema	Sluggish	Absent	>20/min tachypnea
Asthma	Sluggish in acute attack	Retractions	>20/min tachypnea
Bronchiectasis	Sluggish if severe	Retractions if severe	>20/min tachypnea
Congestive heart failure	Sluggish	Retractions	>20/min tachypnea

PALPATION

Condition	Thoracic Expansion	Tactile Fremitus	Tracheal Position
Healthy adult	3–5 cm	Moderate (normal)	Midline
Atelectasis (obstructed bronchus)	Decreased	Increased	Shifts to affected side
Atelectasis (patent bronchus)	Decreased	Increased	Shifts to affected side
Bronchitis	Possibly decreased	Moderate or increased	Midline
Consolidation (pneumonia)	Decreased	Increased	Shifts to affected side
Emphysema	Decreased	Decreased	Midline

continued

Table 14-4 Comparison of Physical Assessment Findings in Selected Respiratory Conditions *continued*

PALPATION *continued*

Condition	Thoracic Expansion	Tactile Fremitus	Tracheal Position
Pleural effusion	Decreased	Decreased	Shifts to unaffected side
Pneumothorax	Decreased	Absent or decreased	Shifts to unaffected side
Pulmonary edema	Decreased	Increased	Midline
Asthma	Decreased in attack	Decreased	Midline
Bronchiectasis	Decreased on affected side	Increased	Midline or deviated toward affected side
Congestive heart failure	May be decreased	Moderate	Midline

PERCUSSION

Condition	General Percussion	Diaphragmatic Excursion
Healthy adult	Resonant	3–5 cm
Atelectasis (obstructed bronchus)	Dull	Decreased
Atelectasis (patent bronchus)	Dull	Decreased
Bronchitis	Resonant	Decreased if severe
Consolidation (pneumonia)	Dull	Decreased
Emphysema	Hyperresonant	Decreased
Pleural effusion	Dull	Decreased
Pneumothorax	Hyperresonant	Decreased
Pulmonary edema	Dull	Decreased
Asthma	Hyperresonant	Decreased
Bronchiectasis	Resonant to dull	Decreased
Congestive heart failure	Resonant	Decreased

AUSCULTATION

Condition	Breath Sounds	Adventitious Sounds	Voice Sounds
Healthy adult	Vesicular in periphery	Absent	Muffled
Atelectasis (obstructed bronchus)	Absent or decreased	Absent	Absent or muffled
Atelectasis (patent bronchus)	Bronchial	Crackles or wheezes	Increased or muffled
Bronchitis	Vesicular or bronchial	Crackles or wheezes	Increased or muffled
Consolidation (pneumonia)	Bronchial	Crackles or occasional friction rub	Increased
Emphysema	Bronchial and decreased	Wheezes	Decreased
Pleural effusion	Absent or decreased	Possible friction rub	Decreased or absent
Pneumothorax	Absent or decreased	Absent	Decreased or absent
Pulmonary edema	Absent or decreased	Crackles	Increased
Asthma	Decreased or absent in severe obstruction	Wheezes	Decreased
Bronchiectasis	Vesicular or bronchial if severe	Crackles or wheezes	Muffled or decreased
Congestive heart failure	Vesicular	Crackles	Muffled

NURSING TIP

Lung Assessment in Older Patients

Frequent rests may be necessary when conducting the thorax and lung assessment in an older patient.

NURSING TIP

Thoracic Changes in the Older Adult

The older patient may be unaware of the changes in the thorax that occur with aging. Reassure the patient that the barrel chest and kyphosis are normal body changes associated with aging.

NURSING TIP

Preventing Respiratory Complications

To minimize respiratory complications, instruct the older adult to:
- Avoid large crowds, especially in enclosed areas, if ill.
- Obtain a flu vaccine as recommended by local health department or primary provider.
- Chew food completely and do not talk while eating.
- Avoid eating in a supine position (if possible).
- Avoid strenuous exercise if not part of normal activity.

GERONTOLOGICAL VARIATIONS

The aging patient undergoes changes that involve the external and internal anatomy of the thorax and lungs and that affect the respiratory process. As a result, the physiology of the respiratory system also becomes altered. The resulting state of the patient depends on the extent of the changes and the condition of the body prior to these changes. The gerontological variations of the respiratory system include four broad areas:

1. Anatomic changes
2. Alveolar gas exchange
3. Regulation of ventilation
4. Lung defense mechanisms

Older adults experience degeneration of the intervertebral discs, stiffening of ligaments and joints, and calcification of the costochondral cartilage. These changes limit chest wall expansion during the respiratory cycle. Muscles atrophy and the diaphragm flattens out. Collectively, these changes make respiratory effort more difficult for the older patient. Strenuous exercise is taxing secondary to the decrease in oxygen uptake and decreased elastic recoil of the lung parenchyma. Most older adults will have barrel chest and some kyphosis. Forced vital capacity decreases, residual volume and functional residual capacity increase, and total lung capacity remains unchanged.

The second major change in the gerontological population is the alveolar gas exchange. The lung's decreased elastic recoil causes the closure of the airways for a portion of the respiratory cycle. This occurs particularly in the lower lobes of the lungs. As a result, the apices and the bases of the lower lobes have a ventilation-perfusion mismatch. Other contributing factors to this loss of alveolar gas exchange are the loss of lung tissue and alveolar capillaries, and pulmonary wall thickening. In essence, this creates a situation in which there is less surface area for diffusion, and this surface area is thicker. In addition, hemoglobin's affinity for oxygen decreases. This leads to a decrease in the partial pressure of oxygen.

The aging patient experiences changes in the regulation of ventilation. The medulla is less sensitive to changes in carbon dioxide and oxygen levels, which normally trigger the respiratory apparatus. Neural output to respiratory muscles is decreased. Both peripheral and central chemoreceptors are affected.

The last area of gerontological variation is in lung defense mechanisms. There is less ciliary activity, which increases susceptibility to infection. The cough reflex decreases. The risk of aspiration increases with this weakened defense mechanism.

NURSING ALERT

Risk Factors for Pneumonia

The following are risk factors for developing pneumonia:
- Smoking
- Emphysema
- Intoxication
- Bedridden status
- Postoperative status
- Immunosuppressed status
- Decreased cough reflex
- Sedated and unconscious condition
- Oxygen therapy that is harboring bacteria

CASE STUDY

The case study illustrates the application and objective documentation of the thorax and lungs assessment.

The Patient with a Pneumothorax

John is a 17-year-old high school football player. In the middle of the third quarter of today's game, he was tackled particularly hard and three members of the opposite team piled in on the tackle.

❖ HEALTH HISTORY

PATIENT PROFILE	17 yo SBM
CHIEF COMPLAINT	"I can't breathe. The pain is terrible. It started after the tackle in the third quarter."
HISTORY OF PRESENT ILLNESS	(Reported by team trainer b/c pt had SOB.) In usual state of good hl until this PM. While playing football was tackled unusually hard, hit & kicked in chest. Pt experienced ®️ sided CP c̄ 5/10 intensity, sharp & stabbing in middle of ®️ chest. Exacerbated by deep breath. Pt rested for 3 plays & pain subsided slightly. Pt was tackled again & experienced SOB. Over next 5 min, CP worsened (10/10) & didn't radiate. Trainer counted RR of 44 bpm. Breathing eased in upright position, pain & breathing aggravated by movement. Pt became pale & sweated profusely. Became "panicked & angry." Ambulance squad transported pt to hospital. O₂ via face mask delivered during transport. (Pt confirmed hx c̄ nod.)
PAST HEALTH HISTORY	(NB: The majority of this information was obtained p̄ pt was stabilized.)
Medical	Denies
Surgical	Wisdom teeth removed 2 yr PTA; Ø complications
Medications	MVI q AM
Communicable Diseases	Denies rheumatic fever, STD, TB
Allergies	Denies allergies to medication, food, animals, environmental conditions
Injuries/Accidents	Broken ®️ arm 7 yr PTA from jumping over fence; cast for 4 wk; Ø complications
Disabilities/Handicaps	Denies
Blood Transfusions	Denies
Childhood Illnesses	Chicken pox 13 yr PTA, Ø complications; doesn't recall any other dz
Immunizations	"Up to date"; no specifics available

continued

FAMILY HEALTH HISTORY

LEGEND

- ⬤ Living female
- ◼ Living male
- ⊗ Deceased female
- ⊠ Deceased male
- ↗ Points to patient

A&W = Alive and well

HTN = Hypertension

MI = Myocardial infarction

MVA = Motor vehicle accident

32 Childbirth — **71** MI HTN   **64** MVA — **70** Glaucoma

48 A&W   **45** Arthritis   **42** A&W — **44** A&W   **4MO** Unknown cause

17 ↗ Pneumothorax

Denies family hx of cystic fibrosis, asthma.

SOCIAL HISTORY

Alcohol Use	Wkend beer drinker: 6 pack × 2 yr
Tobacco Use	Denies
Drug Use	Admits to experimenting with pot & other "pills" in the summer when not in training
Sexual Practice	Refuses to answer
Travel History	Europe 2 yr PTA
Work Environment	N/A
Home Environment	No reply
Hobbies/Leisure Activities	Wt lifts 1 hr qd; runs 3 miles qod when not in training; listens to music
Stress	School, football performance, dating
Education	11th grade
Economic Status	Dependent on parents
Military Service	N/A
Religion	Christian
Ethnic Background	Denies any affiliation
Roles/Relationships	Son
Characteristic Patterns of Daily Living	Deferred

continued

HEALTH MAINTENANCE ACTIVITIES	
Sleep	6–8 hr night
Diet	Reports balanced diet "to keep me fit for football"; follows regimen prescribed by coach
Exercise	See Hobbies/Leisure Activities
Stress Management	Running
Use of Safety Devices	Wears prescribed football padding & helmet; denies use of seat belt
Health Check-Ups	Annual physical by school MD for football
PHYSICAL ASSESSMENT	
Inspection	
Shape of Thorax	AP diameter:transverse diameter = 1:2; $\ominus$ barrel chest, pectus carinatum, pectus excavatum, kyphosis, scoliosis
Symmetry of Chest Wall	Shoulder & scapula ht equal; Ø masses
Presence of Superficial Veins	Ø
Costal Angle	<90°
Angle of the Ribs	45° c̄ sternum
Intercostal Spaces	$\oplus$ bulging Ⓡ chest wall; Ø retractions
Muscles of Respiration	Breathing diaphragmatically c̄ sternocleidomastoid & trapezius muscles
Respirations	Rate: 42/min Pattern: Irregular Depth: Shallow Symmetry: Ⓛ chest expansion > Ⓡ Audibility: Loud Patient position: Sitting Mode of breathing: Mouth breathing c̄ nasal flaring
Sputum	None
Palpation	
General Palpation	Pulsations: Ø pulsations Masses: Ø masses Thoracic tenderness: Over entire Ⓡ chest Crepitus: $\oplus$, inferior to Ⓡ clavicle
Thoracic Expansion	Anterior expansion 2.5 cm, posterior expansion 3.0 cm, moderate Ⓛ chest expansion, minimal Ⓡ chest expansion
Tactile Fremitus	Moderate on Ⓛ chest ant & post; absent on Ⓡ chest ant & post

continued

Tracheal Position	Deviated to Ⓛ
Percussion	
General Percussion	Resonant Ⓛ chest ant & post; hyperresonant Ⓡ chest ant & post
Diaphragmatic Excursion	3.5 cm on Ⓛ at T10 & T12; unable to obtain on Ⓡ
Auscultation	
General Auscultation	Vesicular sounds in Ⓛ periphery, bronchial over trachea, bronchovesicular at edge of Ⓛ scapula; absent breath sounds over entire Ⓡ lung field
Breath Sounds	Ø crackles, wheezes, pleural friction rub, stridor
Voice Sounds	Muffled voice sounds on Ⓛ; absent voice sounds on Ⓡ
Special Technique	Fractured rib assessment: c/o pain on Ⓡ, ribs 4–7
Assistive Devices	Currently on 100% face mask

LABORATORY DATA

ABG	On Admission (100% face mask)	15 min. after chest tube placement (100% face mask)	3 hr. after chest tube placement (40% face mask)	Normal Range
pH	7.60	7.55	7.44	7.35–7.45
PaO_2	58 mm Hg	72 mm Hg	89 mm Hg	80–100 mm Hg
$PaCO_2$	30 mm Hg	34 mm Hg	37 mm Hg	35–45 mm Hg
HCO_3	18 mEq/L	20 mEq/L	22 mEq/L	22–26 mEq/L
O_2 saturation	88%	90%	96%	95–100%

DIAGNOSTIC DATA

Chest X-Ray   General impression: No previous film available with which to compare the presenting film. Anterior right ribs 3–7 are fractured and there is a hairline fracture on the fifth rib on the left. No signs of sclerosing or healing consistent with an acute fracture. All other anterior skeletal structures intact. Right lung with 75% pneumothorax. Slight tracheal deviation to the left with minimal left mediastinal shift.

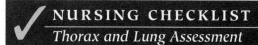

NURSING CHECKLIST
Thorax and Lung Assessment

Inspection
- Shape of Thorax
- Symmetry of Chest Wall
- Presence of Superficial Veins
- Costal Angle
- Angle of the Ribs
- Intercostal Spaces
- Muscles of Respiration
- Respirations
    - Rate
    - Pattern
    - Depth
    - Symmetry
    - Audibility
    - Patient position
    - Mode of breathing
- Sputum

Palpation
- General Palpation
    - Pulsations
    - Masses
    - Thoracic tenderness
    - Crepitus
- Thoracic Expansion
- Tactile Fremitus
- Tracheal Position

Percussion
- General Percussion
- Diaphragmatic Excursion

Auscultation
- General Auscultation
- Breath Sounds
- Voice Sounds

Special Techniques
- Locating the Site of a Fractured Rib
- Forced Expiratory Time

Assistive Devices
- Oxygen
- Incentive Spirometer
- Endotracheal Tube
- Tracheostomy Tube
- Mechanical Ventilation

REVIEW QUESTIONS AND ACTIVITIES

1. It is helpful to visualize the locations of the different anatomic landmarks and lobes of the lungs when describing respiratory pathology. To assist you in this activity, you will need a volunteer and a washable marker. First, have your volunteer remove his or her shirt. Count the ribs on the left and the right thoraxes and number them with the marker. Mark the level of the sternal angle and the diaphragm. Next, identify and mark the anatomic landmarks described in the text. Trace the outlines of the three lobes of the right lung and the two lobes of the left lung. Move posteriorly and count the spinous process. Mark the vertebra prominens. Trace the outlines of the lungs.

2. Describe the inspection assessment findings that you would expect to see in the patient with severe emphysema. Provide rationale for each finding.

3. Explain the pathophysiology for increased tactile fremitus in pulmonary edema, and decreased tactile fremitus in pleural effusion.

4. Resonance, hyperresonance, and dullness are possible percussion findings in the pulmonary assessment. State the condition(s) when each percussion note can be found and provide rationale for each.

5. Your patient is experiencing an acute episode of asthma. Describe the assessment findings that you would expect in inspection, palpation, percussion, and auscultation.

6. Bronchophony is performed on a patient with a suspected lung infiltration. Describe what you expect to find and provide scientific rationale.

7. Match the following breath sounds:
   a. Bronchial _____ peripheral lung
   b. Bronchovesicular _____ trachea
   c. Vesicular _____ between scapula, first and second ICS lateral to the sternum

Questions 8–10 refer to the following situation:
   Marta Radaszkiewicz is an 81-year-old woman who presents with respiratory difficulty. Her respiratory rate is 35 breaths per minute and she is expectorating moderate amounts of sputum. She is diagnosed with left lower lobe pneumonia.

8. A respiratory rate of 35 breaths per minute is called:
   a. Eupnea
   b. Bradypnea
   c. Tachypnea
   d. Apnea

   The correct answer is (c).

9. The color of sputum most commonly found in pneumonia is:
   a. Mucoid
   b. Pink
   c. Black
   d. Rust

   The correct answer is (d).

10. Which of the following assessment findings may be found in a patient with pneumonia?
   a. Increased tactile fremitus
   b. Tracheal shift to the unaffected side
   c. Resonant percussion
   d. Decreased voice sounds

   The correct answer is (a).

Heart and Peripheral Vasculature

1. Identify the anatomic landmarks of the chest and periphery.
2. Describe the characteristics of the most common cardiovascular chief complaints.
3. Elicit a health history from a patient with cardiovascular pathology.
4. Perform a cardiovascular assessment on a healthy adult.
5. Perform a cardiovascular assessment on a patient with cardiovascular pathology.
6. Provide scientific rationale for abnormal cardiovascular assessment findings.
7. Describe the changes that occur in the cardiovascular system in the elderly.

The heart's primary function is to pump blood to all parts of the body. The circulating blood not only brings oxygen and nutrients to the body's tissues but also helps to take away the body's waste products. The body's activities determine the amount of blood that is pumped. The heart will beat faster or slower and the blood vessels will expand or relax in order to properly distribute the blood that the body demands.

ANATOMY AND PHYSIOLOGY

Heart

In a resting, healthy adult, the heart contracts 60 to 100 times while pumping 4 to 5 liters of blood per minute. An individual's heart is only about the size of his or her clenched fist. The human heart is remarkably efficient considering its size in relation to the rest of the body.

The heart is located in the thoracic cavity between the lungs and above the diaphragm in an area known as the mediastinum (refer to Figure 15-1). The **base** of the heart is the uppermost portion, which includes the left and right atria as well as the aorta, pulmonary arteries, and the superior and inferior venae cavae. These structures lie behind the upper portion of the sternum. The **apex**, or lower portion of the heart, extends into the left thoracic cavity, causing the heart to appear as if it is lying on its right ventricle.

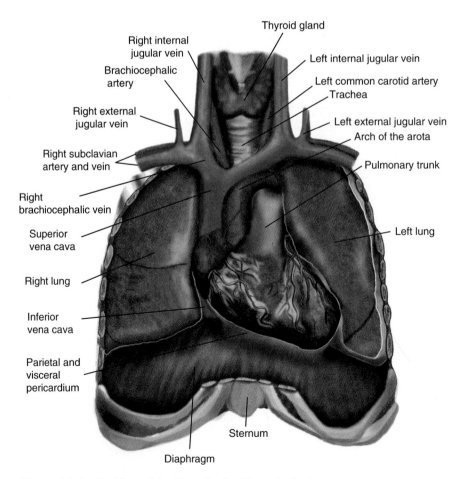

Figure 15-1   Position of the Heart in the Thoracic Cavity

Pericardium

The heart and roots of the great vessels lie within a sac called the pericardium, which is composed of serous and fibrous layers. The fibrous layer is the outermost layer and is connected to the diaphragm and sternum by ligaments and tendons. Its major role is to limit the stretching of the myocardial muscle, especially in the setting of strenuous activity or hypervolemia.

There are two serous layers of the pericardium: the **parietal** layer, which lies close to the fibrous tissues, and the **visceral** layer, which lies against the actual heart muscle. This visceral layer is often referred to as the epicardium. Between the two serous layers is a small space that contains approximately 20 to 50 ml of pericardial fluid. This pericardial fluid serves to facilitate the movement of the heart muscle and protect it via its lubricant effect.

Chambers of the Heart

The heart is divided into four chambers, which are separated laterally by walls known as the vertical **septa**. These vertical septa divide the heart into the right and the left atria (interatrial septum) and the right and the left ventricles (interventricular septum). The right atrium is the collection point for the blood returning from the systemic circulation for reoxygenation in the lungs. The left atrium receives its freshly oxygenated blood via the four pulmonary veins, which are the only veins in the body that carry oxygenated blood.

The walls of the left ventricle are three times thicker than those of the right ventricle because of its greater workload as it pumps blood through the high-pressure systemic arterial system. Left ventricular pressures are five times greater than those in the right ventricle. Figure 15-2 shows the configuration of the heart's chambers, the pressures, and normal oxygen content of the blood contained therein.

Heart Valves

As blood empties into the two atria, the **atrioventricular (A-V) valves** prevent it from prematurely entering the ventricles. The A-V valve between the right atrium and the right ventricle is known as the tricuspid valve, named for its three flaps or cusps. The A-V valve between the left atrium and the left ventricle is the bicuspid valve, named for its two flaps or cusps; it is commonly known as the mitral valve. When the tricuspid and mitral valves are closed, blood cannot flow from the atria into the ventricles. In a normal heart, they open only as atrial pressures increase with progressive filling.

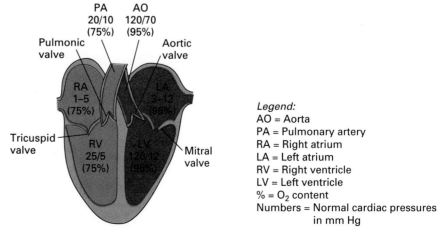

Figure 15-2   The Configuration, Normal Pressures, and Oxygen Content of the Heart Chambers

The semilunar valves are also known as outflow valves because blood exits the heart through them. Blood flows from the right ventricle to the pulmonary vasculature for oxygenation by way of the pulmonic valve. Blood is pumped from the left ventricle into the systemic and coronary circulation through the aortic valve.

⚠ NURSING ALERT

Warning Signs of Imminent Cardiovascular Problems

- Change in color of lips, face, or nails
- Chest pain
- Diaphoresis (extreme)
- Dizziness
- Dyspnea
- Edema
- Extremity pain
- Fatigue
- Feeling of doom
- Numbness in the extremities
- Pain that limits self-care
- Palpitations
- Syncope
- Tingling in the extremities

Coronary Circulation

The exterior surface of the heart muscle contains a very important and intricate blood supply. Two major coronary arteries arise from the small openings in the aorta known as the sinuses of Valsalva, located just behind the aortic valve. Figure 15-3 demonstrates the position of the coronary arteries as they exit from the aorta to cover the myocardium with an arterial network. The left and right coronary arteries run superficially across the heart muscle, but the smaller branches of these two main arteries actually penetrate deeply into the myocardium, carrying with them a rich, nutritive blood supply. Blood flow to the coronary arteries is greatest during diastole because the force of the ventricular contraction during systole actually impedes flow through the sinuses of Valsalva.

The myocardium is extremely dependent on a constant supply of oxygen that is delivered through the coronary arterial system. The heart's oxygen requirements increase when it is stimulated by conditions such as exercise. If the coronary blood supply is not sufficient to meet the needs of the heart, the result may be **ischemia** (local and temporary lack of blood supply to the heart), injury (beyond ischemia but still reversible), or an **infarction** (necrosis) of the heart muscle itself. Myocardial ischemia is often manifested as chest, neck, or arm pain known as **angina**.

The left main coronary artery branches into the left circumflex coronary artery and the left anterior descending coronary artery (LAD). The left main coronary artery may be referred to as the "widowmaker" because of the lethal effect of any obstruction to blood flow prior to its branch point.

The LAD supplies blood to the anterior wall and apex of the left ventricle as well as to the anterior portion of the interventricular septum. The smaller arterial branches that supply the septum also nourish the ventricular conduction system, including the bundle of His and the right and left bundle branches. The left circumflex branch supplies arterial blood to the left atrium and to the lateral and posterior portions of the left ventricle. In some individuals, the sinoatrial (S-A) node and the A-V node are also supplied by this branch.

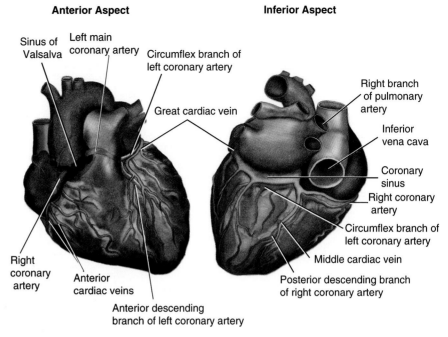

Figure 15-3 The Coronary Arteries and Major Veins of the Heart (Anterior and Inferior Views)

The right coronary artery (RCA) supplies nutrients and oxygen to the right atrium, the right ventricle, and the inferior wall of the left ventricle. In most individuals, the RCA supplies the S-A and the A-V nodes as well as the posterior portion of the interventricular septum. In inferior wall infarction, the RCA is most likely the vessel that has been occluded. In anterior wall infarction, the LAD branch would be the most likely source of occlusion with resulting complications in the ventricular conduction system, such as bundle branch blocks or ventricular dysrhythmias.

Venous drainage from the myocardium is carried by the coronary sinus, anterior cardiac veins, and thebesian veins. About 75% of the venous blood empties into the right atrium via the coronary sinus. The thebesian veins carry only a small portion of the unoxygenated blood that is emptied directly into all four chambers of the heart.

Cardiac Cycle

Figure 15-4 illustrates the electrical and mechanical events in the heart. Physical assessment findings can be correlated with these electrophysiological mechanisms.

The cardiac cycle consists of two phases: systole and diastole. In **systole**, the myocardial fibers contract and tighten to eject blood from the ventricles (for the purpose of this chapter, any mention of systole will mean ventricular

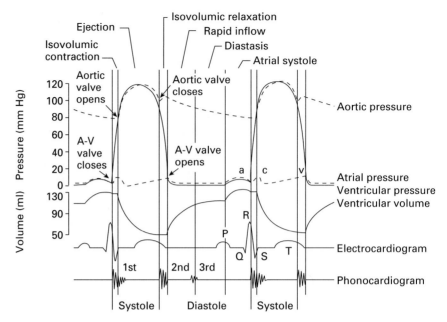

Figure 15-4 Events of the Cardiac Cycle *Reproduced with permission from Guyton, A. C. (1995). Textbook of medical physiology (9th ed.). Philadelphia: W. B. Saunders Company.*

 NURSING TIP

Heart Smart Diet

Teach your patients to eat "heart smart" as recommended by the AHA, and to follow a diet low in total fat, saturated fat, cholesterol, and sodium.

1. Total fat intake <30% of calories.
   - Saturated fatty acid intake <10% of calories (sources: animal fats, coconut oil, and palm oil).
   - Polyunsaturated fatty acid intake <10% of calories (sources: corn, soybean, and sunflower oil).
   - Monounsaturated fatty acids = 10% to 15% of calories (sources: canola and olive oil).
2. Cholesterol intake <300 mg/day (sources: beef, pork, poultry, fish, dairy products, and eggs).
3. Sodium intake <3,000 mg/day.
4. If overweight, lose weight to lower blood cholesterol level and blood pressure and to improve glucose tolerance.
5. When decreasing the total fat content of the diet, eat more carbohydrates such as those found in vegetables, fruits, and cereals.

systole unless specifically called atrial systole). **Diastole** is a period of relaxation and reflects the pressure remaining in the blood vessels after the heart has pumped.

Systole is divided into three phases, beginning with the isovolumic (or isometric) contraction phase, which marks the onset of a ventricular contraction. During this phase, the pressure is increasing but no blood is entering or leaving the ventricle. As the pressure rises in the left ventricle, the mitral valve closes (similar events occur in the right ventricle with the tricuspid valve). Closure of these A-V valves produces the first heart sound, known as S_1 (depicted as "1st" on the phonocardiogram [a recording of the heart sounds] curve in Figure 15-4).

Once the pressure in the left ventricle exceeds that in the aorta, and the pressure in the right ventricle exceeds that in the pulmonary artery, the semilunar (aortic and pulmonic) valves open and blood is rapidly ejected. This rapid ejection phase is also referred to as early systole. It is followed by a third phase of reduced ejection, which is also known as late systole.

Ventricular diastole begins with the isovolumic, or isometric, relaxation phase. During this phase, ventricular ejection ceases and the pressure in the left ventricle is reduced to less than that in the aorta. This permits a backflow of blood from the aorta to the left ventricle, causing the aortic valve to close (similar events occur in the pulmonary artery to cause the pulmonic valve to close). The closure of the semilunar valves produces the second heart sound, known as S_2 (depicted as "2nd" on the phonocardiogram curve in Figure 15-4). When the A-V and semilunar valves are closed, the pressure in the left ventricle falls rapidly.

Atrial pressures then rise as a result of the large amount of blood accumulating in the atria because of the closed A-V valves. When systole is over and the ventricular pressures fall, the high pressure in the atria forces the A-V valves to open to allow for rapid ventricular filling (rapid inflow) during early diastole. Filling then slows during a phase called diastasis or mid-diastole. Seventy percent of ventricular filling occurs in a passive manner during these early and mid-diastolic filling periods.

The final phase of diastole is known as atrial systole. The atria contract to complete the remaining 20% to 30% of ventricular filling, which is often referred to as **atrial kick**. After atrial systole, the cardiac cycle starts all over again.

The **electrocardiogram (EKG)** in Figure 15-4 shows the P, Q, R, S, and T waves. These waves are electrical voltages produced by the heart and recorded by EKG leads placed on the body. When the atria depolarize, the P wave is produced on the EKG. During this period, the pressure in the atria exceeds that in the ventricles, thus forcing the blood from the atria into the ventricles. Approximately 0.16 seconds after the appearance of the P wave, the QRS complex on the EKG occurs as the ventricles are electrically depolarized. As the ventricles begin to repolarize, the T wave appears on the EKG. The downslope of the T wave indicates the end of ventricular repolarization and the beginning of a relaxation period. Note that the EKG contains an **isoelectric line**, or flat line, after the T wave, indicating a period of electrical rest.

🌸 NURSING TIP

Sexual Activity following Cardiac Compromise

Teach your patients the following about sex after cardiac surgery or myocardial infarction (MI), as recommended by the American Heart Association (AHA):

1. Resume sexual activity as soon as you feel ready; however, check with your health care provider first. Most patients who have had an MI are able to resume sex after 4 weeks; heart surgery patients usually resume sex 2 to 3 weeks after leaving the hospital.
2. Although most patients resume sex with the same frequency as before the hospitalization, others may be less active. Begin with lower energy forms of sexual expression, such as touching, holding, and caressing, if this will raise your comfort level.
3. Seek medical care or sexual counseling if you are afraid to resume sex because of anxiety, depression, cardiac symptoms, or lack of desire.
4. Medications such as those used for chest pain, irregular heart beats, high blood pressure, edema, anxiety, and depression can affect sexual desire and performance. If a sexual problem occurs, continue taking the medication and consult your physician.
5. If recovering from an MI, you may be more aware of your breathing, heart beat, muscle tightening, or tension; this awareness is normal.

Excitation of the Heart

The **sinoatrial (S-A) node** is the normal pacemaker of the heart and is located about 1 mm below the right atrial epicardium at its junction with the superior vena cava. It initiates a rhythmic impulse approximately 70 times per minute. The infranodal atrial pathways conduct the impulse initiated in the S-A node to the **atrioventricular (A-V) node** via the myocardium of the right atrium. The three infranodal pathways are the anterior, the middle, and the posterior tracts. Meanwhile, the Bachmann's bundle conducts the impulse from the S-A node to the left atrium. In the absence of a signal from the S-A node, the A-V node has its own intrinsic rate of 40 to 60 impulses per minute. The A-V node, also known as the A-V junction, delays the impulse received from the atria before transmitting it to the ventricles in order to give them time to fill prior to the next systole. The impulse then travels very rapidly from the A-V node to the bundle branch system via the bundle of His. The bundle branch system is composed of the right bundle branch (RBB) and the left bundle branch (LBB). The RBB carries the impulse down the right side of the interventricular septum into the right ventricle. The LBB separates into three fascicles that relay the impulse to the left ventricle. Finally, the Purkinje fibers arising from the distal portions of the bundle branches transmit the impulse into the subendocardial layers of both ventricles. Barring interference with the connections described above, the final transmission of the impulse allows

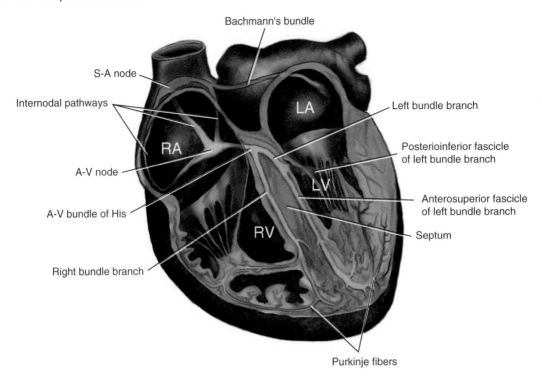

Bachmann's bundle

S-A node

Internodal pathways

A-V node

A-V bundle of His

Right bundle branch

LA

RA

LV

RV

Left bundle branch

Posterioinferior fascicle
of left bundle branch

Anterosuperior fascicle
of left bundle branch

Septum

Purkinje fibers

Figure 15-5 Excitation of the Heart. The cardiac impulse is transmitted from the S-A node to the A-V node via the internodal pathways and Bachmann's bundle, and then on to the bundle of His and down the left and right bundle branches to the Purkinje fibers, which distribute the impulse to the rest of the ventricles.

🌿 NURSING TIP

Exercise and Cardiovascular Health

Teach your patients the following about exercise:

- Always consult with a physician before starting an exercise program to determine how much exercise is right for you. This may be determined through stress, bicycle, or treadmill tests.
- Avoid activities that have caused previous cardiac problems.
- Avoid strenuous activity in extremes of temperature or after a heavy meal because this may predispose to angina.
- Stop any exercise and notify the physician if dizziness, faintness, lightheadedness, or angina occurs.

---

depolarization of the ventricles to occur followed by a normal systole. Figure 15-5 depicts the normal conduction pathways of the heart. If A-V node disease causes transmission of the electrical signal to be blocked, the intrinsic rate of the ventricles kicks in at a rate of fewer than 40 beats per minute.

Peripheral Vasculature

The circulatory system consists of arterial pathways, which are the distribution routes, and venous pathways, or the collection system that returns the blood to a central pumping station, the heart. Figure 15-6 demonstrates the journey of the blood through the systemic and pulmonary circuits.

Arterial walls are composed of three coats or linings. The innermost lining is known as the tunica intima and is composed of the endothelium and some connective tissue. The tunica media is the middle layer and is composed of both smooth muscle and an elastic type of connective tissue. The outer layer, the tunica externa or adventitia, has a more fibrous connective tissue that is arranged longitudinally.

As the arterial system branches and subdivides on its way to the periphery, the diameters of the vessels decrease. Arterioles are the smallest group of arteries, with a diameter of less than 0.5 mm. It is here that the rapid velocity of blood flow found in the larger arteries begins to decrease. Blood flow becomes even slower in the capillaries arising from each arteriole. The walls of the capillaries are only one cell thick, which, coupled with the slow rate of blood flow, provides optimal conditions for the exchange of nutrients and wastes and the transfer of fluid volume between the plasma and the interstitium.

After leaving the capillaries, the blood flows into the low-pressure venous system beginning with vessels known as venules. Veins are similar in construction to arteries, but they have much less elasticity, thinner walls, and greater diameters. One-way valves are found in most veins where blood is carried against the force of gravity, such as in the lower extremities. Arteries do not have valves.

As blood passes from the arterial system through the capillaries, there is a change from the pulsatile character of arterial flow to a steady flow in the venous system. Arterial pulsations are caused by the intermittent contractions of the left ventricle. Figures 15-7 and 15-8 illustrate the arterial and venous networks of blood flow.

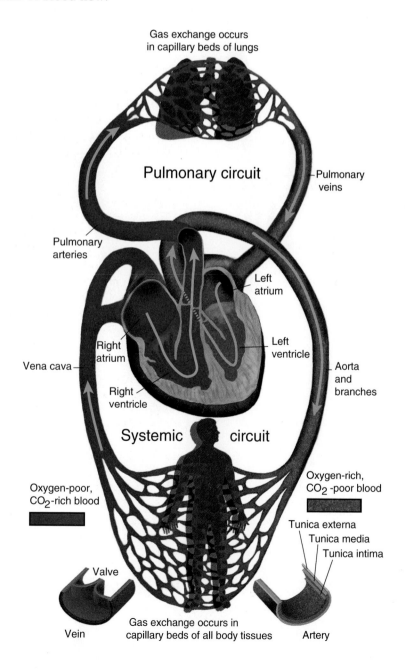

Figure 15-6 The Systemic and Pulmonary Circuits. The systemic pump consists of the left side of the heart, and the pulmonary circuit pump represents the right side of the heart.

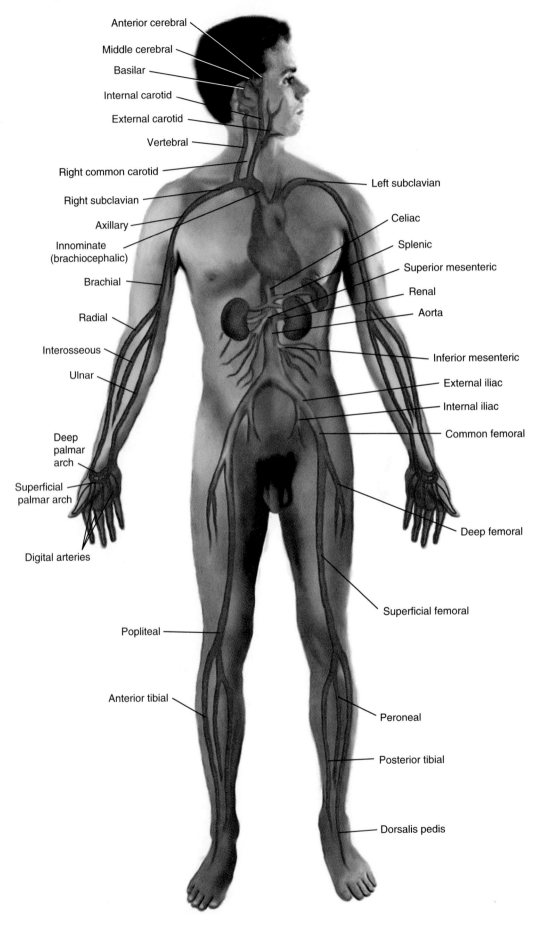

Figure 15-7 Arterial System Anatomy

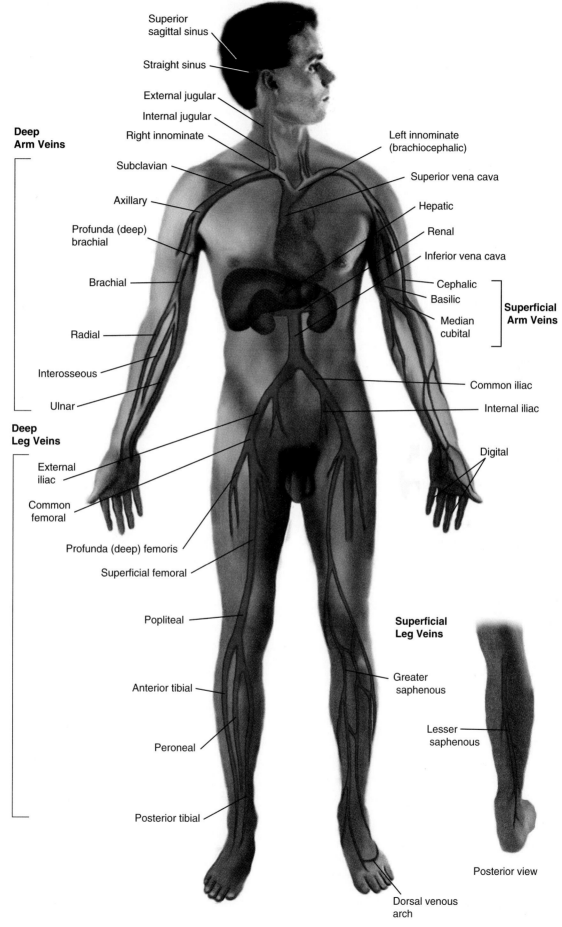

Figure 15-8   Venous System Anatomy

❖ HEALTH HISTORY

The heart and peripheral vasculature health history provides insight into the link between a patient's life/lifestyle and heart and peripheral vasculature information and pathology.

PATIENT PROFILE	*Diseases that are age-, sex-, and race-specific for the heart and peripheral vasculature are listed. Table 15-1 differentiates the common cardiovascular disorders.*
Age	Rheumatic fever (5–15) Raynaud's disease (18–50) Mitral valve prolapse (20–50) Hypertension (HTN) (20–70) Valve **stenosis** (narrowing or constriction of a diseased heart valve) or **regurgitation** (backward flow of blood through a heart valve) (30–50) Coronary artery disease (CAD) (40–60) Dilated or congestive cardiomyopathy (40–60) Myocardial infarction (MI) (40–60) Arteriosclerosis (50–70) Cerebrovascular accident (CVA) (50–70) Abdominal aortic aneurysm (AAA) (60–70)
Sex	
Female	Higher mortality rate after a severe MI; marked rise in CAD after menopause; atrial septal defect (ASD); Raynaud's disease
Male	Marked predisposition to CAD; ventricular septal defect (VSD)
Race	
African American	CVA, CAD, HTN, diabetes mellitus
Hispanic and Filipino	HTN
American Indian	CVA, CAD
CHIEF COMPLAINT	*Common chief complaints for the heart and peripheral vasculature are defined and information on the characteristics of each sign/symptom is provided.*
Chest Pain	Subjective sense of discomfort in the thorax; also referred to as angina if it is caused by myocardial ischemia; all chest pain is not angina; Table 15-2 differentiates different origins of chest pain
Radiation	Arm, shoulder, neck, jaw, teeth
Quality	Crushing, heavy, tight, stabbing, burning, squeezing, aching, smothering, or perceived as indigestion
Associated Manifestations	Nausea and vomiting, shortness of breath (SOB), restlessness, anxiety, weakness, feeling of impending doom, diaphoresis, faintness, dizziness
Aggravating Factors	Exercise, stress

continued

Alleviating Factors	Medication (e.g., nitroglycerin), rest, position change
Setting	While dreaming, eating, excited, stressed, exercising, or resting; hot or cold environment
Timing	Early morning is more common but can be any time of the day
Syncope	Fainting caused by a transient decrease in cerebral blood flow
Associated Manifestations	Nausea, perspiration, palpitations, yawning, seizures, flushed face, cessation of breathing during episode, aura prior to episode
Aggravating Factors	Exercise, medications, fever, lack of food
Alleviating Factors	Rest
Setting	Heavy activity, hot environment, buttoning the collar of a shirt
Timing	Early morning, after medication, after exercise, arising from a supine or sitting position
Palpitations	Irregular heart beats; the sensation of a rapidly throbbing or fluttering heart
Quality	Skipped heart beats, throbbing, pounding, fluttering
Associated Manifestations	Anxiety, weakness, nausea, SOB, chest pain, perspiration, fainting
Aggravating Factors	Smoking, caffeine, exercise
Alleviating Factors	Rest
Setting	Resting, smoking, exercising, drinking or eating food containing caffeine
Timing	After exercise or at rest
Peripheral Edema	Swelling of the extremities, usually the feet and hands
Quality	Imprints on swollen areas after applying pressure
Associated Manifestations	Recent weight gain, pain in upper right half of abdomen, swollen abdomen, shoes tighter, rings difficult to remove from fingers
Aggravating Factors	Continuous standing, high salt intake
Alleviating Factors	Lying down or elevating the feet
Extremity Pain	Sense of discomfort usually occurring in the legs or feet; claudication
Quality	Temperature change in feet or leg
Associated Manifestations	Swelling in the affected extremity, discoloration of the skin, tenderness, change in skin temperature
Aggravating Factors	Continual standing, walking, exercise, cold weather, smoking, stress
Alleviating Factors	Rest, elevation, dangling the extremity to a dependent position if the pain is caused by arterial insufficiency (but pain actually worsens with venous insufficiency)
Setting	Walking, exercise
Timing	Late night, early morning

continued

PAST HEALTH HISTORY	*The various components of the past health history are linked to heart and peripheral vasculature pathology and heart- and peripheral-vasculature-related information.*
Medical	
Cardiac Specific	AAA, angina, cardiogenic shock, cardiomyopathy, chest trauma, congenital anomalies, congestive heart failure (CHF), CAD, endocarditis, hyperlipoproteinemia, HTN, MI, myocarditis, pericarditis, peripheral vascular disease (PVD), rheumatic fever, valvular disease
Noncardiac Specific	Bleeding or blood disorder, diabetes mellitus, gout, Marfan's syndrome, pheochromocytoma, primary aldosteronism, renal artery disease, CVA, thyroid disease
Surgical	Ablation of accessory pathways, aneurysm repair, cardiac catheterization, chest surgery for trauma, congenital heart repair, coronary artery bypass graft (CABG), coronary stents, directional coronary atherectomy (DCA), electrophysiology studies (EPS), heart transplant, implantable or internal cardioverter/defibrillator (ICD) placement, myotomy or myectomy, percutaneous laser myoplasty, pacemaker insertion, percutaneous transluminal coronary angioplasty (PTCA), pericardial window, pericardiectomy, pericardiotomy, peripheral vascular grafting and bypass, valve replacement
Medications	Antianginals, antidysrhythmics, anticoagulants, antihypertensives, antilipemics, diuretics, inotropics, thrombolytic enzymes, vasodilators
Communicable Diseases	Rheumatic fever (valvular dysfunction), untreated syphilis (aortic regurgitation, aortitis, and aortic aneurysm), viral myocarditis (cardiomyopathy)
Childhood Illnesses	Rheumatic fever: Valvular dysfunction
Allergies	Aspirin (most patients who are recovering from an MI receive aspirin), intravenous pyelogram (IVP) dye or seafood (both contain iodine compounds used in the dye that is injected during a cardiac catheterization)
Injuries/Accidents	Chest trauma (falls, motor vehicle accidents, blunt force)
FAMILY HEALTH HISTORY	*Heart and peripheral vasculature diseases that are familial are listed.* Aneurysm, CVA, CAD, HTN, hypertrophic cardiomyopathy, Marfan's syndrome, mitral valve prolapse (MVP), MI, Raynaud's disease, rheumatic fever, sudden cardiac death
SOCIAL HISTORY	*The components of the social history are linked to heart and peripheral vasculature factors/pathology.*
Alcohol Use	Prolonged use of alcohol can interfere with the normal pumping function and electrical activity of the heart, leading to **cardiomegaly** (enlargement of the heart), poor left ventricular contractility, ventricular dilatation, palpitations, peripheral edema, fatigue, and SOB.

continued

	Thiamine deficiencies that usually occur concurrently with alcohol abuse may contribute to dysrhythmias and heart failure.
	Excessive alcohol intake may play a role in the pathogenesis of dilated cardiomyopathy, angina, CAD, and beriberi heart disease. On the other hand, the use of alcohol in moderation, up to 2 ounces a day, is inversely related to the development of CAD due to the protective effect of the increased HDL cholesterol.
Tobacco Use	Nicotine increases catecholamine release, leading to elevated cardiac output, heart rate, and blood pressure. Nicotine also inhibits the development of collateral circulation, causes peripheral vasoconstriction, thickens cardiac arterioles, causes platelet aggregation, leads to dysrhythmias, and neutralizes heparin thus increasing the risk of thrombus formation. The tobacco habit contributes to the pathogenesis of CAD, angina, and atherosclerosis.
Drug Use	Intravenous drug use: Increased risk for contracting infective endocarditis because of the use of nonsterile needles and the embolization of localized infections from the injection site
	Amphetamines, cocaine, and heroin: Tachycardia, severe hypertension, coronary vasospasm, MI, and dysrhythmias
Sexual Practice	Effect of intercourse on the heart (such as exertional chest pain) or eliciting a vagal response (which may occur with anal intercourse), thus making the patient prone to syncope and other sequelae
Travel History	Arsenic poisoning: Systemic arterial disease, including gangrene and PVD; traced to the elevated arsenic content in drinking water and soil in Taiwan and Chile
	Chagas' disease: Severe dysrhythmias, mitral regurgitation or insufficiency, and cardiomegaly; caused by a protozoan parasite endemic to Central America, South America, and the Southwestern United States
Work Environment	Table 15-3 lists toxic substances that can cause profound cardiac pathology.
Home Environment	A dirty fireplace may cause a smoky environment that leads to the worsening of chest pain.
Hobbies/Leisure Activities	Any activity that involves exertion may contribute to a decline in status in a patient with cardiovascular pathology.
Stress	Atherosclerosis, tachycardia, HTN, dysrhythmias, sudden death
HEALTH MAINTENANCE ACTIVITIES	*This information provides a bridge between the health maintenance activities and heart and peripheral vasculature function.*
Sleep	Dyspnea, orthopnea, or paroxysmal nocturnal dyspnea (PND)
Diet	Liquid protein diet has been associated with sudden death due to electrolyte imbalances.
	Foods high in vitamin K may reduce the effectiveness of anticoagulants.
	Awareness of the sodium content of the tap water in your area (home water softeners often contain sodium)

continued

Caffeine (in coffee, tea, soft drinks, chocolate, over-the-counter medications) is a sympathomimetic amine that increases the blood pressure and heart rate, elevates the serum catecholamine level, and can lead to dysrhythmias (especially premature atrial contractions).

Exercise

Physical exercise may have either deleterious or beneficial effects on the heart, depending on the type of activity performed, the amount, and the condition of the exerciser. The aim of an individual's cardiovascular fitness program should be the attainment of the THR (also known as perceived rate of exertion) to increase cardiovascular tone. In general, it is believed that aerobic exercise or sustained physical activity for at least 15 to 30 minutes per day, three or four times per week, positively affects one's cardiovascular conditioning.

Stress Management

Exercise, time management, pet therapy, reading, listening to music, eating, biofeedback, yoga, imagery, massages, transcendental meditation, and participation in a variety of support groups

Use of Safety Devices

Patients with older pacemakers should avoid areas with microwaves; cellular phones (especially digital cellular phones) may cause interference with pacemakers.

Health Check-Ups

EKG, chest x-ray, blood pressure, pulse, serum triglyceride, serum cholesterol

PATIENT CLASSIFICATION

The New York Heart Association (NYHA) has outlined four classifications for patients with cardiac pathologies. Class I indicates that the patient has no symptoms with ordinary physical activity. Class II means that the patient has some symptoms with normal activity and may have a slight limitation of activity. Class III states that a patient has symptoms with less than ordinary activity and has a marked limit of activity. Class IV indicates that the patient has symptoms with any physical activity or even at rest.

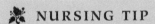

NURSING TIP

Managing Anger

When confronted with a stressful situation, teach your patients to:
- Always keep things in perspective.
- Learn to "cool off" when confronted with a stressful situation (e.g., count to 10).
- Walk away from potentially stressful situations if they feel that they may lose control.
- Use humor liberally in situations that would otherwise lead to exasperation.
- Consider the consequences: letting it out and clearing the air once in a while may be better than keeping anger and frustration bottled up inside.

NURSING ALERT

Risk Factors for Cardiovascular Disease

Fixed (patient cannot alter)
Age, gender, race, family history

Major Modifiable (patient can significantly reduce risk of cardiovascular disease by controlling these factors)
HTN, hyperlipidemia, tobacco use, glucose intolerance, physical inactivity, diet

Minor Modifiable (patient can decrease risk of cardiovascular disease to a lesser degree)
Psychophysiological stress, sedentary living, obesity

Table 15-1 Cardiovascular Disorders

DISORDER	DEFINITION	COMMON FINDINGS
Aneurysm	Localized abnormal dilation of a blood vessel	AAA: dulled abdominal or lower back pain; nausea and vomiting; ruptured AAA – severe, sudden, and continuous pain that radiates to back Thoracic aortic aneurysm (TAA): sudden, tearing pain in chest radiating to shoulders, neck, and back; dysphagia; dyspnea
Aortic regurgitation or insufficiency	Backflow of blood from the aorta to the left ventricle during diastole because of an incompetent valve	Dyspnea; PND; orthopnea; palpitations; angina; fatigue; syncope; diastolic murmur
Aortic stenosis	A narrowing or constriction of the aortic valve causing an obstruction to the ejection of blood from the left ventricle during systole	Syncope; fatigue; weakness; palpitations; angina; systolic murmur
Atherosclerosis (coronary artery disease)	A type of arteriosclerosis; localized accumulations of lipid-containing material within the blood vessels	Angina; MI; CHF; sudden cardiac death; dysrhythmias
Atrial septal defect (ASD)	A communicating defect of the septum between the right and left atria initially causing a left-to-right shunt followed by a right-to-left shunt	Fatigue; dyspnea; palpitations; murmur
Cardiac tamponade	Compression of the heart resulting from the accumulation of excess fluid in the pericardium	Beck's triad (hypotension, distended neck veins, and distant heart sounds); pulsus paradoxus
Cardiogenic shock	A shock of cardiac origin caused by pump failure	Pulmonary congestion; peripheral edema; hypotension; tachycardia; decreased pulse pressure; cool, pale, and clammy skin
Cardiomyopathy • congestive or dilated • hypertrophic • restrictive	Heart muscle disease	CHF-type symptoms; cardiomegaly with dilated or congestive form; familial history with hypertrophic form
Cerebrovascular accident	Brain damage that results from decreased blood flow; a CVA can have an embolic, thrombotic, or hemorrhagic cause	Decreased neurological function; headaches; hemiparesis; hemiplegia; aphasia; coma; cranial nerve findings
Coarctation of the aorta (COA)	A congenital narrowing of the aorta	Headaches; epistaxis; heave over left ventricle; blood pressure in upper extremities is greater than in the lower extremities; systolic murmur that may be auscultated over the back
Congestive heart failure	A condition whereby pump failure makes the heart unable to maintain a cardiac output sufficient to meet the metabolic needs of the body; the left ventricle, the right ventricle, or both may fail	Left-sided: anxiety, diaphoresis, rales, S_3, fatigue; right-sided: dependent pitting edema, hepatomegaly, weight gain, hepatojugular reflux
Deep vein thrombosis (DVT) and thrombophlebitis	The formation of a blood clot in a deep vein (most commonly in the leg or pelvis); inflammation of a vein due to a blood clot	Unilateral edema; calf pain or tenderness; temperature and color changes in the affected leg; cyanosis in the foot
Endocarditis (bacterial)	Infection of the endocardial surface or the heart valves	Fever; chills; fatigue; anorexia; nausea and vomiting; arthralgia; back pain; dyspnea; splinter hemorrhages of the nails; petechiae
Hypertension	Elevated blood pressure	Systolic blood pressure (SBP) >140 mm Hg; diastolic blood pressure (DBP) >100 mm Hg; most often asymptomatic; headaches or epistaxis; see Chapter 9 for further clarification
Marfan's syndrome (annuloaortic ectasia)	A syndrome of congenital collagen deficiency affecting the connective tissues	Patient may be tall and thin with hyper-extensive joints and long arms, legs, and fingers; aortic dissection; aortic regurgitation; mitral regurgitation; dysrhythmias

continued

Table 15-1 Cardiovascular Disorders *continued*

DISORDER	DEFINITION	COMMON FINDINGS
Mitral regurgitation or insufficiency	The backflow of blood from the left ventricle to the left atrium during systole and resulting from an incompetent valve	CHF-type symptoms; history of rheumatic fever, infection, trauma, or mitral valve prolapse; systolic murmur
Mitral stenosis	A narrowing or constriction of the mitral valve causing an obstruction of blood flow from the left atrium to the left ventricle during diastole	CHF-type symptoms; history of rheumatic heart disease or congenital heart defect; diastolic murmur; thrill at apex
Myocardial infarction	The necrosis of cardiac muscle due to cessation of blood supply	Nausea and vomiting; diaphoresis; shortness of breath; abnormal heart and lung sounds; angina; dysrhythmias; CHF; cardiogenic shock
Myocarditis	Inflammation of the heart's muscular tissue	History of rheumatic fever; viral or parasitic infection; irregular pulse; tenderness over the pericardium; may lead to dilated cardiomyopathy
Patent ductus arteriosus (PDA)	An opening between the aorta and the pulmonary artery that fails to close after birth; initially results in a left-to-right shunt followed by right-to-left shunt	CHF-type symptoms; bounding pulses; cyanosis; clubbing; prominent apical pulse; fatigue
Pericarditis	An inflammation of the pericardium; origin may be viral, malignant, or autoimmune	Precordial pain that increases with inspiration or in the supine position; pain may be relieved by leaning forward; fever; fatigue; pulsus paradoxus; pericardial friction rub
Peripheral vascular disease	Vascular disorders of the arteries and veins that supply the extremities (usually refers to arterial disease)	Intermittent claudication; pain in the toes; ulcers that don't heal; impotence; loss of pulses; severe extremity pain; paresthesia
Pulmonary regurgitation or insufficiency	The backflow of blood from the pulmonary artery to the right ventricle because of an incompetent valve	Dyspnea on exertion (DOE); fatigue; diastolic murmur
Pulmonary stenosis	A narrowing or constriction of the pulmonary artery causing an obstruction to the ejection of blood from the right ventricle	DOE; fatigue; right-sided heart failure symptoms; systolic murmur
Raynaud's disease	A condition caused by abnormal blood vessel spasms in the extremities, especially in response to cold temperatures	Finger or toe becomes pale, cold, and numb, then becomes red, hot, and tingling
Tetralogy of Fallot	A cyanotic congenital heart defect that combines pulmonary stenosis with a high ventricular septal defect (VSD) and an aorta that overrides the VSD and receives blood from both the right and the left ventricles	Cyanosis; heart failure unlikely to occur
Tricuspid regurgitation or insufficiency	The backflow of blood from the right ventricle to the right atrium because of an incompetent valve	Dyspnea; fatigue; systolic murmur
Tricuspid stenosis	A narrowing or constriction of the tricuspid valve causing an obstruction of blood flow from the right atrium to the right ventricle	Dyspnea; fatigue; diastolic murmur; right-sided CHF
Ventricular aneurysm	The dilatation of a portion of necrosed ventricular wall after an MI	Tachydysrhythmias; CHF-type symptoms; clot formation; arterial emboli; rupture: cardiac tamponade; systolic murmur
Ventricular septal defect	A communicating defect of the septum between the right and the left ventricles causing a left-to-right shunt initially and then a right-to-left shunt when irreversible	Fatigue; dyspnea; systolic murmur

Table 15-2   Differentiating Chest Pain

All of these conditions (excluding musculoskeletal) are life threatening and require immediate attention.

CARDIAC ISCHEMIA

Pain: burning, squeezing or aching, heaviness, smothering

- Not reproducible by palpation of the chest wall, may be relieved with rest or oxygen, and may or may not be accompanied by EKG changes.
- Myocardial ischemia may lead to myocardial infarction; when in doubt, assume a cardiac cause and follow your institution's chest pain protocol.

AORTIC (THORACIC) DISSECTION

Pain: sudden, sharp, and tearing, and radiates to shoulders, neck, back, and abdomen.

- Neurological complications: hemiplegia, sensory deficits secondary to carotid artery occlusion.

PULMONARY EMBOLUS

Pain: sudden onset, sharp or stabbing, varies with respiration

- May also present with dyspnea, tachypnea, fever, tachycardia, diaphoresis.

PNEUMOTHORAX

Pain: sudden onset, tearing or pleuritic, worsened by breathing

- May also have dyspnea, tachycardia, decreased breath sounds, and a deviated trachea. Refer to Chapter 14 for further information.

PNEUMONIA

Pain: stabbing that is exacerbated by coughing and deep breathing

- Presents with fever, chills, productive cough, tachypnea. Refer to Chapter 14 for further information.

ESOPHAGEAL RUPTURE

Pain: sudden onset upon swallowing

- May mimic signs and symptoms of a pneumothorax.
- Consider esophageal rupture when a patient has experienced penetrating trauma, a severe epigastric blow, or a first or second rib fracture.

MISCELLANEOUS: MUSCULOSKELETAL

Pain: reproducible by chest wall palpation

- May be relieved by position changes.

Table 15-3   Work-Related Exposures to Cardiotoxic Substances

PHYSICAL

- Extremes of oxygen pressure, barometric pressure, gravity, acceleration, noise, temperature, and humidity

BIOLOGICAL

- Laboratory-acquired infections
- Work in endemic areas

CHEMICAL

- Arsenic
- Carbon disulfide
- Carbon monoxide
- Cobalt
- Fibrogenic dust found in asbestos
- Fluorocarbons found in solvents and propellants
- Halogenated hydrocarbons
- Heavy metals such as lead

EQUIPMENT

- Stethoscope
- Sphygmomanometer
- Watch with second hand
- Tape measure

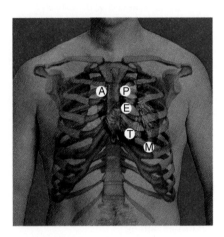

Figure 15-9 The Cardiac Landmarks.
A = Aortic Area; P = Pulmonic Area;
E = Erb's Point; T = Tricuspid Area;
M = Mitral Area

✓ NURSING CHECKLIST
General Approach to Heart Assessment

1. Explain to the patient what you are going to do.
2. Ensure that the room is warm, quiet, and well lit.
3. Expose the patient's chest only as much as is needed for the assessment.
4. Position the patient in a flat, supine position.
5. Stand to the patient's right side. The light should come from the opposite side of where you are standing so that shadows can be accentuated.

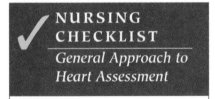

E	**Examination**
N	**Normal Findings**
A	**Abnormal Findings**
P	**Pathophysiology**

ASSESSMENT OF THE PRECORDIUM

The cardiovascular physical assessment has two major components:

1. Assessment of the **precordium** (the area on the anterior surface of the body overlying the heart, great vessels, pericardium, and some pulmonary tissue) and
2. Assessment of the periphery.

Inspection, palpation, and auscultation should be performed in a systematic manner, using certain cardiac landmarks. Percussion has limited usefulness in the cardiovascular assessment because x-rays and other diagnostic tests provide the same information in a much more accurate manner. The cardiac landmarks (see Figure 15-9) are defined as follows:

1. The aortic area is the second intercostal space (ICS) to the right of the sternum.
2. The pulmonic area is the second ICS to the left of the sternum.
3. The midprecordial area, Erb's point, is located in the third ICS to the left of the sternum.
4. The tricuspid area is the fifth ICS to the left of the sternum. Other terms for this area are the right ventricular area or the septal area.
5. The mitral area is the fifth ICS at the left midclavicular line. Other terms for this area are the left ventricular area or the apical area.

These cardiac landmarks are the locations where the heart sounds are heard best, not where the valves are actually located. The mitral area correlates anatomically with the apex of the heart; the aortic and pulmonic areas correlate anatomically with the base of the heart. Assessment of the heart should proceed in an orderly fashion from the base of the heart to the apex, or from the apex of the heart to the base.

Inspection
Aortic Area

E 1. Lightly place your index finger on the angle of Louis.
   2. Move your finger laterally to the right of the sternum to the rib. This is the second rib.
   3. Move your finger down beneath the second rib to the ICS. The aortic area is located in the second ICS to the right of the sternum.

N *No pulsations should be visible.*

A A pulsation in the aortic area is abnormal.

P A pulsation in the aortic area may indicate the presence of an aortic root aneurysm. The aneurysm's dilation may become bigger when the patient experiences hypertension. A rupture can occur at any time but the risk is greater when the aneurysm becomes 5 cm or more in diameter.

Pulmonic Area

E 1. Lightly place your index finger on the left second ICS.
   2. The pulmonic area is located at the second ICS to the left of the sternum.

N *No pulsations should be visible.*

A A pulsation or bulge in the pulmonic area is an abnormal finding.

P Pulmonary stenosis, which is usually congenital, impedes blood flow from the right ventricle into the lungs, causing a bulge. The right side of the heart then dilates and the right ventricle becomes hypertrophied in order to accommodate the load.

Midprecordial Area

E 1. Lightly place your index finger on the left second ICS.
2. Continue to move your finger down the left rib cage, counting the third rib and the third ICS.
3. The midprecordial area, or Erb's point, is located at the third ICS, left sternal border. Both aortic and pulmonic murmurs may be heard here.

N *No pulsations should be visible.*

A The presence of a pulsation or a systolic bulge in the midprecordial area is not normal.

P A left ventricular aneurysm can produce a midprecordial pulsation. Ventricular aneurysms can develop several weeks following an acute MI. With an MI, the hydraulic stress on the infarcted area may cause the damaged ventricular wall to bulge and become extremely thin during systole.

A A retraction in the midprecordial area is abnormal.

P Pericardial disease can produce retractions in this area (retractions occur when there is a pulling in some of the tissues of the precordium, depending on the activities of the heart).

Tricuspid Area

E 1. Lightly place your index finger on the left third ICS.
2. Continue to move your finger down the left rib cage, counting the fourth rib, the fourth ICS, and the fifth rib followed by the fifth ICS.
3. The tricuspid area is located at the fifth ICS, left of the sternal border.

N *No pulsations should be visible.*

A A visible systolic pulsation in the tricuspid area is abnormal.

P A visible systolic pulsation can result from right ventricular enlargement secondary to an increased stroke volume. Anxiety, hyperthyroidism, fever, and pregnancy are clinical situations that produce an increased stroke volume.

Mitral Area

E 1. Lightly place your index finger on the left fifth ICS.
2. Move your finger laterally to the midclavicular line. This is the mitral landmark. In a large-breasted patient, have the patient displace the left breast upward and to the left so you can locate the mitral landmark.

N *Normally, there is no movement in the precordium except at the mitral area, where the left ventricle lies close enough to the skin's surface that it visibly pulsates during systole. The apical impulse at the mitral landmark is generally visible in about half of the adult population. This pulsation is also known as the point of maximal impulse (PMI) and occurs simultaneously with the carotid pulse.*

A **Hypokinetic** (decreased movement) pulsations at the mitral area are considered abnormal.

P Conditions that place more fluid between the left ventricle and the chest wall, such as a pericardial effusion or cardiac tamponade, produce a hypokinetic or absent pulsation. In obese individuals, excess subcutaneous tissue dampens the apical impulse. Low output states such as shock produce a less palpable apical impulse from the reduced blood volume and decreased myocardial contractility. Keep in mind that absent pulsations are normal in half of the adult population.

A **Hyperkinetic** (increased movement) pulsations are always abnormal when located at the mitral area.

P High-output states such as mitral regurgitation, thyrotoxicosis, severe anemia, and left-to-right heart shunts are potential causes of hyperkinetic pulsations.

NURSING TIP

PMI Versus Apical Impulse

The term *PMI* has fallen out of favor because it can be a misnomer if cardiac pathology causes a stronger impulse in a different region. Any movement other than the apical impulse is abnormal and should be described in terms of type, location, and timing in relation to the cardiac cycle.

E **Examination**
N **Normal Findings**
A **Abnormal Findings**
P **Pathophysiology**

428 UNIT III Physical Assessment

Assessing Patients with Cardiovascular Assistive Devices

The patient with cardiovascular disease may need the assistance of special equipment to maintain an optimal cardiovascular system. The presence of cardiovascular assistive devices must be noted during the inspection process. Consider the following to assist you in observing these devices:

1. Artificial cardiac pacemakers (e.g., temporary external chest pacing, temporary internal pacing, permanent pacemaker); ICD.
   - The pacemaker is on. Check the settings.
   - The ICD is on. Check the settings.
   - Check for external pacer wires. Wires should be protected from electrical hazards per your facility's policy.
   - The insertion site is free of infection.
   - Check your facility's policy for verifying and controlling the settings.

2. Hemodynamic monitoring (e.g., arterial pressure line [a-line]; central venous pressure [CVP] line; right atrial pressure [RAP] line; left atrial pressure [LAP] line; pulmonary artery [PA] catheter [Swan-Ganz]).
   - Check the goal of the line (fluid, monitoring).
   - The monitor's alarms are on. The appropriate limits are set.
   - The transducer level is at the patient's right atrium (phlebostatic axis — fourth ICS, midaxillary line).
   - The pressure bag(s) is pumped to 300 mm Hg.
   - Change the flush bag(s) if necessary.
   - The line is safely secured to the patient or the bed (it is not just dangling).
   - The insertion site is free of infection.

3. Antiembolic stockings
   - Determine whether the stockings are knee-high or thigh-high.
   - Ensure that they are the correct size (see the manufacturer's directions for correct sizing).
   - The patient has palpable or audible pulses in the lower extremities.
   - The stockings have been removed at least once per day to assess the patient's skin.

4. Chest tubes
   - Determine where the chest tube is.
   - Determine whether the chest tube is for air or fluid.
   - Determine whether the chest tube is on wall suction or water seal.
   - If the chest tube is on suction, the chest drainage system is bubbling and the water-seal chamber is fluctuating.
   - The chest tube connections are secured.
   - The chest tube is kink-free.
   - The insertion site is free of subcutaneous emphysema.
   - The insertion site is free of infection.

5. EKG monitoring
   - The leads are placed correctly.
   - The monitor's alarms are on. The appropriate limits are set.
   - The patient's skin is intact where the EKG pads are.

6. Intravenous (IV) catheters
   - Determine whether the catheter is inserted peripherally or centrally.
   - The insertion site is free of infection.
   - Determine what the fluid is.
   - Determine whether there are any additives in the fluid.
   - Determine the rate of the IV.
   - Determine when the IV can be discontinued.

7. Pneumatic compression stockings
   - Determine whether the patient has some sort of stocking between the legs and the plastic enclosures.
   - The device is on.
   - The stockings have been removed at least once per day to assess the patient's skin.

8. Pulse oximetry
   - The monitor's alarms are on. The appropriate limits are set.
   - Determine the settings.
   - The patient's skin is intact where the probe is located.
   - The patient's fingernail polish has been removed where the probe is located.

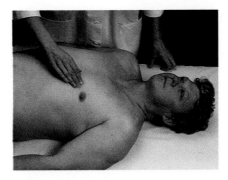

Figure 15-10   Palpating for Pulsations

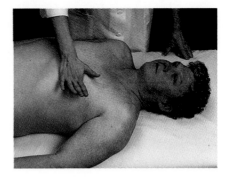

Figure 15-11   Palpating for Thrills

🅝 NURSING ALERT

Discontinuing an IV

An IV should be discontinued when any of the following signs occur (despite a good blood return): the site is swollen, cool, or hot to touch, is reddened, phlebitic, streaking, or painful.

Palpation

Inspection and palpation of the heart go hand in hand. Again, you must be systematic in this part of the assessment and palpate the cardiac landmarks starting at either the base or the apex of the heart. During palpation, assess for the apical impulse, pulsations, **thrills** (vibrations that feel similar to what one feels when a hand is placed on a purring cat), and **heaves** (lifting of the cardiac area secondary to an increased workload and force of left ventricular contraction; also referred to as lift). The patient should be in a supine position for this portion of the assessment.

E   Palpate the cardiac landmarks for:

    1. Pulsations: Using the finger pads, locate the cardiac landmark and palpate the area for pulsations (see Figure 15-10).

    2. Thrills: Using the palmar surface of the hand, at the base of the fingers (also known as the ball of the hand), locate the cardiac landmark and palpate the area for thrills (see Figure 15-11).

    3. Heaves: Follow step 2 and palpate the area for heaves.

Aortic Area

E   Palpate the aortic area for pulsations, thrills, and heaves.
N   *No pulsations, thrills, or heaves should be palpated.*
A   Palpation of a thrill in the aortic area is abnormal.
P   Aortic stenosis and aortic regurgitation create turbulent blood flow in the left ventricle, which may be palpated as a thrill.

Pulmonic Area

E   Palpate the pulmonic area for pulsations, thrills, and heaves.
N   *No pulsations, thrills, or heaves should be palpated.*
A   Palpation of a thrill in the pulmonic area is abnormal.
P   Pulmonic stenosis and pulmonic regurgitation create turbulent blood flow in the right ventricle, which may be palpated as a thrill.

E	**Examination**
N	**Normal Findings**
A	**Abnormal Findings**
P	**Pathophysiology**

Midprecordial Area

E Palpate the midprecordial area for pulsations, thrills, and heaves.

N *No pulsations, thrills, or heaves should be palpated.*

A Palpation of pulsations in the midprecordial area is abnormal.

P Both a left ventricular aneurysm and an enlarged right ventricle can produce a pulsation in the midprecordial area.

Tricuspid Area

E Palpate the tricuspid area for pulsations, thrills, and heaves.

N *No pulsations, thrills, or heaves should be felt.*

A Palpation of a thrill in the tricuspid area is abnormal.

P Tricuspid stenosis and tricuspid regurgitation create turbulent blood flow in the right atrium, which may be palpated as a thrill.

A Palpation of a heave in the tricuspid area is abnormal.

P Right ventricular enlargement may produce a heave in the tricuspid area secondary to an increased workload.

Mitral Area

E Palpate the mitral area for pulsations, thrills, and heaves. If a pulsation (apical impulse) is not palpable, turn the patient to the left side and palpate in this position (see Figure 15-12). This position facilitates palpation because the heart shifts closer to the chest wall.

N *The apical impulse is palpable in approximately half of the adult population. It is felt as a light, localized tap that is 1 to 2 cm in diameter. The amplitude is small and it can be felt immediately after the first heart sound, lasting for about one-half of systole. This impulse may be exaggerated in young patients. A thrill is not found in the normal adult population. A heave is absent in the healthy adult.*

A A thrill palpated at the fifth ICS at the left midclavicular line is considered abnormal.

P Mitral stenosis and mitral regurgitation may produce a thrill from the turbulent blood flow found in the left atrium.

A A visible heave, or sustained apex beat, displaced laterally to the left sixth ICS at the anterior axillary line is abnormal. It is usually more than 3 cm in diameter and has a large amplitude.

P Left ventricular hypertrophy produces a laterally displaced apical impulse because of the increased size of the left ventricle in the thorax and the subsequent shifting of the heart. In addition, the hypertrophied muscle works harder during a contraction to produce a heave or sustained apex. This frequently occurs in conditions such as aortic stenosis, systemic hypertension, and idiopathic hypertrophic subaortic stenosis (a form of hypertrophic cardiomyopathy).

A Hypokinetic pulsations, usually less than 1 to 2 cm in diameter and of small amplitude, are abnormal.

P Conditions that place more fluid between the left ventricle and the chest wall, such as a pericardial effusion or cardiac tamponade, produce a hypokinetic or absent pulsation. In obesity, the excess subcutaneous tissue dampens the apical impulse. Low-output states such as shock produce a less palpable apical impulse from the reduced blood volume and decreased myocardial contractility.

A Hyperkinetic pulsations, usually greater than 1 to 2 cm in diameter and of increased amplitude, are abnormal.

P High-output states such as mitral regurgitation, thyrotoxicosis, severe anemia, and left-to-right heart shunts are potential causes of hyperkinetic pulsations.

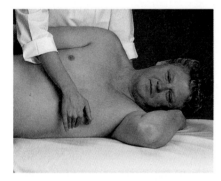

Figure 15-12 Palpating the Apical Impulse with the Patient on the Left Side

E	Examination
N	Normal Findings
A	Abnormal Findings
P	Pathophysiology

Auscultation

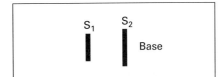

A. Normal S_2

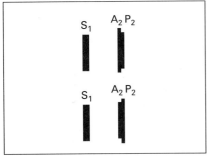

B. Intensified A_2, Diminished A_2

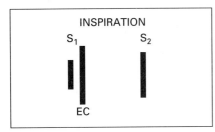

C. Aortic Ejection Click

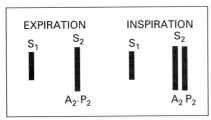

D. Normal Physiological Split of S_2

Figure 15-13 Summation of Heart Sounds

E	**Examination**
N	**Normal Findings**
A	**Abnormal Findings**
P	**Pathophysiology**

NURSING CHECKLIST
General Approach to Heart Auscultation

1. Explain to the patient what you are going to do.
2. Expose the patient's chest only as much as is needed for the assessment.
3. Position the patient in a supine or sitting position. The left lateral position may be used for auscultation of the mitral and tricuspid areas.
4. Stand to the patient's right side.
5. Use the correct headpiece of the stethoscope. The diaphragm transmits high-frequency sounds whereas the bell is used for low-pitched sounds. Keep in mind when using the bell that it should rest lightly on the skin. If too much pressure is applied, the bell will act like a diaphragm.
6. Warm the headpiece in your hands prior to touching it to the patient.
7. Listen to all four of the valvular cardiac landmarks at least twice. During the first auscultation, identify S_1 and S_2, and then listen for a possible S_3 and S_4. During the second auscultation, listen for murmurs and friction rubs. As you gain expertise, you may be able to listen for S_1, S_2, S_3, S_4, murmurs, and friction rubs all at the same time.
8. Listen for at least a few cardiac cycles (10 to 15 seconds) in each area.

Aortic Area

E Place the diaphragm of the stethoscope on the aortic landmark and listen for S_2.

N *S_2 is caused by the closure of the semilunar valves. S_2 corresponds to the "dub" sound in the phonetic "lub-dub" representation of heart sounds. S_2 heralds the onset of diastole. S_2 is louder than S_1 at this landmark (refer to Figure 15-13A).*

A The components of S_2 are A_2 (aortic) and P_2 (pulmonic). A greatly intensified or diminished A_2 is considered abnormal (refer to Figure 15-13B).

P Arterial hypertension, which increases the pressure in the aorta, may be suspected in the case of a greatly intensified A_2. Aortic stenosis, where the aortic valve is calcified or thickened, may be the cause of a diminished A_2.

A An ejection **click** is an abnormal systolic sound that is high pitched and can radiate in the chest wall. It is created by the opening of the valve and it does not vary with the respiratory cycle. An ejection click follows S_1 (refer to Figure 15-13C).

P An ejection click can be auscultated in aortic stenosis, where the calcified valve produces this sound on opening.

Pulmonic Area

E Place the diaphragm of the stethoscope on the chest wall at the pulmonic landmark and listen for S_2.

N *S_2 is also heard in the pulmonic area. S_2 is louder than S_1 at this landmark as depicted in Figure 15-13A. It is softer than the S_2 auscultated in the aortic area because the pressure on the left side of the heart is greater than that on the right. There is a normal physiological splitting of S_2 that is heard best at the pulmonic area. The components of a split S_2 are A_2 (aortic) and P_2 (pulmonic) (see Figure 15-13D). The aortic component occurs*

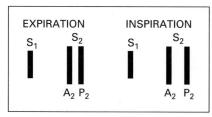

E. Wide Splitting of S_2

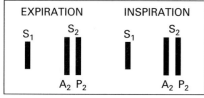

F. Fixed Splitting of S_2

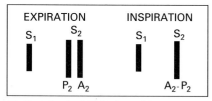

G. Paradoxical Splitting of S_2

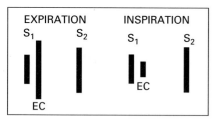

H. Pulmonic Ejection Click

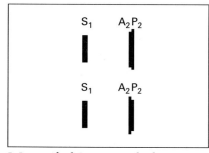

I. Intensified P_2, Diminished P_2

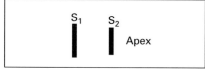

J. Normal S_1

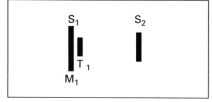

K. Normal Physiological Split of S_1

Figure 15-13 Summation of Heart Sounds *continued*

slightly before the pulmonic component during inspiration. The physiology of a split S_2 is that during inspiration, because of the more negative intra-thoracic pressure, the venous return to the right side of the heart increases. Thus, pulmonic closure is delayed because of the extra time needed for the increased blood volume to pass through the valve. Normally, the A_2 component of the split S_2 is louder than the P_2 component due to the greater pressures in the left side of the heart.

A When a split S_2 occurs that is abnormally wide, the aortic valve closes early and the pulmonic valve closes late. There is a split on both inspiration and expiration, but a wider split on inspiration, as shown in Figure 15-13E.

P Delayed closure of the pulmonic valve may be due to a delay in the electrical stimulation of the right ventricle such as seen with right bundle branch block.

A Fixed splitting, a wide splitting that does not change with inspiration or expiration, is abnormal (refer to Figure 15-13F). The pulmonic valve consistently closes later than the aortic valve. The right side of the heart is already ejecting a large volume, so filling cannot be increased during inspiration.

P Right ventricular failure that results in a prolonged right ventricular systole or a large atrial septal defect can lead to fixed splitting.

A In paradoxical splitting, the aortic valve closes after the pulmonic valve because of the delay in left ventricular systole. This occurs during expiration and disappears with inspiration. It is considered abnormal (see Figure 15-13G).

P Left bundle branch block, aortic stenosis, patent ductus arteriosus, severe hypertension, and left ventricular failure are conditions in which paradoxical splitting may be auscultated.

A A pulmonic ejection click always indicates an abnormality (refer to Figure 15-13H).

P A pulmonic ejection click is caused by the opening of a diseased pulmonic valve. It is heard loudest on expiration and is quieter on inspiration. It occurs early in systole and it does not radiate.

A A P_2 that is louder than or equal in volume to A_2 is abnormal, as is a greatly diminished P_2 (see Figure 15-13I).

P A loud P_2 is expected in pulmonary hypertension, where the pressures in the pulmonary artery are abnormally high; pulmonic stenosis, where the pulmonic valve is calcified or thickened, may be the cause of a diminished P_2.

Midprecordial Area

Erb's point is where both aortic and pulmonic murmurs may be auscultated. Refer to the discussion on murmurs later in this chapter for additional information.

Tricuspid Area

E Place the diaphragm of the stethoscope on the chest wall at the tricuspid landmark to listen for S_1.

N *S_1 in the tricuspid area is softer than the S_1 auscultated in the mitral area because the pressure in the left side of the heart is greater than that in the right. S_1 is louder than S_2 at this landmark (refer to Figure 15-13J). There is a normal physiological splitting of S_1 that is best heard in the tricuspid area (Figure 15-13K). This split occurs because the mitral valve closes slightly before the tricuspid valve due to greater pressures in the left side of the heart. The components of a split S_1 are M_1 (mitral) and T_1 (tricuspid). Physiological splitting disappears when the patient holds his or her breath.*

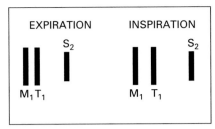

L. Wide Split of S₁

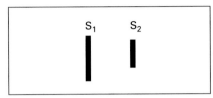

M. Loud S₁

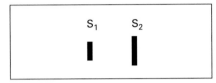

N. Soft S₁

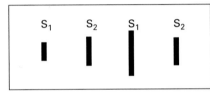

O. Variable S₁

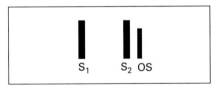

P. Opening Snap

Figure 15-13 Summation of Heart Sounds *continued*

E Examination
N Normal Findings
A Abnormal Findings
P Pathophysiology

A A split S_1 with an abnormally wide split is pathological (refer to Figure 15-13L). The split is wider than usual during inspiration and is still heard on expiration.

P A split S_1 is usually due to electrical malfunctions such as right bundle branch block or mechanical problems such as mitral stenosis. In mitral stenosis, the tricuspid valve can close before the mitral valve closes because of calcification of the diseased mitral valve.

Mitral Area

E 1. Place the diaphragm of the stethoscope over the mitral area to identify S_1.

2. If you are unable to distinguish S_1 from S_2, palpate the carotid artery with the hand closest to the head while auscultating the mitral landmark. You will hear S_1 with each carotid pulse beat.

N *S_1 is heard the loudest in the mitral area. S_1 is caused by the closure of the mitral and tricuspid valves. S_1 corresponds to the "lub" sound in the phonetic "lub-dub" representation of heart sounds. S_1 is louder than S_2 at this landmark (refer to Figure 15-13J). S_1 also heralds the onset of systole. At normal or slow heart rates, systole (the time occurring between S_1 and S_2) is usually shorter than diastole. Diastole constitutes two-thirds of the cardiac cycle and systole constitutes the other third. The intensity of S_1 depends on:*

1. *The adequacy of the A-V cusps in halting the ventricular blood flow*
2. *The mobility of the cusps*
3. *The position of the cusps and the rate of ventricular contraction*

A An abnormally loud S_1 occurs when the mitral valve is wide open when systolic contraction begins, then slams shut (Figure 15-13M).

P A loud S_1 occurs in mitral stenosis, short PR interval syndrome (0.11 to 0.13 seconds), or in high-output states such as tachycardia, hyperthyroidism, and exercise.

A A soft S_1 is abnormal (refer to Figure 15-13N).

P A soft S_1 can occur as a result of rheumatic fever, where the mitral valve has only limited motion.

A A variable abnormal S_1 occurs when diastolic filling time varies. Both a soft and a loud S_1 can be auscultated (see Figure 15-13O).

P A variable S_1 can occur with complete heart block, where the atria and the ventricles are beating independently, and in atrial fibrillation, where the ventricles are beating irregularly.

A An opening **snap** is an early diastolic sound that is high-pitched. It is abnormal (refer to Figure 15-13P).

P An opening snap is caused by the opening of a diseased valve and can be auscultated in mitral stenosis. The sound does not vary with respirations and can radiate throughout the chest. It follows S_2 and can be differentiated from an S_3 because it occurs earlier than an S_3.

A In tachycardia, the heart rate increases, diastole shortens, and systole and diastole become increasingly difficult to distinguish. Tachycardia is abnormal.

P Tachycardia can occur in exercise, fever, anxiety, pregnancy, and conditions that lead to hypertrophy, such as heart failure.

Mitral and Tricuspid Area (S₃)

Auscultation of the mitral and tricuspid areas is repeated for low-pitched sounds, specifically an S_3 (otherwise known as a ventricular diastolic **gallop**, or extra heart sound). An S_3 is an early diastolic filling sound that originates in the ventricles and is therefore heard best at the apex of the

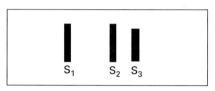

Q. S_3

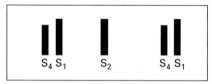

R. S_4

S. Summation Gallop

Figure 15-13 Summation of Heart Sounds *continued*

heart. A right-sided S_3 (tricuspid area) is heard louder during inspiration because the venous return to the right side of the heart increases with a more negative intrathoracic pressure. An S_3 sound occurs just after an S_2 (Figure 15-13Q).

E   1. Place the bell of the stethoscope lightly over the mitral landmark. When the S_3 originates in the left ventricle, it is heard best with the patient in a left lateral decubitus position and exhaling.
   2. When originating in the right ventricle, an S_3 can best be heard by placing the bell of the stethoscope lightly over the third or fourth ICS at the left sternal border.
   3. Auscultate for 10 to 15 seconds for a left- or right-sided S_3.

N   *An S_3 heart sound can be a normal physiological sound in children and in young adults. After the age of 30, a physiological S_3 is very infrequent. An S_3 can also be normal in high-output states such as the third trimester of pregnancy.*

A   In an adult, an S_3 heart sound may be one of the earliest clinical findings of cardiac dysfunction. A loud, persistent S_3 can be an ominous sign. The average life expectancy after a persistent S_3 sound is detected is approximately 4 to 5 years.

P   An S_3 is caused by rapid ventricular filling. An S_3 sound may occur with ventricular dysfunction, excessively rapid early diastolic ventricular filling, and restrictive myocardial or pericardial disease. It often indicates congestive heart failure and fluid overload.

Mitral and Tricuspid Area (S_4)

An S_4 heart sound, or atrial diastolic gallop, is a late diastolic filling sound associated with atrial contraction. An S_4 can be either left- or right-sided and is therefore heard best in the mitral or tricuspid area. An S_4 is a late diastolic filling sound that occurs just before S_1 (Figure 15-13R).

Sometimes, the S_3 and the S_4 heart sounds can occur simultaneously in mid-diastole, thus creating one loud diastolic filling sound. This is known as a summation gallop (Figure 15-13S).

E   1. Place the bell of the stethoscope lightly over the mitral area.
   2. Place the bell of the stethoscope lightly over the tricuspid area.
   3. Auscultate for 10 to 15 seconds for a left- or right-sided S_4.

N   *An S_4 heart sound may occur with or without any evidence of cardiac decompensation. A left-sided S_4 is usually louder on expiration. A right-sided S_4 is usually louder on inspiration.*

A   The presence of an S_4 can be indicative of cardiac decompensation.

P   An S_4 heart sound can be auscultated in conditions that increase the resistance to filling because of a poorly compliant ventricle (e.g., MI, CAD, CHF, and cardiomyopathy) or in conditions that result in systolic overload (e.g., HTN, aortic stenosis, and hyperthyroidism).

Murmurs

Murmurs are distinguished from heart sounds by their longer duration. Murmurs are produced by turbulent blood flow in the following situations:

1. Flow across a partial obstruction
2. Increased flow through normal structures
3. Flow into a dilated chamber
4. Backward or regurgitant flow across incompetent valves
5. Shunting of blood out of a high-pressure chamber or artery through an abnormal passageway

A. Crescendo

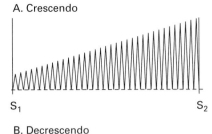

B. Decrescendo

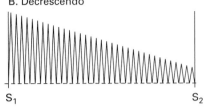

C. Crescendo-decrescendo

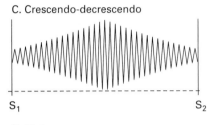

D. Plateau

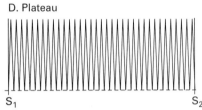

Figure 15-14 Characteristic Patterns of Murmurs

Table 15-4	Grading Heart Murmurs
GRADE	**CHARACTERISTICS**
I	Very faint; heard only after a period of concentration
II	Faint; heard immediately
III	Moderate intensity
IV	Loud; may be associated with a thrill
V	Loud; stethoscope must remain in contact with the chest wall in order to hear; thrill palpable
VI	Very loud; heard with stethoscope off of chest wall; thrill palpable

E	**Examination**
N	**Normal Findings**
A	**Abnormal Findings**
P	**Pathophysiology**

When assessing for a murmur, analyze the murmur according to the following seven characteristics:

1. Location: area where the murmur is heard the loudest (e.g., mitral, pulmonic, etc.).
2. Radiation: transmission of sounds from the specific valves to other adjacent anatomic areas. For example, mitral murmurs can often radiate to the axilla.
3. Timing: phase of the cardiac cycle in which the murmur is heard. Murmurs can be either systolic or diastolic. If the murmur occurs simultaneously with the pulse, it is a systolic murmur. If it does not, it is a diastolic murmur. Murmurs can further be characterized as **pansystolic** or **holosystolic**, meaning that the murmur is heard throughout all of systole. Murmurs can also be characterized as early, mid-, or late systolic or diastolic murmurs.
4. Intensity: Refer to Table 15-4 for the six grades of loudness or intensity. The murmur is recorded with the grade over the roman numeral "VI" to show the scale being used (e.g., III/VI).
5. Quality: harsh, rumbling, blowing, or musical.
6. Pitch: high, medium, or low. Low-pitched murmurs should be auscultated with the bell of the stethoscope whereas high-pitched murmurs should be auscultated with the diaphragm of the stethoscope.
7. Configuration: pattern that the murmur makes over time (refer to Figure 15-14). The configuration of a murmur can be described as **crescendo** (soft to loud), **decrescendo** (loud to soft), crescendo-decrescendo (soft to loud to soft), and plateau (sound is sustained).

E
1. The patient should be in the same position for murmur auscultation as that which was used for the first auscultation (i.e., supine or sitting).
2. Auscultate each of the following cardiac landmarks for 10 to 15 seconds:
   a. Aortic and pulmonic areas, with the diaphragm of the stethoscope
   b. Mitral and tricuspid areas, with the diaphragm of the stethoscope
   c. Mitral and tricuspid areas, with the bell of the stethoscope
3. Label the murmur using the characteristics of location, radiation, timing, configuration, intensity, pitch, and quality. Refer to Table 15-4 for information on grading heart murmurs.

N *No murmur should be heard; however, a physiological or functional murmur in children and adolescents may be innocent. These murmurs are usually systolic, short, grade I or II, vibratory, heard at the left sternal border, and do not radiate. No cardiac symptoms accompany the murmur.*

A Abnormal murmurs of stenosis can be found in each of the four valvular cardiac landmarks.

P Stenosis occurs when a valve that should be open remains partially closed. It produces an increased **afterload**, or pressure overload. Stenosis may develop from rheumatic fever, congenital defects of the valves, or calcification associated with the aging process.

A Abnormal murmurs of regurgitation or insufficiency can be auscultated in each of the four valvular cardiac landmarks.

P Regurgitation or insufficiency occurs when a valve that should be closed remains partially open. An insufficient valve causes volume overload, or increased **preload**. Regurgitation frequently results from the effects of rheumatic fever and congenital defects of the valves.

Pericardial Friction Rub

E
1. Position the patient so that he or she is reclining in the sitting position, in the knee-chest position, or leaning forward.

E Examination
N Normal Findings
A Abnormal Findings
P Pathophysiology

2. Auscultate from the sternum (third to fifth ICS) to the apex (mitral area) with the diaphragm of the stethoscope for 10 to 15 seconds.

3. Characterize any sound according to its location, radiation, timing, quality, and pitch.

N *No pericardial friction rub should be auscultated.*

A A pericardial friction rub is always an abnormal finding. It is heard best during held inspiration or expiration. It does not change with the respiratory cycle. Refer to Table 15-5 for additional information on pericardial friction rubs.

P Pericardial friction rubs are caused by the rubbing together of the inflamed visceral and parietal layers of the pericardium. They may be present in conditions such as **pericarditis** (inflammation of the pericardium) and renal failure.

Prosthetic Heart Valves

E/N *Prosthetic heart valves can be located in any of the four heart valves, although mitral and aortic valve replacements are the most common. Refer to the aortic and mitral valve auscultation discussions.*

A Prosthetic heart valves produce abnormal heart sounds. Furthermore, mechanical prosthetic valve sounds can usually be heard without the use of a stethoscope.

P Mechanical prosthetic valves (caged-ball, tilting disk, and bileaflet valves) produce "clicky" opening and closing sounds. Homograft (human tissue) and heterograft (animal tissue) valves produce sounds that are similar to those of the human valves; however, they usually also produce a murmur.

Table 15-5 Murmurs and Pericardial Friction Rub

HEART SOUND	LOCATION/RADIATION	QUALITY/PITCH	CONFIGURATION
Systolic Murmurs			
Aortic stenosis	Second right ICS; may radiate to neck or left sternal border	Harsh/medium	Crescendo/decrescendo
Pulmonic stenosis	Second or third left ICS; radiates toward shoulder and neck	Harsh/medium	Crescendo/decrescendo
Mitral regurgitation	Apex; fifth ICS, left midclavicular line; may radiate to left axilla and back	Blowing/high	Holosystolic/plateau
Tricuspid regurgitation	Lower left sternal border; may radiate to right sternum	Blowing/high	Holosystolic/plateau
Diastolic Murmurs			
Aortic regurgitation	Second right ICS and Erb's point; may radiate to left or right sternal border	Blowing/high	Decrescendo
Pulmonic regurgitation	Second left ICS; may radiate to left lower sternal border	Blowing/high	Decrescendo
Mitral stenosis	Apex; fifth ICS, left midclavicular line; may get louder with patient on left side; does not radiate	Rumbling/low	Crescendo/decrescendo
Tricuspid stenosis	Fourth ICS, at sternal border	Rumbling/low	Crescendo/decrescendo
Pericardial Friction Rub	Third to fifth ICS, left of sternum; does not radiate	Leathery, scratchy, grating/high	Three components: 1. Ventricular systole 2. Ventricular diastole 3. Atrial systole

Note: Timing is described as systolic or diastolic; intensity is described in Table 15-4.

ASSESSMENT OF THE PERIPHERAL VASCULATURE

Assessment of the periphery is the second major component of a comprehensive cardiovascular assessment. The components of the assessment of the periphery include:

1. Inspection of the jugular venous pressure (JVP)
2. Inspection of the hepatojugular reflux
3. Palpation and auscultation of the arterial pulses
4. Inspection and palpation of peripheral perfusion
5. Palpation of the epitrochlear node

✓ **NURSING CHECKLIST**
General Approach to Peripheral Vasculature Assessment

1. Explain to the patient what you are going to do.
2. Use a drape and uncover only those areas that are necessary as the assessment is done.
3. Position the patient in a supine or sitting position.

Inspection of the Jugular Venous Pressure

Identify the internal and external jugular veins (refer to Figure 15-15) with the patient in a supine position with the head elevated to 30° or 45° so that the jugular veins are visible. Tangential lighting (lighting across the veins rather than on top of the veins) will facilitate the assessment. Both sides of the neck should be assessed. The external jugular veins are more superficial than the internal jugular (IJ) veins and traverse the neck diagonally from the center of the clavicle to the angle of the jaw. The IJ veins are larger and are located deep below the sternocleidomastoid muscle adjacent to the carotid arteries. The pulsations of the IJ veins can be difficult to identify visually because the veins are deep and the pulsations can be confused with the adjacent carotid arteries.

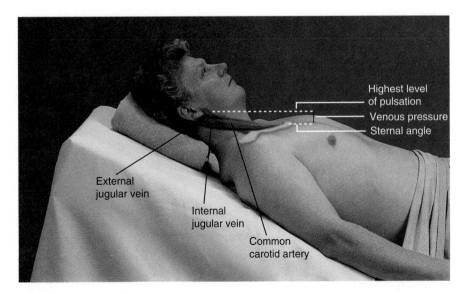

Figure 15-15   Inspection of Jugular Venous Pressure

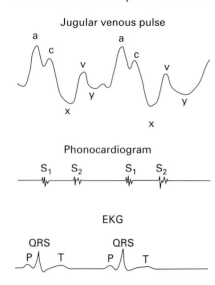

Figure 15-16 Jugular Venous Pulse Waves in Relation to the Phono-cardiogram and Electrocardiogram

Jugular vein pulsations consist of two or three waves (refer to Figure 15-16). These waves are called the *a*, *c*, and *v* waves. The *a* wave is produced by the contraction of the right atrium and it reflects the backflow of blood into the venae cavae as the right atrium ejects blood into the right ventricle. The *a* wave occurs just before S_1.

The *c* wave occurs at the end of S_1 and is produced when the right ventricle begins to contract. The *c* wave is caused by both the slight backflow of blood into the right atrium when the ventricular contraction occurs and by the bulging of the tricuspid valve backward toward the right atrium because of increased right ventricular pressure.

The *v* wave results from the slow buildup of blood in the right atrium during the ventricular contraction (when the tricuspid valve is closed) and occurs during late systole. The *v* wave disappears when the tricuspid valve opens and blood flows rapidly into the right ventricle.

Two negative slopes, the *x* and *y* descents, also occur in the jugular venous pulse. The *x* descent occurs after the *c* wave and reflects the fall of the right atrial pressure when the tricuspid valve closes and the right atrium relaxes. The *y* descent follows the *v* wave and occurs when the tricuspid valve opens and blood flows rapidly from the right atrium into the right ventricle.

These waves and descents are clearly noted when the patient has a direct central venous pressure (CVP) line and the right atrial pressure waves are depicted on an oscilloscope.

Information about the CVP can be obtained directly via a catheter inserted into one of the jugular veins (the IJ veins are the veins of choice for cannulation because they do not have valves and they provide a more direct route to the right atrium) or indirectly as discussed below.

E   **1.** To indirectly estimate a patient's CVP (see Figure 15-15):

  a. Place the patient at a 30° to 45° angle (the highest position where the neck veins remain visible).

  b. Measure the vertical distance in centimeters from the patient's sternal angle to the top of the distended neck vein. This will give you the JVP.

  c. Knowing that the sternal angle is roughly 5 cm above the right atrium, take the JVP measurement obtained in the previous step and add 5 cm to get an estimate of the CVP. For example, a JVP of 2 cm at a 45° angle estimated on a patient's right side is equivalent to a CVP of 5 + 2, or 7, cm.

 2. Direct CVP measurements in the patient with a central venous cannula should be obtained with the patient in the supine position or reclining at no more than a 45° angle.

  a. Do not forget to level the transducer at the patient's right atrium (phlebostatic axis – fourth ICS, midaxillary line) prior to obtaining any CVP reading.

  b. When recording CVP measurements, chart the angle of the patient when the measurement was taken.

N   *CVP readings of 0 to 9 cm are considered normal. Normally, the jugular veins are:*

 1. Most distended when the patient is flat because gravity is eliminated and the jugular veins fill

 2. 1 to 2 cm above the sternal angle when the head of the bed is elevated to a 45° angle

 3. Absent when the head of the bed is at a 90° angle

A   A CVP greater than 9 cm is considered abnormal.

P   An elevated CVP can be due to an increased right ventricular pressure, increased blood volume, or an obstruction to right ventricular flow.

A   Bilateral jugular venous distension (JVD) is abnormal.

P   JVD indicates an increased CVP.

E   **Examination**

N   **Normal Findings**

A   **Abnormal Findings**

P   **Pathophysiology**

A   Unilateral JVD is abnormal.

P   Unilateral JVD indicates a local vein blockage.

A   JVD with the head of the bed elevated to a 90° angle is abnormal.

P   JVD at a 90° angle indicates more serious pathology such as severe right ventricular failure, constrictive pericarditis, or cardiac tamponade.

A   An increased *a* wave is abnormal.

P   An increased *a* wave can occur with stenosis of the tricuspid valve (because the right atrium has difficulty emptying blood into the right ventricle) or when the right ventricle is enlarged and the right atrium needs to more forcefully contract to fill it. An increased *a* wave can also occur in complete heart block because the right atrium contracts at its own pace against a closed tricuspid valve.

A   An enlarged *v* wave is abnormal.

P   An enlarged *v* wave can occur with tricuspid regurgitation or insufficiency. It is exaggerated when the tricuspid valve allows blood to flow back from the right ventricle to the right atrium during systole, thus causing the *x* slope to be replaced by a large *c–v* wave. It can also occur with right-sided heart failure, where the right ventricle becomes so enlarged that it forces the tricuspid valve to stretch and allow blood back into the right atrium.

Inspection of the Hepatojugular Reflux

Hepatojugular reflux is a test that is very sensitive in detecting right ventricular failure. This procedure is performed if the CVP is normal but right ventricular failure is suspected.

E   1.   Place the patient flat in bed, or elevated to a 30° angle if the jugular veins are visible. Remind the patient to breathe normally.

2.   Using single or bimanual deep palpation, press firmly on the right upper quadrant for 30 to 60 seconds. Press on another part of the abdomen if this area is tender.

3.   Observe the neck for an elevation in JVP (see Figure 15-17).

N   *Normally, this pressure should not elicit any change in the jugular veins.*

A   A rise of more than 1 cm in JVP is abnormal.

P   A rise in JVP that occurs with this technique is suggestive of right-sided congestive heart failure or fluid overload. The heart simply cannot accept the increase in venous return.

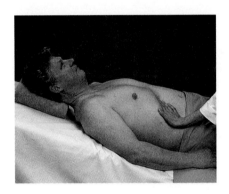

Figure 15-17   Hepatojugular Reflux

Palpation and Auscultation of Arterial Pulses

Information concerning the function of the right ventricle is gained via the assessment of the venous pulses; however, assessment of the arterial pulses provides information about the left ventricle. The pulses to be evaluated are the temporal carotid, brachial, radial, femoral, popliteal, posterior tibial, and the dorsalis pedis. The arteries that are most frequently examined are the radial arteries due to their easy accessibility. In a cardiac arrest situation, the carotid pulse is the artery of choice for palpation.

E   1.   The arterial pulse assessment is best facilitated with the patient in a supine position with the head of the bed elevated at 30° to 45°. If the patient cannot tolerate such a position, then the supine position alone is acceptable.

2.   Using your dominant hand, palpate the pulses with the pads of the index and middle fingers. The number of fingers used will be determined by the amount of space where the pulse is located.

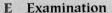

E   Examination
N   Normal Findings
A   Abnormal Findings
P   Pathophysiology

NURSING TIP

Documenting Pulses

You can document the amplitude of a patient's pulses by drawing a small stick figure and labeling the pulses accordingly (refer to Figure 15-18) or by recording the pulses in tabular format (see page 791, Chapter 24).

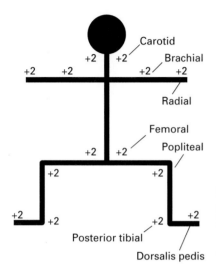

Figure 15-18 Stick Figure Depicting Arterial Pulse Assessment (temporal pulse is not routinely shown on the stick figure)

NURSING ALERT

Palpation of Carotid Pulses

The carotid pulses should not be palpated together because excessive stimulation can elicit a vagal response and slow down the heart. Palpating both carotid pulses at the same time could also cut off circulation to the patient's head.

E	**Examination**
N	**Normal Findings**
A	**Abnormal Findings**
P	**Pathophysiology**

3. Evaluate the pulse in terms of:
  a. Rate
  b. Rhythm: If there is an irregularity in the pulse rate, then auscultate the heart.
  c. Amplitude: Refer to Chapter 9 for grading scales.
  d. Symmetry: Palpate the pulses on both sides of the patient's body simultaneously (with the exception of the carotid pulses).
4. Using the bell of the stethoscope, auscultate the temporal, carotid, and femoral pulses for **bruits**, which are blowing sounds heard when blood flow becomes turbulent as it rushes past an obstruction. Ask the patient to hold his or her breath during auscultation of the carotid pulse because respiratory sounds can interfere with auscultation.

N *Refer to Chapter 9, pages 209 and 210, for normal pulse rate, rhythm, and amplitude. When assessing symmetry, the pulses should be equal bilaterally. No bruits should be auscultated in the carotid or femoral pulses.*

A/P Figure 15-19 illustrates abnormal pulses with possible etiologies.

A Asymmetrical pulses are abnormal.

P Variations in the symmetry of pulses can occur because of anatomic differences in the depths and locations of the arteries.

A Auscultation of bruits at the temporal, carotid, and femoral areas is abnormal.

P Bruits in both of these areas can be caused by an obstruction related to atherosclerotic plaque formation, a jugular vein–carotid artery fistula, or high-output states such as anemia or thyrotoxicosis.

SPECIAL TECHNIQUE

Orthostatic Hypotension Assessment

When an individual stands, blood pools in the lower part of the body and the blood pressure falls transiently. However, in the healthy individual, **baroreceptors** (receptors located in the walls of most of the great arteries) located in the carotid sinus area sense the decrease in blood pressure and initiate reflex vasoconstriction and increased heart rate. These mechanisms bring the blood pressure back to normal. When this mechanism fails, **orthostatic hypotension** may ensue and an evaluation must be made. When assessing for orthostatic hypotension, take the patient's blood pressure and heart rate with the patient in supine, sitting, and standing positions. This set of orthostatic vital signs is commonly referred to as **tilts**.

E **1.** First check the blood pressure in a supine position. In this position, the patient should be flat for at least 5 minutes. (This time ensures that no reflex mechanisms from the upright position are influencing the blood pressure.) Record the blood pressure and the heart rate as the first set of tilts.
  2. Next, assist the patient to a sitting position with the feet dangling. Wait 1 to 3 minutes. (There is no consensus in the literature regarding how long to wait after a position change before obtaining the next set of vital signs.) Retake the blood pressure and heart rate. This waiting period allows time for the reflex mechanisms to activate and ensure a normal blood pressure. Record the blood pressure and the heart rate as the second set of tilts. Also, ask the patient about any symptoms of weakness or dizziness related to the position change. If the patient becomes weak or dizzy, assist the patient back to a supine position.
  3. Finally, assist the patient to a standing position. Measure the blood pressure and heart rate again after 1 to 3 minutes. Again, ask the patient about any symptoms of weakness or dizziness related to the position change. If the patient becomes weak or dizzy, assist the patient back to a supine position.

continued

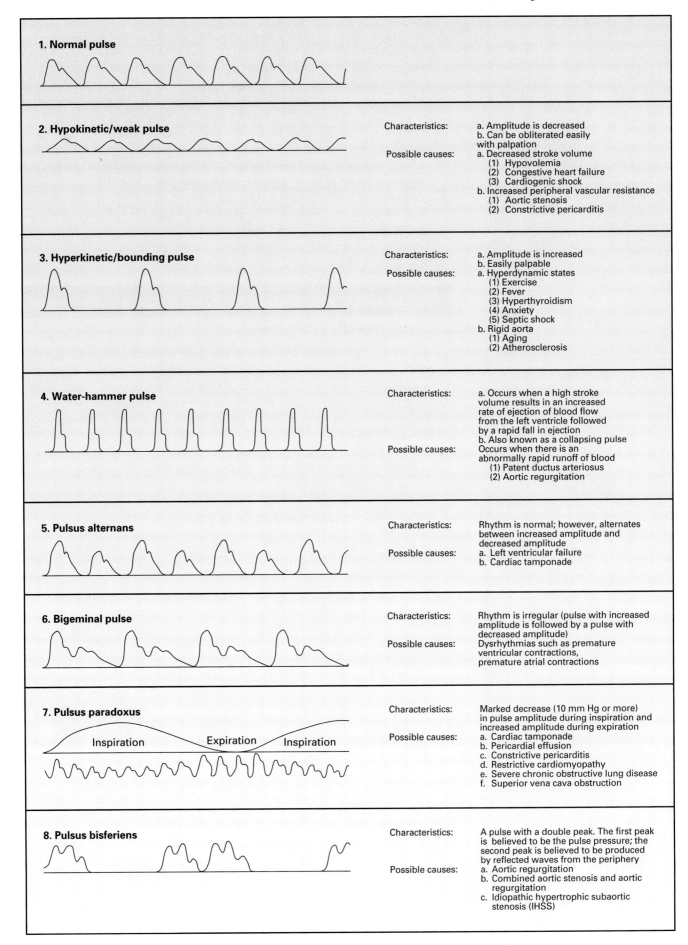

Figure 15-19   Alterations in Arterial Pulses

N *Wide discrepancies in the literature exist regarding the magnitude of the orthostatic response. The latest studies reveal that there is no relationship between orthostatic vital signs and volume status, yet tilts are still frequently used as indicators of intravascular volume status. Many normal patients may have what has been considered in the past to be positive tilts consistent with hypovolemia even though they are not hypovolemic.*

A Orthostatic vital signs that have been considered positive in the past include a systolic or a diastolic blood pressure decrease of more than 10 mm Hg or a heart rate increase of more than 20 beats per minute. However, tilts have fallen out of favor with many for the reason previously stated.

P Orthostatic hypotension can occur in patients who are hypovolemic, have a neurogenic problem, or are experiencing side effects from a prescribed medication.

✸ SPECIAL TECHNIQUE

Assessing for Pulsus Paradoxus

During inspiration, the blood flow into the right side of the heart is increased, the right ventricular output is enhanced, and pulmonary venous capacitance is increased resulting in less blood reaching the left ventricle. These mechanisms account for a decrease in both the left ventricular stroke volume and arterial pressure. An exaggerated form of this mechanism is referred to as **pulsus paradoxus**.

E 1. Place the patient in a supine position. Instruct the patient to breathe normally.
   2. Apply the blood pressure cuff.
   3. Inflate the cuff to 20 mm Hg above the patient's last systolic blood pressure reading.
   4. Slowly deflate the cuff until the first systolic sound is heard.
   5. Observe the patient's respirations because the systolic sound may disappear during normal inspiration.
   6. Slowly deflate the cuff again and note the point at which all of the systolic sounds are heard regardless of respirations.

N *The difference between the first systolic sound and the point at which all the systolic sounds are heard is the paradox. The paradox should be less than or equal to 10 mm Hg.*

A A paradox greater than 10 mm Hg is considered abnormal.

P Pulsus paradoxus can occur in conditions such as cardiac tamponade, pericardial effusion, constrictive pericarditis, restrictive cardiomyopathy, severe chronic obstructive lung disease, and superior vena cava obstruction because all of these conditions can result in a decreased blood return to the left ventricle.

🌹 NURSING TIP

Peripheral Perfusion

Refer to Chapter 10 for **E**, **N**, **A**, and **P** on color, clubbing, capillary refill, skin temperature, edema, skin texture, and hair distribution.

E Examination
N Normal Findings
A Abnormal Findings
P Pathophysiology

Inspection and Palpation of Peripheral Perfusion

Peripheral perfusion can be impaired with any pathological state that affects the flow of blood through the peripheral arteries and veins. Components of peripheral perfusion assessment include: peripheral pulse, color, clubbing, capillary refill, skin temperature, edema, ulcerations, skin texture, hair distribution, and special techniques for the assessment of arterial and venous blood flow.

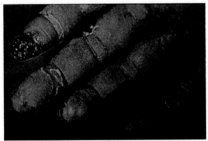

A. Raynaud's Disease   *Courtesy of Marvin Ackerman, M.D., Scarsdale, NY*

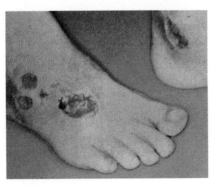

B. Venous Ulceration   *Courtesy of Delmar Publishers, Albany, NY*

Figure 15-20   Ulcerations

E	**Examination**
N	**Normal Findings**
A	**Abnormal Findings**
P	**Pathophysiology**

E 1. Inspect the fingers, toes, or points of trauma on the feet and legs for ulceration. Inspect the sides of the ankles for ulceration.
   2. Special techniques for assessing the venous system (discussed in more detail later):
      a. Homan's sign
      b. Manual compression
      c. Retrograde filling or Trendelenburg test
   3. Special techniques for examining the arterial system (discussed in more detail later):
      a. Pallor
      b. Color return (CR) and venous filling time (VFT)
      c. Allen Test

N *Ulcerations: No ulcerations should be noted.*

A Arterial ulcerations are abnormal.
   1. Location: occurs at toes or points of trauma on the feet or the legs.
   2. Characteristics: well-defined edges; black or necrotic tissue; a deep, pale base, and lack of bleeding; hairlessness or disruption of the hair along with shiny, thick, waxy skin.
   3. Pain: exceedingly painful; claudication related to arterial disease is relieved by rest; pain at rest is relieved by dependency.

P The location and characteristics of ulceration are due to inadequate arterial flow, such as in peripheral vascular disease and diabetes mellitus. Most distal arterial beds are prone to ulceration. The pain is caused by ischemia.

P Arterial ulcers on the tips of the fingers, toes, or nose can be caused by Raynaud's disease (see Figure 15-20A). Arteriolar spasms lead to pallor and pain in the affected area, followed by cyanosis, with numbness, tingling, and burning; rubor also develops. Over time, the affected area may develop an ulcer. Attacks occur bilaterally and last minutes to hours.

A Venous ulcerations are abnormal (refer to Figure 15-20B):
   1. Location: occurs at the sides of the ankles.
   2. Characteristics: uneven edges and ruddy granulation of tissue; thin, shiny skin that lacks the support of subcutaneous tissue; disruption of hair pattern, or hairlessness.
   3. Pain: deep muscular pain (associated with inadequate venous flow) with acute DVT; aching and cramping are relieved with elevation.

P Ulcers are due to inadequate venous flow that results when communication between the superficial and deep veins is compromised. Both the characteristics and the pain are related to inadequate venous blood flow.

❖ **SPECIAL TECHNIQUE**

Assessing the Venous System

Homan's Sign
It is important to note that because a Homan's sign has a low sensitivity (an indication of the frequency of a positive test result in a population with the disease) for thrombophlebitis, the use of this test has fallen out of favor with some health care providers. A positive Homan's sign is present in less than 20% of all DVT cases.

E 1. With the patient's knee slightly bent, sharply dorsiflex the patient's foot and ask the patient if this maneuver elicits pain in the calf.
   2. Repeat this technique with the other foot.

N *There should be no complaints of calf pain when this is evaluated.*

A A positive Homan's sign may be abnormal.

continued

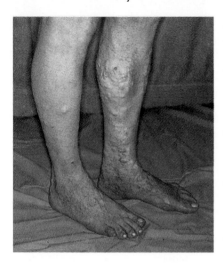

Figure 15-21 Varicose Veins
Courtesy of the Armed Forces Institute of Pathology

⚡ NURSING ALERT

Risk Factors for Varicose Veins

Varicose veins affect approximately 10% of the adult population and occur four times more often in women than in men. The pathogenesis of varicose veins remains unknown; however, it is not uncommon to find varicose veins in patients who have a family history of varicose veins, whose occupations require long periods of standing, or who are obese or pregnant.

Some measures to prevent unnecessary pressure on the leg veins include avoiding heavy lifting, excessive weight gain, and crossing the legs; wearing support pantyhose; stopping smoking; elevating feet when sitting; and exercising.

E	**Examination**
N	**Normal Findings**
A	**Abnormal Findings**
P	**Pathophysiology**

P A positive Homan's sign may indicate thrombophlebitis or DVT. Early detection of thrombophlebitis is essential because it can lead to life-threatening complications such as pulmonary emboli, which occurs when a thrombus breaks loose from the vein and travels to the lung. Three factors can disrupt the balance between blood-clotting activators and inhibitors. Known as Virchow's triad, they are: stasis of blood flow, an injured venous wall, and hypercoagulability. All three of these factors can predispose a patient to thrombosis. Thrombosis can occur in either deep or superficial veins.

Manual Compression
Manual compression tests the competency of the saphenous vein's valves.
E 1. Palpate the dilated vein with one hand.
2. Use the other hand to compress the same vein 20 cm higher in the leg.
3. Note if an impulse is felt.
N *If the valves are competent, you will not feel the impulse because competent valves block transmission of the impulse.*
A An impulse felt with manual compression is abnormal.
P Varicose veins are dilated, tortuous veins that are caused by incompetent valves (see Figure 15-21). They are most prevalent in the saphenous veins of the lower extremities.

Retrograde Filling, or Trendelenburg, Test
The retrograde filling, or Trendelenburg, test assesses the competency of the valves in the communicating and saphenous veins (evaluating varicose veins).
E 1. Raise the patient's leg 90° to drain the venous blood.
2. Place a tourniquet or your hands around the upper thigh to occlude the patient's saphenous vein.
3. Instruct the patient to stand so that venous filling can be noted.
4. Release the compression and watch venous filling again.
N *Normal veins fill from below the occlusion and within 35 seconds as blood flows down from the arteries to the veins. Following release of the hands or tourniquet, there should be no additional filling because competent valves prevent the backflow of blood.*
A A varicose vein that fills from above in the retrograde filling, or Trendelenburg, test is not normal.
P This occurs in varicose veins because of the backward flow of blood through incompetent valves. If sudden additional filling occurs when the hands or tourniquet are removed, it is another indication that varicosities occur because of incompetent valves.

✳ SPECIAL TECHNIQUE

Assessing the Arterial System

Pallor
E 1. Instruct the patient to raise the extremities.
2. Note the time it takes for pallor, or lack of color, to develop.
N *Normally no pallor develops within 60 seconds.*
A Pallor that develops quickly in the extremities when the extremities are lifted is abnormal.
P Pallor that develops quickly is indicative of arterial insufficiency. The quicker the pallor develops, the more severe the disease.

Color Return and Venous Filling Time
E 1. To drain the patient's feet of venous blood, elevate the supine patient's legs approximately 12 inches and ask the patient to move his or her feet up and down at the ankles for approximately 1 minute.

continued

2. Next, place the patient in a sitting position on the edge of the bed, with the legs dangling over the side.

3. Note the time it takes for the color to return to the legs and for the superficial veins to refill.

N *Normal color return (CR) is 10 seconds and venous filling time (VFT) is 15 seconds.*

A A delayed CR of 15 to 25 seconds or a VFT of 20 to 30 seconds is abnormal.

P These scores indicate moderate ischemia.

A A delayed CR of 40 seconds or more or a VFT of 40 seconds or more is abnormal.

P These scores indicate severe ischemia.

Allen Test

The Allen test is used to assess the patency of the radial and ulnar arteries (refer to Figure 15-22). This test is usually performed prior to radial artery cannulation because radial artery cannulation is commonly associated with radial artery thrombosis. If the radial artery becomes occluded with a thrombus, continued viability of the hand depends on collateral blood flow from the ulnar artery.

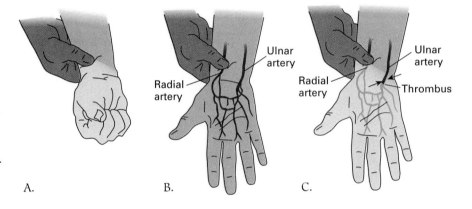

Figure 15-22 The Allen Test. A. Pallor is initiated by compressing the radial artery with the fist clenched. B. A patent ulnar artery reveals the return of palm perfusion despite radial artery compression. C. An occluded ulnar artery results in continued pallor of the hand while the radial artery is still compressed.

E **1.** Compress the patient's radial artery and ask the patient to clench the fist so that blanching occurs. If the patient is unable to cooperate, then clench the fist passively for the patient.

2. After blanching occurs, instruct the patient to release the fist.

3. Note the color return of the patient's palms.

4. Repeat this test on the ulnar arteries.

N *If the radial artery is compressed, the blood flow through the ulnar artery should be sufficient to maintain the normal palm color after the patient unclenches the fist. Also, if the ulnar artery is compressed, the blood flow through the radial artery should be sufficient to maintain the normal palm color.*

A If the color does not return to normal within 6 seconds after the patient unclenches the fist, then obstruction of either the radial or the ulnar arteries may be present.

P Atherosclerosis or a thrombus can cause either artery to be not patent.

Palpation of the Epitrochlear Node

The epitrochlear node drains lymph from the ulnar surface of the forearm and hand and from the middle, ring, and little fingers.

E **1.** Place the patient in a sitting position.

2. Support the patient's hand with your hand.

3. With the other hand, reach behind the elbow and place your finger pads in the groove between the biceps and the triceps muscles, superior to the medial condyle of the humerus.

E	**Examination**
N	**Normal Findings**
A	**Abnormal Findings**
P	**Pathophysiology**

4. Palpate the epitrochlear node for size, shape, consistency, tenderness, and mobility.

N *Normally, the epitrochlear node is not palpable.*

A An enlarged lymph node is abnormal.

P An infection in the forearm or hand can lead to a palpable and tender epitrochlear node.

P Malignancies can cause an enlarged, hard, and nontender epitrochlear node.

GERONTOLOGICAL VARIATIONS

As adults age, their cardiovascular systems undergo physiological changes that in many instances are complicated by disease processes. In the normal individual, the size of the cardiac muscle begins to decrease with age. As fibrotic and sclerotic changes take place in the atria and the ventricles, cardiac output can fall by as much as 35% at rest after the age of 70. Skeletal changes that sometimes occur in the elderly, such as kyphosis or collapsed vertebrae from osteoporosis, can alter the position of the heart within the thoracic cavity, giving rise to changes in the electrocardiographic data. Obesity that results in an increased abdominal girth with subsequent diaphragmatic elevation can also displace the heart within the chest.

With the aging process, intracardiac valves may develop calcifications or fibrosis that results in systolic or diastolic murmurs. If the left ventricle has thickened or enlarged, thus losing its compliance, an S_4 heart sound can be heard on auscultation. Changes in the conduction system resulting from electrolyte imbalances, from debilitating states or pharmacotherapy, or from thickened myocardial fibers can cause cardiac irritability leading to a variety of dysrhythmias.

Vascular integrity is also susceptible to the aging process. The arterial system becomes increasingly rigid as the vessels become fibrotic. If a pathological process such as atherosclerosis is added, the insult to the vascular tree becomes even greater. Elasticity is lost, the vessel lumen is narrowed, and peripheral vascular resistance is increased, thus impeding blood flow. Other conditions that cause vascular spasm, such as smoking, contribute to a decrease in vascular flow. In the venous system, there is intimal thickening with dilation and loss of valvular competency. Venous return to the heart is affected, and edema or varicosities may develop. The baroreceptors located in the aortic arch and the carotid sinuses are also affected by vascular integrity. In the presence of impaired compliance, these structures are altered in their abilities to respond to changes in blood pressure.

In addition to cardiovascular changes associated with the aging process, diseases affecting other body systems may also affect the heart and vessels. For example, right-sided heart failure may be precipitated by chronic obstructive lung disease, and diabetes mellitus can have deleterious effects on the peripheral vasculature.

Alterations in cerebral perfusion related to atherosclerosis or arteriosclerotic heart disease can cause patients to become confused or forgetful, thus making history taking difficult. The patient may tire easily because of his or her decreased cardiac output and thus may require periods of rest during the interview and assessment.

It is interesting to note that more elderly people die of cardiovascular problems than of any other single disease. Among elderly persons with hypertension in addition to CAD, the mortality rate is even higher. Finally, eight of the top ten drugs prescribed for geriatric patients are either cardiac or diuretic drugs. Age-related changes may delay the peak effect of cardiovascular drugs, thus creating the possibility for additional cardiovascular problems in the elderly patient.

E	**Examination**
N	**Normal Findings**
A	**Abnormal Findings**
P	**Pathophysiology**

CASE STUDY

The case study illustrates the application and objective documentation of the heart and peripheral vasculature assessment.

The Patient with Congestive Heart Failure

Mrs. Weinstein is a 72-year-old white female admitted to the coronary care unit (CCU) with SOB, which has been increasing in severity over the past 4 days.

❖ HEALTH HISTORY

PATIENT PROFILE	72 yo widowed WF
CHIEF COMPLAINT	"I've been having SOB & I noticed that my legs now swell."
HISTORY OF PRESENT ILLNESS	Pt describes her present SOB as being similar to that she had for 1 wk $\bar{p}$ inferior wall myocardial infarction (IWMI) 4 mo PTA; tx $\bar{c}$ "some med." Describes SOB as suffocating feeling that quickly tires her out. SOB alleviated by resting, sitting upright, aggravated by walking up stairs, doing light housework. When climbing steps, feels out of breath $\bar{p}$ 6 steps (1/2 distance to top). Rests for brief time & continues up stairs. Takes 2nd break at top. Last wk was able to climb stairs $\bar{s}$ difficulty. Admits she didn't refill Rx for KCl (tasted bad) and furosemide (frequent urination). Since yesterday, shoes feel tighter & unable to get rings off; feet swollen, elevating them ↓ swelling. Gained 8 lb in past 8 wk. Admits to ↑ smoking this past wk due to stress of being indoors b/c of snowstorm; canceled appt $\bar{c}$ cardiologist. Sleeps on 3 pillows × 3 nights. Denies sputum, chest pain, palpitations, leg pain, or abd pain.
PAST HEALTH HISTORY	
Medical	IWMI per HPI; in CCU at St. Agnes Hospital; hospitalization complicated by CHF requiring additional wk in hospital (doesn't recall tx); dx $\bar{c}$ HTN 15 yr ago by general practitioner & told to eliminate salt from diet (admits she was not compliant); told by "some MD" many yrs ago that her cholesterol level was ↑.
Surgical	Denies
Medications	Digoxin 0.125 mg po qd × 4 mo; denies side effects; doesn't take radial pulse prior to administration; admits omitting med when she can't afford it or bad weather prevents her from purchasing it Furosemide 20 mg po bid × 4 mo Enteric-coated ASA 325 mg po q AM × 4 mo $\bar{c}$ meal; denies complications; can't remember why she needs to take it KCl 20 mEq po bid × 4 mo; "upsets my stomach" Alka seltzer 2 tabs po prn for upset stomach
Communicable Diseases	Denies
Allergies	Lidocaine (caused ringing in the ears in CCU)

continued

Injuries/Accidents	Denies
Disabilities/Handicaps	Denies
Blood Transfusions	Denies ever receiving blood or blood products but is proud she has donated blood in the past
Childhood Illnesses	Recalls "having the usual: measles, mumps, & chicken pox"; denies having had any other dz
Immunizations	Can't remember having PPD & thinks she had tetanus shot in last 10 yr; doesn't get flu shot q yr

FAMILY HEALTH HISTORY

LEGEND

◯ Living female

▢ Living male

⊗ Deceased female

⊠ Deceased male

⟋ Points to patient

─//─ = Divorced

A&W = Alive & well

CA = Cancer

CHF = Congestive heart failure

Chol = Cholesterol

HTN = Hypertension

IDDM = Insulin-dependent diabetes mellitus

MI = Myocardial infarction

MVA = Motor vehicle accident

Denies family hx of aneurysm, CVA, mitral valve prolapse, rheumatic fever, & hypertrophic cardiomyopathy.

SOCIAL HISTORY

Alcohol Use	6 oz whiskey qd × 10 yr; denies having drinking problem; denies ↓ LOC p̄ drinking; denies knowledge of thiamine deficiency
Tobacco Use	55 pk/yr hx of smoking high-tar & nicotine cigarettes, chews snuff throughout day; ↑ usual 1 ppd to 2 ppd c̄ snowstorm; denies quitting or desire to quit; denies palpitations c̄ smoking
Drug Use	Denies
Sexual Practice	Denies sexual contact since widowed 10 yr ago
Travel History	Denies travel outside continental USA
Work Environment	Never employed outside of home
Home Environment	Resides in 2-story townhouse; kitchen & living areas on 1st floor; only bathroom & bedroom on 2nd floor

continued

Hobbies/Leisure Activities	Likes to watch TV
Stress	States she is impatient, has a fast pace c̄ activities, & has rapid, loud speech; states that snow & her inability to leave the house & go to synagogue have made her very anxious this past wk
Education	Finished high school
Economic Status	"Gets by c̄ Medicare & Social Security"
Military Service	Denies
Religion	Judaism; unable to attend synagogue this past wk c̄ snow
Ethnic Background	Jewish
Roles/Relationships	Lives alone & has no children; has no neighbors she can rely on; denies any close relationships; doesn't use any community support systems
Characteristic Patterns of Daily Living	Awakens 0700; eats breakfast at 0800; watches TV all AM; eats lunch at 1300; naps at 1400 (sleeps for 1 hr); watches TV rest of afternoon; eats dinner at 1800; watches TV until she feels sleepy; takes bath at 2200; goes to bed at 2300

HEALTH MAINTENANCE ACTIVITIES

Sleep	8 hr/night
Diet	Admits to salting foods heavily during cooking & eating; eats processed foods & very little fresh fruits & vegetables
Exercise	Denies any exercise
Stress Management	Denies
Use of Safety Devices	Denies use of seat belt
Health Check-Ups	Denies seeking medical attention until IWMI 4 mo ago; since that time, has kept "about half" of her f/u appt; states that when weather is bad or she has no transportation, the appt are not kept nor are they rescheduled; doesn't know BP reading

RISK FACTORS

Fixed	Age & family hx
Major Modifiable	HTN, hyperlipoproteinemia, smoking, & ↑ salt intake
Minor Modifiable	Sedentary lifestyle, stress, & ETOH intake

PATIENT CLASSIFICATION	NYHA Class III

continued

PHYSICAL ASSESSMENT

Assessment of the Precordium

Inspection

Aortic area: Neg
Pulmonic area: Neg
Midprecordial area: Neg
Tricuspid area: Neg
Mitral area: Visible apical impulse in 6th Ⓛ ICS, Ⓛ anterior axillary line

Palpation

Aortic area: Neg
Pulmonic area: Neg
Midprecordial area: Neg
Tricuspid area: Neg
Mitral area: Apical impulse located at 6th Ⓛ ICS, Ⓛ anterior axillary line; ∅ thrill; ∅ heave

Auscultation

Aortic area: ⊕S_2
Pulmonic area: ⊕S_2
Midprecordial area: Neg
Tricuspid area: ⊕S_1, ⊕S_3, ⊖S_4
Mitral area: ⊕S_1, ⊕S_3, ⊖S_4
Murmurs: Neg
Pericardial friction rub: Neg

Assessment of the Peripheral Vasculature

Inspection of JVP (Indirect)

15 cm at 45°; 12 cm at 90°

Inspection of the Hepatojugular Reflux

↑ 3 cm at 30°

Palpation and Auscultation of Arterial Pulses

Arterial pulses
  Rate: 110 bpm
  Rhythm: Irregular
  Amplitude:

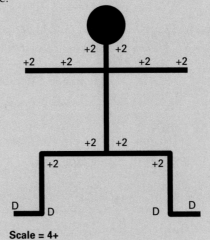

Scale = 4+

D = not palpable secondary to edema; pulse obtained c̄ Doppler ultrasonic transducer

continued

Symmetry: All symmetrical
Bruits: Ø carotid bruit; Ø femoral bruit

Inspection and Palpation of Peripheral Perfusion

Color: Pale extremities
Clubbing: None
Capillary refill: 5 sec
Skin temperature: Cool, clammy
Edema: 3+/4+ pitting edema in ankles bilaterally
Ulcerations: Neg
Skin texture: Shiny, dry, scaly
Hair distribution: Hair absent from midcalf down bilaterally

Palpation of the Epitrochlear Node

Nonpalpable

Special Technique

Pulsus paradoxus: Neg

DIAGNOSTIC DATA

Chest X-Ray

Consistent with CHF

EKG

Atrial fibrillation with a rapid ventricular response (ventricular rate of 110 bpm); old IWMI; everything else is WNL

Echocardiogram

Mildly dilated left ventricle that is consistent with CHF

CVP

On admission, a central line was inserted and the pressure readings obtained at a 45° angle were as follows:
1:00 AM: 17 cm H_2O
3:00 AM: 20 cm H_2O
5:00 AM: 21 cm H_2O
7:00 AM: 20 cm H_2O

LABORATORY DATA

	Pt's Values	Normal Range
Serum Cholesterol	389 mg/dl	140–220 mg/dl
Triglycerides	212 mg/dl	35–135 mg/dl
HDL	35 mg/dl	38–85 mg/dl
LDL	188 mg/dl	<130 mg/dl
Potassium	3.6 mEq/L	3.5–5.0 mEq/L

✓ NURSING CHECKLIST
Heart and Peripheral Vasculature Assessment

Assessment of the Precordium
- Inspection
  - Aortic Area
  - Pulmonic Area
  - Midprecordial Area
  - Tricuspid Area
  - Mitral Area
- Palpation
  - Aortic Area
  - Pulmonic Area
  - Midprecordial Area
  - Tricuspid Area
  - Mitral Area
- Auscultation
  - Aortic Area
  - Pulmonic Area
  - Midprecordial Area
  - Tricuspid Area
  - Mitral Area
  - Mitral and Tricuspid Area (S_3)
  - Mitral and Tricuspid Area (S_4)
  - Murmurs
  - Pericardial Friction Rub
  - Prosthetic Heart Valves

Assessment of the Peripheral Vasculature
- Inspection of the Jugular Venous Pressure
- Inspection of the Hepatojugular Reflux
- Palpation and Auscultation of Arterial Pulses
- Inspection and Palpation of Peripheral Perfusion
  - Peripheral Pulse
  - Color
  - Clubbing
  - Capillary Refill
  - Skin Temperature
  - Edema
  - Ulcerations
  - Skin Texture
  - Hair Distribution
- Palpation of the Epitrochlear Node

Special Techniques
- Orthostatic Hypotension Assessment
- Assessing for Pulsus Paradoxus
- Assessing the Venous System
  - Homan's Sign
  - Manual Compression
  - Retrograde Filling, or Trendelenburg, Test
- Assessing the Arterial System
  - Pallor
  - Color Return and Venous Filling Time
  - Allen Test

Assistive Devices
- Artificial Cardiac Pacemakers
- Hemodynamic Monitoring
- Antiembolic Stockings
- Chest Tubes
- EKG Monitoring
- Intravenous Catheters
- Pneumatic Compression Stockings
- Pulse Oximetry

REVIEW QUESTIONS AND ACTIVITIES

1. Your patient is complaining of chest pain. What questions should you ask?

2. Distinguish the risk factors that are fixed versus those that are both major and minor modifiable for cardiovascular disease.

3. When assessing the precordium, what are the five cardiac landmarks you should use? Does it matter whether you start at the base or the apex?

4. Whenever you hear a colleague state that his or her patient has an extra heart sound or murmur, ask if you can listen to it. Also, always ask the patient whether you can listen. Try to take advantage of any opportunity you can to identify heart sounds when you are working with patients.

5. Your patient has a grade III/VI systolic murmur heard best at the fifth ICS, left midclavicular line. What could be some causes of the murmur?

6. What are at least four characteristics to look for when evaluating pulses?

Questions 7–9 refer to the following situation:

Mr. Henry is admitted to your critical care unit with chest pain, DOE, and pitting edema. His chest x-ray confirms a diagnosis of heart failure.

7. What heart sound is a common finding in the patient with heart failure?
   a. S_3
   b. S_4
   c. Pericardial friction rub
   d. Pleural friction rub

The correct answer is (a).

8. While auscultating Mr. Henry's heart sounds, you detect a murmur at the patient's fifth ICS, left midclavicular line. You would suspect this to be:
   a. An aortic valve murmur
   b. A pulmonic valve murmur
   c. A tricuspid valve murmur
   d. A mitral valve murmur

The correct answer is (d).

9. The murmur that you have auscultated has a moderate intensity and you do not palpate a thrill. You would grade this murmur as a:
   a. Grade I/VI
   b. Grade II/VI
   c. Grade III/VI
   d. Grade VI/VI

The correct answer is (c).

Abdomen

1. Specify the physiological function of the normal gastrointestinal anatomic organs.
2. Assess the health status of a patient with a gastrointestinal complaint.
3. Demonstrate the techniques of gastrointestinal assessment.
4. Relate abnormal physical gastrointestinal findings to potential pathological processes.
5. Outline the gastrointestinal variations associated with the aging process.

Assessing the abdomen requires a complete understanding of anatomic and abdominal assessment norms. Examination of the abdomen provides significant information about the various functions of the gastrointestinal, cardiovascular, and genitourinary systems.

ANATOMY AND PHYSIOLOGY

Abdominal Cavity

The abdomen is the largest cavity of the body. It is located between the diaphragm and the symphysis pubis. It is oval-shaped and contains several vital organs. The posterior wall of the cavity includes the lumbar vertebrae, the sacrum, and the coccyx. The iliac bones and the lateral portion of the ribs shape the sides of the abdominal cavity (Figures 16-1 and 16-2). These bony structures are held together by muscular tissue that surrounds the entire abdominal cavity. The anterior wall is formed by flat muscles and fascia, reinforced by the abdominal rectus muscle.

Peritoneum

The endothelial lining of the abdominal cavity consists of membranes called peritoneal serous membranes. The serous layer that lines the walls of the cavity itself is called the parietal peritoneum and that which covers the organs is called the visceral peritoneum. The potential space between the two layers is referred to as the peritoneal cavity. In the male, this cavity is completely closed, whereas in the female, openings exist for the fallopian tubes.

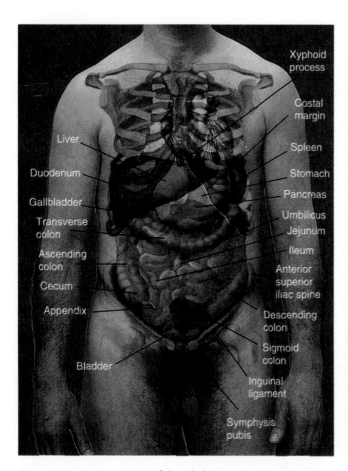

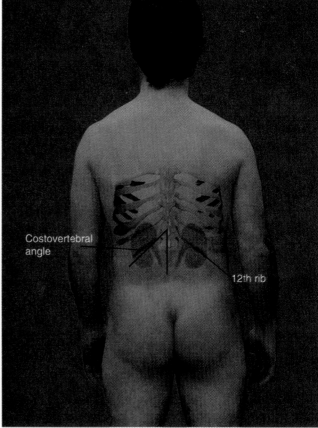

Figure 16-1 Structures of the Abdomen: Anterior View

Figure 16-2 Structures of the Abdomen: Posterior View

The organs covered with peritoneum and held in place by mesentery are referred to as intraperitoneal organs. The intraperitoneal organs are the spleen, gallbladder, stomach, liver, bile duct, small intestine, and large intestine. In contrast, the organs situated behind the peritoneum and without mesenteric attachment are known as retroperitoneal organs. The retroperitoneal organs are the pancreas, kidneys, ureters, and bladder.

Abdominal Vasculature

The aorta is the largest artery in the body. Below the level of the diaphragm, the descending aorta becomes the abdominal aorta, giving rise to arterial vessels that supply the abdominal wall and gastrointestinal organs with blood (see Figure 16-3). At about the fourth lumbar vertebra, the aorta bifurcates to become the right and left common iliac arteries.

Anatomic Mapping

Anatomic maps serve as a frame of reference during assessment of the abdomen. The abdominal cavity can be subdivided using two methods: quadrants or nine regions.

The most commonly used assessment approach in clinical practice is the four-quadrant technique. For accuracy in documentation, the abdominal surface is divided into four sections by imaginary vertical and horizontal lines intersecting at the umbilicus (refer to Figure 16-4). Commit to memory the location of abdominal organs according to quadrants (see Table 16-1).

Another strategy for pinpointing the location of abdominal assessment findings is via nine abdominal anatomic regions (see Figure 16-5).

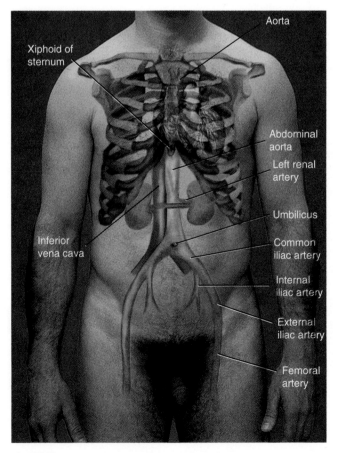

Figure 16-3   Abdominal Vasculature

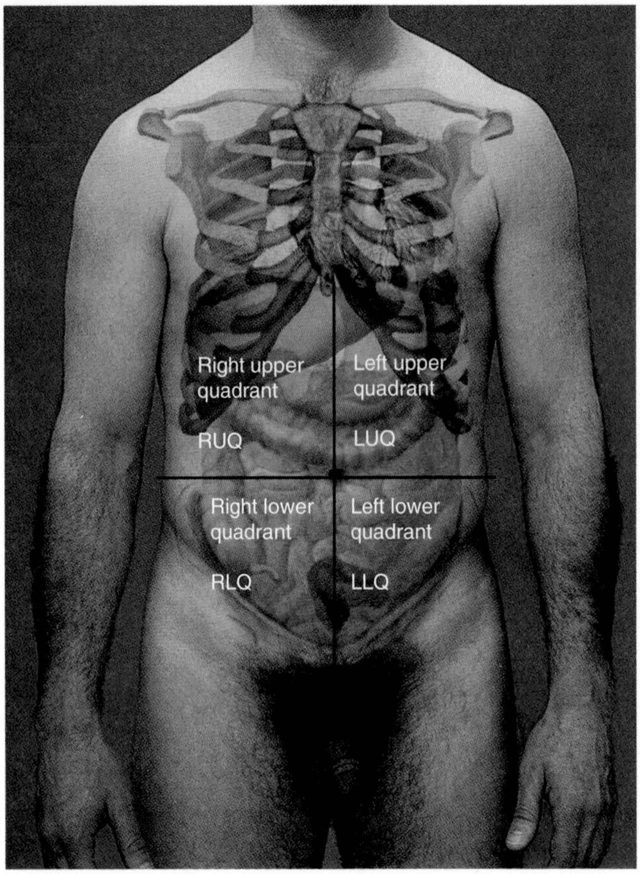

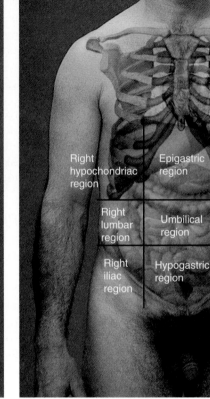

Figure 16-4 Abdominal Quadrants

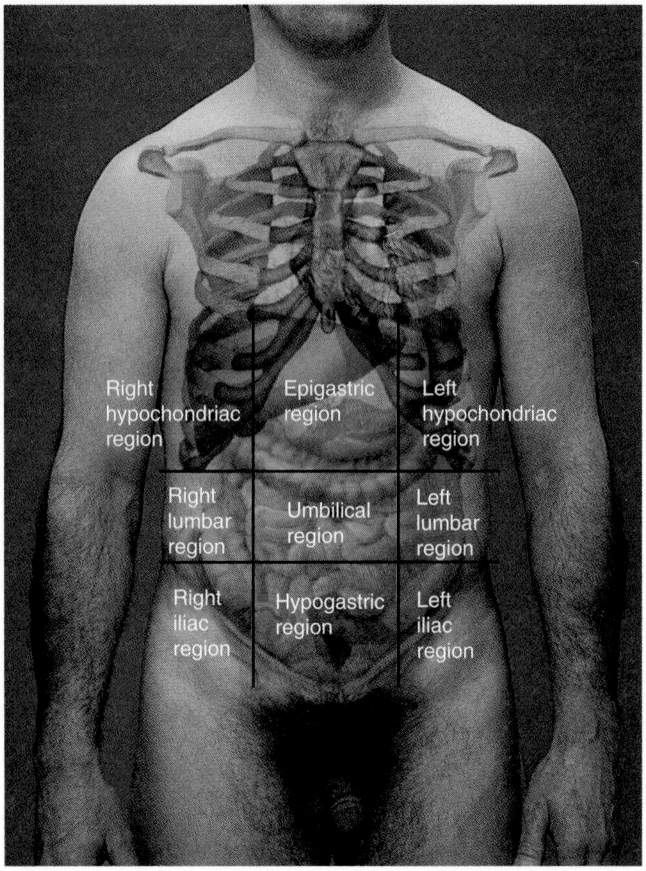

Figure 16-5 Nine Abdominal Anatomic Regions

Table 16-1 Four-Quadrant Anatomic Map	
RIGHT UPPER QUADRANT (RUQ)	**LEFT UPPER QUADRANT (LUQ)**
• Liver	• Left lobe of liver
• Gallbladder	• Stomach
• Pylorus	• Spleen
• Duodenum	• Pancreas (body)
• Pancreas (head)	• Portion of left kidney and adrenal gland
• Portion of right kidney and adrenal gland	• Splenic flexure of colon
• Hepatic flexure of colon	• Sections of transverse and descending colons
• Section of ascending and transverse colons	
RIGHT LOWER QUADRANT (RLQ)	**LEFT LOWER QUADRANT (LLQ)**
• Appendix	• Sigmoid colon
• Cecum	• Section of descending colon
• Lower pole of right kidney	• Lower pole of left kidney
• Right ureter	• Left ureter
• Right ovary (female)	• Left ovary (female)
• Right spermatic cord (male)	• Left spermatic cord (male)

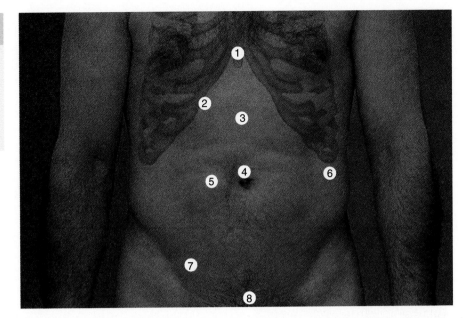

Figure 16-6 Abdominal Assessment Landmarks: 1. Xiphoid Process; 2. Costal Margin; 3. Abdominal Midline; 4. Umbilicus; 5. Rectus Abdominis Muscle; 6. Anterior Superior Iliac Spine; 7. Inguinal Ligament (Poupart's Ligament); 8. Symphysis Pubis

Abdominal Viscera (Organs)

Stomach

The stomach is a J-shaped pouchlike organ located in the left upper quadrant of the abdomen beneath the diaphragm; it lies to the right of the spleen and is partially covered by the liver.

The stomach functions as a reservoir where the complex mechanical and chemical processes of digestion occur. Little absorption of foodstuffs occurs in the stomach. Foodstuffs are liquified via gastric secretions into a semisolid substance called chyme. The usual capacity of the stomach is 1 to 1.5 L. In a regulated manner, chyme is released into the small intestine's duodenum for further digestion and absorption.

Small Intestine

The small intestine is a tubular-shaped organ extending from the pyloric sphincter to the ileocecal valve at the opening of the large intestine. The majority of foodstuffs are digested and absorbed in the small intestine. The convoluted loops of intestine are relatively mobile and can measure from 10 feet to 30 feet, depending on the degree of muscular relaxation of the intestinal wall and the size of the individual. Portions of the small intestine can be found in all four abdominal quadrants. The three segments of the small intestine are the duodenum, the jejunum and the ileum. The duodenum is the first and shortest section. It plays a significant role in digestion because hormonal secretions are released and both the common bile and main pancreatic ducts open into the duodenum. The jejunum, the second component, is composed of circular mucosal folds that provide surface area for nutrient absorption. The ileum absorbs bile salts and vitamin B_{12}. The ileum terminates at the ileocecal valve.

Large Intestine

The large intestine is a tubular-shaped organ extending from the ileocecal valve to the anus. It has a greater diameter than the small intestine and can vary considerably in length, depending on the size of the individual, but generally is 5 feet in length.

The four segments of the large intestine are the ascending, transverse, descending, and sigmoid colons. The cecum is the blind pouch that is continuous with the ascending colon, the large intestine located in the lower right quadrant of the abdomen.

The work of the large intestine is to form stool from cellulose, indigestible fibers, fat, bacteria, cellular debris, and inorganic materials, and then carry these intestinal contents to the end of the gastrointestinal tract. An additional function of the large intestine is the absorption of water and electrolytes. Water absorption occurs primarily in the ascending colon under the influence of the osmotic pressure gradient produced by sodium ions. The large intestine has limited digestive function.

Liver

The liver is the largest solid organ in the body. It lies directly below the diaphragm. The liver is located in the right upper quadrant, but extends across the midline into the left upper quadrant. In the right upper quadrant, the superior aspect of the liver is at the fifth rib, or at the nipples. The lower border does not extend more than 1 to 2 cm below the right costal margin.

The functions of the liver are complex and varied, and can be divided into:
- Storage (carbohydrates, amino acids, vitamins, minerals, and blood)
- Detoxification and filtration (drugs, hormones, and bacteria)
- Metabolism (carbohydrates, proteins, fat, ammonia to urea)
- Synthesis and secretion (bile production — 600 to 1,000 ml/day, formation of lymph, bile salts, plasma proteins, fibrinogen, blood-clotting substances, and antibodies)

Gallbladder

The gallbladder is a pear-shaped sac located in the right upper quadrant of the abdomen. It is attached to the inferior surface of the liver.

The primary role of the gallbladder is to store and concentrate the bile produced by the liver. Bile contributes to fat digestion and absorption. The gallbladder stores approximately 30 to 50 ml of bile and releases bile in the presence of cholecystokinin, pancreozymin, and parasympathetic stimulation. As the gallbladder contracts, bile is released through the cystic duct into the common bile duct, which drains into the duodenum.

Pancreas

The pancreas is an elongated accessory organ of digestion. It lies in a transverse position along the posterior abdominal wall. It is located in the upper right and upper left quadrants of the abdomen. The pancreas is both an exocrine gland that secretes bicarbonate and pancreatic enzymes (which aid in digestion), and an endocrine gland that secretes the hormones insulin, glucagon, and gastrin.

Spleen

The spleen is the largest lymph organ in the body. It is oval in shape and is composed of white pulpy lymphoid tissue and red pulp containing capillaries and venous sinuses. It is located behind the fundus of the stomach, below the diaphragm and above the left kidney and splenic flexure. The spleen is found in the upper left quadrant of the abdomen.

The spleen is part of the reticuloendothelial system and serves the body as a filter and a reservoir for red blood cell mass. During events that can cause vasoconstriction, such as hemorrhage or exercise, the spleen contributes needed blood to the general circulation. As a filter, the spleen rids the body of old or deformed red blood cells and platelets.

Vermiform Appendix

The vermiform appendix extends off the lower cecum in the right lower quadrant. This fingerlike appendage fills with digestive materials from the cecum. The vermiform appendix frequently does not empty completely, causing obstruction and subsequent infection.

Kidneys, Ureters, and Bladder

The kidneys are bean-shaped organs that lie tucked against the posterior abdominal wall. The left kidney is slightly larger in some individuals. Because of the superior placement of the liver over the right kidney, that kidney tends to hang about a half inch lower than the left, between T12 and L3.

The primary function of the kidneys is to rid the body of waste products and to maintain homeostasis through regulation of the acid–base balance, fluid and electrolyte balance, and arterial blood pressure.

Urine leaves the kidneys via the ureters. Peristaltic waves move the waste products to the bladder. The bladder stores the urine. Normally the bladder holds 200 to 400 cc of urine; however, its capacity is greater.

Lymph Nodes

The inguinal area contains deep and superficial lymph nodes. Only the superficial nodes are palpable. These lymph nodes are grouped into superior and inferior chains. The superior chain of lymph nodes is located horizontally near the inguinal ligament. The inferior chain of lymph nodes lies vertically below the junction of the saphenous and femoral veins (Figure 16-7).

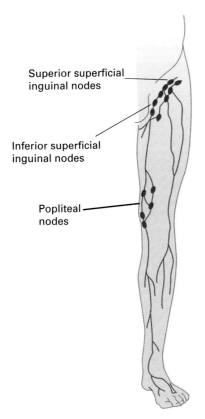

Superior superficial inguinal nodes

Inferior superficial inguinal nodes

Popliteal nodes

Figure 16-7 Inguinal Lymph Nodes

❖ HEALTH HISTORY

The abdominal health history provides insight into the link between a patient's life/lifestyle and abdominal information and pathology.

PATIENT PROFILE	*Diseases that are age- and sex-specific for the abdomen are listed.*
Age	Appendicitis (young child–30) Peptic ulcer disease (>30, with an increased incidence in the elderly) Cholecystitis (40–50) Gastrointestinal secretory deficiencies (40–50s) Diabetes mellitus (type II >45) Colonic diverticulosis (>50) Bladder cancer (50–70) Gastrointestinal malignancies (60–80s, although cancers of the rectum, stomach, and liver tend to occur earlier) Pancreatic cancer (60–70s) Mesenteric arterial insufficiency or infarct (more prevalent in the elderly, especially those with arteriosclerotic or atherosclerotic disease)
Sex	
Female	Gallbladder disease
Male	Pancreatic cancer, cirrhosis, duodenal ulcer disease, cancer of the kidney or bladder, diverticulosis, gastric cancer

continued

CHIEF COMPLAINT	Common chief complaints for the abdomen are defined and information on the characteristics of each sign/symptom is provided.
Nausea	An uncomfortable sensation in the stomach and abdominal region
Quality	Retching (dry heaves)
Associated Manifestations	Vomiting, medication use, fever, chills, foods eaten, fluids consumed, diarrhea, pregnancy
Aggravating Factors	Noxious odors
Alleviating Factors	Flat soda, dry crackers, sleep
Timing	Early morning, bedtime, middle of the night, after eating, after missed menstrual period
Vomiting	Expulsion of contents from the upper gastrointestinal tract via contraction of abdominal wall muscles and relaxation of the esophageal sphincter
Quality	Color (bright red: fresh blood; coffee grounds appearance: "old" blood that has had time to mix with digestive juices; dark brown or black: bile; other colors may occur secondary to food intake), projectile
Associated Manifestations	Nausea, medications, fever, chills, abdominal pain, headache, foods eaten, fluids consumed, diarrhea, pregnancy
Aggravating Factors	Noxious odors
Alleviating Factors	Flat soda, dry crackers, sleep, antiemetic medications
Timing	Early morning, bedtime, middle of the night, after eating, after missed menstrual period
Anorexia	Lost or decreased interest and desire for food
Quantity	Amount of food consumed in relation to patient's normal intake
Associated Manifestations	Physical weakness, fatigue, nausea, cramps, dietary intolerances, weight loss, abdominal distension, abdominal fullness, anxiety, depression
Aggravating Factors	Smoking, sleeplessness, odors, pain, emotional status
Timing	Early morning, afternoon, bedtime, continuous, days, weeks, months, during pregnancy
Dysphagia	Difficulty swallowing; associated with damage to the 9th or 10th cranial nerve, causing paralysis of the swallowing mechanism or disorders of the throat, neck, or esophagus
Associated Manifestations	Weight loss, choking, or difficulty breathing when swallowing
Aggravating Factors	Solid or liquid foods
Alleviating Factors	Position, throat lozenges

continued

Timing	Associated with specific times and meals during the day
Diarrhea	Frequent watery stools resulting in the loss of essential electrolytes
Quality	Color, presence of blood, odor
Associated Manifestations	Abdominal cramping, pain, physical weakness, weight loss, or fever
Aggravating Factors	Food, medications, stress
Alleviating Factors	Diet (bananas, rice, apples, toast), medications, fluids with electrolyte supplement, physical rest
Constipation	Infrequent stools resulting in the passage of dry, hard fecal waste
Quality	Color, odor, appearance of blood
Associated Manifestations	Physical discomfort, rectal fullness, nausea, bloating
Aggravating Factors	Food, medications, stress
Alleviating Factors	High-fiber diet, medications, physical activity, increased fluid intake
Abdominal Distension	Protuberance of the abdomen
Quantity	Degree of distension and frequency (may need to measure abdomen)
Associated Manifestations	Constipation, abdominal discomfort, ascites, enlarged liver, enlarged spleen
Aggravating Factors	Food, medications, stress
Alleviating Factors	Diet, medications, physical activity
Abdominal Pain	Discomfort in the abdomen; may be visceral, parietal, or referred pain (see Table 16-2, page 467)
Quality	Dull, burning, sharp, cramping (severe cramping is referred to as colic pain), aching, gradual, sudden
Associated Manifestations	Bleeding, flank pain, weight loss, nausea and vomiting, fever or chills, changes in bowel habits
Aggravating Factors	Position, stress, eating, smoking, medications, alcohol or drug use
Alleviating Factors	Antacids, histamine-2 antagonists, rest, diet, stress management
Setting	Home environment, work environment, mealtimes, social occasions involving alcohol or drug use
Timing	Pre- or postprandial, night time, seasonal, stressful situations, menstruation
Increased Eructation	Belching, or the oral expression of air (gas) from the stomach
Quantity	Marked increase over patient's normal status
Associated Manifestations	Ingestion of milk products, certain foods, carbonated beverages, beer

continued

Increased Flatulence	Passage of excess gas via the rectum
Quantity	Marked increase over patient's normal status
Associated Manifestations	Ingestion of certain foods (onions, cabbage, beans, cauliflower, corn, wheat, barley, rye)
Aggravating Factors	Food or medications
Alleviating Factors	Avoidance of particular foods that are fermentable
Timing	Following meals
Dysuria	Painful urination
Location	Suprapubic, near urinary meatus
Quality	Burning, stabbing
Associated Manifestations	Abdominal/flank/testicular pain, fever, chills, current bacterial infection, hematuria, dribbling, urethral discharge, decreased urinary flow, urgency, hesitancy, nocturia
Aggravating Factors	Presence of prostatic stones or renal calculi
Alleviating Factors	Medications (antibiotics, pyridium, analgesics), passage or surgical removal of stone, transurethral resection of the prostate
Setting	New sexual partner in the last 6 months, a sexual partner known to have other sexual partners, unprotected intercourse
Timing	At start of urination, midstream, throughout stream, sense of urgency, pregnancy
Nocturia	Night arousal to void
Associated Manifestations	Hesitancy, decrease in force of urinary stream, postvoid dribbling, urge incontinence
Aggravating Factors	Enlarged prostate, diabetes mellitus, diuretics, urinary tract infection, alcohol ingestion, anticholinergic medications, over-the-counter decongestants and cough medicines
Alleviating Factors	Adrenergic antagonists, 5–alpha-reductase inhibitors, transurethral resection of prostate, elimination of causative medications
PAST HEALTH HISTORY	*The various components of the past health history are linked to abdominal pathology and abdomen-related information.*
Medical	
Abdomen Specific	Malignancies, inflammation of the peritoneum, cholecystitis, appendicitis, pancreatitis, small bowel obstruction, colitis, hepatitis, diverticulosis, peptic ulcer disease, Crohn's disease, acute renal failure, chronic renal failure, gallstones, kidney stone, rectal bleeding, hemorrhoids, parasitic infections, food poisoning, cirrhosis, infectious mononucleosis, hyper- or hypoadrenalism

continued

Nonabdomen Specific	Pulmonary tuberculosis, malaria, heart disease, thyroid or parathyroid disease, upper respiratory infections, allergies, postnasal discharge, sinusitis, stress, sexually transmitted disease (STD), puberty, menopause, diabetes mellitus, ectopic pregnancy, cystic fibrosis, endometriosis, malabsorption syndromes
Surgical	Cholecystectomy, gastrectomy, Billroth I or II, ileostomy, colostomy, appendectomy, colectomy, nephrectomy, pancreatectomy, ileal conduit, portal caval shunt, splenectomy, hiatal hernia repair, umbilical hernia repair, femoral or inguinal hernia repair, removal of renal calculi, partial hepatectomy, liver transplant, renal transplant
Medications	Histamine-2 antagonists, antibiotics, lactulose, antacids, vitamins, antiparasitics, anticholinergics, minerals, tranquilizers, steroids, antidiarrheals, electrolytes, laxatives, stool softeners, insulin, sulfonamides, chemotherapeutics, antiemetics, pancreatic enzymes, antiflatulents
Communicable Diseases	STD, HIV infection, infectious hepatitis, tuberculosis, infectious mononucleosis, and intestinal parasites HIV opportunistic infections: enteric pathogens — *Cryptosporidium* causes weight loss from malabsorption syndrome and persistent debilitating diarrhea. Kaposi's sarcoma lesions can cause bowel occlusion, leading to constipation.
Allergies	Ingestion of certain food types or medications may cause gastric irritation, nausea, and vomiting.
Injuries/Accidents	Abdominal trauma such as ruptured or bruised organs, gunshot wounds, or knife stabbings; swallowing of foreign bodies or noxious substances
FAMILY HEALTH HISTORY	*Abdominal diseases and disorders that are familial are listed.* Malignancies of the stomach, liver, or pancreas, peptic ulcer disease, diabetes mellitus, familial polyposis, inflammatory bowel disease, irritable bowel syndrome, polycystic kidney disease, colitis
SOCIAL HISTORY	*The components of the social history are linked to abdomen factors/pathology.*
Alcohol Use	Altered nutrition, impaired gastric absorption, at risk for upper and lower gastrointestinal bleeding, cirrhosis of liver
Drug Use	Opioids reduce peristalsis and are associated with the development of constipation.
Travel History	Infectious diarrhea may be produced by bacteria such as *Escherichia coli*, and parasites that may not be indigenous to the patient's usual environment.
Work Environment	Improper food preparation and handling, water contamination, and poor sanitation can lead to hepatitis and *Escherichia coli* infections.

continued

Hobbies/Leisure Activities	Sports often associated with traumatic injuries, such as lacrosse, football, and boxing
Stress	Psychogenic factors that cause stress or anxiety can contribute to the development of duodenal peptic ulcers and gastric ulcers. Peptic ulcers form because of excessive acid secretion or the presence of *Helicobacter pylori*. Gastric ulcers result from reduced mucosal resistance to the digestion process.
Economic Status	Bacterial and parasitic diseases from poor sanitation
HEALTH MAINTENANCE ACTIVITIES	*This information provides a bridge between the health maintenance activities and abdominal function.*
Sleep	Nocturnal pain with peptic ulcer disease; hiatal hernia discomfort in recumbent position
Diet	Healthy diet as a means of avoiding problems (fruits, vegetables, fiber, alcohol in moderation, decreased intake of fat, and prepared foods); gallbladder attacks after fatty meals; caffeinated beverages, coffee, tea, and alcohol irritate gastrointestinal tract.
Exercise	Regular exercise facilitates gastrointestinal functioning.
Stress Management	High stress levels are associated with stress ulcers.
Use of Safety Devices	Shoulder and lap restraints in automobiles to prevent abdominal injuries; appropriate sports safety equipment to protect abdominal region
Health Check-Ups	Blood chemistry: Elevated glucose might indicate onset of diabetes mellitus. Blood count: Anemia could reflect silent gastrointestinal bleeds. Urinalysis: Dark color may signify bilirubin in urine. Stool guaiac: Annually after age 40 Colonoscopy: Biannually after age 50

🌹 NURSING TIP

Referred Abdominal Pain

Abdominal pain can be difficult to assess because the location of abdominal pain may not be directly attributive to the area of the causative factors. In referred pain, the sensory cortex perceives pain via nerve fibers where the internal abdominal organs were located in fetal development. Pain originating from the liver, spleen, pancreas, stomach, and duodenum may be referred (refer to Figure 16-8).

Table 16-2	Differentiating Abdominal Pain		
	VISCERAL PAIN	**PARIETAL PAIN**	**REFERRED PAIN**
Origin	Originates in the abdominal organs	Originates in the parietal peritoneum	Originates from abdominal organs to nonabdominal locations or nonabdominal sites, chest, spine, or pelvis; refer path to abdominal region
Cause	Hollow structures become painful when they contract forcefully or when distended, e.g., intestines; solid organs become painful when stretched	Inflammation	Nerve innervation
Characteristics	Poorly localized, usually begins as dull pain, but when it becomes intense, is associated with nausea, vomiting, pallor, and diaphoresis	Precisely localized; usually severe from the onset and intensifies with movement	Well localized; pain is from a disorder in another site. Duodenal pain: back and right shoulder. Pancreatic pain: back and left shoulder

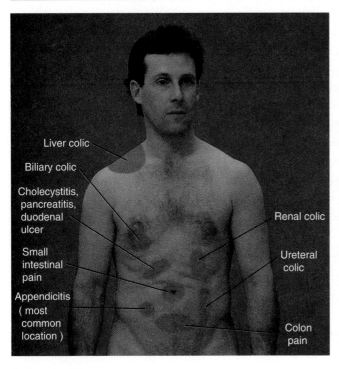

A. Anterior View

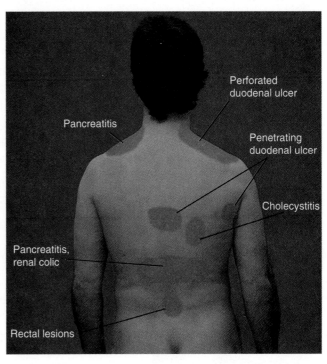

B. Posterior View

Figure 16-8   Areas of Referred Pain

EQUIPMENT

- Drapes for patient
- Small pillows for under knee
- Tape measure or small ruler with centimeter markings
- Marking pencil
- Gooseneck lamp for tangential lighting
- Stethoscope
- Sterile safety pin or sterile needle

ASSESSMENT OF THE ABDOMEN

The order of abdominal assessment is inspection, auscultation, percussion, and palpation. Auscultation is performed second because palpation and percussion can alter bowel sounds.

🌹 NURSING TIP

Abdominal Inspection

1. Position tangential light lengthwise across the patient's abdomen at a right angle.
2. Position yourself on a horizontal plane looking at the patient's abdomen, or slightly higher.

NURSING TIP

7 F's of Abdominal Distension

Seven possible causes of abdominal distension are:
- Fat
- Fluid (ascites)
- Flatus
- Feces
- Fetus
- Fatal growth (malignancy)
- Fibroid tumor

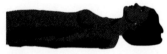

Flat

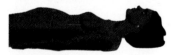

Rounded

Scaphoid

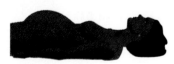

Protuberant

Figure 16-9 Abdominal Configurations

E	**Examination**
N	**Normal Findings**
A	**Abnormal Findings**
P	**Pathophysiology**

NURSING CHECKLIST
General Approach to Abdominal Assessment

1. Greet the patient and explain the assessment technique.
2. Ensure that the room is at a warm, comfortable temperature to prevent patient chilling and shivering.
3. Use a quiet room that will be free from interruptions.
4. Utilize an adequate light source. This includes both a bright overhead light and a freestanding lamp for tangential lighting.
5. Ask the patient to urinate before the exam.
6. Drape the patient from the xiphoid process to the symphysis pubis, then expose the patient's abdomen.
7. Position the patient comfortably in a supine position with knees flexed over a pillow or position the patient so that the arms are either folded across the chest or at the sides to ensure abdominal relaxation.
8. Visualize the underlying abdominal structures during the assessment process in order to accurately describe the location of any pathology.
9. Have the patient point to tender areas; assess these last. Mark these and other significant findings (scars, dullness, etc.) on the body diagram in the patient's chart.
10. Watch the patient's face closely for signs of discomfort or pain.
11. Help the patient relax by using an unhurried approach, diverting attention with questions, etc.
12. Stand to the right side of the patient for the examination.

Inspection

Contour

E View the contour of the patient's abdomen from the costal margin to the symphysis pubis.

N *In the normal adult, the abdominal contour is flat (straight horizontal line from costal margin to symphysis pubis) or rounded (convexity of abdomen from costal margin to symphysis pubis). See Figure 16-9.*

A Assessment reveals a large convex symmetrical profile from the costal margin to the symphysis pubis.

P A large convex abdomen can result from one of the 7 F's.

A A concave symmetrical profile from the costal margin to the symphysis pubis is abnormal.

P A scaphoid abdomen reflects a decrease in fat deposits, a malnourished state, or flaccid muscle tone.

A A convex abdomen that has a marked increase at the height of the umbilicus is abnormal.

P A protuberant abdomen results from a wide range of disorders. Taut stretching of the skin across the abdominal wall may occur. Refer to the Nursing Tip on this page for a discussion of the 7 F's.

Symmetry

E 1. View the symmetry of the patient's abdomen from the costal margin to the symphysis pubis.
   2. Move to the foot of the examination table and recheck the symmetry of the patient's abdomen.

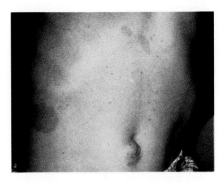

Figure 16-10 von Recklinghausen's Disease *Courtesy of the Armed Forces Institute of Pathology*

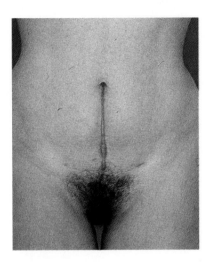

Figure 16-11 Abdominal Scar (Hysterectomy)

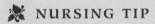

NURSING TIP

Abdominal Scars

The most common scars are from an appendectomy, a hysterectomy, or a cesarean section. Refer to Chapter 10 for characteristics of scars. Always observe a new scar for abnormalities, including bleeding or discharge. Whenever an abdominal scar is located, document the location, size, and condition in a diagram in the patient's chart.

E	**Examination**
N	**Normal Findings**
A	**Abnormal Findings**
P	**Pathophysiology**

N *The abdomen should be symmetrical bilaterally.*
A Assessment reveals an asymmetrical abdomen.
P Asymmetry may be caused by a tumor, cysts, bowel obstruction, enlargement of abdominal organs, or scoliosis. Bulging at the umbilicus can indicate an umbilical hernia.

Rectus Abdominis Muscles

E **1.** Instruct the patient to raise the head and shoulders off the examination table.
    2. Observe the rectus abdominis muscles for separation.
N *The symmetry of the abdomen remains uniform; no ridge is observed parallel to the umbilicus or between the rectus abdominis muscles.*
A A ridge between the rectus abdominis muscles is observed.
P This abnormality is known as diastasis recti abdominis and is attributed to marked obesity or past pregnancy. The observed separation of rectus abdominis muscles is caused by increased intra-abdominal pressure and is not considered to be harmful or ominous.

Pigmentation and Color

E View the color of the patient's abdomen from the costal margin to the symphysis pubis.
N *The abdomen should be uniform in color and pigmentation.*
A Uneven skin color or pigmentation is abnormal.
P The presence of jaundice suggests liver dysfunction. The yellow discoloration of the skin in light-skinned patients is due to the accumulation of bilirubin in the blood. The average level for visible jaundice is 2 mg/dl.
P In light-skinned individuals, the observation of a blue tint at the umbilicus suggests free blood in the peritoneal cavity, known as **Cullen's sign**. Such bleeding can occur either following rupture of a fallopian tube secondary to an ectopic pregnancy or with acute hemorrhagic pancreatitis.
P Irregular patches of tan skin pigmentation (café au lait spots) may be attributed to von Recklinghausen's disease (Figure 16-10), a familial condition associated with the formation of neurofibromas.
A Engorged abdominal veins are abnormal.
P The appearance of engorged or dilated veins around the umbilicus is called **caput medusae**. It is associated with circulatory obstruction of the superior or the inferior vena cava. In some instances, this condition is related to obstruction of the portal vein or to emaciation.

Scars

E Inspect the abdomen for scars from the costal margin to the symphysis pubis.
N *There should be no abdominal scars present.*
A Scars are present (Figure 16-11).
P The site of the scars discloses useful information about the patient's surgical history. Dense, irregular, collagenous scars are keloids, which are more common in dark-skinned individuals and may be associated with traumatic injuries or burns. The presence of surgical scars may indicate internal adhesions.

Striae

E Observe the abdominal skin for **striae**, or abdominal atrophic lines or scars.
N *No evidence of striae is present.*
A Striae are present (refer to Figure 16-12).

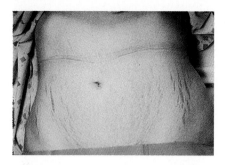

Figure 16-12 Abdominal Striae

⚡ NURSING ALERT

Risk Factors for Hepatitis A

- Overcrowded living quarters
- Poor personal hygiene (poor handwashing, especially after defecation)
- Poor sanitation (sewage disposal)
- Food and water contamination
- Ingestion of shellfish caught in contaminated water

⚡ NURSING ALERT

Risk Factors for Hepatitis B

- IV drug use with shared needles
- Receipt of multiple transfusions of blood and blood products (oncology and hemodialysis patients, hemophiliacs)
- Frequent contact with blood (health care workers such as nurses, doctors, phlebotomists, and laboratory personnel)

E	Examination
N	Normal Findings
A	Abnormal Findings
P	Pathophysiology

P Striae, atrophic lines or streaks, occur when there has been rapid or prolonged stretching of the skin. Abdominal striae, also known as linea albicantes, may be caused by abdominal tumors, obesity, ascites, or pregnancy. Following pregnancy, striae are a normal finding. Refer to Chapter 13 for characteristics of striae.

Respiratory Movement

E Observe the abdomen for smooth, even respiratory movement.

N *There is no evidence of respiratory retractions. Normally, the abdomen rises with inspiration and falls with expiration.*

A Abnormal respiratory movements and retractions are observed.

P The origin of abnormal respirations due to an abdominal disorder may include appendicitis with local peritonitis, pancreatitis, biliary colic, or a perforated ulcer.

Masses or Nodules

E Observe the abdominal skin for nodules or masses.

N *No masses or nodules are present.*

A Abdominal masses or nodules are present.

P The presence of abdominal masses or nodules may indicate tumors, metastases of an internal malignancy, or pregnancy.

Visible Peristalsis

E Observe the abdominal wall for surface motion.

N *Ripples of peristalsis may be observed in thin patients. Peristalsis movement slowly traverses the abdomen in a slanting downward direction.*

A Strong peristaltic contractions are observed.

P Peristaltic waves may indicate intestinal obstruction.

Pulsation

E Inspect the epigastric area for pulsations.

N *In the patient with a normal build, a nonexaggerated pulsation of the abdominal aorta may be visible in the epigastric area. In heavier patients, pulsation may not be visible.*

A Marked, strong abdominal pulsations are observed.

P Widened pulse pressure and strong epigastric pulsations may indicate an aortic aneurysm. An exaggerated pulsation can also occur in aortic regurgitation and in right ventricular hypertrophy.

Umbilicus

E Observe the umbilicus in relation to the abdominal surface.

N *The umbilicus is depressed and beneath the abdominal surface.*

A The umbilicus protrudes above the abdominal surface.

P Umbilical hernia in the adult is the protrusion of part of the intestine through an incomplete umbilical ring. Umbilical hernia is confirmed by inserting the index finger into the navel and feeling an opening in the fascia.

P The umbilicus that appears as a nodule may be the manifestation of abdominal carcinoma with metastasis to the umbilicus. This physical finding is known as Sister Mary Joseph's nodule.

P Intra-abdominal pressure from ascites, masses, or pregnancy can cause the umbilicus to protrude.

NURSING CHECKLIST

Assessing Patients with Abdominal Tubes and Drains

For all tubes, drains, and intestinal and urinary diversions, note color, odor, amount, consistency, and the presence of blood in any drainage. Check for an obstruction if there is no drainage. The skin around the device should be intact without excoriation.

Tubes

1. Enteral Tubes
   - Nasogastric, nasoduodenal, or nasojejunal.
   - Check the residual amount on a frequent basis. If greater than 100 cc, stop the feeding; restart the feeding based on further inspection of residual amounts.

2. Nasogastric Suction Tubes
   - Levin or Salem sump.
   - Ensure that the suction setting (intermittent or continuous) is set at the appropriate suction level.

3. Intestinal Tubes
   - Miller-Abbott, Cantor, Johnston, or Baker.
   - Ensure that tube is advancing with peristalsis as expected.
   - Ensure that the suction setting is at the appropriate suction level.

4. Gastrostomy
   - Continuous versus intermittent feeding.
   - With intermittent feedings, clamp is applied when not in use.
   - Tube should be secured to abdomen.
   - Check that dressing is applied.

Drains

1. Abdominal Cavity Drain (Jackson-Pratt, Hemovac)
   - To self-suction or wall suction; if wall suction, ensure that it is set at appropriate level.

2. Biliary Drain (T-Tube)
   - Tube is below insertion site.

Intestinal Diversions

1. Colostomy
   - Stoma is pink.
   - Skin barrier should be used around stoma if appliance is worn.
   - Evacuation method: natural or irrigation.

2. Ileostomy
   - Stoma is pink.
   - Skin barrier is used and appliance is worn.
   - If patient has Kock pouch, nipple valve is pink; frequency of drainage.

Urinary Diversions

1. Ileal Conduit
   - Stoma is pink.
   - Skin barrier is used with appliance.

2. Ureteral Stents
   - Stent is secured to collection bag.
   - No bleeding from insertion site.

3. Indwelling Catheter
   - Balloon inflated.
   - Catheter secured to patient to prevent dislodgement.
   - Urinary collecting bag is closed.
   - Drainage tube is below level of bladder and without kinks.

NURSING TIP

Nasogastric Tube Suction

Prior to assessing the abdomen, if the patient has a nasogastric tube, discontinue any suction in order to avoid interfering with auscultation findings. Remember to turn the suction on after your assessment.

NURSING TIP

Abdominal Auscultation

- Ensure that your hands and the stethoscope are warm to promote patient comfort.
- Use the diaphragm of the stethoscope to auscultate bowel sounds because they are high pitched.

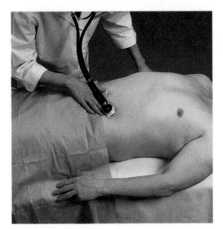

Figure 16-13 Technique of Abdominal Auscultation

◎ THINK ABOUT IT

Bowel Sounds

You auscultate Ms. Enriquez's bowel sounds and do not hear any after listening for 30 seconds in the RLQ. You are aware that you should auscultate the abdomen for 5 minutes in each quadrant if necessary. How would you proceed? What assessment findings would you document?

⚠ NURSING ALERT

Palpation Contraindication

Never palpate over areas where bruits are auscultated. Palpation may cause rupture. Refer the patient to a physician immediately.

E	**Examination**
N	**Normal Findings**
A	**Abnormal Findings**
P	**Pathophysiology**

Auscultation

Bowel Sounds

E 1. Place the diaphragm lightly on the abdominal wall beginning at the RLQ.
2. Listen to the frequency and character of the bowel sounds. It is necessary to listen for at least 5 minutes in an abdominal quadrant before concluding that bowel sounds are absent.
3. Move diaphragm to RUQ, LUQ, LLQ (see Figure 16-13).

N *Bowel sounds are heard as intermittent gurgling sounds throughout the abdominal quadrants. Usually, they are high-pitched sounds and occur 5 to 30 times per minute. Bowel sounds result from the movement of air and fluid through the gastrointestinal tract. Normally, bowel sounds are always present at the ileocecal valve area (RLQ).*

*Normal hyperactive bowel sounds are called **borborygmi**. They are loud, audible, gurgling sounds. Borborygmi may be due to hyperperistalsis ("stomach growling") or the sound of flatus in the intestines.*

A Absent bowel sounds are abnormal.

P Absent bowel sounds are indicative of late intestinal obstruction, both mechanical and nonmechanical in nature. Mechanical obstruction of the bowel may result from extraluminal lesions such as adhesions, hernias, and masses. In nonmechanical obstruction, the gastrointestinal lumen remains unobstructed, but the muscles of the intestinal wall cannot move its contents. This type of obstruction can be caused by physiological, neurogenic, or chemical imbalances that result in paralytic ileus.

A Hypoactive bowel sounds are abnormal.

P Hypoactive or diminished bowel sounds indicate decreased motility of the bowel and can occur with peritonitis and nonmechanical obstruction. Other causes include inflammation, gangrene, electrolyte imbalances, and intraoperative manipulation of the bowel.

A Hyperactive bowel sounds are abnormal.

P Hyperactive or increased bowel sounds signify increased motility of the bowel and can result from gastroenteritis, diarrhea, laxative use, and subsiding ileus.

P Auscultation of high-pitched tinkling hyperactive bowel sounds is indicative of partial obstruction. These sounds are caused by the powerful peristaltic action of the bowel segment attempting to eject its contents through a narrow, constricted area. Frequently, patients complain of abdominal cramping.

Vascular Sounds

E 1. Place the bell of the stethoscope over the abdominal aorta, renal arteries, iliac arteries, and femoral arteries (see Figure 16-14).
2. Listen for bruits over each area (see Figure 16-15).

N *No audible bruits are auscultated.*

A Audible bruits are auscultated.

P A bruit over an abdominal vessel indicates turbulence of blood flow and suggests a partial obstruction. Bruits can occur with abdominal aortic aneurysm, renal stenosis, and femoral stenosis.

Venous Hum

E Using the bell of the stethoscope, listen for a **venous hum**, or a continuous, medium-pitched sound, in all four quadrants.

N *Venous hums are normally not present in adults.*

A A continuous pulsing or fibrillary sound is auscultated.

P A venous hum in the periumbilical area is usually due to obstructed portal circulation. Portal hypertension caused by cirrhosis of the liver impedes portal circulation.

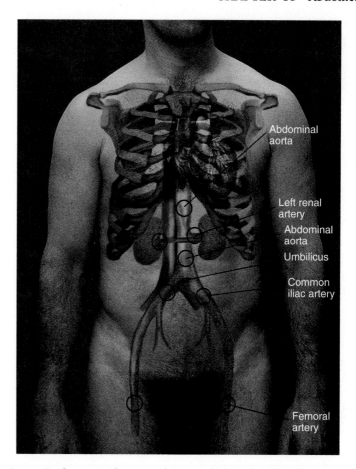

Figure 16-14 Stethoscope Placement for Auscultating Abdominal Vasculature

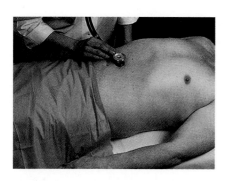

Figure 16-15 Auscultation for Aortic Bruits with Bell of Stethoscope

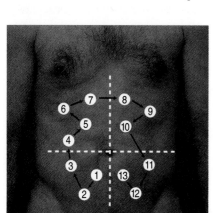

Figure 16-16 Direction of Pattern of Abdominal Percussion

Friction Rubs

E **1.** Using the diaphragm of the stethoscope, listen for friction rubs over the right and left costal margins, the liver, and the spleen.
  2. Listen for friction rubs in all four quadrants.
N *No friction rubs should be present.*
A Friction rubs are high-pitched sounds that resemble the sound produced by two pieces of sandpaper being rubbed together. The sound increases with inspiration.
P Friction rubs occur when tumors, inflammation, or infarct cause the visceral layers of the peritoneum to rub together over the liver and the spleen.

Percussion

General Percussion

E **1.** Percuss all four quadrants in a systematic manner. Begin percussion in the RLQ, moving upward to the RUQ, crossing over to the LUQ, and moving down to the LLQ (see Figure 16-16).
  2. Visualize each organ in the corresponding quadrant; note when tympany changes to dullness.
N *Tympany is the predominant sound heard because air is present in the stomach and in the intestines. It is a high-pitched sound of long duration. Dullness is normally heard over organs such as the liver or a distended bladder. Dull sounds are high-pitched and of moderate duration.*
A Dullness over areas where tympany normally occurs, such as over the stomach and intestines, is considered abnormal.
P Dullness may be caused by a mass or tumor, pregnancy, ascites, or a full intestine.

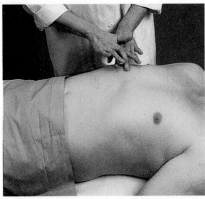

A. Determining Lower Liver Border

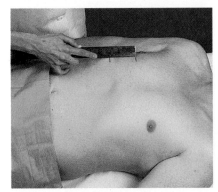

B. Measuring Liver Span

Figure 16-17 Percussing Liver Span

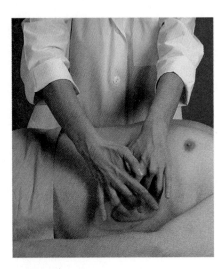

Figure 16-18 Percussion of the Spleen

E	**Examination**
N	**Normal Findings**
A	**Abnormal Findings**
P	**Pathophysiology**

Liver Span

E 1. Stand to the right side of the patient.
2. Begin at the right midclavicular line below the umbilicus and percuss upward to determine the lower border of the liver (refer to Figure 16-17A).
3. With a marking pen, mark where the sound changes from tympany to dullness.
4. Then, at the right midclavicular line, percuss downward from an area of lung resonance to one of dullness.
5. With a tape measure or ruler, measure the two marks in centimeters (see Figure 16-17B).

N *Normally, the distance between the two marks is 6 to 12 cm. There is a direct correlation between body size and the size of the liver. The mean span for a man is 10.5 cm.and for a woman it is 7.0 cm.*

A A liver span greater than 12 cm or less than 6 cm is considered abnormal.

P The liver span is increased when the liver becomes enlarged. Hepatomegaly can occur with various liver diseases such as hepatitis, cirrhosis, cardiac or renal congestion, cysts, or metastatic tumors.

P The liver span can be falsely increased when the upper border is obscured by the dullness of lung consolidation or pleural effusion.

P The liver span can be decreased in the later stages of cirrhosis when the disease causes liver atrophy.

P The liver span can be falsely decreased when gas in the colon, tumors, or pregnancy push the lower border of the liver upward.

Liver Descent

E 1. Percuss the liver descent by asking the patient to take a deep breath and to hold it (because on inspiration, the diaphragm moves downward).
2. Again, percuss the lower border of the liver at the right midclavicular line by percussing from tympany to dullness. Have the patient exhale.
3. Repercuss the liver-lung border.
4. Mark where the change in sound takes place.
5. Measure the difference in centimeters between the two lower borders of the liver.

N *Normally, the area of lower border dullness descends 2 to 3 cm.*

A The liver descent is considered abnormal if it is greater or less than 2 to 3 cm.

P The liver descent is greater than 2 to 3 cm due to hepatomegaly, as in cirrhosis.

P The liver descent is less than 2 cm due to abdominal tumors, pregnancy, or ascites.

Spleen

E 1. Percuss the lower level of the left lung slightly posterior to the midaxillary line and continue downward (see Figure 16-18).
2. Percuss downward until dullness is ascertained. In some individuals, the spleen is positioned too deeply to be discernable by percussion.

N *Normally, the upper border of dullness is found 6 to 8 cm above the left costal margin. Splenic dullness may be heard from the 6th to the 10th rib.*

A Dullness beyond the 8 cm line is indicative of splenic enlargement. However, a full stomach or a feces-filled intestine may mimic the dullness

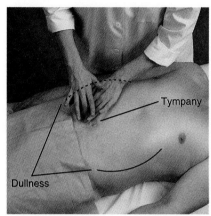

A. Patient Supine

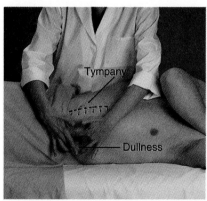

B. Patient on Left Side

Figure 16-19 Percussion for Ascites: Shifting Dullness

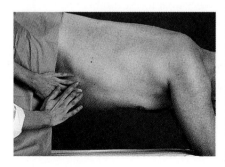

Figure 16-20 Percussion for Ascites: Puddle Sign

of splenic enlargement. Moreover, gastric or colonic air may obscure the dullness of the spleen.

P Splenic enlargement can be due to portal hypertension resulting from liver disease; other potential causes are thrombosis, stenosis, atresia, angiomatous deformities of the portal or splenic vein, cysts, or aneurysm of the splenic artery.

Stomach

E Percuss for a gastric air bubble in the LUQ at the left lower anterior rib cage and left epigastric region.

N *The tympany of the gastric air bubble is lower in pitch than the tympany of the intestine.*

A An increase in size of the gastric air bubble is abnormal.

P This increase in size accompanied by gastric distension can suggest gastric dilation.

✵ SPECIAL TECHNIQUE

Percussion for Ascites

Assess the patient for **ascites**, or excess accumulation of fluid in the abdominal cavity. There are two methods for this assessment: **shifting dullness** and **puddle sign**.

Shifting Dullness

E 1. Standing to the right, with the patient supine, percuss over the top of the abdomen, beginning at the midline.
  2. Percuss outward toward the right side of the patient, following a downward direction (see Figure 16-19A).
  3. Mark on the abdomen where percussion changes from tympany to dullness because this change is indicative of settled fluid in the flanks of the abdominal cavity.
  4. Turn the patient onto the right side.
  5. Repercuss the upper side of the abdomen, moving downward.
  6. If the percussion sound changes from tympany to dullness above the prior-marked fluid line, this shifting dullness is positive for ascites.
  7. Repeat the same assessment technique on the left side of the patient. Change the patient's position from the right to the left side (refer to Figure 16-19B).
  8. Mark where the percussion changes from tympany to dullness.

N *There should be no change from tympany to dullness.*

A There is a marked change from tympany to dullness as you percuss outward and downward. Ascites is present in the abdominal cavity.

P Ascitic fluid sinks with gravity, which accounts for the dullness in dependent areas. Ascites is found in cirrhosis and in other liver diseases.

Puddle Sign

E 1. Ask the patient to kneel and assume the knee-chest position for several minutes.
  2. Percuss the umbilical area (see Figure 16-20).

N *The umbilical area should remain tympanic.*

A The umbilical area percusses dull.

P The ascitic fluid pools in the dependent area of the umbilicus because of gravity.

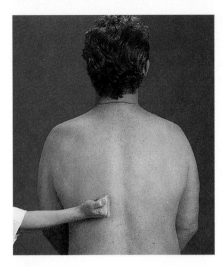

Figure 16-21A Direct Fist Percussion of Left Kidney

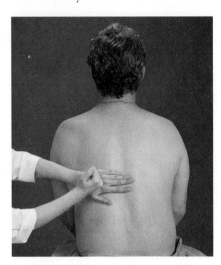

Figure 16-21B Indirect Fist Percussion of Left Kidney

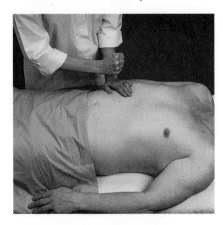

Figure 16-22 Indirect Fist Percussion of Liver

E	**Examination**
N	**Normal Findings**
A	**Abnormal Findings**
P	**Pathophysiology**

> ### ⚡ NURSING ALERT
>
> **Risk Factors for Ascites**
>
> - Increased vascular resistance to hepatic outflow
> - Increased hepatic lymph flow and extravasation of fluid into the peritoneal cavity
> - Portal hypertension and increased capillary filtration pressure
> - Hypoalbuminemia and decreased colloid osmotic pressure of the serum
> - Disordered kidney function
> - Hyperaldosteronism
> - Excessive secretion of antidiuretic hormone

Fist Percussion

Fist percussion is done over the kidneys and liver to check for tenderness.

Kidney

E 1. Place the patient in a sitting position.
   2. Strike the costovertebral angle with a closed fist (direct fist percussion, see Figure 16-21A) or
   2A. Place the palmar surface of one hand over the costovertebral angle. Strike that hand with the ulnar surface of the fist of the other hand (indirect fist percussion, see Figure 16-21B).
   3. Ask the patient what was felt. Observe the patient's reaction.
   4. Repeat on the other side.

Liver

E 1. Place the patient in a supine position.
   2. Place the palmar surface of one hand over the lower right rib cage (where the liver was percussed).
   3. Strike that hand with the ulnar surface of the fist of the other hand (see Figure 16-22).
   4. Ask the patient what was felt. Observe the patient's reaction.

N *No tenderness should be elicited by either maneuver.*

A Tenderness or pain that can be elicited over the costovertebral angle or over the liver is abnormal.

P Costovertebral angle tenderness can occur in conjunction with pyelonephritis. Liver tenderness can occur in conjunction with cholecystitis or hepatitis.

Bladder

E 1. Percuss upward from the symphysis pubis to the umbilicus.
   2. Note where the sound changes from dullness to tympany.

N *A urine-filled bladder is dull to percussion. A recently emptied bladder should not be percussable above the symphysis pubis.*

A It is abnormal to percuss a bladder that has recently been emptied. The urine that remains in the bladder after urination is called residual urine. A bladder may also be dull to percussion when the patient has difficulty voiding.

P The inability to completely empty the bladder occurs in the elderly, in postoperative, bedridden, and acutely ill patients, and in patients with neurogenic bladder dysfunction.

P Difficult voiding can occur in conjunction with benign prostatic hypertrophy (see Chapter 21 for additional information), urethral pathology, and some medications (antipsychotics: phenothiazine; anticholinergics: atropine; antihypertensives: hydralazine).

Palpation

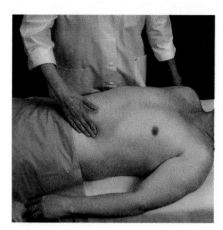

Figure 16-23 Light Palpation of Abdomen

Light Palpation

E 1. With your hands and forearm on a horizontal plane, use the pads of the approximated fingers to depress the abdominal wall 1 cm (see Figure 16-23).
   2. Avoid short, quick jabs.
   3. Lightly palpate all four quadrants in a systematic manner.

N *The abdomen should feel smooth with consistent softness.*

A Light palpation reveals changes in skin temperature, tenderness, or large masses.

P Tenderness and elevated skin temperature can be due to inflammation. Large masses can be due to tumors, feces, or enlarged organs.

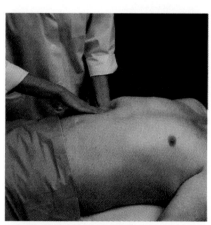

A. One-Handed Method

Abdominal Muscle Guarding

To determine whether muscle guarding is involuntary:

E 1. Perform light palpation of the rectus muscles during expiration.
   2. Note muscle tensing.

N *Muscle guarding, or tensing of the abdominal musculature, is absent during expiration. The abdomen is soft. Normally, during expiration the patient cannot exercise voluntary muscle tensing.*

A Muscle guarding of the rectus muscles occurs during expiration.

P Involuntary muscle guarding suggests irritation of the peritoneum, as in peritonitis.

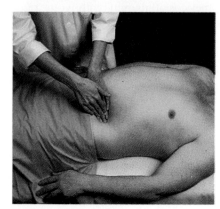

B. Bimanual Method

Figure 16-24 Deep Palpation

Deep Palpation

In performing deep palpation of all four quadrants, you can use either a one-handed or a two-handed method.

E 1. With the one-handed method, use the palmar surface of the extended fingers to depress the skin approximately 2 to 3 inches in the RLQ (see Figure 16-24A).
   2. A two-handed approach is used when palpation is difficult because of obesity or muscular resistance. With the bimanual technique, the nondominant hand is placed on top of the dominant hand. The bottom hand is used for sensation, and the top hand is used to apply pressure (see Figure 16-24B).
   3. Identify any masses and note location, size, shape, consistency, tenderness, pulsation, and degree of mobility.
   4. Continue palpation of RUQ, LUQ, and LLQ.

🌺 NURSING TIP

Ascites

It is often helpful to monitor the amount of ascites by measuring the patient's abdomen at its largest diameter. In order for there to be consistency among nurses, it is advised that marks be drawn on the patient's abdomen showing placement of the tape measure.

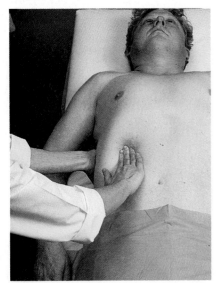

Figure 16-25   Palpation for Ascites: Fluid Wave

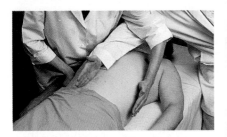

A. Bimanual Method

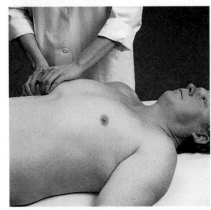

B. Hook Method

Figure 16-26   Palpation of the Liver

N   *No organ enlargement should be palpable nor should there be any abnormal masses, bulges, or swelling. Normally, only the aorta and the edge of the liver are palpable. When the large colon or the bladder is full, palpation is possible but is atypical.*

A   The gallbladder, liver, spleen, fecal-filled colon, or flatus-filled cecum should not be palpable. Masses, bulges, and swellings are also considered abnormal.

P   Organomegaly can be caused by many pathological states such as cholecystitis, hepatitis, or cirrhosis; masses, bulges, or swelling can be due to tumors, fluids, feces, flatus, or fat.

✺ SPECIAL TECHNIQUE

Fluid Wave

E   **1.** With the patient in a supine position, stand at the patient's right side.
   2. Have the patient or a second nurse firmly place the ulnar side of the right hand midline on the abdomen to prevent displacement of fat.
   3. Place your right hand on the patient's right hip or flank area. Reach across the patient with your left hand and deliver a blow to the patient's left hip or flank area (refer to Figure 16-25).
   4. Assess if a fluid wave is felt on the right hand of the patient or the other nurse.

N   *No fluid wave should be felt.*

A   A fluid wave is easily felt if a large amount of ascites is present. This sign is often negative until the ascites is obvious. In addition, the fluid wave is sometimes positive in people without ascites.

P   The factors that contribute to the development of ascites are outlined on page 476.

Liver

Liver palpation can be performed by one of two methods: the bimanual method or the hook method.

Bimanual Method

E   **1.** Stand at the patient's right side, facing the patient's head.
   2. Place the left hand under the patient's right flank at about the 11th or 12th rib.
   3. Press upward with the left hand to elevate the liver toward the abdominal wall.
   4. Place the right hand parallel to the midline at the right midclavicular line below the right costal margin or below the level of liver dullness.
   5. Instruct the patient to take a deep breath.
   6. Push down deeply and under the costal margin with your right fingers. On inspiration, the liver will descend and contact the hand (see Figure 16-26A)
   7. Note the level of the liver.
   8. Note the size, shape, consistency, and any masses.

Hook Method

E   **1.** Stand at the patient's right side, facing the patient's feet.
   2. Place both hands side by side on the right costal margin below the border of liver dullness.
   3. Hook the fingers in and up toward the costal margin and ask the patient to take a deep breath and hold it.
   4. Palpate the liver's edge as it descends (see Figure 16-26B).
   5. Note the level of the liver.
   6. Note the size, shape, consistency, and any masses.

NURSING ALERT

Risk Factors for Liver Cancer

- Cirrhosis
- Hepatitis B
- Cigarette smoking
- Alcohol use
- Exposure to toxic substances such as arsenic or vinyl chloride
- Primary malignancy

N *A normal liver edge presents as a firm, sharp, regular ridge with a smooth surface. Normally, the liver is not palpable, although it may be felt in extremely thin adults.*

A If the liver is palpable below the costal margin both medially and laterally, it is abnormal.

P An enlarged liver can be due to congestive heart failure, hepatitis, encephalopathy, cirrhosis, cysts, or cancer.

A A liver that is enlarged and has an irregular border and nodules and is hard is abnormal.

P These findings suggest liver malignancy. Tenderness may or may not be present.

NURSING ALERT

Liver Encephalopathy

Early recognition of signs and symptoms of liver encephalopathy may minimize complications.
- Slowed mentation or mental confusion
- Asterixis (liver flap)
- Uncoordinated muscle movements
- Elevated values for serum BUN, ammonia, liver enzymes, and osmolarity. Increased values reflect systemic effects of liver dysfunction. Monitor glucose and electrolytes to maintain electrolyte balance.

✸ SPECIAL TECHNIQUE

Murphy's Sign

E 1. With the patient supine, stand at the patient's right side.
2. Palpate below the liver margin at the lateral border of the rectus muscle.
3. Have the patient take a deep breath.

N *No pain is elicited.*

A Pain is present with palpation. The patient may stop inhaling to guard against the pain. This is known as **Murphy's sign**.

P Murphy's sign is positive in inflammatory processes of the gallbladder, such as cholecystitis.

NURSING ALERT

Risk for Spleen Rupture

Palpate the spleen gently because an enlarged spleen will be very tender and may rupture.

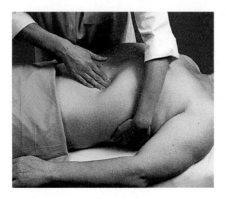

Figure 16-27 Palpation of the Spleen

E	Examination
N	Normal Findings
A	Abnormal Findings
P	Pathophysiology

Spleen

Use the bimanual technique to palpate the spleen.

E 1. Stand at the patient's right side.
2. Reach across and place the left hand beneath the patient and over the left costovertebral angle. Press upward to lift the spleen anteriorly toward the abdominal wall.
3. With the right hand, press inward along the left costal margin while asking the patient to take a deep breath (see Figure 16-27).
3A. The procedure can be repeated with the patient lying on the right side, with the hips and knees flexed. This position will facilitate the spleen coming forward and to the right because the spleen is located retroperitoneally.
4. Note the size, shape, consistency, and any masses.

N *The spleen should not be palpable.*

A Because of its retroperitoneal position in the body, the spleen becomes palpable only when it has become enlarged to three times its normal size. An enlarged spleen is usually very tender.

P Splenomegaly can be due to inflammation, congestive heart failure, cancer, cirrhosis, or mononucleosis.

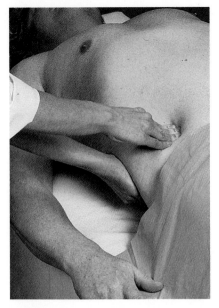

Figure 16-28 Palpation of the Right Kidney

> **⚡ NURSING ALERT**
>
> **Risk for Aortic Rupture**
>
> Do not palpate an aorta that you suspect has an aneurysm. Notify the patient's physician immediately if you suspect an abdominal aortic aneurysm because it may dissect and cause renal failure, loss of limbs, and, eventually, death if left untreated.

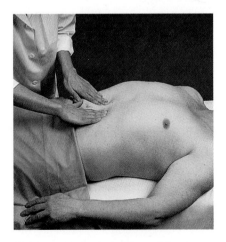

Figure 16-29 Palpation of the Aorta

E	**Examination**
N	**Normal Findings**
A	**Abnormal Findings**
P	**Pathophysiology**

Kidneys

E 1. Stand at the patient's right side.
2. Place one hand on the right costovertebral angle on the patient's back.
3. Place the palpating hand below and parallel to the costal margin.
4. As the patient takes a deep breath, press hands firmly together and try to feel the lower pole of the kidney (see Figure 16-28).
5. At the peak of inspiration, press the fingers together with greater pressure from above than from below.
6. Ask the patient to exhale and to hold the breath briefly.
7. Release the pressure of your fingers.
8. If the kidney has been "captured," it can be felt as it slips back into place.
9. Note the size, shape, and consistency. Note any masses.
10. For the left kidney, reach across the patient and place the left hand under the patient's left flank.
11. Apply downward pressure with the right hand below the left costal margin and repeat steps 4 through 9.

N *The kidneys should not be palpable in the normal adult. However, the lower pole of the right kidney may be felt in very thin individuals. Kidneys are more readily palpable in the elderly due to loss of muscle tone and muscle bulk.*

A Enlarged kidneys are abnormal. The right kidney may be difficult to distinguish from an enlarged liver. Left kidney enlargement may be difficult to distinguish from an enlarged spleen.

P Enlarged, palpable kidneys can be caused by hydronephrosis, neoplasms, or polycystic disease.

> **🌹 NURSING TIP**
>
> **Kidney Palpation**
>
> The distinguishing features between an enlarged liver and an enlarged kidney include:
> 1. The edge of the liver tends to be sharper and to extend medially and laterally, whereas the pole of the kidney is more rounded.
> 2. In addition, the edge of the liver cannot be "captured," whereas an enlarged kidney can be.
>
> Distinguishing features between an enlarged left kidney and an enlarged spleen include:
> 1. A palpable notch on the medial edge of the organ favors the spleen.
> 2. Percussion of the spleen produces dullness because the bowel is displaced downward; however, resonance is heard over the left kidney because of the intervening bowel.

Aorta

E 1. Press the upper abdomen with one hand on each side of the abdominal aorta, slightly to the left of the midline.
2. Assess the width of the aorta (refer to Figure 16-29).

N *The aorta width is 2.5 to 4.0 cm, and the aorta pulsates in an anterior direction.*

A Aorta width greater than 4.0 cm is abnormal. Lateral pulsation of the aorta is also abnormal.

P A widened aorta and lateral pulsations suggest an abdominal aortic aneurysm.

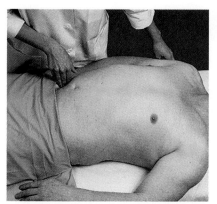

A. Apply Firm Pressure to the Abdomen

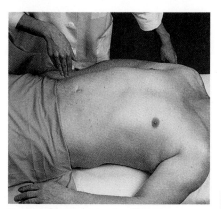

B. Quickly Release the Pressure

Figure 16-30   Rebound Tenderness

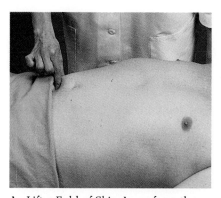

A. Lift a Fold of Skin Away from the Underlying Muscle

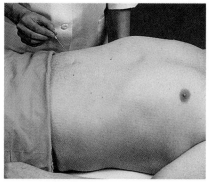

B. Stimulate the Skin with a Sterile Needle

Figure 16-31   Assessment of Cutaneous Hypersensitivity

✼ SPECIAL TECHNIQUE

Rebound Tenderness

Rebound tenderness is assessed if pain has been elicited during palpation, or the patient has reported pain. Rebound tenderness is an abnormal finding frequently associated with peritoneal inflammation or appendicitis. Be prepared to recognize that rebound tenderness assessment could elicit a strong pain response from the patient. It is imperative to test for rebound tenderness away from the site where pain is initially determined and to conclude abdominal assessment with this test. If other tests are positive, omit this assessment.

E   1. Apply several seconds of firm pressure to the abdomen, with the hand at a 90° angle (perpendicular to the abdomen) and the fingers extended (see Figure 16-30A).
     2. Quickly release the pressure (see Figure 16-30B).

N   *Pain is not elicited.*

A   As the abdominal wall returns to its normal position, the patient complains of pain at the pressure site (direct rebound tenderness) or at another site (referred rebound tenderness).

P   Rebound tenderness may indicate peritoneal irritation. The rebound effect of the internal structures indented by this technique causes sharp pain in the area of inflammation.

P   Pain in the RLQ can indicate appendicitis. This location is known as **McBurney's point**.

✼ SPECIAL TECHNIQUE

Rovsing's Sign

Rovsing's sign is a differential technique to elicit referred pain, reflective of peritoneal inflammation secondary to appendicitis.

E   1. Press deeply and evenly in the LLQ for 5 seconds.
     2. Note the patient's response.

N   *No pain should be elicited.*

A   Abdominal pain felt in the RLQ is abnormal and is a positive Rovsing's sign.

P   This sign is based on the concept that changes in intraluminal pressure will be transmitted through the intestine when the ileocecal valve is competent. Pressing the LLQ traps air within the large intestine and increases the pressure in the cecum. When the appendix is inflamed, this increase in pressure causes pain.

✼ SPECIAL TECHNIQUE

Cutaneous Hypersensitivity

On stimulation with a sterile pin or by lifting a fold of skin away from the musculature, **cutaneous hypersensitivity** zones of sensory nerves initiate a painful response. The irritative stimulus detects specific zones of peritoneal irritation.

E   1. Lift a fold of skin away from the underlying muscle (refer to Figure 16-31A) or stimulate the skin by gently jabbing the abdominal surface with a sterile pin (refer to Figure 16-31B).
     2. Observe for pain response.

N   *No adverse reaction should be noted.*

A   The patient experiences an exaggerated sense of pain.

P   Cutaneous hypersensitivity indicates a zone of peritoneal irritation. Localized pain in all or part of the RLQ may accompany appendicitis. Midepigastrium pain could signal a peptic ulcer.

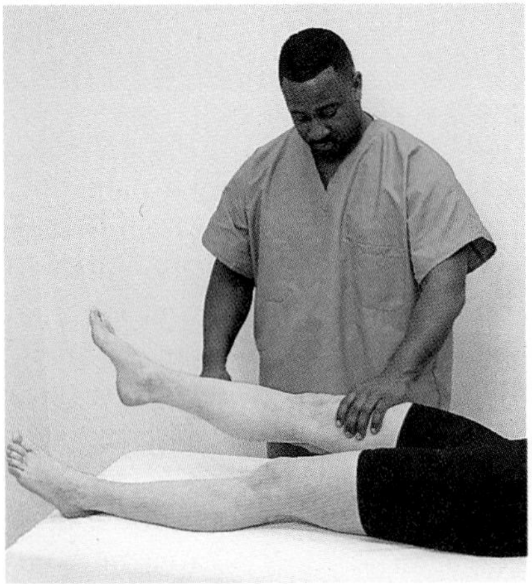

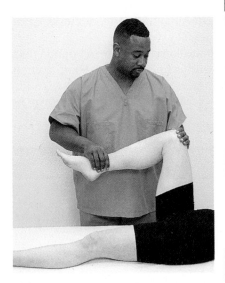

Figure 16-32   Iliopsoas Muscle Test

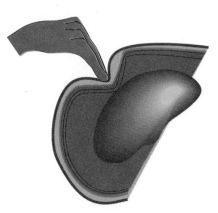

Figure 16-33   Obturator Muscle Test

![Abdominal Ballottement illustration]

Figure 16-34   Abdominal Ballottement

E	Examination
N	Normal Findings
A	Abnormal Findings
P	Pathophysiology

✸ SPECIAL TECHNIQUE

Iliopsoas Muscle Test

When a patient presents with acute abdominal pain, an inflamed or perforated appendix may be distinguished via irritation of the lateral iliopsoas muscle.

E   1. Place your hand over the right thigh and push downward as the patient raises the leg, flexing at the hip (see Figure 16-32).
   2. Observe for pain response in the RLQ as described by the patient.

N   *Normally, the patient should experience no pain.*

A   The patient experiences pain in the RLQ.

P   This pain indicates an inflammation of the iliopsoas muscle in the groin and is caused by an inflamed appendix.

✸ SPECIAL TECHNIQUE

Obturator Muscle Test

Another differential technique used to help determine if the patient is experiencing appendicitis is eliciting the **obturator sign**. This test can be used when pelvic abscess is suspected. Both conditions may cause irritation of the obturator internus muscle.

E   1. Flex the right leg at the hip and knee at a right angle.
   2. Rotate the leg both internally and externally (see Figure 16-33).
   3. Observe for pain response.

N   *No pain is elicited with this maneuver.*

A   Pain is elicited in the hypogastric area.

P   This pain indicates irritation of the obturator muscle and can be caused by a ruptured appendix or pelvic abscess.

✸ SPECIAL TECHNIQUE

Ballottement

Ballottement is a palpation technique used to displace excess fluid in the abdominal cavity in order to locate an organ or mass.

E   1. Extend the fingers of the right hand in a straight line, perpendicular to the abdominal surface.
   2. Stiffen the fingers.
   3. Jab the abdominal surface in the desired area (see Figure 16-34).
   4. Determine if the intended organ is felt at the fingertips.

N   *Excluding during pregnancy, internal organs are not felt during this assessment technique.*

A   Internal masses, or organs such as the liver or spleen, are palpated.

P   The presence of ascites transmits external pressure to an internal organ or mass. The resulting impact felt on palpation is known as ballottement. It determines the presence of a free-floating abdominal mass, which can indicate a cancerous process in the abdominal cavity. Pain should not be elicited. A painful response would indicate inflammation and require further investigation.

Bladder

E   1. Using deep palpation, palpate the abdomen at the midline, starting at the symphysis pubis and progressing upward to the umbilicus (see Figure 16-35).
   2. If the bladder is located, palpate the shape, size, and consistency.

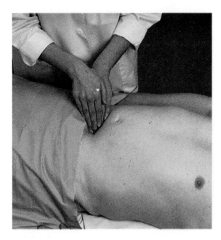

Figure 16-35 Palpation of the Bladder

N *An empty bladder is not usually palpable. A moderately full bladder is smooth and round, and it is palpable above the symphysis pubis. A full bladder is palpated above the symphysis pubis, and it may be close to the umbilicus.*

A A bladder that is nodular or asymmetrical to palpation is abnormal.

P A nodular bladder may indicate a malignancy. An asymmetrical bladder may result from a tumor in the bladder or an abdominal tumor that is compressing the bladder.

A It is abnormal to palpate a bladder that has been recently emptied.

P Refer to page 478 for additional information.

Inguinal Lymph Nodes

E 1. Place the patient in a supine position, with the knees slightly flexed.
2. Drape the genital area.
3. Using the finger pads of the second, third, and fourth fingers, apply firm pressure and palpate with a rotary motion in the right inguinal area.
4. Palpate for lymph nodes in the left inguinal area.

N *It is normal to palpate small, movable nodes less than 1 cm in diameter. Palpable nodes are nontender.*

A Presence of inguinal lymph nodes greater than 1 cm in diameter or elicitation of nonmovable, tender lymph nodes is abnormal.

P Large, palpable nodes can be attributed to localized or systemic infections. More serious pathology includes processes associated with cancer or lymphomas.

GERONTOLOGICAL VARIATIONS

In the process of aging, the abdominal musculature diminishes in mass and loses much of its tone. The mucosal lining of the gastrointestinal tract becomes less elastic, and changes in gastric motility result in alterations in digestion and absorption. Gastric acid secretion decreases and pepsin secretion is thought to diminish.

Gastrointestinal complaints such as gas or epigastric discomfort constitute many of the reasons for the elderly to seek care. Although many of these complaints may be functional in nature, other cues should be investigated. Prolonged gastric irritation from gastric acid or excessive use of medications such as aspirin may cause occult bleeding that goes undetected until profound anemia occurs.

With an increase in age comes an increase in the incidence of malignant disease. Constipation is a frequent digestive complaint of the elderly. Changes in bowel habits may be benign manifestations of diet, medications, a loss of sphincter tone, or lack of exercise. However, in the elderly, these symptoms could signify the presence of gastric or colonic malignancies. As the intestinal wall weakens, diverticuli (outpouching) can develop and sometimes progress to inflammation and obstruction. Chronic ulcerative colitis and Crohn's disease, usually thought of as occurring in a younger population, occur with equal incidence after the age of 50.

There is little evidence that the liver function changes significantly with age. However, weight, blood flow, and regenerative capacity decrease progressively with age. The decrease in liver mass and blood flow alters the pharmacokinetic effects of various drugs.

Persistent jaundice in the elderly is generally thought to be due to malignant obstruction of the biliary system. Multiple-drug therapy (such as Aldomet and isoniazid) may cause hepatitis-like reactions that mimic viral hepatitis. Cholelithiasis, which occurs in one-third of the population between the ages of 70 and 80, is also a frequent cause of jaundice.

❧ NURSING TIP

Avoiding Gastrointestinal Distress

Advise older patients with frequent gastrointestinal distress to:
- Eat six small meals a day.
- Avoid spices, alcohol, caffeine, and citric acid juices.
- Avoid aspirin and ibuprofen.

E	Examination
N	Normal Findings
A	Abnormal Findings
P	Pathophysiology

The small and large intestines are subject to acute and chronic ischemia when atherosclerosis is extensive. Vascular occlusions that are embolic in origin, from the heart for example, can cause life-threatening infarctions of the gut. Nonocclusive intestinal infarctions may also result in the presence of congestive heart failure.

CASE STUDY

The case study illustrates the application and objective documentation of abdominal assessment.

The Patient with Liver Failure

Arnold Klovstad presents to the emergency department with difficulty breathing.

❖ HEALTH HISTORY

PATIENT PROFILE	57 yo MWM
CHIEF COMPLAINT	"I've been having trouble catching my breath all wk. I've been very tired. I'm not hungry, but I seem to be gaining wt & my ankles are swollen."
HISTORY OF PRESENT ILLNESS	Pt claims a 14 yr h/o ETOH abuse. Despite regular medical check-ups, condition deteriorated over past yr. Been hospitalized for chronic liver dz 2 × this yr. Last ETOH drink 10 mo PTA. Attends local AA chapter q wk × 10 mo. Describes sl to mod difficulty breathing in recumbent position. By end of wk, sleep was intermittent b/c of continued recumbent dyspnea. ↓ appetite c̄ fatigue, physical weakness, inability to complete ADL, wt gain, ↑ abd size c̄ fullness. Denies epigastric pain, NVD, hematemesis, abd pain.
PAST HEALTH HISTORY	
Medical	Alcoholic liver dz dx 4 yr ago GI bleed 3 yr PTA, controlled by gastric lavage; d/c home on 10th hospital day Hemorrhoids 10 yr ago; Ø tx
Surgical	Fx Ⓛ femur (resulted from a fall while intoxicated) 7 yr ago; open reduction internal fixation, uncomplicated postsurgical course; received home care, PT × 4 wk p̄ d/c; fully recovered c̄ in 6 mo Appendectomy 40 yr PTA T & A 51 yr PTA
Medications	1 MVI qd po Thiamine 100 mg qd po Folate 1 tab qd po Maalox tab prn for epigastric discomfort
Communicable Diseases	Denies
Allergies	ASA (states he breaks out in hives)
Injuries/Accidents	See surg hx
Disabilities/Handicaps	Denies

continued

Blood Transfusions	Denies
Childhood Illnesses	"Usual childhood diseases"
Immunizations	Received heptavax series (finished 2 yr ago), refuses flu shot during winter

FAMILY HEALTH HISTORY

LEGEND

◯ Living female

▢ Living male

⊗ Deceased female

⊠ Deceased male

╱ Points to patient

—//— = Divorced

A&W = Alive & well

AAA = Abdominal aortic aneurysm

CA = Cancer

HTN = Hypertension

MI = Myocardial infarction

PUD = Peptic ulcer disease

47 Alcoholic cirrhosis —//— 53 Colon CA   43 Ruptured AAA — 68 HTN pneumonia

68 Alcoholic cirrhosis esophageal varices — 74 Arthritis HTN

67 A&W   64 PUD   60 MI   57 Alcoholic cirrhosis Hemorrhoids — 52 A&W

19 A&W

Denies family hx of malignancies of stomach, liver, or pancreas; DM; familial polyposis; inflammatory bowel dz; irritable bowel syndrome; polycystic kidney dz; colitis.

SOCIAL HISTORY

Alcohol Use	6 beers/d × 10 yr; 1/5 L vodka qd × 4 yr
Tobacco Use	Smokes 1 PPD × 35 yr; enjoys smoking & doesn't want to quit
Drug Use	Denies use of illegal drugs or abuse of Rx drugs
Sexual Practice	Monogamous sexual relationship c̄ wife × 32 yr
Travel History	No foreign travel
Work Environment	Car insurance auditor/claims; employed c̄ same company × 23 yr; describes work as stressful, but interesting; denies occupational health hazards related to work or environment other than occasional exposure to car fumes
Home Environment	Lives in 18 yo duplex that has all modern conveniences; smoke & CO detectors installed in house; cleaning supplies kept in closet, paint kept in garage
Hobbies/Leisure Activities	Until last yr, belonged to bowling league, but due to onset of fatigue & weakness has given this up; enjoys watching sports on TV
Stress	Potential ↓ in income due to physical disabilities; concern about future well-being of family in the event of his premature death
Education	2 yr college degree

continued

Economic Status	Describes self as "middle class"; "modest savings in the bank"
Military Service	None
Religion	Presbyterian; denies that his religious orientation interferes with receiving hl care
Ethnic Background	Swedish; denies any effect that his ethnicity has on hl care practices
Roles/Relationships	Lives c̄ wife & 19 yo son; describes family as "very strained," his illness has been the source of numerous arguments c̄ wife; socializes c̄ several neighbors; previously involved in community activities, states he is now too embarrassed to socialize because of his big abd: "I look pregnant"
Characteristic Patterns of Daily Living	Wakes at 0630, showers, shaves, smokes, & dresses; attempts to eat breakfast at 0700; reads the newspaper. Leaves for work at 0800 via bus (usual travel time 30 min), smokes ā work starts at 0900. Coffee & cigarette break at 1030. Eats lunch from 1300–1400, usually fast food; describes lunch as his largest meal now. Leaves work at 1730 & usually arrives home by 1830. Dinner at 1900, pt comments his appetite is poor in evening. Frequently socializes in evening c̄ neighbors, enjoys late night TV. Goes to bed around MN. Until 10 mo ago, consumed vodka & OJ c̄ dinner & throughout the evening.
HEALTH MAINTENANCE ACTIVITIES	
Sleep	In the past, states there were times when he could not remember going to bed "due to intoxication"; prior to last wk, slept ≅ 6–7 hr/night, same on wkend.
Diet	Eats 3 meals/d & snacks b/t meals; does not follow prescribed low-protein/low-Na diet; "I can't remember what I was told, maybe I should learn it again"; states diet is lacking in milk food group; describes Chinese food as his favorite meal
Exercise	Does not follow an exercise routine
Stress Management	Smoking & talking about his worries
Use of Safety Devices	Consistently wears seat belt, car has dual airbags; denies any occurrence of drinking & driving c̄ in last yr
Health Check-Ups	Maintains appt c̄ GP; neg TB test 4 mo ago; sees dentist q yr, teeth cleaned q 6 mo; sees ophthalmologist q 2 yr; denies practice of testicular self-examination
PHYSICAL ASSESSMENT	
Inspection	
Shape	Distended
Symmetry	Symmetrically round
Rectus Abdominis Muscle	Intact, no separation
Pigmentation and Color	Uniform color, s̄ jaundice; neg Cullen's sign, caput medusae in umbilical area

continued

Scars	7 cm incision RLQ
Striae	Along Ⓡ & Ⓛ lateral aspects of abd
Respiratory Movement	Smooth & even
Masses/Nodules	Ø
Visible Peristalsis	Ø
Pulsation	Ø
Umbilicus	Protrudes above abd surface
Auscultation	
Bowel Sounds	⊕ 4 quads, c̄ hyperactivity in RLQ & LLQ
Vascular Sounds	Ø aortic, femoral, renal bruits
Venous Hum	⊕ over umbilical area
Friction Rub	⊕ liver, ⊕ spleen
Percussion	
General	Dullness Ⓡ & Ⓛ lateral aspects of abd c̄ tympany over umbilical area
Liver Span	14 cm in Ⓡ MCL
Liver Descent	5 cm
Spleen	Unable to discern 2° to ascites
Stomach	Unable to discern 2° to ascites
Fist Percussion (Indirect)	Neg CVA tenderness, neg liver tenderness
Bladder	Unable to discern 2° to ascites
Special Techniques	⊕ shifting dullness, ⊕ puddle sign
Palpation	
Light Palpation	No generalized tenderness; Ø masses
Abdominal Muscle Guarding	Neg
Deep Palpation	Difficult to palpate 2° to ascites Liver: Blunt border 4 cm below Ⓡ costal margin Spleen: Nonpalpable Kidneys: Nonpalpable Aorta: Nonpalpable Bladder: Nonpalpable Inguinal Lymph Nodes: Neg
Special Techniques	⊕ Fluid wave Neg rebound tenderness Ballottement: nodular liver

continued

LABORATORY DATA

Serum Electrolytes:	Pt's Values	Normal Range
Potassium	3.0 mEq/L	3.5–5.0 mEq/L
Chloride	99 mEq/L	95–105 mEq/L
Sodium	130 mEq/L	135–145 mEq/L
Calcium	7.9 mEq/L	8–11 mEq/L
Serum Enzymes:		
Alanine aminotransferase (ALT) or SGPT	74 IU/L	4–24 IU/L
Aspartate aminotransferase (AST) or SGOT	58 IU/L	0–36 IU/L
Lactic dehydrogenase (LDH)	116 IU/L	30–90 IU/L
Serum Ammonia	118 mg/dl	40–110 mg/dl
Serum Bilirubin:		
Total serum bilirubin	2.4 mg/dl	0.3–1.3 mg/dl
Direct bilirubin	1.6 mg/dl	0.1–0.4 mg/dl
Indirect bilirubin	2.0 mg/dl	0.2–0.8 mg/dl
Stool Specimen	⊖ for occult blood	⊖

✓ **NURSING CHECKLIST**
Abdominal Assessment

Inspection
- Contour
- Symmetry
- Rectus Abdominis Muscles
- Pigmentation and Color
- Scars
- Striae
- Respiratory Movement
- Masses or Nodules
- Visible Peristalsis
- Pulsation
- Umbilicus

Auscultation
- Bowel Sounds
- Vascular Sounds
- Venous Hum
- Friction Rubs

Percussion
- General Percussion
- Liver Span
- Liver Descent
- Spleen
- Stomach
- Fist Percussion
  - Kidney
  - Liver
- Bladder

Palpation
- Light Palpation
- Abdominal Muscle Guarding
- Deep Palpation
- Liver
  - Bimanual Method
  - Hook Method
- Spleen
- Kidneys
- Aorta
- Bladder
- Inguinal Lymph Nodes

continued

Special Techniques
- Percussion for Ascites
  - Shifting Dullness
  - Puddle Sign
- Fluid Wave
- Murphy's Sign
- Rebound Tenderness
- Rovsing's Sign
- Cutaneous Hypersensitivity
- Iliopsoas Muscle Test
- Obturator Muscle Test
- Ballottement

Abdominal Tubes and Drains
- Tubes
  - Enteral Tubes
  - Nasogastric Suction Tubes
  - Intestinal Tubes
  - Gastrostomy
- Drains
  - Abdominal Cavity Drain
  - Biliary Drain
- Intestinal Diversions
  - Colostomy
  - Ileostomy
- Urinary Diversions
  - Ileal Conduit
  - Ureteral Stents
  - Indwelling Catheter

REVIEW QUESTIONS AND ACTIVITIES

1. It is helpful to visualize the location of the different anatomic landmarks of the abdomen. Match the following abdominal organs with the appropriate quadrant.
   a. Right upper quadrant
   b. Right lower quadrant
   c. Left upper quadrant
   d. Left lower quadrant
      1. _____ Spleen
      2. _____ Appendix
      3. _____ Gallbladder
      4. _____ Cecum
      5. _____ Liver
      6. _____ Body of the pancreas
      7. _____ Stomach
      8. _____ Duodenum

2. Describe how you would best assist a ticklish patient during palpation.

3. You determine your patient has rebound tenderness; explain what conditions are commonly associated with your finding.

4. Explain the pathophysiological reasons for the following abnormal abdominal sounds:
   a. Venous hum
   b. Friction rub
   c. Hyperactive bowel sounds
   d. Hypoactive bowel sounds

5. Describe the palpation assessment findings you would expect to see in the patient with:
   a. Enlarged liver
   b. Enlarged spleen

Questions 6–8 refer to the following situation:

Frieda Vandersluis is a 45-year-old divorced mother of two children. She presents to the clinic with a chief complaint of sharp right-upper-quadrant abdominal pain. Episodes of pain have occurred following meals within the last 2 days. Average duration of pain is 2 hours, followed by a persistent, dull, aching abdominal pain.

- Inspection reveals a distended, symmetrical abdomen with separation of rectus abdominis muscles. Abdominal striae are evident. Abdominal rigidity with guarding is noted.
- On auscultation, bowel sounds are evident in all four quadrants. No abdominal bruit is ascertained.
- With percussion, tympany is elicited over the stomach and intestines, dull sounds are heard over the abdominal organs, and RUQ pain response is initiated.
- Palpation revealed involuntary muscle guarding; order of palpation was changed to assess the RUQ last. Positive Murphy's sign. Negative Rovsing's sign and iliopsoas muscle test.

6. The Rovsing's sign and iliopsoas muscle test are useful to rule out:
   a. Appendicitis
   b. Cholecystitis
   c. Duodenal ulcer
   d. Hepatic congestion

   The correct answer is (a).

7. A positive Murphy's sign indicates an inflammatory process associated with:
   a. Ascites
   b. Appendicitis
   c. Cholecystitis
   d. Pelvic abscess

   The correct answer is (c).

8. What additional assessment technique might be useful for this patient?
   a. Fluid wave
   b. Ballottement
   c. Puddle sign
   d. Liver fist percussion

   The correct answer is (d).

17

Musculoskeletal System

1. Perform inspection and palpation of the musculoskeletal system.
2. Perform a measurement of limb length and circumference.
3. Describe the average range of motion movements of the major skeletal joints.
4. Measure range of joint motion with a goniometer.
5. Assess muscle strength of the arms and legs using the Muscle Strength Grading Scale.
6. Document the findings of musculoskeletal assessment.

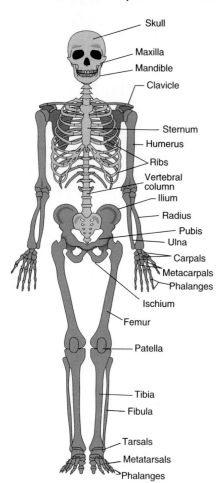

Appendicular skeleton (blue)
Axial skeleton (grey)

Figure 17-1   Adult Skeleton: Anterior View

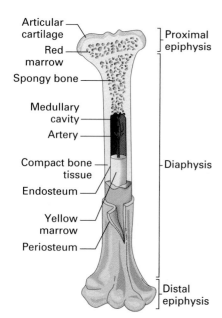

Figure 17-2   Structure of a Long Bone

The musculoskeletal system provides the ability to maintain and change body position in response to both internal and external stimuli. Muscle tone and bone strength allow an individual to maintain an upright and erect posture position. Muscle contraction and joint movement allow an individual to move toward positive stimuli and away from noxious stimuli. Alterations in the musculoskeletal system will affect the individual's ability to complete activities of daily living, occupation, and recreation.

ANATOMY AND PHYSIOLOGY

The musculoskeletal system consists of an intricate framework of bones, joints, skeletal muscles, and supportive connective tissue (cartilage, tendons, and ligaments). Although the primary purpose of the musculoskeletal system is to support body position and promote mobility, it also protects underlying soft organs and allows for mineral storage. In addition, it produces select blood components (platelets, red blood cells, and white blood cells). Only those aspects of the musculoskeletal system that are responsible for body position and mobility are discussed in this chapter.

Bones

The adult human skeleton is composed of 206 bones (refer to Figure 17-1). Bone is ossified connective tissue. The skeleton is divided into the central **axial skeleton** (facial bones, skull, auditory ossicles, hyoid bone, ribs, sternum, and vertebrae) and the peripheral **appendicular skeleton** (limbs, pelvis, scapula, and clavicle). A bone's size and shape are directly related to the mobility and weight-bearing function of that bone. In some cases, bone size and shape are also related to the protection of underlying internal organs and tissues (e.g., the ribs in relation to the lungs, heart, and thoracic aorta).

Shape and Structure

Bones have long, short, flat, rounded, and irregular shapes. The long bone is a shaft (**diaphysis**) with two large ends (**epiphyses**). The two epiphyses each articulate with another bone to form a joint. A 1 to 4 cm layer of cartilage covers each epiphysis in order to minimize stress and friction on the bone ends during movement and weight bearing. The thickness of the cartilage layer varies, depending on the amount of stress placed on that joint. The interior of the diaphysis is the **medullary cavity**, which contains the bone marrow (refer to Figure 17-2).

Short bones are found in the hands (carpals) and feet (tarsals). Flat bones, such as the skull and parts of the pelvic girdle, are associated with the protection of nearby soft body parts. Rounded, or sesamoid, bones are often encased in the fascia or in a tendon near a joint, such as is the patella. Irregular bones include the mandible, vertebrae, and the auditory ossicles of the inner ear.

Muscles

There are over 600 muscles in the human body, and they can be characterized as one of three types. Cardiac and smooth muscles are involuntary, meaning that the individual has no conscious control over the initiation and termination of the muscle contraction. The largest type of muscle, and the only type of voluntary muscle, is called skeletal muscle. Skeletal muscle provides for mobility by exerting a pull on the bones near a joint. In addition, skeletal muscle provides for body contour and contributes to overall body weight.

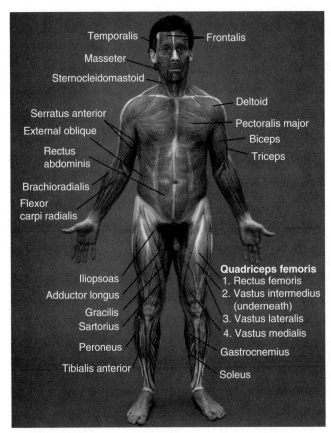

A. Anterior View

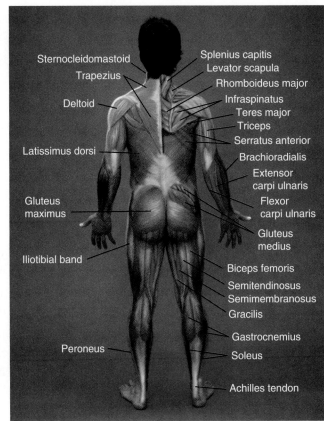

B. Posterior View

Figure 17-3 Muscles of the Body

Figure 17-3 illustrates the major muscles. It is estimated that 40% to 50% of adult body weight is due to the weight of the skeletal muscles.

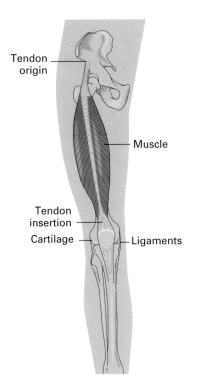

Figure 17-4 Connective Tissue Structures of the Leg

Tendons

A strong connective tissue sheath (**epimysium**) acts as the outer covering of the muscle belly. The ends of the epimysium extend beyond the muscle belly to form the **tendons** of the muscle. The tendon attaches the muscle to a bone (refer to Figure 17-4).

Bursae

Bursae are sacs filled with fluid. Bursae act as cushions between two nearby surfaces (e.g., between tendon and bone or between tendon and ligament) to reduce friction. They can also develop in response to prolonged friction or pressure.

Joints

A **joint** is a union between two bones. Joints secure the bones firmly together but allow for some degree of movement between the two bones. Contraction of overlying skeletal muscle will act to alter the angle of the two bones by pulling the distal bone toward or away from the proximal bone. Terms used for joint range of motion are described in Table 17-1.

Of the three classifications of skeletal joints found in the adult human skeleton (synarthroses, amphiarthroses, and diarthroses), only the synovial joint (diarthroses) is considered freely movable. Examples of each joint are provided

TERM	DESCRIPTION	CHANGE IN JOINT ANGLE
Flexion	Bending of a joint so that the articulating bones on either side of the joints are moved closer together	Decreased
Extension	Bending the joint so that the articulating bones on either side of the joint are moved farther apart	Increased
Hyperextension	Extension beyond the neutral position	Increased beyond the angle of extension
Adduction	Moving the extremity medially and toward the midline of the body	Decreased
Abduction	Moving the extremity laterally and away from the midline of the body	Increased
Internal rotation	Rotating the extremity medially along its own axis	No change
External rotation	Rotating the extremity laterally along its own axis	No change
Circumduction	Moving the extremity in a conical fashion so that the distal aspect of the extremity moves in a circle	No change
Supination	Rotating the forearm laterally at the elbow so that the palm of the hand turns laterally to face upward	No change
Pronation	Rotating the forearm medially at the elbow so that the palm of the hand turns medially to face downward	No change
Opposition	Moving the thumb outward to touch the little finger of the same hand	No change
Inversion	Tilting the foot inward, with the medial side of the foot lowered	No change
Eversion	Tilting the foot outward, with the lateral side of the foot lowered	No change
Dorsiflexion	Flexing the foot at the ankle so that the toes move toward the chest	Decreased
Plantar flexion	Moving the foot at the ankle so that the toes move away from the chest	Increased
Elevation	Raising a body part in an upward direction	No change
Depression	Lowering a body part	No change
Protraction	Moving a body part anteriorly along its own axis (parallel to the ground)	No change
Retraction	Moving a body part posteriorly along its own axis (parallel to the ground)	No change
Gliding	One joint surface moves over another joint surface in a circular or angular nature	No change

Table 17-1 Descriptive Terms for Joint Range of Motion

Table 17-2   Classification of Skeletal Joints

CATEGORY	DEGREE OF MOVEMENT	EXAMPLES
Diarthroses (synovial)	Freely movable	Shoulder, elbow, wrist, thumb, hip, knee, ankle, and proximal cervical vertebrae
Amphiarthroses	Slightly movable	Vertebrae, manubriosternal joint, radioulnar joint, and symphysis pubis
Synarthroses	Immovable	Epiphyseal growth plate (adult), skull sutures (child), between the distal ends of the radius and ulnar, between the distal ends of the tibia and fibula, and the attachment of the root of a tooth to the alveolar process of the maxilla or mandible

Table 17-3   Categories of the Major Synovial Joints

CATEGORY	DESCRIPTION	EXAMPLES
Uniaxial Joints		
Hinge joint	Angular movement in one axis and in one plane	Elbow, fingers, knee
Pivot joint (trochoid)	Rotary movement in one axis; a ring rotates around a pivot, or a pivotlike process rotates within a ring	Radioulnar joint, atlanto-odontal joint of the first and second cervical vertebrae
Biaxial Joints		
Saddle joint (sellar)	Articulating surface of one bone is convex and articulating surface of second bone is concave	Metacarpal bone of thumb, trapezium bone of carpus
Condyloid joint	Angular motion in two planes without axial rotation	Wrist between the distal radius and the carpals
Multiaxial Joints		
Ball and socket (spheroidal) joint	Round end of bone fits into cuplike cavity of another bone; provides movement around three or more axes, or in three or more planes	Shoulder, hip
Gliding joint	Gliding movement	Vertebrae, tarsal bones of ankle

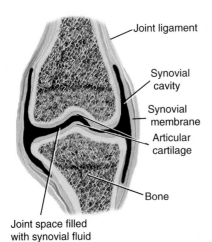

Joint ligament

Synovial cavity

Synovial membrane

Articular cartilage

Bone

Joint space filled with synovial fluid

Figure 17-5   Synovial Joint

in Table 17-2. Table 17-3 shows categories of the major synovial joints. The synovial joint allows body movement.

A synovial membrane lines the interior of the joint space (refer to Figure 17-5). The primary purpose of the synovial membrane is to secrete fluid for joint lubrication, nourishment, and waste removal. Normally, the joint space contains only 1 to 3 ml of synovial fluid. Excessive synovial joint fluid is called a **synovial effusion**.

Ligaments

Ligaments are composed of strong, fibrous, connective tissue. They connect bones to each other at the joint level and encase the joint capsule (refer to Figure 17-4). Ligaments may be seen as oblique to or parallel to a joint (e.g., knee) or encircling the joint (e.g., hip). Ligaments support purposeful joint movement and prevent joint movement that is detrimental to that type of joint.

❖ HEALTH HISTORY

The musculoskeletal health history provides insight into the link between a patient's life/lifestyle and musculoskeletal information and pathology.

PATIENT PROFILE   *Diseases that are age-, sex-, and race-specific for the musculoskeletal system are listed.*

Age   Osteosarcoma (10–20 and 50–60)
Ankylosing spondylitis (20–40)
Bursitis (20–40)
Rheumatoid arthritis (onset 20–40 unless juvenile form of the disease)
Systemic lupus erythematosus (SLE) (25–35)
Fibrosarcoma (after 30)
Low back pain (30–50)
Gout (onset over 30, postmenopausal female)
Type I osteoporosis (menopausal female)
Carpal tunnel syndrome (pregnant or menopausal female)
Degenerative joint disease or osteoarthritis (onset after 55 in the female and before 45 in the male)
Type II osteoporosis (onset 50–70)
Multiple myeloma (50–70)
Paget's disease (50–70)

Sex

Female   Type I osteoporosis, rheumatoid arthritis, scoliosis, carpal tunnel syndrome, SLE, postmenopausal gout, polymyalgia rheumatica, scleroderma, myasthenia gravis, multiple sclerosis (MS), osteoporosis, senile kyphosis

Male   Type II osteoporosis, ankylosing spondylitis, gout, Paget's disease, Reiter's syndrome, Dupuytren's contracture, psoriatic arthritis, muscular dystrophy (MD), amyotrophic lateral sclerosis (ALS), rhabdomyosarcoma, osteosarcoma, low back pain

Race

Caucasian   Rheumatoid arthritis, primary osteoarthritis, polymyalgia rheumatica, type I osteoporosis, Paget's disease, Dupuytren's contracture, ALS, ankylosing spondylitis

African American   SLE, rheumatoid arthritis

CHIEF COMPLAINT   *Common chief complaints for the musculoskeletal system are defined and information on the characteristics of each sign/symptom is provided.*

Pain   The subjective sense of discomfort in the axial or appendicular skeleton

Location   Muscle, bone, tendon, ligament, or joint

Quantity   Degree of interruption in the patient's usual activities of daily living (ADL) (changes in ambulation, bathing, dressing, food preparation, working, sitting, transfer to a sitting or standing position, climbing stairs, lifting, pushing, and pulling)

continued

Associated Manifestations	Inflammation, skin abrasion, laceration, bruising, hematoma, stiffness, deformity, muscle spasm, paresthesia, decreased joint mobility, restriction of weight bearing and movement, excessive weakness or fatigue, mental depression, insomnia, guarding of the painful area, crying, moaning, facial grimacing, anxiety, social withdrawal, agitation, restlessness, altered time perception, rocking motion of body, diaphoresis, tachycardia, elevated blood pressure, tachypnea
Aggravating Factors	Muscle contraction, muscle spasm, joint movement, partial or full weight bearing, obesity, dependent position, cold and damp weather, anxiety, noncompliance to physical or occupational therapy guidelines
Alleviating Factors	Restriction of movement, position change, nonweight bearing, limb elevation and rest, ice, heat, analgesics, anti-inflammatory agents, steroids, muscle relaxants, local anesthetic agents, whirlpool therapy, transcutaneous electrical nerve stimulation (TENS), acupuncture, acupressure, assistive devices for use during weight bearing and mobility, splints
Timing	Sudden, insidious, intermittent, continuous
Weakness	The subjective sense of an overall decrease in strength and endurance
Location	Local or diffuse, central or peripheral
Quantity	Effect on ADL
Associated Manifestations	Fatigue, muscle atrophy, decreased sensation, decreased joint mobility, decreased muscle strength, discomfort
Aggravating Factors	Overexertion, fatigue, immobility, noncompliance to physical or occupational therapy guidelines, malnutrition, fluid or electrolyte imbalance, physical or emotional stress
Alleviating Factors	Rest, adequate nutrition and hydration, electrolyte replacement therapy, physical and occupational therapy geared toward muscle strengthening exercises and adaptive techniques
Limited Movement	Decrease in mobility caused by a problem with impulse transmission to the muscle, stimulation of a muscle, the ability of that muscle to contract sufficiently to move the joint, or bone stability
Location	Diffuse, or localized to a specific joint
Quantity	Range of joint motion compared to maximum potential or previous measurement
Associated Manifestations	Pain, inflammation, stiffness, muscle atrophy, weakness, deformity, palpable joint crepitus or joint effusion
Aggravating Factors	Overexertion, immobility, excessive weight gain, noncompliance to medication regime (e.g., anti-inflammatory agents), noncompliance to physical and occupational therapy guidelines
Alleviating Factors	Physical and occupational therapy, anti-inflammatory agents, analgesics, ice, heat, rest, reduction of fractures, correction of dislocation or subluxation

continued

Stiffness	The subjective sense of inflexibility
Location	Diffuse, or localized to a specific joint
Quantity	Effect on ADL
Associated Manifestations	Joint inflammation, muscle atrophy, deformity, contracture, immobility, pain, palpable joint crepitus, limited range of joint motion
Aggravating Factors	Immobility, aging, overexertion (especially without adequate warming up and cooling down sessions during exercise), noncompliance to medication regime (e.g., anti-inflammatory agents), noncompliance to physical and occupational therapy guidelines
Alleviating Factors	Physical and occupational therapy, exercise, anti-inflammatory agents, analgesics, heat, rest, massage, muscle relaxants
Setting	Cold and damp environment
Timing	Sudden or insidious, time of day (e.g., morning stiffness for more than 30 minutes is associated with rheumatoid arthritis), in relation to vigorous or excessive physical exercise
Deformity	The congenital or acquired alteration in the configuration of the axial or appendicular skeleton
Location	General (e.g., decreased overall body size) or localized (e.g., disruption in limb length and alignment due to a fracture)
Quality	Degree of cosmetic alteration, degree of musculoskeletal dysfunction (adverse changes in mobility, weight bearing, and the ability to maintain body posture and position)
Associated Manifestations	Enlarged skull, jaw protrusion, forehead protrusion, abnormal joint angle, limb malalignment, missing or extra digits, missing limb, discrepancy in limb length or width, abnormal posture, muscle atrophy, joint contractures, footdrop
Aggravating Factors	Certain body positions or movements
Alleviating Factors	Surgery, skeletal or skin traction, manual reduction of a fracture or dislocation, limb elevation, ice, physical therapy, splint, cast, brace
Timing	Sudden or insidious, temporary or permanent
PAST HEALTH HISTORY	*The various components of the past health history are linked to musculoskeletal pathology and musculoskeletal-related information.*
Medical	
Musculoskeletal Specific	Rheumatoid arthritis, osteoarthritis, osteoporosis, Paget's disease, gout, ankylosing spondylitis, osteogenesis imperfecta, loosening or malfunction of joint prosthesis, aseptic necrosis, chronic low back pain, herniated nucleus pulposus, chronic muscle spasms or cramps, scoliosis, rhabdomyolosis, poliomyelitis, polymyalgia rheumatica, osteomalacia, rickets, Marfan's syndrome, scleroderma, spina bifida,

continued

	congenital deformity, MD, MS, myasthenia gravis, ALS, Guillain Barré syndrome, Reiter's syndrome, carpal tunnel syndrome, compartment syndrome, fat emboli syndrome, bone malignancy, bone metastasis, paralysis
Nonmusculoskeletal Specific	Immunosuppression, necrotizing faciitis, gas gangrene, tetanus, sickle cell anemia, SLE, Lyme disease, blood dyscrasias (including hemophilia), diabetes mellitus with or without peripheral neuropathy, hypo- or hypercalcemia, hypo- or hyperpituitarism, hyper- or hypoparathyroidism, hyper- or hypothyroidism, peripheral vascular disease with or without claudication, malnutrition, obesity, menopause
Surgical	Joint aspiration, therapeutic joint arthroscopy, joint arthroplasty, joint replacement, synovectomy, meniscectomy, arthrodesis, open reduction and internal fixation (ORIF), discectomy, laminectomy, spinal fusion, chemonucleolysis, Harrington rod placement or other spinal instrumentation, repair of torn rotator cuff, debridement, limb or digit amputation, reattachment of a limb or digit
Medications	Narcotic analgesics, non-narcotic analgesics, anti-inflammatory agents, antigout agents, muscle relaxants, steroids, estrogen supplements, hormone replacements, calcitonin, calcium supplements, vaccinations (especially polio and tetanus), intra-articular injections (local anesthetics, steroids)
Communicable Diseases	Poliomyelitis
Injuries/Accidents	Fracture, dislocation, subluxation, tendon tear, tendonitis, muscle contusion, joint strain or sprain, spinal cord injury, torn rotator cuff, traumatic amputation of a digit or limb, crush injury, back injury (including herniated vertebral disc), sports-related injury (e.g., golf elbow, pitcher's shoulder), cartilage damage. Refer to Table 17-4 for age-related trauma.
Disabilities/Handicaps	Amputation, hemiplegia, paraplegia, quadriplegia, need for brace or splint, limb in a cast, need for supportive devices, muscle atrophy
Childhood Illnesses	Poliomyelitis, juvenile arthritis
FAMILY HEALTH HISTORY	*Musculoskeletal diseases that are familial are listed.*
	Rheumatoid arthritis, osteoporosis, ankylosing spondylitis, gout, Paget's disease, Dupuytren's contracture, SLE, Marfan's syndrome, osteomalacia, congenital defect
SOCIAL HISTORY	*The components of the social history are linked to musculoskeletal factors/pathology.*
Alcohol Use	Increased use associated with increased risk of osteoporosis
Tobacco Use	Increased use associated with increased risk of osteoporosis

continued

Work Environment	Manual movement of heavy objects (lifting, pushing, pulling), duties requiring repetitive motions (e.g., keyboard use), duties requiring prolonged standing or ambulation, use of hazardous equipment, availability and use of safety equipment (e.g., lifting equipment, availability of back support vest or brace)
Home Environment	Design of home (e.g., number of floors, width of doorways, stairs, location of bedroom and bathroom)
Hobbies/Leisure Activities	Basketball, wrestling, gymnastics, hockey, ballet, aerobics, use of free weights and exercise machines, baseball, football, lacrosse, rugby, cycling, running, horseback riding, skiing, hiking, tennis, racquetball, swimming, camping, gardening, painting, needlepoint, carpentry, rollerblading, skateboarding
HEALTH MAINTENANCE ACTIVITIES	*This information provides a bridge between the health maintenance activities and musculoskeletal function.*
Sleep	Sleeping positions, need for pillow support, need for firm mattress
Diet	Intake of dairy products and protein, use of dietary supplements or vitamins
Exercise	Prevents disuse atrophy, promotes bone growth (especially weight-bearing exercise), can aggravate existing musculoskeletal conditions and cause musculoskeletal trauma
Use of Safety Devices	Use of back support vest or lifting equipment for movement of heavy objects (e.g., Hoyer lift, forklift), safety shields when using hazardous equipment, protective padding (wrist or knee guards)

Table 17-4   Common Age-Related Trauma

AGE RANGE	COMMON TRAUMA
10 to 20	Sports-related injuries, motorcycle accidents, high-energy falls (e.g., downhill skiing or cycling)
20 to 50	Sports-related injuries, stress or overuse injuries (e.g., stress fractures, tendonitis), pedestrian accidents
50 to 65+	Recreation-related injuries, falls, pathological fractures, pedestrian accidents

 NURSING TIP

Weakness Rating Scale

A 0–10/10 scale can be used to obtain the patient's subjective rating of the intensity of the weakness. When a 0–10/10 scale is being utilized, 0 represents complete absence of weakness and 10 represents weakness necessitating complete bed rest.

NURSING TIP

Stiffness Rating Scale

When assessing a patient's ability to complete ADL, question the patient's family as well as the patient. The changes in activities of daily living over time may be too subtle to have been noticed by the patient, or the patient may have developed compensatory measures so that these activities can still be accomplished (although they may take longer to complete). A 0–10/10 scale can be used to obtain the patient's subjective rating of the intensity of the stiffness. When utilizing a 0–10/10 scale, 0 represents the complete absence of stiffness and 10 represents total inflexibility.

NURSING TIP

Assessing Musculoskeletal Pain

Musculoskeletal pain may be of an acute or a chronic nature. Acute pain is associated with a recent onset and a short duration. Chronic pain has a malignant or nonmalignant etiology and lasts longer than 6 months. Pain is the most common musculoskeletal complaint verbalized to health care providers.

NURSING TIP

Ensuring Home Safety

To ensure a safe home environment, encourage patients (especially those who have an increased risk for injury in the home) to avoid:

- Loose or unsecured rugs (e.g., scatter rugs, rugs on stairways)
- Stairways without banisters or stairways with loose banisters
- Stairs with a slippery surface
- Dim lighting, especially near stairways or steps
- Ill-fitting shoes, loose nonlaced shoes, shoes with high heels, or shoes with slippery soles
- Household clutter beneath waist level
- Electrical or phone cords that are too long and fall on the floor
- Only one phone or a phone that is not easily accessible during most of the day
- Wet or waxed floors
- Unleashed small pets
- Bathtubs or shower stalls without a nonskid surface
- Lack of grab bars in the bathroom near the toilet and tub or shower stall
- Objects that are not within easy reach
- Wet or icy outdoor steps and sidewalks

EQUIPMENT

- Measuring tape: cloth tape measure that will not stretch
- **Goniometer:** protractor-type instrument with two movable arms to measure the angle of a skeletal joint during range of motion
- Sphygmomanometer and blood pressure cuff
- Felt-tip marker

ASSESSMENT OF THE MUSCULOSKELETAL SYSTEM

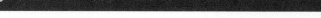

NURSING CHECKLIST

General Approach to Musculoskeletal Assessment

1. Assist the patient to a comfortable position.
2. Offer pillows or folded blankets to support a painful body part.
3. If necessary because of a painful body part or limited mobility, provide the patient assistance in disrobing. Allow the patient extra time to remove clothing.
4. To maximize patient comfort during the physical assessment, maintain a warm temperature in the exam room.
5. Be clear in your instructions to the patient if you are asking the patient to perform a certain body movement or to assume a certain position. Demonstrate the desired movement if necessary.
6. Notify the patient before touching or manipulating a painful body part.
7. Inspection, palpation, range of motion, and muscle testing are performed on the major skeletal muscles and joints of the body in a cephalocaudal, proximal-to-distal manner. Always compare paired muscles and joints.
8. Examine nonaffected body parts before examining affected body parts.
9. Avoid unnecessary or excessive manipulation of a painful body part. If the patient complains of pain, stop the aggravating motion.
10. If necessary because of a painful body part or limited mobility, provide the patient assistance in dressing after the physical assessment. Allow the patient extra time to get dressed.
11. Some musculoskeletal disorders may affect the patient more during certain parts of the day. Arrange for the follow-up appointment to be during the patient's time of optimal function.

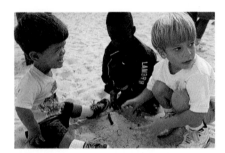

Figure 17-6 Dwarfism

General Assessment
Overall Appearance

E **1.** Obtain height and weight. Refer to Chapter 7.
   2. Observe the patient's ability to tolerate weight bearing on the lower limbs during standing and ambulation. Assess the amount of weight bearing placed on each of the lower limbs. Refer to Table 17-5 for a description of weight-bearing terms.
   3. Identify obvious structural abnormalities (e.g., atrophy, scoliosis, kyphosis, amputated limbs, contractures).
   4. Note indications of discomfort (e.g., restricted weight bearing or movement, frequent shifting of position, facial grimacing, excessive fatigue).

N *Body height and weight should be appropriate for age and gender. Refer to Chapter 7. The patient should be able to enter the assessment area via independent ambulation. Structural defects should be absent. There should be no outward indications of discomfort during rest, weight bearing, or joint movement. There should be a distinct and symmetrical relationship among the limbs, torso, and pelvis.*

A An excessively tall or short or overweight or underweight patient is abnormal.

P Marfan's syndrome affects multiple systems. The musculoskeletal changes are increased height for age due to an increased length of the distal limbs, extra digits, joint instability, pectus excavatum, and kyphosis.

P Dwarfism, a congenital disorder, is manifested by a decrease in body size. It is regarded as proportionate if both limb and trunk size are smaller than average. The decrease in size may affect only the limbs, which then appear out of proportion to the torso size (see Figure 17-6).

P Severe osteoporosis and ankylosing spondylitis can result in height loss due to vertebral compression fractures and thoracic kyphosis.

P Obesity is considered to be a factor in both degenerative joint disease and low back pain.

A Any weight-bearing status other than full weight bearing is abnormal.

P Low back pain may cause a patient to lean forward or toward the affected side.

A Structural defects are abnormal.

P **Acromegaly**, due to hyperpituitary function, may result in an enlarged skull with jaw protrusion, and an increase in the size of the hands, feet, and long bones. The increased length of the long bones can contribute to increased height.

Table 17-5 Weight-Bearing Status	
DEGREE OF WEIGHT BEARING	**DESCRIPTION**
Nonweight bearing	Patient does not bear weight on the affected extremity. The affected extremity does not touch the floor.
Touchdown weight bearing	Patient's foot of the affected extremity may rest on the floor, but no weight is distributed through that extremity.
Partial weight bearing	Patient bears 30% to 50% of his or her weight on the affected extremity.
Weight bearing as tolerated	Patient bears as much weight as can be tolerated on the affected extremity without undue strain or pain.
Full weight bearing	Patient bears weight fully on the affected extremity.

Reprinted with permission from Maher, A. (1994). Orthopedic nursing. *Philadelphia: W.B. Saunders.*

P A missing limb can be due to a congenital defect, surgery, or trauma.

P Pectus excavatum and pectus carinatum are abnormal findings. Refer to Chapter 14.

P Scoliosis and kyphosis are abnormal findings. They are discussed later in this chapter on page 538.

Posture

E 1. Stand in front of the patient.
2. Instruct the patient to stand with the feet together.
3. Observe the structural and spatial relationship of the head, torso, pelvis, and limbs. Assess for symmetry of the shoulders, scapulae, and iliac crests.
4. Ask the patient to sit; observe posture.

N *In the standing position, the torso and head are upright. The head is midline and perpendicular to the horizontal line of the shoulders and pelvis. The shoulders and hips are level, with symmetry of the scapulae and iliac crests. The arms hang freely from the shoulders. The feet are aligned and the toes point forward. The extremities are proportional to the overall body size and shape, and the limbs are also symmetrical with each other. The knees face forward, with symmetry of the level of the knees. There is usually less than a 2-inch interval between the knees when the patient stands with the feet together, facing forward. When full growth is reached, the arm span is equal to the height. In the sitting position, both feet should be placed firmly on the floor surface, with toes pointing forward.*

A Forward slouching of the shoulders produces a false thoracic kyphosis.

P These findings can be caused by poor posture habits.

Gait and Mobility

E 1. Instruct the patient to walk normally across the room.
2. Ask the patient to walk on the toes and then on the heels of the feet.
3. Ask the patient to walk by placing one foot in front of the other, in a "heel-to-toe" fashion (tandem walking).
4. Instruct the patient to walk forward, then backward.
5. Ask the patient to side step to the left, then to the right.
6. Instruct the patient to ambulate forward a few steps with the eyes closed.
7. Observe the patient during transfer between the standing and sitting position.

N *Walking is initiated in one smooth, rhythmic fashion. The foot is lifted 1 to 2 inches off the floor and then propelled 12 to 18 inches forward in a straight path. As the heel strikes the floor, body weight is then shifted onto the ball of that foot. The heel of the foot is then elevated off the floor before the next step forward. The patient remains erect and balanced during all stages of gait. Step height and length are symmetrical for each foot. The arms swing freely at the side of the torso but in opposite direction to the movement of the legs. The lower limbs are able to bear full body weight during standing and ambulation. Prior to turning, the head and neck turn toward the intended direction, followed by the rest of the body. The patient should be able to transfer easily to various positions.*

A Indications of gait disturbance include hesitancy or multiple attempts to initiate ambulation, unsteadiness, staggering, grasping for external support, high stepping, foot scraping due to inability to raise the foot completely off the floor, persistent toe or heel walking, excessive pointing of the toes inward or outward, asymmetry of step height or length, limping, stooping during walking, wavering gait, shuffling gait, waddling gait, excessive swinging of the shoulders or pelvis, and slow or rapid step speed. Table 17-6 provides examples of abnormal gait patterns.

⚡ NURSING ALERT

Guarding Against Patient Falls

Use caution when assessing the patient with limited ability, poor coordination, poor balance, or a sensory deficit (e.g., visual loss, hearing loss, limb amputation, peripheral neuropathy, hemiplegia). Some of the positions and movements that are necessary may place the patient at increased risk for falling during the assessment. Be prepared to support the patient on short notice to prevent a fall. If necessary, omit those components of the musculoskeletal assessment that would place the patient at high risk for injury, or seek the assistance of a second nurse.

E Examination
N Normal Findings
A Abnormal Findings
P Pathophysiology

Table 17-6	Examples of Abnormal Gait Patterns	
TYPE OF ABNORMAL GAIT	**ETIOLOGY**	**DESCRIPTION**
Antalgic	Degenerative joint disease of the hip or knee	Limited weight bearing is placed on an affected leg in an attempt to limit discomfort.
Short leg	Discrepancy in leg length, flexion contracture of the hip or knee, congenital hip dislocation	A limp is present during ambulation unless shoes have been adapted to compensate for length discrepancy.
Spastic hemiplegia	Cerebral palsy, unilateral upper motor neuron lesion (e.g., stroke)	Extension of one lower extremity with plantar flexion and foot inversion; arm is flexed at the elbow, wrist, and fingers. The patient walks by swinging the affected leg in a semicircle. The foot is not lifted off the floor. The affected arm does not swing with the gait.
Scissors	Multiple sclerosis, bilateral upper motor neuron disease	Adduction at the knee level produces short, slow steps. Gait is uncoordinated, stiff, and jerky. The foot is dragged across the floor in a semicircle.
Cerebellar ataxia	Cerebellar disease	Gait is broad based and uncoordinated, and the patient appears to stagger and sway during ambulation.
Sensory ataxia	Disorders of peripheral nerves, dorsal roots, and posterior column that interfere with proprioceptive input	Stance is broad based. Patient lifts feet up too high and abruptly slaps them on the floor, heel first. The patient watches the floor carefully to help ensure correct foot placement because the patient is unaware of position in space.
Festinating	Parkinson's disease	Decreased step height and length, but increased step speed, resulting in "shuffling" (feet barely clearing the floor). Patient's posture is stooped and patient appears to hesitate both in initiation and in termination of ambulation. Rigid body position, with flexion of the knees during standing and ambulation.
Steppage or footdrop	Peroneal nerve injury, paralysis of the dorsiflexor muscles, damage to spinal nerve roots L5 and S1 from poliomyelitis	Hip and knee flexion are needed for step height in order to lift the foot off the floor. Instead of placing the heel of the foot on the floor first, the whole sole of the foot is slapped on the floor at once. May be unilateral or bilateral.
Apraxic	Alzheimer's disease, frontal lobe tumors	Patient has difficulty with walking despite intact motor and sensory systems. The patient is unable to initiate walking, as if stuck to the floor. After walking is initiated, the gait is slow and shuffling.
Trendelenburg	Developmental dysplasia of hip, muscular dystrophy	During ambulation, pelvis of the unaffected side drops when weight bearing is performed on the affected side. When both hips are affected, a "waddling" gait may be evident.

Adapted with permission from Maher, A. (1994). Orthopedic nursing. *Philadelphia: W.B. Saunders.*

P Causes of abnormal gait include muscle weakness, joint deterioration, malalignment of the lower limbs, paralysis, lack of coordination or balance, fatigue, and pain.

P Limited mobility due to stiffness is associated with degenerative joint disease, rheumatoid arthritis, Paget's disease, and Parkinson's disease.

P Severe thoracic kyphosis will alter the body's center of gravity and affect balance during both standing and ambulation.

P Pathological fracture of the femoral shaft during the stress of weight bearing may occur during standing or ambulation. Pathological fracture can occur if the bone has been significantly weakened by malignancy, osteoporosis, Paget's disease, or osteomalacia.

A When rising from or sitting in a chair, the patient may have to lean on the armrest for external support. The patient may also tend to rock forward and push off from the armrest for propulsion upward into the standing position. Discomfort felt while bearing the body's weight in the standing position may be reduced in the sitting position. In Table 17-7, transfer techniques that will assist you in documenting the type of patient transfer are described.

E	**Examination**
N	**Normal Findings**
A	**Abnormal Findings**
P	**Pathophysiology**

Table 17-7 Transfer Techniques	
TECHNIQUE	**DESCRIPTION**
Independent	The patient is safe with transfers and requires no assistance.
Standby assist of 1	The patient is basically independent but may need verbal cues or observation.
Contact guard of 1	The patient transfers well with hands-on contact by a nurse. This method is used if the patient's judgment is questionable or for patients with slightly decreased balance.
Minimal assistance of 1	The patient requires minimal physical assistance from a nurse to stand or sit (e.g., for lower extremity placement on footrest of wheelchair).
Maximal assistance of 1	The patient requires maximal physical assistance and many verbal cues from a nurse to transfer (e.g., for extremity placement, trunk placement).
Maximal assistance of 2	Same as for the previous example but requires two nurses. This necessitates good body mechanics and often calls for assistive devices (e.g., Hoyer lift, total lift).

Reprinted with permission from Maher, A. (1994). Orthopedic nursing. *Philadelphia: W.B. Saunders.*

P Because of stiffness and discomfort, the patient with degenerative joint disease of the hip joint often has difficulty rising from a sitting position without assistance.

Inspection

Muscle Size and Shape

E 1. Survey the overall appearance of the muscle mass.
2. Ask the patient to contract the muscle without inducing movement (isometric muscle contraction), relax the muscle, and then repeat the muscle contraction.
3. Look for any obvious muscle contraction.

N *Muscle contour will be affected by the exercise and activity patterns of the individual. Muscle shape may be accentuated in certain body areas (e.g., the limbs and upper torso) but should be symmetrical. There may be hypertrophy in the dominant hand. During muscle contraction, you should be able to visualize sudden tautness of the muscle area. Muscle relaxation will be associated with termination of muscle tautness. There is no involuntary movement.*

Hypertrophy refers to an increase in muscle size and shape due to an increase in the muscle fibers. Hypertrophy is detected as a unilateral or bilateral increase in the contour of the muscle. During contraction, the borders of the muscle will become accentuated. An increase in muscle strength will accompany the increase in muscle size (refer to Figure 17-7A). Bilateral hypertrophy is common among athletes involved in weight lifting or other activities that require repetitive motion against opposing resistance. Hypertrophy of the proximal arms is often seen in patients who are dependent on a wheelchair for mobility yet are able to propel the wheelchair manually.

A **Atrophy** describes a reduction in muscle size and shape. Atrophy is evidenced by the appearance of thin, flabby muscles. The contour of the skeletal muscle is less distinct than usual. The muscle will appear relaxed, even during voluntary isometric contraction. Atrophy may be local or diffuse (refer to Figure 17-7B).

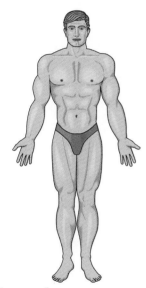

A. Hypertrophy

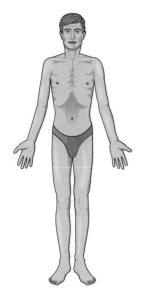

B. Atrophy

Figure 17-7 Variances of Muscle Size and Shape

Table 17-8	Involuntary Muscle Movements
TYPE	**DESCRIPTION**
Fasciculation	Visible twitching of a group of muscle fibers that may be stimulated by the tapping of a muscle.
Fibrillation	Ineffective, uncoordinated muscle contraction that resembles quivering.
Spasm	Sudden muscle contraction. A cramp is a muscle spasm that is strong and painful. Clonic muscle spasms are contractions that alternate with a period of muscle relaxation. A tonic muscle spasm is a sustained contraction with a period of relaxation.
Tetany	Paroxysmal tonic muscle spasms, usually of the extremities. The face and jaw may also be affected by spasm. Tetany may be associated with discomfort.
Chorea	Rapid, irregular, and jerky muscle contractions of random muscle groups. It is unpredictable and without purpose. It can involve the face, upper trunk, and limbs. Sometimes, the patient tries to incorporate the movement into voluntary movement, which may appear grotesque and exaggerated. The patient may have difficulty with chewing, speaking, and swallowing.
Tremors	A period of continuous shaking due to muscle contractions. Although the quality of the tremors will be influenced by the cause, the amplitude and the frequency should remain the same. Tremors may be fine or coarse, rapid or slow, continuous or intermittent. They may be exacerbated during rest and attempts at purposeful movements, or by certain body positions.
Tic	Sudden, rapid muscle spasms of the upper trunk, face, or shoulders. The action is often repetitive and may decrease during purposeful movement. It can be persistent or limited in nature.
Ballism	Jerky, twisting movements due to strong muscle contraction.
Athetosis	Slow, writhing, twisting type of movement. The patient is unable to sustain any part of the body in one position. The movements are most often in the fingers, hands, face, throat, and tongue, although any part of the body can be affected. The movements are generally slower than in chorea.
Dystonia	Similar to athetosis but differing in the duration of the postural abnormality, and involving large muscles such as the trunk. The patient may present with an overflexed or overextended posture of the hand, pulling of the head to one side, torsion of the spine, inversion of the foot, or closure of the eyes along with a fixed grimace.
Myoclonus	A rapid, irregular contraction of a muscle or group of muscles, such as the type of jerking movement that occurs when drifting off to sleep.
Tremors at rest	Asymmetrical and coarse movements that disappear or diminish with action. They tend to diminish or cease with purposeful movement.
Action tremors	Symmetrical or asymmetrical movements that increase in states of fatigue, weakness, drug withdrawal, hypocalcemia, uremia, or hepatic disease. This type of tremor may be induced in a normal individual when he or she is required to maintain a posture that demands extremes of power or precision. Action tremors are also called postural tremors.
Intention tremors	These tremors may appear only on voluntary movement of a limb and may intensify on termination of movement.
Asterixis	This is a variant of a tremor. The rate of limb flexion and extension is irregular, slow, and of wide amplitude. The outstretched limb temporarily loses muscle tone.

P Generalized atrophy is directly related to prolonged immobility of the body as a whole (**disuse atrophy**), unless isometric exercises were routinely performed during the period of immobility. It is accentuated by poor nutrition.

P Generalized atrophy may also be noted in grossly obese patients who lead sedentary lifestyles.

P Local atrophy is often detected in the limb or limbs affected by hemiparesis, paraplegia, or quadriplegia. It is also seen following the removal of a limb cast or splint.

A There is involuntary muscle movement.

P Refer to Table 17-8.

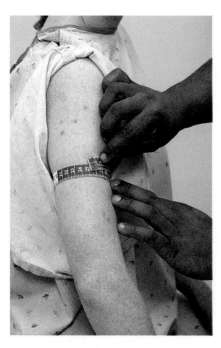

Figure 17-8 Measuring Limb Circumference

✴ SPECIAL TECHNIQUE

Measuring Limb Circumference

Limb circumference is measured when a limb looks larger or smaller than its counterpart during inspection.

E During muscle relaxation or nonweight bearing, measure the limbs at exactly the same distance from a nearby joint (e.g., the knee or elbow) at the site of maximal limb diameter (see Figure 17-8).

N *Bilateral measurements should be within 1 to 3 cm of each other. A slight increase in the girth of the dominant arm is normal.*

A A discrepancy in limb girth of 3 cm or more is abnormal.

P Atrophy results from disuse of a limb, as may occur in stroke.

P Swelling following trauma to soft tissue or bone (e.g., crush injury or fracture) results in an increased limb circumference.

P Unilateral hypertrophy can result from selected activities that use one side of the body more than the other (e.g., tennis arm).

P Unilateral hypertrophy may also be the result of compensating for a deficit in the corresponding limb. For example, a patient with hemiparesis of a limb will present with some degree of hypertrophy of the nonaffected arm muscles.

P A unilateral increase in calf girth may indicate a deep vein thrombosis. Calf girth alters prior to the development of a positive Homan's sign.

Joint Contour and Periarticular Tissue

E **1.** Observe the shape of the joint while the joint is in its neutral anatomic position.

   2. Visually inspect the 2 to 3 inches of skin and subcutaneous tissue surrounding that joint. Assess the periarticular area for erythema, swelling, bruising, nodules, deformities, masses, skin atrophy, or skin breakdown.

N *Joint contour should be somewhat flat in extension, and smooth and rounded in flexion. You should be unable to detect any difference between periarticular tissue and the skin and subcutaneous tissue of the rest of the body. Bilateral joints should be symmetrical in position and appearance. There should be no observable erythema, swelling, bruising, nodules, deformities, masses, skin atrophy, or skin breakdown.*

A Enlargement of the joint is an abnormal finding.

P Joint inflammation can result from inflammatory disorders such as rheumatoid arthritis and gout.

P Trauma to the joint and its extra-articular structures will also result in joint inflammation.

E	**Examination**
N	**Normal Findings**
A	**Abnormal Findings**
P	**Pathophysiology**

A Deformity of the joint capsule is an abnormal finding.

P Immobility results in joint contractures, which cause the joint to be permanently fixated in one position. The acquired joint position may be one within its normal range of joint motion or an abnormal joint position.

P Joint destruction from rheumatoid arthritis may result in a joint becoming fixated in one position.

P Joint dislocation or subluxation will alter the normal contour of a joint. **Dislocation** refers to a complete dislodgment of one bone out of the joint cavity. **Subluxation** is a partial dislodgment of a bone from its place in the joint cavity.

A Alteration in periarticular skin and subcutaneous tissue is an abnormal finding.

P Trauma to the joint results in inflammation and bruising of the periarticular tissue. Joint trauma may include strain, sprain, contusion, dislocation, subluxation, or fracture within or near the joint capsule.

P The patient with rheumatoid arthritis often presents with periarticular skin atrophy and subcutaneous nodules near a joint (e.g., elbow).

P Synovial effusion within the joint capsule may cause a bulging appearance that extends into the periarticular area.

Palpation

Muscle Tone

E 1. Palpate the muscle by applying light pressure with the finger pads of the dominant hand.
2. Note the change in muscle shape as the muscle belly (wide central aspect of the muscle) tapers off to become a tendon.
3. Ask the patient to alternately perform muscle relaxation and isometric muscle contraction. Note the change in palpable muscle tone between relaxation and isometric contraction.
4. Palpate the muscle belly during contraction induced by voluntary movement of a nearby joint.
5. Perform passive range of motion to all extremities and note whether these movements are smooth and sustained.

N *Muscle tone refers to the partial muscle contraction state that is maintained in order for the muscle to respond quickly to the next stimulus. On palpation, the muscle should feel smooth and firm, even during the phase of muscle relaxation. Normal muscle tone provides light resistance to passive stretch. During muscle contraction, especially against moderate external resistance to nearby joint movement, you will be able to palpate a significant overall increase in the firmness of the muscle belly. Muscle tone increases during anxiety or excitable states. Tone decreases during rest and sleep. You will be able to palpate the muscle belly and detect a change in its shape as it tapers down to become a tendon. The hypertrophied muscle will have a distinctive contour. You will detect muscle tautness even during the phase of relaxation.*

A **Hypotonicity** (flaccidity) is a decrease in muscle tone. When the muscle is palpated, it feels flabby and soft to the touch. When a flaccid limb is held away from the body and then released, it falls quickly with gravity.

P Etiology of flaccidity may include diseases involving the muscles, anterior horn cells, or peripheral nerves.

A **Spasticity** refers to an increase in muscle tension on passive stretching (especially rapid or forced stretching of the muscle). It is often noted with extreme flexion or extension.

P Upper motor neuron dysfunction is associated with spasticity.

A The atrophied muscle will feel small and flabby, even during the phase of muscle contraction.

P Refer to page 507.

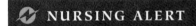

NURSING ALERT

Assessing the Patient with Fragile Bones

Use a gentle approach when assessing the patient with severe osteoporosis or bone metastasis because pathological fracture can occur with minor stress.

E	**Examination**
N	**Normal Findings**
A	**Abnormal Findings**
P	**Pathophysiology**

A A muscle spasm represents persistent muscle contraction without relaxation. The muscle belly will feel taut and the patient may complain of discomfort over the muscle area. The spasm may also result in involuntary joint movement or a change in body position.

P Spasm follows fracture and may alter the distance between the bone fragments. Spasm is also common in the affected limbs of patients with paralysis, electrolyte imbalance, peripheral vascular disease, and cerebral palsy.

A Crepitus refers to a grating or crackling sensation caused by two rough musculoskeletal surfaces rubbing together. Crepitus is more commonly detected with joint movement than it is with muscle contraction.

P Crepitus detected during palpation of muscle contraction, especially in a nonarticulating area, may indicate shaft fracture due to trauma or loss of bone density. Muscle spasm following fracture may bring bone fragments in contact with each other, resulting in crepitus.

A Muscle masses detected on palpation are to be considered an abnormal finding.

P Muscle rupture (e.g., of the long head of the biceps muscle) will present as an inappropriate muscle mass above the joint. The muscle mass may be accentuated by muscle contraction.

P Tendon rupture may also result in an inappropriate muscle mass. An example is a complete rupture of the Achilles tendon, resulting in a mass noted in the calf area.

P Displaced fracture (e.g., of the femoral shaft near the hip joint) will often result in palpation of the displaced bone near a muscle.

P Complete dislocation (e.g., of the hip joint) will also result in palpation of the displaced bone near a muscle.

Joints

E **1.** With the joint in its neutral anatomic position, begin palpating the joint by applying light pressure with the finger pads of the dominant hand 5 to 7 cm away from the center of the joint.

2. Palpate from the periphery inward to the center of the joint.

3. Note any swelling, pain, tenderness, warmth, or nodules.

N *When the major skeletal joints are palpated in their neutral anatomic positions, the external joint contour will feel smooth, strong, and firm. The shape of the joint corresponds to that specific joint type. The area surrounding the joint (periarticular tissue) is free from swelling, pain, tenderness, warmth, or nodules. As the joint is moved through its normal range of motion, it should be able to articulate in proper alignment without any visible or palpable deformity. Palpation of joint movement produces a smooth sensation, without tactile detection of grating or popping. A synovial membrane is not palpable under normal circumstances.*

A Bony enlargement or bony deformities of the joint are considered abnormal findings. Refer to Table 17-9, which provides a tool for grading joint swelling, tenderness, and limitations.

P Urate deposits associated with gout will result in a reactive synovitis, producing joint enlargement. Urate crystals accumulate in the joint as a result of a prolonged elevation of serum uric acid. The affected joint will be extremely warm and tender to the touch. Although the great toe is most commonly affected, gout can also affect other joints.

A Subcutaneous nodules detected in the periarticular area are abnormal.

P Rheumatoid arthritis is associated with subcutaneous nodules over the bony prominences and extensor joint surfaces (e.g., olecranon area of the elbow). These nodules are painless, firm but movable, and of normal skin color. They are more of a cosmetic concern than a threat to nearby joint function, although the overlying skin is at risk for breakdown due to irritation or pressure.

E	**Examination**
N	**Normal Findings**
A	**Abnormal Findings**
P	**Pathophysiology**

Table 17-9 Grading of Joint Swelling, Tenderness, and Limitation			
GRADE	**SWELLING (S)**	**TENDERNESS (T)**	**LIMITATION (L)**
0	None	None	None
1	Mild	Mild, but tolerable tenderness upon palpation	25% decrease in joint range of motion
2	Moderate	Moderate tenderness upon palpation (which the patient can tolerate but prefers not to)	50% decrease in joint range of motion
3	Marked	Light pressure or palpation induces an intolerable tenderness	75% decrease in joint range of motion
4	Maximum	Slight skin motion or sensation induces an intolerable tenderness	Complete loss of joint range of motion

0 = normal   2 = moderate abnormality   4 = maximum abnormality
1 = mild abnormality   3 = marked abnormality

Example: S3/T3/L4 = marked joint swelling with intolerable joint tenderness upon light pressure and with complete loss of joint range of motion.

P Tophi nodules may be detected in the patient with chronic gout, and they represent soft tissue reaction to uric acid crystal deposition. They are often found on the great toes.

A Palpable, audible, severe crepitus that presents as more of a coarse than a fine sensation is abnormal.

P Crepitus is often palpated in joints affected by acute rheumatoid arthritis and degenerative joint disease due to the contact of bone surfaces.

P Bony overgrowth, muscle contracture, dislocation, and subluxation are associated with joint crepitus.

A Any tenderness felt on light touch or joint palpation is considered abnormal. You must differentiate between tenderness on palpation of the joint at rest versus palpation during joint movement (refer to Table 17-9).

P Increased joint capsule pressure with a significant joint effusion may induce discomfort with light touch or pressure to the joint in the neutral position.

P Localized joint tenderness may be detected in the presence of joint contusion, infection, or synovitis.

A Periarticular warmth, with temperature exceeding overall body temperature, indicates an underlying problem.

P Joint inflammation (e.g., due to acute rheumatoid arthritis or recent trauma) and gout produce significant joint warmth because of the increased localized perfusion associated with the inflammatory process.

Range of Motion (ROM)

E 1. Ask the patient to move the joint through each of its various ROM movements.
2. Note angle of each joint movement.
3. Note any pain, tenderness, or crepitus.
4. If the patient is unable to perform active ROM, then passively move each joint through its ROM.
5. Always stop if the patient complains of pain, and never push a joint beyond its anatomic angle.
6. Use a goniometer to determine exact ROM in joints with limited ROM. Refer to the Special Technique on page 511.

E	**Examination**
N	**Normal Findings**
A	**Abnormal Findings**
P	**Pathophysiology**

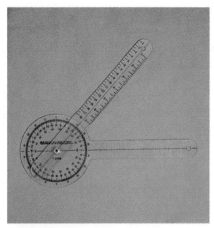

A. Goniometer

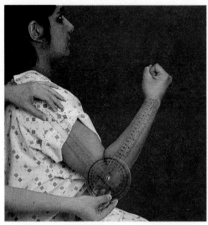

B. Use of Goniometer

Figure 17-9 Goniometer and Its Use

E Examination
N Normal Findings
A Abnormal Findings
P Pathophysiology

✿ SPECIAL TECHNIQUE

Using a Goniometer

E **1.** With the joint in its neutral position, place the center of the goniometer over the joint so that the two distal arms of the goniometer are in alignment with the proximal and distal bones adjacent to that joint.

2. Move the joint through its ROM and note the degree of the joint angle visible on the center of the goniometer (see Figure 17-9).

N *Refer to the specific sections on joints for the ROM for each joint movement.*

A Abnormalities of joint function are indicated by the inability of the patient to voluntarily and comfortably move a joint in the directions and to the degrees that are considered the norms for that joint.

P Degenerative joint disease, rheumatoid arthritis, and joint trauma are some of the many musculoskeletal disorders that prevent the affected joint from moving through its normal ROM.

Muscle Strength

Each muscle group is assessed for strength via the same movements as are performed in range of motion.

E **1.** Note whether muscle groups are strong and equal.

2. Always compare right and left sides of paired muscle groups.

3. Note involuntary movements.

N *Normal muscle strength allows for complete voluntary range of joint motion against both gravity and moderate to full resistance. Muscle strength is equal bilaterally. There is no observed involuntary muscle movement.*

A A decrease in skeletal muscle strength is significant if complete range of joint motion is either impossible or possible only without resistance or gravity.

P Local decrease in muscle strength will accompany muscle atrophy of the limbs secondary to disuse.

Table 17-10 Muscle Strength Grading Scale		
FUNCTIONAL ABILITY DESCRIPTION	**SCALE (%)**	**0–5/5 SCALE**
Complete range of joint motion against both gravity and full manual resistance from the nurse.	100%	5/5 Normal (N)
Complete range of joint motion against both gravity and moderate manual resistance from the nurse.	75%	4/5 Good (G)
Complete range of joint motion possible only without manual resistance from the nurse.	50%	3/5 Fair (F)
Complete range of joint motion possible only with the joint supported by the nurse to eliminate the force of gravity and without any manual resistance from the nurse.	25%	2/5 Poor (P)
Muscle contraction detectable but insufficient to move the joint even when the forces of both gravity and manual resistance have been eliminated.	10%	1/5 Trace (Tr)
Complete absence of visible and palpable muscle contraction.	0%	0/5 None (0)

P Diffuse reduction in muscle strength is associated with general atrophy, severe fatigue, malnutrition, muscle relaxant medications (e.g., valium), long-term steroid use, and deteriorating neuromuscular disorders. These deteriorating neuromuscular diseases include but are not limited to ALS, MD, MS, myasthenia gravis, and Guillain Barré syndrome.

A One-sided muscle weakness or paralysis is considered abnormal.

P Unilateral weakness or paralysis is indicative of **hemiparesis (hemiplegia)** from a cerebrovascular accident, brain tumor, or head trauma.

Examination of Joints

Temporomandibular Joint

E 1. Stand in front of the patient.
   2. Inspect the right and left temporomandibular joints (see Figure 17-10).
   3. Palpate the temporomandibular joints (refer to Figure 17-11).
      a. Place your index and middle fingers over the joint.
      b. Ask the patient to open and close the mouth.
      c. Feel the depression into which your fingers move with an open mouth.
      d. Note the smoothness with which the mandible moves.
      e. Note any audible or palpable click as the mouth opens.
   4. Assess ROM. Ask the patient to:
      a. Open the mouth as wide as possible.
      b. Push out the lower jaw (see Figure 17-12A).
      c. Move the jaw from side to side (refer to Figure 17-12B).
   5. Palpate the strength of the masseter and temporalis muscles as the patient clenches the teeth. This assesses cranial nerve V.

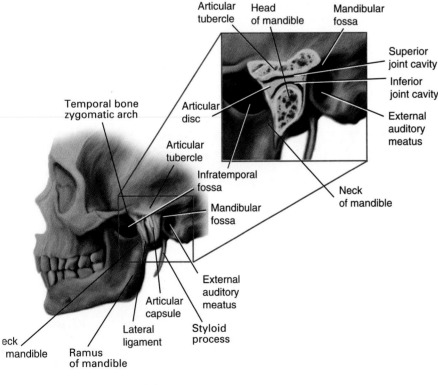

Figure 17-10 Anatomy of the Temporomandibular Joint (Sagittal Section)

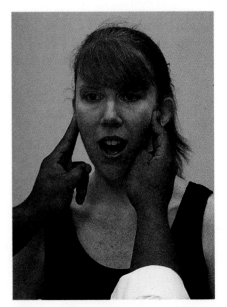

Figure 17-11 Palpation of the Temporomandibular Joint

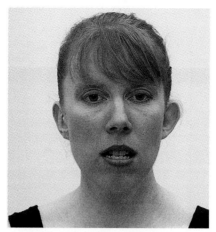 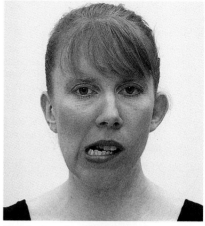

A. Pushing Out the Lower Jaw   B. Moving the Jaw From Side to Side

Figure 17-12   Range of Motion of the Temporomandibular Joint

N *It is normal to hear or palpate a click when the mouth opens. The mouth can normally open 3 to 6 cm with ease. The lower jaw protrudes without deviating to the side and moves 1 to 2 cm with lateral movement.*

A Pain, limited ROM, and crepitus can occur in temporomandibular joint dysfunction.

P Temporomandibular joint dysfunction can occur secondary to malocclusion, arthritis, dislocation, poorly fitting dentures, and myofacial dysfunction.

✻ SPECIAL TECHNIQUE

Assessing for Chvostek's Sign

E **1.** The patient can be assessed in the standing, sitting, or supine position.
    2. While the patient is facing forward, tap the side of the face just below the temple area, using the middle or index finger (see Figure 17-13).
    3. Observe for ipsilateral changes in facial expression immediately after tapping the face.
    4. Repeat the procedure on the other side of the face.

N *There will be no change in the patient's facial expression when the temple area is stimulated.*

A A positive Chvostek's sign, indicated by ipsilateral muscle spasm of the mouth and cheek, is abnormal. The muscle spasm will occur in an upward direction, toward the temple.

P A positive Chvostek's sign is suggestive of neuroexcitability associated with hypocalcemia and tetanus infection.

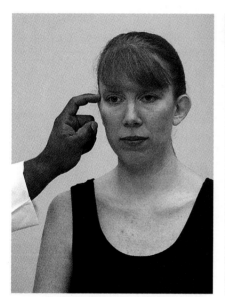

Figure 17-13   Assessing for Chvostek's Sign

Cervical Spine

⚡ NURSING ALERT

Preventing Neck Injury

Never move the head and neck of a patient with a suspected neck injury. Movement can result in permanent spinal cord injury. Refer the patient to an orthopedist or a neurosurgeon immediately.

Use caution when applying mild to moderate resistance during neck assessment, especially when the patient has a known musculoskeletal disorder.

E **1.** Stand behind the patient.
    2. Inspect the position of the cervical spine.
    3. Palpate the spinous processes (see Figure 17-14) of the cervical spine and the muscles of the neck.

E **Examination**
N **Normal Findings**
A **Abnormal Findings**
P **Pathophysiology**

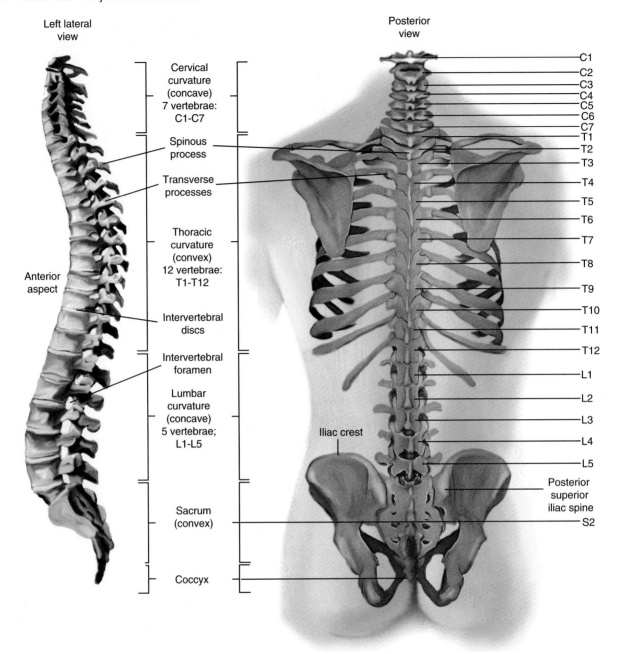

Left lateral view

Posterior view

Cervical curvature (concave) 7 vertebrae: C1-C7

Spinous process

Transverse processes

Thoracic curvature (convex) 12 vertebrae: T1-T12

Anterior aspect

Intervertebral discs

Intervertebral foramen

Lumbar curvature (concave) 5 vertebrae; L1-L5

Sacrum (convex)

Coccyx

C1
C2
C3
C4
C5
C6
C7
T1
T2
T3
T4
T5
T6
T7
T8
T9
T10
T11
T12
L1
L2
L3
L4
L5

Iliac crest

Posterior superior iliac spine

S2

Figure 17-14 Anatomy of the Spine

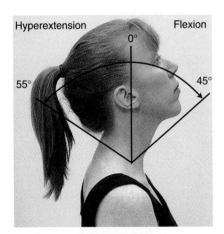

Hyperextension

Flexion

0°

55°

45°

A. Flexion, Hyperextension

Figure 17-15 Range of Motion of the Cervical Spine

4. Stand in front of the patient.
5. Assess the ROM of the cervical spine. Ask the patient to:
   a. Touch the chin to the chest (flexion).
   b. Look up at the ceiling (hyperextension) (see Figure 17-15A).
   c. Move each ear to the shoulder on its respective side without elevating the shoulder (lateral bending) (see Figure 17-15B).
   d. Turn the head to each side to look at the shoulder (rotation) (see Figure 17-15C).
6. Assess strength of the cervical spine by repeating the movements in step 5d while applying opposing force. This also assesses the function of cranial nerve XI.

N *The cervical spine's alignment is straight and the head is held erect. The normal ROM for the cervical spine is: flexion — 45°, hyperextension — 55°, lateral bending — 40° to each side, rotation — 70° to each side. Hypertrophy of the neck muscles due to weight-lifting exercises will produce the appearance of a thick neck.*

A A neck that is not erect and straight is abnormal.

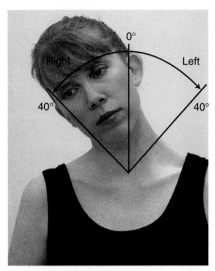

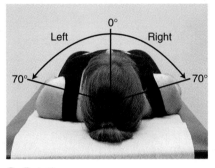

B. Lateral Bending

C. Rotation

Figure 17-15 Range of Motion of the Cervical Spine *continued*

P Degenerative joint disease of the cervical vertebrae may result in lateral tilting of the head and neck.

P Torticollis is discussed on page 275.

A A change in the size of the neck is abnormal.

P Klippel-Feil syndrome is the congenital absence of one or more cervical vertebrae along with fusion of the upper cervical vertebrae and bilateral elevation of the scapulae, resulting in a shortened neck appearance. It may be accompanied by a low hairline, webbing of the neck, and decreased neck mobility.

A Inability of the patient to perform ROM, and pain and tenderness on palpation are abnormal.

P Arthritis, neck injury, disc degeneration (among aging patients or from occupational stress), degenerative joint disease, and spondylosis can cause these cervical spine signs or symptoms.

Shoulders

E 1. Stand in front of the patient.
  2. Inspect the size, shape, and symmetry of the shoulders (refer to Figure 17-16).
  3. Move behind the patient and inspect the scapula for size, shape, and symmetry.
  4. Palpate the shoulders and surrounding muscles.
     a. Move from the sternoclavicular joint along the clavicle to the acromioclavicular joint.
     b. Palpate the acromion process, subacromial area, greater tubercle of the humerus, the anterior aspect of the glenohumeral joint, and the biceps groove.
  5. Assess ROM of the shoulders. Ask the patient to:
     a. Place arms at the side, elbows extended, and move the arms forward in an arc (forward flexion).

E	**Examination**
N	**Normal Findings**
A	**Abnormal Findings**
P	**Pathophysiology**

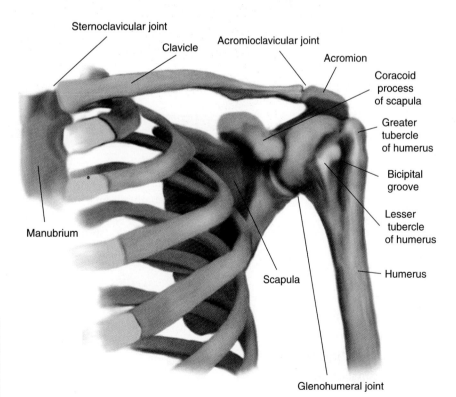

Figure 17-16 Anatomy of the Shoulder Joint

b. Move the arms backward in an arc as far as possible (hyperextension) (see Figure 17-17A).

c. Place arms at side, elbows extended, and move both arms out to the sides in an arc until the palms touch together overhead (abduction) (see Figure 17-17B).

d. Move one arm at a time in an arc toward the midline and cross it as far as possible (adduction).

e. Place hands behind the back and reach up, trying to touch the scapula (internal rotation) (see Figure 17-17C).

f. Place both hands behind the head with elbows flexed (external rotation) (see Figure 17-17D).

g. Shrug the shoulders. This assesses cranial nerve XI function.

6. Assess strength of the shoulders by applying opposing force to the ROM movements in step 5g.

N *The shoulders are equal in height. There is no fluid palpable in the shoulder area. Crepitus is absent. The normal ROM for the shoulder is: forward flexion — 180°, hyperextension — 50°, abduction — 180°, adduction — 50°, internal rotation — 90°, external rotation — 90°.*

A Increased outward prominence of the scapula (winging) is an abnormal finding.

P Scapular winging is indicative of serratus anterior muscle injury or weakness.

A Decreased movement, pain with movement, swelling from fluid, and asymmetry are abnormal.

P These findings are associated with degenerative joint disease, arthritic syndromes, and injury. Swelling from fluid is usually best seen anteriorly.

P Bursitis of the shoulder can result from overuse of the shoulder in repetitive activity (either a new activity such as leaf raking and car polishing or a familiar activity such as swimming).

P An acromioclavicular joint separation (separated shoulder) causes pain in the acromioclavicular joint. Swelling frequently occurs at the distal end of the clavicle.

P Shoulder subluxation and dislocation are common athletic injuries. Patients with recurrent subluxations may feel the glenohumeral joint pop out of the socket and pop back in without medical intervention. With an anterior dislocation, fluid is usually seen anteriorly, whereas with a posterior dislocation, fluid is usually best seen posteriorly.

E	Examination
N	Normal Findings
A	Abnormal Findings
P	Pathophysiology

❋ SPECIAL TECHNIQUE

Drop Arm Test

The drop arm test assesses for rotator cuff damage.

E 1. Manually abduct the patient's affected arm.

2. Ask the patient to slowly lower the raised arm to the side while maintaining extension of the arm.

3. Observe the speed at which the patient lowers the arm.

N *The patient will be able to slowly lower the arm to the side while maintaining the arm in extension.*

A An abnormal drop arm test is manifested by the inability of the patient to slowly lower the arm to the side (e.g., the arm quickly falls to the side of the torso), or by severe pain occuring in the shoulder while the arm is slowly lowered to the side.

P An abnormal drop arm test is indicative of a rotator cuff tear. It is caused by trauma to the shoulder.

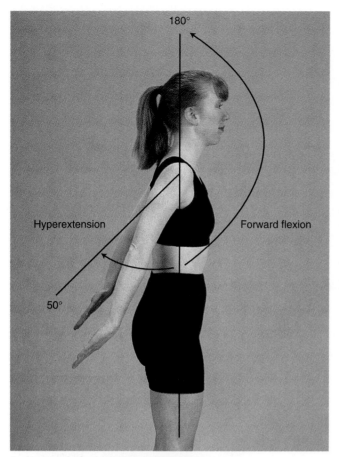

A. Forward Flexion, Hyperextension

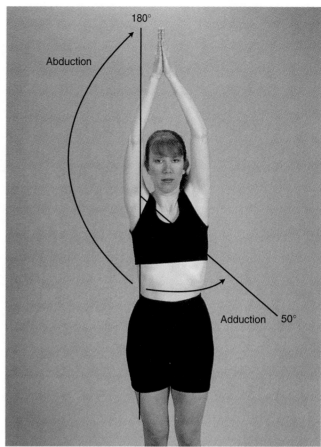

B. Abduction, Adduction

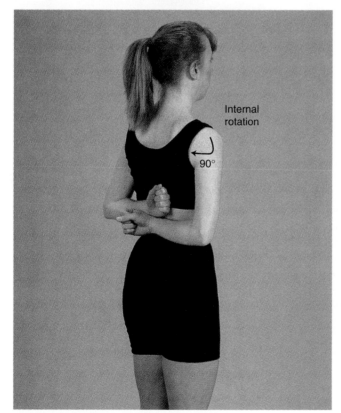

C. Internal Rotation

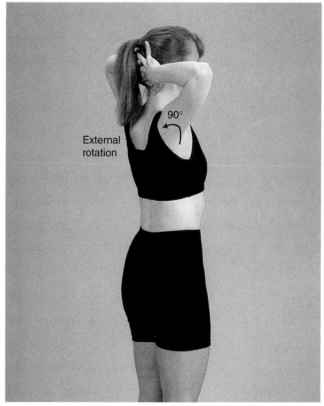

D. External Rotation

Figure 17-17 Range of Motion of the Shoulder Joint

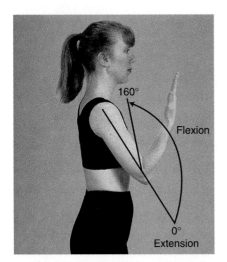

A. Flexion, Extension

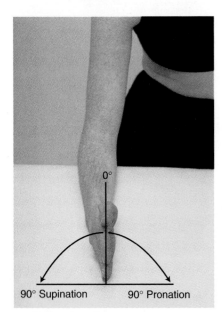

B. Supination, Pronation

Figure 17-19   Range of Motion of the Elbow Joint

E	**Examination**
N	**Normal Findings**
A	**Abnormal Findings**
P	**Pathophysiology**

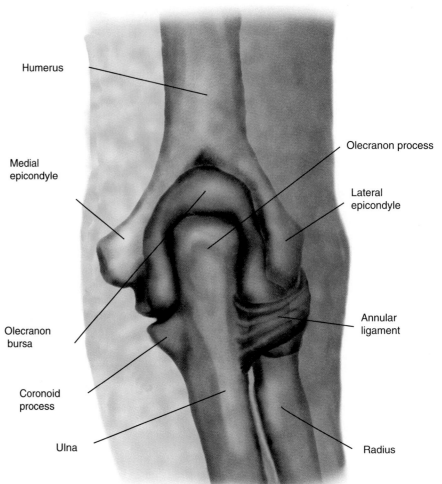

Figure 17-18   Anatomy of the Elbow Joint (Posterior View, Right Elbow)

Elbows

E   1. Stand to the side of the elbow being examined.

2. Support the patient's forearm on the side that is being examined (approximately 70°).

3. Inspect the elbow in flexed and extended (see Figure 17-18) positions. Note the olecranon process and the grooves on each side of the olecranon process.

4. Using your thumb and middle fingers, palpate the elbow. Note the olecranon process, the olecranon bursa, the groove on each side of the olecranon process, and the medial and lateral epicondyles of the humerus.

5. Assess ROM of the elbows. Ask the patient to:

   a. Bend the elbow (flexion) (see Figure 17-19A).

   b. Straighten the elbow (extension).

   c. Hold the arm straight out, bent at the elbow, and turn the palm upward toward the ceiling (supination) (see Figure 17-19B).

   d. Turn the palm downward toward the floor (pronation).

6. Assess strength of the elbow:

   a. Stabilize the patient's arm at the elbow with your nondominant hand. With your dominant hand, grasp the patient's wrist.

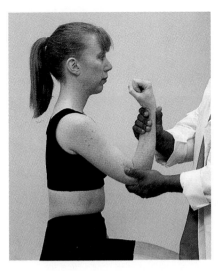

Figure 17-20 Muscle Strength of the Elbow

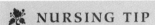

NURSING TIP

Suspected Radial Head Fractures

Any patient, particularly an elderly person, who complains of elbow pain after suffering a fall must be carefully assessed for a radial head fracture.

E **Examination**
N **Normal Findings**
A **Abnormal Findings**
P **Pathophysiology**

b. Ask the patient to flex the elbow (pulling it toward the chest) while you apply opposing resistance (see Figure 17-20).

c. Ask the patient to extend the elbow (pushing it away from the chest) while you apply opposing resistance.

N *The elbows are at the same height and are symmetrical in appearance. The normal ROM for the elbow is: flexion — 160°, extension — 0°, supination — 90°, pronation — 90°.*

A Elbows that are not symmetrical are abnormal. The forearm is not in its usual alignment. Pain is present.

P These findings occur in a dislocation or a subluxation of the elbow. They usually occur from sports-related injuries, falls, or motor vehicle accidents.

A Localized tenderness and pain with elbow flexion, extension, or both are abnormal.

P Epicondylitis (tennis elbow) occurs from repetitive motions such as swinging a tennis racquet, hammering, using a screwdriver, and other activities involving repetitive movements of the forearm.

P Radial head fractures usually result from falls. Frequently, the elbow is flexed in a 90° position.

P A flexion contracture of the elbow may be seen in a patient with hemiparesis following a cerebrovascular accident.

A Red, warm, swollen, and tender areas in the grooves beside the olecranon process are abnormal. Synovial fluid may be palpable and is soft or boggy.

P Inflammatory processes such as gouty arthritis, bursitis, rheumatoid arthritis, and SLE can cause these clinical manifestations.

P Olecranon bursitis is classified as an overuse syndrome. It usually results from repetitive motions rather than from an acute injury.

SPECIAL TECHNIQUE

Assessing for Trousseau's Sign

E **1.** Place the patient in a sitting or a supine position.
2. Apply a blood pressure cuff to the patient's upper arm.
3. Inflate the blood pressure cuff to 10 mm Hg above the patient's systolic blood pressure for 1 to 3 minutes.
4. Observe for twitching of the hand and fingers on the side being tested.

N *There will be no visible twitching of the hand and fingers during cuff inflation.*

A A positive Trousseau's sign, indicated by visible ipsilateral twitching of the hand and fingers during cuff inflation, is abnormal.

P A positive Trousseau's sign is suggestive of neuroexcitability associated with hypocalcemia and tetanus infection.

Wrists and Hands

E **1.** Stand in front of the patient.
2. Inspect the wrists and the palmar and dorsal aspects of the hands. Note the shape, position, contour, and number of fingers (see Figure 17-21).
3. Inspect the **thenar eminence** (the rounded prominence at the base of the thumb).
4. Support the patient's hand in your two hands, with your fingers underneath the patient's hands and your thumbs on the dorsum of the patient's hand.

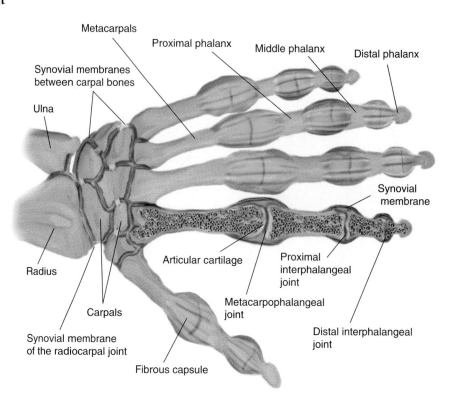

Figure 17-21 Anatomy of the Wrist and Hand

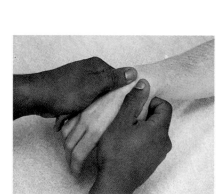

Figure 17-22 Palpating the Wrist Joint

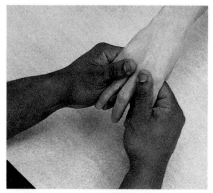

A. Metacarpophalangeal Joint

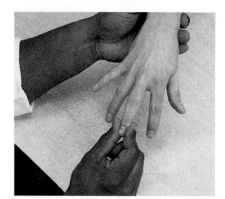

B. Interphalangeal Joint

Figure 17-23 Palpating the Hand Joints

5. Palpate the joints of the wrists by moving your thumbs from side to side. Feel the natural indentations (see Figure 17-22).

6. Palpate the joints of the hand:
   a. Use your thumbs to palpate the metacarpophalangeal joints, which are immediately distal to and on each side of the knuckle (see Figure 17-23A).
   b. Between your thumb and index finger, gently pinch the sides of the proximal and distal interphalangeal joints (see Figure 17-23B).

7. Assess the ROM of the wrists and hands. Ask the patient to:
   a. Straighten the hand (extension) and bend it up at the wrist toward the ceiling (hyperextension).
   b. Bend the hand down at the wrist toward the floor (flexion) (see Figure 17-24A).
   c. Bend the fingers up at the metacarpophalangeal joint toward the ceiling (hyperextension).
   d. Bend the fingers down at the metacarpophalangeal joint toward the floor (flexion) (see Figure 17-24B).
   e. Place the hands on a flat surface and move them side to side (radial deviation is movement toward the thumb, and ulnar deviation is movement toward the little finger) without moving the elbow (see Figure 17-24C).
   f. Make a fist with the thumb on the outside of the clenched fingers.
   g. Spread the fingers apart.
   h. Touch the thumb to each fingertip. Touch the thumb to the base of the little finger.

8. Assess the strength of the wrists. Ask the patient to:
   a. Place the arm on a table with the forearm supinated. Stabilize the forearm by placing your nondominant hand on it.
   b. Flex the wrist while you apply resistance with your dominant hand (see Figure 17-25).
   c. Extend the wrist while you apply resistance.

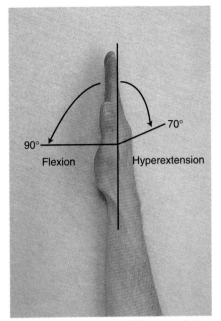

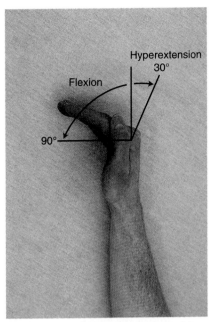

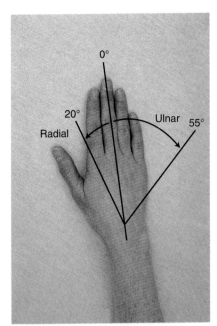

A. Hyperextension and Flexion of the Wrist

B. Flexion and Hyperextension of the Fingers

C. Radial and Ulnar Deviation of the Wrist

Figure 17-24 Range of Motion of the Wrist and Hand Joints

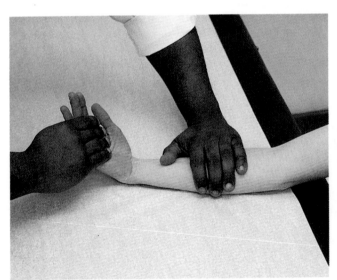

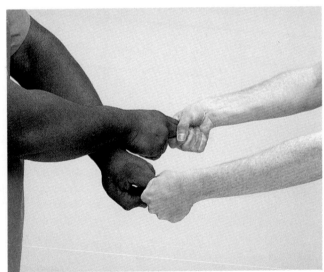

Figure 17-25 Muscle Strength of the Wrist

Figure 17-26 Muscle Strength of the Hand

9. Assess the strength of the fingers. Ask the patient to:
   a. Spread the fingers apart while you apply resistance.
   b. Push the fingers together while you apply resistance.
10. Assess the strength of the hand grasp. Ask the patient to:
    a. Grasp your dominant index and middle fingers in the patient's dominant hand and your nondominant index and middle fingers in the patient's nondominant hand (see Figure 17-26).
    b. Squeeze your fingers as hard as possible.
    c. Release their grasp.

E **Examination**
N **Normal Findings**
A **Abnormal Findings**
P **Pathophysiology**

N *There are five fingers on each hand. The normal range of motion for the wrists is: extension — 0°, hyperextension — 70°, flexion — 90°, radial deviation — 20°, ulnar deviation — 55°. The normal range of motion for the metacarpophalangeal joints is: hyperextension — 30° and flexion — 90°.*

A Extra fingers, loss of fingers, or webbing between fingers is abnormal.

P **Polydactyly** is the congenital presence of extra digits (see Figure 17-27A). **Syndactyly** is the congenital webbing or fusion of fingers or toes (see Figure 17-27B).

A Bony enlargement or bony deformities of the joints of the hand are abnormal.

P Osteoarthritis is associated with bony enlargement of the proximal interphalangeal joint (**Bouchard's node**) and the distal interphalangeal joint (**Heberden's node**) of the finger. These enlargements are hard and nontender. Bony enlargement may be masked by subcutaneous swelling. Bony enlargement is usually symmetrical (see Figure 17-28).

P Rheumatoid arthritis results in ulnar deviation (see Figure 17-29A), swan neck deformity (Figure 17-29B), and boutonniere deformities of the fingers. The patient frequently complains of pain, especially early in the morning. The joints may feel boggy on palpation. ROM may be restricted.

A A round, cystic growth near the tendons of the wrist or joint capsule is abnormal.

P A **ganglion** is a benign growth that is usually nontender and more prominent on the dorsum of the hand and wrist. Its etiology is unknown (see Figure 17-30).

A Flexion of the fingers is abnormal.

P Dupuytren's contracture is a flexion contracture that affects the little finger, ring finger, and middle finger. Pain does not normally accompany this disorder. It is caused by the progressive contracture of the palmar fascia from an unknown etiology (see Figure 17-31).

A Muscular atrophy of the thenar eminence is abnormal.

P This disorder occurs in median nerve compression such as in carpal tunnel syndrome.

A Severe flexion ankylosis of the wrist is abnormal.

P Ankylosis can be caused by rheumatoid arthritis or severe disuse (see Figure 17-32).

A Wrist drop, demonstrated by the inability of the patient to flex the fisted hand downward at the wrist, is abnormal.

P Radial nerve injury may cause wrist drop.

A Inability of the patient to prevent moving of spread fingers together is abnormal.

P Ulnar nerve injury causes weakness of the fingers.

A Weakness of opposition of the thumb and ipsilateral finger against resistance is abnormal.

P Median nerve disorders, such as carpal tunnel syndrome, affect thumb opposition. Weak thumb opposition usually occurs from injuries where the hand is outstretched during a fall or from a twisting motion.

NURSING TIP

Significance of Hand Grasp Strength

Although some nurses measure hand grasp strength as part of assessment, the true significance of this measurement may be in representing the patient's ability to respond to a command. A strong hand grasp around an object (e.g., the nurse's fingers or hand) as demonstrated by patients with brain disorders may actually represent a reflex action. When assessing muscle strength, arm muscle strength should thus always be considered more representative of muscle strength than is hand grasp strength.

E **Examination**
N **Normal Findings**
A **Abnormal Findings**
P **Pathophysiology**

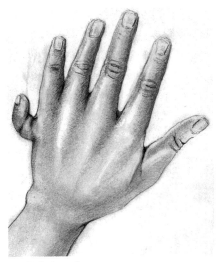

A. Polydactyly

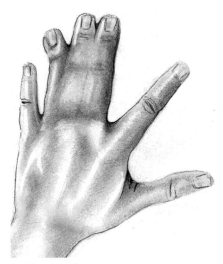

B. Syndactyly

Figure 17-27 Finger Abnormalities

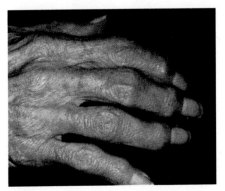

Figure 17-28 Bouchard's Nodes and Heberden's Nodes *Courtesy of Delmar Publishers, Albany, NY*

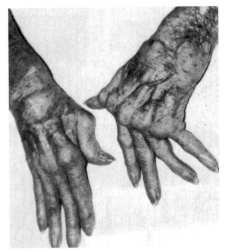

A. Ulnar Deviation *Courtesy of Delmar Publishers, Albany, NY*

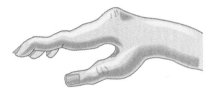

B. Swan Neck Deformity

Figure 17-29 Bony Deformities of the Hand

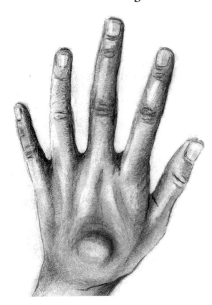

Figure 17-30 Ganglion

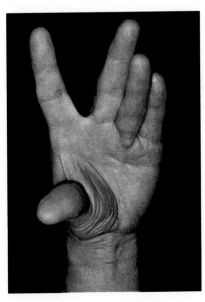

Figure 17-31 Dupuytren's Contracture

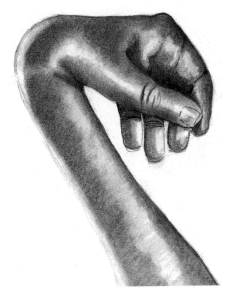

Figure 17-32 Flexion Ankylosis

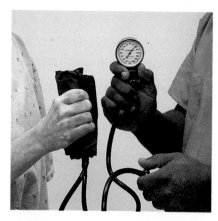

Figure 17-33 Assessing Grip Strength Using a Blood Pressure Cuff

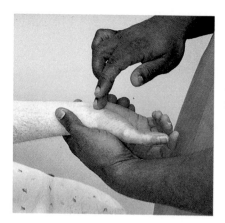

Figure 17-34 Assessing for Tinel's Sign

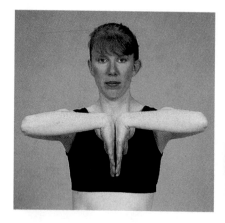

Figure 17-35 Assessing for Phalen's Sign

E	Examination
N	Normal Findings
A	Abnormal Findings
P	Pathophysiology

✹ SPECIAL TECHNIQUE

Assessing Grip Strength Using a Blood Pressure Cuff

E
1. Roll up a blood pressure cuff into a ball and inflate the cuff to 20 mm Hg.
2. Ask the patient to squeeze the inflated cuff (to determine the strength of the hand grasp action).
3. Note the increase in mm Hg during the grasp (refer to Figure 17-33).
4. Assess the strength of the other hand.

N *A healthy individual can usually achieve 150 mm Hg during a strong hand grasp action.*

A A hand grasp that measures below 150 mm Hg is abnormal.

P Neurological pathology, such as in stroke, myasthenia gravis, as well as musculoskeletal disease such as MS, and rheumatoid arthritis can lead to decreased grip strength.

✹ SPECIAL TECHNIQUE

Assessing for Tinel's Sign

E
1. Place the patient in a sitting position with the arm flexed at the elbow and the palm facing up.
2. Using the index or middle finger of the dominant hand, briskly tap the center of the patient's wrist (median nerve) (see Figure 17-34).
3. Ask the patient to describe the sensations that occur in the forearm, hands, thumb, or fingers.
4. Repeat the technique on the other wrist.

N *There will be no tingling or burning noted in the hand, thumb, or fingers.*

A A positive Tinel's test, indicated by a tingling or pricking sensation that occurs in the hand, thumb, and index and middle fingers when the median nerve is tapped, is abnormal.

P A positive Tinel's test is indicative of median nerve compression (carpal tunnel syndrome).

✹ SPECIAL TECHNIQUE

Assessing for Phalen's Sign

E
1. Place the patient in a sitting position with the arms flexed at the elbow and the backs of the hands pressed together (see Figure 17-35).
2. Ask the patient to maintain the wrist flexion of 90° for at least 1 minute.
3. Ask the patient to describe the sensations that occur in the hands and fingers.

N *There will be no change in the sensation of the hands and fingers.*

A A positive Phalen's test, indicated by sensations of numbness and paresthesia in the palmar aspect of the hand and in the fingers (especially the first three fingers), is abnormal. These sensations disappear when the wrist joint is returned to its neutral anatomic position.

P A positive Phalen's test is indicative of carpal tunnel syndrome.

Hips

Trendelenburg Test

E 1. Ask the patient to stand on one foot, with the knee of the non-weight-bearing leg flexed to raise the foot off the floor.
    2. Assess the symmetry of the iliac crests while the patient is standing on one leg.
    3. Repeat this technique on the other leg.

N *The iliac crest on the side opposite the weight-bearing leg elevates slightly.*

A It is abnormal for the iliac crest on the nonweight-bearing leg to drop.

P This finding is a positive Trendelenburg test and it is indicative of hip dislocation. The weakness of the gluteus medius muscle causes the hip on the unaffected side to drop.

E 1. While the patient is standing, inspect the iliac crests (refer to the Special Technique for the Trendelenburg test), size and symmetry of the buttocks, and number of gluteal folds (see Figure 17-36).
    2. Observe the patient's gait, if not previously assessed (refer to General Assessment).
    3. Assist the patient to a supine position on the examination table with the legs straight and the feet pointing toward the ceiling.
    4. Palpate the hip joints.
    5. Assess ROM of the hips. Ask the patient to:
       a. Raise the leg straight off the examination table with the knee extended (hip flexion with knee straight). The other leg should remain on the table (see Figure 17-37A).

E	**Examination**
N	**Normal Findings**
A	**Abnormal Findings**
P	**Pathophysiology**

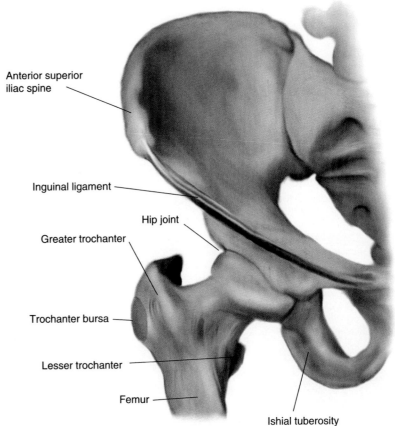

Anterior superior iliac spine

Inguinal ligament

Hip joint

Greater trochanter

Trochanter bursa

Lesser trochanter

Femur

Ishial tuberosity

Figure 17-36 Anatomy of the Hip Joint

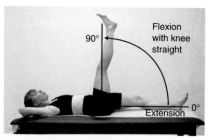

A. Flexion with Knee Straight

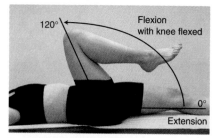

B. Flexion with Knee Flexed

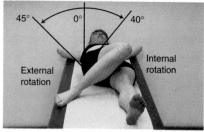

C. Internal Rotation and External Rotation

b. With the knee flexed, raise the leg off the examination table toward the chest as far as possible (hip flexion with knee flexed). The other leg should remain on the table (see Figure 17-37B). This is called the Thomas test.

c. Flex the hip and knee. Move the flexed leg medially as the foot moves outward (internal rotation) (see Figure 17-37C).

d. Flex the hip and knee. Move the flexed leg laterally as the foot moves medially (external rotation) (see Figure 17-37D).

e. With the knee straight, swing the leg away from the midline (abduction) (see Figure 17-37E).

f. With the knee straight, swing the leg toward the midline (adduction).

g. Roll over onto the abdomen and assume a prone position.

h. From the hip, move the leg back as far as possible while maintaining the pelvis on the table (hyperextension) (see Figure 17-37F). This can also be performed while the patient is standing.

6. Assist the patient to a supine position.

7. Assess strength of the hips.

a. Place the palm of your hand on the anterior thigh, above the knee. Instruct the patient to raise the leg against your resistance (see Figure 17-38A). Repeat on the other leg.

b. Place the palm of your hand posteriorly above and behind the knee. Instruct the patient to lower the leg against your resistance. Repeat on the other leg.

c. Place your hands on the lateral aspects of the patient's legs at the level of the knee. Instruct the patient to move the legs apart against your resistance (see Figure 17-38B).

d. Place your hands on the medial aspects of the patient's legs just above the knee. Instruct the patient to move the legs together against your resistance.

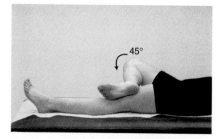

D. Position of the Leg for Full External Rotation

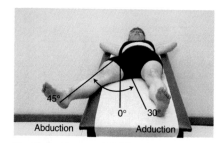

E. Abduction and Adduction

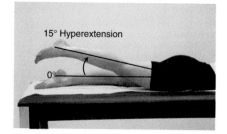

F. Hyperextension

Figure 17-37 Range of Motion of the Hip Joint

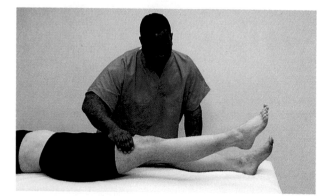

A. Flexion with Opposing Force

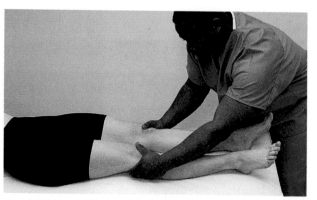

B. Abduction with Opposing Force

Figure 17-38 Muscle Strength of the Hip

N *The normal ROM for the hips is: flexion with knee straight — 90°, flexion with knee flexed — 120°, internal rotation — 40°, external rotation — 45°, abduction — 45°, adduction — 30°, hyperextension — 15°.*

A A leg that is externally rotated and painful on movement is abnormal.

P These findings occur in hip fractures, which usually result from falls (especially in elderly persons). The affected leg may also be shorter. Refer to the Special Technique for guidelines on measuring limb length.

A A positive Thomas test, when the patient is unable to flex one knee and hip while simultaneously maintaining the other leg in full extension, is abnormal. There may be slight to moderate hip and knee flexion of the extended leg.

P Flexion contractures of the hip joint, such as in long term degenerative joint diseases, will result in a positive Thomas test. This test will identify hip flexion contractures that are masked by lumbar lordosis.

✸ SPECIAL TECHNIQUE

Measuring Limb Length

E 1. Place the patient in a supine position on the examination table with the legs extended.
2. Measure the leg from the anterior superior iliac spine to the medial malleolus (see Figure 17-39).
3. Repeat on the other limb.
4. Compare measurements.

N *Limb length measurements should be within 1 to 3 cm of each other.*

A A more than 3-cm difference in the length of limbs is abnormal.

P Unilateral discrepancy in lower limb length may be a congenital defect.

P Sudden unilateral decrease in limb length occurs with fracture and dislocation of the hip and leg.

P A displaced proximal femoral shaft fracture (hip fracture) can result in limb shortening and internal or external rotation. Internal rotation is common if the patient fell forward during the fall, and external rotation is common if the patient fell onto the buttocks. The patient is unable to straighten the leg into its neutral anatomic position.

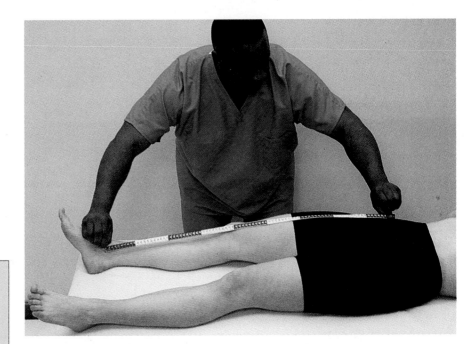

E Examination
N Normal Findings
A Abnormal Findings
P Pathophysiology

Figure 17-39 Measuring Limb Length

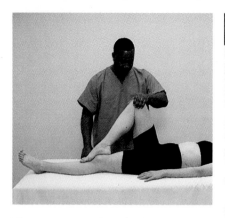

Figure 17-40 Patrick's Test

✹ SPECIAL TECHNIQUE

Patrick's Test

E **1.** Place the patient in a supine position on the examination table.
  2. Position the heel of the right foot on the knee of the left leg.
  3. Lower the right leg toward the examination table by placing moderate manual pressure on the right knee (see Figure 17-40).
  4. Note if pain occurs with movement, and the distance the knee can be lowered.
  5. Repeat on the opposite leg.

N *You are able to lower the leg being tested to the point that the knee touches the examination table or at least is parallel to the opposite leg. Pain should not occur as the leg is being lowered toward the examination table.*

A It is abnormal to be unable to lower the leg being tested (i.e., the leg being tested remains higher than the other leg) or if pain occurs in the lower back or inguinal area as the leg is being lowered toward the examination table.

P A positive Patrick's test may be indicative of degenerative hip joint disease.
P Spasm of the iliopsoas muscle may also cause a positive Patrick's test.

Knees

E **1.** With the patient standing, note the position of the knees in relation to each other and in relation to the hips, thighs, ankles, and feet.
  2. Ask the patient to sit on the examination table with the knees flexed and resting at the edge of the table.
  3. Inspect the contour of the knees. Note the normal depressions around the patella (see Figure 17-41).

E Examination
N Normal Findings
A Abnormal Findings
P Pathophysiology

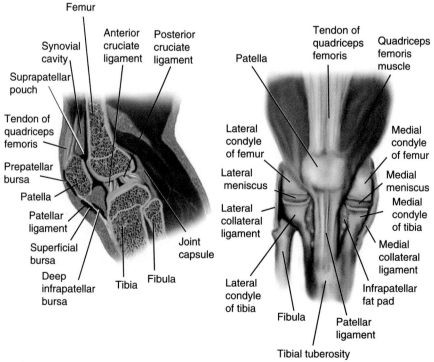

A. Sagittal Section   B. Anterior View

Figure 17-41 Anatomy of the Right Knee Joint

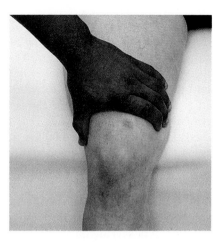

Figure 17-42 Palpating the Knee

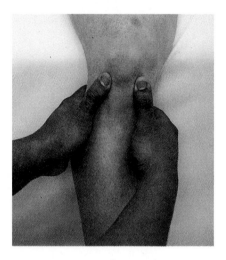

Figure 17-43 Palpating the Tibiofemoral Joint

4. Inspect the suprapatellar pouch and the prepatellar bursa.
5. Note the quadriceps muscle, located on the anterior thigh.
6. Palpate the knees. The patient may assume a supine position if this is more comfortable.
   a. Grasp the anterior thigh approximately 10 cm above the patella, with your thumb on one side of the knee and the other four fingers on the other side of the knee (see Figure 17-42).
   b. As you palpate, gradually move your hand down the suprapatellar pouch.
7. Palpate the tibiofemoral joints. It is best to have the knee flexed to 90° when performing this assessment.
   a. Place both thumbs on the knee, with the fingers wrapped around the knee posteriorly.
   b. Press in with the thumbs as you palpate the tibial margins (see Figure 17-43).
   c. Palpate the lateral collateral ligament.
8. If knee fluid is suspected, test for the bulge sign and ballottement. Refer to the Special Techniques on pages 530 and 531.
9. Assess ROM of the knees. Ask the patient to stand and:
   a. Bend the knee (flexion) (see Figure 17-44).
   b. Straighten the knee (extension). The patient may also be able to hyperextend the knee during this movement.
10. Assess strength of the knees with the patient seated and the legs hanging off the table.
    a. Ask the patient to bend the knee. Place your nondominant hand under the knee and place your other hand over the ankle.
    b. Instruct the patient to straighten the leg against your resistance (see Figure 17-45).
    c. Ask the patient to place the foot on the bed and the knee at approximately 45° of flexion. Place one hand under the knee and place the other hand over the ankle.
    d. Instruct the patient to maintain the foot on the table despite your attempts to straighten the leg.

N *The knees are in alignment with each other and do not protrude medially or laterally. The normal ROM for the knees is: flexion — 130°, extension — 0°; in some cases, hyperextension is possible up to 15°.*

E	**Examination**
N	**Normal Findings**
A	**Abnormal Findings**
P	**Pathophysiology**

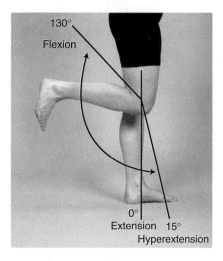

Figure 17-44 Range of Motion of the Knee Joint: Flexion, Extension, and Hyperextension

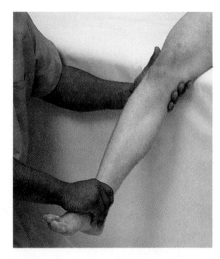

Figure 17-45 Strength of Knee Joint

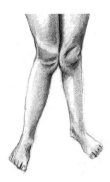

Figure 17-46 Genu Valgum

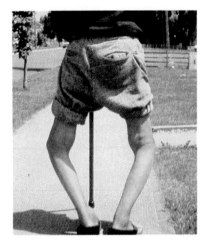

Figure 17-47 Genu Varum *Courtesy of Delmar Publishers, Albany, NY*

A Alteration in lower limb alignment is considered an abnormal finding.

P **Genu valgum** (knock knees) is inward deviation toward the midline at the level of the knees. Both legs are usually affected by the disorder. It is detected as an increased distance between the medial malleoli when the femoral condyles are close together and the patella are facing forward. The knees appear closer together than is normal. Genu valgum can be congenital or acquired (rickets) (refer to Figure 17-46).

P **Genu varum** (bow legs) is outward deviation away from the midline at the level of the knees. Both legs are usually affected by the disorder. It is detected as an increased distance between the femoral condyles when the medial malleoli are close together and the patella are facing forward. The knees appear farther apart than is normal. Genu varum can be congenital or acquired. This syndrome is common in horse jockeys due to the stretching of the nearby ligaments. It may also be seen in rickets, rheumatoid arthritis, and osteomalacia due to the body's attempt to bend bone shape in order to tolerate the weight of the upper body (refer to Figure 17-47).

✳ **SPECIAL TECHNIQUE**

Assessing for Bulge Sign

The bulge sign tests for small effusions (4 to 8 ml) in the knee.

E **1.** Place the patient in a supine position with the legs extended.
   2. Firmly milk upward the medial aspect of the patella several times. This displaces any fluid (refer to Figure 17-48A).
   3. Press or tap the lateral aspect of the knee.
   4. Observe the hollow on the medial aspect of the knee for a bulge of fluid (refer to Figure 17-48B).

N *Normally there is no fluid return to the knee. This is a negative bulge sign.*

A The return of fluid to the medial aspect of the patella is abnormal.

P A positive bulge sign is present in joint effusion.

E	**Examination**
N	**Normal Findings**
A	**Abnormal Findings**
P	**Pathophysiology**

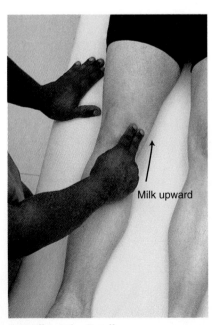

Milk upward

A. Milking the Patella

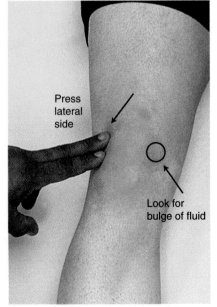

Press lateral side

Look for bulge of fluid

B. Observing for Fluid

Figure 17-48 Assessing for Bulge Sign

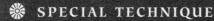

SPECIAL TECHNIQUE

Patellar Ballottement

Ballottement is performed to detect large effusions in the knee.

E   **1.** Place the patient either in a supine position with the legs extended or sitting up with the knees flexed at 90° and hanging over the edge of the examination table.
  2. Firmly grasp the thigh (with your thumb on one side and the four fingers on the other side) just above the patella. This compresses fluid out of the suprapatellar pouch.
  3. With your other hand, push the patella back toward the femur (see Figure 17-49).
  4. Feel for a click.

N   *There is no palpable click. Normally, the patella is close to the femur because there is no excess fluid.*

A   A palpable click is abnormal.

P   When fluid is present between the femur and the patella, the patella "floats" on top of the femur. As the patella is pushed back, fluid is displaced and a palpable click is felt when the patella hits the femur.

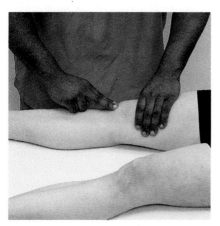

Figure 17-49   Patellar Ballottement

SPECIAL TECHNIQUE

Assessing for Apley's Sign

This test is performed to identify a loose and movable object within the knee joint:

E   **1.** Place the patient into a prone position on the examination table.
  2. Manually flex the knee to a 90° angle so that the lower leg is perpendicular to the table.
  3. With the dominant hand, apply firm downward pressure on the foot while simultaneously rotating the lower leg inward and then outward (see Figure 17-50).
  4. Assess for limited knee joint movement or audible clicks during knee joint movement.
  5. Repeat on the other knee.

N   *The patient will be able to flex the knee joint to a 90° angle and no audible clicks will be heard during joint movement.*

A   A positive Apley's sign of the knee joint is indicated by limited movement of the knee joint (locking of the knee joint) or audible clicks.

P   A positive Apley's sign is suggestive of a loose object, such as torn cartilage, within the knee joint.

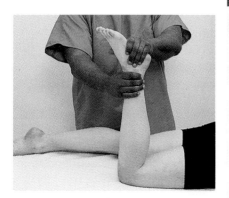

Figure 17-50   Assessing for Apley's Sign

SPECIAL TECHNIQUE

Assessing for McMurray's Sign

This test is performed to assess the integrity of the meniscus of the knee.

E   **1.** Place the patient in a supine position on the examination table and stand on the affected side.
  2. Manually flex the hip and knee. Hold the patient's heel with one hand and stabilize the knee with the other hand (see Figure 17-51).
  3. Using the hand that is holding the heel, internally rotate the leg while applying resistance to the medial aspect of the knee joint. This assesses the medial meniscus.
  4. Move the knee to a position of full extension. Note if full extension of the knee joint can be achieved or tolerated by the patient.

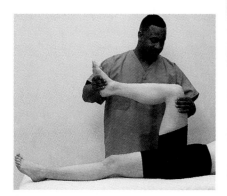

Figure 17-51   Assessing for McMurray's Sign

continued

5. Flex the hip and knee and externally rotate the leg. While stabilizing the knee joint, apply resistance to the lateral aspect of the knee joint. This assesses the lateral meniscus.

6. Assess for an audible or palpable click of the knee joint.

N *The patient will be able to extend the leg at the knee joint and there will be no audible or palpable click detected.*

A A positive McMurray's sign is indicated when the patient is unable to extend the leg at the knee joint or when an audible or palpable click is detected.

P A positive McMurray's sign is suggestive of torn meniscus cartilage of the knee. The patient may also state that full extension of the knee joint is impossible, that the knee joint "locks into place," or that "it feels like something is in the knee joint." If the torn meniscus cartilage is obstructing the articulating function of the joint, knee joint extension will be limited.

✷ SPECIAL TECHNIQUE

Drawer Test

This test is performed to assess the stability of the anterior and posterior cruciate ligaments of the knee.

E 1. Assist the patient to a supine position on the examination table.

2. Instruct the patient to flex the right knee to 90° and to flex the right hip joint to 45°, placing the right foot flat on the examination table.

3. Sit on the patient's right foot to stabilize it in place.

4. Observe for "sagging" of the tibia, resulting in visible concavity below the patella (gravity drawer test, or "sag" sign).

5. Place both hands on the patient's right tibia, with the thumb of the right hand on the medial aspect of the knee, and the left thumb on the lateral aspect of the knee (see Figure 17-52).

6. Attempt to move the tibia forward (anterior drawer test) and then backward (posterior drawer test).

7. Repeat on the left leg.

N *You will not be able to pull the tibia forward more than 6 mm or to move the tibia backward at all. Concavity should not be detected distal to the patella.*

A An abnormal result is indicated by the ability to move the tibia forward more than 6 mm or to move the tibia backward.

P Forward movement of the tibia more than 6 mm indicates a tear in the anterior cruciate ligament of the knee. A false positive result may occur if the patient has instability of the posterior cruciate ligament of the knee.

P "Sagging" of the tibia or backward movement of the tibia indicates a tear in the posterior cruciate ligament of the knee.

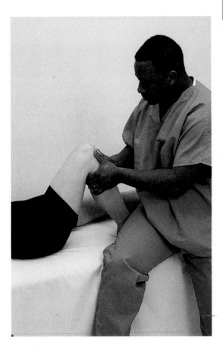

Figure 17-52 Drawer Test

✷ SPECIAL TECHNIQUE

Lachman's Test

This test is performed to assess for stability of the anterior cruciate ligament of the knee. It is considered the most reliable assessment technique for detecting instability of the anterior cruciate ligament.

E 1. Place the patient in a supine position on the examination table with the unaffected knee flexed to approximately 30°. The affected leg should be fully extended and in contact with the examination table.

continued

E	**Examination**
N	**Normal Findings**
A	**Abnormal Findings**
P	**Pathophysiology**

2. Stabilize the femur of the affected leg by holding the leg above the knee joint with the right hand.

3. Grasp the affected lower leg beneath the knee with the left hand and move the tibia forward.

4. Note any changes in the infrapatellar slope.

N   *When the tibia is moved forward, the infrapatellar tendon slope should still be noticeable.*

A   It is abnormal for the infrapatellar tendon slope to no longer be noticeable when the tibia is moved forward.

P   A positive Lachman's test is indicative of damage to the anterior cruciate ligament of the knee.

Ankles and Feet

> ### 🌸 NURSING TIP
>
> **Assessing a Patient's Shoes**
>
> Examine the patient's shoes and observe for wear in unusual areas. This provides information on the patient's weight bearing. Keep this in mind as you watch the patient stand and walk.

E   **1.** Inspect the ankles and feet (see Figure 17-53) as the patient stands, walks, and sits (bearing no weight).

2. Inspect the alignment of the feet and toes with the lower leg.

3. Inspect the shape and position of the toes.

4. Assist the patient to a supine position on the examination table.

5. Stand by the patient's feet.

6. Palpate the ankle and foot.

    a. Grasp the heel with the fingers of both hands. Use your thumbs to palpate the anterior, lateral, and medial aspects of the ankle (see Figure 17-54).

    b. Use your finger pads to palpate the Achilles tendon.

    c. Palpate with your thumb and index finger each metatarsophalangeal joint.

    d. Between your thumb and index finger, palpate the medial and lateral surfaces of each interphalangeal joint.

E	Examination
N	Normal Findings
A	Abnormal Findings
P	Pathophysiology

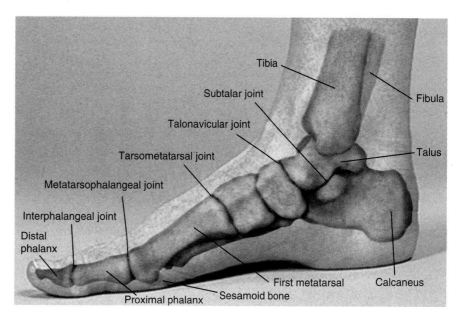

Figure 17-53   Anatomy of the Ankle and Foot

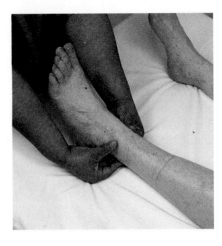

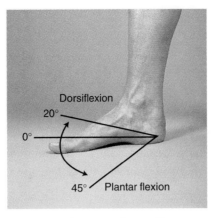

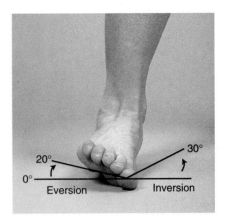

A. Plantar Flexion and Dorsiflexion   B. Eversion and Inversion

Figure 17-54 Palpation of the Ankle   **Figure 17-55** Range of Motion of the Ankle and Foot

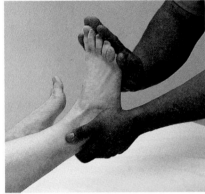

Figure 17-56 Strength of the Ankle and Foot

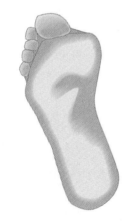

Figure 17-57 Hallux Valgus

E	**Examination**
N	**Normal Findings**
A	**Abnormal Findings**
P	**Pathophysiology**

7. Assess ROM of the ankles and feet. Ask the patient to:
  a. Point the toes toward the chest by moving the ankle (dorsiflexion) (see Figure 17-55A).
  b. Point the toes toward the floor by moving the ankle (plantar flexion).
  c. Turn the soles of the feet outward (eversion) (see Figure 17-55B).
  d. Turn the soles of the feet inward (inversion).
  e. Curl the toes toward the floor (flexion).
  f. Spread the toes apart (abduction).
  g. Move the toes together (adduction).
8. Assess strength of the ankles and feet.
  a. Assist the patient to a supine position on the examination table with the legs extended and the feet slightly apart.
  b. Stand at the foot of the examination table.
  c. Place your left hand on top of the patient's right foot and place your right hand on top of the patient's left foot.
  d. Ask the patient to point the toes toward the chest (dorsiflexion) despite your resistance.
  e. Place your left hand on the sole of the patient's right foot and place your right hand on the sole of the patient's left foot.
  f. Ask the patient to point the toes down (plantar flexion) despite your resistance. This technique can also be performed one foot at a time as demonstrated in Figure 17-56.

N *The foot is in alignment with the lower leg. The normal ROM for the ankles and feet is: dorsiflexion — 20°, plantar flexion — 45°, eversion — 20°, inversion — 30°, abduction — 30°, and adduction — 10°.*

A An alteration in the shape and the position of the foot is considered abnormal.

P **Pes varus** describes a foot that is turned inward toward the midline.

P **Pes valgus** occurs when the foot is turned laterally away from the midline.

P **Pes planus** (flat foot) refers to a foot with a low longitudinal arch.

P **Pes cavus** refers to a foot with an exaggerated arch height.

P In **hallux valgus** (bunion), the big toe is deviated laterally while the first metatarsal is deviated medially. The metatarsophalangeal joint enlarges and becomes inflamed from the pressure. A bursa may form at this point. Hallux valgus can be congenital or caused by narrow shoes and arthritis (see Figure 17-57).

P Tight shoes can also cause **hammertoe**. In hammertoe, there is a flexion of the proximal interphalangeal joint and hyperextension of the distal metatarsophalangeal joint. A corn or callus can develop from undue pressure at the point of flexion (see Figure 17-58).

P A **corn** is a conical area of thickened skin. It extends into the dermis and can be painful. Corns are caused by pressure on the affected area,

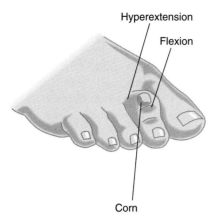

Figure 17-58 Hammertoe with Corn

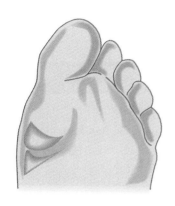

Figure 17-59 Callus

particularly over bony prominences. Tight shoes and hammertoe can cause corns.

P A **callus** is a thickening of the skin due to prolonged pressure. It usually occurs on the sole of the foot and is not painful (see Figure 17-59).

A A swollen, red, warm, and painful metatarsophalangeal joint is abnormal.

P The first metatarsophalangeal joint is usually affected in acute gouty arthritis.

A Decreased ROM of the ankle is abnormal.

P The patient with an ankle sprain or fracture secondary to injury or trauma complains of pain on palpation and ROM. Crepitus may be present in an ankle fracture. Ankle sprain cannot always be differentiated from ankle fracture without the use of x-rays. Refer these patients to an orthopedist.

 SPECIAL TECHNIQUE

Assessing Status of Distal Limbs and Digits

When you suspect distal limb or digit hypoperfusion due to trauma, injury, or pathology, conduct the following assessment:

E 1. Uncover the distal aspects of both limbs being assessed. A bilateral assessment allows for comparison of the affected and unaffected limbs. When assessing an injured limb, assess the limb areas proximal and distal to the site of injury.
2. Assess for swelling.
3. Assess the vascular status of the distal limb and its digits (peripheral pulses, skin color, skin temperature, and capillary refill).
4. Ask the patient to perform specific movements of the distal limb on command.
   a. To assess the ulnar nerve, ask the patient to perform abduction of the fingers.
   b. To assess the radial nerve, ask the patient to perform hyperextension of the thumb or wrist.
   c. To assess the median nerve, ask the patient to perform opposition of the thumb to the little finger of the same hand.
   d. To assess the peroneal nerve, ask the patient to perform dorsiflexion of the toes and ankle.
   e. To assess the tibial nerve, ask the patient to perform plantar flexion of the toes and ankle.
5. When assessing sensation, instruct the patient to close the eyes to prevent biased results. Use the thumb and index finger of the dominant hand to pinch certain areas of the distal limb.
   a. To assess the ulnar nerve, pinch the finger pad of the little finger.
   b. To assess the radial nerve, pinch the web space between the thumb and the index finger.
   c. To assess the median nerve, pinch the distal aspect of the index finger.
   d. To assess the peroneal nerve, pinch the lateral aspect of the great toe and the medial surface of the second toe.
   e. To assess the tibial nerve, pinch the medial and lateral surfaces of the sole of the foot.

N *The individual with normal perfusion to the limbs and digits will appear comfortable during rest and muscle contraction. Pain will not occur with movement of the distal limb or digits. Limb perfusion will be manifested by strong peripheral pulses, warm skin temperature, and a brisk capillary refill. There will be complete motor and sensory function of the distal limb and digits. The patient will not experience any numbness or tingling.*

A Neurovascular deterioration, manifested by the "5 P's" (pain, pallor, decreased perfusion, paresthesia, and paralysis) is abnormal.

continued

P Neurovascular deterioration can occur in compartment syndrome. It is a severe complication of musculoskeletal trauma in which swelling is limited due to a confined space. Pain is the most significant and the earliest clinical manifestation of acute compartment syndrome. It occurs distal to the site of injury and is induced by the contraction of the muscle compartment being compressed. Pain results from stretching of a muscle that is experiencing vascular compromise.

P Inadequate arterial flow is a complication of digit or limb replantation following traumatic amputation.

P Arterial occlusion may also be detected as a complication of fracture or dislocation.

A Inadequate venous flow from the distal limb or digits, manifested by cyanosis, mottling, skin temperature that is warmer than usual, immediate capillary refill, and a distended or tense tissue turgor, is abnormal.

P Inadequate venous flow is a complication of digit or limb replantation following traumatic amputation.

✳ SPECIAL TECHNIQUE

Thompson Test

E **1.** Assist the patient to a prone position with the feet hanging over the edge of the examination table.
     2. Manually squeeze the calf muscles of the leg.
     3. Observe for plantar flexion of the foot being examined.

N *When the calf muscles are squeezed, you should be able to visualize plantar flexion of the foot on the leg being examined.*

A A positive Thompson test is manifested by the absence of plantar flexion when the calf muscles are squeezed.

P A positive Thompson test is suggestive of a ruptured Achilles tendon.

Spine

E **1.** Ask the patient to stand and to leave the back of the gown open.
     2. Stand behind the patient so that you can visualize the posterior anatomy.
     3. Inspect the position and alignment of the spine from a posterior and a lateral position.
     4. Draw an imaginary line:
       a. From the head down through the spinous processes (see Figure 17-60A).
       b. Across the top of the scapula (see Figure 17-60B).
       c. Across the top of the iliac crests.
       d. Across the bottom of the gluteal folds.
     5. Palpate the spinous processes with your thumb.
     6. Palpate the paravertebral muscles.
     7. Assess ROM of the spine. Ask the patient to bend forward from the waist and touch the toes (flexion) (see Figure 17-61A).
     8. If necessary, stabilize the patient's pelvis with your hands during the ROM assessment. Ask the patient to:
       a. Bend to each side (lateral bending) (see Figure 17-61B).
       b. Bend backward (hyperextension).
       c. Twist the shoulders to each side (rotation) (see Figure 17-61C).

✿ NURSING TIP

Differentiating Back Pain

Keep in mind that tenderness of the costovertebral angle can indicate a musculoskeletal problem or a kidney problem. Integrate the information obtained during the health history with clinical findings to guide your nursing interventions.

E Examination
N Normal Findings
A Abnormal Findings
P Pathophysiology

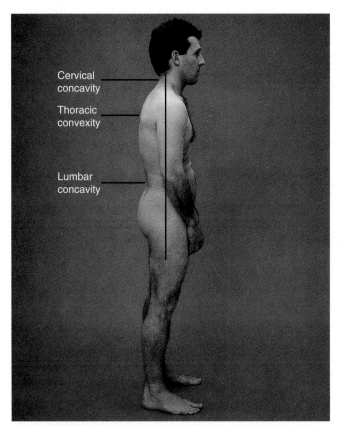

Cervical concavity

Thoracic convexity

Lumbar concavity

A. Lateral View

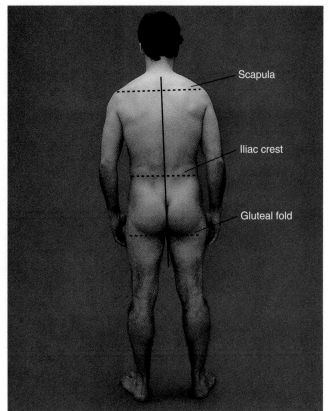

Scapula

Iliac crest

Gluteal fold

B. Posterior View

Figure 17-60 Alignment of Spinal Landmarks

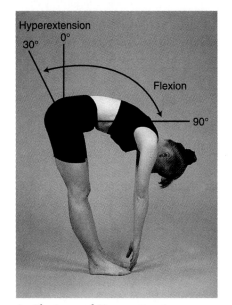

Hyperextension
0°
30°

Flexion

90°

A. Flexion and Hyperextension

35°   0°   35°

Right   Left

B. Lateral Bending

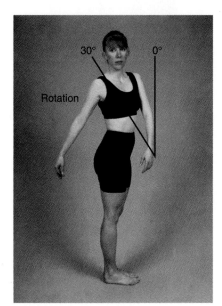

30°   0°

Rotation

C. Rotation

Figure 17-61 Range of Motion of the Spine

E	Examination
N	Normal Findings
A	Abnormal Findings
P	Pathophysiology

N *The normal spine has a cervical concavity, a thoracic convexity, and a lumbar concavity. An imaginary line can be drawn from the head straight down the spinous processes to the gluteal cleft. The imaginary lines drawn from the scapula, iliac crests, and gluteal folds are symmetrical with each other. The normal ROM of the spine is: flexion — 90°, hyperextension — 30°, lateral bending — 35°, and rotation — 30°. As the patient flexes forward, the concavity of the lumbar spine disappears and the entire back assumes a convex C shape.*

A From a posterior view, **scoliosis** (lateral curvature of the thoracic or lumbar vertebrae) may be detectable (see Figure 17-62A, B) and is an abnormal finding. The curvature is visible despite voluntary attempts at proper posture. This is structural scoliosis. The curvature becomes accentuated on forward flexion from the waist. Scoliosis may also be accompanied by asymmetry of the clavicles, uneven shoulder and iliac crest levels, and a visible prominence of a scapula. One leg may be longer than the other, and limb length should be measured. If the lateral curvature is allowed to progress beyond 55°, cardiopulmonary problems can occur. Surgery may be indicated if the curve exceeds 40°.

P Structural scoliosis occurs most frequently in adolescence, especially in females.

A Functional scoliosis, which manifests itself only in a standing position, is abnormal.

P Functional scoliosis is due to unequal leg length or poor posture.

A **Kyphosis**, an excessive convexity of the thoracic spine (see Figure 17-62C), is abnormal. The patient with kyphosis presents with the chin tilted downward onto the chest and with abdominal protrusion. There is also a decrease in the interval between the lower rib cage and the iliac crests. This appearance is due to forward and downward hunching of the head, neck, shoulders, and upper back.

P Kyphosis is seen in elderly patients and in patients with osteoporosis, ankylosing spondylitis, and Paget's disease.

A **Lordosis**, an excessive concavity of the lumbar spine (see Figure 17-62D), is abnormal.

P Lordosis is accentuated in obesity and pregnancy due to the change in the center of gravity.

A A **list**, a leaning of the spine (see Figure 17-62E), is abnormal. If an imaginary line is drawn straight down from T1, the gluteal cleft is lateral to it. In scoliosis, the imaginary line rests in the gluteal cleft, and the spine deviates from this straight line.

P A list can result from a herniated vertebral disc and painful paravertebral muscle spasms.

A It is abnormal to have iliac crests that are unequal in height.

P Scoliosis and congenital or acquired limb length discrepancies lead to iliac crests that are not equal in height.

A Decreased ROM is abnormal. This is usually accompanied by pain.

P These clinical findings are found in back injury, osteoarthritis, and ankylosing spondylitis.

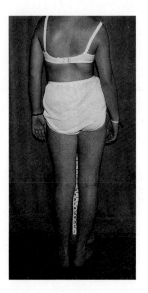

A. Scoliosis   *Courtesy of the Armed Forces Institute of Pathology*

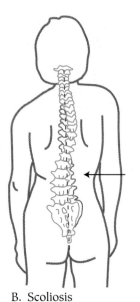

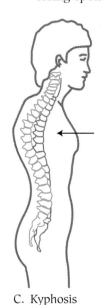

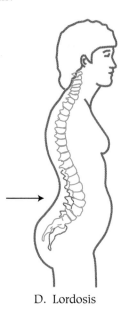

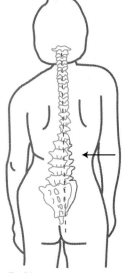

B. Scoliosis   C. Kyphosis   D. Lordosis   E. List

Figure 17-62   Abnormalities of the Spine

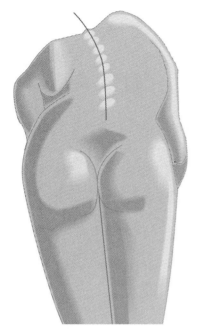

Figure 17-63 Scoliosis Screening

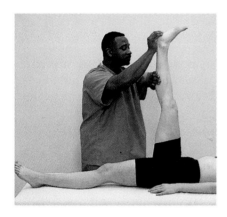

Figure 17-64 Straight Leg Raising Test

E	**Examination**
N	**Normal Findings**
A	**Abnormal Findings**
P	**Pathophysiology**

✳ **SPECIAL TECHNIQUE**

Assessing for Scoliosis

E 1. Instruct the patient to disrobe down to the underclothing.
　　 2. Have the patient stand upright with the feet together.
　　 3. Stand behind the patient and stabilize the patient's pelvis by holding both hips at the iliac crest level.
　　 4. Instruct the patient to flex forward from the waist, allowing the arms and head to hang loosely.
　　 5. Palpate each spinous process and place a dot on each with a felt-tip pen.
　　 6. With the patient in a flexed position and then in an upright position draw an imaginary line through the dots.
N *The imaginary line through the dots should be straight in both the upright and flexed positions (see Figure 17-63).*
A/P Refer to the section on spine abnormalities and pathophysiology.

✳ **SPECIAL TECHNIQUE**

Straight Leg Raising Test (Lasègue's Test)

This test is performed to assess for a herniated disc of the lumbar vertebrae.
E 1. Assist the patient to a supine position on the examination table.
　　 2. Place one hand on the heel of the right foot and place the other hand behind the upper calf area of the same leg.
　　 3. Maintain the foot in its neutral anatomic position.
　　 4. Raise the leg to the angle at which low back pain occurs.
　　 5. With the extended leg still raised to its maximum height, manually dorsiflex the foot (see Figure 17-64).
　　 6. Repeat the technique on the left leg.
N *The patient will be able to flex the hip joint and raise the straight leg to a hip flexion angle of 90°. There will be no low back pain with lifting of the extended leg or with dorsiflexion of the foot while the leg is raised.*
A A positive straight leg raising test is abnormal. The patient will be unable to raise the extended leg to a 90° angle of hip joint flexion. Low back pain will occur with any lifting of the straight leg, and this discomfort will increase when the foot is dorsiflexed while the leg is in the raised position.
P Irritation of the nerve roots of the lumbosacral area causes pain in the sciatic nerve. Pain at less than 40° generally means an irritated nerve root caused by a herniated vertebral disc. Pain may also occur in the other leg.

✳ **SPECIAL TECHNIQUE**

Milgram Test

E 1. Place the patient in a supine position on the examination table with both legs fully extended and resting on the table.
　　 2. Instruct the patient to raise both legs at least 2 inches off the examination table while maintaining the legs in extension for at least 30 seconds.
N *The patient will be able to hold the extended legs in the raised position for at least 30 seconds.*
A The inability to maintain the straight legs in the raised position for at least 30 seconds is suggestive of pressure on the spinal nerves and is abnormal.
P A positive Milgram test is often indicative of a herniated intervertebral disc.

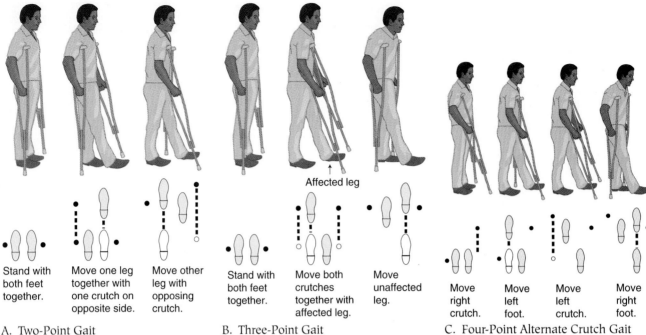

A. Two-Point Gait

Stand with both feet together.

Move one leg together with one crutch on opposite side.

Move other leg with opposing crutch.

B. Three-Point Gait

Affected leg

Stand with both feet together.

Move both crutches together with affected leg.

Move unaffected leg.

C. Four-Point Alternate Crutch Gait

Move right crutch.

Move left foot.

Move left crutch.

Move right foot.

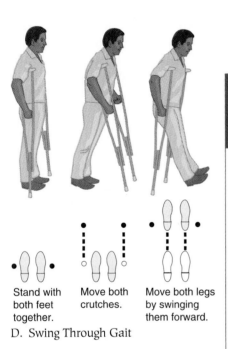

D. Swing Through Gait

Stand with both feet together.

Move both crutches.

Move both legs by swinging them forward.

Figure 17-65 Crutch Gaits

NURSING CHECKLIST
Assessing Patients with Musculoskeletal Assistive Devices

Assistive devices may be necessary to support musculoskeletal structure and function. The need for such devices automatically indicates an underlying musculoskeletal disorder. For each assistive device, determine the reason for its use.

Crutches

Determine the following:

1. Amount of weight bearing allowed on affected lower limb
2. Appropriate crutch height
3. Type of crutch gait and appropriateness for the amount of weight bearing on affected leg
   - Two-point crutch gait (partial weight bearing) (refer to Figure 17-65A).
   - Three-point crutch gait (partial or nonweight bearing) (see Figure 17-65B).
   - Four-point alternate crutch gait (partial or full weight bearing) (refer to Figure 17-65C).
   - Swing gait (nonweight bearing) (see Figure 17-65D).
4. Condition of crutches (padded handles, rubber tips)
5. Ease of transfer into and out of a chair
6. Ease of stair climbing with the crutches
7. Patient wearing flat, properly fitted shoes with nonskid surfaces
8. Signs or symptoms of skin breakdown or distal limb hypoperfusion

continued

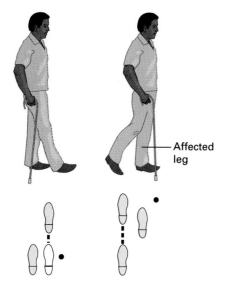

Figure 17-66 Proper Cane Stance

— Affected leg

Cane

Determine the following:

1. Shape of handle (C or T)
2. Number of points on contact surface
3. Appropriateness for patient's height
4. Cane used on unaffected side (see Figure 17-66)
5. Refer to numbers 4–8 in the section on crutches

Walker

Determine the following:

1. Amount of weight bearing allowed on the lower limb
2. Type of walker (e.g., rolling or pickup walker)
3. Appropriateness for patient's height
4. Patient's ability to grip and propel the walker forward with rolling walker; patient's ability to grip, lift, and propel the walker forward with pickup walker
5. Refer to numbers 4–8 in the section on crutches

Brace, Splint, Immobilizer

Determine the following:

1. Location of device (e.g., limb, neck, torso, lower back, or pelvis)
2. Joint position maintained by device (e.g., extension, flexion, or abduction)
3. Joint motion allowed by device
4. If a movable device is used, is the hinge joint of the device aligned with the skeletal joint?
5. Padding under pressure points of device
6. Amount of weight bearing allowed on the affected leg (lower leg device)
7. Refer to numbers 7 and 8 in the section on crutches

Cast

Determine the following:

1. Plaster or nonplaster (e.g., synthetic, fiberglass)
2. Location of cast (e.g., limb, neck, torso, pelvis, body)
3. Joint position maintained (e.g., extension, flexion, or abduction)
4. Joint motion allowed
5. Edges of the cast covered ("petaled") with tape to prevent skin irritation
6. Amount of weight bearing allowed (lower leg cast)
7. Damage to cast (e.g., cracked, flaking or crumbling, dented, wet, softening)
8. Visible discoloration on the cast (e.g., from underlying wound drainage or bleeding)
9. Significant odor around the cast (e.g., a musty or foul smell)
10. Refer to number 8 in the section on crutches

Skin Traction

Determine the following:

1. Location of traction (e.g., cervical vertebrae, limb, pelvis)
2. Type of skin traction (e.g., cervical, Buck's traction, Russell's traction)
3. Amount of traction weight being applied to the affected body part (e.g., 10 lb)

continued

4. Traction weights free falling
5. Traction rope unfrayed, taut, and unobstructed through the pulley
6. Body position being maintained in traction (e.g., extension)
7. Immobilzed body part aligned with rest of body
8. Continuous, scheduled, intermittent, or only as needed basis application of skin traction
9. Refer to number 8 in the section on crutches

Skeletal Traction
Determine the following:
1. Location of traction (e.g., cervical vertebrae, limb, pelvis)
2. Type of skeletal traction being used (e.g., running traction, balanced suspension traction)
3. Amount of skeletal traction being applied to the affected body part (e.g., 10 lb)
4. Countertraction applied (e.g., weight of the patient's body, position of the patient's bed, or traction weights); amount of countertraction applied to the affected limb (e.g., 10 lb)
5. Refer to numbers 4–8 in the section on skin traction
6. Appearance of the skeletal pin or wire sites (e.g., dry, encrusted, inflamed, draining)
7. Drainage from the skeletal pin or wire sites
8. Refer to number 8 in the section on crutches

External Fixation
Determine the following:
1. Refer to numbers 1 and 8 in the section on crutches
2. Refer to numbers 1, 6, and 7 in the section on skin traction
3. Refer to numbers 1, 6, and 7 in the section on skeletal traction
4. Looseness of screws, bolts, or bars

GERONTOLOGICAL VARIATIONS

Bone density decreases due to an increased rate of bone reabsorption, which exceeds the rate of bone cell replenishment. Bone density loss is accentuated in the elderly female due to the estrogen deficiency that accompanies menopause. Although components of bone tissue become calcified with age, the loss of bone density results in a weaker bone that is more susceptible to fracture. For example, the elderly patient with osteoporosis is at risk for hip or wrist fracture from a minor fall. Other changes seen as a result of bone density loss include thoracic kyphosis and a reduction in height. Thoracic kyphosis will cause a change in the patient's center of gravity, making the patient more prone to loss of balance and to falls.

With age, muscle fibers deteriorate and are replaced by fibrous connective tissue. Muscle atrophy is accompanied by a reduction in muscle mass, a loss of muscle strength against resistance, and a reduction in overall body mass.

The elderly patient may be less able to perform heavy physical activity or activities of daily living, especially if these activities are prolonged in duration. The severity of muscle atrophy will be influenced by the patient's activity level and by peak muscle mass. Because muscle atrophy with aging is a gradual process, some elderly patients are able to compensate for the loss in muscle strength, and changes in activities of daily living may be minimal. The ability to maintain an active lifestyle, including physical exercise, will act to prevent disuse muscle atrophy and will maximize muscle strength.

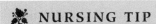 **NURSING TIP**

Reducing the Risk of Osteoporosis

Increased dietary intake of calcium; calcium supplements; estrogen supplements; calcitonin therapy; and moderate weight-bearing exercises may be helpful in minimizing the effect of osteoporosis by strengthening bone in the elderly. Unfortunately, the severity of osteoporosis in the later years is affected by the peak bone density achieved in young adulthood. Therapeutic modalities implemented in the later years may thus have limited effect.

Cartilage ages better than bone or muscle. A decrease in the water content of hyaline cartilage occurs with age, resulting in a reduction of joint flexibility and possible irregularities on the surface of the articulating cartilage. There is also a reduction in the ability of cartilage to repair itself following trauma or surgery. Articulating cartilage will deteriorate slightly due to a lifetime of wear and tear.

A decrease in the water content of the intervertebral discs occurs with age, resulting in a reduction of vertebral flexibility. Thinning of the discs, which results in a decrease in height, makes the elderly patient prone to back pain and injury.

The degree of thoracic kyphosis, muscle atrophy, articulating cartilage deterioration, and vertebral inflexibility seen with aging will directly affect the mobility of the elderly patient. During ambulation, a reduction in step height and length is common and results from joint inflexibility and reduced muscle strength. Steps may become slower or more rapid in speed (e.g., "shuffling"). Transfers in and out of a sitting position will be more difficult because of vertebral inflexibility and reduced muscle strength. Stair climbing will also be affected by the reduction in muscle strength. The elderly patient may require some degree of external support to rise from a chair, to ambulate, or to climb stairs.

⚡ NURSING ALERT

Elder Abuse and Neglect

There is an increased incidence of physical abuse and neglect among the elderly. Etiological factors may include stress related to financial difficulties, multiple family members residing in limited space, the lack of nearby family members, and the stress of dealing with an elderly relative with dementia or incontinence. Possible indications of physical abuse include unexplained bruises, swelling, hematomas, burns, fractures, poor hygiene, and poor nutritional status. Health care providers are obligated to investigate these symptoms further when they are unexplained or when the explanation is inappropriate for the location and severity of the trauma. Be familiar with your institution's policy on elder abuse.

꩜ THINK ABOUT IT

Recognizing Possible Elder Abuse and Neglect

A 78-year-old female with Alzheimer's disease is admitted through the emergency department with a diagnosis of probable aspiration pneumonia. Chest x-ray reveals pulmonary infiltrates consistent with the diagnosis of pneumonia but also reveals multiple old rib fractures. Further assessment of the patient indicates cachexia, poor general hygiene, urinary and fecal incontinence, fecal impaction, decubiti of the sacral area, bruising of both arms in a "grip" fashion, and multiple bruises and abrasions of the buttocks and lower legs. The patient moans in pain frequently during the physical assessment. Follow-up limb x-rays reveal an old healed fracture of the left humerus. The patient is a widow and has been living with her divorced daughter for the last year. The daughter is the patient's only child as well as the patient's primary caregiver. During the day, the daughter works full time and the patient is cared for by hired help. The hired caregiver claims that the patient "falls frequently during the day."
- What is your initial reaction to these clinical findings?
- Do the findings of the physical assessment indicate possible physical abuse or neglect? Explain.
- What would you say to the patient's daughter?
- What questions would you ask the patient?

CASE STUDY

The case study illustrates the application and objective documentation of the musculoskeletal assessment.

The Patient with Severe Degenerative Joint Disease of the Hip

Mrs. Rose Testa had a right total hip joint replacement yesterday due to degenerative joint disease. The health history was conducted prior to Mrs. Testa's surgery.

❖ HEALTH HISTORY

PATIENT PROFILE

58 yo MWF

CHIEF COMPLAINT

"My ® hip is too painful to even stand or walk on now, even though I am using a cane & taking the medication that my doctor prescribed for me."

HISTORY OF PRESENT ILLNESS

Pt was in good hl until she noticed pain in ® hip 5 yr ago. X-rays revealed degenerative joint dz (osteoarthritis) of ® hip. Pain radiates to ® buttock & upper ® thigh, c̄ occasional pain in knees if standing >15 min. Pain is deep, boring, & disruptive (8/10 c̄ mvt & weight bearing, & 4/10 at rest s̄ weight bearing). Pt has ® hip joint stiffness, ↓ mobility of ® hip joint, weakness of ® leg muscles, grating sensation when hip is moved, & fatigue c̄ prolonged standing or ambulation, even c̄ cane. Hip pain is aggravated by joint mvt, prolonged sitting, or cold & damp weather. Pain worse in afternoon & early PM, especially p̄ an active day. In last yr, hip pain has progressed so rapidly that it is now problematic & disruptive to her lifestyle. Pt is scheduled to undergo ® total hip joint replacement sgy.

PAST HEALTH HISTORY

Medical

Benign x̄ for hip

Surgical

Appendectomy 23 yr PTA s̄ complications

Medications

Aspirin (ASA) 650 mg po qid prn c̄ food
Motrin (ibuprofen) 400 mg qid po prn c̄ food
Multivitamin (MVI) 1 tablet po qd
Occasional use of OTC cold medication & antacids
Stopped taking ASA & Motrin 2 wk PTA (in anticipation of sgy)

Communicable Diseases

Rubella, mumps, & chicken pox as child

Allergies

Denies

Injuries/Accidents

3" laceration of ® hand last yr during food preparation c̄ lg kitchen knife; laceration required suturing & tetanus booster

Disabilities/Handicaps

Denies

Blood Transfusions

Denies

continued

Childhood Illnesses	See communicable dz
Immunizations	Current tetanus; annual flu vaccine

FAMILY HEALTH HISTORY

LEGEND

- ⬤ Living female
- ◼ Living male
- ⊗ Deceased female
- ◼ Deceased male
- ↗ Points to patient

A&W = Alive & well
HTN = Hypertension
MVA = Motor vehicle accident

80 Hard of hearing HTN — 72 MVA

60 A&W   12 Drowned   2 Pneumonia   58 Degenerative hip disease   61 A&W

30 A&W   27 A&W   25 A&W

Denies family hx of rheumatoid arthritis, osteoporosis, ankylosing spondylitis, gout, Paget's dz, and Dupuytren's contracture.

SOCIAL HISTORY

Alcohol Use	1–2 glasses of wine per month c̄ dinner
Tobacco Use	1/2 ppd unfiltered cigarette smoker ×25 yr; quit smoking c̄ husband 15 yr ago
Drug Use	Denies
Sexual Practice	Heterosexual; sexual activity has ↓ 2° hip discomfort; any position induces severe Ⓡ hip pain
Travel History	Frequent traveler to Europe & Caribbean in the past; hip pain has made traveling difficult in recent yr
Work Environment	Recently taken early retirement; now a homemaker
Home Environment	Lives in 2 story house c̄ 10 steps to enter 1st floor & 20 steps b/t 2 floors of house; kitchen & LR are on 1st floor; last yr, pt started to use guest bedroom & bath on 1st floor; laundry area is in basement; last yr, pt arranged for someone to come in 1 ×/wk to do heavy house cleaning, laundry; pt still does light housekeeping & cooking; husband does grocery shopping & children help c̄ other chores prn
Hobbies/Leisure Activities	Devoted gardener ā hip pain made it too difficult to kneel & bend over; c̄ husband, would take walk q PM in good weather & golf on wkends, but had to terminate these habits; pt & husband play cards few nights/wk
Stress	Pt is worried that her degenerative joint dz will progress & make her completely dependent on family
Education	Retired elementary school teacher, who completed 4 yr of college

continued

Economic Status	Denies financial difficulties or concerns; receives monthly pensions; husband is still employed
Military Service	Denies
Religion	Roman Catholic; "I find comfort in my faith during difficult times."
Ethnic Background	Italian descent
Roles/Relationships	Maintains matriarchal role in family. Her children value her opinion & consult her on important decisions. She states that they are all very "close."
Characteristic Patterns of Daily Living	Awakes at 6:30 q AM, eats breakfast $\bar{c}$ husband, which she prepares. Showers & dresses. On "bad days" she needs to rest. Performs light house cleaning in AM & rests at lunch. Eats lunch alone & reads in afternoon. Husband arrives home at 5:30. They frequently eat out or get takeout for dinner 2° hip pain. She reads $\bar{p}$ dinner & goes to bed at 9:30 PM.

HEALTH MAINTENANCE ACTIVITIES

Sleep	9 hr per night; sleep is often interrupted by hip pain
Diet	3 balanced meals/d; admits to snacks b/t meals especially in last yr 2° immobility
Exercise	Due to hip pain, does not engage in any exercise regimen. "I'm lucky if I can just make it through the day."
Stress Management	"I just worry & get myself all in a tizzy."
Use of Safety Devices	Uses C-shaped cane × 1/yr; wears flat shoes $\bar{c}$ nonskid surface; rugs tacked down in house, stairway bannisters tightened, & grab bars installed in bathroom; avoids walking outside in icy or wet weather
Health Check-Ups	Annual physical exam, including Pap smear & mammogram

PHYSICAL ASSESSMENT

General Assessment

Overall Appearance	HT: 65" (1½" ht loss since onset of menopause) WT: 165 lb Partial wt bearing on Ⓡ leg; Ø obvious deformities
Posture	Head & torso erect, feet sl apart $\bar{c}$ sl thoracic kyphosis
Gait and Mobility	Antalgic gait, slow speed; cane for external support during standing & ambulation; requires external support from 2nd person or object (e.g., armrest) to sit or rise from chair

continued

Inspection

Muscle Size and Shape   Mod atrophy of Ⓡ gluteus maximus, quadriceps, semitendinosus, semimembranosus, gracilis, & gastrocnemius muscles; all other muscles s̄ atrophy; Ø involuntary mvt

Joint Contour and Periarticular Tissue   Skin intact, s̄ rashes, deformities, erythema, ecchymosis, swelling, enlargement, masses, or nodules

Palpation

Muscle Tone   ↓ in muscle tone of Ⓡ gluteus maximus, quadriceps, semitendinosus, semimembranosus, gracilis, & gastrocnemius muscles during muscle contraction & relaxation; size, shape, & tone of other muscles WNL. Ø masses, tenderness, spasms

Joints   Contour smooth; Ø masses; Ø periarticular erythema, swelling, warmth, masses, nodules or tenderness; mild Ⓡ hip joint tenderness c̄ rest & flexion; crepitus over Ⓡ hip joint c̄ flexion

Range of Motion   ↓ Ⓡ hip mvt during sitting, standing, & ambulation; unable to perform hyperextension of Ⓡ hip 2° pain & stiffness; all other joints c̄ full ROM

Muscle Strength   Ⓡ leg = 3/5; strength of all other muscles = 5/5

Special Techniques

Goniometer   Ⓡ hip: flexion c̄ knee straight = 45°
  abduction = 15°
  internal & external rotation = 10°

Limb Length and Circumference   Ⓡ leg = 78 cm, Ⓛ leg = 80.5 cm; Ⓡ thigh = 40 cm, Ⓛ thigh = 43 cm

Status of Distal Limbs and Digits   Pink skin color, warm skin temp, brisk cap refill, intact mvt & sensation in feet & toes, 2+/4+ pedal pulses

Use of Assistive Devices   C-shaped cane c̄ 4 point contact surface (rubber tipped) that is appropriate for ht; uses on affected side; wearing sneakers

Laboratory Data

Blood   CBC c̄ WBC differential, PLT count, serum electrolytes, PT, PTT, bleeding time, BUN, serum creatinine, & serum glucose WNL

Urine   Urinalysis WNL

Diagnostic Data

Electrocardiogram   12 lead EKG: Regular rhythm & rate; no dysrhythmias

X-Rays   Anterior/Posterior & Lateral Chest X-Ray: No pathology
Anterior/Posterior & Lateral Right Hip X-Ray: Significant deterioration of the joint, with loss of articulating cartilage

NURSING CHECKLIST
Musculoskeletal Assessment

General Assessment
- Overall Appearance
- Posture
- Gait and Mobility

Inspection
- Muscle Size and Shape
- Joint Contour and Periarticular Tissue

Palpation
- Muscle Tone
- Joints

Range of Motion

Muscle Strength

Examination of Joints
- Temporomandibular Joint
- Cervical Spine
- Shoulders
- Elbows
- Wrists and Hands
- Hips
- Knees
- Ankles and Feet
- Spine

Special Techniques
- Measuring Limb Circumference
- Using a Goniometer
- Assessing for Chvostek's Sign
- Drop Arm Test
- Assessing for Trousseau's Sign
- Assessing Grip Strength Using a Blood Pressure Cuff
- Assessing for Tinel's Sign
- Assessing for Phalen's Sign
- Trendelenburg Test
- Measuring Limb Length
- Patrick's Test
- Assessing for Bulge Sign
- Patellar Ballottement
- Assessing for Apley's Sign
- Assessing for McMurray's Sign
- Drawer Test
- Lachman's Test
- Assessing Status of Distal Limbs and Digits
- Thompson Test
- Assessing for Scoliosis
- Straight Leg Raising Test (Lasègue's Test)
- Milgram Test

continued

Assistive Devices
- Crutches
- Cane
- Walker
- Brace, Splint, Immobilizer
- Cast
- Skin Traction
- Skeletal Traction
- External Fixation

REVIEW QUESTIONS AND ACTIVITIES

1. Differentiate between weight bearing as tolerated, partial weight bearing, and touchdown weight bearing.

2. Describe the possible joint movements and degrees of range of motion for the following joints: shoulder, elbow, hip, and knee.

Questions 3–5 refer to the following situation:

Ms. Sykhammountry is an avid tennis player who plays on the tennis team at her sports club. She is complaining of left shoulder pain that has left her unable to play for the past week. You abduct her left arm (dominant arm) and ask her to lower it slowly while maintaining arm extension. Ms. Sykhammountry complains of pain with this movement and lowers the arm quickly.

3. What injury do you suspect Ms. Sykhammountry has sustained?
   a. Radial head fracture
   b. Carpal tunnel syndrome
   c. Rotator cuff tear
   d. Flexion ankylosis

   The correct answer is (c).

4. What normal finding would you expect to see in this patient's arms related to her tennis playing?
   a. Unilateral hypertrophy
   b. Bilateral atrophy
   c. Increased limb length
   d. Decreased limb circumference

   The correct answer is (a).

5. You are assessing range of motion in Ms. Sykhammountry's shoulder joint. You ask her to place her arms at her side, elbows extended, and to move the arms forward in an arc. This movement of the shoulder is called:
   a. Internal rotation
   b. Adduction
   c. Hyperextension
   d. Forward flexion

   The correct answer is (d).

6. You suspect an injury to Mrs. Chan's anterior cruciate ligament. Which of the following tests would you perform to assess the knee?
   a. Straight leg raising test
   b. Lachman's test
   c. Trendelenburg test
   d. Phalen's test

   The correct answer is (b).

7. Match the following joints with their normal anatomic joint ROM:
   a. Knee flexion   ____ 20°
   b. Dorsiflexion of foot   ____ 30°
   c. Inversion of foot   ____ 40°
   d. Internal rotation of shoulder ____ 90°
   e. Lateral bending of cervical spine ____ 130°
   f. Elbow flexion   ____ 160°

8. You note that Mr. Terninski complains of a pricking sensation as you tap the median nerve. This clinical finding indicates:
   a. A negative Phalen's test for compartment syndrome
   b. A positive drawer test for meniscus damage
   c. A negative Chvostek's sign for hypocalcemia
   d. A positive Tinel's sign for carpal tunnel syndrome

   The correct answer is (d).

9. Describe the assessment findings you would expect for inspection, palpation, ROM, and muscle strength for a patient with severe rheumatoid arthritis.

10. Describe five abnormal gait patterns and the etiology of each.

Mental Status and Neurological Techniques

COMPETENCIES

COMPETENCIES

1. Discuss the divisions of the nervous system and their functions.
2. Relate blood flow to the brain to the functional area supplied.
3. Describe the characteristics of the most common neurological complaints.
4. Document a complete health history as it relates to the neurological system.
5. Perform a mental status assessment and document the results.
6. Assess the neurological system in a systematic manner and document the results.
7. Explain the pathophysiology of any abnormal results obtained.

T he nervous system controls all body functions and thought processes. The complex interrelationships among the various divisions of the nervous system permit the body to maintain homeostasis, to receive, interpret, and react to stimuli, and to control voluntary and involuntary processes, including cognition.

ANATOMY AND PHYSIOLOGY

Macrostructure

The scalp and skull are two protective layers covering the brain. The scalp performs a unique function in that it moves freely, helping to protect and cushion the head from traumatic injury. The skull is a rigid, bony cavity that has a fixed volume of approximately 1,500 ml.

Meninges

There are three layers of meninges (protective membranes), known as the dura mater, arachnoid mater, and pia mater, located between the brain and the skull (see Figure 18-1). The dura mater is the thick, tough, outermost layer. Below the dura mater is a small, serous space known as the subdural space.

The arachnoid mater lies between the dura mater and the pia mater. Below the arachnoid mater is the subarachnoid space, where cerebrospinal fluid (CSF) is circulated. Portions of the arachnoid mater, called arachnoid villi, project into the subarachnoid space (also shown in Figure 18-1). These serve to absorb CSF.

The pia mater is thin and vascular. It is the innermost layer of the meninges. The pia mater helps form the choroid plexuses, which are vascular structures located in the ventricles of the brain that form CSF.

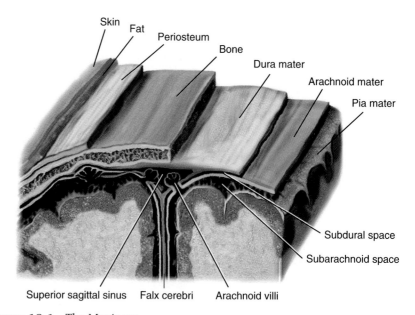

Figure 18-1 The Meninges

Central Nervous System

The brain and the spinal cord make up the central nervous system (CNS). The brain is divided into four main components: the cerebrum, the diencephalon, the cerebellum, and the brain stem. Each of these areas is subdivided into various anatomic areas.

Cerebrum

The cerebrum is the largest portion of the brain. It is incompletely divided into right and left hemispheres by the longitudinal fissure. The two hemispheres are connected by the corpus callosum, which serves as a communication link between the left and right hemispheres.

The cerebral cortex, or the outermost layer of the cerebrum, contains gray matter. Higher cognitive functioning is dependent on the cerebral cortex and its interaction with other parts of the nervous system. The cerebral cortex is involved in memory storage and recall, conscious understanding of sensation, vision, hearing, and motor function. The basal ganglia are located deep within the cerebral hemispheres and function intricately with the cerebral cortex and the cerebellum in regulating motor activity.

Each cerebral hemisphere is divided into four lobes: the frontal, parietal, temporal, and occipital lobes. The locations and functions of each of the cerebral lobes are illustrated in Figure 18-2. A fifth lobe called the limbic lobe is anatomically part of the temporal lobe and is involved in emotional behavior and self-preservation.

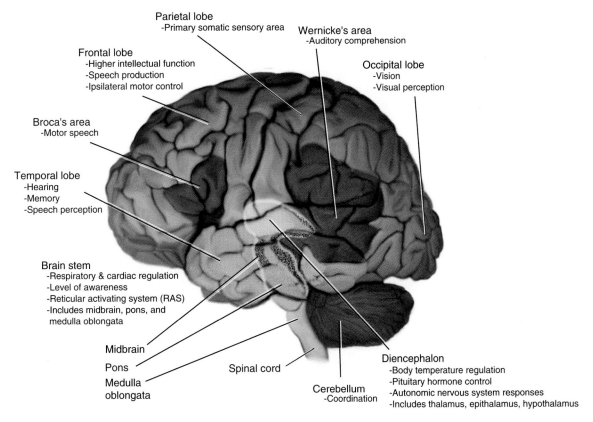

Figure 18-2   The Locations and Functions of the Cerebral Lobes, Brain Stem, and Cerebellum

Diencephalon

The diencephalon, a relay center for the brain, is composed of the thalamic structures: the thalamus, the epithalamus, and the hypothalamus. The hypothalamus is important in body temperature regulation, pituitary hormone control, and autonomic nervous system responses. It also plays a role in behavior via its connections with the limbic system.

Cerebellum

The cerebellum lies inferior to the occipital lobe and behind the brain stem. It is divided into two lateral lobes and a medial part called the vermis. The vermis is the part of the cerebellum concerned primarily with maintenance of posture and equilibrium. Each cerebellar hemisphere is responsible for coordination of movement of the ipsilateral (same) side of the body.

Brain Stem

The brain stem is located immediately below the diencephalon and is divided into the midbrain, the pons, and the medulla oblongata. The reticular formation, a complex network of sensory fibers in the brain stem, contains centers that control respiratory, cardiovascular, and vegetative functions. The ascending reticular activating system (RAS) is located in the brain stem and extends to the cerebral cortex. The RAS is mostly excitatory and is essential for arousal from sleep, maintaining attention, and perception of sensory input.

The midbrain contains the nuclei of cranial nerves III (oculomotor) and IV (trochlear), which are associated with control of eye movements. The pons is located between the midbrain and the medulla oblongata. Sensory and motor nuclei of cranial nerves V (trigeminal), VI (abducens), VII (facial), and VIII (acoustic) are located in the pons. The medulla oblongata is located between the pons and the spinal cord. It contains the nuclei of cranial nerves IX (glossopharyngeal), X (vagus), XI (spinal accessory), and XII (hypoglossal). Also located in the medulla oblongata are the centers for reflexes such as sneezing, swallowing, coughing, and vomiting, as well as the centers regulating the respiratory and cardiovascular systems.

Spinal Cord

The spinal cord is a continuation of the medulla oblongata. It exits the skull at the foramen magnum and begins at the upper border of the atlas (C1), continuing downward to the conus medullaris, a tapered ending of the cord at about the level of the first or second lumbar vertebrae (see Figure 18-3A). From the conus medullaris is a connective tissue filament, the filum terminale, which continues down to its attachment at the coccyx (see Figure 18-3B).

A cross-section of the spinal cord will show that the central part of the cord is gray matter. The gray matter is in the shape of an H. White matter surrounds the gray matter.

The gray matter is made up of nerve cell bodies and short segments of unmyelinated fibers. The posterior portion of the H is called the dorsal horn, and the anterior portion is the ventral horn. Small lateral horns are also present in thoracic and upper lumbar sections of the spinal cord.

The dorsal horn contains cell bodies of sensory (afferent) neurons, which receive and transmit sensory messages from the afferent fibers in the spinal nerve. The ventral horn contains cell bodies of motor (efferent) neurons, which send axons into the spinal nerves and innervate skeletal muscles, carrying signals from the brain and the spinal cord.

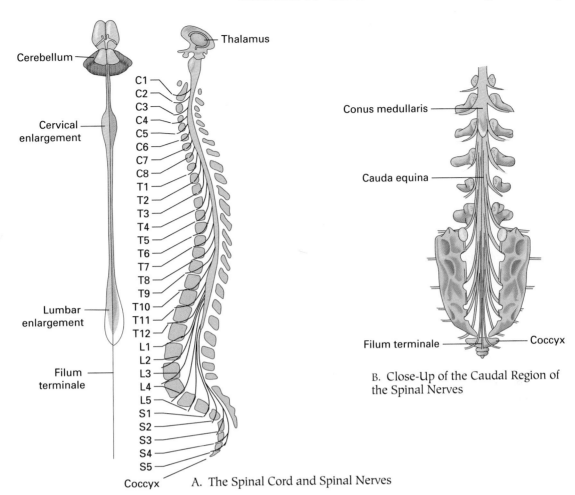

Figure 18-3 The Spinal Cord

B. Close-Up of the Caudal Region of the Spinal Nerves

A. The Spinal Cord and Spinal Nerves

Motor Pathways of the CNS

There are three motor pathways in the CNS: the corticospinal or pyramidal tract, the extrapyramidal tract, and the cerebellum (refer to page 554).

Pyramidal Tract The corticospinal pathway descends from the motor area of the cerebral cortex, through the midbrain, the pons, and the medulla. At the level of the medulla, 90% of the fibers of the corticospinal tract cross (decussate) to travel down the opposite side of the spinal cord, becoming the lateral corticospinal tract. The remaining fibers travel down the spinal cord in a tract known as the anterior corticospinal tract. Fibers of the lateral corticospinal tract synapse in the anterior horn (gray matter) at all levels of the cord just before they leave the cord (see Figure 18-4). The motor neurons above this synapse in the anterior horn are known as upper motor neurons. Upper motor neurons connect the cerebral cortex with the anterior horn and are entirely contained within the CNS. Lower motor neurons are motor neurons below the level of the upper motor neurons. Lower motor neuron cell bodies are located in the anterior horn, where they connect with the corticospinal tract. Lower motor neurons innervate skeletal muscle at the myoneural junction. They are responsible for purposeful, voluntary movement.

Extrapyramidal Tract This pathway includes all motor neurons in the motor cortex, basal ganglia, brain stem, and spinal cord that are outside the corticospinal, or pyramidal, tract (henceforth referred to as extrapyramidal). The extrapyramidal tract is responsible for controlling body movement, particularly gross automatic movements (e.g., walking), and for controlling muscle tone.

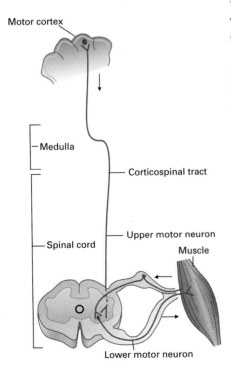

Figure 18-4 Motor Pathways of the CNS

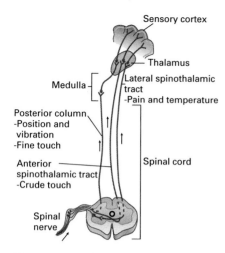

Figure 18-5 Sensory Pathways of the CNS

Sensory Pathways of the CNS

The sensory portion of the peripheral nervous system consists of afferent neurons divided into somatic afferent and visceral afferent neurons. Somatic afferent fibers originate in skeletal muscles, joints, tendons, and skin. Visceral fibers originate in the viscera. Both types of afferent fibers carry impulses from both the external and the internal environments to the CNS.

Afferent fibers containing impulses, or messages, enter the spinal cord through the dorsal roots. From the spinal cord the message travels via the spinothalamic tracts or the posterior column to the thalamus and sensory cortex. The thalamus receives the message and interprets a general sensation. The impulse synapses with another sensory neuron to the sensory cortex, where the message is fully interpreted (see Figure 18-5).

Spinothalamic Tracts In the spinal cord, the spinothalamic tracts synapse with a second sensory neuron and then decussate to the opposite side. The message is then carried up the tract. The lateral spinothalamic tract carries pain and temperature sensations, and the anterior spinothalamic tract carries the sensation of crude or light touch.

Posterior Column The posterior column carries position, vibration, and fine-touch sensations. The nerve impulse enters the spinal cord and travels upward to the medulla, where a synapse with a second sensory neuron occurs. The neuron decussates to the opposite side of the medulla and continues on to the thalamus and sensory cortex.

Blood Supply

Blood is supplied to the brain by two pairs of arteries, the internal carotid arteries (anterior circulation) and the vertebral arteries (posterior circulation). At the base of the brain lies the circle of Willis, an arterial anastomosis that links the anterior and posterior blood supplies (see Figure 18-6). The functional areas supplied by each of the main cerebral arteries are listed in Table 18-1.

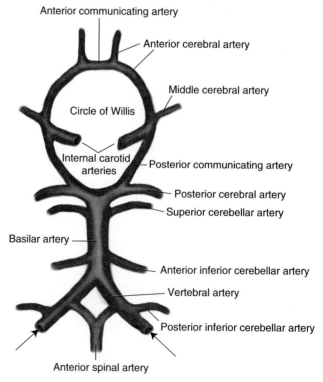

Figure 18-6 Major Arteries of the Brain

Table 18-1 Cerebral Blood Supply	
ARTERY	**FUNCTIONAL AREA**
Anterior cerebral artery	Medial and inferior surfaces of each hemisphere: • Frontal lobe • Parietal lobe
Middle cerebral artery	Lateral surface of each hemisphere: • Frontal lobe • Temporal lobe • Parietal lobe • Occipital lobe
Posterior cerebral artery	Medial and inferior surfaces of each hemisphere: • Temporal lobe • Medial occipital lobe • Midbrain
Basilar artery	• Midbrain • Upper brain stem • Medulla oblongata
Cerebellar arteries	• Pons • Midbrain • Cerebellum

Peripheral Nervous System

The peripheral nervous system consists of nervous tissue found outside the CNS, including the spinal nerves, cranial nerves, and the autonomic nervous system.

Spinal Nerves

The 31 pairs of spinal nerves include eight cervical, twelve thoracic, five lumbar, five sacral, and one coccygeal. Each spinal nerve is made up of a dorsal (afferent) root and a ventral (efferent) root. Each afferent spinal nerve root innervates a specific area of the skin, called a **dermatome**, for superficial cutaneous sensations. Figure 18-7 illustrates both the anterior and the posterior dermatomal distributions. Spinal nerves leaving the right side of the cord supply the right side of the body, and those leaving the left side supply muscles on the left side.

Each of the eight cervical nerves exits above its corresponding vertebra. Each of the spinal nerves below the cervical portion exits below its corresponding vertebra. The spinal cord is not as long as the vertebral column, so the lumbar and sacral nerves are comparatively long. These longer roots are called the cauda equina, meaning "horse's tail" (refer to Figure 18-3B).

Cranial Nerves

There are 12 pairs of cranial nerves. They are designated in order of their position with Roman numerals I through XII. Some cranial nerves have purely motor functions and some have only sensory functions. Others have mixed sensory and motor functions. Table 18-2 summarizes the functions of the cranial nerves.

Autonomic Nervous System

The autonomic nervous system (ANS) is divided into two functionally different subdivisions: the sympathetic and parasympathetic nervous systems. The

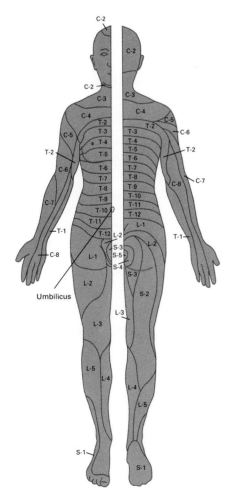

Figure 18-7 Anterior and Posterior Dermatomal Distributions

Table 18-2 Functions of the Cranial Nerves	
NAME AND NUMBER	**FUNCTION**
Olfactory (I)	Smell
Optic (II)	Visual acuity, visual fields, funduscopic examination
Oculomotor (III)	Cardinal fields of gaze (EOM movement), eyelid elevation, pupil reaction, doll's eyes phenomenon
Trochlear (IV)	EOM movement
Trigeminal (V)	Motor: strength of temporalis and masseter muscles Sensory: light touch, superficial pain and temperature to face, corneal reflex
Abducens (VI)	EOM movement
Facial (VII)	Motor: facial movements Sensory: taste anterior two-thirds of tongue *Parasympathetic: tears and saliva secretion
Acoustic (VIII)	Cochlear: gross hearing, Weber and Rinne tests Vestibular: vertigo, equilibrium, nystagmus
Glossopharyngeal (IX)	Motor: soft palate and uvula movement, gag reflex, swallowing, guttural and palatal sounds Sensory: taste posterior one-third of tongue *Parasympathetic: carotid reflex, chemoreceptors
Vagus (X)	Motor and Sensory: same as CN IX *Parasympathetic: carotid reflex, stomach and intestinal secretions, peristalsis, involuntary control of bronchi, heart innervation
Spinal Accesory (XI)	Sternocleidomastoid and trapezius muscle movements
Hypoglossal (XII)	Tongue movement, lingual sounds

Cannot be directly assessed.
EOM = extraocular muscle; CN = cranial nerve.

ANS functions without voluntary control to maintain the body in a state of homeostasis. Most organs that are under the influence of the ANS have dual innervation of both sympathetic and parasympathetic systems.

The sympathetic nervous system, sometimes called the thoracolumbar system, controls "fight or flight" actions. The parasympathetic nervous system (craniosacral) is responsible for "general housekeeping" of the body. Refer to Table 18-3 for specific system responses to autonomic stimulation.

Reflexes

A reflex action, a specific response to an adequate stimulus, occurs without conscious control. The stimulus can occur in a joint, muscle, or the skin, and is transmitted to the CNS by one or more afferent, or sensory, neurons. The impulse enters the spinal cord through the dorsal roots of a spinal nerve, where it synapses. Following synapse in the cord, the anterior motor neurons send an impulse on efferent neurons to the endplates of the skeletal muscle, causing the effector muscle to react (see Figure 18-8).

A monosynaptic reflex, such as the patellar reflex, involves two neurons: one afferent and one efferent. Polysynaptic reflexes involve many neurons in addition to the afferent and efferent limbs of the reflex arc. Reflexes are classified into three main categories: muscle stretch, or deep tendon reflexes (DTR); superficial reflexes; and pathological reflexes.

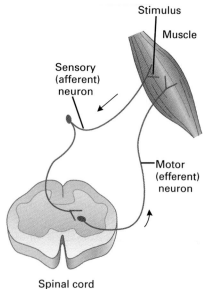

Figure 18-8 Monosynaptic Reflex Arc

Table 18-3 Sympathetic versus Parasympathetic Response		
SYSTEM	**SYMPATHETIC RESPONSE**	**PARASYMPATHETIC RESPONSE**
Neurological	Pupils dilated Heightened awareness	Pupils normal size
Cardiovascular	Increased heart rate Increased myocardial contractility Increased blood pressure	Decreased heart rate Decreased myocardial contractility Vasodilatation
Respiratory	Increased respiratory rate Increased respiratory depth Bronchial constriction	Bronchial relaxation
Gastrointestinal	Decreased gastric motility Decreased gastric secretions Increased glycogenolysis Decreased insulin production Sphincter contraction	Increased gastric motility Increased gastric secretions Sphincter dilatation
Genitourinary	Decreased urine output Decreased renal blood flow	Normal urine output

❖ HEALTH HISTORY

The neurological health history provides insight into the link between a patient's life/lifestyle and neurological information and pathology.

PATIENT PROFILE
Diseases that are age-, sex-, and race-specific for the neurological system are listed.

Age
Multiple sclerosis (MS) (20–40)
Myasthenia gravis (20–30)
Syringomyelia (30)
Huntington's chorea (30–40)
Parkinson's disease (>50)
Alzheimer's disease (middle age–old age)

Sex

Female
Myasthenia gravis, MS, meningiomas, pseudotumor cerebri, migraine headaches

Male
Cervical spine injuries, cluster headache, dyslexia (boys)

Race

African American
Intracerebral hemorrhage (due to increased incidence of hypertension)

CHIEF COMPLAINT
Common chief complaints for the neurological system are defined and information on the characteristics of each sign/symptom is provided.

Headache
Diffuse pain in various parts of the head, not confined to the area of distribution of any nerve. Migraine headache (vascular headache) is the most common type of recurrent headache.

continued

Location	Hemicranial, frontal, temporal, occipital, retrobulbar, orbital, maxillary region
Radiation	Neck, shoulders, face, teeth, eyes, back
Quality	Throbbing, sharp, stabbing, steady
Associated Manifestations	Nausea, vomiting, nasal congestion, watery eyes, papilledema, photophobia, hyperacusis, visual disturbances, numbness or tingling, any associated neurological trauma, infection, stresses, family history
Aggravating Factors	Flickering lights, weather changes, stress, fatigue, menstruation, exertion, sneezing, coughing, bending over, caffeine, alcohol, foods containing tyramine, anxiety
Alleviating Factors	Medications, quiet environment, rest, cold compress
Timing	Minutes, hours, days, episodic, continuous
Seizure	A transient disturbance of cerebral function caused by an excessive discharge of neurons
Location	Body parts involved
Quality	General or localized
Quantity	Number of minutes or seconds, weekly, monthly, every few months
Associated Manifestations	Incontinence, injury (tongue, cheeks, limbs), memory loss, cyanosis, respiratory arrest; postictal headache, somnolence, or confusion
Aggravating Factors	Television viewing, bright lights, sleep deprivation, stress, flashing lights, fever in children or infants, alcohol
Alleviating factors	Medications
Setting	Sequence of events: warning (aura) such as headache, abdominal discomfort, euphoria or depression, visual hallucination; phases: tonic, clonic, postictal, fugue states
Timing	First occurrence, age at onset of seizures, associated trauma or presumed cause, sleeping hours, first awakening, menses
Syncope	Abrupt loss of consciousness of brief duration due to decreased oxygen or glucose supply to the brain
Quality	Total versus partial loss of consciousness
Quantity	Duration of seconds, minutes, or hours; daily, monthly
Associated Manifestations	Nausea, diaphoresis, dimmed vision, increased salivation, gastrointestinal bleeding, dyspnea, chest pain, hemiparesis, transient focal deficits, seizures, migraine headache, associated illness (myocardial infarction, insulin-dependent diabetes mellitus)

continued

Aggravating Factors	Injury, intense emotion, carotid occlusion, cardiovascular disorders, exertion, anemia, hypoglycemia, insulin peak, crowded space, decreased atmospheric oxygen
Alleviating Factors	Cool air, change in position, oxygen, glucose, medication, volume infusions
Setting	Hot, stuffy room; standing still for long periods of time
Pain	A sensation of discomfort, distress, or suffering
Location	Anatomic location (e.g., lower back, head)
Quality	Aching, stabbing, throbbing, cramping
Associated Manifestations	Crying, hysteria, muscular tenseness, depression, shortness of breath, diaphoresis, splinting or protective behaviors, focal deficits, limited range of motion
Aggravating Factors	Stress, excessive exercise, lifting, coughing or sneezing, posture changes, trauma, illness, extreme temperatures, humidity
Alleviating Factors	Medications, heat, cold, distraction, physical therapy
Timing	Minutes to constant; early morning, late day; daily, monthly
Paresthesia	Abnormal sensations such as numbness, pricking, tingling
Associated Manifestations	Pain, stiffness, changes in gait, pulseless extremities, pallor, injury, ulcers, muscle wasting, traumatic injury
Aggravating Factors	Activity, extreme cold, diabetes mellitus
Alleviating Factors	Medication, warmth, position changes
Disturbances in Gait	Abnormal way of moving on foot, walking, or running
Quality	Ataxic, spastic, bizarre, shuffling, hemiplegic, scissors, clumsy, festinating, steppage
Associated Manifestations	Vertigo, visual impairments, blackouts, stroke, focal weakness, muscle wasting, abnormal movements or posture, spasticity, falling
Aggravating Factors	Fatigue, alcohol ingestion, vitamin D deficiency
Alleviating Factors	Rest, assistive devices
Setting	Level ground versus uneven terrain
Visual Changes	Changes in visual acuity, visual fields, color perception, depth perception
Quality	Blindness in particular field of vision; scotoma; perception of flashing, bright lights; blurriness
Associated Manifestations	Vertigo, dizziness, nausea, weakness, headache
Aggravating Factors	Darkness, fatigue, bright light, reading, alcohol ingestion, medication

continued

Alleviating Factors	Rest, medications, glasses
Timing	Abrupt, gradual, constant, intermittent, morning, evening
Vertigo	The sensation of moving in space or objects moving around the person; also may be referred to as dizziness, lightheadedness
Quality	Spinning sensations, dizziness, or lightheadedness
Associated Manifestations	Nausea, vomiting, headache, tinnitus, deafness, discharge from ear, cranial nerve palsies, hemiparesis, seizure, loss of consciousness, chest pain, falling
Aggravating Factors	Motion, movement of head, changes in atmospheric pressure (weather), heights, amusement rides, anxiety, alcohol ingestion, pain, medications
Alleviating Factors	Medications, lying down, maintaining a still posture
Setting	Amusement rides, glassed-in elevators, rising from a seated or supine position
Timing	Sudden, gradual; seconds, minutes, days, months; constant, intermittent
Memory Disorders	Change in ability to remember events or facts
Quality	Recent or remote memory loss
Associated Manifestations	Irritability, anxiety, agitation, confabulation, associated trauma
Aggravating Factors	Distraction, anxiety, medications, alcohol ingestion, drug abuse, unfamiliar environment, sleep deprivation, anesthesia, hypoxia, electrolyte imbalance
Alleviating Factors	Visual or auditory cues, familiarity with environment, oxygen, electrolyte replacement, narcotic reversal, detoxification
Setting	Unfamiliar environment
Timing	Night time, upon awakening
Difficulty with Swallowing or Speech	Inability to swallow food or drink, choking, or aspiration; changes in enunciation of words, volume of speech, content of speech, or comprehension of written or verbal language
Associated Manifestations	Excessive drooling and saliva, paresis, dysarthria, weight loss, dehydration, irritability, depression, disease or damage to the CNS, such as stroke, cerebral palsy
Aggravating Factors	Fatigue, position, prolonged tracheal intubation, alcohol intake
Alleviating Factors	Rest, quiet environment, thickened liquids, soft foods, varied communication tools
Setting	Loud, chaotic environment; after prolonged intubation

continued

PAST HEALTH HISTORY	*The various components of the past health history are linked to neurological pathology and neurology-related information.*
Medical	
Neurologic Specific	Amyotrophic lateral sclerosis (ALS), multiple sclerosis (MS), tumors, Guillain Barré syndrome, cerebral aneurysm, arteriovenous malformations (AVM), cerebrovascular accident (CVA), migraines, Alzheimer's disease, myasthenia gravis, congenital defects, metabolic disorders, childhood seizures
Non-Neurologic Specific	Hypertension, heart disease, cardiac surgery, invasive procedures, diabetes mellitus, leukemia, hypoglycemia
Surgical	Craniotomy, laminectomy, carotid endarterectomy, transsphenoidal hypophysectomy, cordotomy, aneurysmectomy or repair
Medications	Antidepressants, antiseizure medications, narcotics, antianxiety medications
Communicable Diseases	Encephalitis, meningitis or poliomyelitis, AIDS dementia, botulism, syphilis, cat scratch disease, rickettsial infections, toxoplasmosis
Injuries/Accidents	Closed head injury, chronic subdural hematoma, spinal cord injury, peripheral nerve damage
FAMILY HEALTH HISTORY	*Neurological diseases that are familial are listed.*
	Congenital defects such as neural tube defects, hydrocephalus, AVM, headaches, epilepsy, Alzheimer's disease, Huntington's chorea, muscular dystrophies, lipid storage diseases, Gaucher's disease, Niemann-Pick's disease
SOCIAL HISTORY	*The components of the social history are linked to neurological factors/pathology.*
Alcohol Use	Patients suffering from chronic alcoholism may exhibit the following abnormal findings: Korsakoff's psychosis, polyneuropathy, Wernicke's encephalopathy, tremor.
Tobacco Use	Increased risk of stroke
Drug Use	Neurological signs of drug use are listed in Table 18-4.
Sexual Practice	Neurosyphilis; impotence secondary to neuropathies, MS, or lower motor neuron lesions
Travel History	Arthropod-born encephalitis (Venezuelan equine, Japanese B, Murray-Valley, Russian spring-summer, Central European, Colorado tick), malaria
Work Environment	Exposure to continuous loud noise, performing repetitive-motion tasks, toxic chemical exposure (carbon dioxide, insecticides)
Home Environment	Exposure to toxic chemicals (carbon dioxide, insecticides), lead paint

continued

Hobbies/Leisure Activities	Use of protective equipment; participation in contact sports or high-risk activities such as football, soccer, hockey, boxing, race car driving, motorcycling; hobbies involving repetitive motion (needlework)
Stress	Headaches
Ethnic Background	
Jewish	Tay-Sachs disease
Northern European	MS
HEALTH MAINTENANCE ACTIVITIES	*This information provides a bridge between the health maintenance activities and neurological function.*
Sleep	Narcolepsy, insomnia
Diet	Beriberi (vitamin B_1), pellagra (niacin)
Exercise	Increased muscle strength, increased coordination
Use of Safety Devices	Helmet, seat belt
Health Check-Ups	Developmental milestones

Table 18-4   Neurological Signs of Drug Ingestion

ASSESSMENT PARAMETER	DRUG				
	Hallucinogens	**Cannabis (Marijuana)**	**Narcotics**	**Sedative-Hypnotics**	**CNS Stimulants**
Pupils	Dilated React to light	Normal	Pinpoint Fixed	Normal	Dilated React to light
Deep tendon reflexes	Hyperactive	Normal	Normal	Hypoactive	Hyperactive
Speech	Normal	Often normal	Normal or dulled	Slurred	N/A
Coordination	Normal	Normal	Normal or unsteady	Ataxia	N/A
Sensorium	Often clear	Usually clear	Dulled	Confusion	May be confused
Sensory perception	Distorted	Distorted	Dulled	Dulled	Heightened
Memory	Unchanged	Transient loss	Unchanged	Impaired	Unchanged
Hallucinations	Any type	Rare	Rare	N/A	N/A
Delusions	Variable	Paranoid	N/A	N/A	Paranoid

N/A = not applicable.

NURSING ALERT

Risk Factors for Stroke

Significant risk factors for stroke include:

- Hypertension
- Diabetes mellitus
- Cocaine use
- Cigarette smoking
- Hyperlipidemia
- Chronic atrial fibrillation and flutter
- Sickle cell disease
- IV drug abuse
- Alcohol abuse
- Obesity
- Oral contraceptive use, especially in women over age 35 who smoke and have hypertension

EQUIPMENT

- Cotton wisp
- Cotton-tipped applicators
- Penlight
- Tongue blade
- Tuning fork: 128Hz or 256Hz, compatible with human hearing ranges.
- Reflex hammer
- Sterile needle, either a 22-gauge needle or a sterile safety pin
- Familiar small objects (coins, key, paperclip)
- Vials containing odorous materials (coffee, orange extract, vinegar)
- Vials containing hot and cold water
- Vials with solutions for tasting: quinine (bitter), glucose solution (sweet), lemon or vinegar (sour), saline (salty)
- Snellen chart or Rosenbaum pocket screener
- Pupil gauge in millimeters

NURSING CHECKLIST
General Approach to Neurological Assessment

1. Greet the patient and explain the assessment techniques that you will be using.
2. Maintain a quiet, unhurried, self-confident demeanor to help relieve any feelings of anxiety or discomfort and to help the patient relax during the assessment.
3. Provide a warm, quiet, and well-lit environment.
4. After the mental status examination, instruct the patient to remove all street clothes, and provide an examination gown for the patient to put on.
5. Begin the assessment with the patient in a comfortable upright sitting position, or for the patient on bed rest, position the patient comfortably, preferably with the head of the bed elevated, or flat, whichever is tolerated best or is within activity orders for the patient.

ASSESSMENT OF THE NEUROLOGICAL SYSTEM

A complete neurological assessment includes an assessment of mental status, sensation, cranial nerves, motor function, cerebellar function, and reflexes. For patients with minor or intermittent symptoms, a rapid screening assessment may be used as outlined in Table 18-5. The findings of the screening assessment will determine the emphasis of a more thorough examination.

Mental Status

Much of the mental status assessment should be done during the interview, with the patient comfortably positioned facing you. Mental status may also be assessed throughout the neurological assessment. Assess physical appearance and behavior, communication, level of consciousness, cognitive abilities, and mentation while conversing with the patient.

🌸 NURSING TIP

Patient History and Mental Status Assessment

1. Begin your assessment as the patient approaches you. Observe gait, posture, mode of dress, involuntary movements, voice, and other features that will help guide and refine your assessment priorities.
2. The history should be holistic because neurological disorders can affect all body systems.
3. The history should be age sensitive:
   - Utilize other family members when the patient is a child
   - Acknowledge adolescents' ability to speak for themselves
   - Do not make assumptions regarding elderly patients' ability to relate their own health histories.
4. Allow the patient to remain clothed during the history and mental status assessment.
5. Consider language and cultural norms when obtaining the history and performing the mental status assessment.

Table 18-5 Neurological Screening Assessment		
ASSESSMENT PARAMETER	**ASSESSMENT SKILL**	**COMMENTS**
Mental status/ level of consciousness	Note general appearance, affect, speech content, memory, logic, judgment, and speech patterns during the history.	If any abnormalities or inconsistencies are evident, perform full mental status assessment.
	Perform Glasgow Coma Scale (GCS) with motor assessment component and pupil assessment.	If GCS <15, perform full assessment of mental status and consciousness. If motor assessment is abnormal or asymmetrical, perform complete motor and sensory assessment.
Sensation	Assess pain and vibration in the hands and feet, light touch on the limbs.	If deficits are identified, perform a complete sensory assessment.
Cranial nerves	Assess CN II, III, IV, VI: visual acuity, gross visual fields, funduscopic examination, pupillary reactions, and extraocular movements. Assess CN VII, VIII, IX, X, XII: facial expression, gross hearing, voice, and tongue.	If any abnormalities exist, perform complete assessment of all 12 cranial nerves.
Motor system	• Muscle tone and strength • Abnormal movements • Grasps	If deficits are noted, perform a complete motor system assessment.

Cerebellar function	Observe the patient's:
	1. Gait on arrival
	2. Ability to:
	  • Walk heel-to-toe
	  • Walk on toes
	  • Walk on heels
	  • Hop in place
	  • Perform shallow knee bends
	3. Check Romberg's sign.
		If any abnormalities exist, perform complete cerebellar assessment.

Reflexes	Assess the muscle stretch reflexes and the plantar response.	If an abnormal response is elicited, perform a complete reflex assessment.

 NURSING TIP

Focusing the Mental Status Assessment

In most cases, the information obtained during the health history is sufficient to assess mental status. A more specific mental assessment should be performed if the following are noted:
• Known brain lesion (stroke, tumors, trauma)
• Suspected brain lesion (new seizures, headaches, behavioral changes)
• Memory deficits
• Confusion
• Vague behavioral complaints (by significant others if patient is unaware of or denies behavioral changes)
• Aphasia
• Irritability
• Emotional lability

Physical Appearance and Behavior

Posture and Movements

E **1.** Observe the patient's ability to wait patiently.
2. Note if patient's posture is relaxed, slumped, or stiff.
3. Observe the patient's movements for control and symmetry.
4. Observe the patient's gait (refer to Chapter 17).

N *The patient should appear relaxed with the appropriate amount of concern for the assessment. The patient should exhibit erect posture, a smooth gait, and symmetrical body movements.*

A Restlessness, tenseness, and pacing are abnormal.
P These may be signs of anxiety or metabolic disorders, which should alert you to further investigate these problems.

A Slumped posture, slow gait, poor eye contact, and slow responses are abnormal findings.
P These may be signs of depression.

A Stooped, flexed, or rigid posture, drooping neck, deformities of the spine, and tics are abnormal findings.
P Patients with kyphosis, scoliosis, Parkinson's disease, cerebral palsy, schizophrenia, muscular atrophy, myasthenia gravis, or stroke may exhibit these signs.

Dress, Grooming, and Personal Hygiene

E **1.** Note the appearance of the patient's clothing, specifically:
a. cleanliness
b. condition
c. age appropriateness
d. weather appropriateness
e. appropriateness for the patient's socioeconomic group
2. Observe the patient's personal grooming (hair, skin, nails, teeth) for:
a. adequacy
b. symmetry
c. odor

N *The patient should be clean and well groomed, and should wear appropriate clothing for age, weather, and socioeconomic status.*

A Poor personal hygiene such as uncombed hair, body odor, or unkempt clothing is abnormal.
P These signs may be indications of depression, schizophrenia, or dementia.

A Excessive, meticulous care and attention to clothing and grooming are abnormal behaviors.
P These signs may indicate obsessive-compulsive behavior.

A Obvious one-sided differences in grooming and dressing or the use of only one side of the body is abnormal.
P Stroke in the parietal lobe may cause the patient to be aware of only one side of the body, which is termed one-sided neglect.

Facial Expression

E Observe for appropriateness of, variations in, and symmetry of facial expressions.

N *Facial expressions should be appropriate to the content of the conversation and should be symmetrical.*

A Extreme, inappropriate, or unchanging facial expressions, or asymmetrical facial movements are abnormal.
P Abnormal facial expressions demonstrate anxiety, depression, or the unchanging facial expression of a patient with Parkinson's disease. They may also indicate a lesion in the facial nerve (CN VII).

🌹 NURSING TIP

Influences on Dress and Grooming

Dress and grooming are influenced by the patient's economic status, age, home situation, and ethnic background. Information obtained during the health history will assist you in determining appropriate dress and grooming for each patient. It is helpful to directly ask the patient about grooming routines and clothing choices when there is a question as to appropriateness.

E	**Examination**
N	**Normal Findings**
A	**Abnormal Findings**
P	**Pathophysiology**

Affect

E 1. Observe the patient's interaction with you, paying particular attention to both verbal and nonverbal behaviors.
2. Note if the patient's affect appears labile, blunted, or flat.
3. Note the variations in the patient's affect with a variety of topics.
4. Note any extreme emotional responses during the interview.

N *The appropriateness and degree of affect should vary with the topics and the patient's cultural norms, and be reasonable, or eurhythmic (normal).*

A Blunted affect, manifested by the patient shuffling into the examination room, slumping into a chair, moving slowly and not making eye contact, is abnormal.

P A blunted affect may indicate depression.

A Unresponsive, inappropriate affect is abnormal.

P A flat, unresponsive affect may indicate depression or schizophrenia.

A Anger, hostility, and paranoia are abnormal responses in most clinical situations.

P These may be the responses of a paranoid schizophrenic individual.

A Euphoric, dramatic, disruptive, irrational, or elated behaviors are abnormal in most clinical situations.

P A manic-depressive patient might display these responses during the manic phase.

Communication

Communication skills should be assessed throughout the entire interview and physical assessment.

E 1. Note voice quality, which includes voice volume and pitch.
2. Assess articulation, fluency, and rate of speech by engaging the patient in normal conversation. Ask the patient to repeat words and sentences after you or to name objects you point out.
3. Note the patient's ability to carry out requests during the assessment, such as pointing to objects within the room as requested. Ask questions that require "yes" and "no" responses.
4. Write simple commands for the patient to read and perform, for example "point to your nose" or "tap your right foot." Reading ability may be influenced by the patient's educational level or visual impairment.
5. Ask the patient to write his or her name, birthday, a sentence the patient composes, or a sentence that you dictate. Note the patient's spelling, grammatical accuracy, and logical thought process.

N *The patient should be able to produce spontaneous, coherent speech. The speech should have an effortless flow with normal inflections, volume, pitch, articulation, rate, and rhythm. Content of the message should make sense. Comprehension of language should be intact. The patient's ability to read and write should match the patient's educational level. Non-native speakers may exhibit some hesitancy or inaccuracy in written and spoken language.*

A **Aphasia**, an impairment of language functioning, is abnormal.

P Aphasias are classified by involved anatomy, behavioral speech manifestations, fluency of speech (fluent: rhythm, grammar, and articulation are normal; nonfluent: speech production is limited and speech is poorly articulated), and comprehension (receptive) versus expression (expressive) deficits. Other categories include amnesic, inability to recall specific types of words, and central, a deficit in the coordination among the speech areas. See Table 18-6 for a summary of the characteristics and pathophysiology of specific aphasias.

🌺 NURSING TIP

Handedness

Note handedness prior to language testing. Handedness and cerebral dominance for language are closely allied. Patients with dominant hemisphere lesions will frequently show communication abnormalities, e.g., aphasia in the righthanded individual almost always indicates left hemisphere disease.

E Examination
N Normal Findings
A Abnormal Findings
P Pathophysiology

Table 18-6 Classification of Aphasias

APHASIA	PATHOPHYSIOLOGY	EXPRESSION	CHARACTERISTICS
Broca's aphasia	Motor cortex lesion, Broca's area	Expressive Nonfluent	Speech slow and hesitant, the patient has difficulty in selecting and organizing words. Naming, word and phrase repetition, and writing impaired. Subtle defects in comprehension.
Wernicke's aphasia	Left hemisphere lesion in Wernicke's area	Receptive Fluent	Auditory comprehension impaired, as is content of speech. Patient unaware of deficits. Naming severely impaired.
Anomic aphasia	Left hemisphere lesion in Wernicke's area	Amnesic Fluent	Patient unable to name objects or places. Comprehension and repetition of words and phrases intact.
Conduction aphasia	Lesion in the arcuate fasciculus, which connects and transports messages between Broca's and Wernicke's areas	Central Fluent	Patient has difficulty repeating words, substitutes incorrect sounds for another (e.g., *dork* for *fork*).
Global aphasia	Lesions in the frontal-temporal area	Mixed Fluent	Both oral and written comprehension severely impaired; naming, repetition of words and phrases, ability to write impaired.
Transcortical sensory aphasia	Lesion in the periphery of Broca's and Wernicke's areas (watershed zone)	Fluent	Impairment in comprehension, naming, and writing. Word and phrase repetition intact.
Transcortical motor aphasia	Lesion anterior, superior, or lateral to Broca's area	Nonfluent	Comprehension intact. Naming and ability to write impaired. Word and phrase repetition intact.

NURSING ALERT

The Patient with Dysphonia

Patients with signs of dysphonia (impaired laryngeal speech) are at high risk for dysphagia (difficulty with swallowing) and therefore aspiration. A thorough assessment of swallowing is warranted before the patient may eat unassisted.

A **Dysarthria**, a disturbance in muscular control of speech, is abnormal.
P Dysarthria is due to ischemia affecting motor nuclei of CN X and CN XII; defects in the premotor or motor cortex that provide motor input for the face, throat, and mouth; or cerebellar disease.
A **Dysphonia**, difficulty making laryngeal sounds, is abnormal and can progress to **aphonia** (total loss of voice).
P Dysphonia is usually caused by lesions of CN X or swelling and inflammation of the larynx.
A **Apraxia**, the inability to convert the intended speech into the motor act of speech, is abnormal.
P Apraxia is due to dysfunction in the precentral gyrus of the frontal lobe.
A **Agraphia**, the loss of the ability to write, is abnormal.
P Agraphia is caused by lesions of Broca's and Wernicke's areas in the dominant side of the brain.
A **Alexia**, the inability to grasp the meaning of written words and sentences (word blindness), is abnormal.
P Alexia is usually due to a lesion of the angular gyrus and the occipital lobe.

E Examination
N Normal Findings
A Abnormal Findings
P Pathophysiology

NURSING ALERT

The Confused Patient

The confused patient should be thoroughly assessed for aphasia. A missed diagnosis because of "confusion" can be fatal if aphasia is present and due to a subdural hematoma. Check for other signs associated with a subdural hematoma, including headache, slow cerebration, decreasing level of consciousness, and ipsilateral pupil dilatation with a sluggish response to light.

Level of Consciousness (LOC)

Consciousness is the level of awareness of the self and the environment. Conscious behavior requires arousal, or wakefulness, and awareness, or cognition and affect. Arousal is controlled by the RAS. The RAS activates the cortex after receiving stimuli from the somatic and special sensory pathways. Awareness is a higher level function of the cerebral cortex, which interprets incoming sensory stimuli. Aspects of awareness at a higher level include judgment and thinking, which are generally assessed as part of the cognitive assessment. Orientation is awareness of self and environment.

E 1. Observe the patient's eyes when entering the room (environmental stimuli). Note whether the patient's eyes are open or whether they open when you enter the room (prior to any verbalization). Note the patient's response to any general environmental stimuli, such as noises or lights.
2. If the patient is not awake, call out the patient's name (verbal stimuli). Observe whether the patient's eyes open, whether he responds verbally and appropriately, and whether he follows verbal commands.
3. If the patient does not respond to verbal stimuli, lightly touch the patient's hand or gently shake the patient awake.
4. If the patient is not responding to environmental or verbal stimuli, proceed to the application of a painful stimulus.
   a. Apply pressure with a pen to the nailbed of each extremity, or
   b. Firmly pinch the trapezius muscle, or
   c. Apply pressure to the supraorbital ridge or the manubrium.
5. Observe the patient's reaction to the painful stimulus. Note whether the patient's eyes open.
6. Observe whether the patient can localize the painful stimulus by reaching for the area being stimulated. Strength of the patient's extremities can be assessed by the strength and distance of movement during his attempt to reach the painful stimulus. Note any abnormal motor responses.
7. Compare the motor responses and strength of the responses of right versus left sides of the patient.
8. Note whether the patient responds verbally to the painful stimulus.
9. Assess orientation by asking questions related to person, place, and time:
   a. Person: name of the patient, name of spouse or significant other
   b. Place: where the patient is now (what town, what state), where the patient lives
   c. Time: the time of day, month, year, season
10. Determine the **Glasgow Coma Scale** (GCS) score, an international method for grading neurological responses of the injured or severely ill patient. It is used for patients who have the potential for rapid deterioration. The GCS assesses three parameters of consciousness: eye opening, verbal response, and motor response.

🌺 NURSING TIP

Application of Painful Stimuli

1. Application of painful stimuli is extremely upsetting to family members and therefore should not be performed in their presence or without a comprehensive explanation.
2. These methods of applying painful stimuli may cause severe bruising if excessive force is used.
   • Apply only the amount of pressure needed to elicit a response.
   • Alternate sites when possible.

🌺 NURSING TIP

Glasgow Coma Scale

Most often, the Glasgow Coma Scale is included in a neurological observation sheet, which also includes vital signs, motor movement and strength, and pupillary size and reactions, to give a more in-depth evaluation of the neurological status of the patient (see Figure 18-9).

E	**Examination**
N	**Normal Findings**
A	**Abnormal Findings**
P	**Pathophysiology**

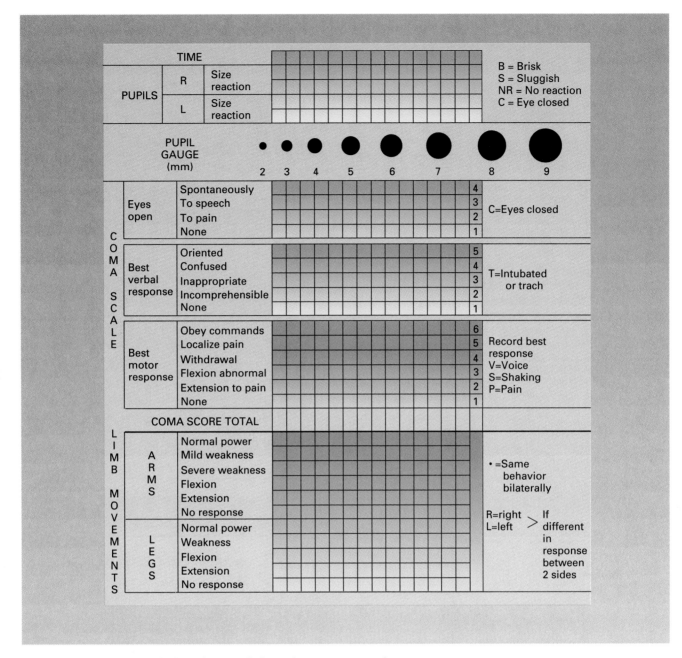

Figure 18-9   Neurological Flow Sheet, Including Glasgow Coma Scale

N   *The patient's best response to each of these categories is what the nurse records on the scale. The sum of the three categories is the total GCS score. The highest score of responsiveness is 15 and the lowest is 3. A score of 15 would indicate a fully alert, oriented individual.*

A/P   Refer to Table 18-7.

E   Examination
N   Normal Findings
A   Abnormal Findings
P   Pathophysiology

NURSING ALERT

Airway Protection

Patients with altered LOC may be unable to protect their airways. A complete airway assessment is required to determine the need for intubation.

Table 18-7   Levels of Consciousness: Abnormalities and Pathophysiology

LOC	RESPONSE TO STIMULI	PUPIL RESPONSE	PATHOPHYSIOLOGY	PROGNOSIS
Confusion GCS = 14	Spontaneous but may be inappropriate Memory faulty Reflexes intact	Normal	Metabolic derangements Diffuse brain dysfunction	Good chance of recovery Must treat primary cause
Lethargy GCS = 13–14	Requires stimulus to respond (verbal, touch) Reflexes intact	Normal to unequal	Metabolic derangements Medications Increased ICP	Good chance of recovery Must treat primary cause
Stupor GCS = 12–13	Requires vigorous, continuous stimuli to respond Reflexes intact	Normal, unequal, or sluggish	Metabolic derangements Medications Increased ICP	Good chance of recovery Must treat primary cause
Permanent vegetative state GCS = 8–10	Responds to pain No cognitive response Reflexes abnormal	Normal	Anoxic ischemic insults	Irreversible
Locked-in syndrome GCS = 6	Awake and aware Responds with eyes only	Normal	Lesion in ventral pons All four extremities and lower cranial nerves paralyzed Myasthenia gravis Acute polyneuritis	Poor prognosis
Coma GCS = 3–6	Abnormal Varied response to pain Reflexes abnormal or absent	Abnormal Dilated or pinpoint	Anoxia Traumatic injury Space-occupying lesion Cerebral edema	Prognosis dependent on length of time in coma
Brain death GCS = 3	No response Reflexes abnormal or absent	Abnormal Dilated or pinpoint	Anoxia Structural damage	Irreversible

LOC = level of consciousness; GCS = Glasgow Coma Scale; ICP = intracranial pressure.

⊙⊙ THINK ABOUT IT

Brain Death

You are caring for J.T., a 20-year-old male who has suffered a massive closed head injury in a motor vehicle accident. The physicians with whom you are working are completing the assessment required for a declaration of brain death.
- Do you know your state's definition of brain death?
- What clinical conditions must be met prior to the declaration of brain death?

J.T. has met the criteria for brain death. You have developed a therapeutic and trusting relationship with his parents and will now assist the physician in presenting the diagnosis to the parents.
- How will you present the concept of brain death to J.T.'s parents, particularly since he looks "normal" except for the ventilator?
- How will you explain death when the patient's heart is still beating?

J.T.'s parents have had time alone with him, and it is now appropriate to approach them with the request for organ donation.
- What is your obligation to offer organ donation to families under state and federal required-request laws?
- Who in your institution approaches families about organ donation?
- Are you able to answer these commonly asked questions?
  - Who pays the medical costs after the pronouncement of death until the harvesting of the organs?
  - If consent to donate is given, can the family still have an open casket funeral?
  - Is the family able to donate only specific organs?
  - Can the donation remain anonymous?
  - Are you *sure* that he is dead?

Cognitive Abilities and Mentation

Assessment of cognitive function includes testing for attention, memory, judgment, insight, spatial perception, calculation, abstraction, thought processes, and thought content.

✓ NURSING CHECKLIST
Assessment of Cognitive Function

You should have on hand:
- Preprinted lists of objects, phrases, and numbers for patient recall and explanation
- Preprinted scoring sheets to record responses
- Answers to long-term memory questions to accurately assess recall
- Alternate tests prepared for patients with language barriers, aphasia, deafness, blindness, etc.
- Paper and pencils for patient to use to respond

Attention

E
1. Pronounce a list of numbers slowly (approximately 1 second apart), starting with a list of two numbers and progressing to a series of five or six numbers. For example: 2, 5; 3, 7, 8; 1, 9, 4, 3; 1, 5, 4, 9, 0.
2. Ask the patient to repeat the numbers in correct order, both forward and backward.
3. Give the patient a different series of the same number of digits if the patient is unable to repeat the first series correctly. Stop after two misses of any length series.
4. "Serial 7's" is another way of assessing attention and concentration. Instruct the patient to begin with the number 100 and to count backwards by subtracting 7 each time: 100, 93, 86, 79, 72, 65, etc.
5. The patient may also try serial 3's (counting backwards from 100 by threes) if unable to perform serial 7's.

N *The patient should be able to correctly repeat the series of numbers up to a series of five numbers. The patient should be able to recite serial sevens or serial threes accurately to at least the 40s or 50s from 100 within 1 minute.*

A If the patient has a short attention span, the patient will not be able to repeat the numbers in sequence or perform serial sevens or threes.

P Dementia, neurological injury or disease, and mental retardation may impair attention.

Memory

E
1. Assess immediate recall in conjunction with attention span as discussed previously.
2. Give a list of three items that the patient is to remember and repeat in 5 minutes. Have the patient repeat the items to check initial understanding. During the 5 minutes, carry on conversation as usual. Ask the patient to repeat the items again after the 5-minute time frame.
3. If the patient is unable to remember one or more of the objects, show a list containing the objects along with others, and check recognition.
4. Record the number of objects remembered over the number of objects given.
5. Long-term memory is memory that is retained for at least 24 hours. Commonly asked questions for testing long-term memory include: name of spouse, spouse's birthday, mother's maiden name, name of the president, or the patient's birthday.

❖ ASK YOURSELF

Serial 7's

Try beginning with the number 100 and counting backwards by subtracting 7 each time. Do this in front of someone you respect.
- How did you feel?
- Imagine how a patient feels when asked to perform this activity.
- How could you make the patient feel more comfortable when performing calculations?

E	**Examination**
N	**Normal Findings**
A	**Abnormal Findings**
P	**Pathophysiology**

N *The patient should be able to correctly respond to questions and to identify all the objects as requested.*

A Memory loss is abnormal.

P Memory loss may be caused by pathologies such as nervous system infection, trauma, stroke, tumors, Alzheimer's disease, seizure disorders, alcohol, and drug toxicity. Memory is located in the temporal lobe and the hippocampus. Damage to these areas, in the form of hemorrhage, ischemia, compression, or herniation, will cause memory impairment.

Judgment

E
1. During the interview, assess whether the patient is responding appropriately to social, family, and work situations that are discussed.
2. Note whether the patient's decisions are based on sound reasoning and decision making.
3. Present hypothetical situations and ask the patient to make decisions as to what his or her responses would be. For example: "What would you do if followed by a police car with flashing lights?" or "What would you do if you saw a house burning?"
4. Interview the patient's family or directly observe the patient to assess judgment more carefully.

N *The patient should be able to evaluate and act appropriately in situations requiring judgment.*

A Impaired judgment, the inability to act appropriately in situations, is abnormal.

P Frontal lobe damage, dementia, psychotic states, and mental retardation may cause the patient to exhibit lack of appropriate judgment.

Insight

Insight is the ability to realistically understand oneself.

E
1. Ask the patient to describe personal health status, reason for seeking health care, symptoms, current life situation, and general coping behaviors.
2. If the patient describes symptoms, ask what life was like prior to the appearance of the symptoms, what life changes the illness has introduced, and whether the patient feels a need for help.
3. Ask the patient to draw a self-portrait; note the emphasis put on specific body parts, the patient's ability to reproduce figures on paper, and the representation of any part of the self-portrait. Note the facial features and the feelings portrayed by the picture.

N *The patient should demonstrate a realistic awareness and understanding of self.*

A Unrealistic perceptions of self are abnormal.

P Lack of insight may occur in the euphoric stages of bipolar affective disorders, endogenous anxiety states, or depressed states.

Spatial Perception

Spatial perception is the ability to recognize the relationships of objects in space.

E
1. Ask the patient to copy figures that you have previously drawn, such as a circle, triangle, square, cross, and a three-dimensional cube.
2. Ask the patient to draw the face of a clock, including the numbers around the dial.
3. Ask the patient to identify a familiar sound while keeping the eyes closed, for example, a closing door, running water, or a finger snap.
4. Have the patient identify right from left body parts.

N *The patient should be able to draw the objects without difficulty and as closely as possible to the original drawing, and to identify familiar sounds and left and right body parts.*

A **Agnosia**, the inability to recognize the form and nature of objects or persons, is abnormal. It may be visual, auditory, or somatosensory. For

E	**Examination**
N	**Normal Findings**
A	**Abnormal Findings**
P	**Pathophysiology**

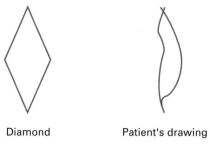

Diamond   Patient's drawing

Figure 18-10   Constructional Apraxia

example, the patient may be unable to name or recognize objects, faces, or familiar objects by touch, or to identify the meaning of nonverbal sounds.

P   Lesions in the right parietal lobe impair the patient's ability to appreciate self in relation to the environment and to conceive three-dimensional objects. Lesions in the occipital lobe will cause visual agnosia, and temporal lesions will cause auditory agnosia.

A   Apraxia, the inability to perform purposeful movements despite the preservation of motor ability and sensation, is abnormal. **Constructional apraxia** is the inability to reproduce figures on paper (see Figure 18-10).

P   Apraxia is usually associated with lesions of the precentral gyrus of the frontal lobe.

Calculation

The patient's ability to perform serial 7's was discussed in the section on attention and is also an assessment of calculation.

E   **1.** Ask the patient to add 3 to 100, then 3 to that number, until he reaches numbers greater than 150.
2. Note the amount of time and difficulty associated with the calculations.

N   *The patient should be able to calculate the correct numbers upon subtraction or addition within educational abilities and with fewer than four errors in less than 1½ minutes.*

A   **Dyscalculia**, the inability to perform calculations, is abnormal.

P   Dyscalculia may be caused by depression or anxiety, dementia, or mental retardation. The most common cause of dyscalculia is focal lesions in the dominant parietal lobe; however, calculation deficits have also been ascribed to focal lesions in the frontal, temporal, and occipital lobes.

Abstract Reasoning

E   **1.** Ask the patient to describe the meaning of a familiar fable, proverb, or metaphor. Use examples that are meaningful within the context of the patient's culture and language. Some examples from American culture are:
  • The squeaky wheel gets the grease.
  • A rolling stone gathers no moss.
  • A stitch in time saves nine.
  • People in glass houses should not throw stones.
  • Don't count your chickens before they hatch.
2. Note the degree of concreteness versus abstraction in the answers.

N   *Patients should be able to give the abstract meanings of proverbs, fables, or metaphors within their cultural understanding.*

A   Conceptual concreteness, the inability to describe in abstractions, to generalize from specifics, and to apply general principles, is abnormal.

P   Alterations of cognitive processes causing concreteness in thought may occur in patients with dementia, frontal tumors, or schizophrenia. Concreteness in thought processes may also indicate low intelligence.

Thought Process and Content

E   **1.** Observe the patient's pattern of thought for relevance, consistency, coherence, logic, and organization.
2. Listen throughout the interview for flaws in content of conversation.

N   *Thought processes should be logical, coherent, and goal oriented. Thought content should be based on reality.*

A   Unrealistic, illogical thought processes and interruptions of the thinking processes, such as blocking, are abnormal. Blocking is demonstrated when an extended pause occurs during a sentence due to a repressed or painful subject matter. Sometimes, the thoughts following are unrelated to what the patient was discussing.

P   Abnormal thought processes are often due to schizophrenia.

NURSING ALERT

Dyscalculia

Significant dyscalculia often accompanies aphasia. If dyscalculia is noted, a reassessment of speech and language ability should be performed.

E   Examination
N   Normal Findings
A   Abnormal Findings
P   Pathophysiology

A Flight of ideas, demonstrated when the patient changes from subject to subject within a sentence, is abnormal. This is frequently due to distractions or word associations with a resultant lack of sense of purpose of the conversation.

P Patients suffering from manic episodes of bipolar affective disorder often demonstrate flight of ideas.

A **Confabulation**, the making up of answers unrelated to facts, is abnormal.

P Confabulation is often related to aging, memory loss, disorientation, Korsakoff's psychosis, and psychopathic disorders.

A **Echolalia**, the involuntary repetition of a word or sentence that was uttered by another person, is abnormal.

P Schizophrenics and patients suffering from dementia often demonstrate echolalia.

A Delusions of persecution, grandiose delusions, hallucinations, illusions, obsessive-compulsiveness, and paranoia are examples of abnormal thoughts.

P Abnormal thought content is demonstrated in patients suffering from schizophrenia or dementia and in patients who use illegal drugs.

Table 18-8 compares and contrasts the various clinical parameters that distinguish dementia, depression, delirium, and acute confusion.

Sensory Assessment

<table>
<tr><td>✓</td><td>NURSING CHECKLIST</td></tr>
</table>

Assessing Sensation

1. Explain the procedure to the patient before starting the assessment.
2. The sensory assessment is carried out with the patient's eyes closed.
3. For a thorough sensory examination, the patient should be in a supine position.
4. The patient should be cooperative and reliable, although the pain assessment may be performed on comatose patients.
5. Note the patient's ability to perceive the sensation.
6. Much of the sensory component of the neurological assessment is subjective; observe the reactions of the patient by watching the face for grimacing, or withdrawal of the stimulated extremity.
7. Compare the patient's sensation on the corresponding areas bilaterally.
8. Note whether any sensory deficits follow a dermatome distribution.
9. The borders of any area exhibiting changes in sensation should be mapped (refer to Figure 18-7).

Sensation should be tested early in the neurological assessment because of the detail involved and because the cooperation of the patient is required. The conclusions of the assessment may be unreliable if the patient becomes fatigued.

The sensory assessment is divided into three sections. First, the exteroceptive sensations (superficial sensations that originate in the sensory receptors in the skin and mucous membranes) are tested. These are the sensations of light touch, superficial pain, and temperature.

Next, the proprioceptive sensations (deep sensations, with sensory receptors in the muscles, joints, tendons, and ligaments) are assessed. **Proprioception** is tested with the modalities of motion and position, and vibration sense.

Finally, the cortical sensations (those that require cerebral integrative and discriminative abilities) are assessed. Stereognosis, graphesthesia, two-point discrimination, and extinction are tested.

E	**Examination**
N	**Normal Findings**
A	**Abnormal Findings**
P	**Pathophysiology**

Table 18-8   Distinguishing Dementia, Depression, Delirium, and Acute Confusion

PARAMETER	DEMENTIA	DEPRESSION	DELIRIUM	ACUTE CONFUSION
Definition	Deterioration of all cognitive function with little or no disturbance of consciousness or perception Onset: gradual	An abnormal emotional state characterized by feelings of sadness, despair, and discouragement Onset: variable	A disorder of perception with heightened awareness, hallucinations, vivid dreams, and intense emotional disturbances Onset: sudden	An inability to think with customary speed, clarity, and coherence Onset: variable
Pathophysiology	Alzheimer's disease Metabolic disorders Stroke Head injury	Inherited: neurochemical abnormalities Situational: acute loss of significant person CVA Parkinson's disease Alzheimer's disease Medications (e.g., steroids)	Withdrawal from alcohol and other drugs Drug intoxications Encephalitis Traumatic injury Febrile states Hypoxia Fluid and electrolyte imbalance	Metabolic disorders Drug intoxication CVA Traumatic injury Febrile states
Attention	Impaired	Intact	Impaired: heightened or dulled	Impaired: dulled
Memory	Short term: impaired first Long term: intact for awhile	Intact	Short term: impaired Long term: intact	Short term: impaired Long term: may be intact
Judgment	Impaired	Intact	Grossly impaired Impulsive Volatile	Impaired
Insight	Impaired	Impaired if in manic phase	Impaired	Impaired
Spatial perception	Impaired	Intact	Intact	May be impaired
Calculation	Impaired	May be intact	May be intact	Impaired
Abstract reasoning	Impaired	Intact	Impaired	Impaired
Thought process and content	Impaired	Intact but may demonstrate flight of ideas	Impaired, hallucinations present	Impaired, incoherent

CVA = cerebrovascular accident.

Exteroceptive Sensation

For the entire exteroceptive sensation assessment, expose the patient's legs, arms, and abdomen.

Light Touch

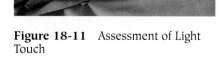

Figure 18-11   Assessment of Light Touch

E   1. Use a wisp of cotton and apply the stimulus with very light strokes (see Figure 18-11). If the skin is calloused, or for thicker skin on the hands and soles, the stimulus may need to be intensified, although care must be taken not to stimulate subcutaneous tissues.
2. Begin with distal areas of the patient's limbs and move proximally.
3. Test the hand, lower arm, abdomen, foot, and leg. Assessment of sensation of the face is discussed in the cranial nerve section.
4. To prevent the patient from being able to predict the next touch, alter the rate and rhythm of stimulation. Also, vary the sites of stimulation, keeping in mind that the right and left sides must be compared.
5. Instruct the patient to respond by saying "now" or "yes" when the stimulus is felt, and to identify the area that was stimulated either verbally or by pointing to it.

N/A/P   Refer to Temperature, pages 578–579.

Superficial Pain

E
1. Use a sharp object: sterile needle, sterile safety pin, or partially opened paperclip.
2. Establish that the patient can identify sharp and dull sensations by touching the patient with each stimulus and asking the patient to describe what is felt. This will help alleviate some of the fears the patient may have about being touched with a sharp object.
3. Hold the object loosely between the thumb and first finger to allow the sharp point to slide if too much pressure is applied.
4. Begin peripherally, moving in a distal to proximal direction and following the dermatomal distribution. If impaired sensation is identified, move from impaired sensation to normal sensation for comparison. Attempt to define the area of impaired sensation (mapping) by proceeding from the analgesic area to the normal area.
5. Alternate the sharp point with the dull end to test the patient's accuracy of shear sensation.
6. Instruct the patient to reply "sharp," "dull," or "I don't know" as quickly as the stimulus is felt and to indicate areas of the skin that perceive differences in pain sensation.
7. Again, compare the two sides, taking care not to proceed too fast or to cue the patient with regularity in the stimulus presentation.

N/A/P Refer to Temperature, following.

Temperature

Assess temperature sensation only if abnormalities in superficial pain sensation are noted.

E
1. Use glass vials containing warm water (40° to 45° C) and cold water (5° to 10° C). Hotter or colder temperatures will stimulate pain receptors.
2. Touch the warm or cold test tubes on the skin, distal to proximal and following dermatome distribution.
3. Instruct the patient to respond "hot," "cold," or "I can't tell" and to indicate where the sensation is felt.

N *The patient should be able to perceive light touch, superficial pain, and temperature accurately, and be able to correctly perceive the location of the stimulus.*

A **Anesthesia** refers to an absence of touch sensation. **Hypesthesia** is a diminished sense of touch; this may also be called hypoesthesia. **Hyperesthesia** is marked acuteness to the sensitivity of touch. **Paresthesia** is numbness, tingling, or pricking sensation. **Dysesthesia** is an abnormal interpretation of a stimulus such as burning or tingling from a stimulus such as touch or superficial pain. All of these findings are abnormal.

P Peripheral nerve lesions may cause anesthesia, hypesthesia, or hyperesthesia, which may be mapped out in the specific sensory distribution of the affected nerve. Lesions of the nerve roots produce areas of anesthesia and hypesthesia limited to the segmental distribution of the roots involved. Lesions in the brain stem or spinal cord can cause anesthesia, paresthesia, or dysesthesia.

A **Analgesia** refers to insensitivity to pain. **Hypalgesia** refers to diminished sensitivity to pain. **Hyperalgesia** is increased sensitivity to pain. These findings are abnormal.

P Lesions of the thalamus and the peripheral nerves and nerve roots can cause analgesia, hypalgesia, and hyperalgesia.

A Total unilateral loss of all forms of sensation is an abnormal finding.

P This is due to an extensive lesion of the thalamus and results in gross disability.

A A "saddle" pattern of sensation loss is abnormal.

P A lesion of the cauda equina produces the "saddle" pattern of sensation loss, the loss of leg reflexes, and the loss of sphincter control. If touch is preserved, the lesion is in or near the conus medullaris.

E	**Examination**
N	**Normal Findings**
A	**Abnormal Findings**
P	**Pathophysiology**

A The loss of touch sensation in the hands and lower legs (glove and stocking anesthesia) is abnormal.

P Glove and stocking anesthesia is common in polyneuritis of any cause.

A Unilateral loss of all exteroceptive sensation is abnormal.

P This is caused by a partial lesion of the thalamus or a lesion laterally situated in the upper brain stem. It may also be caused by hysteria.

Proprioceptive Sensation

Motion and Position

E 1. Grasp the patient's index finger with your thumb and index finger. Hold the finger at the sides (parallel to the plane of movement) in order not to exert upward or downward pressure with your fingers and thus give the patient any clues as to which direction the finger is moving. The patient's fingers should be relaxed.

2. Have the patient shut the eyes and show the patient what "up" and "down" feel like by moving the finger in those directions.

3. Use gentle, slow, and deliberate movements. Begin with larger movements that become smaller and less perceptible.

4. Instruct the patient to respond "up," "down," or "I can't tell" after each time you raise or lower the finger.

5. Repeat this several times. Vary the motion in order not to establish a predictable pattern.

6. Repeat steps 2 through 5 with the finger of the patient's opposite hand, and then with the great toes.

7. If there appears to be a deficit in motion sense, proceed to the proximal joints such as wrists or ankles, and repeat the test.

N *The patient should be able to correctly identify the changes of position of the body.*

A Inability to perceive direction of movement is abnormal.

P Peripheral neuropathies will interfere with position sense. A lesion of the posterior column will cause an ipsilateral loss of position sense. Lesions of the sensory cortex, the thalamus, or the connections between them (thalamocortical connections) may also disrupt position sense.

Vibration Sense

E 1. Strike the prongs of a low-pitch tuning fork against the ulnar surface of your hand or your knuckles, and place the base of the fork firmly on the patient's skin over bony prominences (see Figure 18-12). Be sure that your fingers touch only the stem of the fork, not the tines.

2. Begin with distal prominences such as a toe or finger, testing each extremity.

3. Instruct the patient to say "now" when the buzzing, vibrating tuning fork is felt, and to report immediately when the vibrations are no longer felt.

4. Be sure that the patient is reporting the vibration sense rather than hearing a humming sound or just feeling pressure from the tuning fork.

5. After the patient can no longer feel the vibrations, determine whether the vibrations can, in fact, still be felt by holding the prongs while the tuning fork is left on the patient.

6. If you detect a deficit in vibratory sense in the peripheral bony prominences, progress toward the trunk by testing ankles, knees, wrists, elbows, anterior superior iliac crests, ribs, sternum, and spinous processes of the vertebrae.

N *Normally, the patient should be able to perceive vibration over all bony prominences.*

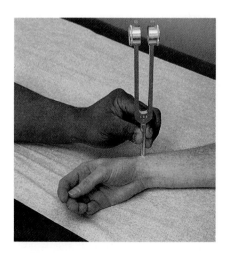

Figure 18-12 Assessment of Vibration

E	**Examination**
N	**Normal Findings**
A	**Abnormal Findings**
P	**Pathophysiology**

A The inability to perceive vibration sense is abnormal.

P Vibratory sense may be lost as a result of polyneuropathies (e.g., diabetic) or spinal cord lesions involving the posterior columns. Vibratory sensation is normally lower in patients over age 65.

Cortical Sensation

Stereognosis

Stereognosis is the ability to identify objects by manipulating and touching them.

E 1. Place a familiar object (dime, button, closed safety pin, key) into the patient's hand (see Figure 18-13).

   2. Ask the patient to manipulate the object, appreciating size and form.

   3. Ask the patient to name the object.

   4. Repeat in the opposite hand with a different object.

N *The patient should be able to identify the objects by holding them.*

A The inability to recognize the nature of objects by touch manipulation, termed **astereognosis**, is abnormal.

P Astereognosis is related to dysfunction of the parietal lobe, where the sensory cortex is located.

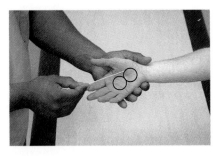

Figure 18-13 Assessment of Stereognosis

Graphesthesia

The ability to identify numbers, letters, or shapes drawn on the skin is termed **graphesthesia**.

E 1. Draw a number or letter with a blunt object (such as a closed pen or the stick of a cotton-tipped applicator) on the patient's outstretched palm. Make sure the number or letter is facing the patient's direction (see Figure 18-14).

   2. Ask the patient to identify what has been written.

   3. Repeat on the opposite side.

N *The patient should be able to identify what number or letter has been written on the palm or other skin surface.*

A **Graphanesthesia** is the inability to recognize a number or letter drawn on the skin and is abnormal.

P Graphanesthesia, in the presence of intact peripheral sensation, indicates parietal lobe dysfunction.

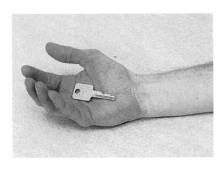

Figure 18-14 Assessment of Graphesthesia

Two-Point Discrimination

Two-point discrimination is tested by simultaneously and closely touching various parts of the body with two identical, sharp objects.

E 1. With two sterile pins, tips of opened paperclips, or broken cotton-tipped applicators, simultaneously touch the tip of one of the patient's fingers, starting with the objects far apart.

   2. Ask the patient whether one or two points are felt.

   3. Continue to move the two points closer together until the patient is unable to distinguish two points. Note the minimum distance between the two points at which the patient reports feeling the objects separately.

   4. Irregularly alternate, using one or two pins throughout the test to verify that the patient is feeling two points.

   5. Repeats steps 1–4 with the fingers of the opposite hand.

   6. Other areas of the body that may be tested include the dorsum of the hand, the tongue, the lips, the feet, or the trunk.

N *The patient should be able to identify two points at 5 mm apart on the fingertips. Other parts of the body vary widely in normal distance of discrimination, such as the dorsum of the hand or feet, where a separation of as much as 20 mm may be necessary for discrimination. The patient may be able to detect two points as close as 2 to 3 mm on the tip of the tongue.*

E	**Examination**
N	**Normal Findings**
A	**Abnormal Findings**
P	**Pathophysiology**

A Distances greater than those described previously that are required to identify two points are abnormal.

P Lesions in the parietal lobe impair two-point discrimination (with intact tactile sensation).

Extinction

Extinction (sensory inattention) is tested by simultaneously touching opposite sides of the body at the identical site. Use cotton-tipped applicators or your fingers.

E 1. Ask the patient if one or two points are felt and where they are felt.
  2. Remove the stimulus from one side while maintaining the stimulus on the opposite side.
  3. Ask the patient if one or two points are felt and where the sensations are felt.

N *The patient should be able to feel both stimuli.*

A The inability to feel the two points simultaneously and to discriminate that one point has been removed is abnormal.

P A lesion in one parietal lobe may prevent the patient from feeling the stimulus on the opposite side of the body even if sensation is intact on that side during routine assessment.

Cranial Nerves

A complete assessment of the 12 cranial nerves is necessary when a baseline assessment is desired, if a tumor of a specific cranial nerve is suspected, or if periodic assessment is needed after surgery or radiation treatments. An abbreviated cranial nerve assessment is an integral part of a neurological screening examination. The screening examination would include cranial nerves II, III, IV, and VI: visual acuity and gross visual fields, funduscopic examination, pupillary reactions, and extraocular movements; cranial nerves VII, VIII, IX, X, and XII: facial musculature and expression, gross hearing, voice, and inspection of the tongue.

Olfactory Nerve (CN I)

E 1. Ask the patient to close the eyes.
  2. Test each side separately by asking the patient to occlude one nostril by pressing against it with a finger.
  3. Ask the patient to inhale deeply in order to cause the odor to surround the mucous membranes and adequately stimulate the olfactory nerve (see Figure 18-15).
  4. Ask the patient to identify the contents of each vial.
  5. Present one odor at a time and alternate them from nostril to nostril.
  6. Allow enough time to pass between presentation of vials to prevent confusion of the olfactory system.
  7. Record the number of substances tested and the number of times the patient was able to correctly identify the contents.
  8. Note whether a difference between the right and the left sides was apparent.

N *The patient should be able to distinguish and identify the odors with each nostril.*

A **Anosmia**, the loss of the sense of smell, is abnormal.

P Total loss of the sense of smell may be caused by trauma to the cribriform plate, sinusitis, colds, or heavy smoking. Unilateral anosmia may be the result of an intracranial neoplasm, such as a meningioma of the sphenoid ridge compressing the olfactory tract or bulb.

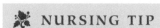

NURSING TIP

Olfactory Assessment

- Determine whether the nasal passages are patent by asking the patient to breathe through first one nostril and then through the other while occluding the opposing nostril by pressing against it with a finger. Assessment of the olfactory nerve may be delayed if the patient has a severe cold.

- Keep aromatic substances such as tobacco, cloves, coffee, orange, peanut butter, or chocolate in closed glass vials until they are presented to the patient.

- Avoid using noxious odors such as alcohol, camphor, ammonia, acetic acid, or formaldehyde, which may stimulate the trigeminal nerve endings in the nasal mucosa.

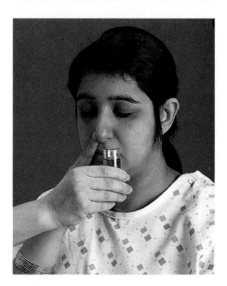

Figure 18-15 Assessment of CN I

Optic Nerve (CN II)

Visual Acuity (ENAP: Refer to Chapter 12.)
Visual Fields (ENAP: Refer to Chapter 12.)
Funduscopic Examination (ENAP: Refer to Chapter 12.)

Oculomotor Nerve (CN III)

Cardinal Fields of Gaze (ENAP: Refer to Chapter 12.)
Eyelid Elevation (ENAP: Refer to Chapter 12.)
Pupil Reactions (Direct, Consensual, Accommodation) (ENAP: Refer to Chapter 12.)

Normal (reflex present)

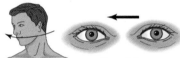

Head rotated   Eyes move to the left
to the right

Abnormal (reflex absent)

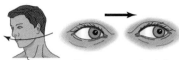

Head rotated   Eyes follow
to the right

Figure 18-16 Assessing the Oculocephalic Reflex

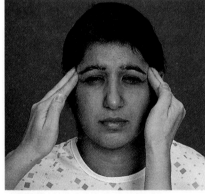

A. Temporalis Muscles

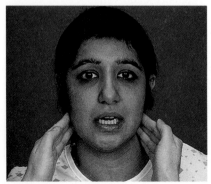

B. Masseter Muscles

Figure 18-17 Assessment of the Motor Component of CN V

✸ SPECIAL TECHNIQUE

Doll's Eyes Phenomenon

Assess doll's eyes phenomenon (oculocephalic reflex) (CN III) in the unconscious patient. This tests the intactness of the vestibular and oculomotor pathways. Doll's eyes phenomenon should not be tested in the patient with suspected neck injury.

E 1. Hold the patient's eyelids open and rotate the head of the patient briskly from the center to one side and then to the opposite side, holding briefly at the end points.
   2. Watch for eye movement.
   3. Further evaluate the oculocephalic reflex by alternately flexing and extending the head with the eyelids held as before.

N *Normally, the eyes should deviate in the direction opposite the head (e.g., head up, eyes look down; head turned to the right, eyes look left) (see Figure 18-16).*

A Loss of doll's eyes phenomenon is abnormal and is demonstrated when the eyes remain fixed with neither lateral nor vertical deviation in response to head movement (refer to Figure 18-16).

P Patients with low brain stem lesions will exhibit abnormal doll's eyes phenomenon.

Trochlear Nerve (CN IV)

Cardinal Fields of Gaze (ENAP: Refer to Chapter 12.)

Trigeminal Nerve (CN V)

Motor Component

E 1. Instruct the patient to clench the jaw.
   2. Palpate the contraction of the temporalis (see Figure 18-17A) and masseter (see Figure 18-17B) muscles on each side of the face by feeling for contraction of the muscles with the finger pads of the first three fingers.
   3. Ask the patient to move the jaw from side to side against resistance from your hand. Feel for weakness on one side or the other as the patient pushes against resistance.
   4. Test the muscles of mastication by having the patient bite down with the molars on each side of a tongue blade and comparing the depth of the impressions made by the teeth. If you can pull the tongue blade out while the patient is biting on it, there is weakness of the muscles of mastication.
   5. Observe for fasciculation and note the bulk, contour, and tone of the muscles of mastication.

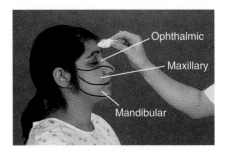

Figure 18-18 Assessment of the Sensory Component of CN V: Light Touch

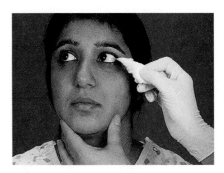

Figure 18-19 Assessment of the Sensory Component of CN V and Motor Component of CN VII: Corneal Reflex

Sensory Component

E
1. Instruct the patient to close the eyes.
2. Test light touch by using a cotton wisp to lightly stroke the patient's face in each area of the sensory distribution of the trigeminal nerve (see Figure 18-18).
3. Instruct the patient to respond by saying "now" each time the touch of the cotton wisp is felt.
4. Test and compare both sides of the face.
5. To assess superficial pain sensation, use a sterile needle or open paperclip. Before testing, show the patient how the sharpness of the needle or paperclip feels compared to the dullness of the opposite, blunt end. Testing with the blunt end will give some reliability to the assessment.
   a. Instruct the patient to respond by saying "sharp" or "dull" when each sensation is felt.
   b. Irregularly alternate the sharp and dull ends, and again test each distribution area of the trigeminal nerve on both sides of the face.
6. Test temperature sensation if other abnormalities have been detected. Use vials of hot and cold water.
   a. Touch the vials to each dermatomal distribution area, alternating hot and cold.
   b. The patient should respond by saying "hot" or "cold."
7. Because sensation to the cornea is supplied by the trigeminal nerve, test the corneal reflex (the motor component is CN VII).
   a. Ask the patient to open the eyes and look away from you.
   b. Approach the patient out of the line of vision to eliminate the blink reflex. You can stabilize the patient's chin with your hand if it is moving.
   c. Lightly stroke the cornea with a slightly moistened cotton wisp (to avoid irritating the cornea, see Figure 18-19). Avoid stroking just the sclera or the lashes of the eye.
   d. Observe for bilateral blinking of the eyes.
   e. Repeat on the opposite eye.

N *The temporalis and masseter muscles should be equally strong on palpation. The jaw should not deviate and should be equally strong during side-to-side movement against resistance. The volume and bulk of the muscles should be bilaterally equal. Sensation to light touch, superficial pain, and temperature should be present on the sensory distribution areas of the trigeminal nerve. The corneal reflex should cause bilateral blinking of eyes.*

A Lesions of the trigeminal nerve may give rise to either reduced sensory perception or to facial pain, both of which are abnormal.

P Aneurysms of the internal carotid artery next to the cavernous sinus may give rise to severe pain in the ophthalmic or mandibular distribution of the trigeminal nerve due to the pressure of the aneurysm on the nerve. Neoplasms that compress the gasserian ganglion or root, such as meningiomas, pituitary adenomas, and malignant tumors of the nasopharynx, may cause facial pain and impairment of sensation. Head injuries, especially basilar skull fractures, may give rise to facial anesthesia and paralysis of the muscles of mastication.

A Trigeminal neuralgia (tic douloureux), characterized by brief, paroxysmal unilateral facial pain along the distribution of the trigeminal nerve, is abnormal. The pain can be provoked by touch or movement of the face, such as in tooth brushing, yawning, chewing, or talking. There is no associated motor weakness.

P Trigeminal neuralgia may occur in patients with multiple sclerosis due to demyelinization of the root of CN V. The patient with a posterior fossa tumor may have trigeminal neuralgia. In most cases, there is no etiology found.

E	**Examination**
N	**Normal Findings**
A	**Abnormal Findings**
P	**Pathophysiology**

A Postherpetic neuralgia is found most often in the elderly. The pain is continuous and is described as a constant, burning ache with occasional stabbing pains. The stabbing pain may begin spontaneously or may be provoked by touch. The pain is unilateral and tends to follow the distribution of the ophthalmic distribution of the trigeminal nerve. It is abnormal.

P Herpes zoster involvement of the trigeminal nerve causes postherpetic neuralgia. Inflammatory lesions are found throughout the trigeminal pathways.

A Tetanus is characterized by tonic spasms interfering with the muscles that open the jaw (trismus). Dysphagia and spasms of the pharyngeal muscles are also observed in tetanus. Tetanus is abnormal.

P Motor root involvement of the trigeminal nerve causes the spasm of the masseter muscles.

Abducens Nerve (CN VI)

Cardinal Fields of Gaze (ENAP: Refer to Chapter 12.)

Facial Nerve (CN VII)

Motor Component

E 1. Observe the patient's facial expressions for symmetry and mobility throughout the assessment.
2. Note any asymmetry of the face, such as wrinkles or lack of wrinkles on one side of the face or one-sided blinking.
3. Test muscle contraction by asking the patient to:
   a. frown
   b. raise the eyebrows
   c. wrinkle the forehead while looking up
   d. close the eyes lightly and then keep them closed against your resistance (see Figure 18-20).
   e. smile, show teeth, purse lips, and whistle
   f. puff out the cheeks against the resistance of your hands
4. Observe for symmetry of facial muscles and for weakness during the above maneuvers.
5. Note any abnormal movements such as tremors, tics, grimaces, or immobility.

N *Normal findings of the motor portion of the facial nerve include symmetry between the right and the left sides of the face as well as the upper and lower portions of the face at rest and while executing facial movements. There should be an absence of abnormal muscle movement.*

A **Bell's palsy** (idiopathic facial palsy), characterized by complete flaccid paralysis of the facial muscles on the involved side, is abnormal. The affected side of the face is smooth, the eye cannot close, the eyebrow droops, the labiofacial fold is gone, and the mouth may droop. Loss of the sensation of taste in the anterior two-thirds of the tongue may occur.

P Bell's palsy is caused by damage to the facial nerve. It is a lower motor neuron paralysis because the damage occurs along the facial nerve from its origin to its periphery.

A Supranuclear facial palsy is characterized by paralysis in the lower one-third to one-half to two-thirds of the face; the upper portion of the face is spared. The nasolabial fold is flat, and the eye on the affected side can close, although more weakly. The patient may be unable to keep the eye closed against resistance applied by the nurse. The muscles of the upper portion of the face remain intact. Supranuclear facial palsy is abnormal.

P Supranuclear facial palsy is due to an upper motor neuron lesion of the facial nerve.

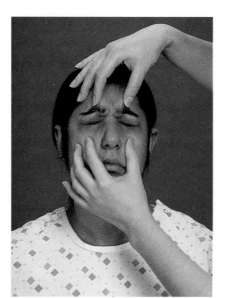

Figure 18-20 Assessment of the Motor Component of CN VII: Opening the Patient's Eyes Against Resistance

E	Examination
N	Normal Findings
A	Abnormal Findings
P	Pathophysiology

Sensory Component

E 1. Sensory assessment of the facial nerve is limited to testing taste. The portions of the tongue that are tested are:

a. the tip of the tongue for sweet and salty tastes

b. along the borders and at the tip for sour taste

c. the back of the tongue and the soft palate for bitter taste

2. Test both sides of the tongue with each solution.

3. The patient's tongue should protrude during the entire assessment of taste, and talking is not allowed. In order for the patient to identify the substance, the words *sweet*, *salty*, *bitter*, and *sour* should be written on a card so the patient can point to what is tasted. Be sure the patient does not see which solution is being tested.

4. Cotton swabs may be used as applicators, using a different one for each solution.

5. Dip the cotton swab into the solution being tested and place it on the appropriate part of the tongue.

6. Instruct the patient to point to the word that best describes taste perception.

7. Instruct the patient to rinse the mouth with water before the next solution is tested.

8. Repeat steps 5, 6, and 7 until each solution has been tested on both sides of the tongue.

N *Normal sensation would be accurate perceptions of sweet, sour, salty, and bitter tastes.*

A **Ageusia**, the loss of taste, and **hypogeusia**, the diminution of taste, are abnormal.

P Age, excessive smoking, extreme dryness of the oral mucosa, lesions of the medulla oblongata, or lesions of the parietal lobe may cause alterations in the sense of taste.

Acoustic Nerve (CN VIII)

Cochlear Division

Hearing. (ENAP: Refer to Chapter 12.)

Weber and Rinne Tests. (ENAP: Refer to Chapter 12.)

Vestibular Division The vestibular division of CN VIII assesses for vertigo.

E 1. During the history, ask the patient if vertigo is experienced.

2. Note any evidence of equilibrium disturbances. Refer to the section on cerebellar assessment.

3. Note the presence of nystagmus.

N *Vertigo is not normally present.*

A Vertigo describes an uncomfortable sensation of movement of the environment or the movement of self within a stationary environment. The sensation of movement is often accompanied by nausea, vomiting, and nystagmus, and is abnormal.

P Vertigo is caused by a disorder of the labyrinth or the vestibular nerve. Causative factors may include migraine headache, which causes a disruption in the supply of the internal auditory artery. Tumors of the cerebellopontine angle may cause vertigo by compressing the vestibular nerve. Head injuries that involve the labyrinth may cause vertigo. Blockage of the eustachian tube during ascent in an airplane may lead to vertigo.

A Ménière's disease, characterized by vertigo that lasts for minutes or hours, low-pitched roaring tinnitus, progressive hearing loss, nausea, and vomiting, is abnormal. The patient also experiences pressure in the ear.

P The main pathological finding is distension of the endolymphatic system, with degenerative changes in the organ of corti.

E	**Examination**
N	**Normal Findings**
A	**Abnormal Findings**
P	**Pathophysiology**

Glossopharyngeal and Vagus Nerves (CN IX and CN X)

The glossopharyngeal and vagus nerves are tested together because of their overlap in function.

E 1. Examine soft palate and uvula movement and gag reflex as described in Chapter 12.

2. Assess the patient's quality of speech for a nasal quality or hoarseness. Ask the patient to produce guttural and palatal sounds, such as *k*, *q*, *ch*, *b*, and *d*.

3. Assess the patient's ability to swallow a small amount of water. Observe for regurgitation of fluids through the nose. If the patient is unable to swallow, observe how oral secretions are handled.

4. The sensory assessment of the glossopharyngeal and vagus nerves is limited to taste on the posterior one-third of the tongue. This assessment was previously discussed in the section on CN VII.

N *Refer to Chapter 12 for normal soft palate and uvula movement and gag reflex findings. The speech is clear, without hoarseness or a nasal quality. The patient is able to swallow water or oral secretions easily. Taste (sweet, salty, sour, and bitter) is intact in the posterior one-third of the tongue.*

A Unilateral lowering and flattening of the palatine arch; weakness of the soft palate; deviation of the uvula to the normal side; mild dysphagia, regurgitation of fluids, and nasal quality of the voice; loss of taste in the posterior one-third of the tongue; and hemianesthesia of the palate and pharynx are abnormal.

P Unilateral glossopharyngeal and vagal paralysis, such as with missile wounds or skull fractures at the base of the skull, will cause these symptoms.

A Marked nasal quality of the voice, difficulty with guttural and palatal sounds, severe dysphagia with liquids, and inability of the palate to elevate on phonation are abnormal.

P Bilateral vagus nerve paralysis will cause these more marked symptoms, and often occurs simultaneously with signs and symptoms of other lower brain stem cranial nerve dysfunction such as in progressive bulbar palsy in amyotrophic lateral sclerosis (ALS).

Spinal Accessory Nerve (CN XI)

E 1. Place the patient in a seated or a supine position. Inspect the sternocleidomastoid muscles for contour, volume, and fasciculation.

2. Place your right hand on the left side of the patient's face. Instruct the patient to turn the head sideways against the resistance of your hand (see Figure 18-21A).

3. Use the other hand to palpate the sternocleidomastoid muscle for strength of contraction. Inspect the muscle for contraction.

4. Repeat steps 2 and 3 in the opposite direction. Compare the strength of the two sides.

5. To assess the function of the trapezius muscle, stand behind the patient and inspect the shoulders and scapula for symmetry of contour. Note any atrophy or fasciculation.

6. Place your hands on top of the patient's shoulders and instruct the patient to raise the shoulders against the downward resistance of your hands (see Figure 18-21B). This can be performed in front of or behind the patient.

7. Observe the movements and palpate the contraction of the trapezius muscles. Compare the strength of the two sides.

N *The patient should be able to turn the head against resistance with a smooth, strong, and symmetrical motion. The patient should also demonstrate the ability to shrug the shoulders against resistance with strong, symmetrical movement of the trapezius muscles.*

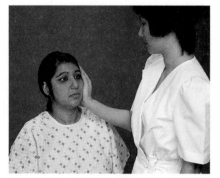

A. Strength of Sternocleidomastoid Muscle

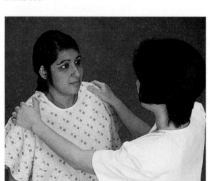

B. Strength of Trapezius Muscles

Figure 18-21 Assessment of CN XI

E	Examination
N	Normal Findings
A	Abnormal Findings
P	Pathophysiology

A Inability to turn the head toward the paralyzed side, and a flat, noncontracting muscle on that side are abnormal findings. The contralateral sternocleidomastoid muscle may be contracted.

P These findings are the result of unilateral paralysis of the sternocleidomastoid muscle due to trauma, tumors, or infection affecting the spinal accessory nerve.

A The inability of the patient to elevate one shoulder, asymmetrical drooping of the shoulder and scapula, and a depressed outline of the neck are abnormal findings. The involved shoulder may also show atrophy and fasciculation of the muscles.

P Unilateral paralysis of the trapezius muscle may be suspected, usually due to trauma, tumors, or infection.

A/P For information on torticollis, refer to Chapter 11.

Hypoglossal Nerve (CN XII)

E **1.** Refer to Chapter 12 for assessment of tongue movement.
      2. Assess lingual sounds by asking the patient to say "la la la."

N *Refer to Chapter 12 for normal tongue movements. Lingual speech is clear.*

A Inability or difficulty in producing lingual sounds is abnormal. The speech sounds lispy and clumsy.

P Lesions of the hypoglossal nerve will cause difficulty in pronunciation of lingual sounds.

Motor System

For ENAP on muscle size, tone, and strength, and involuntary movements, refer to Chapter 17. See following for additional A & P.

A Extrapyramidal rigidity is evident when resistance is present during passive movement of the muscles in all directions and lasts throughout the entire range of motion. It may involve both flexor and extensor muscles and is abnormal.

P Extrapyramidal rigidity is due to lesions located in the basal ganglia.

A **Decerebrate rigidity** (decerebration) is characterized by rigidity and sustained contraction of the extensor muscles and is abnormal. The arms are adducted, extended, and hyperpronated. The legs are stiffly extended and the feet are plantar flexed (see Figure 18-22A). The back and neck may be arched and the teeth clenched (opisthotonos).

P Decerebration may be found in unconscious patients with deep, bilateral diencephalic injury that progresses to midbrain dysfunction. Decerebrate rigidity may also occur due to midbrain and pontine damage, which occurs with compression of these structures due to expanding cerebellar or posterior fossa lesions. Severe metabolic disorders that depress diencephalic and forebrain function may also cause decerebration.

A **Decorticate rigidity** (decortication) is characterized by hyperflexion of the arms (flexion of the arm, wrist, and finger, adduction of the arms) and hyperextension, internal rotation, and plantar flexion of the legs (see Figure 18-22B). It is abnormal.

P Decorticate rigidity is found in unconscious patients with cerebral hemisphere lesions that interfere with the corticospinal tract.

Pronator Drift

E **1.** Have the patient extend the arms out in front with palms up for 20 seconds.
      2. Observe for downward drifting of an arm.

N *There should be no downward drifting of an arm.*

A Downward drifting of an arm is abnormal.

P Downward drifting of an arm may indicate hemiparesis, such as in stroke.

E **Examination**
N **Normal Findings**
A **Abnormal Findings**
P **Pathophysiology**

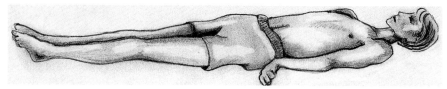

A. Decerebrate Rigidity

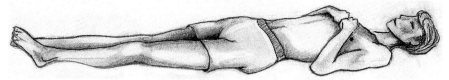

B. Decorticate Rigidity

Figure 18-22 Motor System Dysfunction

Cerebellar Function (Coordination, Station, and Gait)

Motor coordination refers to smooth, precise, and harmonious muscular activity. Movement requires the coordination of many muscle groups. Coordination is an integrated process, involving complicated neural integration of the motor and premotor cortex, basal ganglia, cerebellum, vestibular system, posterior columns, and peripheral nerves.

Equilibratory coordination refers to maintenance of an upright stance and depends on the vestibular, cerebellar, and proprioceptive systems. Nonequilibratory coordination refers to smaller movements of the extremities and involves the cerebellar and proprioceptive mechanisms.

Incoordination is categorized into three different types of syndromes: cerebellar, vestibular, and posterior column syndromes. Incoordination is not considered to be secondary to involuntary movements, paresis, or alterations of muscle tone.

Station refers to the patient's posture, and gait refers to the patient's manner of walking.

Coordination

E 1. Instruct the patient to sit comfortably facing you, with eyes open and arms outstretched.
2. Ask the patient to first touch the index finger to the nose, then to alternate rapidly with the index finger of the opposite hand.
3. With the patient's eyes closed, have the patient continue to rapidly touch the nose with alternate index fingers (see Figure 18-23).
4. With the patient's eyes open, ask the patient to again touch finger to nose. Next, ask the patient to touch your index finger, which is held about 18 inches away from the patient.
5. Change the position of your finger as the patient rapidly repeats the maneuver with one finger.
6. Repeat steps 4 and 5 with the other hand.
7. Observe for intention tremor or overshoot or undershoot of the patient's finger.
8. To assess rapid alternating movements, ask the patient to rapidly alternate patting the knees, first with the palms and then alternating palms with the backs of the hands (rapid supinating [Figure 18-24A] and pronating [Figure 18-24B] of the hands).

NURSING TIP

Patients Who Require Eyeglasses for Coordination

Ensure that patients who wear eyeglasses have their glasses on prior to assessing their coordination.

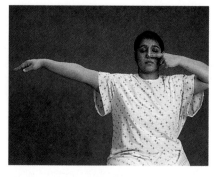

Figure 18-23 Assessment of Coordination: Fingertip-to-Nose Touch

E **Examination**
N **Normal Findings**
A **Abnormal Findings**
P **Pathophysiology**

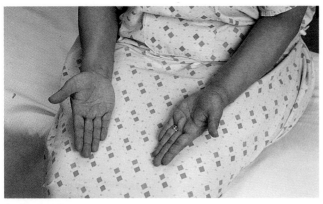

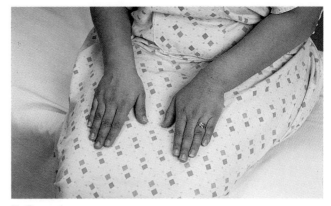

A. Supination   B. Pronation

Figure 18-24   Assessment of Coordination: Rapid Alternating Hand Movements

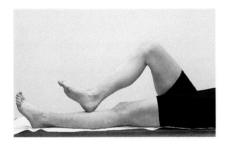

Figure 18-25   Assessment of Coordination: Heel Slide

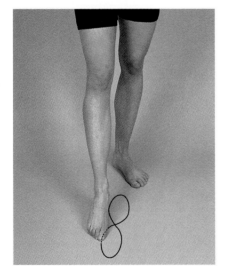

Figure 18-26   Assessment of Coordination: Figure Eight

E	**Examination**
N	**Normal Findings**
A	**Abnormal Findings**
P	**Pathophysiology**

9. Ask the patient to repeatedly touch the thumb to each of the fingers of the hand in rapid succession from index to the fifth finger, and back.

10. Repeat step 9 with the other hand.

11. Observe coordination and the ability of the patient to perform these in rapid sequence.

12. With the patient in a seated or supine position, ask the patient to place the heel just below the knee on the shin of the opposite leg and to slide it down to the foot (see Figure 18-25).

13. Repeat with the opposite foot.

14. Observe coordination of the two legs.

15. Ask the patient to draw a circle or a figure 8 with a foot either on the ground or in the air (see Figure 18-26).

16. Repeat with the other foot.

17. Observe for coordination and regularity of the figure.

18. Test the lower extremities for rapid alternating movement by asking the patient to rapidly extend the ankle ("tap your foot") or to rapidly flex and extend the toes of one foot.

19. Repeat with the opposite foot.

20. Note rate, rhythm, smoothness, and accuracy of the movements.

N *The patient is able to rapidly alternate touching finger to nose and moving finger from nose to your finger in a coordinated fashion. The patient is able to perform alternating movements in a purposeful, rapid, coordinated manner. The patient demonstrates the ability to purposefully and smoothly run heel down shin with equal coordination in both feet and to draw a figure 8 or circles with the foot.*

A **Dyssynergy**, the lack of coordinated action of the muscle groups, is abnormal. The patient is unable to carry out smooth, coordinated movements. The patient's movements appear jerky, irregular, and uncoordinated.

A **Dysmetria**, impaired judgment of distance, range, speed, and force of movement, is abnormal. The patient misjudges distance and overshoots.

A **Dysdiadochokinesia**, the inability to perform rapid alternating movements, is abnormal. The patient is unable to abruptly stop one movement and begin another opposite movement.

P Cerebellar disease causes all of these abnormal findings.

Station   (ENAP: Refer to Chapter 17.)

Gait

E 1. Refer to Chapter 17 for gait assessment technique.
   2. Ask the patient to walk on tiptoes, then on heels.
   3. Ask the patient to walk in a straight line, touching heel to toe (tandem walking). The arms should be held at the side and the eyes should be open.
   4. Note the patient's ability to maintain balance.
   5. Ask the patient to hop in place first on one foot and then on the other.

N *Refer to Chapter 17 for normal gait findings. The patient should be able to walk unaided on tiptoes and heels, and walk heel to toe in a straight line without losing balance. The patient should also be able to maintain balance while hopping on one foot, with bilateral equal strength.*

A/P Refer to Chapter 17.

✳ SPECIAL TECHNIQUE

Romberg's Test

E 1. Ask the patient to stand erect, feet together and arms at side, first with eyes open, then closed.
   2. Note the patient's ability to maintain balance with eyes first open then closed.

N *The patient should be able to maintain balance with eyes open or closed for 20 seconds and with minimum swaying.*

A Romberg's test is positive if the patient becomes unsteady and tends to fall when the eyes are closed.

P In cerebellar disease, Romberg's test is negative, as the patient remains unsteady with the eyes open or closed. In posterior column disease with proprioceptive loss, the patient becomes appreciably more unsteady with eye closure.

NURSING ALERT

Romberg's Test

Stand close to the patient during this test in order to catch the patient if he or she begins to fall.

NURSING TIP

Deep Tendon Reflex Reinforcement

Even when the deep tendon reflex (DTR) is stimulated correctly, the patient may not exhibit a DTR because of conscious thought. If this occurs, reinforcement may be necessary. Reinforcement is a technique used to distract conscious thought of the DTR by concentrating on another action. Examples include the patient clenching the teeth, grasping the thigh with the hand not being assessed, and grasping and pulling the wrists with the contralateral hand.

Reflexes

✓ NURSING CHECKLIST
Assessing Reflexes

1. When testing reflexes, the patient should be relaxed and comfortable.
2. Position the patient so the extremities are symmetrical.
3. To elicit true reflexes, distract the patient by talking about another topic.
4. Hold the reflex hammer loosely between the thumb and index finger and strike the tendon with a brisk motion from the wrist. The reflex hammer should make contact with the correct point on the tendon in a quick, direct manner.
5. Observe the degree and speed of response of the muscles after the reflex hammer makes contact. Grading of DTR is as follows:
   * 0: absent
   * + (1+): present but diminished
   * ++ (2+): normal
   * +++ (3+): mildly increased but not pathological
   * ++++ (4+): markedly hyperactive, clonus may be present
6. Compare reflex responses of the right and the left sides. The normal response to taps in the correct area should elicit a brisk (++ or +++) contraction of the muscles involved.

E Examination
N Normal Findings
A Abnormal Findings
P Pathophysiology

Deep Tendon Reflexes

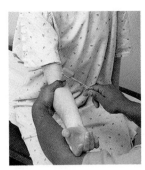

A. Biceps

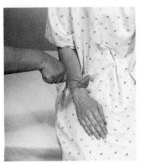

B. Brachioradialis

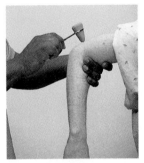

C. Triceps

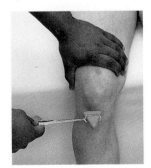

D. Patellar

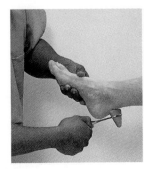

E. Achilles

Figure 18-27 Assessment of Deep Tendon Reflexes

Biceps

E
  1. Flex the patient's arm to between 45° and 90°.
  2. Support the patient's forearm on your forearm.
  3. Place your thumb firmly on the biceps tendon just above the crease of the antecubital fossa (Figure 18-27A).
  4. Wrap your fingers around the patient's arm and rest them on the biceps muscle to feel it contract.
  5. Tap the thumb briskly with the pointed end of the reflex hammer.

N *Observe for contraction of the biceps muscle and flexion of the elbow. Innervation of the biceps reflex is through the musculocutaneous nerve with segmental innervation of C5, C6.*

A/P Refer to Achilles, page 592.

Brachioradialis

E
  1. Flex the patient's arm to 45°.
  2. Support the patient's relaxed arm either on the lap or semipronated on your forearm.
  3. With the blunt end of the reflex hammer, strike the tendon of the brachioradialis above the styloid process of the radius (a few centimeters above the wrist on the thumb side) (Figure 18-27B).

N *Observe for flexion and supination of the forearm. An exaggerated reflex may also show flexion of the wrist and fingers and adduction of the forearm. Innervation of this reflex is through the radial nerve, with segmental innervation of C5, C6.*

A/P Refer to Achilles, page 592.

Triceps

E
  1. Flex the patient's arm to between 45° and 90°.
  2. Support the patient's arm either on the lap or on your hand as shown in Figure 18-27C.
  3. With the pointed end of the reflex hammer, tap the triceps tendon just above its insertion above the olecranon process (elbow).

N *Observe for contraction of the triceps muscle and extension of the arm. Innervation of the triceps reflex is through the radial nerve, with segmental innervation of C7, C8.*

A/P Refer to Achilles, page 592.

Patellar

E
  1. Ask the patient to sit in a chair or at the edge of the examination table.
  2. Place your hand over the quadriceps femoris muscle to feel contraction.
  3. With the other hand, tap the patellar tendon just below the patella with the blunt end of the reflex hammer (Figure 18-27D).
  4. If the patient cannot tolerate a sitting position, lift the flexed knee off the table with one hand, supporting it with your hand under the knee so the foot is hanging freely.

N *There should be contraction of the quadriceps muscle and extension of the leg. Innervation of the patellar reflex is through the femoral nerve, with segmental innervation of L2, L3, L4.*

A/P Refer to Achilles, page 592.

Achilles

E
  1. Ask the patient to sit with the feet dangling and partially dorsiflexed.
  2. With the blunt end of the reflex hammer, tap the Achilles tendon just above its insertion in the heel.
  3. If the patient is lying down, flex the leg at the knee and externally rotate the thigh. Place a hand under the foot to produce dorsiflexion. Hold the foot in your nondominant hand as shown in Figure 18-27E. Apply the stimulus as described in step 2.

N *The normal response is contraction of the muscles of the calf (gastrocnemius, soleus, and plantaris) and plantar flexion of the foot. Innervation of the Achilles reflex is through the tibial nerve, with segmental innervation of L5, S1, S2.*

A Absent or decreased deep tendon reflexes is abnormal.

P Diminished deep tendon reflexes usually result from interference in the reflex arc, and an absence may indicate a break in the reflex arc. Deep tendon reflexes are lost in deep coma, narcosis, or deep sedation. Hypothyroidism, sedative or hypnotic drugs, and infectious diseases may also diminish reflexes. Patients with increased intracranial pressure frequently show decreased or absent deep tendon reflexes. Spinal shock also causes loss of these reflexes.

A Hyperactive deep tendon reflexes are abnormal. Hyperactive deep tendon reflexes are characterized by an increase in speed of response and enhancement of the vigor of movement. The muscle contraction is sustained, with a minimal stimulus needed to elicit the response. Sometimes the adjacent muscles may also contract. Clonus may be present.

P Hyperactivity is associated with a loss of inhibition of the higher centers in the cortex and reticular formation and in lesions of the pyramidal system. Muscle stretch reflexes are also exaggerated in light coma, tetany, and tetanus.

Superficial Reflexes

Abdominal

E 1. Drape and place the patient in a recumbent position, arms at sides and knees slightly flexed. Stand to the right of the patient.
2. Use a moderately sharp object to stroke the skin, such as the wooden tip of a cotton-tipped applicator or a split tongue blade.
3. To elicit the upper abdominal reflex, stimulate the skin of the upper abdominal quadrants. From the tip of the sternum, stroke in a diagonal (downward and inward) fashion (see Figure 18-28).
4. Repeat step 3 on the opposite side.
5. To elicit the lower abdominal reflex, stimulate the skin of the lower abdominal quadrants. From the area below the umbilicus, stroke in a diagonal (downward and inward) fashion to the symphysis pubis.
6. Repeat step 5 on the opposite side.

N *Observe for contraction of the upper abdominal muscles upward and outward with a deviation of the umbilicus toward the stimulus. The upper abdominal reflex is innervated by the intercostal nerves through T7, T8, T9. Observe for contraction of the lower abdominal muscles and contraction of the umbilicus toward the stimulus. The lower abdominal reflex is innervated by the lower intercostal, iliohypogastric, and ilioinguinal nerves through segments T10, T11, T12.*

A/P Refer to Bulbocavernosus, page 593.

Plantar

E 1. With the handle of the reflex hammer, stroke the outer aspect of the sole of the foot from the heel across the ball of the foot to just below the great toe (see Figure 18-29).
2. Repeat on the opposite foot.

N *Observe for plantar flexion of the toes. The plantar reflex is innervated by the tibial nerve with segmental innervation of L5, S1, S2.*

A/P Refer to Bulbocavernosus, page 593.

Cremasteric

E 1. The male patient should be lying down with the thighs exposed and the testicles visible.

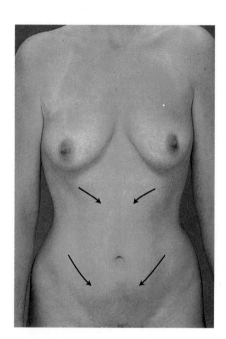

Figure 18-28 Assessment of Superficial Reflexes: Direction of Stimulus for Abdominal Reflexes

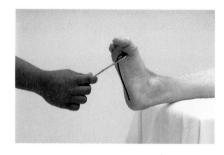

Figure 18-29 Assessment of Superficial Reflexes: Plantar

E	Examination
N	Normal Findings
A	Abnormal Findings
P	Pathophysiology

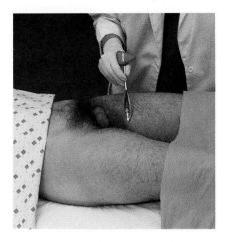

Figure 18-30 Assessment of Superficial Reflexes: Cremasteric

2. Stroke the skin of the inner aspect of the thigh near the groin from above downward (see Figure 18-30).

3. Repeat step 2 on the opposite side.

N *Observe contraction of the cremasteric muscle with corresponding elevation of the ipsilateral testicle. Innervation of the cremasteric reflex is through the ilioinguinal and genitofemoral nerves with segmental innervation of T12, L1, L2.*

A/P Refer to Bulbocavernosus, following.

Bulbocavernosus

E **1.** Pinch the skin of the foreskin or the glans penis.

2. Observe for a contraction of the bulbocavernosus muscle in the perineum at the base of the penis.

N *Contraction of the bulbocavernosus muscle occurs. The presence of this reflex in a paraplegic patient after acute spinal cord injury indicates that the initial stage of spinal shock is passed. The bulbocavernosus reflex is innervated by segments S3 and S4.*

A Decreased or absent superficial reflexes are abnormal.

P Superficial reflexes are diminished or absent with dysfunction of the reflex arc as in the muscle stretch reflexes. Superficial reflexes are complex because they involve the parietal areas and the motor centers of the premotor area and the pyramidal system. Lesions in the pyramidal tracts will cause decrease or absence of superficial reflexes. These reflexes may also be lost in deep sleep and coma.

Pathological Reflexes

All the reflexes described following are abnormal findings and are not usually assessed unless the patient's clinical presentation warrants it.

Grasp

E **1.** With your fingers, gently stroke the palm of the patient's hand.

2. The patient's fingers should flex or the hand should close.

3. Innervation is through the median and ulnar nerves, with segmental innervation in C6 and T1.

A The presence of this reflex is abnormal after infancy.

P This reflex is significant in pathological processes, in which a unilateral grasp reflex indicates a frontal lesion on the contralateral side. Bilateral grasp reflex means diffuse bifrontal dysfunction.

Snout

E **1.** With the reflex hammer, briskly tap the upper or lower lip.

2. Observe for a puckering of the lips.

A This reflex is abnormal after infancy.

P This reflex is seen in corticobulbar lesions and amyotrophic lateral sclerosis.

Glabellar

E **1.** With your finger, tap the patient on the forehead between the eyebrows.

2. Observe for a hyperactive blinking response.

A The presence of this reflex is abnormal.

P Patients with lesions of the corticobulbar pathways from the cortex to the pons, patients with Parkinson's disease, and patients with glioblastoma of the corpus callosum will have this reflex.

❖ ASK YOURSELF

Grasp Reflex

Families often accidentally illicit this reflex when they attempt to hold the comatose patient's hand. How would you explain to family members that this is not a sign of improvement in the patient's condition?

E **Examination**

N **Normal Findings**

A **Abnormal Findings**

P **Pathophysiology**

Sucking

E   **1.** Stroke the lower lip with a tongue blade.
    2. Observe for a pouting of the lips accompanied by a chewing, sucking, or swallowing response.
A   The presence of this reflex is abnormal after infancy.
P   Adults with bifrontal disease may exhibit this reflex.

Clonus

E   **1.** Have the patient assume a recumbent position. Stand to the side.
    2. Support the patient's knee in a slightly flexed position.
    3. Quickly dorsiflex the foot and maintain it in that position.
    4. Assess for **clonus** (a rhythmic oscillation of involuntary muscle contraction).
A   Sustained clonus is an abnormal finding.
P   Sustained clonus, in combination with muscle spasticity and hyperreflexia, indicates upper motor neuron disease. Table 18-9 summarizes the findings associated with upper and lower motor neuron dysfunction.

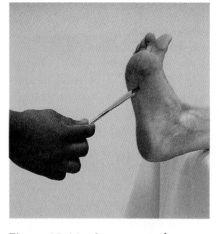

Figure 18-31   Assessment of Pathological Reflexes: Babinski

Babinski

E   With the handle of the reflex hammer, stroke the patient's sole as you did for the plantar reflex. Use a slow and deliberate motion.
A   A positive Babinski's reflex is noted when the patient's toes abduct (fan) and the great toe dorsiflexes (see Figure 18-31).
P   Patients with lesions in the pyramidal system, such as in stroke or trauma, display a positive Babinski's reflex.

Hoffmann's Sign

E   **1.** Hold the patient's hand dorsiflexed at the wrist and with the fingers slightly flexed. The hand should be completely relaxed.
    2. Partially extend the patient's middle finger and flex the distal phalanx over your fingers.
    3. Sharply flick the nail of the middle finger, causing a quick flexion of the distal phalanx and a sudden release.
A   A positive Hoffmann's sign consists of a quick flexion and adduction of the thumb and the index finger.
P   This response indicates hyperreflexia, seen in pyramidal tract disease.

Trömner's Sign

E   **1.** Hold the patient's relaxed hand by grasping the proximal or middle phalanx of the middle finger with your thumb and index finger.
    2. With the index finger of your other hand, tap the patient's distal phalanx on the palmar surface.

E	Examination
N	Normal Findings
A	Abnormal Findings
P	Pathophysiology

Table 18-9	Comparison of Upper Motor Neuron and Lower Motor Neuron Lesions	
PARAMETER	**UPPER MOTOR NEURON**	**LOWER MOTOR NEURON**
Muscle tone	Spasticity	Flaccidity
Muscle bulk	Late atrophy from disease; no fasciculations	Atrophy; fasciculations
Pronator drift	Positive	Absent
Deep tendon reflexes	Hyperreflexia	Hyporeflexia or absent
Babinski's reflex	Positive	Absent
Clonus	Present	Absent

A   Trömner's sign is indicated by flexion and adduction of the thumb and index finger, or sometimes, flexion of all five fingers.

P   This response occurs in conjunction with lesions of upper motor neurons.

Chaddock's Sign

E   By stroking with the blunt handle of the reflex hammer, stimulate the lateral aspect of the dorsum of the foot, continuing around the lateral malleolus.

A   Chaddock's sign manifests as dorsiflexion of the great toe.

P   This response indicates pyramidal tract dysfunction.

Oppenheim's Sign

E   1. Using heavy pressure applied with the thumb and index finger, stroke the anteromedial surface of the tibia.
    2. Begin below the knee and stroke down toward the ankle.

A   Oppenheim's sign is indicated by a slow dorsiflexion of the great toe.

P   Refer to Chaddock's sign.

Gordon's Sign

E   Firmly squeeze or apply deep pressure to the calf muscles.

A   Gordon's sign is indicated by dorsiflexion of the great toe.

P   Refer to Chaddock's sign.

❋ SPECIAL TECHNIQUE

Meningeal Irritation

To assess the patient for signs of meningeal irritation, look for nuchal rigidity, Kernig's sign, and Brudzinski's sign, all abnormal findings. Other signs and symptoms include violent headache, photophobia, fever, nausea and vomiting, decreasing level of consciousness, and convulsions. Definitive diagnosis is obtained through cultures of cerebrospinal fluid.

Nuchal Rigidity

Nuchal rigidity is the tendency by the patient to maintain the head in an immobile, extended position. The patient resists movement of the neck. Severe pain and spasms occur with movement.

E   1. Place the patient in a supine position.
    2. Flex the patient's neck.

A   The patient resists the movement.

P   Nuchal rigidity can be caused by meningeal irritation such as in meningitis. Meningitis is an infectious process of the meninges caused by bacteria, viruses, mycobacteria, fungi, or spirochetes. The organisms enter the subarachnoid space, causing an acute inflammatory response.

P   Irritation of the subarachnoid space due to subarachnoid hemorrhage may cause meningeal irritation.

Kernig's Sign

E   1. Place the patient in a recumbent position.
    2. Lift the patient's leg and flex the knee at a right angle.
    3. Attempt to extend the patient's knee by pushing down on it.

A   A positive Kernig's sign is a resistance to extension and pain (due to spasm of the hamstring), preventing extension of the leg.

P   Kernig's sign is caused by stretching of irritated nerve roots and meninges.

Brudzinski's Sign

E   1. Place one hand under the patient's neck and the other hand on top of the patient's chest to prevent elevation of the body.

continued

E	Examination
N	Normal Findings
A	Abnormal Findings
P	Pathophysiology

2. Flex the patient's neck with a deliberate motion.

A Brudzinski's sign is positive if the patient responds with flexion of one or both legs up to the pelvis. The arms may also flex.

P Refer to nuchal rigidity.

GERONTOLOGICAL VARIATIONS

The nervous system in the aging adult is particularly vulnerable to illness and to dysfunction of other body systems. The brain is dependent on blood flow for oxygen and nutrients. Changes in the cardiovascular system that lead to a decreased oxygen supply to the brain, such as arteriosclerosis of the cerebral arteries, thus affect cerebral functions such as mental acuity, sensory interpretation, and motor ability.

Neuronal changes occur with aging. The myelin sheath surrounding the nerve begins to degenerate, decreasing nerve conduction rate. The axons become smaller. Biochemically, the amount of neurotransmitter produced in the neuron is diminished, and the activity of the enzymes that degrade the neurotransmitter increases. Changes in neurotransmitters are known to affect sleep, temperature control, and mood. Depression, for example, is associated with decreased levels of the neurotransmitter norepinephrine, a common finding among the elderly.

Total brain weight, the number of synapses, and the number of neurons diminish with aging, beginning at age 50. Most of the loss occurs in the cerebral cortex and the cerebellum, and less so in the brain stem. The brain atrophies, causing a widening of the sulci and gyri, especially in the frontal lobes. The tendency of the brain to atrophy increases the size of the subdural space, leaving the cortical bridging veins vulnerable to trauma, bleeding, and the formation of a chronic subdural hematoma. The ventricles increase in size and the amount of cerebrospinal fluid increases to fill the space.

Sensory changes in the elderly are related to vision, hearing, vestibular alterations, and proprioception. The elderly have decreased visual acuity, visual fields, color sensitivity, and pupillary size, and diminished pupillary responses to light. The elderly person's hearing also diminishes due to ossification of the ossicles and degenerative changes in the auditory nerve. Elderly persons also demonstrate difficulties with balance as well as changes in coordination and equilibrium.

Cognitive changes characteristic of aging include decreased memory, primarily short-term memory, increased learning time, and changes in affect, mood, and orientation. Dementia may be a chronic or reversible problem. Delirium or acute mental confusion may be seen in elderly patients suffering from infection, dehydration, or CNS damage. As previously mentioned, depression, another problem among the elderly, may have a neurological base.

✿ NURSING TIP

Progression of Alzheimer's Disease

Alzheimer's disease is associated with an excessive accumulation of neurofibrillary tangles, as well as a large number of senile plaques, particularly in the hippocampus (area of memory). The cortex becomes thin and diffusely atrophied, the ventricles become enlarged, and the level of acetylcholine (neurotransmitter) decreases. These changes are usually seen in middle-aged to elderly persons. With the increasing aging population, it is imperative that you be familiar with the stages of Alzheimer's disease (refer to Table 18-10).

E Examination
N Normal Findings
A Abnormal Findings
P Pathophysiology

Table 18-10 Progression of Alzheimer's Disease		
STAGE	**CHARACTERISTICS**	**INTERVENTIONS**
Stage I Goal: Preservation of function	Decreased spontaneity Slower reaction time Mild depression Angers easily Memory changes: names, naming things Difficulty with spatial orientation (maps) Decreased energy Decreased initiative	Provide time to respond. Provide cues. Relieve anxiety. Give step-by-step directions orally and in writing. Recognize fear of the unfamiliar. Talk through situations. Provide names of people patient might expect to see.
Stage II Goal: Compensating for deficits	Worsening of stage I signs Difficulty with decisions Agnosia Apraxia Dyscalculia Avoidance of situations leading to failure	Assess ability for self-care in emergencies. Refer to home health care. Look for signs of injury (burns, bruises): may need to use microwave rather than stove. Provide orientation cues (pictures, calendar, notes).
Stage III Goal: Safety	Worsening of all of the above signs Marked change in behavior Limited attention span Ideational apraxia Wandering Hygiene deteriorates Psychosis Short-term memory loss	Orient continually. Free environment of hazards. Arrange for adult day care. Administer psychotropic drugs as prescribed. Reduce combativeness: • Step-by-step approach to tasks • Do not offer choices • Allow participation in tasks Speak at eye level with no barriers between you.
Stage IV Goal: Meet all physical needs (total nursing care)	Worsening of all of the above signs Apathy Increased agitation Spasticity **Perseveration**: repetitive motions such as chewing or tapping Hyperorality Incontinence Public genital displays and masturbation	Do not argue with paranoid or delusional conversation. Acknowledge patient's feelings. Toilet frequently. Provide meticulous skin care. Increase exercise to reduce wandering. Intervene to increase sleep but do not give sleep medications. Assess swallow and cue patient if needed to complete the swallowing process.

CASE STUDY

The case study illustrates the application and objective documentation of the neurological assessment.

The Patient with a Stroke

Dr. Barr is a 50-year-old internist who is employed by a busy clinic in the middle of a large midwestern city.

❖ HEALTH HISTORY

PATIENT PROFILE	50 yo MWM
CHIEF COMPLAINT	Unresponsive
HISTORY OF PRESENT ILLNESS	(Reported by wife b/c pt is unresponsive) Wife reported that husband was in good hl until 5 mo PTA, when he suffered transient ischemic attack (TIA); 1st TIA occurred $\bar{p}$ he had come home from work & was sitting watching TV; he suddenly experienced heaviness & weakness in ® arm & felt that a "curtain" had been drawn over OU; sensations lasted 1 min, then resolved completely. Pt experienced 2nd TIA 1 mo later & sought med attn. Evaluated by internist at that time: Doppler studies showed ↓ blood flow of Ⓛ carotid artery; Ⓛ carotid artery bruit auscultated; Ø neuro deficits noted; BP 186/100; serum cholesterol 310 mg/dl. Internist recommended hospitalization for evaluation of carotid arteries by arteriogram & prescribed Hygrotin, Lasix, ASA, & Persantine. Wife stated that husband was noncompliant $\bar{c}$ med tx & refused arteriogram b/c he was "too busy." Today he c/o being stressed & collapsed at work.
PAST HEALTH HISTORY	(Obtained from patient's wife)
Medical	No major illnesses
Surgical	Cervical discectomy & fusion 20 yr PTA, arthrotomy of Ⓛ knee 4 yr PTA; Ø complications
Medications	Hygrotin 100 mg qd, Lasix 40 mg q AM, ASA 85 mg qd, Persantine 50 mg tid
Communicable Diseases	Ø
Allergies	Hay fever
Injuries/Accidents	Ø
Disabilities/Handicaps	Ø
Blood Transfusion	Ø
Childhood Illnesses	Chickenpox age 10, mumps age 8
Immunizations	Unknown

continued

FAMILY HEALTH HISTORY

LEGEND

 Living female

 Living male

 Deceased female

 Deceased male

⟋ Points to patient

A&W = Alive & well

HTN = Hypertension

TIA = Transient ischemic attack

```
        ☒ 80 ──────────────┬──────────────── ⊗ 65
        Old age            │                 Lymphoma
                           │
   ⊗ 49 ──────┬────── ☒ 50          ⊗ 51
  Arthritis   │       ↑ Chol          A&W
              │         TIA
              │         HTN
   ⊙ 16  ⊙ 14  ☒ 11
   A&W   A&W   A&W
```

No known family hx of DM, heart dz, CVA, anemia, asthma, neurological disorders.

SOCIAL HISTORY

Alcohol Use — Occasional glass of wine c̄ dinner

Tobacco Use — "Closet smoker" at the office, consuming 2–3 cigarettes/d × 25 yr.

Drug Use — ∅

Sexual Practice — Married, monogamous

Travel History — East coast, fall 1988

Work Environment — Internal medicine clinic

Home Environment — House in city, water & sewage services, electricity; dog

Hobbies/Leisure Activities — Plumbing, home improvement activities, bicycling, vacation home at lake

Stress — Work, minimum 12 hr days, supporting wife & 3 children

Education — Through med school

Economic Status — Financially comfortable

Military Service — 3 yr active duty (Air Force) p̄ college; remained in USA

Religion — Episcopalian

Ethnic Background — Norwegian American

Roles/Relationships — Husband, father, physician, volunteer c̄ American Red Cross

Characteristic Patterns of Daily Living — Awakens at 0530, walks dog 1/2 mile, breakfast c̄ wife, reports to clinic by 0830. Provides primary care to 10 pt by 1200, spends 1 hr on administrative duties, eats lunch in car en route to hospital for PM rounds. Attends administrative meetings in PM, returns home by 1930 & has dinner c̄ wife. Reads mail & professional literature & retires by 2330.

continued

HEALTH MAINTENANCE ACTIVITIES

Sleep

5–6 hr/night

Diet

Does not follow low-fat diet

Exercise

2 hr/wk of bicycling during summer mos, otherwise limited to walking dog

Stress Management

See Hobbies/Leisure Activities

Use of Safety Devices

Seat belt

Health Check-Ups

Can't recall

PHYSICAL ASSESSMENT

Mental Status

1. Physical appearance and behavior:
   a. Posture and movements: supine in bed, Ⓡ shoulder lower than Ⓛ, Ⓡ sided hemiparesis
   b. Dress, grooming, and personal hygiene: hospital gown; clean hair, skin, nails
   c. Facial expression: asymmetrical, Ⓡ facial droop
   d. Affect: flat, withdrawn

2. Communication: low volume, slurred, hesitant, inappropriate words at times, intact comprehension of spoken word, nods "yes" & "no"

3. Level of consciousness: oriented to person, only; GCS: Eyes – 3; Verbal – 3; Motor – 6; total = 12

4. Cognitive abilities/mentation:
   a. Attention: short, easily distracted
   b. Memory: impaired recent memory; immediate recall and long-term memory intact
   c. Judgment: deferred
   d. Insight: deferred
   e. Spatial perception: intact to familiar sounds; unable to draw due to hemiparesis & responsiveness
   f. Calculation: unable to perform serial 7's
   g. Abstract reasoning: unable to abstract
   h. Thought processes and content: inconsistent & incoherent

Sensory

1. Exteroceptive sensation:
   a. Light touch: intact on Ⓛ; Ⓡ upper & lower extremities unable to detect
   b. Superficial pain: intact on Ⓛ; unable to detect on Ⓡ upper & lower extremities
   c. Temperature: deferred

2. Proprioceptive sensation:
   a. Motion and position: absent on Ⓡ, intact on Ⓛ
   b. Vibration sense: deficit on Ⓡ, intact on Ⓛ

3. Cortical sensation:
   a. Stereognosis, graphesthesia, two-point discrimination, extinction: intact Ⓛ side, impaired on Ⓡ

continued

Cranial Nerves

I: deferred

II: Ⓡ homonymous hemianopsia; visual acuity 20/50 OU; funduscopic deferred

III, IV, & VI: EOM–impairment in conjugate gaze to Ⓡ, Ø nystagmus; pupils equal, round, briskly react to light (PERRL) at 4 mm to 3 mm, Ø accommodation, Ⓡ ptosis

V: ↓ strength masseter & temporalis on Ⓡ, WNL on Ⓛ; ↓ sensation to superficial pain & light touch on Ⓡ, intact on Ⓛ

VII: Ⓡ facial droop lower face & mouth

VIII: gross hearing intact; Rinne: AC>BC, Weber: Ø lateralization

IX & X: NPO, uvula midline, gag not assessed

XI: Ⓡ shoulder shrug flaccid

XII: tongue midline, bilaterally strong

Motor

1. Size: = bilaterally

2. Tone: firm & supple on Ⓛ, ↓ on Ⓡ

3. Strength: LUE 5/5, RUE 2/5, LLE 5/5, RLE 3/5

4. Involuntary movements: none

5. Pronator drift: unable to test

Cerebellar

1. Coordination:
   a. Finger to nose: impaired both sides
   b. Rapid alternating movements: impaired on Ⓡ
   c. Heel to shin: unable to place Ⓡ & Ⓛ heels on shin

2. Station: not tested
   a. Romberg: deferred

3. Gait: not tested

Reflexes

Deep tendon reflexes

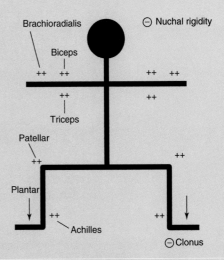

Superficial: deferred
Pathological: + Babinski

LABORATORY DATA

Lumbar puncture: normal exam

continued

	Pt's Values	Normal Range
Color	Clear	Clear, colorless
Pressure	150 mm H_2O	50–180 mm H_2O
Protein	30 mg/dl	15–50 mg/dl
WBC	3 cells/cm	0–5 cells/cm
RBC	0	None
Glucose	60 mg/dl	50–80 mg/dl
Gram Stain	Negative	Negative for organisms
Culture and Sensitivity	Negative	No growth

DIAGNOSTIC DATA   Computerized Tomography (CT Scan): An area of decreased density is noted on the distribution of the left middle cerebral artery with a shift of midline structures to the right.

✓ **NURSING CHECKLIST**
Mental Status Assessment and Neurological Techniques

Mental Status Assessment
- Physical Appearance and Behavior
  - Posture and Movements
  - Dress, Grooming, and Personal Hygiene
  - Facial Expression
  - Affect
- Communication
- Level of Consciousness
- Cognitive Abilities and Mentation
  - Attention
  - Memory
  - Judgment
  - Insight
  - Spatial Perception
  - Calculation
  - Abstract Reasoning
  - Thought Process and Content

Sensory Assessment
- Exteroceptive Sensation
  - Light Touch
  - Superficial Pain
  - Temperature
- Proprioceptive Sensation
  - Motion and Position
  - Vibration Sense
- Cortical Sensation
  - Stereognosis
  - Graphesthesia
  - Two-Point Discrimination
  - Extinction

Cranial Nerves Assessment
- Olfactory Nerve (CN I)
- Optic Nerve (CN II)
  - Visual Acuity
  - Visual Fields
  - Fundoscopic Examination
- Oculomotor Nerve (CN III)
  - Cardinal Fields of Gaze
  - Eyelid Elevation
  - Pupil Reactions

continued

- Trochlear Nerve (CN IV)
  - Cardinal Fields of Gaze
- Trigeminal Nerve (CN V)
  - Motor Component
  - Sensory Component
- Abducens Nerve (CN VI)
  - Cardinal Fields of Gaze
- Facial Nerve (CN VII)
  - Motor Component
  - Sensory Component
- Acoustic Nerve (CN VIII)
  - Cochlear Division
    Hearing
    Weber Test
    Rinne Test
  - Vestibular Division
- Glossopharyngeal Nerve (CN IX)
- Vagus Nerves (CN X)
- Spinal Accessory Nerve (CN XI)
- Hypoglossal Nerve (CN XII)

Motor System Assessment
- Muscle Size
- Muscle Tone
- Muscle Strength
- Involuntary Movements
- Pronator Drift

Cerebellar Function
- Coordination
- Station
- Gait

Reflexes
- Deep Tendon Reflexes
  - Biceps
  - Brachioradialis
  - Triceps
  - Patellar
  - Achilles
- Superficial Reflexes
  - Abdominal
  - Plantar
  - Cremasteric
  - Bulbocavernosus
- Pathological Reflexes
  - Grasp
  - Snout
  - Glabellar
  - Sucking
  - Clonus
  - Babinski
  - Hoffmann's Sign
  - Trömner's Sign
  - Chaddock's Sign
  - Oppenheim's Sign
  - Gordon's Sign

Special Techniques
- Doll's Eyes Phenomenon
- Romberg's Test
- Meningeal Irritation
  - Nuchal Rigidity
  - Kernig's Sign
  - Brudzinski's Sign

REVIEW QUESTIONS AND ACTIVITIES

1. Practice assessing attention with a friend. This will assist you in sequencing numbers and asking for repetition. Can you do serial 7's?

2. You are providing care to a patient admitted for a minor surgical procedure. The patient has Alzheimer's disease and is in stage III. How will you help the patient cope with hospitalization?

3. Your patient has sensory deficits in a "saddle" pattern. Map the area of deficit.

4. Match the cranial nerve tested in column A to the assessment parameter listed in column B.

Column A	Column B
I	Gag reflex
III	Shoulder shrug
V	Pupil response
X	Odor identification
XI	Corneal reflex (afferent)

5. The patient with Parkinson's disease exhibits multiple abnormalities of expression, posture, gait, and muscle tone. Describe the abnormalities that may be noted.

6. Practice reflex assessment with a friend. Are the reflexes normal, hyperreflexive, or hyporeflexive?

Questions 7–10 refer to the following situation:

Mrs. Gold is a 72-year-old female brought to your emergency room by her family after they found her mumbling incoherently this morning. On examination, you note that Mrs. Gold's speech patterns are difficult to understand and that she cannot name objects, is having difficulty repeating simple phrases, and cannot write her name. Mrs. Gold seems to comprehend your directions both orally and in writing.

7. Mrs. Gold's aphasia appears to be:
   a. Receptive/fluent
   b. Receptive/nonfluent
   c. Expressive/fluent
   d. Expressive/nonfluent

   The correct answer is (d).

8. Mrs. Gold is most likely suffering from pathology in which of the communication areas?
   a. Broca's area
   b. Wernicke's area
   c. Extensive frontal–temporal areas
   d. Arcuate fasciculus connecting Broca's and Wernicke's areas

   The correct answer is (a).

9. Mrs. Gold is also having difficulty producing the sounds *b, m, w, l, t,* and *d.* Her speech is slurred and unclear. Mrs. Gold is suffering from:
   a. Alexia
   b. Dysphonia
   c. Agraphia
   d. Dysarthria

   The correct answer is (d).

10. To further assess the speech difficulties experienced by Mrs. Gold, it will be *most* important to completely assess which of the following?
    a. Cranial nerves
    b. Sensation
    c. Motor system
    d. Cerebellar function

    The correct answer is (a).

Female Genitalia

COMPETENCIES

1. Describe the anatomy and physiology of the female genitalia, including age-relevant transformations.
2. Demonstrate the techniques necessary for assessment of the female genitalia, including patient positioning, external and internal inspection, speculum procedures, and palpation methods.
3. Identify normal findings as well as atypical findings of the vulva, vagina, and cervix.
4. Identify anatomic landmarks during bimanual vaginal, uterine, and rectovaginal examinations.
5. Describe procedures for genital and anal smears and cultures.

Assessment of the genitalia is often the last phase of a woman's physical assessment. Deaths attributed to uterine and cervical cancers have declined by more than 50% since the 1960s. This decline in morbidity and mortality rates can be attributed to early detection by physical assessment and Papanicolaou Test (Pap smears) and, to a lesser extent, increased patient knowledge of routine screening techniques. However, previous experiences of painful or embarrassing examinations may contribute to the patient's apprehension of the assessment process. By using a few common sense techniques to diminish patient discomfort and by empowering the patient through education and participation in the assessment process, you can encourage the patient in the management of her own health care. The female reproductive system is an area in which you have a major impact on patient health through routine screening, education, and integrating the patient in the process of self-care.

ANATOMY AND PHYSIOLOGY

External Female Genitalia

The components of the external female genitalia are collectively referred to as the vulva. They consist of the mons pubis, labia majora, labia minora, clitoris, vulval vestibule and its glands, urethral meatus, and vaginal introitus (refer to Figure 19-1).

The **mons pubis** is a pad of subcutaneous fatty tissue lying over the anterior symphysis pubis. At puberty, a characteristic triangular pattern of coarse, curly hair known as **escutcheon** develops over the mons pubis. The function of the mons pubis is to protect the pelvic bones, especially during coitus.

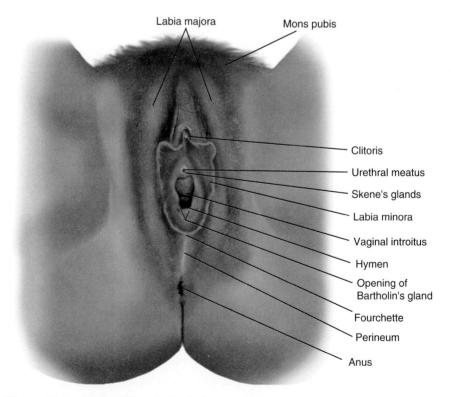

Figure 19-1 External Female Genitalia

The **labia majora** are two longitudinal folds of adipose and connective tissue. They extend from the clitoris anteriorly and gradually narrow to merge and form the posterior commissure of the perineum. The outer surface of the labia majora becomes pigmented, wrinkled, and hairy at puberty. The inner surface is smoother, softer, and contains sebaceous glands. The function of the labia majora is to protect the vulva components that it surrounds.

Tucked within the labia majora are the **labia minora**, which enclose the vestibule. They are two thin folds of skin that extend to form the prepuce, or hood, of the clitoris anteriorly and a transverse fold of skin forming the **fourchette**, or frenulum, posteriorly. The labia minora contain sebaceous glands, erectile tissue, blood vessels, and involuntary muscle tissue but no adipose tissue or hair follicles. The secretions of the sebaceous glands are bactericidal and aid in lubricating the vulval skin and protecting the skin from urine. Both the labia majora and the labia minora contain genital corpuscles that transmit erotic sensation.

The **clitoris** is a cylinder-shaped erectile body approximately 2.5 cm in length and 0.5 cm in diameter, but normally less than 2.0 cm of the body is visible on inspection. It is located at the superior aspect of the vulva and between the labia minora. The clitoris contains erectile tissue and has a significant supply of nerve endings.

As noted earlier in the discussion of the labia minora, the **vestibule** is the area between these two skin folds. The vestibule is a boat-shaped area that contains the urethral meatus, openings of the Skene's glands, hymen, openings of the Bartholin's glands, and vaginal introitus.

The external urethral meatus is located in the superior aspect of the vestibule, approximately 2.5 cm inferior to the clitoris. It is characterized as an elongated dimple or slit. Surrounding the urethral meatus are **Skene's glands**, also known as paraurethral glands, which provide lubrication to protect the skin. These tiny glands open in a posterolateral position to the urethral meatus, but they are not readily visible.

The **vaginal introitus** or orifice is situated at the inferior aspect of the vulval vestibule and is the entrance to the vagina. The size and shape of the vaginal introitus may vary. Surrounding the vaginal introitus is the **hymen**, an avascular, thin fold of connective tissue. It may be annular or crescentic in shape. The hymen may be broken by first-time sexual intercourse, strenuous physical activity, the use of tampons, masturbation, or menstruation, or it may be congenitally absent. Once the hymenal ring is perforated, small, irregular tags of tissue may be visible at the vaginal opening.

In the cleft between the labia minora and the hymenal ring lie the **Bartholin's glands**, also known as the greater vestibular glands. Bartholin's glands are small, pea-shaped glands located deep in the perineal structures. The ductal openings are not usually visible. The glands secrete a clear, viscid, odorless, alkaline mucus that improves the viability and motility of sperm along the female reproductive tract.

The **perineum** is located between the fourchette and the anus. Its composition of muscle, elastic fibers, fascia, and connective tissue gives it an exceptional capacity for stretching during childbirth. The **anal orifice** is located at the seam of the gluteal folds, and it serves as the exit to the gastrointestinal tract.

Internal Female Genitalia

The components of the internal female genitalia are the vagina, uterus, fallopian tubes, and ovaries (see Figure 19-2).

The **vagina** is a pink, hollow, muscular tube extending from the cervix to the vulva. It is located posterior to the bladder and anterior to the rectum, and

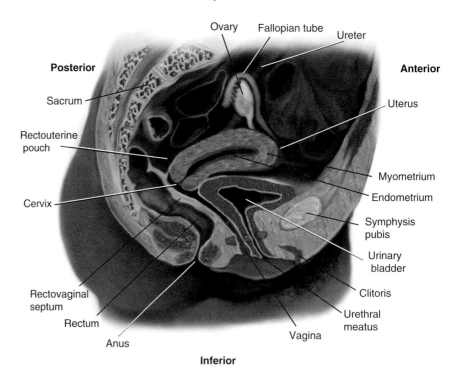

Figure 19-2 Left-Sided Sagittal Section at Midline of Internal Pelvic Organs

it slopes backward at an angle of approximately 45° with the vertical plane of the body. The cervix projects into the anterior wall of the vagina, thus making the anterior wall shorter than the posterior wall. This projection creates pouchlike recesses around the cervix. These recesses are divided into anterior, posterior, and lateral **fornices**. Abdominal organs such as the uterus, ovaries, appendix, cecum, colon, ureters, and distended bladder can be palpated through the thin walls of these fornices.

The vaginal walls consist of an outer layer of longitudinal and circular muscle fibers and a stratified squamous epithelium arranged in folds called rugae. Lactic acid is formed by the normal vaginal flora in conjunction with glycogen, which is contained in the superficial cells of the vagina. This maintains the vaginal pH and assists in the prevention of vaginal infections.

The **uterus** is an inverted pear-shaped, hollow, muscular organ in which an impregnated ovum develops into a fetus. The inferior aspect is the **cervix**; the superior aspect is the **fundus**. The most common position of the uterus is anteverted, but it may also be anteflexed, retroverted, retroflexed, or in mid-position, because the uterine body is very mobile (see Figure 19-3). The mature nonpregnant uterus weighs about 60 gm and is approximately 5.5 to 8.0 cm long, 3.5 to 4.0 cm wide, and 2.0 to 2.5 cm thick. The uterus of a parous patient, or one who has given birth, may be enlarged by 2 to 3 cm in any of the above dimensions.

Anatomically, the uterus can be divided into three parts: the body, the isthmus, and the cervix (see Figure 19-4). The body consists of the fundus, a raised, dome-shaped area on the superior portion of the uterus, and the cornu, the points of insertion of the fallopian tubes. The uterine body has three layers: an outer layer of peritoneum; a middle layer of muscle, called the myometrium; and an inner layer of columnar epithelium, mucous glands, and stroma, called the endometrium. It is this innermost layer that is shed and regenerated under normal hormonal influence during the menstrual cycle. The outer layer of the

peritoneum forms a deep recess called the **rectouterine pouch**, or pouch of Douglas. It is the lowest point in the pelvic cavity and encompasses the lower posterior wall of the uterus, the upper portion of the vagina, and the intestinal surface of the rectum.

The **isthmus** is a constricted area between the body of the uterus and the cervix. The cervix is an open-ended canal approximately 2 to 3 cm in length and diameter. Its internal os (opening) is at the isthmus and its external os extends into the vagina. The os of the **nulliparous** woman, one who has not given birth, will be closed and tight. The os of a **parous** woman, one who has given birth to one or more neonates, may be open by 1 cm and the orifice may be elongated. The endocervical canal is lined with mucus-secreting columnar epithelium. The ectocervix, which protrudes into the vagina, is covered with the same squamous epithelial cells that line the vagina. The point at which the two types of cells merge is the **squamocolumnar junction**. Its exact location varies with age but is clinically important because it is the point at which most cervical cancer originates.

The **adnexa** of the uterus consists of the fallopian tubes, the ovaries, and their supporting ligaments. The **fallopian tubes** extend from the cornu of the uterus to the ovaries and are supported by the broad ligaments. The tubes are approximately 8 to 14 cm long. The distal, funnel-shaped end of the fallopian tube is called the infundibulum. It has moving, fingerlike projections called fimbriae, which help direct ova from the ovary into the tube, where fertilization takes place. The fallopian tubes are lined with ciliated squamous epithelium. The movement of the cilia and the peristaltic waves of the muscular layer of the tube propel the ovum toward the uterus, where implantation occurs.

The **ovaries** are a pair of almond-shaped glands, approximately 3 to 4 cm in length, in the upper pelvic cavity. **Oogenesis**, the development and formation of an ovum, and hormonal production are the ovaries' principal functions. The **rectovaginal septum** separates the rectum from the posterior aspect of the vagina.

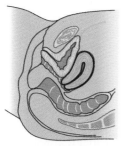

Anteverted (most common)

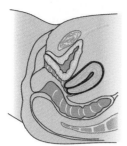

Midposition (midplane)

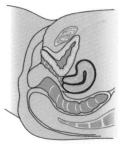

Anteflexed

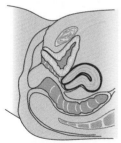

Retroflexed (palpable only during rectovaginal exam)

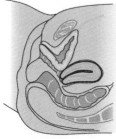

Retroverted (palpable only during rectovaginal exam)

Figure 19-3   Positions of the Uterus

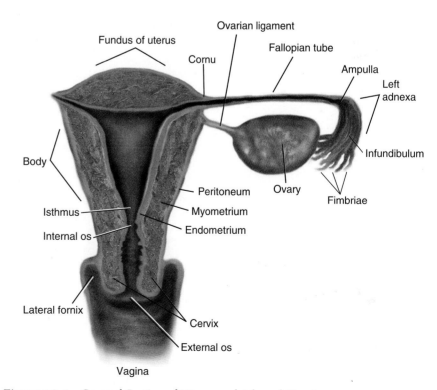

Figure 19-4   Coronal Section of Uterus and Adnexal Structures

THE FEMALE REPRODUCTIVE CYCLE

The female reproductive cycle consists of two interrelated cycles called the ovarian and the menstrual cycles. These cycles occur synchronously under neurohormonal control from the hypothalamus and the anterior pituitary gland.

The ovarian cycle consists of two phases: the follicular phase and the luteal phase. During the follicular phase, the actions of the follicle-stimulating hormone (FSH) and the luteinizing hormone (LH) from the anterior pituitary gland stimulate the ripening of one ovarian follicle called the graafian follicle. The remaining follicles are suppressed by LH. Ovulation occurs when high levels of LH cause the release of the ovum from the graafian follicle. During the luteal phase, LH stimulates the development of the corpus luteum. This yellow pigment that fills the graafian follicle produces high levels of progesterone and low levels of estrogen. The basal body temperature rises, indicating that ovulation has occurred.

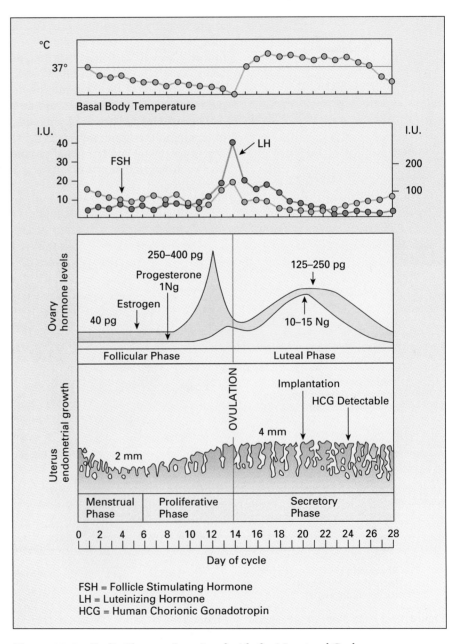

Figure 19-5 Cyclic Changes Associated with the Menstrual Cycle

Table 19-1 Sexual Maturity Rating for Female Genitalia

DEVELOPMENTAL STAGE	DESCRIPTION
Stage 1 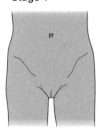	No pubic hair, only body hair (vellus hair)
Stage 2 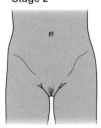	Sparse growth of long, slightly dark, fine pubic hair, slightly curly and located along the labia (ages 11 to 12)
Stage 3 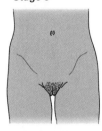	Pubic hair becomes darker, curlier, and spreads over the symphysis (ages 12 to 13)
Stage 4 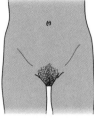	Texture and curl of pubic hair is similar to that of an adult but not spread to thighs (ages 13 to 15)
Stage 5 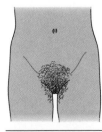	Adult appearance in quality and quantity of pubic hair; growth is spread to inner aspect of thighs and abdomen

The menstrual cycle begins if implantation does not occur. The corpus luteum degenerates and the levels of progesterone and estrogen decrease, causing the endometrium to degenerate and shed. The menstrual flow lasts from 2 to 7 days and the cycles continue every 25 to 34 days, with the average being 28 days. The first day of the cycle is the first day of menstruation. The menstrual flow consists of blood and mucus and normally does not exceed 150 ml. Menstrual blood lacks fibrin; therefore, it does not clot. If clots do occur, they usually form in the vagina and are a combination of red blood cells, glycoproteins, and mucus. Cyclic changes associated with the menstrual cycle are shown in Figure 19-5.

The proliferative phase of the menstrual cycle occurs when the endometrial lining begins to regenerate under the influence of estrogen. Changes in the cervical mucosa also occur during this phase. The cervical mucus becomes clearer, thinner, and threadlike.

If conception and implantation of the fertilized ovum occur, the corpus luteum is maintained by the presence of human chorionic gonadotropin (HCG), which is secreted by the implanting blastocyst. HCG is the hormone tested in at-home pregnancy kits.

The female reproductive cycle begins at **menarche**, the onset of menstruation, which occurs between 9 and 16 years of age, and ends at menopause, which occurs between 45 and 55 years of age. The onset of puberty, which occurs between the ages of 8 and 9, is marked by significant increases in estrogen production and the development of secondary sex characteristics such as breast enlargement, hair distribution on the mons pubis, and contour changes of the hips and abdomen. Tanner's stages of pubic hair development provide objective criteria for the evaluation of developmental changes in the appearance of female genitalia (refer to Table 19-1).

❧ NURSING TIP

Patient Education on the Reproductive Cycle

Educating the patient about the reproductive cycle and its effects on the body will help the patient to better understand her own body's functioning and assist her in planning for gynecological examinations and birth control measures. The cervical mucus becomes clearer, thinner, and threadlike, indicating the onset of ovulation. The patient can perform her own **spinnbarkeit** test, the point at which the mucus can be drawn to a maximal length, by stretching vaginal mucus between her thumb and index finger. Tell the patient it is normal to feel low abdominal or flank pain when the ovum is released during ovulation. Rise in basal body temperature indicates that ovulation has occurred. Spotting may also be present after ovulation.

❖ HEALTH HISTORY

The female genitalia health history provides insight into the link between a patient's life/lifestyle and female genitalia information and pathology.

continued

PATIENT PROFILE	*Diseases that are age- and race-specific for the female genitalia are listed.*

Age	Sexually transmitted diseases (STDs) (increased incidence 15–25)
	Uterine myomas (30–50)
	Cervical cancer (40–60)
	Vulval cancer (postmenopause)
	Uterine prolapse (postmenopause)
	Cystocele (postmenopause)
	Rectocele (postmenopause)
	Atrophic vaginitis (postmenopause)
	Endometrial cancer (diagnosis is usually made between 55 and 69)
	    (American Cancer Society, 1994)
	Vaginal cancer (over 60)
	Ovarian cancer (risk increases with age; highest rates are between
	    65 and 84) (American Cancer Society, 1994)

Race	African American: incidence of invasive cervical cancer is double that among Caucasian Americans (American Cancer Society, 1994)
CHIEF COMPLAINT	*Common chief complaints for the female genitalia are defined and information on the characteristics of each sign/symptom is provided.*
Uterine Bleeding	The presence of bleeding from the endometrium
Quality	Odor, consistency, color
Quantity	Amount (number and size of tampons or pads used in 24 hours), duration and frequency of flow
Associated Manifestations	Abdominal pain or cramping, passage of clots or tissue
Aggravating Factors	Stress, anxiety, medications, rapid weight loss or gain, obesity, sexual intercourse
Alleviating Factors	Medication, dilatation and curettage, surgery
Setting	Traumatic abortion or dilatation and curettage
Timing	Relationship to menses, to use of intrauterine device (IUD)
Vaginal Discharge	The presence of a leaky discharge of fluid from the vagina
Quality	Color, consistency, odor
Quantity	Number and size of tampons or pads used in 24 hours
Associated Manifestations	Itching, presence of discharge in sexual partner, **dyspareunia** (painful sexual intercourse), dysuria, abdominal pain or cramping

Aggravating Factors	Tight pants, wet bathing suits, antibiotics, birth control pills, diet,
	    pregnancy, deodorant tampons, bubble bath, chemical douches,
	    lubricated condoms, contraceptive creams, preexisting disease such as
	    diabetes mellitus, increased number of sexual partners

Alleviating Factors	Position, loose-fitting pants, cotton underpants and pantyhose with
	    cotton crotch, medication, daily bathing of vaginal area with mild,
	    nonperfumed soap

continued

Timing	Post coitus, while taking antibiotics
Urinary Symptoms	Changes in the normal voiding pattern and in characteristics of the urine
Quality	Color: straw, amber, blood stained; consistency: clear, cloudy, presence of particles; odor
Quantity	Polyuria, oliguria or anuria
Associated Manifestations	Flank pain, abdominal pain or cramping, abdominal distention, vaginal discharge, urgency and frequency in voiding, stress incontinence, pneumaturia, fever
Aggravating Factors	Douches, intravaginal devices, traumatic coitus, alcohol, caffeine, spices, delaying urination
Alleviating Factors	Medication, warm baths, hydration
Setting	Post coitus
Timing	At beginning, throughout, or end of stream
Pelvic Pain	The subjective sense of discomfort in the pelvis
Quality	Stabbing, burning, cramping, aching, throbbing, drawing, pulling
Associated Manifestations	Abdominal distension, pelvic fullness, vaginal discharge or bleeding, gastrointestinal symptoms, menstruation, fever
Aggravating Factors	Exercise, sexual activity, cultural perception
Alleviating Factors	Rest, medication, surgery
Setting	During coitus
Timing	Sudden or gradual onset, association with activity, duration, recurrence, relation to menstrual cycle
PAST HEALTH HISTORY	*The various components of the past health history are linked to female genitalia pathology and female genitalia-related information.*
Medical	
Female Genitalia Specific	Refer to Table 19-2.
Nonfemale Genitalia Specific	Diabetes mellitus, thyroid disease, incontinence, constipation, urinary tract infections
Surgical	Hysterectomy, myomectomy, salpingectomy, oophorectomy, dilatation and curettage, laparoscopy, vulvectomy, tubal ligation, colpotomy, cesarean section
Medications	Antibiotics may increase incidence of *Candida* vaginosis and lessen the effectiveness of oral contraceptives.
Communicable Diseases	STD: gonorrhea, syphilis, herpes, HIV/AIDS, hepatitis, *Chlamydia*, condyloma human papillomavirus

continued

Allergies	Numerous feminine hygiene products may cause allergic reactions or increase the incidence of *Candida* vaginosis. Be aware of any latex allergies; condoms and diaphragms are usually made of latex. The spermicide nonoxynol 9 may also cause allergic reactions.
Injuries/Accidents	Abdominal trauma, rape, sexual abuse, vaginal trauma or injuries
Disabilities/Handicaps	Paraplegic and quadriplegic patients are at increased obstetric risk depending on level of injury, tone of uterus, and competency of cervix.
Childhood Illnesses	Fetal diethylstilbestrol (DES) exposure
FAMILY HEALTH HISTORY	*Female genitalia diseases that are familial are listed.*
	Cancers of the reproductive organs, mother received DES while pregnant with patient, transfer of STDs during delivery, placental transfer of HIV/AIDS, multiple pregnancies, congenital anomalies
SOCIAL HISTORY	*The components of the social history are linked to female genitalia factors/pathology.*
Alcohol Use	There is a significant positive correlation between alcohol use and date rape in college-aged groups.
Tobacco Use	There is an increased incidence of strokes in women who concurrently smoke and use oral contraceptives. Smoking is a risk factor for cervical cancer.
Sexual Practice	Often, sexual favors are exchanged for narcotics, leading to increased rates of STDs. Prostitution increases the risk of STDs, HIV/AIDS, hepatitis, and cervical carcinoma (an increase in the number of partners increases the risk of human papillomavirus, which can lead to dysplasia, and of cervical cancer).
Home Environment	Poor sanitation may lead to numerous forms of vaginitis; overcrowding is an ideal condition for mite infestation.
Hobbies/Leisure Activities	Wearing wet bathing suits for extended periods of time may increase the likelihood of *Candida* vaginosis. Strenuous equestrian sports increase the likelihood of external genitalia trauma from saddle injuries.
Stress	Stress can have significant effects on menstruation, causing **amenorrhea** (absent menses) and exacerbating genital herpes simplex.
HEALTH MAINTENANCE ACTIVITIES	*This information provides a bridge between the health maintenance activities and female genitalia function.*
Sleep	Lack of sleep or extreme fatigue can lead to amenorrhea.
Diet	Increased levels of refined sugars, salt, and caffeine enhance PMS symptomology. Extreme dieting can affect menstruation and lead to amenorrhea.

continued

Exercise	Exercise may diminish **dysmenorrhea** (pain or cramping during menses) and **menorrhagia** (heavy menses).
Use of Safety Devices	Condom use
Health Check-Ups	Date of last Pap test and results

 NURSING TIP

Late Onset of Menarche

Late onset of menarche can result from a multiplicity of pathologies. If you encounter a patient who has not experienced the onset of menstruation by 16 to 18 years of age, evaluate the patient for the following:

1. Inadequate nutrition or eating disorders
2. Chronic diseases such as Crohn's disease
3. Environmental stressors
4. Intensive athletic training
5. Hypothyroidism
6. Use of opiates or steroids.

Table 19-2   Female Reproductive Health History

MENSTRUAL HISTORY

Age of menarche, last menstrual period (LMP), length of cycle, regularity of cycle, duration of menses, amenorrhea, menorrhagia, presence of clots or vaginal pooling, number and type of tampons or pads used during menses, dysmenorrhea, spotting between menses.

PREMENSTRUAL SYNDROME (PMS)

Symptoms occur from 3 to 5 days before the onset of menses with cessation of symptoms after second day of cycle. Symptoms include: breast tenderness; bloating; moodiness; cravings for salt, sugar, or chocolate; fatigue; weight gain; headaches; and joint pain.

OBSTETRIC HISTORY

Refer to Chapter 22.

MENOPAUSE HISTORY

Menopause (cessation of menstruation), spotting, associated symptoms of menopause (such as hot flashes, palpitations, numbness, tingling, drenching sweats, mood swings, vaginal dryness, itching), treatment for symptoms (including estrogen replacement therapy), feelings about menopause.

VAGINAL DISCHARGE

Refer to chief complaint section.

HISTORY OF UTERINE BLEEDING

Refer to chief complaint section.

SEXUAL FUNCTIONING

Sexual preference, number of partners, interest, satisfaction, dyspareunia, inorgasmia.

REPRODUCTIVE MEDICAL HISTORY

Vaginal infections, yeast infections, salpingitis, endometritis, endometriosis, cervicitis, fibroids, ovarian cysts, cancer of the reproductive organs, infertility, Pap smear records.

METHOD OF BIRTH CONTROL

Type, frequency of use, methods to prevent STDs, any associated problems with birth control or STD prevention methods, such as a reaction to the spermicides used with the vaginal sponges and diaphragms.

 NURSING TIP

Maintaining Gynecological Health

Encourage patients to adopt healthy gynecological practices:

1. Avoid douches and feminine hygiene sprays, or use sparingly because both products disrupt the natural vaginal flora.
2. Do not leave tampons in the vagina for longer than 8 hours at a time because of the increased risk of toxic shock syndrome.
3. Always wash and wipe the vaginal area from front to back to prevent contamination of the vagina and urethra with fecal material.
4. Thoroughly wash diaphragms, pessaries, and sexual aid devices before and after each use.

EQUIPMENT

Assemble items before placing the patient on the examination table; materials should be arranged in order of use and within easy reach.

- Examination table with stirrups
- Stool, preferably mounted on wheels
- Large hand mirror
- Gooseneck lamp
- Clean gloves
- Linens for draping
- Vaginal specula (see Figure 19-6):
  - Graves' bivalve specula, sizes medium and large, useful for most adult sexually active women
  - Pederson bivalve speculum, sizes small and medium, useful for nonsexually active women, children, menopausal women
- Cytological materials (see Figure 19-7):
  - Ayre spatulas
  - Cytobrushes
  - Cotton-tipped applicators
  - Microscope slides, cover slips, Thayer-Martin culture plates labeled with the patient's name, identification number, and date specimen was collected
  - Cytology fixative spray
  - Reagents: normal saline solution, potassium hydroxide (KOH), acetic acid (white vinegar)
- Warm water
- Water-soluble lubricant

✿ NURSING TIP

Sensitivity During the Gynecological Assessment

Genital assessment produces feelings of fear, anxiety, indignity, and loss of control in many women. These feelings may be reduced by the sensitivity of the nurse before, during, and after the assessment. Remember that you are assessing a person, not just a body part. Respect a patient's wishes regarding privacy. Take into consideration cultural issues; for example many Middle Eastern women will remain veiled during an assessment.

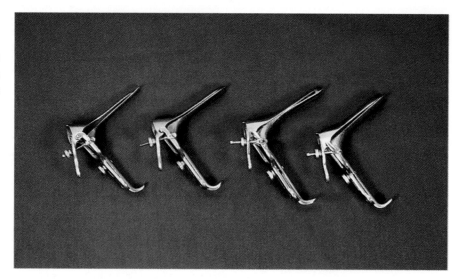

Figure 19-6 Vaginal Specula

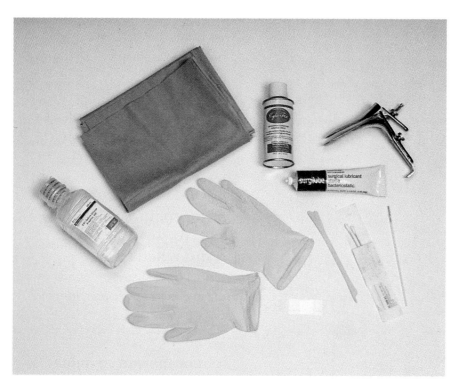

Figure 19-7 Cytological Materials Needed for Gynecological Examination

ASSESSMENT OF THE FEMALE GENITALIA

Assessment of the female reproductive system consists of inspection and palpation only, and includes assessment of the abdomen (refer to Chapter 16), inspection of the external genitalia, palpation of the external genitalia, speculum assessment of the internal genitalia, collection of specimens for laboratory analysis, inspection of the vaginal walls, bimanual examination, and rectovaginal assessment (refer to Chapter 21 for the complete rectal examination.) The assessment process requires somewhat uncomfortable positioning for the patient; therefore, it should be completed as quickly and as efficiently as possible.

NURSING CHECKLIST
General Approach to Female Genitalia Assessment

Prior to the assessment:

1. Instruct the patient not to use vaginal sprays, to douche, or to have coitus 24 to 48 hours before the scheduled physical assessment. The products of coitus and commercial sprays and douches may affect the Pap smear and other vaginal cultures.

2. Encourage the patient to express any anxieties and concerns about the physical assessment. Reassure the patient by acknowledging anxieties and validating concerns. Virgins need reassurance that the pelvic assessment should not affect the hymen.

3. Show the speculum and other equipment to the patient and allow her to touch and explore any items that do not have to remain sterile.

4. Inform the patient that the assessment should not be painful but may be uncomfortable at times, and tell her to inform you if she is experiencing any pain.

5. Instruct the patient to empty her bladder and then to undress from the waist to the ankles.

6. Ensure that the room is warm enough to prevent chilling, and provide additional draping material as necessary.

7. Place drapes or sheep skin over the stirrups to increase patient comfort.

8. Warm your hands with warm water prior to gloving.

9. Ensure that privacy will be maintained during the assessment. Provide screens and a closed door.

During the assessment:

1. Inform the patient of what you are going to do before you do it. Tell her she may feel pressure when the speculum is opened and a pinching sensation when the Pap smear is done.

2. Adopt a nonjudgmental and supportive attitude.

3. Maintain eye contact with the patient as much as possible to reinforce a caring relationship.

4. Use a mirror to show the patient what you are doing and to educate her about her body. Help her with positioning the mirror during the examination so she will feel comfortable using this technique at home to assess her genitalia.

5. Offer the patient the opportunity to ask questions about her body and sexuality.

6. Encourage the patient to use relaxation techniques such as deep breathing or guided imagery to prevent muscle tension during the assessment.

After the assessment:

1. Assess whether the patient needs assistance in dressing.

2. After the patient is dressed, discuss the experience with her, invite questions and comments, listen carefully, and provide her with information regarding the assessment and any laboratory information that is available.

3. Tell the patient she may experience a small amount of spotting following the Pap smear.

❀ NURSING TIP

Preparing for a Gynecological Examination

If you are a beginning nurse or if you have not performed a gynecological examination:

- Ask another nurse to assist you with the first few examinations.
- Familiarize yourself with the equipment. Practice opening and closing the speculum. Plastic specula make significant audible clicking sounds when opening and closing, so you should prepare the patient for this event.
- Review the anatomy and physiology of the female genitalia; visualize the underlying structures of the anatomic landmarks.
- Review and practice any procedures to be done. Some nurses find it difficult to prepare slides and cultures without assistance if they are novices to these procedures.
- Know your institution's policies regarding the option of having a female nurse present if a male nurse is performing the gynecological exam.

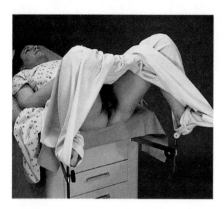

Figure 19-8 Patient Positioning and Draping for Gynecological Examination

Inspection of the External Genitalia

1. With the patient seated, place a drape over the patient's torso and thighs until positioning is completed.

2. Instruct the patient to first sit on the examination table between the stirrups, facing away from the head of the table.

3. Assist the patient in assuming a dorsal recumbent or lithotomy position on the examination table. Assist the patient in placing her heels in the stirrups, thus abducting her legs and flexing her hips.

4. Don clean gloves.

5. Assist the patient as she moves her buttocks down to the lower end of the examination table so that the buttocks are flush with the edge of the table. If the patient desires, raise the head of the examination table slightly to elevate her head and shoulders. This position allows you to maintain eye contact with the patient and prevents abdominal muscle tension (see Figure 19-8).

6. Readjust the drape to cover the abdomen, thighs, and knees; adjust the stirrups as necessary for patient comfort. Push the drape down between the patient's knees so you can see the patient's face.

7. Sit on a stool at the foot of the examination table facing the patient's external genitalia.

8. Adjust your lighting source and provide the patient with a mirror. Instruct her on how to hold the mirror in order to view the examination prior to touching the patient's genitalia.

9. Finally, remember to inform the patient of each step of the assessment process before it is performed, and be gentle.

Pubic Hair Distribution

E Observe the pattern of pubic hair distribution. Sexual maturity ratings can be determined at this time for adolescent patients.

N *The distribution of the female pubic hair should be shaped like an inverse triangle. There may be some growth on the abdomen and upper inner thighs. A diamond-shaped pattern from the umbilicus may be due to cultural or familial differences.*

A A diamond-shaped pattern from the umbilicus, not associated with cultural or familial differences, is abnormal.

P This distribution pattern may occur with hirsutism, which is indicative of an endocrine disorder.

Presence of Parasites

E 1. Inform the patient that you will touch the inside of her thigh before you touch her genitals.
    2. With gloved fingers, separate the pubic hair and observe for parasites.

N *There should be no parasites present.*

A The presence of pubic lice or nits in the pubic hair or flecks of residual blood on the external genitalia is an abnormal finding.

P Pubic lice (pediculosis pubis) is the infestation of the hairy regions of the body, usually the pubic area, but it sometimes involves the hairy aspects of the abdomen, chest, and axillae.

Skin Color and Condition

Mons Pubis and Vulva

E 1. Observe the skin coloration and condition of the mons pubis and vulva.

E Examination
N Normal Findings
A Abnormal Findings
P Pathophysiology

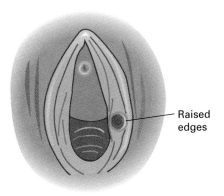

Figure 19-9 Syphilitic Chancre

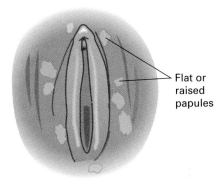

Figure 19-10 Secondary Syphilis (Condyloma Latum)

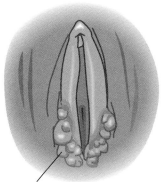

Figure 19-11 Venereal Warts (Condyloma Acuminatum)

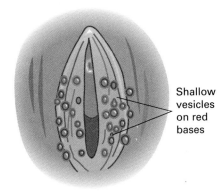

Figure 19-12 Genital Herpes

2. Using the thumb and index finger of the dominant hand, separate the labia majora.

3. Observe both the labia majora and the labia minora for coloration, lesions, or trauma.

N *The skin over the mons pubis should be clear except for nevi and normal hair distribution. The labia majora and minora should appear symmetrical with a smooth to somewhat wrinkled, unbroken, slightly pigmented skin surface. There should be no ecchymosis, excoriation, nodules, swelling, rash, or lesions. An occasional sebaceous cyst is within normal limits. These cysts are nontender, yellow nodules that are less than 1 cm in diameter.*

A Ecchymosis over the mons pubis or labia is abnormal.

P This may be due to blunt trauma that may have resulted from an accident or intentional abuse.

A Edema or swelling of the labia is an abnormal finding.

P This may be due to hematoma formation, Bartholin's cyst, or obstruction of the lymphatic system.

A Broken areas on the skin surface are abnormal.

P These may be due to ulcerations or abrasions secondary to infection or trauma.

A Rash over the mons pubis and labia is abnormal.

P Rashes have multiple etiologies including contact dermatitis and infestations.

A A reddish, round ulcer with a depressed center, and raised, indurated edges (**chancre**) is an abnormal finding (see Figure 19-9).

P A chancre appears during the primary stages of syphilis at the site where the *Treponema* enters the body. The chancre lasts for 4 weeks and then disappears.

A Flat or raised, round, wartlike papules that have moist surfaces covered by gray exudate (condylomata lata) are abnormal (see Figure 19-10).

P These lesions occur during the secondary stage of syphilis.

A White, dry, painless growths that have narrow bases are suggestive of condyloma acuminatum (see Figure 19-11) and are abnormal.

P These warts are caused by the human papillomavirus.

A Small, shallow, red vesicles that fuse together to form a large ulcer that may be painful and itch (see Figure 19-12) are abnormal.

P These ulcers are indicative of herpes simplex lesions.

A A painless mass that may be accompanied by pruritus or a mass that develops into a cauliflowerlike growth is an abnormal finding.

P This type of mass is highly suggestive of malignancy.

A Venous prominences of the labia may be abnormal.

P Varicose veins may develop due to a congenital predisposition, prolonged standing, pregnancy, or aging.

Clitoris

E **1.** Using the dominant thumb and index finger, separate the labia minora laterally to expose the prepuce of the clitoris (see Figure 19-13).

2. Observe the clitoris for size and condition.

N *The clitoris is approximately 2.0 cm in length and 0.5 cm in diameter and without lesions.*

A Hypertrophy of the clitoris is an abnormal finding.

P This may indicate female pseudohermaphroditism due to androgen excess.

A A reddish, round ulcer with a depressed center and raised, indurated edges (chancre) is an abnormal finding.

P Refer to the chancre discussion preceding.

Urethral Meatus

E **1.** Using the dominant thumb and index finger, separate the labia minora laterally to expose the urethral meatus. Do not touch the urethral meatus; this may cause pain and urethral spasm.

Figure 19-13 Inspecting the External Genitalia

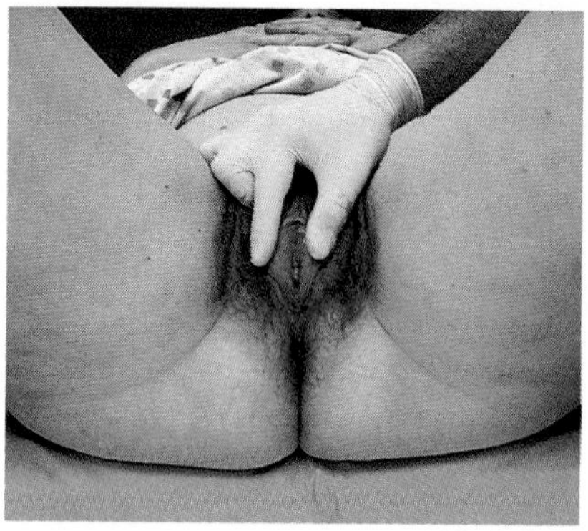

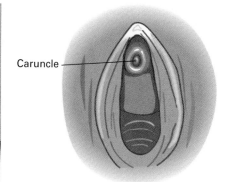

Figure 19-14 Urethral Caruncle

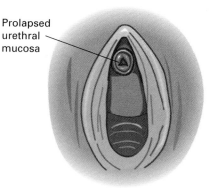

Figure 19-15 Prolapse of the Urethral Mucosa

ASK YOURSELF

Patients with Recurrent STDs

Ask yourself how you feel about patients who come in for treatment of recurrent STDs. Will your personal feelings influence the quality of nursing care you provide? How would you feel if such a patient showed no interest in learning about ways to avoid contracting STDs?

NURSING TIP

Dealing with STDs

It is helpful to assess your attitudes toward sexual practices and STDs. Remember to maintain a nonjudgmental approach, avoid imposing your values on the patient, and avoid talking down to the patient.

E	**Examination**
N	**Normal Findings**
A	**Abnormal Findings**
P	**Pathophysiology**

2. Observe the shape, color, and size of the urethral meatus.

N *The urethral opening is slitlike in appearance and midline; it is free of discharge, swelling, or redness and is about the size of a pea.*

A Discharge of any color from the meatus is an abnormal finding.

P Discharge indicates possible urinary tract infection.

A Swelling or redness around the urethral meatus is an abnormal finding.

P Swelling indicates possible infection of the Skene's glands, urethral caruncle (small, red growth that protrudes from the meatus, shown in Figure 19-14), urethral carcinoma, or prolapse of the urethral mucosa (see Figure 19-15).

Vaginal Introitus

E
1. Keep the labia minora retracted laterally to inspect the vaginal introitus.
2. Ask the patient to bear down.
3. Observe for patency and bulging.

N *The introitus mucosa should be pink and moist. Normal vaginal discharge is clear to white and free of foul odor; some white clumps may be seen that are mass numbers of epithelial cells. The introitus should be patent and without bulging.*

A Pale color and dryness of the introitus are abnormal.

P Possible etiologies include atrophy from topical steroids and the aging process.

A Foul-smelling discharge that is any color other than clear to slightly pale white is abnormal. Malodorous white, yellow, green, or gray discharge that may be purulent are some possible findings.

P Gonorrhea, *Chlamydia*, *Candida* vaginosis, *Trichomonas* vaginitis, bacterial vaginosis, atrophic vaginitis, or cervicitis are possible infectious processes or vectors (refer to Table 19-3).

A An external tear or impatency of the vaginal introitus is abnormal.

P Possible causes include trauma and fissure of the introitus. An external tear may indicate trauma from sexual activity or abuse, and a fissure may indicate a congenital malformation or childbirth trauma.

A Bulging of the anterior vaginal wall indicates a **cystocele** (see Figure 19-16) and is abnormal.

P The upper two-thirds of anterior vaginal wall along with the bladder push forward into the introitus due to weakened supporting tissues and ligaments.

A Bulging of the anterior vaginal wall, bladder, and urethra into the vaginal introitus indicates a **cystourethrocele** (see Figure 19-17) and is abnormal.

P The etiology is usually a weakening of the entire anterior vaginal wall. A fissure may define the urethrocele and cystocele.

A Bulging of the posterior vaginal wall with a portion of the rectum indicates a **rectocele** (see Figure 19-18) and is abnormal.

P This is caused by a weakening of the entire posterior vaginal wall.

Table 19-3	Description of Vaginal Discharges				
DISCHARGE	**NORMAL PHYSIOLOGICAL DISCHARGE**	**NONSPECIFIC VAGINITIS (NSV)**	**TRICHOMONAS**	**CANDIDA**	**GONOCOCCAL**
Color	White	Gray	Grayish yellow	White	Greenish yellow
Odor	Absent	Fishy	Fishy	Absent	Absent
Consistency	Nonhomogenous	Homogenous	Purulent, often with bubbles	Cottage cheeselike	Mucopurulent
Location	Dependent	Adherent to walls	Often pooled in fornix	Adherent to walls	Adherent to walls
Anatomic Appearance					
Vulva	Normal	Normal	Edematous	Erythematous	Erythematous
Vaginal Mucosa	Normal	Normal	Usually normal	Erythematous	Normal
Cervix	Normal	Normal	May show red spots	Patches of discharge	Pus in os

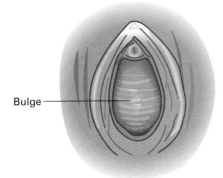

Bulge

Figure 19-16 Cystocele

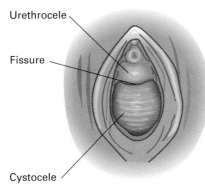

Urethrocele

Fissure

Cystocele

Figure 19-17 Cystourethrocele

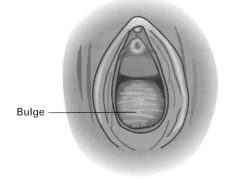

Bulge

Figure 19-18 Rectocele

Perineum and Anus

E 1. Observe for color and shape of the anus.
2. Observe texture and color of the perineum.

N *The perineum should be smooth and slightly darkened. A well-healed episiotomy scar is normal after vaginal delivery. The anus should be dark pink to brown and puckered. Skin tags are not uncommon around the anal area.*

A A fissure or tear of the perineum is an abnormal finding.

P Possible causes include trauma, abscess, or unhealed episiotomy.

A Venous prominences of the anal area indicate external hemorrhoids and are abnormal.

P An external hemorrhoid is the varicose dilatation of a vein of the inferior hemorrhoidal plexus and is covered with modified anal skin.

⚡ NURSING ALERT

The Sexually Abused Patient

No patient, regardless of age, should be excluded from evaluation for sexual abuse. Physical signs of sexual abuse include bruising of the mons pubis, labia, or perineum, and vaginal or rectal tears. The presence of STDs in the very young or the very old patient suggests abuse. Emotional signs such as lack of eye contact during the examination, extreme anxiety or guarding during the assessment, or refusing to assume certain positions may all indicate a history of abuse. Document all signs of suspected sexual abuse.

Know your institution's and state's policy regarding the reporting of sexual abuse. Most states have mandatory reporting policies for sexual abuse in children and teenagers. Some states require mandatory reporting of abuse in the elderly.

Assure the patient that she is safe with you and refer her to the appropriate social services or sexual assault services.

Palpation of the External Genitalia
Labia

E 1. Palpate each labium between the thumb and the index finger of your dominant hand.

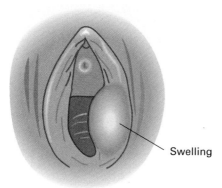

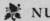
Swelling

Figure 19-19   Bartholin's Gland Infection

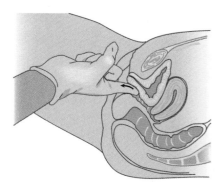

Figure 19-20   Milking the Urethra

E   Examination
N   Normal Findings
A   Abnormal Findings
P   Pathophysiology

2. Observe for swelling, induration, pain, or discharge from a Bartholin's gland duct.

N   *The labium should feel soft and uniform in structure with no swelling, pain, induration, or purulent discharge.*

A   Swelling, redness, induration, or purulent discharge from the labial folds with hot, tender areas are abnormal findings (see Figure 19-19).

P   These findings indicate a probable Bartholin's gland infection. Causative organisms include gonococci and *Chlamydia trachomatis*.

Urethral Meatus and Skene's Glands

E   1. Insert your dominant index finger into the vagina.
2. Apply pressure to the anterior aspect of the vaginal wall and milk the urethra (see Figure 19-20).
3. Observe for discharge and patient discomfort.

N   *Milking the urethra should not cause pain or result in any urethral discharge.*

A   Pain on contact and discharge from the urethra are abnormal findings.

P   These findings indicate a Skene's gland infection or urinary tract infection.

🌸 NURSING TIP

Examining Urethral Discharge

If discharge is noted from the urethra, swab the discharge with a cotton-tipped applicator and spread the sample on a microscope slide for further evaluation.

Vaginal Introitus

E   1. While your finger remains in the vagina, ask the patient to squeeze the vaginal muscles around your finger.
2. Evaluate muscle strength and tone.

N   *Vaginal muscle tone in a nulliparous woman should be tight and strong; in a parous woman, it will be diminished.*

A   Significantly diminished or absent vaginal muscle tone and bulging of vaginal or pelvic contents are abnormal findings.

P   Weakened muscle tone may result from injury, age, childbirth, or medication. Bulging results from cystocele, rectocele, or uterine prolapse.

Perineum

E   1. Withdraw your finger from the introitus until you can place only your dominant index finger posterior to the perineum and place the dominant thumb anterior to the perineum.
2. Assess the perineum between the dominant thumb and index finger for muscular tone and texture.

N   *The perineum should be smooth, firm, and homogenous in the nulliparous woman, and thinner in the parous woman. A well-healed episiotomy scar is also within normal limits for a parous woman.*

A   A thin, tissuelike perineum, fissures, or tears are abnormal.

P   A thin perineum is indicative of atrophy, and fissures and tears may indicate trauma or an unhealed episiotomy.

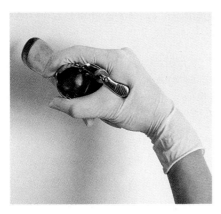

Figure 19-21 Holding the Speculum

Speculum Examination of the Internal Genitalia

Cervix

E 1. Select the appropriate-sized speculum. This selection should be based on the patient's history, size of vaginal introitus, and vaginal muscle tone. See page 616 for description of specula.

2. Lubricate and warm the speculum by rinsing it under warm water. Do not use other lubricants because they may interfere with the accuracy of cytological samples and cultures.

3. Hold the speculum in your dominant hand with the closed blades between the index and middle fingers. The index finger should rest at the proximal end of the superior blade. Wrap the other fingers around the handle, with the thumbscrew over the thumb (see Figure 19-21).

4. Insert your nondominant index and middle fingers, ventral sides down, just inside the vagina and apply pressure to the posterior vaginal wall. Encourage the patient to bear down. This will help to relax the perineal muscles.

5. Encourage the patient to relax by taking deep breaths. Be careful not to pull on pubic hair or pinch the labia.

6. When you feel the muscles relax, insert the speculum at an oblique angle on a plane parallel to the examination table until the speculum reaches the end of the fingers that are in the vagina (see Figure 19-22A).

7. Withdraw the fingers of your nondominant hand.

8. Gently rotate the speculum blades to a horizontal angle and advance the speculum at a 45° downward angle against the posterior vaginal wall until it reaches the end of the vagina (see Figures 19-22 B and C).

9. Using your dominant thumb, depress the lever to open the blades and visualize the cervix (see Figure 19-22D).

10. If the cervix is not visualized, close the blades and withdraw the speculum 2 to 3 cm and reinsert it at a slightly different angle to ensure that the speculum is inserted far enough into the vagina.

E	Examination
N	Normal Findings
A	Abnormal Findings
P	Pathophysiology

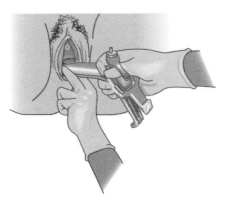

A. Opening of the Vaginal Introitus

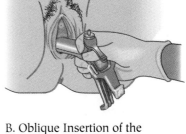

B. Oblique Insertion of the Speculum

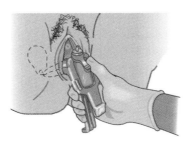

C. Final Advancement of the Speculum

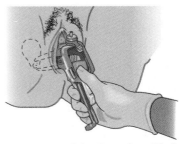

D. Opening of the Speculum Blades

Figure 19-22 Speculum Examination

11. Once the cervix is fully visualized, lock the speculum blades into place. This procedure varies based on the type of speculum being used.
12. Adjust your light source so that it shines through the speculum.
13. If any discharge obstructs the visualization of the cervix, clean it away with a cotton-tipped applicator.
14. Inspect the cervix and the os for color, position, size, surface characteristics such as polyps or lesions, discharge, and shape.

Color

N *The normal cervix is a glistening pink; it may be pale after menopause or blue (**Chadwick's sign**) during pregnancy.*

A Cyanosis not associated with pregnancy is abnormal.

P Possible causes include venous congestion of the area or systemic hypoxia as in congestive heart failure.

A Redness or a friable appearance is an abnormal finding.

P Possible causes include infection and inflammation, such as *Chlamydia* or gonorrhea.

Position

N *The cervix is located midline in the vagina with an anterior or posterior position relative to the vaginal vault and projecting approximately 2.5 cm into the vagina.*

A Lateral positioning of the cervix is an abnormal finding.

P Possible causes include tumor or adhesions that would displace the cervix.

A Projection of the cervix into the vaginal vault greater than normal limits is suspect.

P Uterine prolapse is caused by weakened vaginal wall muscles and pelvic ligaments, and may push the cervix into the vaginal vault.

Size

N *Normal size is 2.5 cm.*

A Cervical size greater than 4 cm is indicative of hypertrophy and is abnormal.

P Inflammation or tumor could result in the morbid enlargement of the cervix.

Surface Characteristics

N *The cervix is covered by the glistening pink squamous epithelium, which is similar to the vaginal epithelium, and the deep pink to red columnar epithelium, which is a continuation of the endocervical lining.*

A A reddish circle around the os may be abnormal.

P This is known as **ectropion** or **eversion**. It occurs when the squamocolumnar junction appears on the ectocervix. It results from lacerations during childbirth or, possibly, from congenital variation.

A Small, round, yellow lesions on the cervical surface indicate **nabothian cysts** (see Figure 19-23), which are abnormal.

P These benign cysts result from the obstruction of cervical glands.

A A bright-red, soft protrusion through the cervical os indicates a cervical polyp (see Figure 19-24) and is abnormal.

P Polyps originate from the endocervical canal; they are usually benign but tend to bleed if abraded.

A Hemorrhages dispersed over the surface and known as strawberry spots are abnormal.

P These may be seen in conjunction with trichomonal infections.

A Irregularities of the cervical surface that may look cauliflowerlike are an abnormal finding.

P Carcinoma of the cervix may manifest as a cauliflowerlike overgrowth (see Figure 19-25).

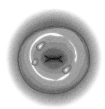

Figure 19-23   Nabothian Cysts

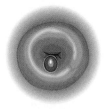

Figure 19-24   Cervical Polyp

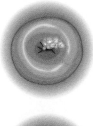

Figure 19-25   Carcinoma of the Cervix

E	Examination
N	**Normal Findings**
A	**Abnormal Findings**
P	**Pathophysiology**

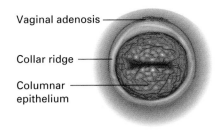

Vaginal adenosis

Collar ridge

Columnar epithelium

Figure 19-26 Fetal Exposure to DES

Normal

Nulliparous   Parous

Lacerations

Unilateral   Bilateral   Stellate
transverse   transverse

Figure 19-27 Shapes of the Cervical Os

A Columnar epithelium covering most of the cervix and extending to the vaginal wall (vaginal adenosis), and a collar-type ridge between the cervix and the vagina are abnormal (see Figure 19-26).
P This denotes fetal exposure to DES.

Discharge

E Note characteristics of any discharge.
N/A/P Refer to Table 19-3.

Shape of the Cervical Os

N *In the nulliparous woman, the os is small and either round or oval. In the parous woman, the os is a horizontal slit.*
A A unilateral transverse, bilateral transverse, stellate, or irregular cervical os is abnormal (see Figure 19-27).
P Possible causes include cervical tears that have occurred during rapid second-stage childbirth delivery, forceps delivery, and trauma.

🗲 NURSING ALERT

Risk Factors for Female Genitalia Cancer

Evaluate each patient for risk factors, and counsel the patient regarding diminishing risk factors that are behavior dependent. Suspected carcinoma of the female genitalia requires an immediate referral.

Cervical Cancer
• Early age at first intercourse
• Multiple sex partners
• Prior history of human papillomavirus
• Tobacco use
• Family history

Endometrial Cancer
• Early or late menarche (before age 11 or after age 16)
• History of infertility
• Failure to ovulate
• Unopposed estrogen therapy
• Use of tamoxifen
• Obesity
• Family history

Ovarian Cancer
• Advancing age
• Nulliparity
• History of breast cancer
• Family history of ovarian cancer

Vaginal Cancer
• Daughters of women who ingested DES during pregnancy

E	**Examination**
N	**Normal Findings**
A	**Abnormal Findings**
P	**Pathophysiology**

🗲 NURSING ALERT

DES Exposure

Most patients with DES exposure were born prior to 1971. These patients are at greater risk for carcinoma of the upper vagina.

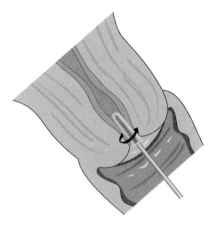

Figure 19-28 Endocervical Smear

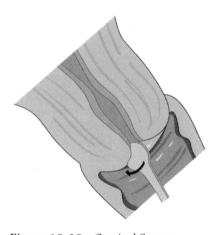

Figure 19-29 Cervical Smear

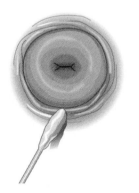

Figure 19-30 Vaginal Pool Smear

Collecting Specimens for Cytological Smears and Cultures

After inspection of the cervix and the cervical os, obtain any laboratory specimens that are indicated.

Collect the Pap smear first, followed by the gonococcal and any other vaginal smears. There are many accepted variations among laboratories regarding the collection and fixing of vaginal specimens. It is prudent to identify the procedure recommended by the laboratory testing the specimens.

Pap Smear

The Pap smear is actually a collection of three specimens that are obtained from three sites: the endocervix, the cervix, and the vaginal pool, or posterior fornix of the vagina. The purpose of the Pap smear is to evaluate cervico-vaginal cells for pathology that may indicate carcinoma. It is recommended that all females over the age of 18 or any female who is sexually active undergo this screening examination on a yearly basis.

A separate slide may be used for each specimen collected from the three areas, or one slide that is divided and labeled in three sections may be used.

Endocervical Smear

E   1. Using your dominant hand, insert the cytobrush through the speculum into the cervical os approximately 1 cm. Many patients find that this procedure causes a cramping sensation, so forewarn your patient that she may feel discomfort during this element of the assessment.

2. Rotate the cytobrush between your index finger and thumb 360° clockwise, then counter clockwise. Keep the cytobrush in contact with the cervical tissue. *Note:* If you have to use a cotton-tipped applicator instead of a cytobrush, leave the applicator in the cervical os for 30 seconds to ensure saturation (see Figure 19-28).

3. Remove the cytobrush and, using a rolling motion, spread the cells on the section of the slide marked *E*, if a sectional slide is being used. Do not press down hard or wipe the cytobrush back and forth because doing so will destroy the cells.

4. Discard the brush.

N/A/P Refer to Vaginal Pool Smear, following.

Cervical Smear

E   1. Insert the bifurcated end of the Ayre spatula through the speculum base. Place the longer projection of the bifurcation into the cervical os. The shorter projection should be snug against the ectocervix.

2. Rotate the spatula 360° one time only (see Figure 19-29).

3. Remove the spatula and gently spread the specimen on the section of the slide labeled *C*, if a sectional slide is being used.

N/A/P Refer to Vaginal Pool Smear, following.

Vaginal Pool Smear

E   1. Reverse the Ayre spatula and insert the rounded end into the posterior vaginal fornix and gently scrape the area. *Note:* a cotton-tipped applicator can also be used to obtain the smear. The cotton-tipped applicator may be the preferred vehicle for obtaining the specimen if vaginal secretions are viscous or dry. By moistening the cotton-tipped applicator with normal saline solution, viscous secretions can be removed with less trauma to the surrounding membranes (see Figure 19-30).

2. Remove the spatula and gently spread the specimen on the section of the slide marked *V*, if a sectional slide is being used.

3. Dispose of the spatula or cotton-tipped applicator.

4. Spray the entire slide or the slides with cytological fixative.

5. Submit the specimens to the appropriate laboratory per your institution's guidelines for cytology specimens.

N *Normal classifications for all cervicovaginal cytology should read "within normal limits" (WNL) using the Bethesda system, which denotes a lack of pathogenesis.*

A A report finding of benign cellular changes is abnormal.

P Benign cellular changes have a multiplicity of causes including fungal, bacterial, protozoan, or viral infections.

A A report finding of "atypical squamous cell of undetermined significance" is abnormal.

P Causes of this finding include inflammatory or infectious processes, a preliminary lesion, or an unknown phenomenon.

A A report finding of epithelial cell abnormalities is aberrant.

P This finding is indicative of squamous intraepithelial lesion, which may or may not be transient; squamous cell carcinoma; or glandular cell abnormalities that are seen in postmenopausal women who are not on hormone replacement therapy.

Gonococcal Culture Specimen

E **1.** Insert a sterile cotton swab applicator 1 cm into the cervical os.
   2. Hold the applicator in place for 20 to 30 seconds.
   3. Remove the swab.
   4. Roll the swab in a large Z pattern over the Thayer-Martin culture plate. Simultaneously rotate the swab as you roll it to ensure that all of the specimen is used (see Figure 19-31).
   5. Dispose of the swab.
   6. Submit the specimens to the appropriate laboratory per your institution's guidelines for culture specimens.

N *Cervicovaginal tissues are normally free of* Neisseria gonorrhoeae.

A It is abnormal to find a large number of gram-negative diplococci present in cervicovaginal secretions.

P *N. gonorrhoeae* are gram-negative diplococci organisms that prefer to invade columnar and stratified epithelium.

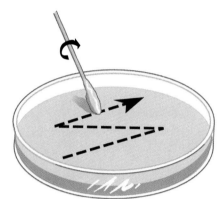

Figure 19-31 Inoculation of Thayer-Martin Culture Plate

Saline Mount or "Wet Prep"

This test is performed for the rapid evaluation of white blood cells, protozoa, etc.

E Spread a sample of the cervical or vaginal pool specimen onto a microscope slide, add one drop of normal saline solution, and apply a cover slip.

N *The sample should have fewer than 10 white blood cells (WBCs) per field.*

A A sample with more than 10 WBCs per field, protozoa, or other organisms is abnormal.

P A large number of WBCs can be indicative of an inflammatory response, *Chlamydia trachomatis*, or a bacterial infection. Protozoa are indicative of trichomoniasis.

KOH Prep

This test is performed for the rapid evaluation of *Candida*.

E Spread a sample of the cervical or vaginal pool specimen onto a microscope slide, add one drop of potassium hydroxide (KOH), and apply a cover slip.

N *Cervicovaginal tissues are normally free of* Candida albicans *except in a small percentage of women.*

A The presence of yeast and pseudohyphae forms (chains of budding yeast) is abnormal.

P The presence of budding yeast is indicative of an overgrowth of *Candida*.

E	**Examination**
N	**Normal Findings**
A	**Abnormal Findings**
P	**Pathophysiology**

Five Percent Acetic Acid Wash

E After completing all other vaginal specimens, swab the cervix with a cotton-tipped applicator that has been soaked in 5% acetic acid.

N *The normal response is no change in the appearance of the cervix.*

A A rapid acetowhitening or blanching with jagged borders is an abnormal finding.

P The cause may be the human papillomavirus, which is the causative agent of genital warts.

Anal Culture

E
1. Insert a sterile cotton swab applicator 1 cm into the anal canal.
2. Hold the applicator in place for 20 to 30 seconds.
3. Remove the swab. If fecal material is collected, discard the applicator and start again.
4. Roll and rotate the swab in a large Z pattern over a Thayer-Martin culture plate.
5. Dispose of the swab.

N *Anal tissues are normally free of* Neisseria gonorrhoeae.

A The presence of a large number of gram-negative diplococci is abnormal.

P This is indicative of *N. gonorrhoeae.*

Inspection of the Vaginal Wall

E
1. Disengage the locking device of the speculum.
2. Slowly withdraw the speculum but do not close the blades.
3. Rotate the speculum into an oblique position as you retract it to allow full inspection of the vaginal walls. Observe vaginal wall color and texture.

N *The vaginal walls should be pink, moist, deeply rugated, and without lesions or redness.*

A Spots that appear as white paint on the walls are abnormal.

P A possible cause is leukoplakia from *Candida albicans.* Repeated occurrences even after treatment may indicate HIV infection.

A Pallor of the vaginal walls is abnormal.

P Possible causes include anemia and menopause.

A Redness of the vaginal walls is abnormal.

P Possible causes include inflammation, hyperemia, and trauma from tampon insertion or removal.

A Vaginal lesions or masses are abnormal findings.

P Possible causes include carcinoma, tumors, and DES exposure.

Bimanual Examination

E
1. Observe the patient's face for signs of discomfort during the assessment process.
2. Inform the patient of the steps of the bimanual assessment, and warn her that the lubricant gel may be cold.
3. Squeeze water-soluble lubricant onto the fingertips of your dominant hand.
4. Stand between the legs of the patient as she remains in the lithotomy position, and place your nondominant hand on her abdomen and below the umbilicus.
5. Insert your dominant index and middle fingers 1 cm into the vagina. The fingers should be extended with the palmar side up. Exert gentle posterior pressure.

E	**Examination**
N	**Normal Findings**
A	**Abnormal Findings**
P	**Pathophysiology**

6. Inform the patient that pressure from palpation may be uncomfortable. Instruct the patient to relax the abdominal muscles by taking deep breaths.
7. When you feel the patient's muscles relax, insert your fingers to their full length into the vagina. Insert your fingers slowly so that you can simultaneously palpate the vaginal walls.
8. Remember to keep your thumb widely abducted and away from the urethral meatus and clitoris throughout the palpation in order to prevent pain or spasm.

Vagina

E Complete steps 1–8 from bimanual examination. Rotate the wrist so that the fingers are able to palpate all surface aspects of the vagina.

N *The vaginal wall is nontender and has a smooth or rugated surface with no lesions, masses, or cysts.*

A The presence of lesion, masses, scarring, or cysts is abnormal.

P These findings may be indicative of benign lesions such as inclusion cysts, myomas, or fibromas. The most common site for malignant lesions of the vagina is the upper one-third of the posterior vaginal wall.

Cervix

E 1. Position the dominant hand so that the palmar surface faces upward.
2. Place the nondominant hand on the abdomen approximately one-third of the way down between the umbilicus and the symphysis pubis.
3. Use the palmar surfaces of the dominant hand's fingerpads, which are in the vagina, to assess the cervix for consistency, position, shape, and tenderness.
4. Grasp the cervix between the fingertips and move the cervix from side to side to assess mobility (see Figure 19-32).

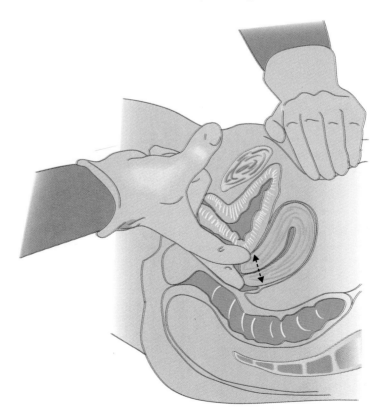

E	**Examination**
N	**Normal Findings**
A	**Abnormal Findings**
P	**Pathophysiology**

Figure 19-32 Assessment of Cervical Mobility

N *The normal cervix is mobile without pain, smooth and firm, symmetrically rounded, and midline.*

A The presence of pain on palpation or the assessment of mobility is a positive **Chandelier's sign** and is abnormal.

P This is indicative of possible pelvic inflammatory disease or ectopic pregnancy.

A Softening of the cervix (Goodell's sign) is a significant finding.

P This sign is seen at the fifth to sixth week of pregnancy.

A Irregular surface, immobility, or nodular surface structure of the cervix indicates abnormality.

P Possible causes include malignancy, nabothian cysts, and polyps.

Fornices

E 1. With the fingertips and palmar surfaces of the fingers, palpate around the fornices.
    2. Note nodules or irregularities.

N *The walls should be smooth and without nodules.*

A The presence of nodules or irregularities is abnormal.

P Possible causes include malignancy, polyps, and herniations if the walls of the fornices are impatent.

Uterus

E 1. With the dominant hand, which is in the vagina, push the pelvic organs out of the pelvic cavity and provide stabilization while the non-dominant hand, which is on the abdomen, performs the palpation (see Figure 19-33).
    2. Press the hand that is on the abdomen inward and downward toward the vagina, and try to grasp the uterus between your hands.

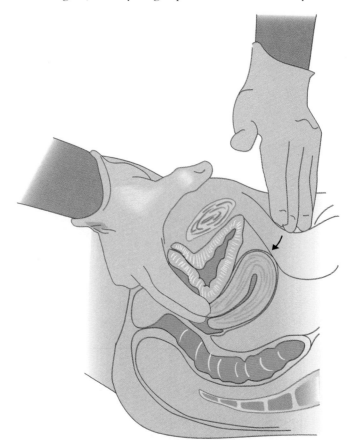

E	Examination
N	Normal Findings
A	Abnormal Findings
P	Pathophysiology

Figure 19-33 Uterine Palpation

3. Evaluate the uterus for size, shape, consistency, mobility, tenderness, masses, and position.
4. Place the fingers of the intravaginal hand into the anterior fornix and palpate the uterine surface.

N *The size of the uterus varies based on parity; it should be pear-shaped in the nongravid patient and more rounded in the parous patient. The uterus should be smooth, firm, mobile, nontender, and without masses. For uterine positions, refer to Figure 19-3. A nonpalpable uterus in the older woman may be a normal finding secondary to uterine atrophy.*

A Significant exterior enlargement and changes in the shape of the uterus are abnormal.

P Uterine enlargement indicates possible intrauterine pregnancy or tumor.

A Presence of nodules or irregularities indicates myomas, which are abnormal.

P Myomas are tumors containing muscle tissue.

A Inability to assess the uterus may be abnormal.

P A retroverted and retroflexed uterus, which can be assessed only via rectovaginal assessment, or a hysterectomy may account for a nonpalpable uterus.

> ### 🌸 NURSING TIP
>
> **Palpating a Retroverted Uterus**
>
> If the uterus is retroverted, the uterus may be palpable from the posterior fornix.

Adnexa

Fallopian tubes are rarely palpable, and palpation of the ovaries depends on patient age and size. Many times, the ovaries are not palpable, and this procedure can be painful to the patient during the luteal phase of the menstrual cycle (postovulation) or due to normal visceral tenderness.

E
1. Move the intravaginal hand to the right lateral fornix, and the hand on the abdomen to the right lower quadrant just inside the anterior iliac spine. Press deeply inward and upward toward the abdominal hand.
2. Push inward and downward with the abdominal hand and try to catch the ovary between your fingertips.
3. Palpate for size, shape, consistency, and mobility of the adnexa.
4. Repeat the above maneuvers on the left side (see Figure 19-34).

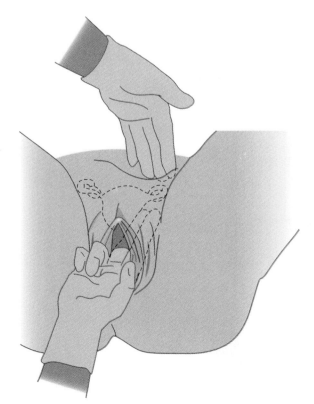

E	**Examination**
N	**Normal Findings**
A	**Abnormal Findings**
P	**Pathophysiology**

Figure 19-34 Palpation of the Left Adnexa

N *The ovaries are normally almond shaped, firm, smooth, and mobile without tenderness.*

A Presence of enlarged ovaries that are irregular, nodular, painful, with decreased mobility, or pulsatile indicate pathology.

P Abnormal adnexal presentation may indicate ectopic pregnancy, ovarian cyst, pelvic inflammatory disease, or malignancy.

Rectovaginal Examination

E 1. Withdraw your dominant hand from the vagina and change gloves. Apply additional lubricant to the fingertips of your dominant hand.
2. Tell the patient you will be inserting one finger into her vagina and one finger into her rectum. Remind her that the lubricant jelly will feel cold and that the rectal examination will be uncomfortable.
3. Insert the dominant index finger back into the vagina.
4. Ask the patient to strain down as if she is having a bowel movement in order to relax the anal sphincter. Assess anal sphincter tone.
5. Insert the middle finger of the dominant hand into the patient's rectum as she strains down (see Figure 19-35). If the rectum is full of stool, carefully remove the stool digitally from the rectum.
6. Advance the rectal finger forward while using the nondominant hand to depress the abdomen. Assess the rectovaginal septum for patency, the cervix and uterus for anomalies such as posterior lesions, and the rectouterine pouch for contour lesions.
7. On completion of the assessment, withdraw the fingers from the vagina and rectum, and if any stool is present on the glove, test for occult blood.

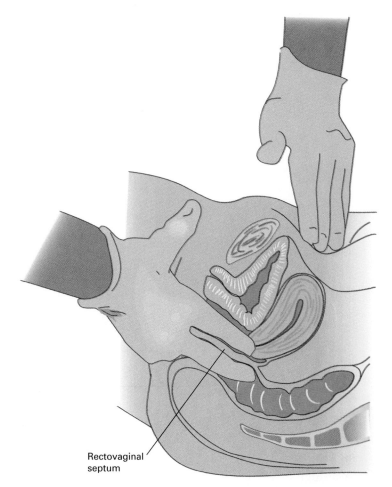

E	Examination
N	Normal Findings
A	Abnormal Findings
P	Pathophysiology

Rectovaginal septum

Figure 19-35 Rectovaginal Examination

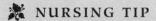 **NURSING TIP**

Examining the Patient with a Hysterectomy

If the patient has had a hysterectomy, follow the same assessment sequence but omit the following items: cervical inspection and palpation, uterine inspection and palpation, endocervical smear, and cervical smear. The vaginal walls and adnexa are evaluated if they were not surgically removed during the hysterectomy.

8. Clean the patient's genitalia and anal area with a tissue and assist her back to a sitting position.

N *The rectal walls are normally smooth and free of lesions. The rectal pouch is rugated and free of masses. Anal sphincter tone is strong. The cervix and uterus, if palpable, are smooth. The rectovaginal septum is smooth and intact. Refer to Chapter 21 for further information on the complete rectal examination.*

A The presence of masses or lesions indicates pathology.

P Possible causes include malignancy and internal hemorrhoids.

A Lax sphincter tone is an abnormal finding.

P Possible causes include perineal trauma from childbirth or anal intercourse and neurological disorders.

☻ THINK ABOUT IT

Gynecological Assessments for Women After Hysterectomies

Some women feel that it is unnecessary to have gynecological examinations after hysterectomies. Many of these women had surgery because of malignancy and therefore are at risk for recurrence. All women who have had this type of surgery must be encouraged to continue seeking annual gynecological examinations. Yearly monitoring helps to determine if malignancy has returned or if other pathologies have developed; for instance, women whose ovaries were not removed in the hysterectomy are still at risk for ovarian cancer.

How can you get this topic out into the public arena? How can you increase women's awareness of the need for annual gynecological check-ups even if they have had hysterectomies?

GERONTOLOGICAL VARIATIONS

The aging woman undergoes definite physical changes in her internal and external genitalia and her reproductive system. These changes begin with menopause, which usually occurs between the ages of 45 and 55. Menopause is characterized by low estrogen levels, which cause the cessation of the menstrual cycle. As aging progresses, a generalized atrophy of the external and internal female reproductive organs evolves.

Atrophy of the external reproductive organs results in a smaller clitoris and smaller labia. The labia also become flatter and lose their pigmentation. The skin of the labia becomes thin, shiny, avascular, and dry. There is a loss of subcutaneous fat in the pubic area, and the pubic hair becomes sparse and turns gray or white.

Atrophy of the internal reproductive organs causes the ovaries and fallopian tubes to diminish in size so that they are rarely palpable. The uterus atrophies so that it may be difficult to palpate. The cervix becomes smaller, paler, and less mobile. The cervical os becomes smaller but should remain palpable. The vagina becomes shorter, narrower, and thinner. The introitus may be constricted due to atrophy. There is a loss of rugae in the vaginal walls, and, therefore, a loss of elasticity in the walls. These changes in the vagina may cause the patient to complain of dyspareunia. Also, a delayed and reduced production of vaginal secretions may cause alterations in sexual response. An increase in the pH of the vaginal secretions and a decrease in the normal vaginal flora leads to an increase in vaginal infections in elderly women.

The pelvic muscles also atrophy, causing a decrease in the support of the pelvic organs. These muscles are often already weakened by trauma from childbirth; therefore, prolapse of the uterus and vaginal walls are common in elderly women.

 NURSING TIP

Maintaining Sexual Function in the Older Woman

Sexually active older women may benefit from:

- Water-soluble lubricant if vaginal secretions are decreased
- Extended foreplay in order to attain orgasm
- A reminder that there is no risk of pregnancy.

CASE STUDY

The case study illustrates the application and objective documentation of the female genitalia assessment.

The Patient with Pelvic Inflammatory Disease

Miss Daly is an 18-year-old white female who was admitted to the hospital with pelvic inflammatory disease.

❖   HEALTH HISTORY

PATIENT PROFILE	18 yo SWF
CHIEF COMPLAINT	"I've had pain in my abd for the last 3 d. It's getting worse."
HISTORY OF PRESENT ILLNESS	States that 2 d $\bar{p}$ LMP finished, developed pain in RLQ; describes pain as dull ache that radiated to Ⓡ side of abd. Pain ↑ $\bar{c}$ mvt, laughing, sneezing, & use of abd muscles. ASA ↓ pain minimally. Was able to sleep that night undisturbed by pain; next day pain became worse (9/10) & wasn't relieved by ASA; walking stick was required for ambulation. c/o malodorous yellowish vaginal d/c × 3 d, $\bar{c}$ mild vaginal itching, malaise, & ↓ appetite; temp of 101°F; denies N, V, D, painful urination, or incontinence.
PAST HEALTH HISTORY	
Medical	
Female Reproductive Health History	Menstrual hx: menarche age 12, 28–30 d cycle $\bar{c}$ mod flow lasting 3–4 d; LMP lasted 5 d & flow was ↑ $\bar{s}$ clots Premenstrual syndrome: denies Obstetrical hx: G: 0 P: 0 A: 0 LC: 0 Menopause hx: N/A Vaginal d/c: per HPI Hx of uterine bleeding: denies Sexual functioning: heterosexual, sexually active for 3 yr, had 7 different partners; denies engaging in anal intercourse; denies dyspareunia, inorgasmia Reproductive medical hx: hospitalized for RUQ pain & liver enlargement at age 17 2° oral contraceptive use; was advised to d/c use by MD. Hepatitis panels ⊖; unable to provide further information regarding tx; last Pap smear 3 mo ago, results were ⊖ Method of birth control: Ortho-Novum × 2 yr until liver enlarged; since then has not used any other method b/c they're "too messy"
Surgical	Tonsillectomy, age 4
Medications	Denies
Communicable Diseases	Gonorrhea × 2 in past 6 mo; tx $\bar{c}$ Ceftriaxone 250 mg & Tetracycline 500 mg, po qid, × 7 d for each occurrence
Allergies	Denies food or drug allergies

continued

Injuries/Accidents	MVA age 15 that required use of cervical collar × 2 mo
Disabilities/Handicaps	Denies
Blood Transfusions	Denies
Childhood Illnesses	Chickenpox age 4, measles age 6
Immunizations	States has "completed all childhood immunizations"

FAMILY HEALTH HISTORY

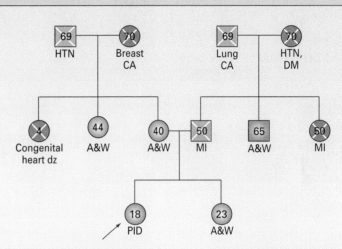

LEGEND

- Living female
- Living male
- Deceased female
- Deceased male
- Points to patient

A&W = Alive & well
CA = Cancer
DM = Diabetes mellitus
dz = Disease
HTN = Hypertension
MI = Myocardial infarction
PID = Pelvic inflammatory disease

Denies family hx of STDs, HIV/AIDS, use of DES by mother while pregnant, CA of reproductive organs.

SOCIAL HISTORY	
Alcohol Use	Drinks beer socially (2–3 cans per night on wkend)
Tobacco Use	Denies
Drug Use	Denies
Sexual Practice	Refer to med hx
Travel History	Denies
Work Environment	Denies
Home Environment	Lives c̄ mother in a 3 BR apt
Hobbies/Leisure Activities	Listening to music
Stress	Finishing school, dating, dealing c̄ her mother
Education	Currently enrolled in 12th grade
Economic Status	Middle class; no source of income x̄ mother; covered by mother's private insurance

continued

Military Service	Denies
Religion	Baptist
Ethnic Background	Southern, Anglo-American
Roles/Relationships	Sister, daughter, student; denies relationship problems
Characteristic Patterns of Daily Living	Awakens at 7:00 AM on school days, catches bus at 7:30 AM; skips breakfast & eats fast food during lunch break. Home from school by 3:00 PM & talks c̄ friends on phone or goes to the mall until dinner. Has dinner c̄ mom, then completes homework or watches TV. Usually in bed by MN.

HEALTH MAINTENANCE ACTIVITIES

Sleep	7 hr per PM
Diet	Mainly fast foods, drinks 4–5 soft drinks c̄ caffeine qd; snacks on chips & pretzels.
Exercise	None x̄ for gym class
Stress Management	Talking c̄ friends
Use of Safety Devices	Wears seat belt when driving; does not use condoms
Health Check-Ups	Annual school physical

PHYSICAL ASSESSMENT

Inspection of the External Genitalia	
Pubic Hair Distribution	Inverse triangle formation, sexual maturity rating — stage 5
Presence of Parasites	Ø
Skin Color and Condition	Mons pubis and vulva: mons pubis s̄ discoloration; vulva sl edematous & beefy red Clitoris: s̄ hypertrophy, s̄ ulcerations Urethral meatus: midline, Ø d/c or swelling Vaginal introitus: yellow d/c at entrance; no lesions, masses, bulging Perineum and anus: perineum pink, intact & s̄ lesions; anus dark pink, no skin tags or external hemorrhoids
Palpation of the External Genitalia	
Labia	Tender

continued

Urethral Meatus and Skene's Glands	No pain or d/c
Vaginal Introitus	Tone strong c̄ no bulging of pelvic contents
Perineum	Intact, firm, & homogenous

Speculum Examination of the Internal Genitalia

Cervix	Color: beefy red Position: midline Size: not enlarged Surface characteristics: no lesions Discharge: malodorous yellow-green purulent d/c from cervical os Shape of the cervical os: small & round
Inspection of the Vaginal Wall	Reddened c̄ inflamed mucosa

Bimanual Examination

Vagina	Nontender, free of lesions & masses
Cervix	Significant motion tenderness (⊕ Chandelier's sign), midline, firm, os admits fingertip
Fornices	Smooth, s̄ herniations or polyps
Uterus	Anteverted, pear shaped, mobile, smooth & firm, mod tenderness, not enlarged
Adnexa	Mobile & round, s̄ masses or lesions, mod tenderness Ⓡ adnexal area, mild tenderness Ⓛ adnexal area, no pulsations
Rectovaginal Examination	Rectovaginal septum intact, no masses or fissures; uterus & cx WNL, strong anal sphincter tone, Ø occult blood

LABORATORY DATA

Complete Blood Count:	Pt's Values	Normal Range
RBC	4.3 M/mm^3	3.6 M/mm^3
Hematocrit	39%	35%–47%
Hemoglobin	13 g/dl	12–16 g/dl
WBC	14 k/mm^3	4–11 k/mm^3
Erythrocyte Sedimentation Rate	23 mm/hr	0–20 mm/hr (Westegren method)
Pregnancy Test: ⊖		
Gonorrhea Culture: ⊕		
Chlamydia Culture: ⊖		
Pap Smear: WNL		
VDRL: ⊖		

NURSING CHECKLIST
Female Genitalia Assessment

Inspection of the External Genitalia
- Pubic Hair Distribution
- Presence of Parasites
- Skin Color and Condition
  - Mons Pubis and Vulva
  - Clitoris
  - Urethral Meatus
  - Vaginal Introitus
  - Perineum and Anus

Palpation of the External Genitalia
- Labia
- Urethral Meatus and Skene's Glands
- Vaginal Introitus
- Perineum

Speculum Examination of the Internal Genitalia
- Cervix
  - Color
  - Position
  - Size
  - Surface Characteristics
  - Discharge
  - Shape of the Cervical Os

Collecting Specimens for Cytological Smears and Cultures
- Pap Smear
- Endocervical Smear
- Cervical Smear
- Vaginal Pool Smear
- Gonococcal Culture Specimen
- Saline Mount or "Wet Prep"
- KOH Prep
- Five Percent Acetic Acid Wash
- Anal Culture

Inspection of the Vaginal Wall

Bimanual Examination
- Vagina
- Cervix
- Fornices
- Uterus
- Adnexa

Rectovaginal Examination

REVIEW QUESTIONS
AND ACTIVITIES

1. Describe anticipated normal findings of inspection and palpation of the external genitalia and rectum. If you are a female nurse, you may wish to use a mirror to examine your own external genitalia.

2. Prior to working with a patient, it is helpful to practice both positioning a patient for a vaginal assessment and handling the equipment. You will need an examination table, drapes, specula, and a volunteer. Your volunteer should remain clothed during this exercise. Practice positioning and draping the patient. Practice manipulating the speculum in one hand.

3. Which speculum would be most suitable for a woman who has never been sexually active? Which speculum would be most suitable for a large woman?

4. Describe the changes to the female genitalia that you would expect after menopause.

5. Which smears compose the Pap smear? Describe how these smears are obtained.

Questions 6 and 7 refer to the following situation:

You are examining a 22-year-old female in your clinic. During inspection of the vaginal introitus, you note a white, cottage cheeselike discharge that has no odor.

6. Based on your finding, you suspect that this patient may have:
   a. Gonorrhea
   b. Vaginitis
   c. Candida
   d. Normal vaginal discharge

   The correct answer is (c).

7. This patient's cervical os is oval in shape. This characteristic suggests that the patient is:
   a. Multiparous
   b. Nulliparous
   c. The mother of twins
   d. Infertile

   The correct answer is (b).

Male Genitalia

1. Identify the anatomic landmarks of the male genitalia.
2. Describe the characteristics of the most common male reproductive chief complaints.
3. Perform inspection, palpation, and auscultation on a healthy adult male and on a male patient with reproductive pathology.
4. Explain the scientific rationale for abnormal findings.
5. Document male reproductive assessment findings.
6. Describe the pathological changes that occur in the male reproductive system with the aging process.

The male reproductive system includes essential and accessory organs, ducts, and supporting structures (see Figure 20-1). The essential organs are the testes, or male gonads. The accessory organs include the seminal vesicles and bulbourethral glands. There are also several ducts, including the epididymis, ductus (vas) deferens, ejaculatory ducts, and urethra. The supporting structures include the scrotum, penis, and spermatic cords. The prostate is discussed in Chapter 21.

ANATOMY

Essential Organs

The **testes**, or testicles, are two oval glands located in the scrotum. Each measures about 5.0 cm (2.0 inches) in length and 2.5 cm (1.0 inch) in width. The testes are partially covered by a serous membrane called the tunica vaginalis (see Figure 20-2). This membrane separates the testes from the scrotal wall. Interior to the tunica vaginalis is a dense, whitish membrane covering each testicle and called the tunica albuginea. This membrane enters the testes and divides each testis into sections called lobules, which contain tightly coiled tubules called the seminiferous tubules. These coiled structures are the main component of testicular mass, and they produce sperm by spermatogenesis.

Accessory Organs

The **seminal vesicles** are two pouches located posteriorly to and at the base of the bladder. They contribute about 60% of the volume of semen. The fluid secreted by the seminal vesicles is rich in fructose and helps provide a source of energy for sperm metabolism. Prostaglandins, which contribute to sperm motility and viability, are also produced by the seminal vesicles.

The **bulbourethral glands**, or Cowper's glands, are pea-sized glands located just below the prostate. Secretions are emptied from the bulbourethral glands at the time of ejaculation. The bulbourethral glands secrete an alkaline substance that protects sperm by neutralizing the acidic environment of the vagina. These glands also provide lubrication at the end of the penis during sexual intercourse.

Ducts

The **epididymis** is a comma-shaped, tightly coiled tube that is located on the top and behind the testis and inside the scrotum. Each epididymis is composed of three parts: the head, which is connected to the testis; the body; and the tail, which is continuous with the vas deferens. Sperm mature and develop the power of motility as they pass through the epididymis.

The **ductus (vas) deferens** is an extension of the tail of the epididymis. Each duct ascends from the scrotum and permits sperm to exit from the scrotal sac upward into the abdominal cavity. The ductus deferens loops over the side and down the posterior surface of the bladder. This is where the duct enlarges into the ampulla of the vas deferens and joins the duct from the seminal vesicles to form the ejaculatory ducts.

The **ejaculatory ducts** are two short tubes posterior to the bladder. They descend through the prostate gland and terminate in the urethra. The ducts eject spermatozoa into the prostatic urethra just prior to ejaculation.

The **urethra** is the terminal duct of the seminal fluid passageway. It measures about 20 cm (8 inches) in length, passes through the prostate gland and penis, and terminates at the external urethral orifice.

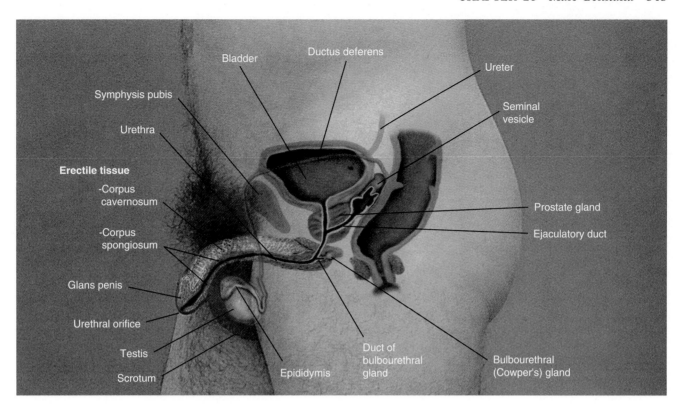

Figure 20-1   Male Genitalia

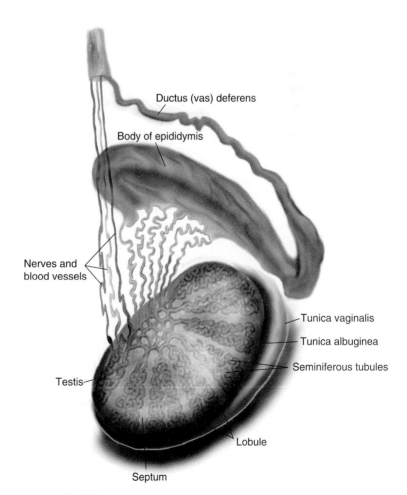

Figure 20-2   Testicle

Supporting Structures

The **scrotum** is a pouchlike supporting structure for the testes and consists of rugated, deeply pigmented, loose skin. Inside, the scrotum is divided by a single septum into two sacs, each containing a single testis. The production and survival of sperm requires a temperature that is 1°C cooler than normal body temperature (37°C). This is achieved by the scrotum's exposed location.

The **penis**, or male organ of copulation, is hairless, slightly pigmented, and cylindrical in shape. It consists of three compartments of erectile tissue. The corpus spongiosum surrounds the urethra and is located ventromedially. The two corpora cavernosa are located on the dorsolateral sides of the corpus spongiosum. Distally, the corpus spongiosum expands to form the **glans penis**, or the bulbous end of the penis. In the uncircumcised male, a fold of loose skin, the **prepuce** (foreskin), covers the glans penis. The corona forms the border between the glans penis and the penile shaft. The penis contains the urethra, a slitlike opening on the tip of the glans. The urethra terminates at the urethral meatus and is the passageway for urine.

The **spermatic cord** is made up of testicular arteries, autonomic nerves, veins that drain the testicles, lymphatic vessels, and the cremaster muscle. The testicles are suspended by the spermatic cord. The left side of the spermatic cord is longer than the right side, causing the left testicle to be lower in the scrotal sac. The cremaster muscle elevates the testes during sexual stimulation and exposure to cold. It also surrounds the testicles. The spermatic cord and ilioinguinal nerves pass through the inguinal canal into the abdomen. The inguinal canal is an oblique passageway in the anterior abdominal wall. The canal is about 4.0 to 5.0 cm (1.5 to 2.0 inches) long. It originates at the deep inguinal ring. The distal opening of the inguinal canal is called the external inguinal ring and is accessible to palpation. Superior to the inguinal canal lies the inguinal ligament, or Poupart's ligament. The inguinal ligament extends from the anterior iliac spine to the pubic tubercle.

Sexual Development

Sexual development can be assessed according to the five stages described by Tanner (see Table 20-1). Most of the changes in the male genitalia occur during puberty.

PHYSIOLOGY

The primary function of the male reproductive system is to produce sperm to fertilize eggs. In order for this to be achieved, there are several essential features of male reproduction that must take place. These are the manufacture of sperm and the deposition of sperm into the female genital tract.

Spermatogenesis

The testes produce sperm by a process called **spermatogenesis**. Specialized cells found between the seminiferous tubules, called the interstitial cells of Leydig, secrete the male hormone testosterone. Testosterone is sometimes called an androgen and is responsible for the development of secondary sexual characteristics and the attainment of reproductive capacity. Testosterone is responsible for male sexual feelings and performance as well as muscle development. The testes prepare for sperm production at approximately 13 years of age.

Table 20-1   Sexual Maturity Rating for Male Genitalia

DEVELOPMENTAL STAGE	PUBIC HAIR	PENIS	SCROTUM
1.	No pubic hair, only fine body hair (vellus hair)	Preadolescent; childhood size and proportion	Preadolescent; childhood size and proportion
2.	Sparse growth of long, slightly dark, straight hair	Slight or no growth	Growth in testes and scrotum; scrotum reddens and changes texture
3.	Becomes darker and coarser; slightly curled and spreads over symphysis	Growth, especially in length	Further growth
4.	Texture and curl of pubic hair is similar to that of an adult but not spread to thighs	Further growth in length; diameter increases; development of glans	Further growth; scrotum darkens
5.	Adult appearance in quality and quantity of pubic hair; growth is spread to medial surface of thighs	Adult size and shape	Adult size and shape

Male Sexual Function

The male sexual act consists of four stages: erection, lubrication, emission, and ejaculation. Erection of the penis is the first stage and is achieved through either physical or psychogenic stimulation of sensory nerves in the genital area. Parasympathetic impulses from the sacral portion of the spinal cord cause a vascular effect. The arterioles dilate and blood fills the corpora cavernosa, causing the penis to expand and become rigid. The corpora cavernosa can hold from 20 to 50 cc of blood. The veins from the tissue are compressed to occlude venous outflow.

Parasympathetic impulses at the same time cause the bulbourethral glands to secrete mucus, which provides lubrication during intercourse. When the sexual stimulus reaches a critical intensity, the reflex centers of the spinal cord send sympathetic impulses to the genital organs, and an orgasm occurs. Emission begins with contraction of the epididymis and the vas deferens, causing expulsion of sperm into the internal urethra. Ejaculation follows with contractions of the penile urethra.

❖ HEALTH HISTORY

The male genitalia health history provides insight into the link between a patient's life/lifestyle and male genitalia information and pathology.

PATIENT PROFILE	*Diseases that are age- and race-specific for the male genitalia are listed.*
Age	Chlamydia trachomatis (14–35) Testicular torsion (15–35) Varicocele (15–35) Testicular cancer (16–35) Gonococcal urethritis (<35) Epididymitis (<35) Hydrocele (>30) Spermatocele (>30) Testicular lymphoma (60+) Erectile dysfunction (60+) Bacteriuria (>65)
Race	
Caucasians	Testicular cancer
CHIEF COMPLAINT	*Common chief complaints for the male genitalia are defined and information on the characteristics of each sign/symptom is provided.*
Urethral Discharge	Excretion of substance from the urethra
Quality	Color: clear, white, purulent, blood-tinged, green, yellow, pink; consistency: thin, moderate, thick, mucoid; foul odor
Quantity	Absent, scant, mild, moderate, copious
Associated Manifestations	Dysuria, painful ejaculation, fever, urethral meatal discharge, change in frequency of urination, pruritus, conjunctivitis, arthritis, dermatological rash
Aggravating Factors	Urethral trauma

continued

Alleviating Factors	Medications (antibiotics, analgesics)
Setting	A new sexual partner in the last 6 months, a partner known to have other partners, unprotected intercourse
Timing	More prominent in the morning before urinating
Palpable Mass	A lump in the male genitalia
Quality	Firm, smooth, stellate, soft, mobile, nonmobile, well circumscribed, poorly circumscribed, "bag of worms," hard, heavy, transilluminating, nontransilluminating, fluctuant, separate from testes
Associated Manifestations	Pain, scrotal enlargement, absence of pain, vague back or abdominal pain, gynecomastia (if mass produces estrogen or human chorionic gonadotropin), nausea, vomiting, generalized edema
Aggravating Factors	Positioning, palpation or pressure, obesity, lifting, edema
Alleviating Factors	Medications, surgical removal or repair, positioning
Setting	Post trauma, recurrent testicular pain
Timing	Mumps orchitis present 7–10 days following parotitis
Erectile Dysfunction	The inability or decrease in ability to achieve and maintain a penile erection or to ejaculate seminal fluid
Quality	Inability to achieve erection (failed nocturnal tumescence test), ability to achieve with failure to maintain erection, inability to achieve complete erection, inability to ejaculate
Associated Manifestations	Anxiety, systemic disease (diabetes mellitus, hypertension, coronary artery disease), decreased libido, phimosis, decreased or absent cremasteric reflex, decreased femoral pulses, trauma, recent transurethral resection of the prostate or prostatectomy surgery
Aggravating Factors	Medications (beta blockers, diuretics, reserpine, monoamine oxidase inhibitors, selective serotonin reuptake inhibitors, Valium, Xanax, chemotherapeutic agents, codeine, Darvon, Percocet), anxiety, unsupportive partner, alcohol, smoking
Alleviating Factors	Medications (hormone therapy, yohimbine, anxiolytics), injections, implants, vascular surgery, sex counseling, avoiding alcohol, stopping smoking, change in diet (avoiding foods high in saturated fat or cholesterol), maintaining ideal body weight, reducing tension and stress, vacuum erectile device
Setting	Uncomfortable physical environment
Timing	Nocturnal tumescence
Penile Lesion	A growth on the penis
Quality	Color: erythematous, hyperpigmented, hypopigmented, pink, brown, black; presentation: flat, raised, indurated, papular, macular, multiple, isolated, ulcerated, warty, exudative (clear, purulent, bloody drainage)

continued

Associated Manifestations	Fever, malaise, inguinal lymphadenopathy, pain, prodromal numbness and tingling at lesion site, myalgias, headache, pruritus, immunosuppression, systemic illness, recurrent herpes simplex virus (HSV), human papillomavirus (HPV)
Aggravating Factors	Stress, systemic illness, immunosuppression
Alleviating Factors	Medications (antivirals, antibiotics), surgical removal, lifestyle changes
Setting	Unprotected intercourse, multiple sexual partners
Timing	Lymphogranuloma venereum: papule appears 1–3 weeks after inoculation; primary HSV: lesions appear 2–7 days after inoculation, vesicles ulcerate in 3–4 days; recurrent HSV: lesions appear a few hours to days after prodromal symptoms, lesions last approximately 10 days
PAST HEALTH HISTORY	*The various components of the past health history are linked to male genitalia pathology and male genitalia-related information.*
Medical	
Male Genitalia Specific	Prior history of sexually transmitted disease (STD), prostatitis, urinary tract infection, nephrolithiasis, cryptorchidism, trauma, cancer, benign prostatic hypertrophy (BPH), congenital or acquired deformity (epispadias, hypospadias), premature ejaculation, impotence, infertility
Nonmale Genitalia Specific	Mumps, rashes, joint pain, conjunctivitis, viral illness, renal disease, congestive heart failure, spinal cord injury, pelvic fracture
Surgical	Prostatectomy, transurethral prostatectomy, circumcision, orchiectomy, correction of malposition of testes, vasectomy, lesion or nodule removal, epispadias repair, hypospadias repair, hernia repair
Medications	Antibiotics, hormone replacements, alpha blockers, 5–alpha-reductase inhibitors
Communicable Diseases	HSV, HPV, molluscum contagiosum, condyloma acuminata, syphilis, penile lesion, chlamydia, gonorrhea, ureaplasma
Allergies	Contact dermatitis from topical preparations, condoms, nonoxynol 9 or other spermicides
Injuries/Accidents	Trauma, testicular torsion
Disabilities/Handicaps	Urinary incontinence, indwelling or intermittent urinary catheter, penile prosthesis, suprapubic urinary catheter
Childhood Illnesses	Mumps: orchitis, infertility

continued

FAMILY HEALTH	*Male genitalia diseases that are familial are listed.*
	Varicocele, testicular cancer, infertility, mother's use of hormones (diethylstilbestrol [DES]) during pregnancy
SOCIAL HISTORY	*The components of the social history are linked to male genitalia factors/pathology.*
Alcohol Use	Impairs gonadotropin release and accelerates testosterone metabolism, causing impotence and loss of libido; large doses can acutely depress the sexual reflexes; chronic alcoholism causes high levels of circulating estrogens, which decrease libido; alcohol intoxication may impair judgment, decreasing incidence of safe sex practices and increasing risk of exposure to STDs
Tobacco Use	Cigarette smoking increases risk of atherosclerotic disease, which may decrease penile blood flow
Drug Use	May impair judgment, increasing the risk for unsafe sex practices and STD exposure Cocaine: priapism with chronic abuse, impotence, increased sexual excitability Barbiturates: impotence Amphetamines: increased libido and delayed orgasm in moderate users, impotence in chronic users
Sexual Practice	Multiple partners, partner with multiple partners, new sexual partner, condom use (frequency and accuracy of use), sexual orientation, anal or oral intercourse
Work Environment	Radiation exposure has been linked to cancer of the male genitalia
HEALTH MAINTENANCE ACTIVITIES	*This information provides a bridge between the health maintenance activities and male genitalia function.*
Sleep	Nocturia secondary to urethritis
Diet	Erectile dysfunction: food high in saturated fat or cholesterol
Exercise	Trauma to the testicle may cause a hydrocele
Use of Safety Devices	Condoms used for vaginal and anal intercourse; supportive device worn while participating in sports
Health Check-Ups	Testicular exam

EQUIPMENT

- Nonsterile gloves
- Penlight
- Stethoscope
- Culturette tube
- Sterile cotton swabs
- Chux
- 1½"–2" gauze wrap
- Five percent acetic acid solution in spray bottle
- Thayer-Martin plate
- Colposcope or 10× power magnifying lens

ASSESSMENT OF THE MALE GENITALIA

✓ NURSING CHECKLIST
General Approach to Male Genitalia Assessment

1. Greet the patient and explain the assessment techniques that you will be using.
2. Ensure that the examination room is at a warm, comfortable room temperature to prevent patient chilling and shivering.
3. Use a quiet room that will be free from interruptions.
4. Ensure that the light in the room provides sufficient brightness to adequately observe the patient.
5. Assess the patient's apprehension level about the assessment and address this with him, reassuring him that this is normal.
6. Instruct the patient to remove his pants and underpants.
7. Place the patient on the examination table in the supine position with the legs spread slightly, and cover with a drape sheet. Stand to the patient's right side **or**
7A. Have the patient stand in front of you while you are sitting.
8. Don clean gloves.
9. Expose the entire genital and groin area.

Inspection

Hair Distribution

E 1. Note hair distribution pattern.
   2. Note the presence of nits or lice.
N *Pubic hair is distributed in a triangular form. It is sparsely distributed on the scrotum and inner thigh and absent on the penis. Genital hair is more coarse than scalp hair. There are no nits or lice.*
A Hair distribution is sparse or hair is absent at the genitalia area. This is called **alopecia** and it is abnormal.
P Alopecia in the genital area may result from genetic factors, aging, or local or systemic disease. These include developmental defects and hereditary disorders, infection, neoplasms, physical or chemical agents, endocrine diseases, deficiency states (nutritional or metabolic), destruction, or damage to the follicles.

Penis

E 1. Inspect the glans, foreskin, and shaft for lesions, swelling, and inflammation. If the patient is uncircumcised, ask him to retract the foreskin so that the underlying area can be inspected. After the assessment, replace the foreskin.
   2. Inspect the anterior surface of the penis first. Then lift the penis to check the posterior surface.
   3. Note the size and shape of the penis.
N *Skin is free of lesions and inflammation. The shaft skin appears loose and wrinkled in the male without an erection. The glans is smooth and without lesions, swelling, and inflammation. The foreskin retracts easily and there is no discharge. There may be a small amount of **smegma**, a white, cottage cheeselike substance, present. The dorsal vein is sometimes visible.*

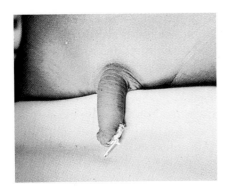

Figure 20-3 Phimosis *Courtesy of Dr. James Mandell, Chief Surgeon, Urology at Albany Medical College, Albany, NY*

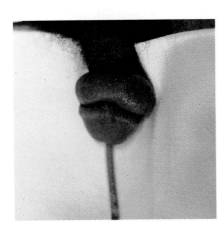

Figure 20-4 Paraphimosis *Courtesy of Dr. James Mandell, Chief Surgeon, Urology at Albany Medical College, Albany, NY*

E	**Examination**
N	**Normal Findings**
A	**Abnormal Findings**
P	**Pathophysiology**

The penis is cylindrical in shape and may vary greatly in size. The glans penis also varies in size and shape and may appear rounded or broad.

A A small papular lesion that enlarges and undergoes superficial necrosis to produce a sharply marginated ulcer on a clean base is abnormal.

P The **chancre** is the lesion of primary syphilis. It contains a multitude of *Treponema pallidum* spirochetes and is highly infectious. The tissue reacts to the organism with infiltration of lymphocytes, fibroblasts, and plasma cells that cause swelling and proliferation of the endothelial tissue, manifesting as a chancre.

A A tender, ulcerated, exudative, papular lesion with an erythematous halo, surrounding edema, and a friable base is abnormal.

P **Chancroid** is caused by inoculation of *Haemophilus ducreyi* through small breaks in epidermal tissue. Acute inflammatory response causes bubo formation.

A Pinhead papules to cauliflowerlike groupings of filiform, skin-colored, pink, or red lesions are abnormal.

P **Condyloma acuminatum** (genital warts) are caused by HPV infection of the epithelial cells. HPV may remain dormant for months to years after infection. There is a high incidence of recurrence of condyloma following appropriate treatment because of the persistence of latent HPV in normal-appearing skin. Some lesions are subclinical and can be identified only by androscopy. Refer to Special Technique page 652.

A Multifocal maculopapular lesions that are tan, brown, pink, violet, or white are abnormal.

P This describes intraepithelial neoplasia. HPV oncogenic types 16, 18, 31, and 33 infection cause epidermal proliferation and koilocytotic, dyskeratotic cells. Female partners may have a history of cervical intraepithelial neoplasm (CIN). The majority of lesions are distributed on the glans penis and prepuce. Changes of squamous cell carcinoma in situ are seen on histological examination.

A Erythematous plaques developing into vesicular lesions that may become pustular are abnormal.

P This describes genital herpes simplex virus infection. Skin-to-skin contact infection of HSV 1 and 2 causes epidermal degeneration, acanthosis, and intraepidermal vesicles. Lesions become ulcerated and eroded and are moist or crusted. Epithelial changes resolve in 2 to 4 weeks and hyper- or hypopigmentation of these areas is common. Postinflammatory scarring is rare. Recurrent herpes lesions are smaller. Diagnosis may be confirmed by Tzanck test for microscopic acanthocytes, viral culture, or serology for HSV antibodies.

A Multiple, discrete, flat pustules with slight scaling and surrounding edema are abnormal.

P *Candida* is a superficial mycotic infection of moist cutaneous sites. Predisposing factors include moisture, diabetes mellitus, antibiotic therapy, and deficiencies in systemic immunity.

A Erythematous plaques with scaling, papular lesions with sharp margins, and occasionally clear centers, and pustules, are abnormal.

P Tinea cruris is a fungal infection of the groin, usually caused by *Epidermophyton floccosum* or *Trichophyton rubrum*. Predisposing factors are a warm, humid environment, tight clothing, and obesity.

A An unusually long foreskin or one that cannot be retracted over the glans penis is abnormal.

P **Phimosis** occurs in uncircumcised males (see Figure 20-3). Inability to retract the foreskin is normal in infancy. In later years, an acquired constricting circumferential scar may follow healing of a split foreskin.

A It is abnormal when the retracted foreskin develops a fixed constriction proximal to the glans (see Figure 20-4). The penis distal to the foreskin may become swollen and gangrenous.

Embarrassing Situations Encountered During the Male Genitalia Assessment

The genitalia examination may cause the patient to feel uncomfortable or embarrassed. How would you handle the following situations if they were to occur during the genitalia assessment?

- The patient has an erection during the examination.
- The patient asks you if you would like to go out with him for dinner.

⚡ NURSING ALERT

Warning Signs of STDs in the Male Patient

1. Penile discharge, bloody or purulent
2. Scrotal or testicular pain
3. Burning or pain during urination
4. Penile lesion

E	Examination
N	Normal Findings
A	Abnormal Findings
P	Pathophysiology

P This is called **paraphimosis**. If the foreskin is retracted and not returned to its original position, paraphimosis can ensue (e.g., a patient's penis is cleansed for indwelling catheter insertion and the foreskin remains retracted). The foreskin acts as a circulatory constrictor, causing decreased blood flow, edema, and potential tissue necrosis.

A A normally formed but diminutive penis is abnormal. There is a discrepancy between the penile size and the age of the individual.

P A **microphallus** penis can result from a disorder in the hypothalamus or pituitary gland. It may be secondary to primary testicular failure due to partial androgen insensitivity. Maternal DES exposure has teratogenic effects caused by defects in nonandrogen-dependent regulatory agents. Microphallus can also be idiopathic in nature.

A It is abnormal when the penis appears larger than what is generally expected for the stated age. This condition is usually evident only before the age of normal puberty.

P Hormonal influence of tumors of the pineal gland or hypothalamus, tumors of the Leydig cells of the testes, tumors of the adrenal gland, or precocious genital maturity may cause penile hyperplasia.

A A continuous and pathological erection of the penis is abnormal.

P The cause of **priapism** is unclear in most patients; however, it does not occur as the result of sexual desire. Some of the cases are associated with leukemia, metastatic carcinoma, or sickling hemoglobinopathies. Priapism is created by the positive imbalance between the arterial blood supply and its return, created by venous drainage.

A Penile curvature, or chordee, is either a ventral or a dorsal curvature of the penis and is abnormal.

P Curvature is usually congenitally caused by a fibrous band along the usual course of the corpus spongiosum. Ventral chordee is seen mostly with **epispadias**, when the urethral meatus opens dorsally on the glans. In cases of congenital penile curvature without epispadias or **hypospadias** (when the urethral meatus opens ventrally on the glans), there is no additional tissue on or in any portion of the corpora cavernosa. This is caused by congenital maldevelopment of the tunica albuginea of the corpora.

P Peyronie's disease is a condition of penile curvature that occurs with erection. The dorsal surface of the corpora cavernosa becomes hardened with palpable, nontender plaques. Its cause is unknown.

✴ SPECIAL TECHNIQUE

Androscopy

The purpose of androscopy is to identify warty skin lesions that are not easily seen by the naked eye. It is indicated with a history of warts or HPV, of sexual contact with partner with warts or HPV, of high-risk sexual behavior, or of STD.

Equipment: clean gloves, 10× power magnifying lens or colposcope, Chux, 1½"–2" gauze wrap, scissors, and five percent acetic acid solution (white vinegar) in spray bottle.

E
1. Explain the procedure to the patient.
2. Have the patient undress from the waist down and sit on Chux at the edge of the examination table.
3. Wash hands. Don gloves.
4. Have the patient lie supine.
5. Wrap the penis and the scrotal area with gauze wrap that has been impregnated with five percent acetic acid solution.

continued

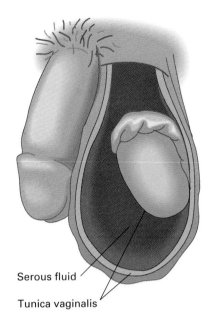

Serous fluid

Tunica vaginalis

Figure 20-5 Hydrocele

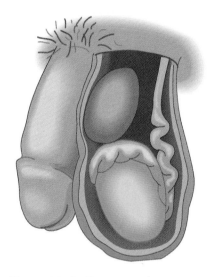

Figure 20-6 Spermatocele

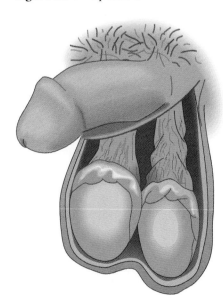

Figure 20-7 Varicocele

6. Allow the area to soak in the saturated gauze for 5 minutes.

7. Remove the gauze from the penis and scrotal areas.

8. Examine the penis and scrotum with a magnifying lens or colposcope.

9. If lesions are present at the underside of the scrotum, an anal androscopy must be performed.

10. Provide a place for the patient to wash and get dressed.

N *The penis and scrotal area should be free of any whitish-appearing areas.*

A Condyloma acuminatum appears as tiny white papules identified with a 10× hand lens or colposcope.

P Refer to page 651.

Scrotum

E 1. Displace the penis to one side in order to inspect the scrotal skin.

2. Lift up the scrotum to inspect the posterior side.

3. Observe for lesions, inflammation, swelling, and nodules.

4. Note size and shape.

N *Scrotal skin appears rugated and thin and appears more deeply pigmented than body color. The skin should hug the testicles firmly in the young male and become elongated and flaccid in the elderly male. All skin areas should be free of any lesions, nodules, swelling, or inflammation. Scrotal size and shape vary greatly from one individual to another. The left scrotal sac is lower than the right.*

A/P Condyloma acuminatum, tinea cruris, and *Candida* are abnormal findings. Refer to page 651.

A Enlargement of or masses within the scrotum are abnormal.

P Scrotal masses can arise from benign or malignant conditions. Scrotal swelling is seen with inguinal hernia, hydrocele, varicocele, spermatocele, tumor, and edema.

A A large, pear-sized mass in the scrotum is abnormal (see Figure 20-5). The scrotal skin is stretched, shiny, and erythematous, which may give the penis a shortened appearance.

P A **hydrocele** is created by the accumulation of fluid between the two layers of the tunica vaginalis. Hydroceles may be idiopathic or due to trauma, inguinal surgery, epididymitis, or testicular tumor.

A A well-defined cystic mass on the superior testis or in the epididymis is abnormal. It is usually <2 cm in diameter (see Figure 20-6). Multiple masses may be present.

P This is called **spermatocele**. Blockage of the efferent ductules of the rete testis causes formation of sperm-filled cysts at the top of the testis or in the epididymis.

A In light-skinned individuals, a scrotal mass with a bluish discoloration is abnormal (see Figure 20-7).

P Dilated veins in the pampiniform plexus of the spermatic cord cause **varicocele** formation and are usually accompanied by a decreased sperm count. Most appear in the left hemiscrotum; the remainder are bilateral. A right-sided varicocele may be indicative of an obstruction at the vena cava. Acute onset of a right-sided varicocele may be pathognomonic for a renal tumor extending into the renal vein or compression of the renal vein. It may increase in size with the Valsalva maneuver and decrease or disappear with supine positioning.

A Round, firm, cystic nodules confined within the scrotal skin are abnormal.

P A sebaceous cyst contains sebum, an oily, fatty matter secreted by the sebaceous glands. The cyst may result from a decrease in localized circulation and closure of sebaceous glands or ducts.

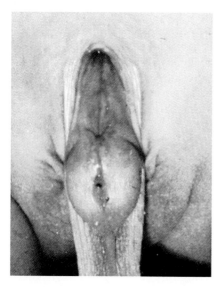

Figure 20-8 Epispadias   *Courtesy of Dr. James Mandell, Chief Surgeon, Urology at Albany Medical College, Albany, NY*

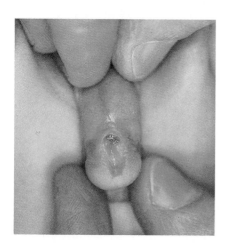

Figure 20-9 Hypospadias   *Courtesy of Dr. James Mandell, Chief Surgeon, Urology at Albany Medical College, Albany, NY*

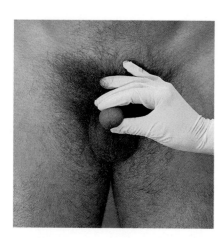

Figure 20-10 Palpation of the Penis

Urethral Meatus

E   1. Note the location of the urethral meatus.
  2. Observe for discharge.
  3. Obtain a culture of any discharge (refer to Special Technique on page 655).

N   *The urethral meatus is located centrally. It is pink and without discharge.*

A   Erythema and swelling at the urethral meatus are abnormal.

P   Urethritis is a localized tissue inflammation resulting from bacterial, viral, or fungal infection as well as from urethral trauma.

A   It is abnormal for the urethral meatus to be displaced dorsally (see Figure 20-8).

P   Epispadias is a congenital abnormality caused by a complete or partial dorsal fusion defect of the urethra.

A   It is abnormal for the urethral meatus to open on the ventral aspect of the glans penis (see Figure 20-9). The urethral meatus may also open at the perineum.

P   Hypospadias is a congenital abnormality, usually associated with chordee. Complications of this defect include urethral meatal stenosis, inability to direct the urine stream, and sexual dysfunction.

❀ NURSING TIP

Penile Discharge

If the patient complains of penile discharge but none is present, ask the patient to milk the penis from the shaft to the glans. This maneuver may express a discharge that can then be cultured.

Inguinal Area

E   1. If the patient is supine, ask the patient to stand.
  2. Stand facing the patient.
  3. Observe for swelling or bulges.
  4. Ask the patient to bear down.
  5. Observe for swelling or bulges.

N   *The inguinal area is free of any swelling or bulges.*

A   A bulge in the inguinal area is abnormal.

P   Hernia pathology is discussed further in the section on palpation.

Palpation

Penis

E   1. Stand in front of the patient's genital area.
  2. Don clean gloves.
  3. Between the thumb and the first two fingers, palpate the entire length of the penis (see Figure 20-10).
  4. Note any pulsations, tenderness, masses, or plaques.

N   *Pulsations are present on the dorsal sides of the penis. The penis is nontender. No masses or firm plaques are palpated.*

A   Vascular insufficiency is evidenced by diminished or absent palpable pulse or pulsations and is abnormal.

P   Systemic disease, localized trauma, and localized disease may adversely affect normal blood flow in the penis.

A   It is abnormal for the penis to be enlarged in a nonerect state. Generalized penile swelling may be present.

P   Fluid accumulation in the loose tissue of the penile integument results from anasarcic states. Obstruction of the penile veins or inflammation of the penis results in local edema. Trauma to the penis may cause swelling secondary to penile contusion and extravasation of blood. Gentle finger pressure may cause pitting.

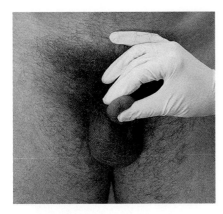

Figure 20-11 Palpation of the Urethral Meatus

Urethral Meatus

E **1.** Stand in front of the patient's genital area.
  2. Between the thumb and forefinger, grasp the glans and gently squeeze to expose the meatus (see Figure 20-11).
  3. If discharge is seen, or if the patient complains of a urethral discharge, a culture should be taken. (Refer to Special Techniques following.)

N *The urethral meatus is free of discharge and drainage.*

A A urethral discharge of pus and mucus shreds is abnormal. The discharge may vary in color, consistency, and amount.

P Bacterial infection of the genitourinary tract causes inflammation and formation of a liquid composed of albuminous substances, leukocytes, shedding tissue cells, and bacteria.

✺ SPECIAL TECHNIQUE

Urethral Culture

The purpose of the urethral culture is to identify the causative organism of penile discharge.

Equipment: sterile cotton swabs, Culturette tube, Thayer-Martin plate.

  1. Explain to the patient what you are going to do and that some discomfort may be involved.
  2. Place the patient in the supine position.
  3. Note the color, consistency, and odor of the discharge.
  4. With the nondominant hand, hold the penis. With the dominant hand, roll a sterile cotton swab in the discharge.
  5. Place the swab in a Culturette tube.
  6. With a second sterile cotton swab, obtain another specimen for a gonorrheal culture.
  7. Roll the swab over a Thayer-Martin plate in a Z pattern.
  8. Label both cultures and send them to the laboratory for analysis.

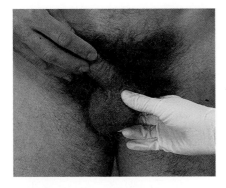

Figure 20-12 Palpation of the Testicle

Scrotum

E **1.** Between the thumb and the first two fingers, gently palpate the left testicle (see Figure 20-12).
  2. Note the size, shape, consistency, and presence of masses.
  3. Palpate the epididymis (see Figure 20-13).
  4. Note the consistency and presence of tenderness or masses.
  5. Between the thumb and the first two fingers, palpate the spermatic cord from the epididymis to the external ring.
  6. Note the consistency and presence of tenderness or masses.
  7. Repeat on the left side.

N *The scrotum contains on each side a testicle and an epididymis. The testicles should be firm but not hard, ovoid, smooth, and equal in size bilaterally. They should be sensitive to pressure but not tender. The epididymis is comma-shaped and should be distinguishable from the testicle. The epididymis should be insensitive to pressure. The spermatic cord should feel smooth and round.*

A A unilateral mass palpated within or about the testicle is abnormal (see Figure 20-14).

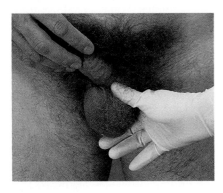

Figure 20-13 Palpation of the Epididymis

E	**Examination**
N	**Normal Findings**
A	**Abnormal Findings**
P	**Pathophysiology**

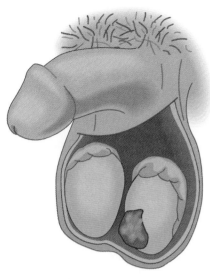

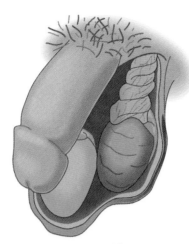

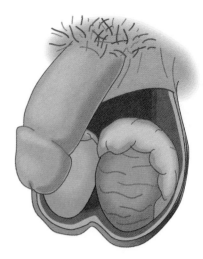

Figure 20-14 Testicular Tumor   **Figure 20-15** Testicular Torsion   **Figure 20-16** Epididymitis

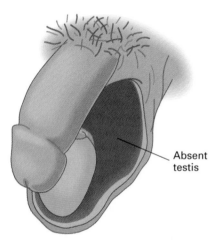

Absent testis

Figure 20-17 Cryptorchidism

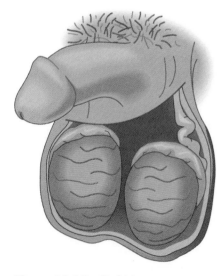

Figure 20-18 Orchitis

P Intratesticular masses should be considered malignant until proven otherwise. They are nodular and associated with painless swelling. The majority of intratesticular masses arise from germinal elements. Extratesticular tumors are uncommon and usually are benign. They can arise from any of the surrounding structures, including the epididymis, the testicular tunica vaginalis, or the spermatic cord.

P Inguinal hernia is discussed on pages 659 and 660.

P Refer to the section on scrotal inspection for a description of spermatocele.

A A large, pear-shaped mass that has a smooth wall is abnormal.

P Refer to the section on scrotal inspection for a description of hydrocele. The entire testicle must be palpated because underlying malignancies cause a small percentage of all hydroceles. Sonography must be performed if the entire testicle is not palpable.

A Palpation of a scrotal mass superior to the testis and that reveals a "bag of worms" is abnormal.

P Refer to the section on scrotal inspection for a description of varicocele.

A It is abnormal for the testicle to be enlarged, retracted, in a lateral position, and extremely sensitive (see Figure 20-15).

P Testicular torsion is a surgical emergency. Twisting or torsion of the testis causes venous obstruction, secondary edema, and eventual arterial obstruction. Doppler ultrasonography reveals absence of perfusion to the testicle.

A Palpation reveals an indurated, swollen, tender epididymis (see Figure 20-16).

P Epididymitis results from the retrograde spreading of pathogenic organisms from the urethra to the epididymis. The majority of infections are caused by bacterial pathogens such as *Chlamydia trachomatis* and *Neisseria gonorrhoeae*. An associated hydrocele may be present. The testis may also be enlarged and tender.

A It is abnormal for one or both testes to be undescended (see Figure 20-17).

P The causes of **cryptorchidism** are not established but may be multiple and related to testicular failure, deficient gonadotrophic stimulation, mechanical obstruction, or gubernacular defects. The undescended testis is usually smaller than its normally descended mate. Unilateral cryptorchidism is more common than is bilateral. The undescended testicle is usually located in the inguinal canal or less commonly intra-abdominally. Spontaneous descent is unusual after one year of age.

A An acute, painful onset of swelling of the testicle along with warm scrotal skin is abnormal (see Figure 20-18). The patient may complain of heaviness in the scrotum.

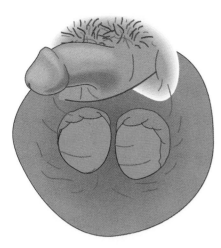

Figure 20-19 Scrotal Edema

E Examination
N Normal Findings
A Abnormal Findings
P Pathophysiology

P **Orchitis** can be caused by mumps, coxsackievirus B, infectious mononucleosis, and varicella. Involvement of the testes is via the hematogenous route. Orchitis is unilateral in the majority of cases, but onset in the second testicle may occur up to one week after that in the first.

A A testicle that is smaller and softer than normal (less than 5.0 cm × 2.5 cm) is abnormal.

P An atrophic testicle may be the result of Klinefelter's syndrome (hypogonadism), hypopituitarism, estrogen therapy, or orchitis.

A In light-skinned individuals, it is abnormal for the scrotum to be enlarged, taut with pitting edema, and reddened (see Figure 20-19).

P Scrotal edema accompanies edema associated with the lower half of the body, such as in congestive heart failure (CHF), renal failure, and portal vein obstruction. Scrotal edema may also be the result of local inflammation. Scrotal contents are usually nonpalpable.

A Acute, painful, scrotal swelling may occur with a history of trauma. This is abnormal.

P Trauma is a major cause of acute scrotal swelling. Scrotal or testicular hematoma formation as well as testicular rupture may be present. A small percentage of all diagnosed testicular tumors are diagnosed through medical attention for trauma; therefore, any intratesticular hematoma must be followed to rule out neoplasm.

🌺 NURSING TIP

Teaching Testicular Self-Examination

Testicular self-examination (TSE) should be taught to the patient during the scrotal examination.

- Ask the patient if monthly testicular self-examination is performed.
- Explain the rationale for the examination. Monthly testicular examination will allow for earlier detection of testicular cancer, which occurs most often in 16 to 35-year-old males.
- Tell the patient to pick a date to perform the exam every month. The best time to perform the examination is after a warm shower when both hands and the scrotum are warm.
- Instruct the patient to gently feel each testicle using the thumb and first two fingers (see Figure 20–20A).
- Remind the patient that the testicles are ovoid and movable, and that they feel firm and rubbery. The epididymis is located on top and behind the testis, is softer, and feels ropelike.
- Instruct the patient to report any changes from these findings, including any lumps and nodules, especially if they are nonmobile.
- Instruct the patient to squeeze the tip of the penis and observe for any discharge (see Figure 20–20B).

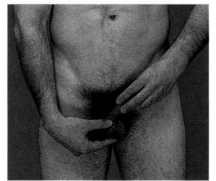
A. Palpating the Testis

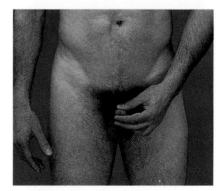
B. Assessing for Penile Discharge

Figure 20-20 Testicular Self-Examination

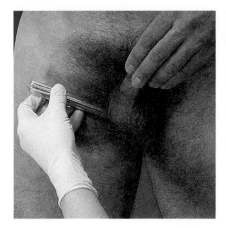

Figure 20-21 Transillumination of the Scrotum

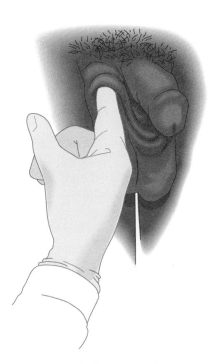

Figure 20-22 Inguinal Palpation

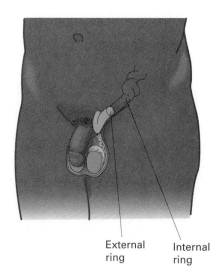

External ring   Internal ring

Figure 20-23 Indirect Inguinal Hernia

✦ SPECIAL TECHNIQUE

Transillumination of the Scrotum

If a scrotal mass or enlargement is detected, the scrotum should be transilluminated.

E 1. Tell the patient what you are going to do and that it should not be painful.
  2. Darken the room.
  3. Using a penlight, apply the light source to the unaffected side behind the scrotum and direct it forward.
  4. Apply the light source to the side of the scrotal enlargement or mass.
  5. Note whether there is transmission of a red glow (see Figure 20–21).

N *A normal testicle does not transilluminate (i.e., there is no red glow).*

A The transmission of a red glow indicates a serous fluid within the scrotal sac. This can occur in hydrocele and spermatocele and is abnormal. Vascular structures such as a hernia and a tumor do not transilluminate.

P Refer to previous discussions of these conditions.

Inguinal Area

E 1. With the index and middle fingers of the right hand, palpate the skin overlying the inguinal and femoral areas for lymph nodes.
  2. Note size, consistency, tenderness, and mobility.
  3. Ask the patient to bear down while you palpate the inguinal area.
  4. Place the right index finger in the patient's right scrotal sac above the right testicle and invaginate the scrotal skin. Follow the spermatic cord until you reach a triangular, slitlike opening (the external inguinal ring).
  5. The finger is placed with the nail facing inward and the finger pad outward (see Figure 20-22).
  6. If the inguinal ring is large enough, continue to advance the finger along the inguinal canal and ask the patient to cough.
  7. Note any masses felt against the finger.
  8. Repeat on the left side using the left hand to perform the palpation.
  9. Palpate the femoral canal. Ask the patient to bear down.

N *It is normal for there to be small (1.0 cm), freely mobile lymph nodes present in the inguinal area. There should not be any bulges present in the inguinal area. There should not be any palpable masses in the inguinal canal. No portions of the bowel should enter the scrotum. There should be no palpable mass at the femoral canal.*

A Unilateral enlargement of the lymph nodes along with erythematous overlying skin that may contain adhesions is abnormal.

P Three of the 15 strains of *Chlamydia trachomatis*, specifically L1, L2, and L3, cause lymphogranuloma venereum (LV). These serovars are more invasive and virulent and selectively infect lymphoid tissue rather than columnar epithelial cells. Firm inguinal masses result when buboes involute.

A Unilateral or bilateral enlargement of the inguinal lymph nodes is abnormal. The nodes may be tender or painless.

P Lymphadenopathy occurs when the immune system responds to bacterial infections, trauma, or carcinoma. Bacterial infections commonly associated with inguinal lymphadenopathy include syphilis, chancroid, and gonorrhea.

A An **indirect inguinal hernia** palpated at the inguinal ring is abnormal (see Figure 20-23). An impulse may be felt on the fingertip when the patient is asked to cough. A larger indirect inguinal hernia may feel like a mass at the inguinal canal.

P Portions of the bowel or omentum protrude at the external inguinal ring. All indirect hernias are congenitally related to a patent processus vaginalis. The severity of a combination of the congenital abnormality and a condition that increases abdominal pressure (e.g., obesity, chronic

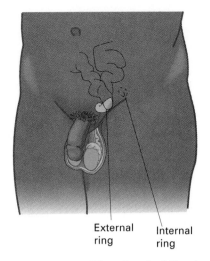

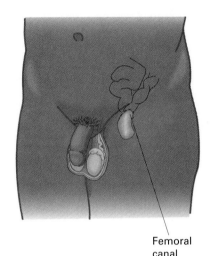

External   Internal
ring   ring

Figure 20-24 Direct Inguinal Hernia

Femoral
canal

Figure 20-25 Femoral Hernia

E	**Examination**
N	**Normal Findings**
A	**Abnormal Findings**
P	**Pathophysiology**

obstructive pulmonary disease [COPD], hard physical labor, ascites) determines the onset and degree of the hernia.

A Oval swelling found at the pubis on inspection represents a **direct
inguinal hernia** and is abnormal (see Figure 20-24). Coughing causes
enlargement on palpation of the mass.

P In direct hernias, portions of the bowel or omentum protrude directly
through the external inguinal ring. Direct hernias are acquired masses that
are influenced by increases in intra-abdominal pressure and weakening of
the inguinal structures as part of the normal aging process. Other related
factors include heavy lifting, obesity, and COPD.

A Palpation of a mass medial to the femoral vessels and inferior to the
inguinal ligament is indicative of a **femoral hernia** and is abnormal (see
Figure 20-25).

P A femoral hernia is caused by protrusion of the omentum or bowel
through the femoral wall. Onset and size of the hernia may be affected
by a congenitally large femoral ring, degradation of collagen and tissue
attenuation associated with aging, increased intra-abdominal pressure,
and presence of preperitoneal fat.

Table 20-2 compares the different types of hernias.

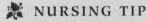 **NURSING TIP**

Reducing a Direct Inguinal Hernia

An attempt should be made by a qualified practitioner to reduce hernia (to
return the bowel to the abdominal cavity) if nausea, vomiting, and tenderness
are absent. Have the patient lie down and gently push the hernia back into the
abdominal cavity. An incarcerated hernia cannot be pushed back into the
abdominal cavity. If nausea, vomiting, and tenderness are present, they may
indicate a strangulated hernia (no blood supply to the affected bowel), which
should be referred to a physician.

Auscultation

Auscultation is performed if a scrotal mass is found on inspection or palpation.

Scrotum

E 1. Place the patient in a supine position.
   2. Stand at the patient's right side at the genitalia area.
   3. Place your stethoscope over the scrotal mass.
   4. Listen for the presence of bowel sounds.

N *No bowel sounds are present in the scrotum.*

A An indirect inguinal hernia is present if bowel sounds are present in the
enlarged scrotum.

Table 20-2 Comparison of Inguinal and Femoral Hernias			
FEATURE	**INDIRECT INGUINAL HERNIA**	**DIRECT INGUINAL HERNIA**	**FEMORAL HERNIA**
Occurrence	More common in infants <1 year and males 16 to 25 years of age.	Middle-aged and elderly men.	More frequent in women.
Origin of Swelling	Above inguinal ligament. Hernia sac enters canal at internal ring and exits at external ring. Can be found in the scrotum.	Above inguinal ligament. Directly behind and through external ring.	Below inguinal ligament.
Cause	Congenital or acquired.	Acquired weakness brought on by heavy lifting, obesity, COPD.	Acquired, due to increased abdominal pressure and muscle weakness.

⚡ NURSING ALERT

Warning Signs of Hernias

- Scrotal or inguinal mass
- Mild aching or discomfort in the scrotal or inguinal area
- Bulging in the groin area with heavy lifting, coughing

If any of these are present, refer the patient for further treatment.

🌹 NURSING TIP

Erectile Function

Treatment for impotence varies greatly, depending on the cause and may include any of the following:

- Patience and a relaxed atmosphere
- Medication: Halotestin, yohimbine HCl
- Surgery
- Penile prosthesis
- Penile injections: papaverine, regitine
- Vacuum erection device

E	**Examination**
N	**Normal Findings**
A	**Abnormal Findings**
P	**Pathophysiology**

P   Loops of bowel extending into the scrotum via an indirect hernia continue to produce bowel sounds unless the hernia is strangulated (lack of blood flow to bowel tissue) and bowel tissue becomes ischemic or necrotic.

GERONTOLOGICAL VARIATIONS

Physiological changes in the male reproductive system occur with aging. Assessment of the external genitalia reveals thinner pubic hair. The penis has an atrophic appearance and the testicles may appear or feel small or atrophied. The scrotal sac loses its elasticity. In most individuals, there is a reduction in testosterone levels by the age of 50.

Testicular degeneration seems to occur in patchy distribution, which allows normal spermatogenesis to be present in the majority of men until 70 years of age. Sperm output may be slightly decreased.

Aging is associated with the development of a variety of disease processes that may have direct effects on gonadal function. Systemic disease (COPD, sarcoidosis, cirrhosis, renal failure, depression, hypo- or hyperthyroidism), for example, can alter hormonal release and metabolism at various levels. Systemic disease can also have direct toxic effects on the testes, cause pituitary damage and hypothalamic disease, and alter hormonal metabolism.

The ability to obtain or maintain an erection is affected by aging. Aging brings a significant delay in erectile attainment, and erection is also often not as complete. An absence or marked reduction of preejaculatory fluid emission is often associated with advancing age.

A marked increase in the prevalence of impotence is associated with increased aging. The most common cause of impotence in the older male is vascular disease, which accounts for half of the cases. Other causes may include diabetes mellitus, hypogonadal states, and psychological stimuli. The older population has a tendency to take more of those medications that can contribute to impotence.

🌹 NURSING TIP

Dealing with Changes in Sexual Function

You must feel comfortable discussing sexual problems and concerns. Be sensitive to the elderly male's possible discomfort and embarrassment during a genital examination and regarding the changes he is experiencing with age. The older male needs to be informed about what are considered to be normal changes in sexual function. If factors causing impotence are not reversible, then alternatives need to be suggested to restore sexual function.

CASE STUDY

The case study illustrates the application and objective documentation of the male genitalia assessment.

The Patient with Urethritis

Mike is a 43-year-old full-time employed construction project manager.

❖ HEALTH HISTORY	
PATIENT PROFILE	43 yo DWM
CHIEF COMPLAINT	"My plumbing hurts. It really hurts when I pee. I'm not sure what's going on."

continued

HISTORY OF PRESENT ILLNESS	Pt c/o intermittent dysuria starting 6 d PTA. Pain (3/10) predominant on initiation of urination; describes pain as "burning & pressure." ↑ fluid intake to "flush my system out." Pt noticed thick, yellow urethral d/c 2 d ago; d/c slight when 1st noticed & now is copious. 2 d PTA, noted ® scrotum was sensitive to pressure & enlarged. Scrotum now painful (6/10) & ↑ in size; c/o feeling "hot c̄ chills." Pt had sexual intercourse c̄ new female partner 7 d PTA (condoms & spermicide not used); ā this, patient had intercourse 2 mo PTA c̄ a different female partner (condoms & spermicide used c̄ q intercourse). Denies traumatic injury to scrotal area.
PAST HEALTH HISTORY	
Medical	HTN & hyperlipidemia dx 4 yr ago; tx c̄ wt loss, doesn't follow low-fat or low-Na⁺ diet; elevated LFTs tx c̄ reduction of alcohol intake
Surgical	Wisdom teeth extracted age 20, Ø complications
Medications	Ø
Communicable Diseases	Hx of gonorrhea (24), tx c̄ PCN injection, denies hx of other STDs
Allergies	Ragweed & spring pollen allergies
Injuries/Accidents	Nose fx 2× in high school & college, Ø complications
Disabilities/Handicaps	Denies
Blood Transfusions	Denies
Childhood Illnesses	Chicken pox (4), mumps (6), rubeola (7), Ø complications
Immunizations	"Up to date," last tetanus 4 yr ago
FAMILY HEALTH HISTORY	

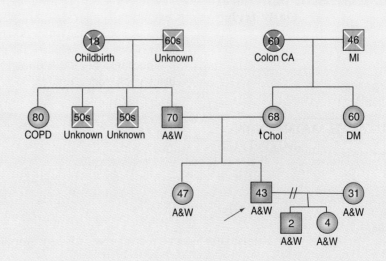

LEGEND

- Living female
- Living male
- Deceased female
- Deceased male
- / Points to patient
- —//— Divorced

A&W = Alive & well
CA = Cancer
Chol = Cholesterol
COPD = Chronic obstructive pulmonary disease
DM = Diabetes mellitus
MI = Myocardial infarction

Denies family hx of varicocele, testicular CA, epididymal tumors.

continued

SOCIAL HISTORY	
Alcohol Use	6 pack+ beer/d × 20 yr (↑ consumption on wkends)
Tobacco Use	Smoked <1 PPD × 2 yr during college, quit 21 yr ago
Drug Use	Daily marijuana use × 20 yr; occasional intranasal cocaine use; prior infrequent use of amphetamines, LSD; denies needle drug use
Sexual Practice	Heterosexual, 2 new partners in last 6 mo, monogamous relationship for 7 yr prior, multiple partners $\bar{a}$ this
Travel History	Mexico 1 yr ago
Work Environment	Office worker employed by lg construction firm for past 2 yr
Home Environment	Divorced 6 mo ago, lives alone in 2 BR apt
Hobbies/Leisure Activities	Watches TV qd, reads newspaper
Stress	Recent divorce, job insecurity, demands at work
Education	Attended 4 yr of college, never completed degree
Economic Status	Middle class, having financial difficulties at present due to expenses related to divorce
Military Service	Denies
Religion	Denies affiliation
Ethnic Background	Denies affiliation
Roles/Relationships	Married × 5 yr, separated from wife 18 mo ago, divorce final 6 mo ago, visitation $\bar{c}$ children occasional wknights & qo wkend; children usually cry when leaving their mother; paying child support. Parents live 30 miles away & visit q wkend.
Characteristic Patterns of Daily Living	Wakes at 0530 & leaves for work by 0630; arrives at work 0730. Has several cups of coffee q AM (no breakfast). Lunch at noon (sandwich, chips, & soda) eaten at desk. Leaves work 1630. Has dinner by himself, $\bar{x}$ for occasional evening $\bar{c}$ his children; eats canned or frozen dinners; $\bar{p}$ dinner watches TV & drinks beer; goes to bed at 2300 but does not usually fall asleep until MN.
HEALTH MAINTENANCE ACTIVITIES	
Sleep	5½–6½ hr (feels tired q AM)
Diet	High fat
Exercise	Ran 2 miles 3×/wk for 2 yr, stopped 6 mo ago
Stress Management	Drinking alcohol

continued

Use of Safety Devices	Wears seat belt while driving, uses condoms occasionally
Health Check-Ups	Last physical examination 4 yr ago, does not perform TSE

PHYSICAL ASSESSMENT

Inspection

Hair Distribution	Triangular distribution of pubic hair; Ø nits or lice
Penis	Erythema at urethral meatus, skin free of lesions & inflammation, rounded glans penis, size equates c̄ developmental stage, Ø penile curvature, circumcised
Scrotum	Rugated, thin scrotal skin, Ⓡ testicular swelling, Ø erythema, Ø masses or nodules, Ⓛ testis slightly lower than Ⓡ
Urethral Meatus	Centrally located c̄ erythema
Inguinal Area	Ø swelling or bulges

Palpation

Penis	Pulsations present on dorsal aspect, Ø masses or firm plaques
Urethral Meatus	≅ 2 cc yellow, thick, mucousy d/c expressed from urethral meatus
Scrotum	Testicles palpated bilaterally s̄ masses or tenderness, Ⓡ epididymis enlarged & tender c̄ guarding to light palpation, Ø swelling or tenderness Ⓛ epididymis; spermatic cords intact s̄ nodules bilaterally; TSE taught to patient
Inguinal Area	Ⓡ inguinal lymph nodes slightly ↑ (1.3 cm) & tender, Ø erythema; Ø lymphadenopathy on Ⓛ; Ø hernial masses

Auscultation

Scrotum	Ø bowel sounds
Special Technique	Urethral culture: cultures sent for gonorrhea, *Chlamydia*, ureaplasma urealyticum, mycoplasma hominis
Special Technique	Transillumination of the scrotum: Ø red glow

LABORATORY DATA

CBC with Differential		Pt's Values	Normal Range
	RBC	4.2 M/mm^3	4.0–5.2 M/mm^3
	WBC	8.5 k/mm^3	4.0–11.0 k/mm^3
	PLT	310 k/mm^3	140–440 k/mm^3
	Hgb	14.2 g/dl	13.0–17.0 g/dl
	Hct	46%	39.0%–51.0%
Urinalysis	WBCs	15–20/hpf	0–3/hpf
	RBCs	2–5/hpf	0–3/hpf

NURSING CHECKLIST
Male Genitalia Assessment

Inspection
- Hair Distribution
- Penis
- Scrotum
- Urethral Meatus
- Inguinal Area

Palpation
- Penis
- Urethral Meatus
- Scrotum
- Inguinal Area

Auscultation
- Scrotum

Special Techniques
- Androscopy
- Urethral Culture
- Transillumination of the Scrotum

REVIEW QUESTIONS AND ACTIVITIES

1. Direct, indirect, and femoral are the three types of hernias. State how each presents, what would be found on examination, and the population among which you would most likely find each.

2. Describe the transillumination technique and what you would expect to see in a patient with a hydrocele and in a patient with a testicular tumor.

3. Your patient is a 24-year-old male who appears very apprehensive about his genital examination. Discuss what you could do to make him feel more comfortable about the examination. Discuss what would be an important part of patient education.

4. A 72-year-old male presents to you with impotence. Describe what factors need to be assessed and what information you would give to the patient about normal reproductive changes related to aging.

5. Explain the differences found in the physical examination related to a hydrocele, a spermatocele, and a varicocele.

Questions 6 and 7 refer to the following situation:
Dillon, a 23-year-old male, presents to your office complaining that his left testicle has been very painful and swollen; he has also had scrotal tenderness for the past 24 hours. He has noticed some pain on urination. The examination reveals a firm, extremely tender left epididymis. The left inguinal lymph nodes are palpable. The testicle is soft and minimally tender. The scrotal skin appears swollen, red, and shiny, and is warm to the touch. Temperature is 101.8°F (oral). Urinalysis shows 10–15 WBCs/hpf.

6. Based on your assessment, what is this patient experiencing?
   a. Left epididymitis
   b. Left varicocele
   c. Urethritis
   d. Left inguinal hernia

   The correct answer is (a).

7. In addition, Dillon may also have which of the following?
   a. Femoral hernia
   b. Hydrocele
   c. Spermatocele
   d. Cryptorchidism

   The correct answer is (b).

8. Everett presents with right inguinal pain. An impulse is felt by your fingertip at the external inguinal ring when the patient coughs. Bowel sounds are auscultated in the scrotum. What do you suspect is the cause of his discomfort?
   a. Indirect inguinal hernia
   b. Direct inguinal hernia
   c. Femoral hernia
   d. None of the above

   The correct answer is (a).

Anus, Rectum, and Prostate

1. Identify anatomic landmarks of the rectum and the prostate gland.
2. Describe the characteristics of the most common rectal and prostatic chief complaints.
3. Perform inspection and palpation on a healthy adult and on a patient with rectal or prostatic pathology.
4. Explain the scientific rationale for abnormal findings.
5. Document rectal and prostatic assessment findings.
6. Describe the changes that occur in the rectum and the prostate with the aging process.

The anorectal examination is an important part of the physical examination. In the male patient, this includes assessment of the anus, rectum, and prostate gland. These assessments are usually performed last and should be performed on a regular basis because they provide vital screening for anorectal and prostate cancers.

ANATOMY AND PHYSIOLOGY

Rectum

The large intestine is composed of the cecum, colon, rectum, and anal canal. The cecum and colon were discussed in Chapter 16. The sigmoid colon begins at the pelvic brim. Beyond the sigmoid colon, the large intestine passes downward in front of the sacrum. This portion is called the **rectum** (see Figure 21-1). The rectum contains three transverse folds, or valves of Houston. These valves work to retain fecal material so it is not passed along with flatus.

Anus

The terminal 3 to 4 cm of the large intestine is called the **anal canal**. The anal canal fuses with the rectum at the anorectal junction, or the dentate line, and together these structures form the **anorectum**. The **anal orifice** is located at the seam of the gluteal folds; it serves as the exit to the gastrointestinal tract and it is marked by corrugated skin. The anal orifice lies 2 cm below the dentate line. The lower 2 cm of the anal canal is lined by **anoderm**, a thin, pale, stratified squamous epithelium, that contains no hair follicles, sweat glands, or sebaceous glands.

In the superior half of the anal canal are **anal columns**, which are longitudinal folds of mucosa (also called columns of Morgagni). The **anal valves** are formed by inferior joining anal columns. There are pockets located superior to the valves and are called the **anal sinuses**. These sinuses secrete mucus

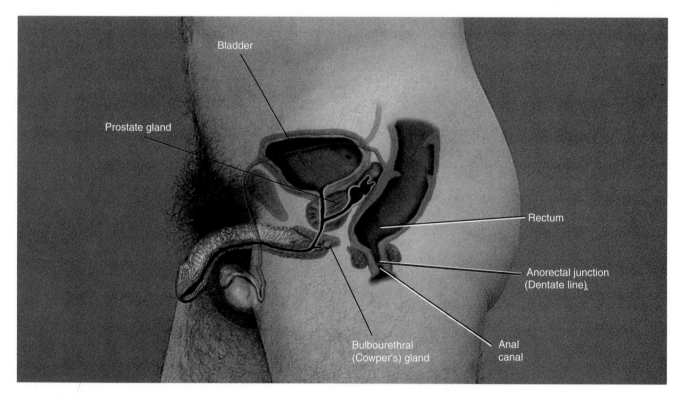

Figure 21-1   The Anorectum and Prostate

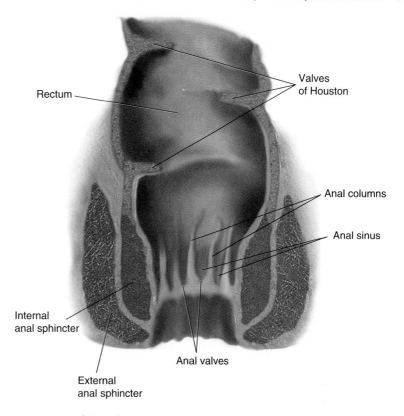

Figure 21-2 Anal Canal

when they are compressed by feces, providing lubrication that eases fecal passage during **defecation** (refer to Figure 21-2).

The anal canal opens to the exterior through the anus. Internal and external anal sphincter muscles surround the anus. Smooth muscle, which is under involuntary control, forms the internal sphincter. Skeletal muscle forms the external sphincter and is under voluntary control, allowing a person to control bowel movements.

The motility of the large intestine is controlled mainly by its nerves. There are two types of nerves: those that lie within the large intestine (the intrinsic nerves) and those that lie outside it (the extrinsic nerves). The rectum has more segmental contractions than does the sigmoid colon. These contractions keep the rectum empty by retrograde movement of contents into the sigmoid colon. As fecal material is forced into the rectum by mass peristaltic movements, the stretching of the rectal wall initiates the defecation reflex. A parasympathetic reflex signals the walls of the sigmoid colon and rectum to contract and the internal anal sphincter to relax. During defecation, the musculature of the rectum contracts to expel the feces.

Prostate

Contiguous with part of the anterior rectal wall in the male is the **prostate** gland. The prostate is an accessory male sex organ the size and shape of a chestnut, approximately 3.5 cm long by 3.0 cm wide. It consists of glandular tissue and muscle, and its small ducts drain into the urethra. The prostate lies just below the bladder and encircles the urethra like a doughnut.

The prostate has five lobes: anterior, posterior, median, and two lateral. The median sulcus is the groove between the lateral lobes. The right and left lateral lobes are accessible to examination.

Prostatic secretions are thin, milky, and alkaline. The secretions are made up of many different components. Citrate, a major component of prostatic fluid, provides a good transport medium for spermatozoa by maintaining the osmotic equilibrium of the seminal fluid. Prostatic fluid composes 15% to 30% of the ejaculate. Prostatic secretions have high levels of prostatic acid phosphatase (PAP) and prostate-specific antigen (PSA).

The prostate is primarily involved in reproduction, but it also provides a certain measure of protection against urinary tract infections. Semen contains high levels of zinc, which is derived from the prostate. Zinc is what provides the antibacterial properties to the prostate.

Within the prostatic cells, testosterone is converted to an androgen called dihydrotestosterone (DHT). DHT is the major androgen responsible for the benign enlargement of the prostate gland.

❖ HEALTH HISTORY

The anus, rectum, and prostate health history provides insight into the link between a patient's life/lifestyle and anal, rectal, and prostatic information and pathology.

PATIENT PROFILE	*Diseases that are age-, sex-, and race-specific for the anus, rectum, and prostate are listed.*
Age	Pilonidal disease (20–35) Crohn's disease of the anorectum (20–40) Anal fissure (20–45) Rectal condylomata acuminata (20–50) Gonococcal proctitis (20–50) Herpes proctitis (20–50) Anal stenosis (>25) Pruritus ani (>25) Anal skin tags (<30) Acute bacterial prostatitis (>30) Anorectal abscess (30–40) Anorectal fistula (30–40) Hemorrhoids (40–65) Prostatic abscess (>40) Fecal incontinence (>40) Benign prostatic hypertrophy (>40) Rectal cancer (>55) Prostate cancer (>55) Fecal impaction (>60) Rectal prolapse (60–80)
Sex	
Female	Rectal prolapse, fecal incontinence
Male	Anorectal abscess, anorectal fistula, pruritus ani, rectal cancer, pilonidal disease, hemorrhoids, gonococcal proctitis, herpes proctitis, benign prostatic hypertrophy, prostatitis, prostate abscess, prostate cancer
Race	
African American	Prostate cancer
Caucasian	Rectal cancer, Crohn's disease of the anorectum, pilonidal disease, benign prostatic hypertrophy

continued

CHIEF COMPLAINT	*Common chief complaints for the anus, rectum, and prostate are defined and information on the characteristics of each sign/symptom is provided.*
Rectal Bleeding	Discharge of blood from the rectum
Quality	Occult, melena, hematochezia, massive hemorrhage
Quantity	Scant, spotty, dripping, massive
Associated Manifestations	Pain, absence of pain, malaise, fever, mass at anus
Aggravating Factors	Defecation, constipation, diarrhea, minor trauma
Alleviating Factors	Increased fiber diet, bulk agents, exercise, increased fluid intake, hemorrhoidectomy
Timing	Constant, intermittent
Rectal Pain	The subjective phenomenon of a sensation indicating real or potential tissue damage in the rectum
Quality	Acute, sharp, tearing, burning, throbbing
Associated Manifestations	Swelling, fever, blood, abdominal pain
Aggravating Factors	Defecation, sitting, movement, foreign bodies
Alleviating Factors	High-fiber diet, bulk agents, exercise, increased fluid intake, warm sitz bath, topical emollients, surgery, removal of foreign body, lying down
Timing	More prominent with defecation; constant or episodic
Anal Incontinence	The involuntary passage of stool
Associated Manifestations	Diarrhea, urgency, rectal prolapse, prolapsed hemorrhoids, gaping anus
Aggravating Factors	Diarrhea, impaction, cognitive impairment, anxiety, physical handicaps, neurological disorders, trauma
Alleviating Factors	Bulk fiber, constipating agents, laxatives, enemas, biofeedback, anal continence plugs
Constipation	The infrequent, difficult passage of stool
Quantity	Fewer than three bowel movements per week
Associated Manifestations	Pain, blood, mucus, hard stool, straining with defecation, flatulence, decreased appetite
Aggravating Factors	Low-fiber diet, lack of exercise, drugs (e.g., narcotics), chronic use of laxatives, ignoring urge to defecate, weak abdominal muscles
Alleviating Factors	High-fiber diet, bulking agents, increased fluid intake, defecation schedule, exercise
Diarrhea	Increased volume, fluidity, or frequency of bowel movements relative to the person's usual pattern

continued

Associated Manifestations	Abdominal pain, blood, steatorrhea, weight changes, appetite changes
Aggravating Factors	Viral infection, bacterial infection, antibiotics, laxatives, fecal impaction, Crohn's disease, ulcerative colitis, lactose intolerance, specific foods (very indivualized), irritable bowel syndrome
Alleviating Factors	Constipating agents, anticholinergics, fluid replacement, certain foods (bananas, rice, apples, toast)
Setting	Stressful situations
Pruritus	Itching of the anal and perianal skin
Associated Manifestations	Erythema, edema, psoriasis, candidiasis, contact dermatitis
Aggravating Factors	Psoriasis, eczema, contact dermatitis, infections, parasites, oral antibiotics, diabetes mellitus, liver disease, obesity, poor hygiene, tight underclothes, wet clothing
Alleviating Factors	Discontinuing current antibiotics and topical agents; eliminating coffee, tea, cola, milk, beer, and wine; discontinuing laxatives; good rectal hygiene; loose clothing; nonmedicated talcum powder; topical fungicides
Palpable Mass	A mass at the anus, in the anal canal, or on the prostate
Quality	Firm, smooth, soft, mobile, nonmobile, nodular, fibrotic
Associated Manifestations	Pain, absence of pain, blood, pus, mucus, fever, hemorrhoids, rectal prolapse
Alleviating Factors	Warm sitz baths, high-fiber diet, bulk agents, surgery
PAST HEALTH HISTORY	*The various components of the past health history are linked to anal, rectal, and prostatic pathology and anal-, rectal-, and prostatic-related information.*
Medical	
Anorectal Specific	Trauma, inflammatory bowel disease, prior history of Sexually Transmitted Disease (STDs), polyps, rectal cancer, hemorrhoids, pruritus ani, constipation, diarrhea, incontinence
Nonanorectal Specific	Radiation, lymphogranuloma venereum, childbirth, arthritis, endocarditis, high serum testosterone, endometrial cancer, ovarian cancer, breast cancer, cervical cancer, HIV infection, penile or vaginal STDs
Prostate Specific	Prostate cancer, prostatitis, benign prostatic hypertrophy
Surgical	
Anorectal	Sigmoidoscopy, colonoscopy, rubber band ligation, injection sclerotherapy, hemorrhoidectomy, drainage of fistula or abscess
Prostate	Prostatectomy, transurethral resection of the prostate (TURP)

continued

Medications	Laxatives, constipating agents, alpha blockers, 5–alpha-reductase inhibitors, antifungals, astringent ointments, suppositories
Communicable Diseases	HIV, *Neisseria gonorrhoeae*, *Treponema pallidum*, *Chlamydia trachomatis*, human papillomavirus (HPV), herpes simplex virus (HSV)
Allergies	Contact dermatitis of perianal area
Injuries/Accidents	Rectal trauma, foreign body in rectum
Childhood Illnesses	Anal stenosis, Hirschsprung's disease (with rectal pull through)
FAMILY HEALTH HISTORY	*Anal, rectal, and prostatic diseases that are familial are listed.*
	Rectal polyps, rectal cancer, pilonidal cyst, prostate cancer
SOCIAL HISTORY	*The components of the social history are linked to anal, rectal, and prostatic factors/pathology.*
Alcohol Use	Excess intake of alcohol associated with pruritus ani; increased amount of alcohol associated with rectal and prostate cancers
Tobacco Use	Cigarette smoking increases the risk for anal carcinoma.
Drug Use	Illicit drug use may distort the user's perception, increasing the risk for unsafe sexual practices and STD exposure
Sexual Practice	Rectal penetration increases the risk for anal carcinoma and anorectal STDs. Use of foreign objects in the rectum can lead to anal valve incompetence.
Work Environment	Excessive sitting causes direct pressure and increases venous pooling, which can lead to hemorrhoids.
Hobbies/Leisure Activities	Weight lifting (hemorrhoids, rectal prolapse)
Stress	Pruritus ani can be exacerbated by stress; diarrhea can be caused by stress; constipation can be caused by depression.
HEALTH MAINTENANCE ACTIVITIES	*This information provides a bridge between the health maintenance activities and anal, rectal, and prostatic function.*
Sleep	Nocturia secondary to an enlarged prostate
Diet	Increased amounts of dietary fats, cured and smoked meats, and charcoal-broiled foods, and decreased amounts of fiber, fruits, and vegetables are associated with prostate and rectal cancers; excessive intake of milk, coffee, tea, cola, and spices is associated with pruritus ani.
Exercise	Exercise promotes regular bowel evacuation.
Use of Safety Devices	Condoms used with vaginal and anal intercourse
Health Check-Ups	Hemoccult cards, colonoscopy, digital rectal exam

EQUIPMENT

- Nonsterile gloves
- Water-soluble lubricant
- Hemoccult cards
- Gooseneck lamp

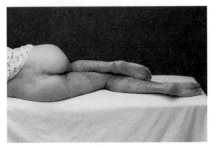

A. Left Lateral Decubitus

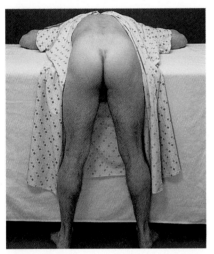

B. Standing

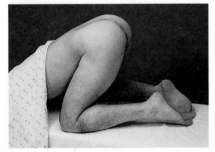

C. Knee-Chest

Figure 21-3 Patient Positions for the Anus, Rectum, and Prostate Examination

ASSESSMENT OF THE ANUS, RECTUM, AND PROSTATE

✓ NURSING CHECKLIST
General Approach to Anus, Rectum, and Prostate Assessment

1. Greet the patient and explain the assessment techniques that you will be using.

2. Ensure that the examination room is at a warm, comfortable temperature to prevent patient chilling and shivering.

3. Use a quiet room that will be free from interruptions.

4. Ensure that the light in the room provides sufficient brightness to adequately observe the patient. It may be helpful to have a gooseneck lamp available for additional lighting when lesions are observed.

5. Instruct the patient to void prior to the assessment.

6. Instruct the patient to remove pants and underpants and to cover up with a drape sheet.

7. Assess the patient's apprehension level about the assessment and reassure the patient that apprehension is normal.

8. For inspection, place the patient in the left lateral decubitus position and visualize the perianal skin (see Figure 21-3A). This position can also be used for palpation.

9. For palpation, have the patient stand at the side or end of the examination table, bending over the table resting the elbows on the table and spreading the legs slightly apart (see Figure 21-3B).

9A. For the patient who cannot stand, have the patient assume the knee-chest position (see Figure 21-3C).

9B. For the female who is undergoing a rectovaginal examination, have her assume the lithotomy position. Refer to Chapter 19.

10. Don nonsterile gloves.

11. Use a systematic approach every time the assessment is performed. Proceed from the anus to the rectum in the female patient. Proceed from the anus to the prostate in the male patient.

❀ NURSING TIP

Rectal Examination of the Female Patient

If a woman is to undergo a rectal examination without a vaginal exam, then the left lateral decubitus, standing, or knee-chest position can be used for the assessment.

❀ NURSING TIP

Skin Assessment During Rectal Examination

As you examine the perineum and the sacrococcygeal area, perform a skin assessment. Refer to Chapter 10 to review this examination.

Inspection

Perineum and Sacrococcygeal Area

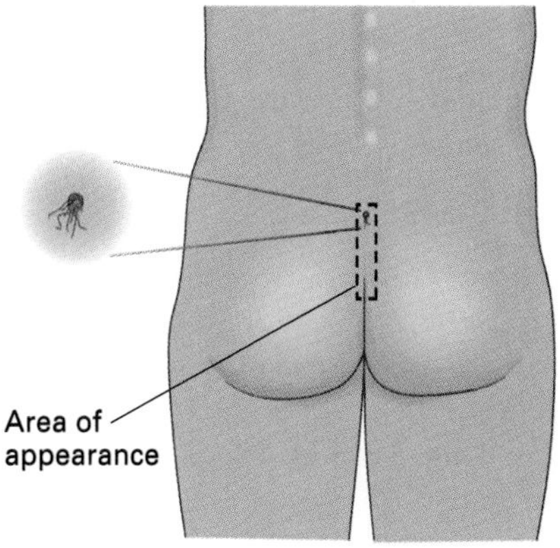

E Inspect the buttocks and sacral region for lesions, swelling, inflammation, and tenderness.

N *This area should be smooth and free of lesions, swelling, inflammation, and tenderness. There should be no evidence of feces or mucus on the perianal skin.*

A It is abnormal for one or several tiny openings to be seen in the midline over the sacral region, often with hair protruding from them (see Figure 21-4).

P Pilonidal disease is an acquired condition of the midline coccygeal skin region induced by local stretching forces. There can be an acute abscess or chronic draining sinuses in the sacrococcygeal area. Small skin pits representing enlarged hair follicles precede development of the draining sinus or abscess. Lesions are often secondarily invaded by hair.

A Areas of hyperpigmentation, coupled with excoriation and thickened skin in the perianal area, are abnormal. The area may be intensely pruritic.

P Pruritis ani is caused by pinworms in children and by fungal infections in adults. The lesions are dull, grayish pink.

A Dry, well-circumscribed, silvery, scaling papules and plaques of various sizes are abnormal.

P In psoriasis, the thick scaling is due to increased epidermal cell proliferation. A family history of psoriasis is common. The cause is unknown.

A Red, pruritic papules or vesicles with S-shaped or straight-line burrows are abnormal.

P Refer to page 259 for a discussion of scabies. The inflammatory lesions usually occur along the belt line and on the lower buttocks.

A Well-demarcated, erythematous, sometimes itchy, exudative patches of varying size and shape and rimmed with small, red-based pustules are abnormal.

P *Candida albicans* occurs in sites where heat and maceration provide a fertile environment. Systemic antibacterial, corticosteroid, or antimetabolic therapy; pregnancy; obesity; diabetes mellitus; blood dyscrasias; and immunologic defects increase susceptibility to candidiasis.

Anal Mucosa

E 1. Spread the patient's buttocks apart with both hands, exposing the anus.
2. Instruct the patient to bear down as though moving the bowels.
3. Examine the anus for color, appearance, lesions, inflammation, rash, and masses.

N *The anal mucosa is deeply pigmented, coarse, moist, and hairless. It should be free of lesions, inflammation, rash, masses, or additional openings. The anal opening should be closed. There should not be any leakage of feces or mucus from the anus with straining and there should not be any tissue protrusion.*

A A spherical, bluish lump that appears suddenly at the anus, and that ranges in size from a few millimeters to several centimeters in diameter (see Figure 21-5) is abnormal. The overlying anal skin may be tense and edematous. Pain and pruritus may be present in the perianal region.

P **Hemorrhoids** result from dilatation of the superior and inferior hemorrhoidal veins. These hemorrhoidal veins form a hemorrhoidal plexus, or cushion, in the submucosal layer of the anorectum. An external hemorrhoid is located below the dentate line. Thrombosed external hemorrhoids (blood clots within subcutaneous hemorrhoidal veins) occur as a result of heavy lifting, childbirth, straining to defecate (which may be due to a low-fiber diet), or other vigorous activity. Bleeding may occur with defecation.

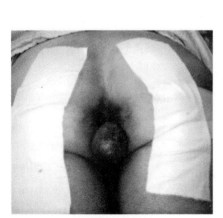

Figure 21-4 Pilonidal Disease

Area of appearance

Figure 21-5 Thrombosed Hemorrhoid *Courtesy of Dr. Haider Goussous, Albany, NY*

E	**Examination**
N	**Normal Findings**
A	**Abnormal Findings**
P	**Pathophysiology**

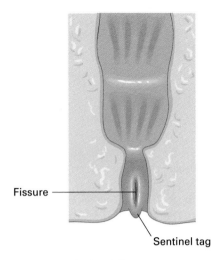

Fissure

Sentinel tag

Figure 21-6 Anal Fissure

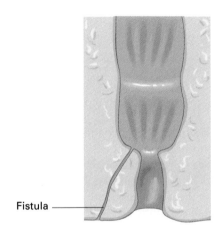

Fistula

Skin surface opening

Figure 21-7 Anorectal Fistula

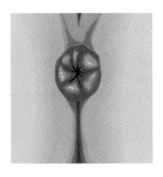

Figure 21-8 Rectal Prolapse

A Excess anal or perianal tissue of varying sizes that is soft, pliable, and covered by normal skin is abnormal.

P Anal skin tags are the result of residual resolved thrombosed external hemorrhoids, pregnancy, or anal operations. In some cases, there is no known cause.

A Linear tears in the epidermis of the anal canal beginning below the dentate line and extending distally to the anal orifice are abnormal (see Figure 21-6). Extreme pain, pruritus, and bleeding may accompany these findings.

P **Anal fissures** are the result of trauma, such as the forced passage of a large, hard stool, and anal intercourse, especially forced intercourse. Fissures occur most often in the area of the posterior coccygeal midline and less frequently in the anterior midline. This is because of weakness in the superficial external sphincter in these sectors. Predisposition to fissure is increased by perianal inflammation that causes the anoderm to lose its normal elasticity. A sentinel skin tag may be visible inferior to the anal fissure and at the anal margin. Sphincter spasms may occur during the examination. The use of a local anesthetic may be necessary to thoroughly examine the area.

A Undrained collections of perianal pus of the tissue spaces in and adjacent to the anorectum are abnormal.

P The most common cause of **anorectal abscesses** is infection of the anal glands, usually located posteriorly and situated between the internal and the external sphincters. These glands normally drain via the internal sphincter through small ducts and into anal crypts. When these ducts are occluded by impacted fecal material or trauma, ductal stasis and abscess formation results. An indurated mass with overlying erythema displaces the anus in cases of superficial abscess.

A An inflamed, red, raised area with purulent or serosanguineous discharge on the perianal skin is abnormal (see Figure 21-7).

P An **anorectal fistula** is a hollow, fibrous tract lined by granulation tissue and having an opening inside the anal canal or rectum and one or more orifices in the perianal skin. Fistulas are usually the result of incomplete healing of drained anorectal abscesses. However, they may occur in the absence of an abscess history. If this is the case, other causes for the fistula must be explored. Additional predisposing factors are inflammatory bowel disease, infectious disease, malignancy, Crohn's disease, radiation therapy, chemotherapy, chlamydial infections, and trauma.

A Soiling of the skin with stool and gaping of the anus are abnormal.

P **Anal incontinence** may be caused by neurological diseases, traumatic injuries, or surgical damage to the puborectalis or sphincter muscles. Perineal or intestinal disorders, diarrhea, fecal impaction, and constipating agents may also cause anal incontinence.

A The protrusion of the rectal mucosa (pinkish red doughnut with radiating folds) through the anal orifice is abnormal (see Figure 21-8).

P **Rectal prolapse** is associated with poor tone of the pelvic musculature, chronic straining at stool, fecal incontinence, and, sometimes, neurological disease or traumatic damage to the pelvis. A complete rectal prolapse involves the entire bowel wall. It is larger, red, and moist looking and has circular folds.

A Erythematous plaques that develop into vesicular lesions that may become pustules and ulcerate are abnormal.

P These lesions are suggestive of HSV. Most anorectal herpes is due to HSV-2, and infections are related to anal intercourse.

A Warts or lesions that are beefy red, irregular, and pedunculated are abnormal findings. The lesions may involve the anoderm but may also extend deep into the anal canal and involve the rectal mucosa. There may be a few scattered lesions or extensive involvement of the entire anus.

NURSING TIP

Documenting Abnormalities of the Anus

When documenting any abnormalities found in the anus, describe them with regard to anatomic location: e.g., posterior toward the patient's back; anterior toward the patient's abdomen; right and left, respectively. Be sure to note patient position and orientation.

 NURSING TIP

Teaching Tip on STD Management

The risk of acquiring an STD increases with the number of sexual partners that one has. Regardless of the type of birth control being used, condoms should always be worn. STDs can occur at any body opening where intercourse has occurred. Once it is known that an STD has been contracted, all sexual partners must be notified.

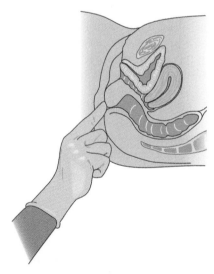

Figure 21-9 Position of the Index Finger for Anorectal Palpation

E	Examination
N	Normal Findings
A	Abnormal Findings
P	Pathophysiology

P Condylomata acuminatum are caused by HPV. Coital trauma allows entry into the anal epidermis in those in whom wart virus is latent in the anorectum. Anal warts may also develop in women via extension of genital warts along the perineum. Of the 50 strains of HPV, types 16, 18, and 31 have been associated with malignant lesions.

A Mucoid or creamy exudate, possibly blood, from the rectum is abnormal.

P Gonococcal proctitis is most often seen in homosexual men as a result of direct inoculation, but it also occurs in women through contamination by vaginal discharge.

A Multiple perianal fissures and edematous skin tags of varying degrees are abnormal.

P Anorectal involvement occurs in the majority of patients with Crohn's disease. Perianal disease may precede the onset of intestinal Crohn's disease by several years. Perianal disease may proceed to anal stricture and incontinence. The development of perianal Crohn's disease has no relation to other extraintestinal manifestations of the disease.

 NURSING TIP

Managing Anal Incontinence

Anal incontinence often responds well to a combination of relatively simple interventions:

• Manage diarrheal stools with bulk fiber and constipating agents. (Solid stools are easier to retain than liquid stools.)
• Clear fecal impactions with enemas or digitally and introduce a treatment plan for constipation.
• Increase fluid intake, daily activity, and dietary fiber.
• Initiate a bowel program of regular defecation, scheduling bowel movements at regular intervals.
• Practice sphincter exercises (contracting and relaxing the anal sphincter several times daily to improve sphincter tone).

⚡ NURSING ALERT

Spotting Rectal Abuse

Suspect rectal abuse if you encounter any of the following in the assessment: bruises around the buttocks and hip area, cuts, tears, or bleeding around the anal mucosa, or refusal by the patient to undergo the rectal examination. Tell the patient about your concern and consult your institution's policy regarding suspected abuse.

Palpation

Anus and Rectum

E To perform anal and rectal wall palpation:

1. Have the patient assume one of the positions described on page 674.
2. Reassure the patient that sensations of urination and defecation are common during the rectal assessment.
3. Lubricate a gloved index finger.
4. Place your finger by the anal orifice and instruct the patient to bear down (Valsalva maneuver) as you gently insert the flexed tip of your gloved finger into the anal sphincter, with the tip of the finger toward the anterior rectal wall (pointed toward the umbilicus) (see Figure 21-9). The anus should never be approached at a right angle (with the index finger extended).

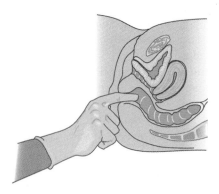

Figure 21-10 Position of the Index Finger in the Anorectum

E	**Examination**
N	**Normal Findings**
A	**Abnormal Findings**
P	**Pathophysiology**

4A. If the patient tightens the sphincter, remove your finger, reassure the patient, and try again, using a relaxation technique such as deep breathing.

5. Feel the sphincter relax. Insert finger as far as it will go (see Figure 21-10). Note anal sphincter tone.

6. Palpate the lateral, posterior, and anterior walls of the rectum in a sequenced manner. The lateral walls are felt by rotating the finger along the sides of the rectum. Palpate for nodules, irregularity, masses, and tenderness.

6A. Ask the patient to bear down again (which may help to palpate masses).

7. Slowly withdraw the finger; inspect any fecal matter on your glove and test it for occult blood. Table 21-1 lists common stool findings and etiologies. Table 21-2 lists the common causes of rectal bleeding.

8. Offer the patient tissues to wipe off any remaining lubricant.

N *The rectum should accommodate the index finger. There should be good sphincter tone at rest and with bearing down. There should be no excessive pain, tenderness, induration, irregularities, or nodules in the rectum or rectal wall.*

A It is abnormal for the anal canal to be tight (making insertion of the index finger very difficult and painful or impossible).

P Anal stenosis can occur congenitally, but this condition usually is acquired. Anorectal operations, diarrheal disease, inflammatory conditions, and the habitual use of laxatives may cause anal stenosis. Chlamydial infections and malignancy must be excluded.

A Internal masses of vascular tissue in the anal canal are abnormal (see Figure 21-11).

P Internal hemorrhoids arise from the superior (internal) hemorrhoidal vascular plexuses above the dentate line; they are covered by mucosa. Internal hemorrhoids are usually painless unless they are thrombosed or prolapsed through the anal orifice. Refer to page 675 for a further discussion of hemorrhoids.

A A soft nodule or nodules in the rectum are abnormal (see Figure 21-12).

P Rectal polyps occur frequently in the general population of the United States. Occasionally, they can be palpated, but more often they are diagnosed by proctoscopy. They vary in size and may be accompanied by rectal bleeding. Rectal polyps are of two types: pedunculated (attached to a stalk) or sessile (adhering to the rectal mucosal wall). A biopsy of the tissue is required to determine if the polyp is benign or malignant.

A A tender, indurated mass in the anorectum is abnormal.

P This may be an anorectal abscess. Refer to page 676.

A An indurated cord palpated in the anorectum is abnormal.

P Anorectal fistula tracts may be palpated from the secondary orifice toward the anus. Digital rectal examination helps to determine the course of the tract. A drop of purulent drainage can be expressed from the opening if the opening is patent.

A A small, symmetrical projection 2 to 4 cm long is abnormal.

Table 21-1 Common Stool Findings and Etiologies	
STOOL FINDING	**ETIOLOGY**
Black, tarry (**melena**)	Upper gastrointestinal bleeding
Bright red	Rectal bleeding
Black	Iron or bismuth ingestion
Gray, tan	Obstructive jaundice
Pale yellow, greasy, fatty (**steatorrhea**)	Malabsorption syndromes (e.g., celiac disease), cystic fibrosis

Table 21-2   Common Causes of Rectal Bleeding

- Cancer of the colon
- Benign polyps of the colon
- Hemorrhoids
- Anal fissure
- Inflammatory bowel disease
- Forced or vigorous anal intercourse
- Traumatic sexual practices

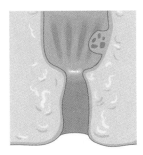

Figure 21-11   Internal Hemorrhoids

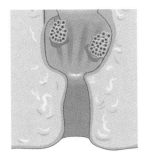

Figure 21-12   Rectal Polyps

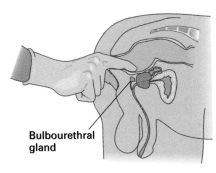

Bulbourethral gland

Figure 21-13   Bidigital Palpation of the Bulbourethral Gland

E	**Examination**
N	**Normal Findings**
A	**Abnormal Findings**
P	**Pathophysiology**

P Rectal prolapse is best assessed with the patient in a squatting position. The anal sphincter is lax and palpation between the finger and thumb reveals only two layers of mucosa. Refer to page 676 for additional information.

A Foreign bodies palpated in the rectum are abnormal.

P Thermometers, enema catheters, vibrators, bottles, and phallic objects may be introduced into the anus by accident, for erotic purposes, for concealment, for self-treatment, or by assault. Complications may include perforation of the rectum, obstruction, and pararectal infections.

A A hard mass in the anal canal is abnormal.

P This finding usually indicates anal carcinoma. There is a strong association between anal carcinoma (squamous cell) and HPV types 16 and 18.

A A firm, sometimes rocklike but often rubbery, puttylike mass is abnormal.

P In fecal impaction, the feces accumulates in the rectum because the colon does not respond to the usual stimuli promoting evacuation, or because accessory stimuli normally provided by eating and physical activity are lacking. Drugs, such as opiates, may compound the problem. Rectal sensitivity may be dulled by habitual disregard of the urge to defecate. The prolonged use of laxatives or enemas may also decrease rectal sensitivity.

⚡ NURSING ALERT

Risk Factors for Rectal Cancer

The primary risk factor for developing rectal cancer is being over 55 years of age. Other principal risk factors for rectal cancer include a family history of colorectal cancer, a personal history of endometrial, ovarian, or breast cancer, previous colorectal cancer, long-standing inflammatory bowel disease, and a diet low in fiber.

✤ ASK YOURSELF

Rectal Assessment

A wide range of situations may be encountered during the rectal assessment. Consider how you would react in each of the following situations:
- Mr. DiCicco presents to you complaining of rectal bleeding and pain. While preparing him for examination, you notice the tip of a thermometer protruding from the rectum.
- Mrs. Kelly visits the office today for her annual Pap smear and pelvic examination. She states, "I am embarrassed to talk about this, but my husband would like me to participate in anal intercourse and I feel the need to discuss this with someone."

Prostate

E To perform prostatic palpation:
1. Position the patient as tolerated (the standing position is preferred).
2. Reassure the patient that sensations of urination and defecation are common during the prostatic assessment.
3. Use a well-lubricated, gloved index finger.
4. Insert the gloved index finger and proceed as described in steps 4 and 5 on pages 677 and 678.
5. Perform bidigital examination of the bulbourethral gland by pressing your gloved thumb into the perianal tissue while pressing your gloved index finger toward it (see Figure 21-13). Assess for tenderness, masses, or swelling.
6. Release pressure of the thumb and index finger. Remove thumb from the perianal tissue and advance your index finger.

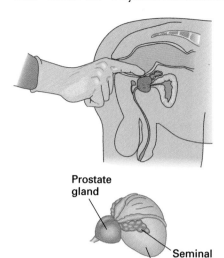

Prostate gland

Seminal vesicle

Bladder

Figure 21-14 Prostatic Palpation

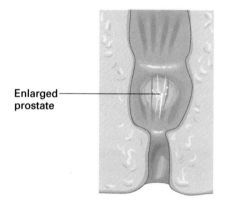

Enlarged prostate

Figure 21-15 Benign Prostatic Hypertrophy

🌺 NURSING TIP

Acute Bacterial Prostatitis

Bacterial prostatitis is associated with a bladder infection caused by the same organism. Obtaining a urine culture will identify the pathogen. Rectal examination should be avoided in known cases of acute bacterial prostatitis because of the possibility of bacteremia.

E Examination
N Normal Findings
A Abnormal Findings
P Pathophysiology

---

7. Palpate the posterior surface of the prostate gland (see Figure 21-14). Note the size, shape, consistency, sensitivity, and mobility of the prostate. Note whether the median sulcus is palpable.

8. Attempt to palpate the seminal vesicles by extending your index finger above the prostate gland. Assess for tenderness and masses.

9. Slowly withdraw the finger; inspect any fecal matter on your glove and test it for occult blood (if not previously performed).

N *The prostate gland should be small, smooth, mobile, and nontender. The median sulcus should be palpable.*

A A soft, nontender, enlarged prostate gland is abnormal (see Figure 21-15).

P The development of benign prostatic hypertrophy (BPH) is related to aging and the presence of testosterone, which converts to dihydrotestosterone and leads to prostatic cell growth. The size of the prostate gland on rectal assessment is not always indicative of the degree of symptoms because the lobes may not be palpable or they may be causing obstruction. In BPH, the median sulcus may not be palpable.

A A firm, tender, or fluctuant mass on the prostate is abnormal.

P A high percentage of patients with prostatic abscess have diabetes mellitus. An abscess is suspected in the patient with acute bacterial prostatitis or urinary tract infection who develops a spiked fever along with rectal pain. Prostatic abscesses are caused mainly by *Escherichia coli*.

A Firm, hard, or indurated nodules on the prostate are abnormal (see Figure 21-16).

P The nodules of prostate cancer may be single or multiple. Early in the disease the nodules may be small, but late in the disease the entire prostate may seem irregular, hard, immobile, and quite large.

A An exquisitely tender and warm prostate is abnormal.

P Bacterial prostatitis is usually caused by *Escherichia coli*. When patients present with a sudden onset of high fever, chills, malaise, myalgias, and arthralgias, acute bacterial prostatitis is suspected.

🔰 NURSING ALERT

Risk Factors for Prostate Cancer

Those men over the age of 55 are at the highest risk for developing prostate cancer. Other risk factors include having a first-degree relative with prostate cancer, being African American, and having high levels of serum testosterone.

Single nodule

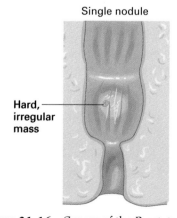

Hard, irregular mass

Multiple nodules

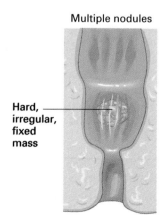

Hard, irregular, fixed mass

Figure 21-16 Cancer of the Prostate

Table 21-3 Causes of Fecal Incontinence in Elderly Patients

- Diarrhea
- Fecal impaction
- Irritable bowel syndrome
- Anorectal carcinoma
- Rectal trauma
- Stroke
- Diabetes mellitus
- Dementia
- Multiple sclerosis
- Rectal prolapse

GERONTOLOGICAL VARIATIONS

There are age-related changes associated with the rectum and prostate. Anorectal function changes due to the loss of muscle elasticity in the rectum. Older adults also have reduced maximum tolerated volumes in the rectum, with higher rectal pressures in response to distension. Rectal prolapse is most commonly seen in elderly women.

Fecal incontinence may develop due to denervation associated with an increase in the motor unit fiber density. Fecal incontinence in elderly individuals is usually the result of impairment of more than one of the factors that ordinarily maintain continence and may be a sign of an underlying acute medical problem. Table 21-3 lists some of the causes of fecal incontinence in elderly individuals.

Constipation is also common and may be caused by a variety of factors, such as lack of exercise, poor diet, medications that affect bowel function, intrinsic slowing of large bowel transit, and decreased fecal water excretion. Patients usually respond to advice on how to prevent constipation.

The prostate undergoes changes related to the aging process. The most obvious change that occurs is that of size. The prostate begins to enlarge after the age of 40, which often leads to the development of benign prostatic hypertrophy. The prostate capsule may contract and prostatic urethral tone may increase, resulting in urinary obstruction.

There are lower levels of zinc in the prostatic fluid of older men, which appear to reduce the amount of prostatic antibacterial factor (PAF), therefore making the older man more susceptible to urinary tract infections. An increase in the prevalence of prostate cancer is also associated with aging.

CASE STUDY

The case study illustrates the application and objective documentation of the anal, rectal, and prostatic assessment.

The Patient with Hemorrhoids

Mr. O'Flynn is a 46-year-old accountant who called you this morning concerning bright-red blood in his stool.

❖ HEALTH HISTORY

PATIENT PROFILE	46 yo MWM
CHIEF COMPLAINT	"I have a lot of fullness & pain around my rectum & I saw blood $\bar{p}$ my BM yesterday."
HISTORY OF PRESENT ILLNESS	Pt arrived home $\bar{p}$ work & had BM; severe pain $\bar{c}$ BM & blood was seen on wiping; noticed pain ($\bar{s}$ radiation) & feeling of "fullness" in rectal area $\bar{p}$ BM. Pt took a hot tub bath, which relieved pain & fullness. Rectal pain & fullness returned later when he sat down. Was able to sleep during the night $\bar{s}$ difficulty. Pain, fullness, & itching present when he awoke in AM but it was not as severe; however, he called in sick to work b/c pain ↑ while sitting. Pt admits to occasional pain $\bar{c}$ BM associated $\bar{c}$ constipation.

continued

PAST HEALTH HISTORY

Medical   Borderline HTN dx 2 yr ago by family MD, controlled by diet; 15 lb overwt; recurrent episodes of constipation

Surgical   Ⓛ knee injury 4 yr ago while skiing, Ⓛ arthroscopy to repair torn cartilage, ∅ complications

Medications   ∅

Communicable Diseases   Denies rheumatic fever, STDs, TB

Allergies   Sulfa drugs cause skin rash over entire body

Injuries/Accidents   Refer to surgical section

Disabilities/Handicaps   Denies

Blood Transfusions   Denies

Childhood Illnesses   Chicken pox age 8; denies any other dz

Immunizations   Tetanus 3 yr ago

FAMILY HEALTH HISTORY

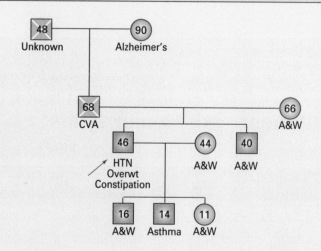

LEGEND

◯ Living female

▢ Living male

⊗ Deceased female

⊠ Deceased male

⟋ Points to patient

A&W = Alive & well

CA = Cancer

CVA = Cerebrovascular accident

HTN = Hypertension

Denies family hx of pilonidal cyst, colorectal CA, rectal polyps, prostate CA.

SOCIAL HISTORY

Alcohol Use   1 beer q PM × 15 yr

Tobacco Use   Denies

Drug Use   Denies

Sexual Practice   Monogamous c̄ wife

Travel History   Annual summer vacations to beach

continued

Work Environment	Employed by a large computer company × 10 yr
Home Environment	Lives c̄ wife & 3 children in town house
Hobbies/Leisure Activities	Watching sports on TV & doing house projects
Stress	Providing for family, job demands
Education	4-yr college degree, MBA
Economic Status	Upper middle class, denies financial difficulties
Military Service	Served 4 yr in U.S. Army, spent 3 yr in Germany
Religion	Roman Catholic
Ethnic Background	Irish
Roles/Relationships	Married for 23 yr, has good relationship c̄ wife; having difficulties at present c̄ 16 yo son & limit setting, good relationships c̄ other children; good working relationship c̄ coworkers & supervisor, has personal friends at work & in neighborhood
Characteristic Patterns of Daily Living	Wakes at 0600 & leaves for work by 0700, arrives at 0800 (coffee & doughnut for breakfast). Has lunch c̄ work friends at cafeteria; leaves work 1700 & arrives home 1830 (usually works 6 d/wk). Entire family sits down for dinner. Spends time alone c̄ wife from 2100–2200.
HEALTH MAINTENANCE ACTIVITIES	
Sleep	8 hr q night, feels rested in AM
Diet	Eats a lot of fast foods (pizza, burgers, etc.), prefers red meats
Exercise	Ø regular exercise program
Stress Management	Discussing problems c̄ family
Use of Safety Devices	Wears seat belt
Health Check-Ups	Annual physical, BP checks q 6 mo, hemoccult checks c̄ physicals, denies colonoscopy
PHYSICAL ASSESSMENT	
Inspection	
Perineum and Sacrococcygeal Area	Skin smooth & even; no lesions, inflammation, or swelling
Anal Mucosa	Single, bluish-colored mass in posterior portion of anus

continued

Palpation

Anus and Rectum   1.5 cm, mobile, smooth, tender mass in posterior portion of anus, no rectal wall masses, sphincter tone intact

Prostate   Nontender, smooth, symmetrical, and mobile $\bar{s}$ enlargement

LABORATORY DATA

Hemoccult   ⊕

CBC

	Pt's Values	Normal Range
RBC	4.8 M/mm³	4.0–5.2 M/mm³
WBC	8.0 k/mm³	4.0–11.0 k/mm³
Platelets	250 k/mm³	140–440 k/mm³
Hgb	15 g/dl	13.0–17.0 g/dl
Hct	46%	39.0%–51.0%

Iron Studies

Serum iron	88 µg/dl	75–175 µg/dl
TIBC	400 µg/dl	240–450 µg/dl

Chemistry Panel

BUN	11 µg/dl	10–20 µg/dl
Creatinine	0.9 µg/dl	0.6–1.2 µg/dl
PSA	1.5 ng/ml	0.2–4.0 ng/ml

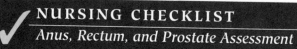

NURSING CHECKLIST
Anus, Rectum, and Prostate Assessment

Inspection
- Perineum and Sacrococcygeal Area
- Anal Mucosa

Palpation
- Anus and Rectum
- Prostate

REVIEW QUESTIONS AND ACTIVITIES

1. Explain the differences in presenting symptoms and physical assessment of thrombosed hemorrhoids and anal fissures.

2. A 26-year-old homosexual male presents to you with rectal bleeding. Describe which rectal conditions you might find and what would be an important part of patient education.

3. Describe what would be found on physical assessment for prostate cancer.

4. Discuss preventive measures that can be taken to avoid some rectal pathologies.

Questions 5 and 6 refer to the following situation:

Mr. Longmueller presents with anorectal pain, pruritus, and bright-red stools. On assessing him, you observe a linear tear in the anoderm.

5. What do you suspect is the cause of Mr. Longmueller's condition?
   a. Prostatic carcinoma
   b. Rectal carcinoma
   c. Anorectal fistula
   d. Anal fissure

   The correct answer is (d).

6. The most likely cause of this patient's abnormal stool color is:
   a. Upper gastrointestinal tract bleeding
   b. Rectal bleeding
   c. Obstructive jaundice
   d. Malabsorption syndrome

   The correct answer is (b).

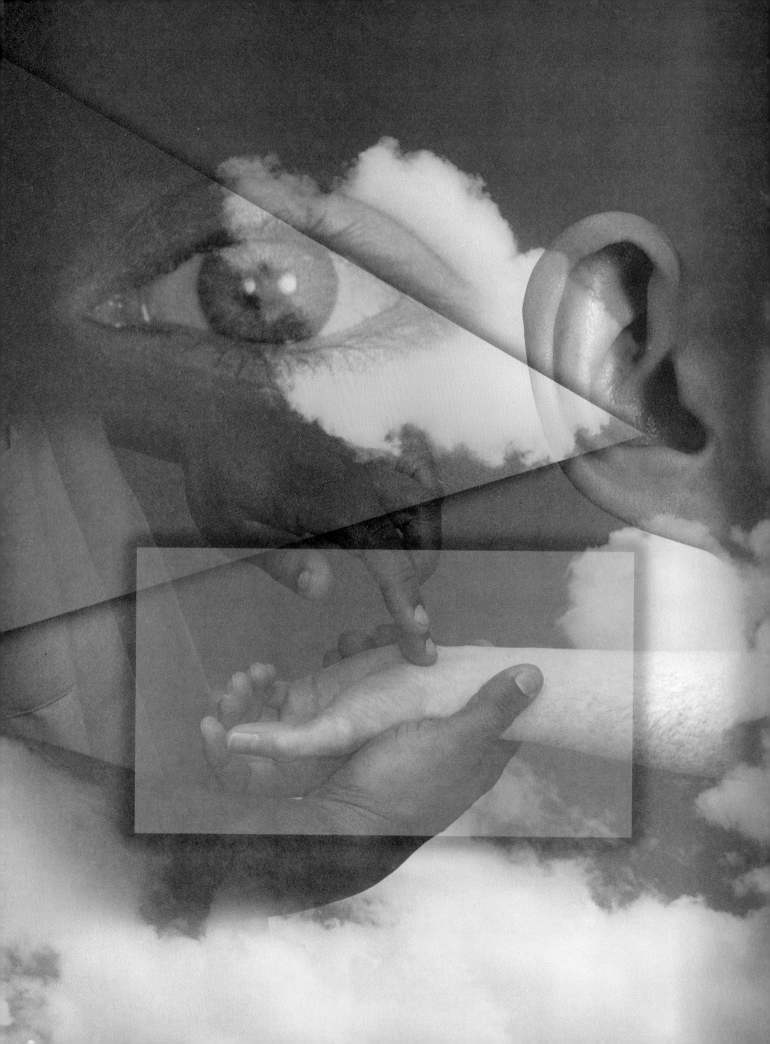

Special Populations

UNIT IV

In dwelling upon the vital importance of sound observation, it must never be lost sight of what observation is for. It is not for the sake of piling up miscellaneous information or curious facts, but for the sake of saving life and increasing health and comfort.

Florence Nightingale

Pregnant Patient

1. Perform a physical assessment on a pregnant woman.
2. Differentiate the normal changes of pregnancy from pathological changes.
3. Describe the characteristics of the most common pregnancy-related complaints.
4. Assess the psychosocial status of a pregnant woman.
5. Assess the learning needs of a pregnant woman.

Pregnancy imposes many physiological, hormonal, and psychological changes on a woman during the 280 days, or approximately 40 (normal range 37 to 40) weeks, of gestation. The pregnancy is subdivided into trimesters of a little more than 13 weeks each, and various symptoms and problems can be specific to certain trimesters. You are encouraged to review Chapters 13 and 19 before beginning this chapter.

The focus when assessing a pregnant patient is the wellness of the mother and the fetus. Much of prenatal care centers around educating and reassuring the pregnant patient and her family regarding physical changes that result from pregnancy. With the availability of accurate home pregnancy tests, a woman may know she's pregnant within 2 weeks of conception, affording an opportunity for early health care interaction. As a nurse, you will often be the primary contact during the pregnancy, and you can play a critical role in helping to ensure a healthy pregnancy. With active listening and a supportive attitude, you can also play an important role in educating the family on what to expect during the next 9 months, as well as educating them about warning signs of possible complications of pregnancy.

ANATOMY AND PHYSIOLOGY

Physiological changes during pregnancy affect every system in the body. These changes occur to maintain maternal health and accommodate the growth of a healthy fetus. This chapter provides an overview of these changes and is not all-inclusive.

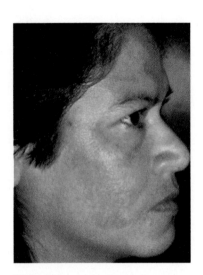

Figure 22-1 Melasma/Chloasma
Courtesy of Timothy Berger, MD, Chief, Department of Dermatology at San Francisco General Hospital, San Francisco, California

Skin and Hair

The skin is subjected to the influence of hormones during pregnancy. There is an increased subdermal fat deposit, along with thickening of the skin. Acne may develop or improve during pregnancy. Other changes include an increase in sweat and sebaceous gland production, which, along with the increase in superficial capillaries and peripheral vasodilation, serves to dissipate heat. Existing pigmentation increases in the nipples, areolae, external genitalia, and the anal region. The face may develop **melasma**, or **chloasma** (see Figure 22-1), known as the mask of pregnancy, which manifests as blotchy, irregular pigmentation. **Linea nigra**, or darkening of the linea alba, may present on the abdomen as a darkened vertical midline between the fundus and the symphysis pubis (see Figure 22-2). Linea nigra regress, or fade, after delivery, but does not totally disappear. **Nevi**, circumscribed, pigmented areas of skin, may be stimulated to grow; and skin tags, molluscum fibrosum gravidarum, may develop from epithelial hyperplasia, especially on the upper body. With connective tissue changes of pregnancy, **striae gravidarum** (stretch marks) often develop on the abdomen, breasts, and upper thighs; after delivery, they regress or fade but do not totally disappear.

Vascular changes reflected in the skin can include the development or enlargement of spider angiomas, hemangiomas, varicosities (including hemorrhoids), and palmar erythema.

Facial hair may increase, but the scalp hair may shed and thin, especially in the postpartum period. The scalp hair may become oily.

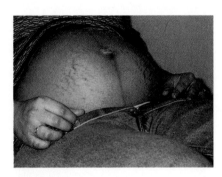

Figure 22-2 Linea Nigra with Striae Gravidarum

🌸 NURSING TIP

Chemical Hair Treatments

Chemical hair treatments such as color and permanents should be avoided during pregnancy, especially in the first trimester, because these chemicals are absorbed into the scalp and the maternal circulation.

Head and Neck

The thyroid gland may increase in size after approximately 12 weeks of gestation (although studies are conflicting as to whether or not there is an increase), related to the increase in vascularity.

Eyes, Ears, Nose, Mouth, and Throat

Corneal thickening and edema (especially in the third trimester) may occur and the pregnant woman may experience visual changes. These changes may be discussed with the patient's ophthalmologist or optometrist, but pregnancy changes in vision are typically not treated because they may resolve shortly after delivery. Contact lens wearers may also experience blurry vision secondary to increased lysozyme in tears, which may lead to an oily sensation.

Increased vascularity and increased mucus production often lead to nasal stuffiness, snoring, congestion and epistaxis, impaired hearing or fullness in the ears, and a decreased sense of smell. The pregnant woman should be reassured that these are normal experiences that usually resolve after delivery.

Increased vascularity and hormonal changes often lead to soft, edematous, and bleeding gums, commonly noticed when brushing teeth. **Ptyalism**, excessive secretion of saliva, may be an annoying symptom and, if marked, may require evaluation for other causes such as goiter. Vocal changes or cough may be noted due to hormonally induced changes in the larynx.

Breasts

Early breast changes may include enlargement, tingling, and tenderness secondary to hormonal changes. As the pregnancy progresses, the breasts continue to enlarge and the mammary glands prepare for lactation after delivery (alveoli increase in both number and size, Montgomery's tubercles enlarge, and lactiferous ducts proliferate). This may cause the breasts to feel more nodular on palpation than in the nonpregnant state. The areolae may darken. The nipples may become darker and more erect. **Colostrum**, a thick, yellow discharge known as early breast milk, may be secreted as early as the second trimester. Veins in the breasts may become more apparent and blue as they become engorged from increased vascularization.

Thorax and Lungs

The demands of the physiological changes of pregnancy and of the fetus lead to increased oxygen consumption and carbon dioxide excretion. This helps to increase oxygen use by the fetus and facilitate the transfer of carbon dioxide from the fetus to the maternal circulation for elimination. With advancing pregnancy, the diaphragm elevates approximately 4 cm and the movement of the diaphragm increases, so that most respiratory effort is diaphragmatic. Stimulated by progesterone, the thoracic cage relaxes and expands by 5 to 7 cm in circumference to accommodate these increased respiratory demands, and may cause discomfort or pain as the intercostal muscles stretch. The tidal volume increases by 30% to 40% during pregnancy, probably due to the stimulatory effects of increased levels of progesterone. These physiological changes often lead to an increased respiratory rate, hyperventilation, or shortness of breath, especially on exertion such as climbing stairs.

Heart and Peripheral Vasculature

The blood volume increases, largely as an increase in plasma, by 30% to 50% (thus, increasing the cardiac output), a process that begins at 12 weeks of gestation and peaks at 28 to 34 weeks. This increase protects the mother from hemorrhage at delivery, increases oxygen transport, increases renal filtration, and dissipates fetal heat production. With cardiac dilatation (maximal by 10 weeks), the mother's heart lies more horizontally and shifts upward and to the left along with the apical impulse. Heart rate increases by 10 to 15 beats per

NURSING TIP

Breast Care During Pregnancy

Teach your patients to properly care for their breasts during pregnancy by:

- Wearing a supportive bra that accommodates the breasts' changing size
- Avoiding nipple stimulation, which may cause either leakage of colostrum or pain in already tender breasts
- Washing the breasts with warm water only, because soap may irritate the skin and sore nipples
- Patting instead of rubbing the breasts dry after bathing
- Wearing nursing pads in the bra and air drying the breasts if colostrum leakage is significant

NURSING TIP

Avoiding Supine Hypotension During Pregnancy

A left side-lying position, with a pillow under the abdomen, behind the back, or between the legs, may provide the most comfort. Committed back sleepers may find comfort by placing a medium-sized pillow such as a body pillow underneath their right sides to displace uterine weight to the left.

NURSING TIP

Decreasing Edema During Pregnancy

Edema may be especially noticeable after prolonged periods of sitting or standing and may be minimized by increased rest on the left side to favor venous return, elevating the feet while sitting, and sitting for no longer than 1 hour at a time without walking.

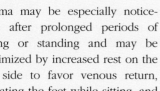
NURSING TIP

Gastrointestinal Health During Pregnancy

Teach your pregnant patients to manage nausea, vomiting, constipation, and indigestion by:
- Eating several small, frequent meals
- Avoiding spicy and fatty foods and carbonated beverages
- Drinking 8 to 10 glasses of water a day
- Increasing dietary fiber or supplemental fiber
- Exercising regularly
- Getting adequate rest
- Using antacids only in moderation and with health care provider approval

NURSING TIP

Maintaining Urinary Health During Pregnancy

Remind your pregnant patients to:
- Drink plenty of fluids, avoiding those with caffeine; 8 to 10 glasses of water each day is best
- Void frequently, especially after intercourse
- Drink cranberry juice (particularly pure concentrated juice)
- Gently wash the external genitalia before and after intercourse
- Always wipe front to back after urination and defecation

minute, a split first heart sound may be heard, physiological systolic murmurs of grade 2/6 may be heard, and blood pressure varies according to position and trimester. Supine hypotension, resulting from the weight of the uterus on the inferior vena cava, is common; it is recommended that pregnant women avoid a supine position starting at 20 weeks, unless there is a left uterine tilt.

Systolic pressure is not significantly different throughout pregnancy, whereas the diastolic pressure may lower by 5 mm Hg in the second trimester and then rise to first trimester levels after midpregnancy. The lower blood pressure in the second trimester occurs as the body adjusts to the changes in the intravascular volume and to the hormonal effects on the vascular walls. Many pregnant women also experience dependent edema partially due to peripheral vasodilation and decreased vascular resistance. This swelling is most commonly seen in the feet but can also occur in the hands and face.

Abdomen

The growing uterus gradually displaces the abdominal contents, leading to decreased tone and motility, decreased bowel sounds, and an increased emptying time for the stomach and intestines. These changes often bring about increased flatulence and constipation and can contribute to the development of hemorrhoids.

Indigestion (heartburn) is often experienced by the pregnant woman due to the relaxation of the esophageal sphincter, subsequent reflux, and slowed gastric emptying. Nausea and vomiting are common early in pregnancy and may even lead to a weight loss in the first trimester.

Increased emptying time and chemical changes in bile composition can put the pregnant woman at increased risk for cholelithiasis, the presence or formation of bilestones or calculi in the gallbladder or duct, and estrogen may augment any tendency to develop cholestasis (arrest of bile excretion).

Some women will also experience a separation of the rectus muscle of the abdominal wall, known as **diastasis recti**, which may be asymptomatic and noticed only as a vertical protrusion midline. Diastasis requires no medical intervention.

Urinary System

Secondary to the increased intravascular volume, the glomerular filtration rate (GFR) increases by approximately 50% and the reabsorption rate of various chemicals, especially sodium and water, changes. Urinary frequency usually increases in the first trimester. **Glycosuria**, glucose in the urine, is common in pregnancy. There is also an increased loss of amino acids that may show as **proteinuria** on a urine dipstick. Dilation of the ureters and renal pelvises, a decrease in bladder tone, and the short female urethra place the pregnant woman at risk for urinary tract infections. In both early and late pregnancy the bladder is encroached upon by the enlarging uterus and fetal presenting parts. **Nocturia**, or excessive night time urination, may disrupt the pregnant woman's sleep pattern.

Musculoskeletal System

The hormones relaxin and progesterone affect all joints in the pregnant woman's body. This leads to a widening (and, occasionally, a separation) of the symphysis pubis at approximately 28 to 32 weeks, increased pelvic mobility to accommodate vaginal delivery, and an unsteady gait known as the "waddle of pregnancy." These hormones also allow the thoracic cage to change shape, which can lead to complaints of upper back or rib pain.

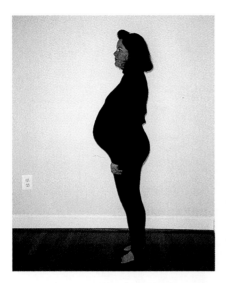

Figure 22-3 Lordosis of Pregnancy

Developing lordosis (see Figure 22-3) of the lumbar spine keeps the center of gravity over the legs and is often associated with lower back pain. Sciatic nerve pain may also present as lower back pain, a shooting pain down the leg, or leg weakness. For unknown reasons, muscle cramps, particularly in the calves, thighs, and buttocks, may develop, especially at night.

Shoe size may increase by as much as one full size as pregnancy progresses, due to edema and relaxation of foot joints. Fat deposits increase throughout the body and are most noticeable on the hips and buttocks.

> ⚡ **NURSING ALERT**
>
> ***Center of Balance During Pregnancy***
>
> Warn the pregnant woman that she is more vulnerable to falls and accidents because of the change in her center of balance. Pregnant women should exercise caution when changing position, moving over uneven surfaces, ascending and descending stairs, and participating in activities such as riding a bicycle.

Neurological System

The most commonly experienced neurological changes of pregnancy include headaches, numbness, and tingling. The more bothersome neuropathies include carpal tunnel syndrome, footdrop, facial palsy, fatigue, and difficulty remaining asleep at night. After ruling out any underlying disorder, reassure the patient that these are temporary symptoms. Headaches may be relieved by small frequent meals, adequate rest, and posture and work environment adjustments. Seizure activity with no prior history may indicate the development of **eclampsia**, or seizures associated with pregnancy-induced hypertension (PIH). Dizziness and lightheadedness may be due to the fetus' pressure on the vena cava. Lapses of memory are common and the etiology is poorly understood.

Female Genitalia

The pelvic organs experience vascular, hormonal, and structural changes. Uterine vessels dilate and at term can hold one-sixth of the maternal circulation with a blood flow of 500 ml/min. With the increased blood flow, the pregnant woman may note a feeling of pelvic congestion as well as vulvar edema. Amenorrhea, secondary to the hormonal changes of pregnancy, is generally the first noticeable symptom.

The pregnant woman's enlarging uterus begins as a pelvic organ, becoming, with bimanual examination, palpably enlarged at 6 to 7 weeks (see Figures 22-4 and 22-5), and progresses to an abdominal organ at approximately 12 weeks of gestation. At 16 weeks the fundus of the uterus is midway between the symphysis pubis and the umbilicus, and at 20 weeks the fundus is typically at the umbilicus.

Between weeks 18 and 32 of gestation, the height of the uterine fundus above the symphysis pubis is measured in centimeters and is used to confirm the gestational age in weeks. After 32 weeks, although still used, this measurement is less accurate.

The round and broad ligaments elongate to accommodate the growing fetus, and may cause the patient lower quadrant pain. **Lightening**, also called dropping, is a decrease in fundal height due to the descent of the presenting fetal part into the pelvis. This typically occurs approximately 3 weeks prior to the onset of labor in a nulliparous woman, and is often indicated by increased pressure in the pelvis and increased frequency of urination. In a multiparous woman, lightening may not occur until after active labor begins.

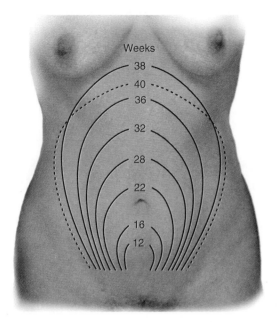

Figure 22-4   Uterine/Abdominal Enlargement of Pregnancy

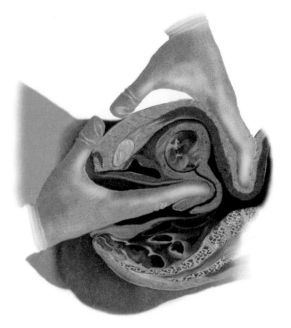

Figure 22-5   Bimanual Examination/Hegar's Sign

 NURSING TIP

Avoiding Vaginal Yeast Infections During Pregnancy

Teach your patients good perineal care during pregnancy:

1. Avoid clothing that fits tightly in the crotch.
2. Choose underwear with a cotton rather than a nylon crotch.
3. Remove a wet bathing suit promptly.
4. Monitor sugar and simple carbohydrates in the diet, if prone to yeast infection.
5. Report recurrent yeast infections, which suggest the possibility of glucose intolerance.

Braxton Hicks contractions, which are irregular and usually painless, begin as early as the first trimester.

The cervix experiences increased vascularity and increased **friability**, or susceptibility to bleeding, especially following a Pap smear or intercourse. Table 22-1 lists additional changes in the cervix and uterus in pregnancy. Mucus production occurs to form an endocervical protective plug, and the vaginal mucosa thickens secondary to hormonal changes. Throughout pregnancy, the vaginal discharge increases and is typically of a white, milky consistency. From 36 weeks on, vaginal discharge may become noticeably thicker and clumps may be present when the mucus plug is expelled. The hormonally induced changes in the vaginal environment lead to an increased risk of yeast infection.

Hematological System

Common hematological changes include increased white blood cell count (WBC), increased total red blood cell (RBC) volume, increased plasma volume, decreased number and increased size of platelets, and increased fibrinogen and clotting factors VII through X. The relatively larger increase in

Table 22-1 Changes in Pelvic Organs		
NAME	**GESTATIONAL AGE**	**DESCRIPTION**
Ladin's sign	5–6 weeks	Softening of cervical-uterine junction
Goodell's sign	6 weeks	Cervical softening
McDonald's sign	7–8 weeks	Easy flexion of fundus on cervix
Chadwick's sign	8 weeks	Cervical bluish hue
Hegar's sign	8 weeks	Softening of uterine isthmus

plasma volume compared to RBC volume leads to physiological anemia of pregnancy. The coagulation changes protect against hemorrhage at birth but may also put the pregnant woman at increased risk for thromboembolic disease.

Endocrine System

The basal metabolic rate (BMR) increases by 15% to 25% due to the increased oxygen consumption and to fetal metabolic demands. This can often lead to feelings of warmth and heat intolerance.

As pregnancy progresses, an increasing resistance to insulin develops, causing pregnancy to be called a "diabetogenic state." Causes for this phenomenon are incompletely understood but are partially related to placental manufacture of the enzyme insulinase. This process occurs to ensure adequate amounts of glucose for fetal demands. Glycosuria may be noted because the distant renal tubules cannot respond to the increased amounts and duration of glucose in the circulatory system. Pregnancy-induced glucose intolerance can be a risk factor for future development of insulin-dependent diabetes mellitus. The maternal immunological system is less resistant to infection due to a decreased cellular immune response.

❖ HEALTH HISTORY

The pregnant patient health history provides insight into the link between a patient's life/lifestyle and pregnancy-related information and pathology. The health history for the pregnant woman is generally taken on a form designed specifically for pregnancy. It may be one of several nationally recognized forms or one created by the individual health care provider. These forms contain information on the patient, from a preconception visit through delivery, as well as on the newborn. They cover the standard health history questions, any prior obstetric history, genetic predispositions, current signs and symptoms including those of pregnancy, any change in normal routine, initial prenatal visit physical assessment, subsequent visits, and laboratory data. This comprehensive approach is essential for directing risk factor assessment and developing a plan of management. Table 22-2 illustrates a typical obstetric history.

PATIENT PROFILE   *Diseases that are age- and race-specific for pregnancy are listed.*

Age   Being under 17 or over 35 puts women at risk for various pregnancy complications such as PIH, gestational diabetes, and genetic disorders.

Race   African Americans: sickle cell trait or disease, increased risk for hypertension and preterm delivery

CHIEF COMPLAINT   *The pregnant patient may have a myriad of complaints as discussed throughout the chapter. The most common chief complaints have been discussed in previous chapters.*

PAST HEALTH HISTORY   *The various components of the past health history are linked to pregnancy pathology and pregnancy-related information.*

Medical   Asthma, diabetes mellitus, cardiac disease, renal disease

Surgical   Uterine surgery, cone or excisional biopsy of the cervix, abdominal surgery leading to internal or external scarring or adhesions

Medications   Certain medications for chronic conditions may be continued during pregnancy, such as methyldopa and hydralazine for hypertension. Other medications may be changed due to the teratogenic effect on the fetus; for example, coumadin would be changed to heparin, and an oral diabetic agent would be changed to insulin. Medications for seizure disorders or psychiatric conditions should be discussed with the health care provider in terms of risk-benefit ratio for both patients, the mother and the fetus, as well as any possible alternate medications for use preconceptually and during pregnancy. Some OTC medications such as acetaminophen are considered safe during pregnancy, but any pregnant (or possibly pregnant) woman should consult her health care provider before taking any medications or therapies.

Communicable Diseases   Rubella, measles, varicella, mumps, human parvovirus (HPV) B19, HIV, hepatitis B (and other varieties). A rubella titer, RPR or VDRL, and hepatitis B surface antigen are routinely drawn on pregnant patients.

continued

HIV testing is recommended, if the patient allows it. Rubella (German measles), especially in the first trimester, and syphilis during pregnancy can cause anomalies and complications. Other infectious diseases may affect the pregnancy depending on their severity and the gestational age at which the disease is contracted; e.g., varicella may present a problem to the fetus if active at the time of delivery. Other infectious diseases to review include tuberculosis, toxoplasmosis, cytomegalovirus (CMV), and herpes and other sexually transmitted diseases (STDs).

Allergies

Symptoms may change with pregnancy; it is best to review all current allergy medications to ensure compatibility with pregnancy.

Injuries/Accidents

Any trauma that leads to abdominal scarring or injury to the pelvic organs themselves may affect the pregnancy; injuries to the back may also be of concern.

Disabilities/Handicaps

Disabilities and handicaps do not generally interfere with pregnancy. Some neuromuscular disorders such as myasthenia gravis may affect muscle response as pregnancy progresses and during labor. Paralysis does not interfere with pregnancy other than with regard to the patient's decreased ability to note significant changes in her physical status, e.g., change in vaginal discharge or increase in uterine contractions.

Childhood Illnesses

Rheumatic heart disease, if mitral valve prolapse (MVP) developed, may put the patient at risk for endocarditis with an extremely long or complicated labor or delivery and could require prophylactic antibiotics with delivery. Knowledge of childhood diseases leading to immunity may decrease anxiety if exposure to those illnesses occurs during pregnancy.

Immunizations

Typically, immunizations should be avoided during pregnancy. Any unavoidable travel to an area with known infectious disease risk requires a discussion of the risk-benefit ratio of immunization. Immune status testing should be encouraged at any preconceptual visit. If immune status is unknown or immune status testing reveals a lack of adequate titers, rubella and varicella immunizations should be given with instructions to avoid pregnancy for 3 months.

FAMILY HEALTH HISTORY

Pregnancy-related conditions and diseases that are familial are listed.

Preterm labor or delivery; PIH; diethylstilbestrol (DES) exposure; multiple births in female relatives of patient's mother; chromosome abnormalities such as Down syndrome; genetic disorders such as Tay-Sachs or Gaucher's diseases or sickle cell disease; inheritable diseases, such as Huntington's chorea; congenital anomalies such as cleft lip or palate; neural tube defects; cardiac deformities; blood disorders; diabetes (gestational, noninsulin dependent, insulin dependent); neuromuscular diseases; psychiatric disorders; any history of abuse, neglect, or substance abuse

Family history of baby's father: genetic, hereditary, or chromosomal disorders, abuse or neglect, substance abuse

SOCIAL HISTORY

The components of the social history are linked to pregnancy factors/pathology.

continued

698 UNIT IV Special Populations

Alcohol Use	Can lead to fetal alcohol syndrome (FAS). The absolute safe level of alcohol consumption is unknown. Problems have been documented with >2 oz of alcohol per day and with binge drinking.
Tobacco Use	Smoking can lead to a small-for-gestational-age (SGA) infant, preterm labor, spontaneous abortions, and lower Apgar scores (refer to Chapter 23). The effects are dose related, and tobacco use during pregnancy should be discontinued. Referral to a smoking cessation program may be beneficial. With a history of smoking or secondary smoke exposure, status should be checked frequently throughout pregnancy.
Drug Use	Drug effects on the fetus vary according to the drug(s) used and the gestational age at time of use. The most common complications are spontaneous abortion, preterm delivery, congenital anomalies, and stillbirth. Some drugs, such as crack cocaine and heroin, lead to an addicted newborn who must then go through withdrawal after birth. Cocaine use is associated with a high incidence of abruptio placenta and preterm delivery.
Sexual Practice	Sexual intercourse should be avoided after the membranes have ruptured.
Travel History	Travel more than 2 hours from home during the last month of pregnancy should be avoided.
Work Environment	Prolonged sitting or standing; heavy lifting; an extremely loud, cold, or wet environment; work with chemicals, lead, or mercury; or a one-way commute greater than 1 hour may put the pregnant woman at risk for preterm labor or congenital anomalies in the newborn.
Home Environment	Stairs may make domestic chores even more difficult for the pregnant woman and may be a significant factor for a high-risk patient who needs to maintain bed rest. The pregnant woman should avoid toxic chemicals; exposure to toxoplasmosis should be avoided by not cleaning cat litter boxes and by wearing gloves and washing hands after gardening. Household chores should be avoided if they either lead to excessive contractions or aggravate pregnancy discomforts.
Hobbies/Leisure Activities	May be continued during the pregnancy unless they present a physical risk
Stress	The patient's perception that she has more stress in her life than she can cope comfortably with should be addressed by practicing relaxation techniques, seeking counseling if needed, and using family and social support systems. Excessive stress may be a risk factor for preterm labor.
Ethnic Background	People of Asian, Asian Indian, or Mediterranean origin (Greece, Italy,Cyprus, Middle Eastern): thalassemia Ashkenazi Jews: Tay-Sachs and Gaucher's diseases French Canadians (and possibly Cajuns): Tay-Sachs disease
HEALTH MAINTENANCE ACTIVITIES	*This information provides a bridge between the health maintenance activities and pregnancy.*
Sleep	Increased demand, complicated frequently by nocturia or difficulty in finding and maintaining a comfortable position

Diet	All meats should be well-cooked and all dairy products should be pasteurized to prevent infections such as toxoplasmosis and listeria.
Exercise	Normal activities may be continued and exercise may help with some of the common complaints such as constipation. Exercise done in moderation is beneficial, but any exercise should be discontinued or modified if pain occurs; intensity and duration may need to be decreased from prepregnant exercise levels (e.g., heart rate should not exceed 150 beats per minute or moderate levels of perceived exertion). Care should be taken to avoid overheating, especially in humid weather, and water intake should be increased as needed. Physically dangerous exercise, such as waterskiing, downhill skiing, and horseback riding, should be discontinued.
Use of Safety Devices	Seat belts are recommended, with the lap portion worn below the pregnant abdomen.
Health Check-Ups	Gynecological evaluations; avoid x-rays

 NURSING TIP

Obstetric Abbreviations

You can classify pregnant patients according to their prior obstetric outcomes by using the following:

G = gravidity
P = parity
A = abortion (either therapeutic or spontaneous; may be listed separately)
LC = living children

Examples:

G: 3 P: 2 A: 1 LC: 2 = 3 pregnancies, 2 live births, 1 abortion, 2 living children
G: 5 P: 3 A: 2 LC: 1 = 5 pregnancies, 3 live births, 2 abortions, 1 living child

Table 22-2 Obstetric History

PRESENT OBSTETRIC HISTORY

Last menstrual period (LMP)

History since LMP (e.g., fever, rashes, disease exposures, abnormal bleeding, nausea and vomiting, medication use, toxic exposures)

Signs and symptoms of pregnancy

Use of fertility drugs

Estimated date of delivery (EDD) or estimated date of confinement (EDC)*

Genetic predispositions

PAST OBSTETRIC HISTORY

Gravidity (number of pregnancies)

Parity (live births): full term (gestational age in weeks), preterm (gestational age in weeks)

Number of living children

Spontaneous abortion

Therapeutic abortion

Pregnancy history:

- Complications during pregnancy
- Duration of gestation
- Date of delivery
- Type of delivery (vaginal versus cesarean section) (if cesarean, reason) (forceps or vacuum extraction) (episiotomy or laceration, and degree)

- Length of labor
- Medications and anesthesia used
- Complications during labor and delivery
- Postpartum complications

Infant weight and sex, Apgar score

Type of feeding (breastfeeding versus bottle feeding)

Breastfeeding: difficulties

*Use Naegele's rule to determine EDD: subtract 3 months from the first day of the LMP, then add 7 days. This is based on a 28-day cycle and may have to be adjusted for shorter or longer cycles. For example, if the LMP is September 1, 9/1 − 3 months = 6/1

6/1 + 7 days = 6/8

The EDD for this patient is June 8.

EQUIPMENT

- Stethoscope
- Doppler and/or **fetoscope** (see Figure 22-6)
- Centimeter tape measure
- Watch with a secondhand
- Nonsterile gloves
- Speculum
- Genital culture supplies
- Pap smear supplies (See Chapter 19)
- Sphygmomanometer
- Urine cup
- Urine dipsticks

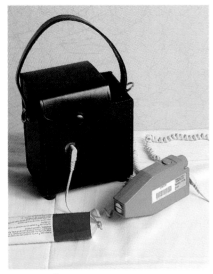

A. Doppler

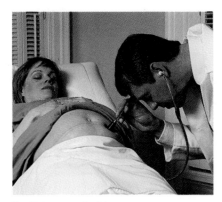

B. Fetoscope in Use

Figure 22-6 Equipment Used for Prenatal Assessment

ASSESSMENT OF THE PREGNANT PATIENT

Assessment of the pregnant patient includes a complete initial assessment as well as subsequent specific follow-up prenatal visits. The initial assessment is done when the pregnant patient first seeks care. Encourage patients to seek prenatal care in the first trimester or as soon as pregnancy is suspected. Optimally, this should be preceded by a visit with the health care provider to assess health status prior to conception. This is especially important for women with preexisting medical problems such as diabetes mellitus, cardiac disease, or seizure disorders. The American College of Obstetricians and Gynecologists (ACOG) recommends the following schedule for prenatal visits: every 4 weeks for weeks 6–28 of gestation, every 2 weeks for weeks 28–36 of gestation, and weekly from 36 weeks until delivery. Patients going beyond the 40th week of gestation (postdates) require additional evaluations. The following examination guidelines discuss how each system examination is different for the pregnant patient than for the nonpregnant patient. Refer to the previous chapters for the specific assessment of each system. The goal of the assessment is not only to confirm pregnancy and gestational age but also to evaluate general health so you can provide any needed intervention and to educate the patient to maintain and promote her health as well as that of the fetus.

✓ **NURSING CHECKLIST**
General Approach to Assessment of the Pregnant Patient

1. Greet the patient and explain how the assessment will proceed.
2. Ensure that the examination room is ready and supplies are at hand.
3. Use a quiet room that will be free from interruptions.
4. Ensure that there is adequate lighting, including a light that is appropriate for the pelvic assessment.
5. Prior to the physical assessment, complete the health history and the nutritional and psychosocial assessments. (This is usually done in an office before proceeding to the examination room.)
6. Ask the patient to void prior to the examination, both for patient comfort and to facilitate uterine and adnexal evaluation (which can be impeded by a full bladder).
7. For the physical assessment, instruct the patient to remove all street clothes, don an examination gown, and cover her lap with a sheet.
8. Perform the initial assessment in a head-to-toe manner. Try to minimize the patient's time in the supine position; i.e., ask questions later. Assist the patient in assuming the lithotomy position via verbal guidance and by assisting in placing her feet in the foot or leg stirrups. Always inform the patient before touching her of what you will be doing and what to expect ("this may pinch," "you may feel some pressure," etc.). Special sensitivity should be given to adolescents and the patient who is having her first pelvic examination. The patient may be dizzy upon sitting up or upon standing. It may be beneficial to assist her to a sitting position or to brace her arm. She should be cautioned not to stand or sit up abruptly.

General Assessment, Vital Signs, and Weight

E   1. Conduct a general assessment, including obtaining vital signs as described in Chapter 9.

   2. Obtain the patient's weight as described in Chapter 7.

N   *Refer to Chapter 9 for normal general assessment, and pages 691 and 692 for vital sign changes that occur in pregnancy. Refer to Chapter 7 for the recommended weight gain in pregnancy.*

A   Hypertension at any time in pregnancy is considered abnormal. In pregnancy, hypertension is defined as a systolic pressure greater than 140 and/or a diastolic pressure greater than 90. Another parameter is a systolic pressure increase of 30 mm Hg and/or a diastolic pressure increase of 15 mm Hg above prepregnancy pressures. This is assessed by taking the blood pressure twice, at least 6 hours apart. If a prepregnancy blood pressure is unknown, the greater than 140/90 criteria is used. Hypertension noted prior to 20 weeks is most likely chronic hypertension. After 20 weeks, hypertension is related to PIH.

P   The pathophysiology of PIH is still being researched. It is widely thought that vasospasms occurring throughout the vasculature contribute to PIH.

A   A weight gain that is more than the recommended amount is abnormal.

P   Excessive weight gain may be due to increased caloric intake, multiple pregnancies, polyhydramnios, and edema secondary to PIH.

A   A weight gain that is less than the recommended amount is abnormal.

P   Weight loss or insufficient weight gain in pregnancy can be due to hyperemesis gravidarum (refer to page 703), decreased caloric intake, and malabsorption syndromes.

Skin and Hair

E   Examine the skin and hair as described in Chapter 10.

N   *Refer to Chapter 10 and to page 690 in this chapter.*

A   **Prurigo** of pregnancy presents as excoriated papules, which are highly pruritic and usually distributed on the hands and feet but in more severe cases, may be noted on the upper trunk. They are most commonly found in mid- to late pregnancy and are abnormal.

P   Etiology is poorly understood, but there is no increase in fetal mortality, and the eruptions fade after delivery.

A   Papular dermatitis of pregnancy may manifest at any time during pregnancy as erythematous, pruritic, widespread, soft papules. These papules are typically 3 to 5 mm in size and are surmounted by smaller, firmer papules or small crusts. There tend to be several new eruptions daily, and those already present heal in 7 to 10 days, possibly with hyperpigmentation. Papular dermatitis is abnormal

P   The pathophysiology of these lesions is poorly understood. Papular dermatitis is associated with an increased risk for fetal loss, which may be significantly reduced by the use of oral prednisone.

A   Erythematous plaques that develop into vesicular lesions that may become pustular are abnormal.

P   Primary herpes (refer to Chapter 10) contracted in the first trimester places the fetus at risk for abnormalities. It is more virulent and likely to cross the placental barrier, leading to fetal abnormalities. Recurrent genital herpes lesions contain fewer viral particles and carry a less severe outcome throughout the pregnancy, most often leading to a cesarean delivery when lesions are noted in and around the vagina.

A   Rashes are generally abnormal and should be further investigated.

P   These should be evaluated for infectious, collagen, or other disease etiology as described in Chapter 10.

E	**Examination**
N	**Normal Findings**
A	**Abnormal Findings**
P	**Pathophysiology**

Head and Neck

E/N   Refer to Chapter 11 and to page 690 of this chapter.

A   The appearance of hyperthyroidism and hypothyroidism is abnormal in pregnancy.

P   Neoplastic disorders such as choriocarcinoma, ovarian teratoma, and hydatidiform mole, as well as a single active thyroid nodule or multinodular goiter should be considered with the diagnosis of hyperthyroidism in the pregnant patient.

Eyes, Ears, Nose, Mouth, and Throat

E/N   Refer to Chapter 12 and to page 691 of this chapter.

A   Arterial constriction of retinal vessels is abnormal.

P   This can occur in PIH.

A   Any growth in the mouth is abnormal.

P   Some women develop pregnancy tumors in their mouths (see Figure 22-7). These growths are usually benign. The vascular proliferation occurs secondary to hormonal changes. They may not resolve at the end of pregnancy.

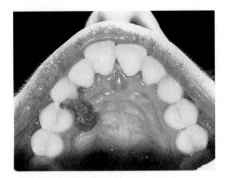

Figure 22-7   Pregnancy Tumor
Courtesy of Dr. Joseph L. Konzelman, School of Dentistry, Medical College of Georgia

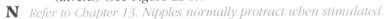

🌸 NURSING TIP

Differentiating PIH from Chronic Hypertension

Retinal examination may help in differentiating chronic hypertension from PIH. With chronic hypertension, hemorrhage, exudates, angiosclerosis, and vascular tortuosity may be noted, while with PIH, arterial constriction may be the only finding.

Breasts

E   **1.** Examine the breasts as described in Chapter 13.
   2. Don gloves.
   3. Assess the shape of each nipple by putting your thumb and index finger on the areola and pressing inward to express any discharge. Note whether the nipple protracts (becomes erect) or retracts (inverts) (see Figure 22-8).

N   *Refer to Chapter 13. Nipples normally protract when stimulated.*

A   Accessory breast tissue, most commonly in the axilla, and secondary nipples on the nipple line are abnormal.

P   This finding is a result of abnormal embryologic development, but does not present a problem in pregnancy. These areas may develop during the pregnancy along with the normal breast tissue. Refer to Chapter 13 for additional information.

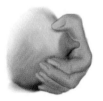

Press just behind areola | Normal nipple protraction

Pseudo-inverted | Inverted

Figure 22-8   Assessing for Protractivity of the Nipple

E	Examination
N	Normal Findings
A	Abnormal Findings
P	Pathophysiology

🌸 NURSING TIP

Nipple Assessment

Assess nipples at the initial visit and again in the third trimester for any changes. The assessment may change as the breasts enlarge with advancing pregnancy. Inverted nipples may be helped by the use of a nursing cup (breast shield) that is held in place by the brassiere; the nipple is pushed forward through the hole in the base of the cup.

Thorax and Lungs

E   Refer to Chapter 14.
N   *Refer to Chapter 14 and to page 691 of this chapter.*
A/P Pathology noted in Chapter 14 would also be considered abnormal for the pregnant patient.

Heart and Peripheral Vasculature

E   Assess the patient as described in Chapter 15.
N   *Refer to Chapter 15 and to pages 691 and 692 of this chapter.*
A   Generalized edema, in contrast to the dependent edema of pregnancy, is abnormal.
P   The most common cause for this is PIH. This disease decreases the colloid osmotic pressure within the vasculature, therefore allowing fluid to leak into the tissues. Other potential causes to be considered are kidney disease and cardiovascular disease such as cardiomyopathy.

Abdomen

E   Assess the patient as described in Chapter 16.
N   *Refer to Chapter 16 and to page 692 of this chapter.*
A   Severe nausea and vomiting (**hyperemesis gravidarum**) leading to a significant weight loss in pregnancy is abnormal.
P   Hyperemesis gravidarum is a disease of unknown etiology. It usually presents in the first trimester and may continue throughout the pregnancy. This is more severe than morning sickness and may persist throughout the day, leading to nutritional deficiencies. There often is associated hyperthyroidism. Other less common causes may include cholestasis, acute fatty liver disease, hepatitis, cirrhosis, appendicitis, and ulcers.
A   Epigastric pain is abnormal.
P   This is usually a result of liver inflammation or necrosis from PIH. It must be differentiated from cholecystitis or other liver disorders. It may be confused with commonly experienced pregnancy heartburn, but epigastric pain is over the liver itself, whereas heartburn is felt more midline.

Urinary System

E   1. Obtain a complete urinalysis at the initial prenatal visit.
    2. Obtain a urine culture if indicated by urinalysis or patient history.
    3. It is common (but not proven to affect outcome) to assess urine for protein, glucose, leukocytes, and nitrates at each subsequent prenatal visit.
N   *The urine may turn a brighter yellow as a result of prenatal vitamins. Trace amounts of protein may be noted. Glycosuria may be noted without pathology, but concern for diabetes mellitus cannot be ignored. Leukocytes and nitrates are normally absent.*
A   Nitrates or large amounts of leukocytes are abnormal.
P   Nitrates, a breakdown product of bacteria, and large amounts of white blood cells (leukocytes) may indicate a urinary tract infection.
A   Dysuria that presents as any of the following is abnormal: difficulty in initiating urinary flow, increased urinary frequency, a feeling of being unable to empty the bladder.
P   Dysuria results most commonly from a bacterial infection, inflammation of the bladder (cystitis), or urinary tract infection.
A   Pain in the flank area (costovertebral angle tenderness) is abnormal.

E	Examination
N	Normal Findings
A	Abnormal Findings
P	Pathophysiology

P The pregnant patient is more prone than the nonpregnant patient to develop pyelonephritis from a lower urinary tract infection secondary to the dilation of the ureters and renal pelvises, along with decreased tone and peristalsis, which lead to stasis. This results from the physiological changes that occur during pregnancy.

A Asymptomatic bacteriuria is abnormal.

P A clean-voided urine specimen containing more than 100,000 organisms of the same species per milliliter of urine is consistent with infection. Asymptomatic bacteriuria sometimes progresses to acute symptomatic infection unless treated. Through poorly understood mechanisms, bacteriuria is associated with an increased rate of preterm labor and birth.

A Proteinuria greater than trace as shown on a urine dipstick is abnormal.

P The most common cause is PIH. The vasospasms that occur also affect the kidneys and their ability to filter substances. Other possible causes are collagen disorders or kidney diseases.

Musculoskeletal System

E Assess the patient as described in Chapter 17.
N *Refer to Chapter 17 and to page 692 in this chapter.*
A/P Pathology described in Chapter 17 is also considered abnormal for the pregnant patient.

Neurological System

E Assess the patient as described in Chapter 18.
N *Refer to Chapter 18 and to page 693 in this chapter.*
A Seizures during pregnancy are abnormal.
P Eclampsia (a subset of PIH) is the most common cause of seizures in the pregnant patient. Other less common causes are stroke, tumors, or epilepsy. The coagulation and vascular changes associated with pregnancy may exacerbate preexisting conditions.
A Hyperreflexia and clonus are abnormal.
P PIH can cause these findings.

Female Genitalia

E 1. For the initial prenatal visit, perform the assessment as described in Chapter 19.
2. Perform cultures as indicated in Table 22-3, page 709.
3. Postdate pregnancies and pregnancies complicated by preterm labor symptoms or preterm labor risk factors may require a cervical assessment at each visit.

N *Refer to Chapter 19 for normal findings of the female genitalia assessment. The multiparous vulva and vagina may appear more relaxed in tone, with a shorter perineum. There is often a visible, white, milky discharge during pregnancy, and the cervix may show more* **ectropion** *(also called eversion and friability). Ectropion is the condition where the columnar epithelium extends from the os past the normal squamocolumnar junction, often producing a red, possibly inflamed appearance. Refer to Table 22-1 on page 694 for additional changes in pelvic organs.*
Manual assessment should show uterine size appropriate for gestational age, and the uterus may be slightly more tender than in a nonpregnant woman. The retroverted and retroflexed uterus may be more difficult to assess. Palpation of the adnexa may demonstrate a slight tenderness and enlargement of the ovulatory ovary secondary to the corpus luteum of pregnancy.

E Examination
N Normal Findings
A Abnormal Findings
P Pathophysiology

A Persistent abdominal pain or tenderness is abnormal and should be evaluated.

P Either finding may indicate many underlying disorders related or unrelated to pregnancy. PIH and abruptio placenta are the most common causes of pain related to pregnancy. PIH pain is secondary to the hepatic involvement in this disease. Abruptio pain is from the retroplacental bleeding of the placental separation. Disorders unrelated to pregnancy include ulcers, cholecystitis, appendicitis, and pancreatitis.

A Painful adnexal masses are abnormal.

P In early pregnancy, these may indicate an **ectopic pregnancy** (pregnancy other than intrauterine, such as in the abdomen or fallopian tube), infection, or cancerous growth. Pain associated with an adnexal mass may be elicited via cervical motion during bimanual assessment.

Uterine Size

Uterine size is determined by palpation on the initial visit if prior to 18 weeks by internal pelvic examination and by fundal height in centimeters for subsequent visits.

Fundal Height by Centimeters

E
1. Place the patient in a supine position.
2. Place the zero centimeter mark of the tape measure at the symphysis pubis in the midline of the abdomen.
3. Palpate the top of the fundus and pull tape measure to the top (see Figure 22-9).
4. Note the centimeter mark.

N *A 16-week uterus is between the symphysis pubis and umbilicus, a 20-week uterus is at the umbilicus (20 cm), and from 18 to 32 weeks the size is equal to the centimeter height of the uterine fundus. After 32 weeks, although still used, this measurement is less accurate.*

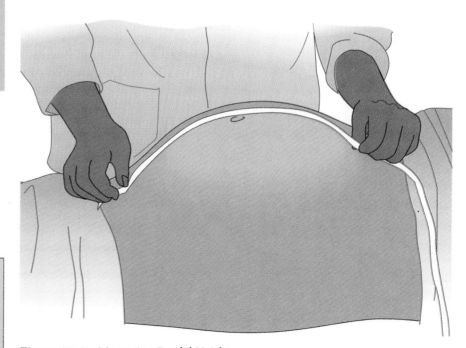

Figure 22-9 Measuring Fundal Height

E	**Examination**
N	**Normal Findings**
A	**Abnormal Findings**
P	**Pathophysiology**

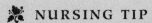

NURSING TIP

FHR AKA FHT

The term *fetal heart tone* (FHT), described in beats per minute, is commonly used in antepartum assessment, whereas, in much of the literature, especially intrapartum discussions, the term *fetal heart rate* (FHR) is used.

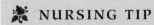

NURSING TIP

Documenting Location of FHT

Document the location of the FHTs by using a cross, with the intersection as the umbilicus, and making an X or writing the numeric count where the rate is heard the strongest.

A Uterine size larger than expected given LMP is abnormal.

P This may indicate hydatidiform mole or molar pregnancy (especially in the absence of fetal heart tones) multiple gestation, inaccurate dating, uterine pathology (fibroid), polyhydramnios, or, in later pregnancy, **macrosomia** (newborn weighing greater than 4,000 gm).

A Uterine size smaller than expected given LMP is abnormal.

P This may indicate a nonviable pregnancy, inaccurate dating, or, later in pregnancy, intrauterine growth retardation (IUGR) or transverse lie of the fetus.

Fetal Heart Rate

E 1. Place the patient in the supine position.
2. Place Doppler or fetoscope on abdomen and move it around until FHTs are heard.
3. Count the FHR for sufficient time to determine rate and absence of an irregularity (optimally 1 minute).

N *During early gestation, the fetal heart is generally heard in the midline area between the symphysis pubis and the umbilicus. It can be heard via Doppler by approximately 12 weeks (and maybe as early as 9 weeks). Use Doppler to auscultate FHT prior to 20 weeks; a fetoscope can be used after 20 weeks. Doppler is commonly used throughout pregnancy, as it is more convenient and also allows the patient to hear FHTs. The normal rate is 110 to 160 bpm. Near-term FHTs are generally heard at maximum intensity in the left or right lower quadrant. If FHTs are best heard above the umbilicus, one should suspect a breech presentation or placenta previa. The fetal heart is best heard through the fetal back, which can be located by performing Leopold's maneuver as described below.*

A FHR below 110 bpm indicates bradycardia, which is abnormal.

P Bradycardia may be a sign of fetal distress or drug use. An FHR of 60 bpm or below may be indicative of a heart block. These conditions may be benign and convert to normal after delivery, but a consultation with a perinatologist is advised for consideration of intervention with the newborn.

A Absence of fetal heart activity is abnormal.

P Absence of fetal heart tones may indicate an ectopic pregnancy, a blighted ovum, fetal demise, or a molar pregnancy.

A FHR above 160 bpm indicates tachycardia, which is abnormal.

P Tachycardia may indicate a cardiac dysrhythmia, maternal fever, or drug use. Prior to approximately 28 weeks of gestation, tachycardia is a natural consequence of the immaturity of the fetal nervous system. In early gestation, the parasympathetic system exerts a greater influence. As the fetus matures, the sympathetic and parasympathetic systems mature and the FHR should remain within the normal range of 110 to 160 bpm.

Leopold's Maneuver

Beginning at 36 weeks, determine fetal presentation using Leopold's maneuver (see Figure 22-10).

First Maneuver

E 1. Place the patient in a supine position with the knees bent.
2. Stand to the patient's right side facing her head.
3. Keeping the fingers of your hand together, palpate the uterine fundus.
4. Determine which fetal part presents at the fundus.

N/A/P Refer to Fourth Maneuver on page 708.

E	**Examination**
N	**Normal Findings**
A	**Abnormal Findings**
P	**Pathophysiology**

NURSING TIP

Fetal Movement

At approximately 18 to 20 weeks, the first fetal movements (FMs) felt in utero, known as **quickening**, are noticed by the pregnant woman as fluttering or kicking, and initially may be difficult to differentiate from other pregnancy symptoms such as gas and ligament stretching. Failure on the part of the pregnant woman to notice fetal movement by approximately 20 weeks should alert you to the possibility of either inaccurate dating or, in the absence of FHTs, nonviable pregnancy. Beginning at approximately 28 weeks for the at-risk pregnancy (e.g., maternal diabetes, previous fetal or newborn demise, multiple fetuses, and PIH) and at approximately 32 weeks for the low-risk pregnancy, fetal kick or movement self-monitoring should be introduced. The pregnant woman's sensation of fetal movement may change in the third trimester, going from "somersaults," to rolling from side to side, to kicks or subtle shifts; however, the actual number of fetal movements should not decrease dramatically. Any decrease in fetal movement requires rapid evaluation.

E Examination
N Normal Findings
A Abnormal Findings
P Pathophysiology

Second Maneuver

E 1. Move both hands to the sides of the uterus.
2. Keep your left hand steady and palpate the patient's abdomen with the right hand.
3. Determine the positions of the fetus' back and small parts.
4. Keep your right hand steady and palpate the patient's abdomen with your left hand.

N/A/P Refer to Fourth Maneuver on page 708.

Third Maneuver

E 1. Place your right hand above the symphysis pubis with your thumb on one side of the fetus' presenting part and your fingers on the other side.
2. Gently palpate the fetus' presenting part.
3. Determine if the buttocks or the head is the presenting part in the pelvis. (This should confirm the findings of the first maneuver.)

N/A/P Refer to Fourth Maneuver on page 708.

Fourth Maneuver

E 1. Change your position so you are facing the patient's feet.
2. Place your hands on each side of the uterus above the symphysis pubis and attempt to palpate the cephalic prominence (forehead). This will assist you in determining the fetal lie (long axis of fetus in relationship to long axis of mother) and attitude (head flexed or extended).

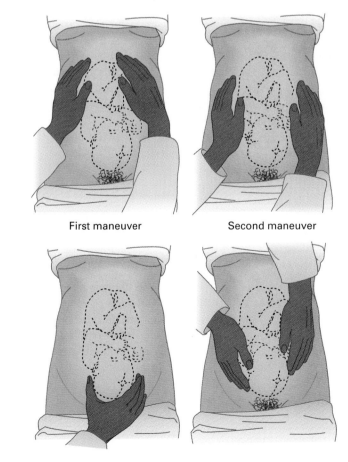

First maneuver   Second maneuver

Third maneuver   Fourth maneuver

Figure 22-10 Leopold's Maneuver

N *The fetus' head is usually the presenting part. It feels firm, round, and smooth. The head can move freely when palpated. If the baby is in a breech position, the buttocks feel soft and irregular. With palpation, the fetus' whole body seems to move but not with as much facility as the head. The fetus' back is firm, smooth, and continuous. The limbs are bumpy and irregular. The long axis is vertical, and the fetal head is flexed. A fetus not in a vertex presentation can affect the type of delivery; e.g., a fetus in a persistent transverse or oblique lie will need to be delivered by cesarean section. A breech fetus may be delivered vaginally or by cesarean section, depending on the health care provider's comfort and experience in doing a vaginal breech delivery. Breech presentation, if uncorrected (i.e., by external version [the manual turning of the fetus by the health care provider]), is associated with an increased rate of perinatal morbidity and mortality, prolapsed umbilical cord, placenta previa, fetal anomalies and abnormalities (which may not manifest immediately after birth), and uterine anomalies.*

A Inability to determine fetal outline is abnormal.

P Polyhydramnios and maternal obesity can lead to an inability to outline the fetus.

Refer to a textbook on obstetrics for more specific information.

Hematological System

E/N See Table 22-3.

Endocrine System

E Refer to Table 22-3 for information on the glucose screen.

N *Refer to Table 22-3.*

A Glucose screen greater than 130–140 mg/dl post glucola or 120 mg/dl post meal test is abnormal.

P Normal physiological changes that occur during pregnancy affect glucose metabolism. In some pregnant women, these changes accentuate and lead to gestational diabetes. These changes affect the known diabetic by altering her need for insulin throughout the pregnancy. The diabetic patient is at an increased risk for PIH, infection, macrosomia or intrauterine growth retardation (IUGR), fetal demise, polyhydramnios, and postpartum hemorrhage.

Nutritional Assessment

Refer to Chapter 7.

Psychosocial Assessment/Learning Needs

The diagnosis of pregnancy can normally lead to very mixed feelings. These feelings can range from ambivalence to anger, fear, or excitement. Crying for no apparent reason and mood swings are common in pregnant patients. Feelings of dependency may also present. Early physical changes such as nausea and fatigue may accentuate these feelings. Among the changes confronting the pregnant patient and her significant others are: role expectations (e.g., lifestyle and career); relationship expectations, definitions, and requirements (e.g., parent versus lover); and physiological changes. Feelings may fluctuate throughout the pregnancy depending on the trimester and can be predicated on a change in medical status, such as the development of a high-risk condition. Early in pregnancy the patient often focuses on herself and how these changes are affecting her physical state and her lifestyle. As pregnancy progresses, the patient usually shifts her focus from herself to the fetus as an individual and to the fetus' well-being. The patient's age, prior history, family history, prior

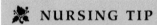

NURSING TIP

Early Glucose Screen

The woman with a positive history for macrosomia or previous pregnancy-induced glucose intolerance (gestational diabetes), or a family history of diabetes mellitus, or who is 35 years of age or older (advanced maternal age) should have an early glucose screen (drawn 1 hour after a 50-gram glucola loading dose) drawn along with her initial prenatal panel.

E   Examination
N   Normal Findings
A   Abnormal Findings
P   Pathophysiology

Table 22-3 Laboratory Tests and Values in Pregnancy

TEST	NORMAL VALUES
Blood type	A, B, O, AB
Rh factor	Positive or negative
Antibody screen	Negative
RPR (rapid plasma reagin) or VDRL (Venereal Disease Research Laboratory)	Nonreactive or negative A positive result requires the more specific MHA-TP microhemagglutination assay or *Treponema pallidum* antibodies.
Rubella	Immune (Nonimmune patients should be cautioned to avoid contact with possible exposure during the first trimester and will require a postpartum immunization.)
Hepatitis B surface antigen	Negative
HIV (many states are mandating that testing be offered)	Negative
CBC to include:	
HGB	12–16 g/dl
HCT	36–47%
MCV	80–100 μm^3
Toxoplasma IgG*	0–5 IU/ml
One hour post 50 gram glucola glucose tolerance test**	130 mg/dl or less
Three hour glucose tolerance test**	
Fasting blood sugar	94 mg/dl or less
One hour post 100 grams glucola	179 mg/dl or less
Two hour post 100 grams glucola	154 mg/dl or less
Three hour post 100 grams glucola	139 mg/dl or less
Genital cultures or probes:	
Chlamydia by DNA probe or culture	Negative
Gonorrhea by DNA probe or culture	Negative
Genital bacterial	Normal flora (negative) for gonorrhea, bacterial vaginosis, and other pathogens

All tests are performed at the initial prenatal visit (except as noted) and when indicated throughout the duration of the pregnancy.

Performed with history of exposure and symptoms.
**Performed at 26–30 weeks.*

Table 22-4 Danger Signs of Pregnancy

- Vaginal bleeding*
- Leaking or gush of watery fluid*
- Abdominal or pelvic pain or cramping*
- Severe headaches or blurring of vision
- Persistent chills or fever greater than 102°F
- Persistent vomiting
- Decreased fetal movement or lack of fetal movement
- Change in vaginal discharge or pelvic pressure before 36–37 weeks*
- Frequent (more than four per hour) uterine contractions or painless tightenings between 20 and 37 weeks*

Associated with preterm labor.

pregnancy experience; whether the pregnancy was planned or accidental; and any known risk factors all serve to affect her state of mind. Social support systems, socioeconomic status, environmental hazards, and culture are also influencing factors.

The learning needs of the pregnant patient also change throughout pregnancy, and your assessments and teaching must change accordingly. Many communities offer pregnancy-related classes that start with early pregnancy and progress through the childbirth process, breastfeeding, infant care, and sibling involvement. The first-trimester classes typically focus on the physiological changes occurring during pregnancy and what the patient must do to develop a healthy infant, e.g., nutrition, rest, exercise, and behaviors to avoid. During the second trimester, emphasis shifts to information on danger signs and symptoms (see Table 22-4). At 24 to 26 weeks, the patient should be provided verbal and written information on signs and symptoms of preterm labor.

Third-trimester classes focus on the preparation for childbirth and the care of a newborn infant. The topic of breastfeeding should be introduced in the first trimester and discussed throughout the pregnancy. The patient should be informed of available childbirth education classes.

Adolescents may need additional support and educational reinforcement. Many school districts offer special programs for pregnant teens in addition to their normal school courses. Such programs typically encompass childbirth preparation and infant care assistance while the teen finishes school.

Learning needs must be assessed on an ongoing basis so that interventions can occur at the appropriate times. A social services consultation may be indicated for certain patients, such as those with a history of physical, emotional, or sexual abuse, those experiencing current drug and or alcohol abuse, and those requiring help with basic housing and food needs. Learning may require reinforcement and educational needs should be reviewed and documented throughout the pregnancy. Appropriate written or visual information should be used to reinforce verbal discussions.

Any couple who suffers fetal loss, whether intrauterine, stillborn, or newborn demise, should be offered supportive follow-up. Many communities have support groups, or couples may seek help from a counselor or religious leader. Couples who experience early miscarriages often find they are not allowed by society to grieve their losses; supportive follow-up should be offered to these couples.

Sexual relations during pregnancy is often viewed as a taboo subject. Intercourse, unless specifically proscribed, is considered safe during pregnancy, although it may not always be easy or comfortable. During the first trimester, there may be no changes in libido for the woman, unless nausea and other physical changes leave her feeling excessively miserable. During the second trimester, the pregnant woman may even experience increased libido, whereas the physical and psychological changes of the third trimester may decrease the woman's interest in sexual relations. As pregnancy advances, the woman may find she is most comfortable on her side, perhaps with a pillow under the abdomen, facing away from her partner. This position may decrease the depth of penetration of the penis. Male partners may express concern about injuring the fetus or the perceived discomfort of the pregnant woman.

CASE STUDY

The case study illustrates the application and objective documentation of the pregnant patient assessment.

The Pregnant Patient

Diana is a 34-year-old woman who tested positive in a home urine pregnancy test. The health history reflects the data obtained during her first prenatal visit.

❖ HEALTH HISTORY

PATIENT PROFILE	34 yo MWF
REASON FOR SEEKING HEALTH CARE	"I performed a home pregnancy test & it was ⊕."
PRESENT HEALTH	Seen c̄ husband, who is father of the baby (FOB), last October for preconceptual counseling, which led to a genetic referral, as pt is at ↑ risk to be a Tay-Sachs carrier; husband has 2 male cousins from maternal aunts c̄ mental retardation; FOB screened ⊖ for Fragile X; pt screened ⊖ for Tay-Sachs. Pt started on prenatal MVI c̄ 0.4 mg folic acid at that time & was instructed to avoid hot tubs, ETOH, tobacco, & meds when possible. Nutritional guidelines were discussed. Pt d/c use of diaphragm 4 mo ago to conceive.

continued

OBSTETRIC HISTORY

Present Obstetric Hx

LMP: April 1
History since LMP: denies fever, rashes, toxic exposures, vaginal bleeding
S/S of Pregnancy: amenorrhea; breast tenderness; nausea q AM c̄
    vomiting 1–2 × especially if goes s̄ eating for a few hr, resolves by
    mid-PM
Use of Fertility Drugs: Ø
EDD: January 8
Genetic Predisposition: refer to present hl

Past Obstetric Hx

G: 1   P: 0   A: 0   LC: 0

PAST HEALTH HISTORY

Medical

Denies

Surgical

T & A age 6 s̄ complications

Medications

Prenatal MVI per present hl; acetaminophen prn for H/A

Communicable Diseases

Denies hx of STDs, TB, measles, mumps, Fifth's dz (HPV B19), hepatitis,
    CMV, toxoplasmosis; denies risk factors for HIV

Allergies

NKA to meds or foods; seasonal environmental allergies

Injuries/Accidents

Denies

Disabilities/Handicaps

Denies

Blood Transfusion

Denies

Childhood Illnesses

Varicella age 6

Immunizations

"Up to date"; last tetanus 6 yr ago

FAMILY HEALTH HISTORY

LEGEND

◯ Living female

▢ Living male

⊗ Deceased female

⊠ Deceased male

╱ Points to patient

A&W = Alive & well
BPH = Benign prostatic
    hypertrophy
CA = Cancer
DM = Diabetes mellitus
HOH = Hard of hearing
HTN = Hypertension
MR = Mental retardation
sz = Seizure

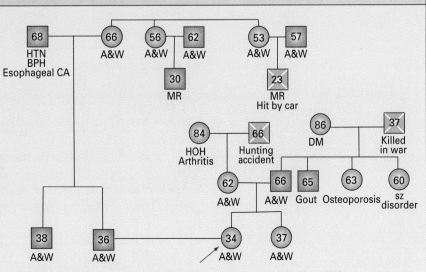

Denies mother or sister had problems c̄ pregnancies; states mother took DES when pregnant
c̄ her. Denies FHH of cerebral palsy, congenital anomalies, cystic fibrosis, Down syndrome,
hemophilia, Huntington's Chorea, MR, MD, neutral tube defect, sickle cell dz or
trait, Tay-Sachs, thalassemia A or B; FOB denies FHH of above.

continued

SOCIAL HISTORY

Alcohol Use	Occasional wine c̄ dinner; Ø ETOH since Oct
Tobacco Use	Denies ever using, FOB does not smoke; denies secondary smoke exposure
Drug Use	Denies she or FOB ever used drugs
Sexual Practice	Monogamous
Travel History	Honeymooned in Caribbean 6 yr ago
Work Environment	Sits, walks, & stands throughout day
Home Environment	High-rise condo in metropolitan area; has all modern amenities
Hobbies/Leisure Activities	Reading, home projects, movies, concerts
Stress	Both she & FOB have "stressful professional careers" but enjoy their work & are supportive of each other
Education	MBA
Economic Status	"Comfortable living"
Military Service	Denies
Religion	Nonpracticing Seventh Day Adventist
Ethnic Background	Pt = French Canadian, FOB = Northern European caucasian
Roles/Relationships	Looking forward to becoming a parent; pt & FOB have participated in counseling to discuss parenting expectations & role changes once baby is born
Characteristic Patterns of Daily Living	Rises at 0630, showers, has breakfast, & drives to work; arrives at 0815; lunches at desk; finishes work 1800–1930, exercises p̄ work, either cooks or picks up dinner; may finish work at home (1–2 hr), reads & goes to bed

HEALTH MAINTENANCE ACTIVITIES

Sleep	6–8 hr/night
Diet	Following nutritional guidelines discussed at preconceptual visit; ↑ her pasteurized dairy & vitamin A- & C-rich fruits & vegetables; added 1–2 daily servings from bread group; limits fats; ↑ fiber intake; vegetables are well washed & meats are well cooked
Exercise	Step aerobics, biking, or jogging for 30–45 min (HR not numerically monitored, but titrated to tolerance & comfort) 4–5 × wk c̄ wt training & stretching

continued

Stress Management	Exercise, hobbies, use of home & work support systems
Use of Safety Devices	Always wears seat belt, usually wears helmet when bike riding
Health Check-Ups	Annual GYN check c̄ Pap smear × 14 yr; BSE monthly × 6 yr

PHYSICAL ASSESSMENT

General Assessment, Vital Signs, and Weight	WDWN ♀ in NAD Vital Signs: 98.8°F (po), 76, 22, 108/60 Weight: 120 lb (prenatal wt: 122 lb)
Skin and Hair	Intact s̄ lesions, rashes, bruises
Head and Neck	Thyroid s̄ enlargement
Eyes, Ears, Nose, Throat	WNL
Breasts	Tender c̄ everted nipples
Thorax and Lungs	WNL, breath sounds clear
Heart and Peripheral Vasculature	Heart: reg rhythm c̄ grade 2/6 SEM at the LSB, Ø edema
Abdomen	↑ bowel sounds, Ø masses or tenderness
Urinary System	u/a sent to lab; ⊖glycosuria, ⊖proteinuria
Musculoskeletal System	s̄ limitations in ROM
Neurological System	WNL
Female Genitalia	External genitalia s̄ lesions or tenderness; cx & vagina s̄ lesions; softening of cx/uterine junction; uterus is upper limits of nl size; sl enlarged (3 cm) & tender Ⓛ ovary
Hematological System	Prenatal panel drawn & sent to lab
Endocrine System	Ø glucola test
Nutritional Assessment	Reports balanced diet; s̄ physical s/s of malnutrition
Psychosocial Assessment/ Learning Needs	Pt & FOB planned for this pregnancy & are looking forward to birth of their child. Pt plans to work 1/2 time once baby is born. Pt is well read on physiological changes that occur in pregnancy & has formulated a list of questions. FOB accompanied wife on visit & shares her enthusiasm & need for information. Couple plans on enrolling in childbirth, infant care, & breastfeeding classes.

✓ **NURSING CHECKLIST**

Assessment of the Pregnant Patient*

Fundal Height

Fetal Heart Rate

Leopold's Maneuvers
- First Maneuver
- Second Maneuver
- Third Maneuver
- Fourth Maneuver

*Only pregnancy-specific assessments are listed.

REVIEW QUESTIONS AND ACTIVITIES

1. Review the technique for Leopold's maneuver and then find a woman who is near term and willing to let you palpate her abdomen. Can you identify the position of the fetus?

2. With the same pregnant woman, practice locating and counting the FHR, with both Doppler and a fetoscope.

3. Describe the assessment of the pregnant patient at the initial visit.

4. Calculate the estimated dates of delivery (EDD) for patients with LMPs of February 22, May 31, and October 5.

Questions 5 and 6 refer to the following situation:

Katrina is a 21-year-old female who is 24 weeks pregnant. She calls you because she is concerned about her baby.

5. Which of the following conditions warrants further investigation?
   a. Chronic fatigue
   b. Temperature of 100°F
   c. Persistent vomiting
   d. Lower back pain

   The correct answer is (c).

6. You examine Katrina later on the same day. Which of the following physical findings is cause for concern?
   a. The uterine fundus is 3 cm above the umbilicus
   b. Lordosis
   c. A thick, yellow discharge from the breasts
   d. A blood pressure of 144/96

   The correct answer is (d).

Pediatric Patient

COMPETENCIES

1. Differentiate the structural and physiological variations of pediatric patients and adults.
2. Identify personal-social, language, and fine and gross motor findings when using the Denver II.
3. Elicit a complete health history from a patient or caregiver using standard components of a pediatric health history.
4. Identify various techniques of approaching patients at different developmental levels before initiating the physical assessment.
5. Perform inspection, palpation, percussion, and auscultation in a head-to-toe assessment of a pediatric patient.

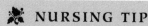
Children are unique individuals who undergo rapid changes from birth through adolescence. Physical growth, motor skills, and cognitive and social development are evidence of the numerous changes family members, friends, and health care professionals observe throughout a child's maturing years. In your assessment of the pediatric patient, you must be aware of these changes as you continually reassess what is considered within normal limits for the child.

PHYSICAL GROWTH

One important set of parameters required for pediatric health assessment is physical growth. The parameters of weight, length or height, and head circumference (dependent on age) are essential in serial physical growth measurements. (Chest circumference is of less importance.) For example, by plotting a child's growth on a chart (see Figures 23-1 and 23-2), you are able to determine normal or abnormal growth curves according to the child's age. Special growth charts are available for genetically transmitted syndromes such as Down or Turner's syndrome.

For infants the average birth weight is 7.5 pounds (3.5 kg), length is 19 to 21 inches (48 to 53 cm), and head circumference is 13 to 14 inches (33.0 to 35.5 cm). Infants should double birth weight at 6 months and triple birth weight by 1 year of age, although it is not uncommon for infants to double birth weight at 4 months. An infant's height increases about 1 inch (2.5 cm) per month for the first 6 months, and then slows to ½ inch (1.3 cm) per month until 12 months. Growth in the toddler period (12–24 months) begins to slow. The birth weight usually quadruples by 2.5 years of age, with an average weight gain during the toddler period of 4 to 6 pounds (1.8 to 2.7 kg) per year. The toddler usually grows 3 inches (7.6 cm).

Preschoolers (2–6 years) each gain an average of 5 pounds (2.3 kg) per year. Height increases between 2.5 and 3 inches (6.4 to 7.6 cm) per year. The preschooler's birth length usually is doubled by 4 years of age. In contrast, the school-age child (6–12 years) grows 1 to 2 inches (2.5 to 5.0 cm) per year and gains 3 to 6 pounds (1.3 to 2.7 kg) annually.

Infancy and adolescence (13–18 years) are two periods of rapid growth in the pediatric patient. Rapid growth in the adolescent is called the growth spurt. Females commonly experience this between ages 10 and 14, whereas in males, it occurs somewhat later, between 12 and 16 years of age.

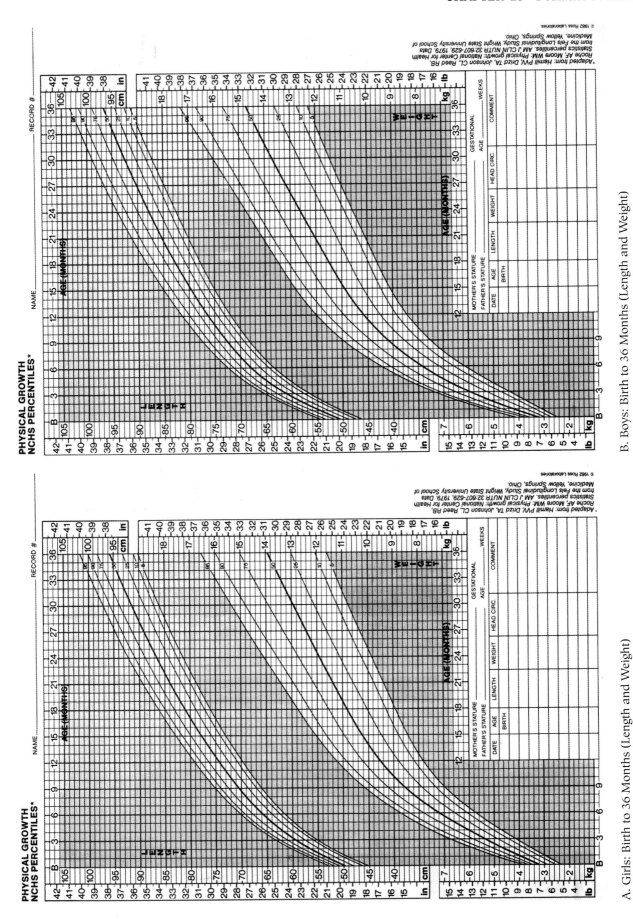

A. Girls: Birth to 36 Months (Length and Weight)

B. Boys: Birth to 36 Months (Length and Weight)

Figure 23-1 Physical Growth NCHS Percentiles *Used with Permission of Ross Products Division, Abbott Laboratories, Columbus, OH 43216. From Ross Laboratories.*
© *1982 Ross Products Division, Abbott Laboratories*

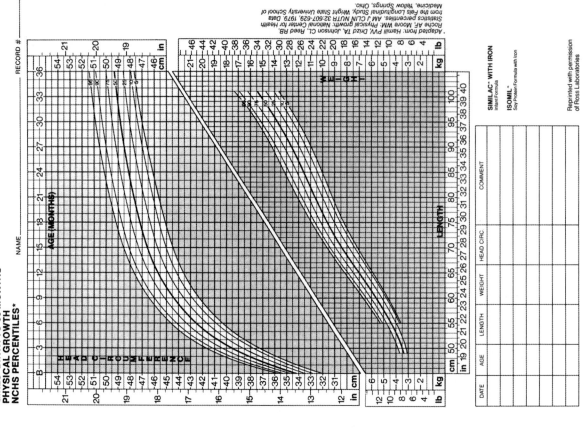

C. Girls: Birth to 36 Months (Head Circumference)

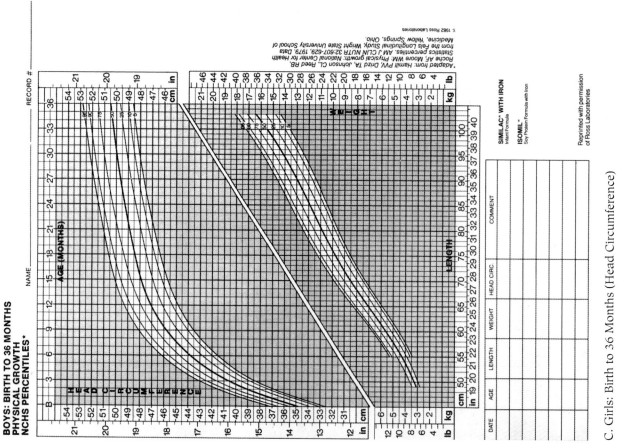

D. Boys: Birth to 36 Months (Head Circumference)

Figure 23-1   Physical Growth NCHS Percentiles   *continued*

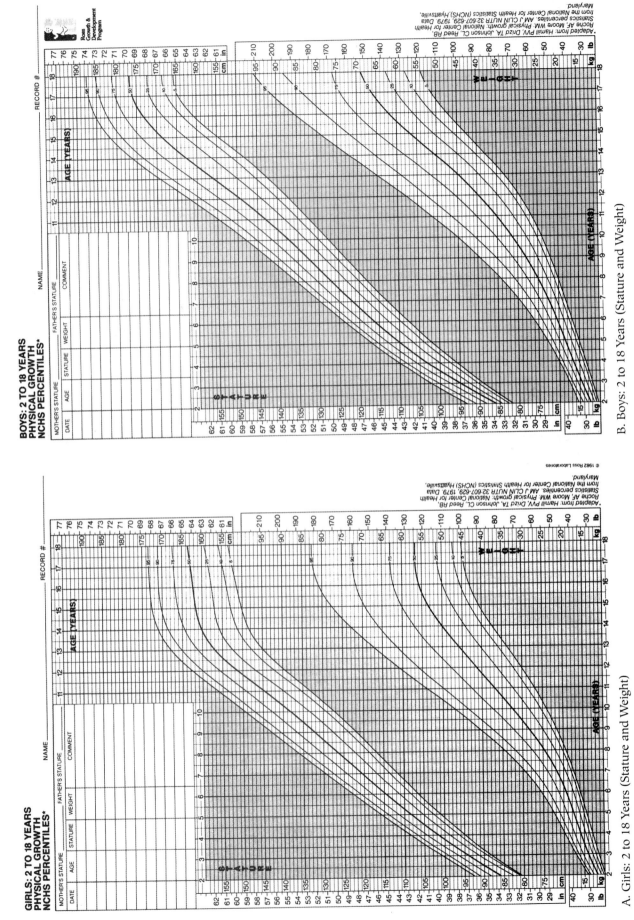

A. Girls: 2 to 18 Years (Stature and Weight)

B. Boys: 2 to 18 Years (Stature and Weight)

Figure 23-2   Physical Growth NCHS Percentiles   *Used with Permission of Ross Products Division, Abbott Laboratories.*
© *1982 Ross Products Division, Abbott Laboratories*

ANATOMY AND PHYSIOLOGY

Structural and Physiological Variations

Children differ from adults and among themselves at various stages of development in their structural and physiological makeups. Following is a list of important variations that occur from birth through a child's maturation.

Vital Signs

- One notable difference in the way children and adults regulate temperature is the inability of infants aged 6 months and younger to shiver in the face of lower ambient temperature. The absence of this important protective mechanism puts infants at risk for hypothermia, bradycardia, and acidosis.
- By age 4, temperature parameters are comparable to those seen in adults.
- Both pulse and respiratory rates in children tend to decline with advancing age and reach levels comparable to those found in adulthood by adolescence.
- In children 1 year of age and older, an easy rule of thumb for determining normal systolic blood pressure is:

  normal systolic BP (mm Hg) = 80 + (2 × age in years).
- Normal diastolic blood pressure is generally two-thirds of systolic blood pressure.

Skin and Hair

- **Lanugo**, a fine, downy hair, can be present on the skin of a newborn. The lanugo is most prominent over the temples of the forehead and on the upper arms, shoulders, back, and pinna of the ears. Dark-skinned newborns have an increased amount of lanugo, which is readily evident as very dark black hair.
- **Vernix caseosa**, a thick, cheesy, protective, integumentary deposit that consists of sebum and shed epithelial cells, is present on the newborn's skin.
- Relative to an adult, a child has a higher ratio of body surface area to body surface mass.

Head

- Suture ridges are palpable until approximately 6 months of age, at which time unionization occurs.
- The posterior fontanel, which is triangular in shape and is formed by the junction of the sagittal and lambdoidal sutures, usually closes by 3 months of age (see Figure 23-3).
- The junction of the sagittal, coronal, and frontal sutures forms the anterior fontanel. It is diamond shaped. This fontanel should close by 19 months of age with the average being between 12 and 18 months (see Figure 23-3).

Eyes, Ears, Nose, Mouth, and Throat

- At birth, the newborn's peripheral vision is intact. Visual acuity is approximately 20/200.
- Newborns do not produce tears until their lacrimal ducts open, at around 2 to 3 months of age.
- The external auditory canal of a child is shorter than that of an adult, and it is positioned upward.
- The eustachian tube is more horizontal, wider, and shorter than that of an adult. These factors increase the likelihood of middle ear infections caused by migration of pathogens from the nasopharynx.

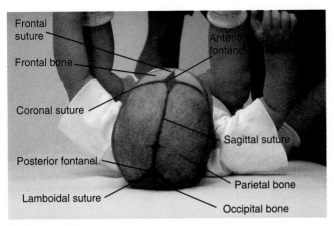

A. Superior View

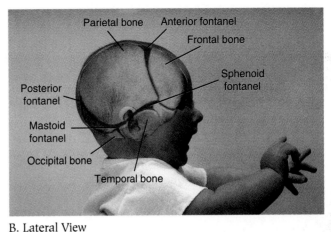

B. Lateral View

Figure 23-3 Infant Head Structures

🌹 **NURSING TIP**

Sleep Position Recommendations

Instruct caregivers to decrease the likelihood of Sudden Infant Death Syndrome (SIDS) by placing infants on the side or back when sleeping.

- Only the ethmoid and maxillary sinuses are present at birth. At approximately 7 years of age, the frontal sinuses develop. The sphenoid sinuses do not develop until after puberty.
- Eruption of the first lower central incisors occurs between 5 and 7 months of age. By 2.5 years of age, toddlers have 20 primary, or deciduous, teeth. Around puberty, permanent teeth and four molars have replaced the primary teeth. Wisdom teeth normally appear between 18 and 21 years of age (refer to Figure 23-4).
- Salivation starts at about 3 months, and the infant drools until the swallowing reflex is more coordinated.

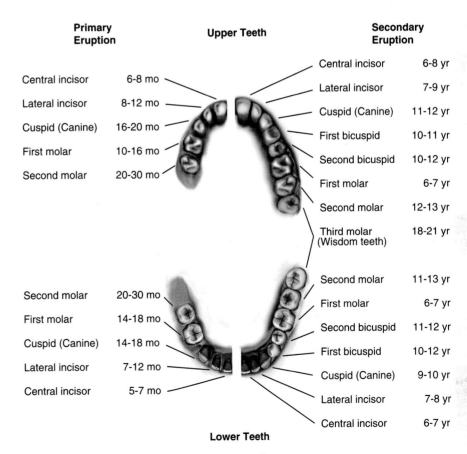

Primary Eruption		Upper Teeth	Secondary Eruption	
Central incisor	6-8 mo		Central incisor	6-8 yr
Lateral incisor	8-12 mo		Lateral incisor	7-9 yr
Cuspid (Canine)	16-20 mo		Cuspid (Canine)	11-12 yr
First molar	10-16 mo		First bicuspid	10-11 yr
Second molar	20-30 mo		Second bicuspid	10-12 yr
			First molar	6-7 yr
			Second molar	12-13 yr
			Third molar (Wisdom teeth)	18-21 yr
			Second molar	11-13 yr
Second molar	20-30 mo		First molar	6-7 yr
First molar	14-18 mo		Second bicuspid	11-12 yr
Cuspid (Canine)	14-18 mo		First bicuspid	10-12 yr
Lateral incisor	7-12 mo		Cuspid (Canine)	9-10 yr
Central incisor	5-7 mo		Lateral incisor	7-8 yr
			Central incisor	6-7 yr

Lower Teeth

Figure 23-4 Deciduous and Permanent Teeth

Breasts

- Breast tissue in the female develops between 9 and 13 years of age. Mature adult breast tissue is achieved between 13 and 16 years of age. Refer to page 344 for Tanner's Sexual Maturity Rating.

Thorax and Lungs

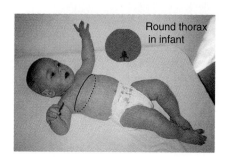

Round thorax in infant

Figure 23-5   Infant Chest Configuration

- A newborn's chest is circular because the anteroposterior and transverse diameters are approximately equal (see Figure 23-5). By 6 years of age, the ratio of anteroposterior to lateral diameters reaches adult values.
- Decreased muscularity is responsible for the thin chest wall in infants.
- Ribs are displaced horizontally in infants.
- The trachea is short in the newborn. By 18 months of age, it has grown from the newborn length of 2 inches (5 cm) to 3 inches (7.6 cm). Toward the latter part of adolescence, the trachea has grown to the adult size, normally 4 to 5 inches (10.2 to 12.7 cm).
- Until 3 to 4 months of age, infants are totally dependent on breathing through their noses.
- During infancy and the toddler period, abdominal breathing is always prevalent over thoracic expansion.

Heart and Peripheral Vasculature

- The infant's, toddler's, and preschooler's heart lies more horizontally than an adult's heart; thus the apex is higher at about the left fourth intercostal space.
- Normally, the three fetal shunts (ductus venosus, foramen ovale, and ductus arteriosus) close at birth or shortly thereafter.
- The cardiac output of an infant is normally 1 liter/minute. Toward the end of the toddler period it increases to 1.5 liters/minute. At the age of 4 years it is 2.2 liters/minute. By 15 years of age cardiac output has reached the adult level of 5.5 liters/minute.
- Infants have a higher circulating blood volume (normally around 85 cc/kg) compared to that of an adult (65 cc/kg).

Abdomen

- At birth, the neonate's umbilical cord contains two arteries and one vein.
- The infant's liver is proportionately larger in the abdominal cavity than is the liver of an adult.

Musculoskeletal System

- Bone growth ends at age 20, when the epiphyses close.

Neurological System

- The neurological system of the infant is incompletely developed. The autonomic nervous system helps maintain homeostasis as the cerebral cortex develops.
- In the first year, the neurons become myelinated, and primitive motor reflexes are replaced by purposeful movement. The myelinization occurs in a cephalocaudal and proximodistal manner (head and neck, trunk, and extremities).

Female Genitalia

- Development of pubic hair in the female begins at puberty, between 9 and 13 years of age. Within about 1 year, the pubic hair becomes dark, coarse, and curly but is not considered fully developed. Axillary hair follows 6 months later. After about age 14, pubic hair distribution approaches adult quantity and consistency. Refer to Tanner's Sexual Maturity Rating on page 611.

Male Genitalia

- The testes usually descend by the age of 1 year.
- Puberty usually starts between the ages of 10 and 13 and can last 3 to 5 years. Testicular enlargement is usually the first area of sexual development to occur. Within about 1 year, the pubic hair becomes dark, coarse, and curly but is not fully developed. Axillary hair follows 6 months later. Facial hair follows approximately 6 months after the emergence of axillary hair. Refer to Tanner's Sexual Maturity Rating on page 645 for additional information.

❖ **ASK YOURSELF**

Adolescent at Risk for Suicide

Sixteen-year-old Jason just moved to a small town from Chicago, Illinois. Before the interview, his mother confides in you that Jason has been acting differently, both socially and physically, since the family move. During your interview with Jason, he tells you he had so many friends before the family moved but has not been able to meet anyone to "hang out with" since Jason proceeds to tell you he just mailed his coin collection and the baseball he caught at a Cubs game to a friend in Chicago.

You summarize the information Jason has given and he replies, "Life is not worth living and I just want to use my father's gun to put an end to this."

1. How would you respond to Jason's last statement?
2. Would you feel obligated to share this information with anyone?

What is your institution's policy on

 NURSING ALERT

Risk Factors for Adolescent Suicide (Boynton, Dunn, & Stephens, 1994)

1. Verbalizing about ways to commit suicide.
2. Giving personal items away to friends and family.
3. Withdrawing from friends and family.
4. Demonstrating difficulty with accepting individual failures or disappointment.
5. Exhibiting an attitude of disgust or discouragement with day-to-day living.

❀ **NURSING TIP**

Assessing for Attention Deficit Hyperactivity Disorder (ADHD)

Pose the following questions to the caregiver if the child is having periods of inattention, impulsiveness, and hyperactivity. If the caregiver answers yes to eight or more questions and the behaviors in question have been demonstrated for 6 or more months, a referral for a more comprehensive evaluation should be made to rule out ADHD.

- Does your child fidget with his hands or feet or squirm in his seat?
- Do you notice your child having difficulty remaining seated?
- Is your child easily distracted?
- Does your child have difficulty waiting in turn?
- Does your child blurt out answers prior to questions being completed?
- Do you have to repeatedly tell your child to do a task?
- Have you observed your child having difficulty staying focused on tasks or in play activities?
- Does your child go from one uncompleted activity to another?
- Do you notice your child having difficulty playing quietly?
- Does your child talk excessively?
- Do you notice your child interrupting others?
- Does your child have difficulty listening to what is said?
- Does your child lose items necessary for school activities or home tasks?
- Does your child take part in any activity that could be detrimental to his physical well-being, such as head banging?

❖ HEALTH HISTORY

The same principles that apply in obtaining an adult health history, such as questioning, listening, observing, and integrating, apply in the pediatric history. Because the historian in a pediatric history is less often the child and most likely the caregiver, it is very important to document the historian's relationship to the child. The following serves only to expand on the adult health history by providing information not previously discussed but relevant to the child.

BIOGRAPHICAL DATA

Patient Name

In addition to the patient's name, obtain the full name of the legal guardian. Occasionally, the caregiver is not the legal guardian, for example, when the child is a ward of the court or state.

Address and Phone Number

Obtain the address and phone number of the caregiver if different from those of the patient.

Source of Information

Other than the patient or caregiver, information can be obtained from medical and school records, diaries, clinic notes, and agencies such as crippled children's services, public health departments, and home health agencies.

CHIEF COMPLAINT

The caregiver is often the individual who seeks health care for the child and provides a description of the perceived problems, especially for infants, toddlers, and young preschoolers whose age and mental status prevent them from offering genuine descriptions of their problem. You must frequently rely on the caregiver's intuition in such cases. The caregiver is usually acutely aware of cues to the child's illness. For instance, changes in sleeping patterns (difficulty falling asleep, reversion to night waking), regression to outgrown behaviors (bedwetting, finicky eating, thumb sucking), and unusual physical complaints in an otherwise healthy child (headaches, stomachaches) are important signs that the child may be experiencing stress or illness, and warrant further investigation. The older preschooler, school-age child, and adolescent are able to provide verbal descriptions of their complaints.

PAST HEALTH HISTORY

Much of the information outlined in the past health history for an adult is applicable to a child. Additional pertinent information should be elicited regarding the birth history, including prenatal, labor and delivery, and postnatal history.

Birth History

Obtaining the birth history may be one of the more sensitive topics of the past health history. You must feel comfortable and show sensitivity when inquiring about whether the pregnancy was planned, the date prenatal care was first sought, and birth order of pregnancy, taking into account miscarriages and abortions.

Prenatal

1. Did you plan your pregnancy for _____ (insert month)?
2. How many weeks after thinking that you were pregnant did you go to a health care provider for a check-up?
3. How many children have you carried to full term?

continued

4. Were there any pregnancies that you were not able to carry to full term? What happened?
5. Did you take any prescribed or over-the-counter medications?
6. Did you drink alcohol or caffeine or smoke cigarettes during pregnancy?
7. Did you take any drugs during pregnancy, such as marijuana, crack cocaine, amphetamines, or hallucinogens such as LSD and mescaline? If so, what were the amounts and frequency of use?
8. Were there any problems or illnesses that either you or your health care provider were worried about during pregnancy (pregnancy-induced hypertension, preterm labor, gestational diabetes, TORCH infection [toxoplasmosis, rubella, cytomegalovirus, and herpes])?

Labor and Delivery

1. How many weeks did you carry the baby before delivering?
2. Was the labor spontaneous or induced?
3. How many hours was the labor?
4. Was the baby delivered vaginally or by cesarean section? If by cesarean section, why?
5. Was any analgesia or anesthetic used?
6. Did you hold your baby immediately after delivery? (This question will provide information about the neonate's condition at delivery.)
7. Immediately following delivery, what was the baby's color?
8. What were the baby's Apgar scores at 1 and 5 minutes? (Refer to page 736.)
9. What were the birth weight and length of the baby?
10. Was the baby's father at the birth with you?
11. Where was the baby born (home, hospital, automobile, or other location)?

Postnatal

1. Did you and your baby go home together? (If answered no, inquire as to the reason for separate discharges.)
2. If hospital delivery, how long was the hospitalization for you and the baby?
3. Did the baby have any breathing or feeding problems during the first week?
4. To your knowledge, did your baby receive any medications during the first week?
5. How would you describe the baby's color at 1 week? (For light-skinned babies, ask if the skin was pale, pale pink, blue, or yellow. For the dark-skinned baby, inquire about the color of the sclera, oral mucosa, and nailbeds.)
6. Was the baby circumcised?
7. Did you start breast- or bottle-feeding your baby?
8. Were there any problems with your choice of feeding?
9. Did you or the baby have a fever after delivery?
10. How did you feel 1 to 2 weeks after delivery?
11. Did you have anyone to help you take care of the baby in the first few weeks after delivery?

Medical

Inquire about the circumstances and outcomes of any hospitalizations or emergency department visits. Keep in mind that some children's caregivers may use the emergency department for episodic health care and may not have regular health care providers.

Injuries/Accidents

Determine if the child has a pattern of frequent injuries or accidents. Repeat trauma may indicate abuse.

continued

Childhood Illnesses	Document past and current exposure to measles, mumps, rubella, pertussis, and chickenpox.
Immunizations	Immunizations provide protection against many contagious diseases of childhood. Maternal antibodies pass through the placenta and breast milk, offering the baby limited protection from disease. Table 23-1 lists a schedule of immunizations recommended by the Advisory Committee on Immunization Practices, (CDC, 1997). Many health care providers follow the immunization schedule as a guide for well-child check-ups. A record of immunizations is often important for school admission and to avoid repeat vaccinations.
FAMILY HEALTH HISTORY	Refer to page 62 from the adult history. In addition, be sure to also ask about a family history of sudden infant death syndrome (SIDS), **attention deficit hyperactivity disorder (ADHD)**, congenital disorders or defects, and mental retardation.
SOCIAL HISTORY	
Sexual Practice	Refer to Nursing Tip on page 761.
Work Environment	Day care facilities and schools are the child's equivalent of a work environment. Inquire about the number of hours the child attends a day care facility per week. Inquire about the child's academic performance. In addition, ask if the child is home alone before or after school.
Home Environment	Ask about potential exposure to lead in chipping paint because lead is harmful to the developing brain and nervous system of fetuses and young children. This group is four to five times more likely to absorb lead by ingestion than are older children (Gerchufsky, 1994). The next series of questions pertains to gun safety. Use the acronym "GUNS" to remember at-risk behaviors. G = Are there *G*uns in your home? U = Are there *U*sers of alcohol or other drugs in the home? N = Do you feel a *N*eed to protect yourself? S = Do any of these *S*ituations apply to you?
Child's Personal Habits	1. Determine what activities the child enjoys. 2. Ask how the child copes with stress and if a security object (blanket, stuffed toy) helps calm the child. 3. Determine if the child is prone to temper tantrums and what type of discipline is used.
HEALTH MAINTENANCE ACTIVITIES	
Sleep	Determine if the child takes naps and if the child shares a bedroom, because children's different sleep habits may lead to interrupted sleep.
Diet	Questions concerning diet need to be tailored to the patient's developmental level. Refer to Chapter 7 for additional information.

continued

Safety   Childproofing the environment, especially for young children, is an essential practice. Incorporate these questions into your interview.

1. Tell me how you have childproofed your home.
2. Do you have gates on the top and bottom of the stairs?
3. Are the slats on the crib less than 2⅜ inches apart?
4. Have you taken the crib mobile down and taken out the bumper pads (applies to infants who are trying to pull up)?
5. Is all sleepwear flame retardant?
6. Is the hot water thermostat turned down to 120° Fahrenheit?
7. Have you installed potty locks to keep the toilet lid down?
8. Do you keep curtain and blind strings out of reach?
9. Have you placed all sharp items such as razors and knives out of reach of the child?
10. Do you monitor your child's bath?
11. Do you always drain the water in the tub after getting out?
12. Have you placed cushioned covering on the tub's water faucet and drain lever ?
13. Do you use a nonskid bath mat in the tub?
14. Are there outlet covers on every outlet in the house?
15. When you are cooking, do you keep the pot or pan handles turned in?
16. Have you removed tablecloths off all tables?
17. Do you keep the phone cord out of reach?
18. Is the slack taken up on all electrical appliance and lamp cords?
19. If you have a raised hearth, have you covered it with bumpers, pads, or towels?
20. Are all of your plants out of reach?
21. Are your deck slats covered with a mesh net?
22. Are slip protectors under all rugs?
23. If you have a pool in the yard, is it fenced in or is a protective cover on the top?
24. Do you empty pails that contain liquid after using them?
25. Are medications, cosmetics, pesticides, gasoline, cleaning solutions, paint thinner, and all other poisonous materials out of the child's reach?
26. Do you have your local poison control telephone number next to each phone?
27. Do you have syrup of ipecac in the house? Do you know why it is used and its expiration date?
28. Do you have smoke detectors close to or in the child's bedroom and on each floor of the house?
29. Do you have a fire extinguisher on each floor?
30. Have you devised and practiced an escape route plan in case of fire?
31. Are you CPR trained?
32. What would you do in case of an emergency?
33. Where do you place your child's car seat — in the front or back seat, facing front or rear? Do you place your child in the car where an air bag is supplied?
34. Does your child use protective gear such as a helmet or knee or elbow pads if participating in an activity in which injuries may occur?
35. Do you keep plastic dry cleaner overwraps, latex balloons (unattended by a caregiver), plastic trash bags, and grocery bags out of the child's reach?

Table 23-1   Recommended Childhood Immunization Schedule, United States (1997)

Vaccines[1] are listed under the routinely recommended ages. Bars indicate range of acceptable ages for vaccination. Shaded bars indicate *catch-up vaccination*: at 11–12 years of age, Hepatitis B vaccine should be administered to children not previously vaccinated, and Varicella Virus vaccine should be administered to unvaccinated children who lack a reliable history of chickenpox.

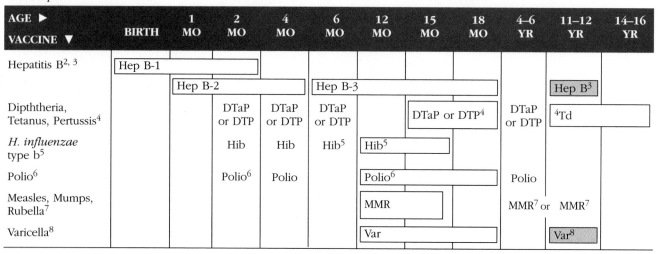

AGE ► VACCINE ▼	BIRTH	1 MO	2 MO	4 MO	6 MO	12 MO	15 MO	18 MO	4–6 YR	11–12 YR	14–16 YR
Hepatitis B[2, 3]	Hep B-1									Hep B[3]	
		Hep B-2			Hep B-3						
Dipththeria, Tetanus, Pertussis[4]		DTaP or DTP	DTaP or DTP	DTaP or DTP		DTaP or DTP[4]			DTaP or DTP	[4]Td	
H. influenzae type b[5]		Hib	Hib	Hib[5]	Hib[5]						
Polio[6]			Polio[6]	Polio		Polio[6]			Polio		
Measles, Mumps, Rubella[7]						MMR			MMR[7] or	MMR[7]	
Varicella[8]						Var				Var[8]	

Approved by the Advisory Committee on immunization Practices (ACIP), the American Academy of Pediatrics (AAP), and the American Academy of Family Physicians (AAFP).

[1]This schedule indicates the recommended age for routine administration of currently licensed childhood vaccines. Some combination vaccines are available and may be used whenever administration of all components of the vaccine is indicated. Providers should consult the manufacturers' package inserts for detailed recommendations.

[2]*Infants born to HBsAg-negative mothers* should receive 2.5 µg of Merck vaccine (Recombivax HB®) or 10 µg of SmithKline Beecham (SB) vaccine (Engerix-B®). The 2nd dose should be administered ≥1 mo after the 1st dose.

Infants born to HBsAg-positive mothers should receive 0.5 ml hepatitis B immune globulin (HBIG) within 12 hrs of birth, and either 5 µg of Merck vaccine (Recombivax HB®) or 10 µg of SB vaccine (Engerix-B®) at a separate site. The 2nd dose is recommended at 1–2 mos of age and the 3rd dose at 6 mos of age.

Infants born to mothers whose HBsAg status is unknown should receive either 5 µg of Merck vaccine (Recombivax HB®) or 10 µg of SB vaccine (Engerix-B®) within 12 hrs of birth. The 2nd dose of vaccine is recommended at 1 mo of age and the 3rd dose at 6 mos of age. Blood should be drawn at the time of delivery to determine the mother's HBsAg status; if it is positive, the infant should receive HBIG as soon as possible (no later than 1 wk of age). The dosage and timing of subsequent vaccine doses should be based upon the mother's HBsAg status.

[3]Children and adolescents who have not been vaccinated against hepatitis B in infancy may begin the series during any childhood visit. Those who have not previously received 3 doses of hepatitis B vaccine should initiate or complete the series during the 11–12 year-old visit. The 2nd dose should be administered at least 1 mo after the 1st dose, and the 3rd dose should be administered at least 4 mos after the 1st dose, and at least 2 mos after the 2nd dose.

[4]DTaP (diphtheria and tetanus toxoids and acellular pertussis vaccine) is the preferred vaccine for all doses in the vaccination series, including completion of the series in children who have received ≥1 dose of whole-cell DTP vaccine. Whole-cell DTP is an acceptable alternative to DTaP. The 4th dose of DTaP may be administered as early as 12 mos of age, provided 8 mos have elapsed since the 3rd dose, and if the child is considered unlikely to return at 15–18 mos of age. Td (tetanus and diphtheria toxoids, adsorbed, for adult use) is recommended at 11–12 yrs of age if at least 5 yrs have elapsed since the last dose of DTP, DTaP, or DT. Subsequent *routine* Td boosters are recommended every 10 yrs.

[5]Three H. influenzae type b (Hib) conjugate vaccines are licensed for infant use. If PRP-OMP (PedvaxHIB® [Merck]) is administered at 2 and 4 mos of age, a dose at 6 mos is not required. After completing the primary series, any Hib conjugate vaccine may be used as a booster.

[6]Two poliovirus vaccines are currently licensed in the US: inactivated poliovirus vaccine (IPV) and oral poliovirus vaccine (OPV). The following schedules are all acceptable by the ACIP, the AAP, and the AAFP, and parents and providers may choose among them:

1. IPV at 2 and 4 mos; OPV at 12–18 mos and 4–6 yrs
2. IPV at 2, 4, 12–18 mos, and 4–6 yrs
3. OPV at 2, 4, 6–18 mos, and 4–6 yrs

The ACIP routinely recommends schedule 1. IPV is the only poliovirus vaccine recommended for immunocompromised persons and their household contacts.

[7]The 2nd dose of MMR is routinely recommended at 4–6 yrs of age or at 11–12 yrs of age, but may be administered during any visit, provided at least 1 mo has elapsed since receipt of the 1st dose, and that both doses are administered at or after 12 mos of age.

[8]Susceptible children may receive Varicella vaccine (Var) during any visit after the 1st birthday, and unvaccinated persons who lack a reliable history of chickenpox should be vaccinated during the 11–12 year-old visit. Susceptible persons ≥13 yrs of age should receive 2 doses, at least 1 mo apart.

The Centers for Disease Control and Prevention (CDC)

⊚⊚ THINK ABOUT IT

Religious Practices Influencing Care Provided to a Young Child

A 3-year-old child arrived at the emergency department by ambulance after being involved in a head-on collision. All family members with the exception of the father and the patient were dead on arrival. The young child sustained extensive trauma to the face as a result of being partially thrown through the front windshield. The father accompanied the child in the ambulance and made it known to the paramedics that the family members were Jehovah's Witnesses and, thus, did not permit blood transfusions. This information was relayed to you on the patient's arrival. The child's blood pressure drops from 80/40 to 50/20 and a hematocrit value of 23% comes back from the laboratory. You are asked to call the blood bank for two units of blood.

1. How would you respond to this request?
2. Do your religious beliefs conflict with this family's beliefs?
3. If you feel you cannot assist with the blood resuscitation, would you feel comfortable asking a fellow coworker to step in for you?
4. What is your institution's policy?

Growth and Development

Refer to Chapter 4 for a summary of motor, language, and sensory tasks that normal children from infancy through adolescence are able to accomplish.

Developmental Assessment

A commonly used tool for assessing neuromuscular development of the child from birth through 6 years of age is the Denver II (see Figure 23-6). The test is composed of four sections: personal-social, fine motor-adaptive, language, and gross motor. There are a total of 125 items described on the test. Some items can be accomplished easily by observing the child without commands from the observer. For instance, the child may be smiling spontaneously, saying words other than "mama" or "dada," or sitting with the head held steady. Certain items can be given an automatic pass mark if the caregiver indicates that the child is able to accomplish the corresponding item, such as drinking from a cup, washing and drying hands, or dressing without help.

Before administering the test, determine the child's chronological age and draw a straight line through the four sections intersecting the age intervals on the top and bottom of the sheet. This line indicates which items are to be tested for the child's chronological age. Begin testing by assessing the item that is three items to the left of the age line. Documentation is reflected by using a "P" for pass, "F" for fail, "R" for refuses, and "NO" for no opportunity. Give up to three trials before documenting the particular item's score on the Denver II. At the end, complete the five Test Behavior questions. A normal test consists of no delays and a maximum of one caution. A caution is failure of the patient to perform an item that has been achieved by 75% to 90% of children the same age. A delay is a failure of any item to the left of the age line. A suspect test is one with one or more delays and/or two or more cautions; in these instances, retest the child in 1 to 2 weeks.

Keep in mind that current illness, lack of sleep, fear and anxiety, deafness, or blindness can affect a child's performance. If these or other logical rationale can explain a child's failure to successfully complete a series of Denver II items during a session, readminister the test in 1 month, providing resolution of the preexisting condition is accomplished, where appropriate. If the child does in fact have a developmental disability, early detection can lead to appropriate intervention and assistance.

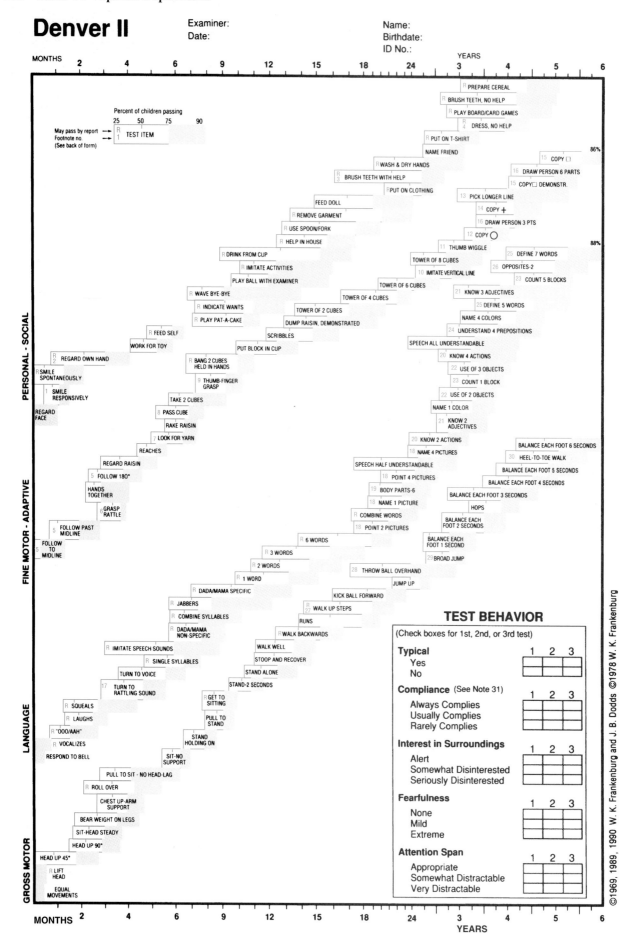

Figure 23-6 Denver II *Reprinted with Permission of DDM*

DIRECTIONS FOR ADMINISTRATION

1. Try to get child to smile by smiling, talking or waving. Do not touch him/her.
2. Child must stare at hand several seconds.
3. Parent may help guide toothbrush and put toothpaste on brush.
4. Child does not have to be able to tie shoes or button/zip in the back.
5. Move yarn slowly in an arc from one side to the other, about 8" above child's face.
6. Pass if child grasps rattle when it is touched to the backs or tips of fingers.
7. Pass if child tries to see where yarn went. Yarn should be dropped quickly from sight from tester's hand without arm movement.
8. Child must transfer cube from hand to hand without help of body, mouth, or table.
9. Pass if child picks up raisin with any part of thumb and finger.
10. Line can vary only 30 degrees or less from tester's line.
11. Make a fist with thumb pointing upward and wiggle only the thumb. Pass if child imitates and does not move any fingers other than the thumb.

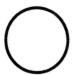

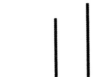

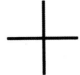

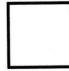

12. Pass any enclosed form. Fail continuous round motions.

13. Which line is longer? (Not bigger.) Turn paper upside down and repeat. (pass 3 of 3 or 5 of 6)

14. Pass any lines crossing near midpoint.

15. Have child copy first. If failed, demonstrate.

When giving items 12, 14, and 15, do not name the forms. Do not demonstrate 12 and 14.

16. When scoring, each pair (2 arms, 2 legs, etc.) counts as one part.
17. Place one cube in cup and shake gently near child's ear, but out of sight. Repeat for other ear.
18. Point to picture and have child name it. (No credit is given for sounds only.)
   If less than 4 pictures are named correctly, have child point to picture as each is named by tester.

 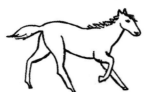 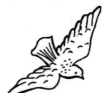 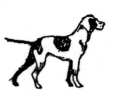 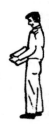

19. Using doll, tell child: Show me the nose, eyes, ears, mouth, hands, feet, tummy, hair. Pass 6 of 8.
20. Using pictures, ask child: Which one flies?... says meow?... talks?... barks?... gallops? Pass 2 of 5, 4 of 5.
21. Ask child: What do you do when you are cold?... tired?... hungry? Pass 2 of 3, 3 of 3.
22. Ask child: What do you do with a cup? What is a chair used for? What is a pencil used for? Action words must be included in answers.
23. Pass if child correctly places and says how many blocks are on paper. (1, 5).
24. Tell child: Put block on table; under table; in front of me, behind me. Pass 4 of 4. (Do not help child by pointing, moving head or eyes.)
25. Ask child: What is a ball?... lake?... desk?... house?... banana?... curtain?... fence?... ceiling? Pass if defined in terms of use, shape, what it is made of, or general category (such as banana is fruit, not just yellow). Pass 5 of 8, 7 of 8.
26. Ask child: If a horse is big, a mouse is __? If fire is hot, ice is __? If the sun shines during the day, the moon shines during the __? Pass 2 of 3.
27. Child may use wall or rail only, not person. May not crawl.
28. Child must throw ball overhand 3 feet to within arm's reach of tester.
29. Child must perform standing broad jump over width of test sheet (8 1/2 inches).
30. Tell child to walk forward, ⚙️⚙️⚙️⚙️➤ heel within 1 inch of toe. Tester may demonstrate. Child must walk 4 consecutive steps.
31. In the second year, half of normal children are non-compliant.

OBSERVATIONS:

Figure 23-6 Denver II   *continued*

EQUIPMENT

- Equipment listed in Chapters 10–21
- Scale (infant or stand-up)
- Appropriate-sized blood pressure cuff
- Snellen E chart
- Allen cards
- Otoscope speculum (2.5 or 4.0 mm)
- Pediatric stethoscope
- Growth chart
- Peanut butter or chocolate
- Small bell
- Brightly colored object
- Denver II materials

E	**Examination**
N	**Normal Findings**
A	**Abnormal Findings**
P	**Pathophysiology**

PHYSICAL ASSESSMENT

✓ NURSING CHECKLIST
General Approach to Pediatric Physical Assessment

1. Assess the patient in a warm, quiet room. To prevent hypothermia, always keep infants under the age of 6 months warm during the examination.

2. Use natural lighting, if available, during the assessment. Fluorescent lighting makes assessing varying degrees of cyanosis and jaundice difficult.

3. To help reduce anxiety and uncooperativeness (especially when assessing young children), have a familiar caregiver present during the assessment.

4. Talk to the child in a soothing voice; even an infant who cannot understand your words will take comfort in a calm and supportive approach.

5. Explain all procedures and allow older infants, toddlers, preschoolers, and younger school-age patients to manipulate medical equipment.

6. To promote the child's feeling of security, allow the infant who cannot sit up and the younger child to sit on the caregiver's lap for as much of the examination as possible.

7. Until the infant or toddler is comfortable, maintain eye contact with the caregiver while the assessment is taking place. Maintaining eye contact with the child who experiences anxiety in the presence of strangers can interfere with completing the examination. Maintain eye contact with caregiver if other means of alleviating the fears are not successful.

8. Interview the older school-age child or adolescent separately, without the caregiver. Talking to the individual without the caregiver present may yield important information not gained during a group interview (e.g., that the patient is using drugs).

9. Respect the patient's modesty.

10. Warm your equipment (e.g., stethoscope).

11. Avoid making abrupt movements because these may startle a child.

12. If the child is sleeping, take advantage of the situation by performing simple procedures (length, head circumference) and system assessments that require a quiet room (such as the cardiac and respiratory assessments) first.

13. Perform all invasive or uncomfortable procedures (ear inspection, hip palpation) last because they may cause discomfort, crying, fear, and increased heart rate.

14. Always provide comfort measures following pain. It is especially helpful to allow the caregiver the opportunity to provide supportive measures. This shows the child that you are genuinely concerned about his or her feelings.

15. To prevent falls, always keep one hand on any infant who is placed on the examination table.

16. Prior to completing the examination, ask the caregiver and patient what questions they have.

Many assessment techniques for the child are similar to those for the adult. Refer to the specific system chapters for detailed explanations of assessment techniques covered in those chapters.

Techniques for approaching the pediatric patient vary from one age group to the next. A basic principle during any physical assessment is building a trusting relationship; this can be done in a variety of ways. First, always explain what will be done prior to each portion of the assessment and answer questions honestly. Second, praise the patient for positive behaviors, e.g., cooperating during assessment of the middle ear. Portraying a caring attitude will greatly influence both the patient's and the caregiver's sense of trust. Show respect for the patient as an individual and allow expression of feelings (whimpering, crying).

Vital Signs
General Approach

1. The act of measuring vital signs is often disturbing to a young patient. Past experiences influence the degree of cooperation you will encounter.
2. Vital signs may be obtained at the beginning of the assessment or during the assessment of a certain system.
3. If the child is particularly anxious, it is best to integrate the assessment of vital signs into the overall assessment.

Temperature

You need to be proficient in measuring axillary, rectal, oral, and tympanic temperatures. Rectal measurement is the method of choice for children under 5 years of age, according to a survey done by Contemporary Pediatrics (Norris, 1985). However, a rectal temperature is not appropriate in all instances, for example, in the patient who presents with a history of diarrhea. Accurate oral temperature is difficult to obtain in most toddlers and preschoolers. Axillary temperature, while quick and painless, is often less reliable than rectal or oral temperatures.

Axillary

E 1. When taking axillary temperature, have the child sit or lie on the caregiver's lap to free your hands for other observations or to prepare for the next area of assessment.
2. Explain to the patient that this type of temperature measurement does not hurt. To pass time, ask the caregiver to read the child a story.

N/A/P Refer to Chapter 9.

Rectal

E 1. Children dislike having rectal temperature taken, so your approach to explanation should be matter of fact: "I need to measure your temperature in your bottom. You need to hold very still while I do this. Your mommy (or other appropriate person) will be right here with you."

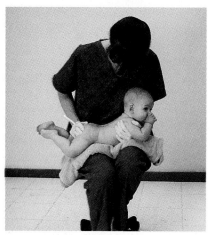

A. Infant in Prone Position

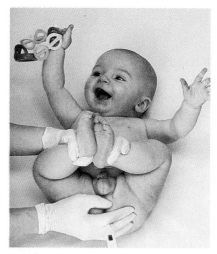

B. Infant in Supine Position

Figure 23-7 Rectal Temperature Measurement

E Examination
N Normal Findings
A Abnormal Findings
P Pathophysiology

---

2. Place the patient in either a side-lying or a prone position on the caregiver's lap or place the patient on the back on the examination table and firmly grasp the feet with your nondominant hand (refer to Figure 23-7).

3. After lubricating the stub-tipped thermometer, insert it gently into the patient's rectum: ½ inch for newborns, ¾ inch for infants, and 1 inch for preschoolers and older patients. Hold the thermometer firmly between your fingers to avoid accidentally inserting it too far.

N/A/P Refer to Chapter 9.

Respiratory Rate

E 1. Try to obtain the rate early in the assessment, when the patient is most cooperative and not crying.

2. If the patient is crying, the measurement will not be accurate and should be retaken.

3. Remember to observe the expansion of the abdomen in infants and toddlers.

N/A/P Refer to Chapter 9.

Physical Growth

Weight

Use the same scale at each visit, if possible, to prevent variations in serial weight checks.

E 1. If using an infant scale, cover it with paper.

2. Balance the scale.

3. Place infants and young toddlers nude on the scale (see Figure 23-8A). Always keep one hand on the child to prevent falls and lift your hand slightly when obtaining the actual weight reading.

4. Preschoolers and young school-age children can wear street clothes to be weighed (see Figure 23-8B). Have the older child undress, don a paper or cloth gown, and step on the standard platform scale.

5. Note and record weight.

N *Refer to growth charts, Figures 23-1A and B on page 717. Usually, neonates lose approximately 10% of birth weight by the third or fourth day after birth, then regain it by 2 weeks of age. This expected change in weight is called **physiological weight loss**, and it is due to a loss of extracellular fluid and **meconium**, a dark-green, sticky, stool-like substance excreted from the rectum within the first 24 hours after birth.*

A A newborn weight less than the 10th gestational age percentile is considered abnormal.

P A newborn whose growth has been retarded in utero is referred to as small for gestational age (SGA). Potential causes include alcohol, drug, or tobacco abuse.

A A newborn weight greater than the 90th gestational age percentile is abnormal.

P A diabetic mother or genetic predisposition may be responsible for producing a large for gestational age (LGA) newborn.

A A weight below the 5th or above the 95th percentiles warrants investigation, as does the patient who falls 2 standard deviations below his or her own established curve. Any such finding is abnormal.

P Possible causes include organic or nonorganic failure to thrive, congenital or cyanotic heart disease, cystic fibrosis (CF), and malabsorption diseases.

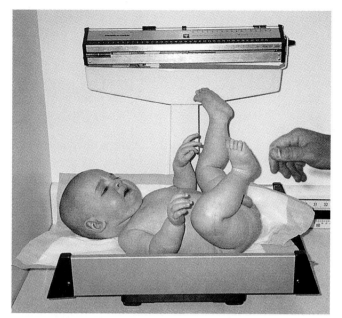

A. Infant

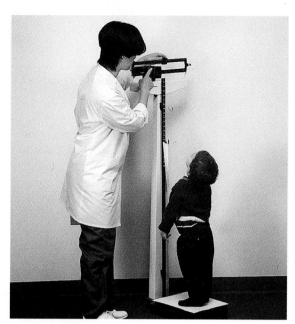

B. Preschooler

Figure 23-8   Measuring Weight in Children

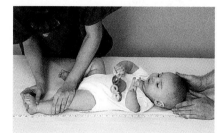

A. Recumbent Length in Infant

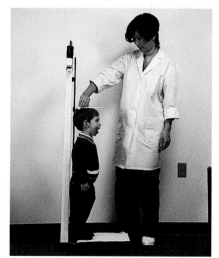

B. Height in Preschooler

Figure 23-9   Measuring Length and Height in Children

E   **Examination**
N   **Normal Findings**
A   **Abnormal Findings**
P   **Pathophysiology**

Length/Height

Recumbent length is measured for children less than 2 years old.

E   1. Position the measuring board flat on the examination table.
    2. Place the child's head at the top of the board and the child's heels at the foot of the board, making sure the legs are fully extended.
    3. Measure and record the length.
    4. If a board is not available, place the child in a supine position and mark lines on the paper at the tip of the head and at the heel (see Figure 23-9A), making sure the legs are fully extended.
    5. Measure between the lines and record.

Height for all other age groups can be measured in the same fashion as for an adult. Figure 23-9 B shows a preschooler's height being measured.

N   *Refer to growth charts in Figures 23-1A and B on page 717.*

A   A height below the 5th or above the 95th percentiles warrants investigation, as does the patient who falls 2 standard deviations below his or her own established curve. Any such finding is abnormal.

P   Possible causes include organic or nonorganic failure to thrive, congenital or cyanotic heart disease, CF, and malabsorption diseases.

> 🌺 **NURSING TIP**
>
> ### Obtaining Length/Height in Children Under 2 Years of Age
>
> 1. If measuring a recumbent length, always plot on the birth-to-36-month chart.
> 2. If measuring height, plot the measurement on a birth-to-36-month growth chart and subtract 1 centimeter, or plot on a 2-to-18-year chart.

Head Circumference

Head circumference is measured in all children less than 2 years of age or in patients with known or suspected hydrocephalus.

E   1. Place the patient in a sitting or supine position.

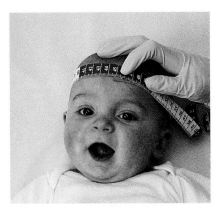

Figure 23-10 Measuring Head Circumference

2. Using a tape measure, measure anteriorly from above the eyebrows and around posteriorly to the occipital protuberance (refer to Figure 23-10).

N *Refer to Figure 23-1C and D on page 718. Normal average head growth is 1.0 to 1.5 cm per month during the first year. Premature infants often have small head circumferences.*

A **Microcephaly**, a condition characterized by a small brain with a resultant small head, is an abnormal finding.

P Microcephaly is a congenital finding associated with a mental deficit. Microcephaly can be caused by a variety of disorders including intrauterine infections, drug or alcohol ingestion (fetal alcohol syndrome) during pregnancy, and genetic defects.

A **Hydrocephalus** (enlarged head) is indicated when an infant's or young child's head circumference is above the 95th percentile and crossing over the patient's established percentile lines from one serial measurement to the next. Hydrocephalus is abnormal. Note if the eyes are looking downward ("setting sun" sign) and the sclera is visible above the iris.

P Hydrocephalus is characterized by an imbalance in cerebrospinal fluid (CSF) production and reabsorption. Hydrocephalus may result from embryological malformations of the nervous system. Congenital hydrocephalus can also be caused by syphilis, rubella, toxoplasmosis, or cytomegalovirus. Bacterial meningitis or tumors are acquired causes of hydrocephalus. The setting sun sign results from progressive enlargement of the lateral and third ventricles related to excessive accumulation of CSF.

Chest Circumference

Chest circumference is measured up to 1 year of age. It is a measurement that by itself provides little information but is compared to head circumference to evaluate the child's overall growth.

E **1.** Stand in front of the supine patient.
    2. Measure the chest circumference by placing the tape measure around the chest at the nipple line (see Figure 23-11).
    3. Measure during exhalation.

N *From birth to about 1 year, the head circumference is greater than the chest circumference. After age 1, the chest circumference is greater than the head circumference.*

A A measured chest circumference below normal limits is abnormal.

P A below-normal chest circumference for age can be attributed to prematurity.

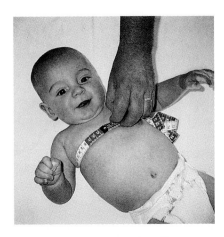

Figure 23-11 Measuring Chest Circumference

Apgar Scoring

The **Apgar scoring** system provides a quick method to assess the need for newborn resuscitation in the delivery room. An Apgar score is given to a newborn at 1 and 5 minutes after birth. Perform steps 1 through 5 at 1 minute following birth; add the score in each category for the total. Repeat at 5 minutes following birth.

E **1.** Auscultate the heart rate for 1 full minute.
    2. Measure the degree of respiratory effort.
    3. Evaluate muscle tone by attempting to straighten each extremity individually.
    4. Evaluate the newborn's reflex irritability. Use a flicking motion of two fingers against the newborn's sole to rate reflex irritability.
    5. Inspect the newborn's color.

N *A score of 8 to 10 demonstrates that the newborn is in good condition. Table 23-2 outlines the scoring system for each of the five areas assessed.*

A A moderately depressed newborn earns a score of 4 to 7. A score of 0 to 3 indicates that the newborn is severely depressed and needs immediate resuscitation. Either finding is abnormal.

E	Examination
N	Normal Findings
A	Abnormal Findings
P	Pathophysiology

Table 23-2 Apgar Scoring

HEART RATE	RESPIRATORY RATE	TONE	REFLEX IRRITABILITY	COLOR
Absent = 0	Apnea = 0	Flaccid = 0	No response = 0	Cyanosis = 0
< 100 = 1	Slow, irregular rate = 1	Some degree of flexion = 1	Grimace = 1	Body pink, extremities acrocyanotic = 1
> 100 = 2	Crying vigorously = 2	Full flexion = 2	Crying = 2	Completely pink = 2

P A low score can be the result of one or numerous problems. Prematurity, central nervous system depression, blood or meconium in the trachea, maternal history of drug abuse, certain drugs that are given to the mother in preparation for delivery and that cross over and cause fetal depression, congenital complete heart block, and congenital heart disease are some of the potential etiologies for a low Apgar score.

Skin

Inspection

Color

E Observe the color of the body, especially at the tip of the nose, the external ear, the lips, the hands, and the feet. These areas are prominent locations for detecting cyanosis or jaundice.

N *The skin of a newborn is reddish in color for the first 24 hours then changes to varying shades of pale pink to pink to brown or black, depending on the child's race. It is normal for dark-skinned newborns to have a ruddy appearance and for light-skinned newborns to exhibit a bluish-purple color of the hands and feet while the rest of the body remains pink. This is called* **acrocyanosis***. It may disappear with warming.* **Mongolian spots***, deep-blue pigmentation over the lumbar and sacral areas of the spine, over the buttocks, and, sometimes, over the upper back or shoulders in newborns of African, Latino, or Asian descent, are extremely common and not to be confused with ecchymosis.*

A A blue hue is abnormal.

P Refer to page 234. Cyanosis in the newborn is often associated with a congenital heart defect because arterial and venous blood mix. In the older child with unrepaired heart disease, cyanosis may be a sign of decreasing levels of oxygen saturation.

A A yellowing of the skin or sclera is abnormal.

P Physiological jaundice of the newborn occurs on the second or third day of life. This type of jaundice results from increased levels of serum bilirubin. The newborn's body is unable to remove the bilirubin, thus producing a yellow cast or hue to the skin of light-skinned infants and to the sclera of both light- and dark-skinned newborns.

P Pathological jaundice of the newborn occurs within the first 24 hours of life. Possible causes of pathological jaundice include Rh/ABO incompatibility and maternal infections (rubella, herpes, syphilis, or toxoplasmosis). The pathophysiological response occurs because there is a deficiency or inactivity of bilirubin glucuronyl transference in the newborn.

P Breast milk jaundice occurs within the first 2 weeks of life, with the onset being 4 to 5 days after birth. The etiology is not clear, but breast milk may contain an inhibitor of bilirubin conjugation.

A It is abnormal when the light-skinned newborn lies on a side and the dependent half becomes red or ruddy and the upper half turns pale in color. In dark-skinned children, the dependent half becomes a ruddy color and the upper half seems normal.

NURSING ALERT

Integumentary Signs of Child Abuse

1. When assessing the skin, observe for injuries in a location the child cannot reach, such as the back.
2. Examine for "item" marks, i.e., marks produced by irons, belts, electrical cords, cigarettes, or teeth.
3. Check for excessive bruising and numerous bruises in various stages of healing.
4. Look for hot water scalding marks, which present as even lines across the skin (usually on the legs or buttocks).
5. Check extremities for limited range of motion and tenderness, which can be related to fractures.

E	**Examination**
N	**Normal Findings**
A	**Abnormal Findings**
P	**Pathophysiology**

P **Harlequin color change** is a benign condition thought to be a result of poor vasomotor control; it occurs between 48 and 96 hours after birth.

Lesions

E/N Refer to Chapter 10.

A Lesions that are usually symmetrical, scaly, erythematous patches or plaques with possible exudation and crusting are abnormal.

P Eczema or atopic dermatitis (AD) is a common abnormal skin disorder involving inflammation of the epidermis and superficial dermis. Inhaled allergens such as pollens, molds, or dust mites, or food allergens are thought to induce mast-cell responses that cause AD.

A Small, erythematous, maculopapular lesions that erupt on the newborn are abnormal.

P Erythema toxicum is a benign rash. The cause is unknown.

A Flat, deep, irregular, localized, pink areas in light-skinned children and deeper-red areas in dark-skinned children are abnormal.

P **Telangiectatic nevi**, commonly known as **stork bites**, appear on the back of the neck, lower occiput, upper eyelids, and upper lip. The cause of telangiectatic nevi is capillary dilatation.

A Diffuse redness, papules, vesicles, edema, scaling, and ulcerations on the area covered by a baby's diaper are abnormal.

P Diaper dermatitis is the result of a bacteria and urea reaction on the skin.

A A dark-black tuft of hair or a dimple over the lumbosacral area is abnormal.

P The neural tube fails to fuse at about the fourth week of gestation and causes a vertebral defect known as spina bifida occulta.

Palpation

Texture

E 1. Use the finger pads to palpate the skin. Refer to Chapter 10.
   2. The technique of palpating the skin of a younger child can be accomplished by playing games. For example, use the finger pads to walk up the abdomen and touch the nose.

N *Skin of the pediatric patient normally is smooth and soft. **Milia**, plugged sebaceous glands, present as small, white papules in the newborn. Milia occur mainly on the head, especially the cheeks and nose. Preterm infants have vernix caseosa.*

A/P Refer to Chapter 10.

Hair
Inspection

Lesions

E/N Refer to Chapter 10.

A Yellow, greasy-appearing scales on the scalp of a light-skinned infant are abnormal. In dark-skinned infants, the scaling is light gray.

P Seborrheic dermatitis (**cradle cap**) is possibly related to increased epidermal tissue growth.

Head
Inspection

Shape and Symmetry

E With the patient sitting upright either in the caregiver's arms or on the examination table, observe the symmetry of the frontal, parietal, and occipital prominences.

E Examination
N Normal Findings
A Abnormal Findings
P Pathophysiology

N *The shape of a child's head is symmetrical without depressions or protrusions. The anterior fontanel normally may pulsate with every heart beat. The Asian infant generally has a flattened occiput, more so than infants of other races.*

A A flattened occipital bone with resultant hair loss over the same area is abnormal.

P A prolonged supine position places pressure on the occipital bone.

Head Control

E 1. Assess head control while the patient is in the position used for assessing shape and symmetry.
2. With the head unsupported, observe the patient's ability to hold the head erect.

N *At 3 months of age, the infant is able to hold the head steady without lag.*

A Lack of head control is evidenced by the infant who is unable to hold the head steady while in a sitting position and is abnormal. Head lag beyond 4 to 6 months of age should be further investigated.

P Documented prematurity, hydrocephalus, and illnesses causing developmental delays are possible causes of head lag.

Palpation

Fontanel

E 1. Place the child in an upright position.
2. Using the second or third finger pad, palpate the anterior fontanel at the junction of the sagittal, coronal, and frontal sutures.
3. Palpate the posterior fontanel at the junction of the sagittal and lambdoidal sutures.
4. Assess for bulging, pulsations, and size. To obtain accurate measurements, the patient should not be crying. Crying will produce a distorted, full, bulging appearance.

N *The anterior fontanel is soft and flat. Size ranges from 4 to 6 centimeters at birth. The fontanel gradually closes between 9 and 19 months of age. The posterior fontanel is also soft and flat. The size ranges from 0.5 to 1.5 centimeters at birth. The posterior fontanel gradually closes between 1 and 3 months of age. It is normal to feel pulsations related to the peripheral pulse.*

A Palpation reveals a bulging, tense fontanel, which is abnormal.

P Signs of increased intracranial pressure are associated with meningitis and an increased amount of CSF.

A A sunken, depressed fontanel is abnormal.

P A sunken, depressed fontanel is a sign of dehydration.

A A wide anterior fontanel in a child older than 2½ years is an abnormal finding.

P An anterior fontanel that remains open after 2½ years of age may indicate disease such as rickets. In rickets, there is a low level of vitamin D relative to decreased phosphate levels.

Suture Lines

E 1. With the finger pads, palpate the sagittal suture line. This runs from the anterior to the posterior portion of the skull in a midline position.
2. Palpate the coronal suture line. This runs along both sides of the head, starting at the anterior fontanel.
3. Palpate the lambdoidal suture. The lambdoidal suture runs along both sides of the head, starting at the posterior fontanel.
4. Ascertain if these suture lines are open, united, or overlapping.

N *Grooves or ridges between sections of the skull are normally palpated up to 6 months of age.*

E	**Examination**
N	**Normal Findings**
A	**Abnormal Findings**
P	**Pathophysiology**

A   Suture lines that overlap or override one another, giving the head an unusual shape, warrant further investigation. See figure 11-7, page 272.

P   **Craniosynostosis** is premature ossification of suture lines, whereby there is early formation and fusion of skull bones. Craniosynostosis may be caused by metabolic disorders or may be a secondary consequence of microcephaly.

Surface Characteristics

E   **1.** With the finger pads, palpate the skull in the same manner as the fontanels and suture lines.
   2. Note surface edema and contour of the cranium.

N   *The skin covering the cranium is flush against the skull and without edema.*

A   A softening of the outer layer of the cranial bones behind and above the ears combined with a ping pong ball sensation as the area is pressed in gently with the fingers is indicative of **craniotabes**, an abnormal finding.

P   Craniotabes is associated with rickets, syphilis, hydrocephaly, or hypervitaminosis A.

A   A localized, subcutaneous swelling over one of the cranial bones of a newborn is referred to as a **cephalhematoma** and is abnormal. This abnormality differs from other surface characteristics in that edema does not cross suture lines with this condition. Varying degrees of swelling can persist up to 3 months.

P   Cephalhematomas acquired during forceps deliveries are due to subperiosteal bleeding and usually resolve within a couple of weeks, but may persist longer.

A   Swelling over the occipitoparietal region of the skull is abnormal.

P   **Caput succedaneum** results from pressure over the occipitoparietal region during a prolonged delivery. It usually resolves within 1 to 2 weeks after birth.

A   **Molding** can occur in conjunction with caput succedaneum.

P   The parietal bone overrides the frontal bone as a result of induced pressure during delivery. It should resolve within 1 week of delivery.

✳ SPECIAL TECHNIQUE

Transillumination of the Skull

Transillumination of the infant's head to rule out hydrocephalus or anencephaly can be performed as a temporary alternative to magnetic resonance imaging (MRI) or computerized tomography (CT) scan if head circumference is not within normal limits.

E   **1.** Support the child in an elevated or sitting position.
   2. Darken the room.
   3. Place a flashlight with a soft, flexible, rubber end directly against the frontal, parietal, and occipital areas of the skull.
   4. Note the size of the light over the various areas.

N   *A normal finding over the frontal and parietal bones is a circle of light no larger than 2 cm around the flashlight. Over the occipital area, a circle of light no larger than 1 cm is considered within normal limits. Normal findings are the same for light- and dark-skinned children.*

A   It is abnormal for the entire cranium to light up.

P   **Anencephaly** is an abnormal finding whereby the cortex or cranium does not develop. The fetal nervous system fails to develop normally. Between the 18th and 24th day of gestation, the neural tube fails to close, resulting in anencephaly. These patients usually do not live more than 24 hours.

E	Examination
N	Normal Findings
A	Abnormal Findings
P	Pathophysiology

Eyes

General Approach

1. From infancy through about 8 to 10 years, you should assess the eyes toward the end of the assessment, with the exception of testing vision, which should be done first. Remember that the child's attention span is short, and attentiveness decreases the longer you evaluate. Children generally are not cooperative for eyes, ears, and throat assessments.

2. Place the young infant, preschooler, school-age, or adolescent patient on the examination table. The older infant or the toddler can be held by the caregiver.

3. Become proficient at performing funduscopic assessments on adults prior to assessing the pediatric patient.

Vision Screening

General Approach

1. The adult Snellen chart can be used on children as young as 6 years, provided they are able to read the alphabet. The Snellen E chart is used for a patient over 3 years of age or any child who cannot read the alphabet.

2. Test every 1 to 2 years through adolescence.

3. If the child resists wearing a cover patch over the eye, make a game out of wearing the patch. For example, the young child could pretend to be a pirate exploring new territory. Use your imagination to think of a fantasy situation.

4. The Allen test (a series of seven pictures on different cards) (Steinslatt, et al., 1994) can be used with children as young as 2 years of age.

Snellen E Chart

E 1. Ask the child to point an arm in the direction the E is pointing.
    2. Observe for squinting.

N *Vision is 20/40 from 2 to approximately 6 years of age, when it approaches the normal 20/20 acuity. Refer the patient to an ophthalmologist if results are 20/40 or greater in a child 3 years of age or 20/30 or greater in a child 6 years or older, or if results are different in each eye.*

A/P Refer to Chapter 12.

Allen Test

E 1. With the child's eyes both open, show each card to the child and elicit a name for each picture. Do not use any pictures with which the child is not familiar. Usually, the only pictures children have difficulty with are the 1940s vintage telephone and the Christmas tree if they belong to a cultural group that does not celebrate this holiday.

    2. Place the 2- to 3-year-old child 15 feet from where you will be standing. Place the 3- to 4-year-old child 20 feet from you.

    3. Ask the caregiver to help cover one of the child's eyes.

    4. With the child's eye covered and the child standing at the appropriate distance listed, show the pictures one at a time, eliciting a response after each showing.

    5. Show the same pictures in different sequence for the other eye.

    6. To record findings, the denominator is always constant at 30, because a child with normal vision should see the picture on the card (target) at 30 feet. To document the numerator, determine the greatest distance at which three of the pictures are recognized by each eye, for example, right eye = 15/30, left eye = 20/30.

N *The child should correctly identify three of the cards in three trials. Two-to three-year-old children should have 15/30 vision. Three- to four-year-old children should be able to achieve a score of 15/30 to 20/30. Each eye should have the same score.*

E	**Examination**
N	**Normal Findings**
A	**Abnormal Findings**
P	**Pathophysiology**

A   If the scores for the patient's right and left eyes differ by 5 feet or more or either or both eyes score less than 15/30, refer the patient to an ophthalmologist.

P   Refer to Chapter 12.

Strabismus Screening

The Hirschberg test and the cover-uncover test screen for strabismus. The latter is the more definitive test.

Hirschberg Test

E/N   Refer to Chapter 12.

A   It is abnormal for the light reflection to be displaced to the outer margin of the cornea as the eye deviates inward (see Figure 23-12).

P   Esotropia is thought to be congenital. Some theories suggest that neurological factors contribute to its development.

A   It is abnormal for the light reflection to be displaced to the inner margin of the cornea as the eye deviates outward.

P   Exotropia can result from eye muscle fatigue or can be congenital.

Cover-Uncover Test

E   Refer to page 741.

N   *Neither eye moves when the occluder is being removed. Infants less than 6 months of age display strabismus due to poor neuromuscular control of eye muscles.*

A   It is abnormal for one or both eyes to move to focus on the penlight during assessment. Assume strabismus is present.

P   Strabismus after 6 months of age is abnormal and indicates eye muscle weakness.

Inspection

Eyelids

E   **1.** Sit at the patient's eye level.
      2. Observe for symmetrical palpebral fissures and position of eyelids in relation to the iris.

N   *The palpebral fissures of both eyes are positioned symmetrically. The upper eyelid normally covers a small portion of the iris, and the lower lid meets the iris. Epicanthal folds are normally present in Asian children.*

A   It is abnormal for a portion of the sclera to be seen above the iris.

P   The sclera is exposed above the iris in hydrocephalus. As the forehead becomes prominent, the eyebrows and eyelids are drawn up, creating a setting sun appearance of the child's eyes.

A   A fold of skin covering the inner canthus and lacrimal caruncle is abnormal.

P   During embryonic development, the fold of skin slants in a downward direction toward the nose. This is found in a child with Down syndrome.

Lacrimal Apparatus

E/N   Refer to Chapter 12.

A   The patient's caregiver reports that the child is unable to produce tears, an abnormal finding.

P   The lacrimal ducts should be open by 3 months of age. Dacryocystitis results when the distal end of the membranous lacrimal duct fails to open or a blockage occurs elsewhere.

Anterior Segment Structures

Sclera

E   Refer to Chapter 12.

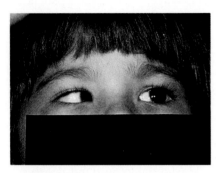

Figure 23-12   Infantile Esotropia
Courtesy of the Armed Forces Institute of Pathology

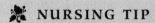
NURSING TIP

Pseudostrabismus

Some infants have an epicanthal fold that gives the false appearance of strabismus. The Hirschberg test reveals a tropia in true strabismus. A tropia is absent in pseudostrabismus.

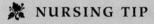
NURSING TIP

Lid Eversion in Children

Lid eversion is not performed in children unless you are assessing for an infection or foreign body. If performed, the technique is the same as for an adult.

E   Examination
N   Normal Findings
A   Abnormal Findings
P   Pathophysiology

N *The newborn exhibits a bluish-tinged sclera related to thinness of the fibrous tissue. The sclera is white in light-skinned children and a slightly darker color in some dark-skinned children.*

A/P Refer to Chapter 12.

Iris

E Conduct the examination in the same manner as for an adult.

N *Up to about 6 months of age, the color of the iris is blue or slate gray in light-skinned infants and brownish in dark-skinned infants. By 12 months of age, complete transition of iris color has occurred.*

A Small white flecks, called **Brushfield's spots**, noted around the perimeter of the iris are abnormal.

P Brushfield's spots are found on the iris of the patient with Down syndrome. The spots develop during embryonic maturation.

Pupils

E Refer to Chapter 12.

N *When the pupils' reaction to light is assessed, a newborn will normally blink and flex the head closer to the body. This is called the optical blink reflex.*

A/P Refer to Chapter 12.

Posterior Segment Structures

General Approach

1. Observe the red reflex, retina, and optic disc.

2. The assessment is easier to accomplish if the infant or toddler is lying supine on an examination table. The assistance of another individual, such as the caregiver, to hold the patient in position is essential. The older patient may be allowed to sit, if cooperative.

Inspection

Red Reflex

E/N Refer to Chapter 12.

A An absent red reflex is abnormal.

P Chromosomal disorders, intrauterine infections, and ocular trauma are possible causes of cataracts in newborns.

A A yellowish or white light reflex (cat's eye reflex) is abnormal.

P Retinoblastoma is a malignant glioma located in the posterior chamber of the eye.

Retina

E/N Refer to Chapter 12.

A A red to dark-red color is abnormal. Some areas may be rounded or flame shaped.

P Hemorrhage is seen in trauma. Bleeding into the optic nerve sheath is found in children who have been physically shaken.

Optic Disc

E/N/A/P Refer to Chapter 12.

E	**Examination**
N	**Normal Findings**
A	**Abnormal Findings**
P	**Pathophysiology**

Ears

Auditory Testing

General Approach

1. Perform auditory testing at about age 3 to 4 years of age or when the child can follow directions. Refer to page 319.

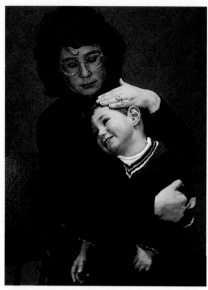

A. Preschooler in a Sitting Position

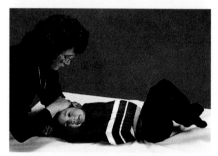

B. Preschooler in a Supine Position

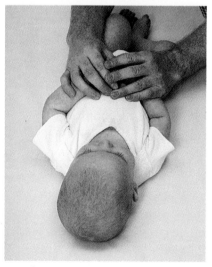

C. Infant

Figure 23-13 Restraining the Child for the Otoscopic Examination

E	Examination
N	Normal Findings
A	Abnormal Findings
P	Pathophysiology

2. Prior to 3 years of age, the following are a few parameters for evaluating hearing.
  a. Does the child react to a loud noise?
  b. Does the child react to the caregiver's voice by cooing, smiling, or turning eyes and head toward the voice?
  c. Does the child try to imitate sounds?
  d. Can the child imitate words and sounds?
  e. Can the child follow directions?
  f. Does the child respond to sounds not directed at him or her?

External Ear

Inspection of Pinna Position

E/N Refer to page 321.

A The top of the ear is below the imaginary line drawn from the outer canthus to the top of the ear.

P Kidneys and ears are formed at the same time in embryonic development. If a child's ears are low set, renal anomalies must be ruled out. Low-set ears can also occur in Down syndrome.

Internal Ear

Inspection

E
  1. A cooperative patient may be allowed to sit for the assessment. A young child may be held as shown in Figure 23-13A.
  2. Restrain the uncooperative young patient by placing him or her supine on a firm surface (see Figure 23-13B). Instruct the caregiver or assistant to hold the patient's arms up near the head, embracing the elbow joints on both sides of either arm. Restrain the infant by having the caregiver hold the infant's hands down (see Figure 23-13C).
  3. With your thumb and forefinger grasping the otoscope, use the lateral side of the hand to prevent the head from jerking. Your other hand can also be used to stabilize the patient's head.
  4. Pull the lower auricle down and out to straighten the canal. This technique is used in children up to about 3 years of age. Use the adult technique after age 3.
  5. Insert the speculum about ¼ to ½ inch, depending on the patient's age.
  6. Suspected otitis media must be evaluated with a pneumatic bulb attached to the side of the otoscope's light source.
  7. Select a larger speculum to make a tight seal and prevent air from escaping from the canal.
  8. If a light reflex is present, focus on the light reflection.
  9. Gently squeeze the bulb attachment to introduce air into the canal. Some nurses prefer to gently blow air through the tubing rather than squeezing air into the canal.
  10. Observe the tympanic membrane for movement.

N/A/P Refer to Chapter 12.

❀ NURSING TIP

False Impression of Otitis Media

If the patient is screaming and crying, a flush or erythema on the tympanic membrane will be present. After allowing the caregiver to comfort the child, attempt to reassess. The flush or erythema can give false impressions of otitis media.

Nose

✸ SPECIAL TECHNIQUE

Assessing for Choanal Atresia

E 1. Select an appropriate-sized catheter (10 to 12 Fr).
2. Place the newborn in a supine position on the examination table.
3. Stand at the newborn's side and use the nondominant hand to hold the newborn's head in a midline position.
4. Use the dominant hand to insert the catheter through the nasal passage and into the nasopharynx.
5. Remove the catheter.
6. Perform the test through the opposite nare to evaluate patency.

N *The catheter does not meet resistance and is able to pass freely to the nasopharynx.*

A Inability to insert the catheter into the nasopharynx coupled with symptoms of snorting respirations, feeding problems, and cyanosis are indicators of choanal atresia, and abnormal.

P An embryological obstruction of bone or membrane causes choanal atresia.

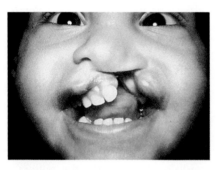

Figure 23-14 Cleft Lip *Courtesy of Dr. Joseph Konzelman, School of Dentistry, Medical College of Georgia*

🌿 NURSING TIP

Fat Intake in Young Children

The caregiver should not restrict or limit fat intake until after 2 years of age because fat is needed for myelin development. After 2 years of age, the caregiver should switch the child to 2% milk; after 6 years of age, a switch to skim milk can be made. Six years of age coincides with the time the brain has achieved its greatest potential for growth (Hahn & Mastrangelo, 1995).

E	**Examination**
N	**Normal Findings**
A	**Abnormal Findings**
P	**Pathophysiology**

Mouth and Throat

Inspection

Lips

E 1. Follow the same technique described in Chapter 12.
2. Observe if the lip edges meet.

N *The lip edges should meet.*

A It is abnormal if the lip edges do not meet.

P Cleft lip is seen as a separated area of lip tissue (see Figure 23-14). It involves the upper lip and sometimes extends into the nostril. A cleft lip is an obvious finding during a newborn assessment. It occurs mainly on the left side and is more frequently found in males. A cleft lip develops during the fifth to sixth week after fertilization. Genetics plays a small role in etiology.

Buccal Mucosa

E Use the same technique as for an adult. If the patient is unable to open the mouth on command, use the edge of a tongue blade to lift the upper lip and move the lower lip down.

N *Refer to Chapter 12.*

A A thick, curdlike coating on the buccal mucosa or tongue is abnormal.

P Thrush can be acquired when a newborn passes through the vagina during delivery.

Teeth

E/N Refer to Chapter 12.

A A lack of visible teeth coupled with roentgenographic findings revealing absence of tooth buds is abnormal.

P Absence of deciduous teeth beyond 16 months of age signifies an abnormality most commonly related to genetic causes.

A It is abnormal for the teeth to turn brownish black, possibly with indentations along the surfaces of the teeth.

P Carbohydrate-rich fluid (from milk or juice) causes severe caries when a child falls asleep with a bottle in the mouth (Jones, Berg, & Coody, 1994).

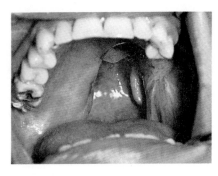

Figure 23-15 Cleft Palate *Courtesy of Dr. Joseph Konzelman, School of Dentistry, Medical College of Georgia*

🌸 **NURSING TIP**

Preventing Choking in Children

The infant's or toddler's airway is small, approximately the size of their "pinky" fingers. Fresh grapes, uncut hot dogs with the skin on, popcorn, and peanuts are common foods that can cause choking. These foods should not be given to young children.

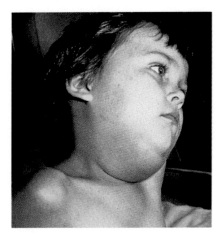

Figure 23-16 Parotitis (Mumps) *Courtesy of the Centers for Disease Control and Prevention (CDC)*

E   Examination

N   Normal Findings

A   Abnormal Findings

P   Pathophysiology

Hard/Soft Palate

E   1. Observe the palate for continuity and shape.

   2. For infants, you will need to use a tongue depressor to push the tongue down. Infants usually cry in response to this action, which allows visualization of the palates.

N   *The roof of the mouth is continuous and has a slight arch.*

A   It is abnormal if the roof of the mouth is not continuous. This anomaly is called cleft palate (see Figure 23-15).

P   Cleft palates vary greatly in size and extent of malformation. The degree of malformation is classified into two groups. A midline malformation may involve the uvula or extend through the soft or hard palates or both. If associated with cleft lip, the malformation may extend through the palates and into the nasal cavity. Cleft palates form between the sixth and tenth week of embryonic development, during fusion of the maxillary and premaxillary processes. Genetics plays a small role in etiology.

A   The roof of the mouth is abnormally arched. On inspection, the shape resembles an upside down letter V.

P   High palates are usually associated with a particular syndrome. Common examples include trisomy 18 and Noonan's syndrome.

A   **Epstein's pearls** in the newborn appear on the hard palate and gum margins and are abnormal. The pearls are small, white cysts that feel hard when palpated.

P   These cysts result from fragments of epithelial tissue trapped during palate formation.

Oropharynx

E   Refer to Chapter 12.

N   *Up to the age of 12 years, a tonsil grade of 2+ is considered normal. Around puberty, tonsillar tissue regresses. Tonsils should not interfere with the act of breathing.*

A   Excessive salivation is an early sign of a tracheoesophageal fistula (TEF). Drooling is accompanied by choking and coughing during the patient's feeding.

P   The esophagus failed to develop as a continuous passage during embryonic formation.

Neck

Inspection

General Appearance

E   1. Observe the neck in a midline position while the patient is sitting upright.

   2. Note shortening or thickness of the neck on both right and left sides.

   3. Note any swelling.

N   *There is a reasonable amount of skin tissue on the sides of the neck. There is no swelling.*

A   Additional weblike tissue found bilaterally from the ear to the shoulder is abnormal.

P   Webbed necks are associated with congenital syndromes. One example is Turner's syndrome, noted in female children.

A   Unilateral or bilateral swelling of the neck below the angle of the jaw is abnormal (see Figure 23-16).

P   Enlargement of the parotid gland occurs in parotitis, or mumps, an inflammation of the parotid gland. There is pain and tenderness in the affected area.

Palpation

Thyroid

E **1.** Use the same technique as for an adult with the exception of using the first two finger pads on both hands.

2. Have the younger child who is unable to swallow on command take a drink from a bottle.

N/A/P The normal findings, abnormal findings, and pathophysiology are the same as for an adult.

Lymph Nodes

E **1.** Because of the infant's short neck, you must extend the chin upward with your hand before proceeding with palpation.

2. With the finger pads, palpate the submental, submandibular, tonsillar, anterior cervical chain, posterior cervical chain, supraclavicular, preauricular, posterior auricular, and occipital lymph nodes.

3. Use a circular motion. Note location, size, shape, tenderness, mobility, and associated skin inflammation of any swollen nodes palpated.

N *Lymph nodes are generally not palpable. Children often have small, movable, cool, nontender nodes referred to as "shotty" nodes. These benign nodes are related to environmental antigen exposure or residual effects of a prior illness and have no clinical significance.*

A Enlargement of the anterior cervical chain is abnormal.

P This occurs in bacterial infections of the pharynx, such as strep throat.

A Enlargement of the occipital nodes or posterior cervical chain nodes is abnormal.

P This can occur in tinea capitis and acute otitis externa.

Breasts

Inspection of the breasts is performed throughout childhood. Palpation is not usually performed on the patient until puberty, unless otherwise indicated.

Thorax and Lungs

General Approach

1. Remove the patient's clothes or gown.

2. Keep the infant warm during the assessment by placing a blanket over the chest until ready for this portion of assessment.

Inspection

Shape of Thorax

E Refer to Chapter 14.

N *The infant has a barrel chest; by age 6, the chest attains the adult configuration.*

A If a school-age child has an abnormal chest configuration, suspect pathology.

P In addition to the conditions discussed in Chapter 14, CF can lead to an altered anteroposterior-transverse diameter.

Retractions

E **1.** In children, it is important to evaluate intercostal muscles for signs of increased work of breathing.

2. If at all possible, perform this examination when the patient is quiet because forceful crying will mimic retractions.

N/A/P Refer to Chapter 14.

E Examination
N Normal Findings
A Abnormal Findings
P Pathophysiology

Palpation

Tactile Fremitus

Fremitus is easily felt when a child cries. If the infant or young patient is not crying, it is advisable to defer this procedure until later in the assessment, perhaps after the throat and ears examinations, which usually produce crying.

Percussion

E Refer to Chapter 14.

N *Normal diaphragmatic excursion in infants and young toddlers is one to two intercostal spaces.*

A/P Refer to Chapter 14.

Auscultation

Breath Sounds

E Use the same assessment techniques as for an adult. Sometimes, it is difficult to differentiate the various adventitious sounds because a child's respiratory rate is rapid; for example, differentiating expiratory wheezing from inspiratory wheezing can be difficult. Mastering the technique takes time and practice.

N *Of the three types of breath sounds — bronchial, bronchovesicular, and vesicular — the bronchovesicular are normally heard throughout the peripheral lung fields up to 5 to 6 years of age, because the chest wall is thin with decreased musculature. Lung fields are clear and equal bilaterally.*

A Crackles are abnormal.

P Conditions such as bronchiolitis, CF, and bronchopulmonary dysplasia produce crackles.

A Wheezing is abnormal; however during infancy and early childhood, it may be common.

P Patients with CF and bronchiolitis may present with wheezing.

> ⚡ **NURSING ALERT**
>
> ***Stridor in Children***
>
> Stridor is indicative of upper airway obstruction, particularly edema in children. Inspiration accentuates stridorous sounds. To prevent medical emergencies such as epiglottitis, prompt attention must be sought for children who present with stridor.

Heart and Peripheral Vasculature

General Approach

1. It is best to perform the cardiac assessment near the beginning of the examination, when the infant or young child is relatively calm.

2. Do not get discouraged during the assessment. The novice nurse is not expected to identify a murmur and location within the cardiac cycle. Be patient because skill will come only with practice.

3. During the assessment, note physical signs of a syndrome such as Down's facies in a child with trisomy 21 or Down syndrome. Many children with Down syndrome have associated atrioventricular (A-V) canal malformations. These defects each involve an atrial septal defect (ASD), ventricular septal defect (VSD), and a common A-V valve.

4. Cardiac landmarks change when a child has dextrocardia. In this condition, the apex of the heart points toward the right thoracic cavity, thus heart sounds are auscultated primarily on the right side of the chest.

> **E** Examination
> **N** Normal Findings
> **A** Abnormal Findings
> **P** Pathophysiology

Inspection

Apical Impulse

E Refer to Chapter 15.

N *In both infants and toddlers, the apical impulse is located at the fourth intercostal space and just left of the midclavicular line. The apical impulse*

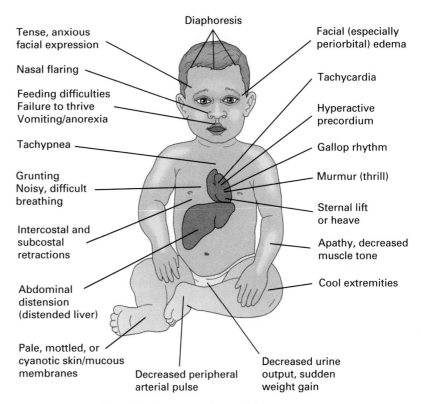

Tense, anxious facial expression

Nasal flaring

Feeding difficulties
Failure to thrive
Vomiting/anorexia

Tachypnea

Grunting
Noisy, difficult
breathing

Intercostal and
subcostal
retractions

Abdominal
distension
(distended liver)

Pale, mottled, or
cyanotic skin/mucous
membranes

Diaphoresis

Facial (especially
periorbital) edema

Tachycardia

Hyperactive
precordium

Gallop rhythm

Murmur (thrill)

Sternal lift
or heave

Apathy, decreased
muscle tone

Cool extremities

Decreased peripheral
arterial pulse

Decreased urine
output, sudden
weight gain

Figure 23-17   Infant with Congestive Heart Failure

of a child 7 years or older is at the fifth intercostal space and to the right of the midclavicular line. The impulse may not be visible in all children, especially in those who have increased adipose tissue or muscle.

A/P   Refer to Chapter 15.

Precordium

E   Observe the chest wall for any movements other than the apical impulse.
N   *Movements other than the apical impulse are abnormal.*
A   Lifting of the cardiac area is abnormal.
P   Heaves are associated with volume overload. A child with congenital heart disease is at risk for developing congestive heart failure (CHF) with associated volume overload. Figure 23-17 depicts the manifestations of CHF in children. Large left-to-right shunt defects, such as a VSD, cause right ventricular volume overload.

Palpation

Thrill

E   1. Palpate as for an adult or use the proximal one-third of each finger and the areas over the metacarpophalangeal joints. Many nurses feel the latter method yields greater sensitivity to the presence of thrills.
   2. Place the hand vertically along the heart's apex and move the hand toward the sternum.
   3. Place the hand horizontally along the sternum, moving up the sternal border about ½ inch to 1 inch each time.
   4. When at the clavicular level, place the hand vertically and assess for a thrill at the heart's base.
   5. Use the finger pads to palpate a thrill at the suprasternal notch and along the carotid arteries.
N   *A thrill is not found in the healthy child.*
A/P   Refer to Chapter 15.

E   Examination
N   Normal Findings
A   Abnormal Findings
P   Pathophysiology

Peripheral Pulses

E 1. Use the same finger to assess each peripheral pulse. The sensation of one finger pad versus another can be different.
   2. Use the finger pads to palpate each pair of peripheral pulses simultaneously, except for the carotid pulse.
   3. Palpate the brachial and femoral pulses simultaneously.

N *Pulse qualities are the same in the adult and the child.*

A A brachial-femoral lag, when femoral pulses are weaker than brachial pulses when palpated simultaneously, is abnormal.

P Coarctation is due to a narrowing of the aorta before, at, or just beyond the entrance of the ductus arteriosus. Thus, blood flow to the lower body is reduced.

Auscultation

Heart Sounds

Auscultating the infant's or the young pediatric patient's heart is difficult because the heart rate is rapid and breath sounds are easily transmitted through the chest wall.

E 1. Have the child lie down. If this position is not possible, the child should be held at a 45° angle in the caregiver's arms.
   2. Use the Z pattern to auscultate the heart. Place the stethoscope in the apical area and gradually move it toward the right lower sternal border and up the sternal border in a right diagonal line. Move gradually from the patient's left to the right upper sternal borders (see Figure 23-18).
   3. Perform a second evaluation with the child in a sitting position.

N *Fifty percent of all children develop an innocent murmur at some time in their lives. Innocent murmurs are accentuated in high cardiac output states such as fever. When the patient is sitting, they are heard early in systole at the second or third intercostal space along the left sternal border and are softly musical in quality; they disappear when the patient lies down. Be aware of sinus arrhythmias during auscultation of the heart's rhythm. On inspiration, the pulse rate speeds up, the pulse rate slows with expiration. To determine if the rhythm is normal, ask the child to hold his or her breath while you auscultate the heart. If the pulse stops, then a sinus arrhythmia is present. S_1 is best heard at the apex of the heart, left lower sternal border. S_2 is best heard at the heart base.*

A A split S_2 sound is abnormal.

P If the S_2 split is fixed with the act of respiration, you can suspect an atrial septal defect. In children, S_2 physiologically splits with inspiration and becomes single with expiration. This phenomenon is due to a greater negative pressure in the thoracic cavity.

A In children, S_3 often sounds like the three syllables of the word "Kentucky," especially when accompanied by tachycardia.

P A loud third heart sound may be present in children with CHF or VSDs.

A Holosystolic murmurs are heard maximally at the left lower sternal border. They begin with S_1 and continue until the second heart sound, S_2, is heard.

P Holosystolic or pansystolic murmurs are heard in children with VSDs, where blood flows from a chamber of higher pressure to one of lower pressure during systole.

A Continuous murmurs heard throughout the cardiac cycle are abnormal.

P Collateral blood flow murmurs are heard radiating throughout the back, such as in pulmonary atresia with a VSD.

P Continuous murmurs are present in coronary artery fistulas.

P Palliative shunt murmurs are normal and should be heard; if they are not heard, there is a possibility of a clotted shunt. These murmurs are heard over the right or left upper chest in the respective area where surgically placed. A palliative shunt is created temporarily until the patient is ready for corrective surgery. A palliative shunt may be needed in a small infant

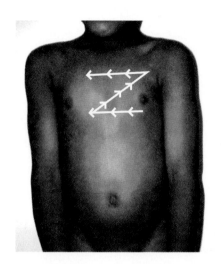

Figure 23-18 Z Auscultation Pattern for Young Children

E	**Examination**
N	**Normal Findings**
A	**Abnormal Findings**
P	**Pathophysiology**

with a combination of tetralogy of Fallot and pulmonary atresia or a hypoplastic pulmonary artery.

✳ SPECIAL TECHNIQUE

Assessing for Coarctation of the Aorta

If coarctation of the aorta is suspected (as when a brachial-femoral lag is present), obtain all four extremity blood pressures and compare the upper and lower extremity readings on each side.

E
1. Place the child on the examination table or caregiver's lap in either a sitting or a supine position.
2. Use the same technique as is used for taking an adult's blood pressure. Remember to use an appropriate-sized cuff. The width of the inflatable cuff should be one-half to two-thirds the length of the upper arm or lower leg.
3. Take the upper extremity blood pressure in the right arm.
4. Because weak or absent leg pulses accompany coarctation, measurements are difficult to obtain. Use a Doppler transducer to intensify the sound of the pulse. Until you feel proficient, the Doppler technique requires two people for accurate measurement; have the caregiver hold the child's leg still while you assess the pulse.
5. Locate the posterior tibial pulse with the Doppler transducer and make an "X" with a pen where the pulse is felt or heard.
6. Place an appropriate-sized cuff on the lower right leg. The lower edge of the cuff should be ½ inch to 1 inch above the presumed posterior tibial pulse location.
7. Apply a small amount of ultrasound gel to the area surrounding the presumed pulse.
8. Turn the Doppler transducer on and adjust the volume control while the attached probe is locating the pulse.
9. When a pulse is identified, proceed with the blood pressure measurement. Only the systolic number is obtained with this technique.
10. Repeat the steps on the left side of body.

N *Upper and lower extremity blood pressures are equal.*

A If the systolic blood pressure in the leg is lower than that in the arm and femoral, popliteal, posterior tibial, or dorsalis pedis pulses are weak or absent, you can assume coarctation of the aorta is present. If undiagnosed, as the child becomes older, the upper extremity pulses are bounding.

P During the fifth or sixth week of embryonic development, the aorta may form abnormally.

Abdomen

General Approach

1. If possible, ask the caregiver to refrain from feeding the infant prior to the assessment because palpation of a full stomach may induce vomiting.
2. Children who are physically able should be encouraged to empty the bladder prior to the assessment.
3. The young infant, school-age child, or adolescent should lie on the examination table. For the toddler or preschooler, have the caregiver hold the child supine on the lap, with the lower extremities bent at the knees and dangling.
4. If the child is crying, encourage the caregiver to help calm the child before you proceed with the assessment.

E	**Examination**
N	**Normal Findings**
A	**Abnormal Findings**
P	**Pathophysiology**

E   Examination
N   Normal Findings
A   Abnormal Findings
P   Pathophysiology

5. Observe nonverbal communication in children who are not able to verbally express feelings. During palpation, listen for a high-pitched cry and look for a change in facial expression or for sudden protective movements that may indicate a painful or tender area.

Inspection

Contour
E   Refer to Chapter 16.
N   *The young child may have a "potbelly."*
A/P   Refer to Chapter 16.

Peristaltic Wave
E/N   Refer to Chapter 16.
A   Visible peristaltic waves seen moving across the epigastrium from left to right are abnormal.
P   Obstruction at the pyloric sphincter causes a condition called pyloric stenosis. The pyloric muscle hypertrophies, causing obstruction during embryonic development.

Auscultation

After performing auscultation of the lungs, it is helpful to proceed to auscultating the abdomen because doing so allows you to complete a good portion of auscultation all at once. If the child is not cooperating, a simple distracting phrase such as "I can hear your breakfast in there" is helpful during auscultation.

Palpation

General Palpation
E/N   Refer to Chapter 16.
A   On palpation, an olive-shaped mass felt in the epigastric area and to the upper right of the umbilicus is abnormal.
P   This is indicative of pyloric stenosis. Refer to peristaltic wave, above.
A   Abdominal distension coupled with palpable stool over the abdomen and the absence of stool in the rectum is abnormal.
P   An aganglionic segment of the colon is responsible for Hirschsprung's disease, which produces abnormal gastrointestinal findings.
A   A sausage-shaped mass that produces intermittent pain when palpated in the upper abdomen is abnormal.
P   There is no clear cause of **intussusception**. Most commonly, the ileocecal region of the intestine telescopes down into the ileum itself. Classic symptoms are vomiting and currant jelly stools.
A   Bowel sounds heard in the thoracic cavity, a scaphoid abdomen, an upward displaced apical impulse, and signs of respiratory distress are abnormal findings in the newborn.
P   Approximately in the eighth week of embryonic development, the diaphragm fails to fuse, creating a **diaphragmatic hernia**. This condition results in protrusion of the intestines into the thoracic cavity.

Liver Palpation
E   For infants and toddlers, use the outer edge of your right thumb to press down and scoop up at the right upper quadrant. For the remaining age groups, use the same technique as for an adult.
N   *The liver is not normally palpated, although the liver edge can be found 1 to 2 cm below the right costal margin in a normal, healthy child. The liver edge is soft and regular.*
A   It is abnormal for the liver edge to be palpated more than 2 cm below the right costal margin and be full with a firm, sharp border.

P Hepatomegaly occurs in several disease states such as viral or bacterial illnesses, tumors, congestive heart failure, and fat and glycogen storage diseases. Viral and bacterial illnesses and tumors cause liver cells to multiply in number, creating an enlarged liver. In heart failure, the hepatic veins and sinusoids enlarge from congestion, resulting in hemorrhage and fibrosis of the liver. In fat and glycogen storage diseases, fat and glycogen accumulate within the liver, and fibrosis ensues.

Musculoskeletal System

General Approach

1. The extent or degree of assessment depends greatly on the patient's or caregiver's complaints of musculoskeletal problems. Be aware that during periods of rapid growth, children complain of normal muscle aches.

2. Try to incorporate musculoskeletal assessment techniques into other system assessments. For instance, while inspecting the integument, inspect the muscles and joints.

3. Inspecting the musculoskeletal system in the ambulatory child is accomplished by allowing the child to move freely about and play in the examination room while you inquire about the health history. Your observations of the child enable you to assess posture, muscle symmetry, and range of motion of muscles and joints.

4. Do not rush through the assessment. Throughout the assessment, incorporate game playing that facilitates evaluation of the musculoskeletal system.

5. Observe range of motion and joint flexibility as the child undresses.

Inspection

Muscles

E 1. Until the lower spine or hips need evaluation, have the child disrobe down to a diaper or underwear.
   2. To evaluate the small infant's shoulder muscles, place your hands under the axillae and pull the infant into a standing position. The infant should not slip through your hands. Be prepared to catch the infant if needed.
   3. Evaluate the infant's leg strength in a semi-standing position. Lower the infant to the examination table so the infant's legs touch the table.
   4. Place the infant older than 4 months in a prone position. Observe the infant's ability to lift the upper body off the examination table using the upper extremities.

N *Degree of joint flexibility and range of motion are the same for the child as for the adult.*

A Increased muscle tone (spasticity) is abnormal.

P Cerebral palsy (CP) results from a nonprogressive abnormality in the pyramidal motor tract. One of the more common contributing factors, perinatal asphyxia, causes abnormal posture and gross motor development and varying degrees of abnormal muscle tone.

A The inability to rise from a sitting to a standing position is abnormal. In attempting to rise from a supine position, the child first turns over onto the abdomen and raises the trunk to a crawling position. Then, with the aid of the arms, the child places the feet firmly on the floor and gradually elevates the upper part of the body by climbing up the legs with the arms.

P This is called Gower's sign. Gower's sign occurs in Duchenne's muscular dystrophy (MD) early in childhood. Genetics is responsible for the abnormality, in the short arm of the X chromosome.

E Examination
N Normal Findings
A Abnormal Findings
P Pathophysiology

Joints

E Refer to Chapter 17.

N *The infant's spine is C-shaped. Head control and standing create the normal S-shaped spine of the adult. Lordosis is normal as the child begins to walk. A toddler's protruding abdomen is counterbalanced by an inward deviation of the lumbar spine.*

A Extra fingers or toes are abnormal.

P Supernumerary digits, or polydactyly, may be found in certain congenital syndromes such as Carpenter's, fetal hydantoin, orofaciodigital, Smith-Lemli-Opitz, trisomy 13, and Vatar's.

A A fusion between two or more digits is abnormal.

P Syndactylism is also associated with certain congenital syndromes such as Aarskog, Apert's, Carpenter's, orofaciodigital, Russell-Silver, and acrocephalosyndactyly. Look for other physical signs of a syndrome if either syndactyly or polydactyly is present.

A It is abnormal for a young male (usually 2 to 12 years old) to present with a painless limp from the affected hip. The limp is accompanied by limited abduction and internal rotation, muscle spasm, and proximal thigh atrophy.

P Legg-Calvé-Perthes disease, also called coxa plana, is caused by an interruption in the blood supply to the capital femoral epiphysis. Avascular necrosis of the femoral head results.

A An exaggerated lumbar curvature of the spine is abnormal after 6 years of age.

P Lordosis can be attributed to bilateral developmental dislocation of the hip or postural factors such as progression of congenital kyphosis, or can occur secondary to contractures of hip flexors.

Tibiofemoral Bones

E 1. Instruct the child to stand on the examination table and with the medial condyles together.
2. Stand at eye level of the patient's knees.
3. Measure the distance between the two medial malleoli.
4. Measure the distance between the two medial condyles.

N *The distance between the medial malleoli is less than 2 inches (5 cm). The distance between the medial condyles is less than 1 inch (2.5 cm). Knock-knee, or genu valgum, is common between 2 and 4 years of age. Bowleg, or genu varum, is normally present in many infants up to 12 months of age.*

A Genu valgum persisting after 6 years of age is abnormal. The distance between the medial condyles is less than 1 inch (2.5 cm) and the distance between the medial malleoli is more than 2 inches (5 cm).

P The cause of genu valgum is usually physiological.

A The measured distance between the two medial condyles is greater than 1 to 2 inches.

P Genu varum persisting after 2 years of age is abnormal and may be caused by rickets.

Palpation

Joints

E/N Refer to Chapter 17.

A Knee pain aggravated by any motion or activity that puts undue pressure on the joint is abnormal. Palpation of a slight elevation of the tibial tuberosity is abnormal.

P The deformed tubercle in Osgood-Schlatter disease is caused by repetitive stress on the area. A fibrocartilage microfracture may cause joint pain.

A Swollen, inflamed, painful joints are abnormal.

P Juvenile rheumatoid arthritis causes synovial inflammation and degeneration of the joint. Its cause is unknown.

E	Examination
N	Normal Findings
A	Abnormal Findings
P	Pathophysiology

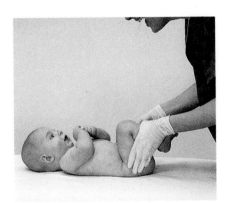

A. Hand Placement

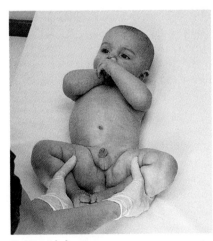

B. Hip Abduction

Figure 23-19 Ortolani Maneuver

E	**Examination**
N	**Normal Findings**
A	**Abnormal Findings**
P	**Pathophysiology**

Feet

E
1. Place the patient on the examination table or caregiver's lap.
2. Stand in front of the child.
3. Hold the right heel immobile with one hand while pushing the forefoot (medial base of great toe) toward a midline position with the other hand.
4. Observe for toe and forefoot adduction and inversion.
5. Repeat on the left foot.

N *The toes and forefoot are not deviated.*

A Medially adducted and inverted toes and forefoot are abnormal.

P **Metatarsus varus (club foot)** usually results from an abnormal intrauterine position of the fetal foot. Heredity also plays a role in the etiology.

Hip and Femur

Ortolani's maneuver is always performed at the very end of the assessment because it may produce crying. The test is performed on one hip at a time. Evaluate the hips up until 12 months of age.

E
1. Place the infant supine on an examination table with the feet facing you.
2. Stand directly in front of the infant.
3. With the thumb, hold the lesser trochanter of the femur and with the middle and third fingers, hold the greater trochanter (see Figure 23-19A). These two fingers should rest over the hip joint.
4. Slowly press outward and abduct until the lateral aspects of the knees nearly touch the table (see Figure 23-19B). The tips of the fingers should palpate each femora's head as it rotates outward.
5. Listen for an audible clunk (Ortolani's sign).
6. With the fingers in the same locations, adduct the hips to elicit a palpable clunk (Ortolani's sign). As each hip is adducted, it is lifted anteriorly into the acetabulum.

N *A clunk is not audible or palpated.*

A Abnormal findings include a positive Ortolani's sign; a sudden, painful cry during the test; asymmetrical thigh skin folds; uneven knee level; and limited hip abduction.

P Epidemiology of **developmental dislocation of the hip (DDH)** is related to familial factors, maternal hormones associated with pelvic laxity, firstborn children, and breech presentations.

Neurological System

General Approach

1. Some aspects of the neurological assessment are different for the infant and the young child as compared to the adult. An infant functions mainly at the subcortical level. Memory and motor coordination are about three-fourths developed by 2 years of age, when cortical functioning is acquiring dominance.

2. Incorporate findings for fine and gross motor skills previously tested during the musculoskeletal assessment. In addition, use the Denver II to assess personal-social and language skills. Refer to normal developmental milestones (see Chapter 4) and extrapolate warning signs of neurological development lag.

3. Because the infant cannot verbally express level of consciousness, instead assess the newborn's ability to cry, level of activity, positioning, and general appearance.

4. Only reflex mechanisms and cranial nerve testing is described in this section. Refer to the adult neurological assessment for all other testing.

Reflex Mechanisms of the Infant

Neonatal reflexes must be lost before motor development can proceed.

Rooting Reflex

E 1. Place the infant supine with the head in a midline position.
2. With your forefinger, stroke the skin located at one corner of the mouth (see Figure 23-20).
3. Observe movement of the head.

N *Up until 3 or 4 months of age, the infant will turn the head toward the side that was stroked. In the sleeping infant, the rooting reflex can be present normally until 6 months of age.*

A An absent rooting reflex from birth through 3 to 4 months is abnormal.

P Central nervous system disease such as frontal lobe lesions accounts for an absent rooting reflex.

Sucking Reflex

E 1. Place the infant in a supine position.
2. With your forefinger, touch the infant's lips to stimulate a response (see Figure 23-21).
3. Observe for a sucking motion.

N *The sucking reflex occurs up to approximately 10 months.*

A Absence of the sucking reflex is abnormal.

P A premature infant or a breast-fed infant of a mother who ingests barbiturates does not exhibit the reflex secondary to CNS depression.

Palmar Grasp Reflex

E 1. Place the infant supine with the head in a midline position.
2. Place the ulnar sides of both index fingers into the infant's hands while the infant's arms are in a semi-flexed position (see Figure 23-22).
3. Press your fingers into the infant's palmar surfaces.

N *Normally, the infant grasps your fingers in flexion.*

A Presence of the palmar grasp reflex after 4 months of age is abnormal.

P The etiology is attributed to frontal lobe lesions.

Tonic Neck Reflex

E 1. Place the infant in a supine position on the examination table.
2. Rotate the head to one side and hold the jaw area parallel to the shoulder.
3. Observe for movement of the extremities.

N *The upper and lower extremities on the side to which the jaw is turned extend, and the opposite arm and leg flex (see Figure 23-23). Sometimes, this reflex does not show up until 6 to 8 weeks of age.*

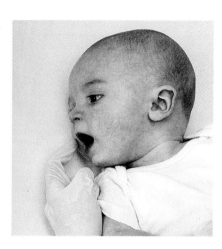

Figure 23-20   Rooting Reflex

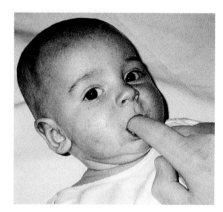

Figure 23-21   Sucking Reflex

E Examination
N Normal Findings
A Abnormal Findings
P Pathophysiology

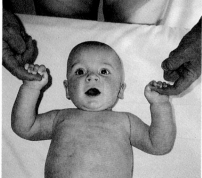

Figure 23-22   Palmar Reflex

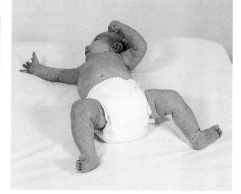

Figure 23-23   Tonic Neck Reflex

A After 6 months of age, the tonic neck reflex is abnormal.

P Cerebral damage is suspected if the tonic neck reflex is seen after 6 months of age.

Stepping Reflex

E 1. Stand behind the infant, grasp the infant under the axillae, and bring the body to a standing position on a flat surface. Use the thumbs to support the back of the head if needed.

2. Push the infant's feet toward a flat surface and simultaneously lean the infant's body forward (see Figure 23-24).

3. Observe the legs and feet for stepping movements.

N *Stepping movements are made by flexing one leg and moving the other leg forward. This reflex disappears at about 3 months of age.*

A Presence of the stepping reflex beyond 3 months of age is abnormal.

P Patients with CP demonstrate a stepping reflex beyond 3 months of age.

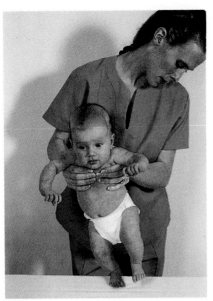

Figure 23-24 Stepping Reflex

Plantar Grasp Reflex

E 1. Position the infant supine on the examination table.

2. Elevate the foot to be examined.

3. Touch the infant's foot on the plantar surface beneath the toes (see Figure 23-25).

4. Repeat on the other side.

N *The toes curl down until 8 months of age.*

A It is abnormal for the plantar grasp reflex to be absent on one or both feet.

P An obstructive lesion such as an abscess or tumor can cause the plantar grasp reflex to be absent on the affected side. Bilateral absence can occur in CP.

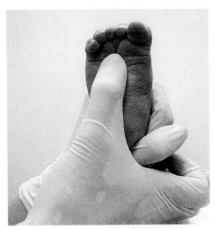

Figure 23-25 Plantar Grasp Reflex

Babinski's Reflex

E 1. Position the infant supine on the examination table.

2. Elevate the foot to be examined.

3. Stroke the plantar surface of the foot from the lateral heel upward with the tip of the thumbnail.

N *A child less than 15 to 18 months of age normally fans the toes outward and dorsiflexes the great toe (see Figure 23-26).*

A After the child masters walking, presence of Babinski's reflex is abnormal.

P Presence of Babinski's reflex after 18 months of age can be indicative of a perinatal insult such as cerebral palsy.

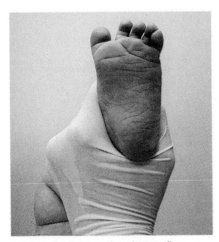

Figure 23-26 Babinski's Reflex

Moro (Startle) Reflex

E 1. Place the infant supine on the examination table.

2. Make a sudden loud noise such as hitting your hand on the examination table.

3. Another technique is to brace the infant's neck and back on the undersurface of your arm while holding the undersurface of the buttocks with the other hand and then mimicing a falling motion by quickly lowering the infant.

N *The infant under 4 months of age quickly extends then flexes the arms and fingers while the maneuver is performed. The thumb and index fingers form a C shape (see Figure 23-27).*

A Presence of the startle reflex after 4 to 6 months of age is abnormal.

P Neurological disease such as CP can be a cause of a positive response after the normal age of disappearance.

E	**Examination**
N	**Normal Findings**
A	**Abnormal Findings**
P	**Pathophysiology**

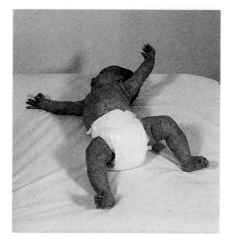

Figure 23-27 Moro Reflex

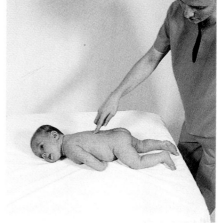

Figure 23-28 Gallant Reflex

Gallant Reflex

E **1.** Place the infant prone, with the infant's hands under the abdomen.
 2. Use your index finger to stroke the skin along the side of the spine (see Figure 23-28).
 3. Observe the stimulated side for any movement.
N *An infant less than 1 to 2 months of age will turn the pelvis and shoulders toward the stimulated side.*
A Lack of response from an infant less than 2 months of age is abnormal.
P A spinal cord lesion is suspected.

Placing Reflex

Do not test the placing and stepping reflexes at the same time because they are two different reflexes.

E **1.** Grasp the infant under the axillae from behind and bring the body to a standing position. Use the thumbs to support the back of the head if needed.
 2. Touch the dorsum of one foot to the edge of the examination table (see Figure 23-29).
 3. Observe the tested leg for movement.
N *The infant's tested leg will flex and lift onto the examination table.*
A Lack of response is abnormal.
P It is difficult to elicit this reflex in breech-born babies and in those with paralysis or cerebral cortex abnormalities.

Landau Reflex

E **1.** Carefully suspend the infant in a prone position, supporting the chest with your hand.
 2. Observe for extension of the head, trunk, and hips.
N *The arms and legs extend during the reflex. The reflex appears at about 3 months of age.*
A Presence of the Landau reflex beyond 2 years of age is abnormal. Also, it is abnormal for the infant to assume a limp position.
P Mental retardation may account for an abnormality.

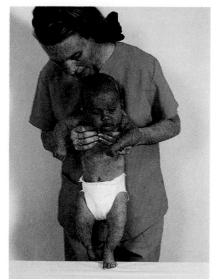

Figure 23-29 Placing Reflex

Cranial Nerve Function

A thorough assessment of cranial nerve function is difficult to perform on the infant less than 1 year old. Difficulty is also encountered with toddlers and preschoolers because they often cannot follow directions or are not willing to cooperate. Testing for the school-age child or the adolescent is carried out in the same manner as for an adult.

E	Examination
N	Normal Findings
A	Abnormal Findings
P	Pathophysiology

Infant (Birth to 12 Months)

E 1. To test cranial nerves (CNs) III, IV, and VI, move a brightly colored toy along the infant's line of vision. An infant older than 1 month responds by following the object. Also evaluate the pupillary response to a bright light in each eye.
2. CN V is tested by assessing the rooting or sucking reflexes.
3. CN VII is tested up until 2 months by assessng the sucking reflex and by observing symmetrical sucking movements. After 2 months of age, an infant will smile, allowing assessment of symmetry of facial expressions.
4. A positive Moro reflex in an infant less than 6 months old is evidence of normal functioning of CN VIII.
5. CNs IX and X are examined by using a tongue blade to produce a gag reflex. Do not test if a positive response was already elicited by using a tongue blade to view the posterior pharynx.
6. To test Cranial Nerve XI, evaluate the infant's ability to lift the head up while in a prone position.
7. CN XII is as assessed by allowing the infant to suck on a pacifier or a bottle, abruptly removing the pacifier or bottle from the infant's mouth, and observing for lingering sucking movements.

N/A/P Refer to Chapter 18.

Toddler and Preschooler (1 to 5 Years)

E 1. The older preschooler is able to identify familiar odors. Most children readily identify the smell of peanut butter and chocolate. Test CN I one side at a time by asking the child to close the eyes and to identify the smell of peanut butter and chocolate. Test each nostril with different substances while occluding the other nostril with your finger.
2. Test vision (CN II) using Allen cards. Refer to page 741.
3. CNs III, IV, and VI are tested in the same fashion as for the infant.
4. CN V is tested by giving the child something to eat and evaluating chewing movements. Sensory responses to light and sharp touch are still not easily interpreted in these age groups.
5. Observe facial weakness or paralysis (CN VII) by making the child smile or laugh. An older preschooler may cooperate by raising the eyebrows, frowning, puffing the cheeks out, and closing the eyes tightly on command.
6. To evaluate CN VIII, ring a small bell out of the child's vision and observe the response to unseen sounds.
7. Test CNs IX and X in the same manner as for the infant.
8. CN XII is difficult to assess in this particular age group.

N/A/P Refer to Chapter 18

Female Genitalia

General Approach

1. Place the up-to-preschool-age child on the caregiver's lap or examination table. Ask caregiver to assist by holding the legs in a froglike position. Place the child older than 4 years on the examination table in a semi-lithotomy position, without the feet in stirrups. Reserve the lithotomy position with the feet in stirrups for the older adolescent.
2. Explain the procedure prior to the assessment. Never ask the caregiver of the infant or young school-age child to leave the room during this portion of the examination because the caregiver is a source of comfort to the child.
3. Drape the older-than-preschool-age child.
4. A vaginal/pelvic exam is not routinely performed on young females. A vaginal assessment is warranted, however, when signs of possible

---

⚡ NURSING ALERT

Allergic Reaction to Inhaled Substances

Be aware of the child's allergies prior to testing CN I. For example, even the smell of peanut butter can cause a severe allergic reaction in some children. In such cases, use a different aromatic source when testing CN I.

E Examination
N Normal Findings
A Abnormal Findings
P Pathophysiology

Sexually Transmitted Disease Education for Adolescents

The following preventive guidelines are essential to discuss during your interview. To fit appropriately into the context of the interview, inquiry is preferable after questioning about sexual relationships and use of contraceptives.

1. If the adolescent is sexually active, discuss his or her feelings on the subject.
2. Talk about the various sexually transmitted diseases (human immunodeficiency virus [HIV], *Chlamydia*, herpes simplex virus [HSV], human papillomavirus [HPV], gonorrhea), including their symptoms and sequelae.
3. Mention that abstinence is the only certain method of preventing sexually transmitted diseases and pregnancy.
4. If the individual cannot comply with abstinence, then discuss proper condom application and use.
5. Encourage the patient to avoid having sex with anyone who claims to be infected.
6. Discuss facilities that offer confidential testing if the individual believes that he or she or a partner has contracted a sexually transmitted disease.

E	Examination
N	Normal Findings
A	Abnormal Findings
P	Pathophysiology

sexual abuse are present. Refer to the Nursing Alert on page 761. The assessment is undertaken by a health care provider who is trained to perform pediatric vaginal examinations and can evaluate these problems.

5. Any female who has reached menarche needs to be evaluated for a pregnant uterus.

Inspection

Perineal Area

E 1. Stand directly in front of the patient.
   2. Assess Tanner's stage. Refer to page 611.
   3. Refer to Chapter 19 for the remainder of the examination.

N *The infant's labia minora are sometimes larger than the labia majora. The hymen is sometimes intact up until the point of sexual activity.*

A It is abnormal for the female infant to display a rudimentary penis in the clitoral area.

P Genital ambiguity occurs during embryonic development as a consequence of genetic causes or androgens or androgen inhibitors that reverse genital characteristics.

A A bloody discharge noted at the vaginal opening or on the diaper is abnormal.

P It is not uncommon to note pseudomenstruation in an infant under 2 weeks of age. Maternal hormones such as estrogen are the cause.

Male Genitalia

General Approach

1. Female nurses may encounter difficulty assessing a reluctant adolescent. Be firm when explaining that this portion of the assessment is a required part of his examination. Infants and toddlers do not object to the assessment.
2. In case the infant or toddler urinates during the examination, have a diaper or disposable cloth available to catch the stream of urine.
3. The older school-age child and the adolescent should be draped in order to maintain modesty.

Inspection

Assess Tanner's stage during inspection. Refer to page 611.

Penis

E 1. Note the position of the urethral meatus.
   2. Note the size of the penis.
   3. If you are not able to determine circumcision status, ask the caregiver if the child was circumcised.

N *The meatus is normally found on the tip of the penis. A disappearing penis phenomenon occurs normally in infants with increased adipose tissue in the area surrounding the penis. Reassure the caregiver that this is normal and will resolve after adipose tissue is lost.*

A It is abnormal for the urethral meatus to be located behind or along the ventral side of the penis.

P During the third month of fetal development, the urethral meatus fails to move toward the glans penis, creating a condition known as hypospadias. Mothers who take hydantoin for epilepsy are at greater risk for having children with hypospadias.

A It is abnormal for the meatal opening to be on the dorsal surface of the penis.

P During the third month of fetal development, the urethral meatus fails to move toward the glans penis, causing an epispadias deformity.

E Examination
N Normal Findings
A Abnormal Findings
P Pathophysiology

Scrotum

E 1. Evaluate scrotal size and color.
　　2. Note if the testes are seen in the scrotal sac.
N *The scrotum appears proportionately large in size when compared to the penis. The sac color is brown or black in dark-skinned children and pink in light-skinned children. Two testes should be present, but, in infants, they may retract into the inguinal canal or abdomen due to various stimuli, including cold and palpation.*
A/P Refer to Chapter 20.

Palpation

Scrotum

E 1. Place the infant in a supine position on the examination table. Instruct the young child to sit cross-legged to inhibit the cremasteric reflex from occurring.
　　2. Locate each testis within the scrotal sac by using the fingers of one hand in a milking motion to descend the testes.
　　3. Palpate and note the size, shape, and mobility of each testis.
N *Refer to Chapter 20.*
A It is abnormal to be unable to palpate the testes.
P **Cryptorchidism** is a failure of the testis to descend into the scrotal sac. One or both testes failing to descend within the inguinal canal occurs during embryonic development.
A An enlargement of the scrotum is abnormal.
P A congenital hydrocele results from failure of the male reproductive tract to develop properly while the fetus is in utero. This mass will transilluminate.

Hernia

E 1. For the infant who is unable to stand, place the infant supine on the examination table. All other children should stand during the examination.
　　2. Use the little finger for the infant's and the index finger for the younger child's examination.
　　3. Follow the inguinal canal as is done on an adult male. Refer to page 658.
　　4. If possible, perform the assessment on a crying infant.
　　5. Have preschoolers and early school-age children attempt to blow up a balloon while you palpate the inguinal areas.
　　6. Palpate the inguinal areas while the older school-age child or adolescent coughs.
N/A/P Refer to Chapter 20.

Anus

As a rule, rectal assessments are not performed on children unless you detect a problem or suspect abuse; in these cases, refer for further evaluation if not trained specifically for this procedure and follow your institution's guidelines.

Inspection

E 1. Ask the child to lie on the abdomen.
　　2. Gently separate the buttocks to allow direct visualization of the anal opening.
　　3. Observe for bleeding, fissures, prolapse, skin tags, hemorrhoids, lesions, and pinworms.
　　4. During separation of the buttocks, observe any movement of the anus.

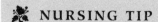

NURSING TIP

Anal Reflex and Sexual Abuse

Anal trauma, such as occurs in sexual assault, manifests as poor anal sphincter control. Consider sexual abuse if a child exhibits an absent or slow anal reflex.

5. Stroke the perianal area with your finger and note any movement. This is called the anal reflex or anal wink.

N *No bleeding, fissures, prolapse, skin tags, hemorrhoids, lesions, or pinworms should be present. An anal reflex is observed.*

A An absent anal reflex is abnormal.

P Conditions such as a spinal cord lesion, trauma, and tumors that interrupt nervous innervation to the anal sphincter cause this finding.

CASE STUDY

The case study illustrates the application and objective documentation of the pediatric assessment.

The Patient with Congenital Heart Disease

Lisa is a 6-month-old infant born with a complete atrioventricular canal (CAVC) defect and Down syndrome. Mrs. Mitchell, Lisa's mother, took her for a routine 6-month check-up.

❖ HEALTH HISTORY

LEGAL GUARDIAN	Rose Mitchell (biological mother and caregiver)
SOURCE OF INFORMATION	Caregiver
PATIENT PROFILE	6-month-old BF
CHIEF COMPLAINT	(Per caregiver): "I have noticed Lisa taking a lot more time to eat & she is always working hard to breathe."
HISTORY OF PRESENT ILLNESS	2 d PTA, Mrs. Mitchell noticed pt was taking 45 min to feed in contrast to her nl 20–30 min. During the feed, pt diaphoretic. Mrs. Mitchell feels pt's respirations are more labored; changing 4 wet diapers/d (had been 7–8).
PAST HEALTH HISTORY	
Birth History	
Prenatal	2 prior spontaneous miscarriages; denies drug, ETOH, tobacco, or caffeine use during pregnancy; viral illness in 1st trimester; sought prenatal care at 2 mo p̄ missed period; unplanned pregnancy for caregivers
Labor and Delivery	38-wk gestation delivered via C-section (failure to progress) p̄ a 24-hr labor, not able to hold baby p̄ birth in delivery room, baby's mucous membranes pale pink, does not remember Apgar scores, birth wt 8 lb, length 22 in.

continued

Postnatal	Pt transported to another facility at 2 d for cardiac catheterization, d/c at 2 wk of age, caregivers visited infant qd in hospital, poor feeding, d/c on NGT (q other feeding), afebrile during hospitalization
Medical	CAVC defect, Down syndrome
Surgical	None
Medications	Digoxin 0.02 mg po bid (q 12°), Lasix 3 mg po bid (q 12°), Aldactone 6.25 mg po qd AM
Communicable Diseases	Mother denies exposure to TB, HIV
Allergies	NKDA, Enfamil $\bar{c}$ Fe produces diarrhea & wt loss
Injuries/Accidents	None
Disabilities/Handicaps	Developmentally delayed
Blood Transfusions	None
Childhood Illnesses	Ø recent exposure to MMR, pertussis, chickenpox
Immunizations	Has had 2 DTP (2 mo, 4 mo), 2 OPVs (2 mo, 4 mo), 2 hepatitis B vaccines (2 mo, 4 mo), 2 Hib (2 mo, 4 mo)

FAMILY HEALTH HISTORY

LEGEND

- ⬤ Living female
- ⬛ Living male
- ⊗ Deceased female
- ⊠ Deceased male
- △ Therapeutic or spontaneous abortion
- ⟋ Points to patient

A&W = Alive & well
CAVC = Complete atrioventricular canal defect
MR = Mental retardation

Paternal uncle died 4 hours $\bar{p}$ birth from complex congenital heart dz. Denies maternal family hx of SIDS, ADHD, and MR.

SOCIAL HISTORY

Alcohol, Tobacco, Drug Use, Sexual Practice	N/A
Travel History	Never left her home town
School Performance	Enrolled in county's early intervention program, has PT & OT 2 ×/wk, mom does PT exercises on remaining days
Home Environment	Family lives in 3 BR home built in 1978; Ø guns in home; neither caregiver drinks ETOH or takes illicit drugs; Ø pets

continued

Hobbies, Leisure Activities, Stress, Education	N/A
Economic Status	Lisa's parents have hl care insurance that covers most expenses
Military Service	N/A
Religion	Baptist
Ethnic Background	Black American
Roles/Relationships	Caregivers married; mom stays at home c̄ infant; FOB assists when home; Ø recent life changes; both caregivers collaborate on hl care decisions
Child's Personal Habits	Does best c̄ mom holding her during stressful periods
Characteristic Patterns of Daily Living	Wakes at 7 AM, takes meds then formula; lies on mat c̄ toys while mother fixes breakfast; 5 ×/wk mother does PT for 30 min, then pt takes formula, naps 45 min, sits in bouncer seat while mother fixes lunch; mother plays c̄ pt until next feed, when pt takes formula; mother sings & reads stories; pt naps 45 min; outdoor walk in stroller; pt takes formula, then sits in swing while mother makes supper; FOB comes home from work & plays c̄ pt; pt sits in bouncer seat c̄ parents at dinner; FOB gives bath, administers meds & gives formula; pt goes to bed at 8 PM.
HEALTH MAINTENANCE ACTIVITIES	
Sleep	11 hr at night, 2 naps (45 min each)
Diet	Bottle-fed c̄ Isomil plus Moducal added to formula to yield 30 calories/oz; was taking 28 oz qd; in past 2 d, has ↓ to 23 oz qd; no solids have been introduced, no MVI given
Exercise	PT
Stress Management	N/A
Use of Safety Devices	Car seat in rear-facing position in back seat only
Safety	House has been childproofed c̄ outlet covers, gates on stairs, poisons & cleaning supplies in locked cabinet, meds in shoe box on highest shelf in closet, table edge protectors, bumpers over hearth's edge, poison control # posted next to phone, smoke detectors upstairs & downstairs, fire extinguisher in kitchen; have not devised escape route for fires; parents both CPR trained ā pt d/c from hospital, would dial 911 for an emergency
Health Check-Ups	At 2 & 4 mo; sees cardiologist q month
DEVELOPMENT	
Motor	Able to roll from side to back, follows moving object c̄ eyes, attempts to hold objects & attempts to hold head up while in prone position

continued

Cognitive	Gurgles & coos
Social	Smiles, pays attention to familiar voices, & recognizes caregiver

PHYSICAL ASSESSMENT

Vital Signs	T: 99.6°F Ⓡ; apical HR: 140; RR: 60; BP: 88/42 mm Hg (RUE, supine)
Physical Growth	Wt: 10 lb 8 oz; length: 25 in; head circumference: 40.0 cm; chest circumference: 39.5 cm
Skin	
Inspection	No erythema, papules, vesicles, edema, scaling, or ulcerations; Mongolian spot 4 × 5 cm noted over lumbar-sacral area
Palpation	Soft, smooth s̄ roughness, dryness, scaliness, or keratic areas; turgor WNL, diaphoretic along hairline & forehead; arms & legs warm & clammy bilaterally
Hair and Nails	
Inspection and Palpation	s̄ alopecia, infestations; cap refill 4 sec UE & LE
Head	
Inspection	Symmetrical, round, no bulges or prominence of forehead or involuntary mvt, face symmetrical, unsteady head control
Palpation	Anterior fontanel soft & flat (1.5 cm × 1.0 cm), posterior fontanel closed, suture lines not overriding, no edema
Eyes	
Vision Screening	Bilateral symmetrical light reflex c̄ Hirschberg test, no malalignment of eyes c̄ cover-uncover test
Inspection	No ptosis, inner epicanthal folds present, producing tears, sclera light & muddy, conjunctiva pale pink, cornea smooth & transparent, iris brown, Brushfield's spots around perimeter of iris (OU), PERRL, ⊕ red reflex, optic discs creamy pink, round, borders regular s̄ hemorrhages
Ears	
Auditory Testing	Reacts to loud noises
Inspection (External Ear)	Top of pinna positioned ⅛" below outer canthus, pinna s̄ lesions or masses
Palpation (External Ear)	No pain c̄ mvt
Inspection (Internal Ear)	No erythema; sm amt cerumen in EAC; bilateral TMs pearly s̄ retraction, bulging, perforation, fluid, or air bubbles; mobility c̄ pneumatic bulb; landmarks intact; ⊕ light reflex

continued

Nose

Inspection   Patent nares c̄ flaring, mucosa pale pink, septum midline, no edema of turbinates

Mouth and Throat

Inspection   Lips pale pink, no fissures/cracking, edges meet; buccal mucosa pale pink s̄ lesions; Ø teeth; tongue pale pink, thick, & midline, protrudes slightly, s̄ fasciculations; high, arched palate; both hard/soft palates intact s̄ lesions; tonsils 1+, no erythema or exudate; uvula midline; oropharynx pink s̄ exudate

Neck

Inspection   Symmetrical, short & thin, s̄ edema; active ROM

Palpation   Thyroid nonpalpable, trachea midline, s̄ lymphadenopathy

Breasts and Regional Lymphatics

Inspection   Tanner stage I; no retractions, erythema, venous distention, edema, ulcerations; areolas circular & even bilaterally, neg masses & ulcerations; nipples circular s̄ retractions/inversions, erythema, d/c, ulcerations or supranumerary nipples

Palpation   Breasts neg for nodes glands, masses, or tenderness; axillary area: nonpalpable nodes, neg tenderness or masses

Thorax and Lungs

Inspection   Thorax rounded, moderate intercostal retractions

Palpation   ↓ Tactile fremitus RLL

Percussion   Diaphragmatic excursion 1 ICS on Ⓛ (hyperresonant), unable to obtain on Ⓡ (dull)

Auscultation   Breath sounds = bilaterally, bronchial sounds over trachea, bronchovesicular breath sounds throughout peripheral lung fields, coarse crackles throughout

Heart and Peripheral Vasculature

Inspection   Apical impulse at 4th ICS to Ⓛ of MCL; Ø heaves, lifts of precordium; Ø clubbing of fingers or toes; neg JVD

Palpation   Neg thrills on precordium, suprasternal notch & carotids; Ø brachial-femoral lag using Ⓡ brachial, Ⓡ femoral artery; pulses 2+/4+ bilaterally

Auscultation   Apical HR even & regular, nl S_1, narrowly split S_2, ⊕ S_3, Ø S_4, III/VI systolic ejection murmur along LSB

continued

Abdomen

Inspection   Rounded & symmetrical c̄ inverted umbilicus, abd musculature continuous, Ø visible peristalsis

Auscultation   Hyperactive BS in 4 quadrants; Ø venous hums, Ø bruits @ femoral, iliac, renal, and aortic areas; Ø peritoneal friction rub

Percussion   Tympanic; neg fluid shift

Palpation   Ø pain or tenderness, Ø masses, liver edge down 3.0 cm from RCM, spleen tip 1.0 cm from LCM, kidneys not palpable

Musculoskeletal

Inspection   AROM & hyperextensibility of all 4 extremities, attempts to hold head up in prone position, unable to lift chest off table in prone position, C-shaped spine

Palpation   Strength: ⅖ of all muscle groups; toes & forefoot not deviated; neg for hip pain & limitation of mvt; neg Ortolani's maneuver

Neurological

Inspection   Alert, smiling, reaching for objects; ⊕ Babinski, ⊕ suck; CN III–XII grossly intact; DTR 2+/4+

Female Genitalia

Inspection   Tanner stage I, labia dark pink s̄ hypertrophy, excoriation, ulcerations; no vaginal d/c; perineum smooth s̄ lacerations; hymen intact

Anus

Inspection   Anal area darker pink in color than perineum; s̄ lesions, bleeding, fissures, prolapse, hemorrhoids

LABORATORY DATA

Chemistry

	Pt's Values	Normal Range
Sodium	139 mEq/L	135–145 mEq/L
Potassium	5.4 mEq/L	3.5–5.0 mEq/L
Chloride	89 mEq/L	95–105 mEq/L
Carbon Dioxide	37.0 mEq/L	18–27 mEq/L
Calcium	11.1 mg/dl	8.0-11.0 mg/dl
Glucose	98 mg/dl	60-100 mg/dl
BUN	14 mg/dl	6.0-23.0 mg/dl
Creatinine	0.5 mg/dl	0.2–0.5 mg/dl

DIAGNOSTIC DATA

Radiological Report

AP and Lateral Chest X-Ray   The overall heart size is enlarged, with the right heart border being unusually rounded, suggesting right atrial prominence. The lungs are grossly hyperinflated, with uneven aeration and patchy infiltrate in the right upper lobe. The pulmonary vascularity is increased and slightly congested. The aortic arch is left-sided.

NURSING CHECKLIST
Pediatric Patient Assessment*

Developmental Assessment
- Denver II

Physical Growth
- Weight
- Length/Height
- Head Circumference
- Chest Circumference

Physical Assessment
- Apgar Scoring
- Head
  - Inspection
    - Head Control
  - Palpation
    - Anterior Fontanel
    - Posterior Fontanel
    - Suture Lines
    - Surface Characteristics
- Eyes
  - Vision Screening
    - Allen Test
- Musculoskeletal System
  - Inspection
    - Tibiofemoral Bones
  - Palpation
    - Feet (Metatarsus Varus)
    - Hip and Femur (Ortolani Maneuver)
- Neurological System
  - Rooting
  - Sucking
  - Palmar Grasp
  - Tonic Neck
  - Stepping
  - Plantar Grasp
  - Babinski
  - Moro (Startle)
  - Gallant
  - Placing
  - Landau

Special Techniques
- Transillumination of the Skull
- Assessing for Choanal Atresia
- Assessing for Coarctation of the Aorta

Only pediatric-specific tests are listed.

REVIEW QUESTIONS AND ACTIVITIES

1. Describe two physiological differences between the pediatric and the adult patient.

2. State two structural variations that would change the technique of assessment in the child.

3. List two environmental problems that put a child at risk for illness or death.

4. State an easy rule of thumb for determining normal systolic blood pressure in patients older than 1 year.

5. Which surface characteristic of the head does not cross suture lines?
   a. Molding
   b. Caput succedaneum
   c. Cephalhematoma
   d. Craniotabes
   The correct answer is (c).

6. What vision screening examination would be most appropriate to administer to a child who cannot read?
   a. Snellen chart
   b. Hirschberg test
   c. Snellen E chart
   d. Cover-uncover test
   The correct answer is (c).

Questions 7–9 refer to the following situation:

Fazal is a 6-month-old infant brought in by his father for a well-baby check. He is awake during the examination.

7. You palpate the area of his head where the sagittal, coronal, and frontal sutures meet. This anatomic landmark is called the:
   a. Anterior fontanel
   b. Mastoid fontanel
   c. Posterior fontanel
   d. Sphenoid fontanel
   The correct answer is (a).

8. With the tip of your thumbnail, you stroke the plantar surface of the foot, from the lateral heel upward. The normal response of a 6-month-old infant to this assessment is:
   a. Turning of the pelvis and shoulders toward the stimulated side
   b. Lifting and flexion of the tested leg
   c. Curling down of the toes
   d: Fanning of the toes outward and dorsiflexion of the great toe
   The correct answer is (d).

9. With your forefinger, you stroke the skin at the right corner of Fazal's mouth. The infant turns his head to the right. You recognize that:
   a. This is the sucking reflex, which is normal for a 6-month-old infant.
   b. This is the rooting reflex, which is abnormal in a 6-month-old infant.
   c. This is the Gallant reflex, which is normal in a 6-month-old infant.
   d. This is the Landau reflex, which is abnormal in a 6-month-old infant.
   The correct answer is (b).

10. Describe the cranial nerve assessment of an infant and a toddler.

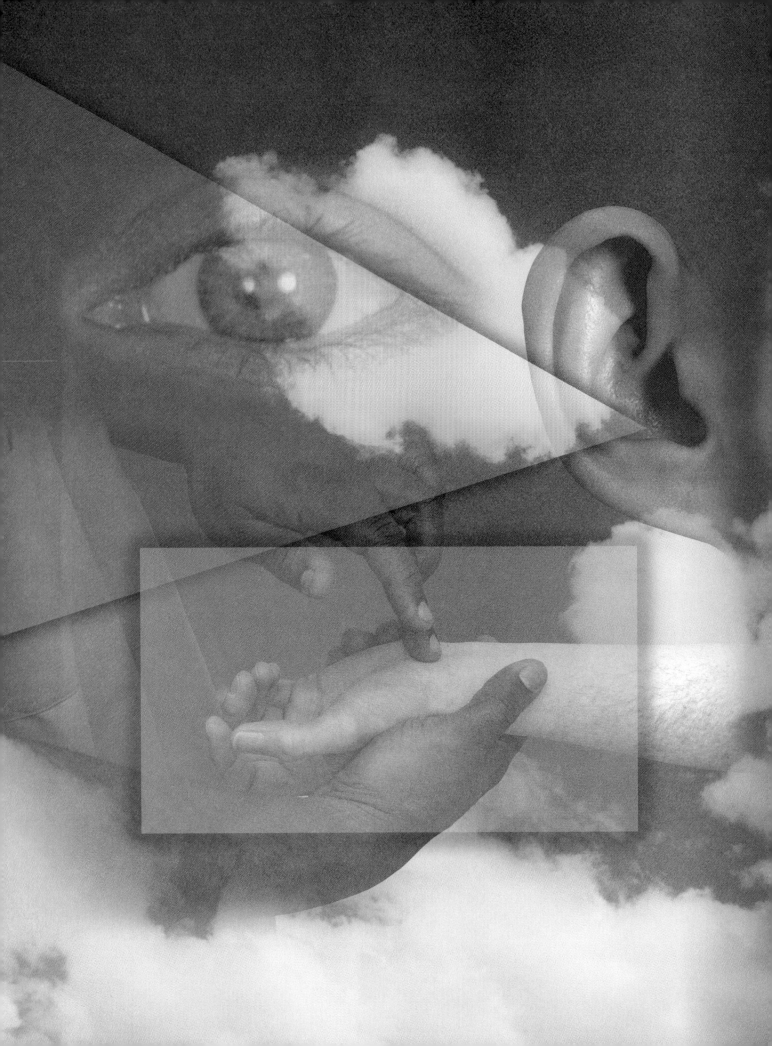

Putting It All Together

24 The Complete Health and Physical Assessment

Conciseness and decision in your movements, as well as your words, are necessary in the sick room, as necessary as absence of hurry and bustle.

Florence Nightingale

The Complete Health and Physical Assessment

1. State the components of the complete health and physical assessment.
2. Conduct a complete health and physical assessment on a patient.
3. Document a complete health and physical assessment.
4. Develop a nursing care plan based on the data from the complete health and physical assessment.

Performing a complete health and physical assessment is a skill that takes time and practice to develop. You must concentrate on perfecting interviewing techniques and assessment skills. You must be able to accurately recognize normal findings in order to appreciate abnormal and pathological findings. Practicing in an academic laboratory setting or on a volunteer patient is a crucial step leading to skill mastery. Learning the assessment techniques system by system, as described in this text, helps you to gradually build on previously developed skills.

Keep in mind that as assessment skills are perfected, the amount of time it takes to perform them will decrease. Plan on spending between 30 and 90 minutes conducting the complete health and physical assessment. If the patient's chief complaint is not of an urgent or critical nature, the patient's first visit to the health care facility is the ideal time to perform a comprehensive assessment. Interval or follow-up visits frequently require partial assessments that document changes from the initial database; these visits require substantially less time.

It is important to develop a routine that is comfortable so that steps in the assessment process will not be overlooked. The patient's physical, emotional, or mental state may necessitate a change in the usual progression of the assessment. Clinical judgment and experience will dictate when specific steps should be omitted, deferred, or repeated.

Once the content of Chapters 9–21 is learned and you are comfortable performing each assessment, it is time to integrate the entire health and physical assessment. This chapter provides a step-by-step approach to guide you through the entire process for an adult patient. With time, you will develop a personal rhythm.

Special techniques are normally inserted in the assessment process at different phases, depending on the techniques to be performed and the patient's condition. Experience will guide you in determining when these special techniques are warranted. They are omitted in the following assessment sequence, which illustrates a "typical" head-to-toe assessment.

🌸 NURSING TIP

Fostering Patient Cooperation

The success of any health history and physical assessment rests, in part, with obtaining and maintaining the patient's cooperation. Guidelines to assist you in this endeavor are:

- Have the patient wait as little as possible prior to the examination; explain any delays that occur.
- Greet the patient first, shake hands, and put the patient at ease.
- Proceed in an efficient and organized manner.
- Encourage the patient to actively participate in the assessment process (e.g., provide information, ask questions, teach).
- Use terms the patient will understand.
- Ask the patient to repeat home care or self-examination instructions and to demonstrate learned skills when appropriate to verify patient understanding.
- Display ease with any disease or condition.
- Be honest; do not offer false reassurance or jump to conclusions.
- Discuss findings first without diagnosing; validate findings when indicated.
- Arrange for the presence of a third party if requested.

✓ NURSING CHECKLIST
General Assessment Reminders

- Understand illness in human terms, not just scientific terms.
- Approach the patient from a holistic viewpoint and try to understand the patient's perspective.
- Remember that nursing is both art and science.
- Follow your judgment; critical thinking incorporates the consideration of objective and subjective data. Always ask, "Why?"
- Act unhurried.
- Act in a professional manner at all times; remember that the patient is simultaneously examining you (mannerisms, facial expressions, hesitations in speech).
- Recognize both the patient's and your potential stressors (work, home, environment, schedules) and try to account for them.
- Acknowledge emotional reactions to illness (anger, fear, anxiety, disbelief, confusion, guilt, shame, blame, hurt, and betrayal).
- Embrace sensitivity to cultural, ethnic, and spiritual issues.
- Show respect for the patient and his or her circumstances.
- Possess a sense of self-awareness to guide your actions.

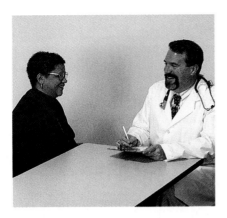

Figure 24-1 Carefully document all interview responses and assessment findings.

👀 THINK ABOUT IT

Documentation Dilemma

You overhear a colleague say to a new orientee, "We won't document that Mr. Ryan fell off the exam table today." How would you proceed?

✤ ASK YOURSELF

Ethical Dilemmas

Have you ever encountered an ethical dilemma in your clinical practice that developed during the history or physical assessment? What action did you take? What resources were available to you? In retrospect, would you have done anything differently?

LEGAL CONSIDERATIONS

The increasingly litigious nature of society has not bypassed the nursing profession. More and more nurses are being named as codefendants in lawsuits. What is legally expected of the nurse is to conduct himself or herself in a reasonably prudent manner at all times. Some specific guidelines are:

- Document all patient interactions (refer to Figure 24-1).
- Respect the patient's confidentiality. Do not discuss any patient's case in a public area or with colleagues who are not on that patient's care team; keep discussions at a strict professional level.
- Report any disease that is considered a public health concern (according to local, state, and federal regulations).
- Respect a patient's right to privacy.
- Respect a patient's right to refuse treatment or assessments (document thoroughly).
- When appropriate, ask the patient for permission to perform various assessments, especially those that may be uncomfortable (breast, thorax, genitalia). If the patient denies permission, explain the importance of the assessment to the patient and repeat the request. If the patient still denies permission, omit the assessment and document the patient's refusal.
- Know your institution's policies and standards of practice, and practice within those guidelines.
- Know your state's Nurse Practice Act and practice within that scope.
- Consult with your nurse manager, risk manager, or institutional attorney when indicated.

These guidelines are neither foolproof nor comprehensive. When in doubt, use common sense.

ETHICAL CONSIDERATIONS

Respect the patient's right to privacy, whether it is physical, emotional, social, psychological, or family related. Be truthful when talking with the patient. Do not tell the patient things that are unfounded just to gain his or her trust. Give the patient assurance that confidentiality will be maintained.

Respect the patient's wishes. For example, if the patient vehemently refuses to answer questions about the family, respect this. Likewise, do not pry into areas that do not relate to the patient's condition or reason for seeking health care.

Many institutions have a multidisciplinary ethics committee. Some institutions employ an ethicist. Many professional nursing organizations issue ethics statements, both general and specific in nature, to help guide nursing actions. Use these or whatever resources are available to you when presented with ethical dilemmas or questions.

In general, treat all patients as you would like to be treated.

HEALTH HISTORY

Conduct the health history. Depending on the patient's reason for the visit, this can be the complete, episodic, interval (follow-up), or emergency health history. Refer to Chapter 3. The patient can be dressed in street clothes for this interview.

Components of the developmental, cultural, and spiritual assessments are continually evaluated during the course of the patient interaction. Thorough assessments of any or all of these special assessments can be completed if dictated by the patient's situation. The inspection component of the nutrition assessment is noted during the health history. Refer to Chapters 4–7. Sit opposite the patient who is sitting or lying in bed.

❀ NURSING TIP

Tips for a Successful Assessment

- Ensure that the examination table is at a comfortable height for you and the patient, with easy access on all sides.
- Respect the patient's modesty.
- Have the patient make as few position changes as possible.
- Ensure that all of the equipment is accessible and arranged in a logical manner.
- Keep interruptions to a minimum.
- Teach self-assessment while the patient is gowned or during specific system examinations.
- Advise the patient about potential discomfort or sensations prior to procedures.
- Ask the patient about pain or other sensations during certain assessments.
- Offer cleaning wipes or tissues to the patient following certain examinations; e.g., the pelvic examination.
- Provide the patient with privacy for redressing.

✓ NURSING CHECKLIST
General Approach to the Physical Assessment

- Develop an approach that is logical but allows flexibility.
- Use clinical judgment to modify the examination sequence and adapt to circumstances.
- Allow time at the conclusion of the examination to discuss relevant findings and to allow the patient to ask questions.
- Assist older or disabled patients to focus on how well they can meet the demands of daily life rather than on their limitations.
- Remember that a physical examination can be tiring, both for you and for the patient.

This text has provided a head-to-toe assessment format in order to discuss body systems in their entirety. However, in practice, a head-to-toe assessment combines systems when assessing most body parts. For example, when assessing the hands, you combine components of the skin, musculoskeletal, and neurological assessments. For this reason, the complete physical examination, which demonstrates how to put it all together, reflects this clinical approach. The sample case study at the end of the chapter documents a standard format of the complete physical assessment.

General Appearance

The patient's general appearance is assessed during the health history. Incorporate the following into this assessment:

Physical Presence

Age: stated age versus apparent age
Stature: posture, proportion of body limbs to trunk
Motor activity: gait, speed, and effort of movement; weight bearing; absence or presence of movement in different body areas
Body and breath odors

Psychological Presence

Dress, grooming, and personal hygiene
Mood and manner
Speech
Facial expressions

Distress

Physical
Psychological
Emotional

Neurological System

1. Assess mental status: level of consciousness, fund of information, attention span, memory, judgment, insight, spatial perception, calculations, abstract reasoning, thought processes, and content.

After the mental status examination, ask the patient to undress and don an examination gown (underwear may be worn). Ask the patient to empty the bladder prior to commencing the assessment process. The urine may be collected for a specimen. Ask the patient to sit on the examination table with the legs hanging over the front. A second drape can be provided to cover the lap and legs. Stand in front of the patient.

Measurements

Record the patient's:
1. Height
2. Weight
3. Temperature
4. Pulse (radial preferred site in adult)
5. Respirations
6. Blood pressure (both arms)
7. Anthropometric measurements (if indicated)

Skin

Throughout the entire head-to-toe assessment, inspect the skin for the following characteristics:
1. Color
2. Bleeding
3. Ecchymosis
4. Vascularity
5. Lesions

Throughout the entire head-to-toe assessment, palpate the skin for:
1. Moisture
2. Temperature
3. Texture
4. Turgor
5. Edema

Head and Face

1. Inspect the shape of the head.
2. Inspect and palpate the head and scalp.
3. Inspect the color and distribution of the hair. Note any infestations; palpate the hair.
4. Inspect the face for expression, shape, symmetry (CN VII), symmetry of eyes, eyebrows, ears, nose, and mouth.
5. Instruct the patient to raise the eyebrows, frown, smile, wrinkle the forehead, show the teeth, purse the lips, puff the cheeks, and whistle (CN VII).

6. Palpate the temporal pulses.
7. Palpate (CN V) and auscultate the temporomandibular joints.

Eyes

1. Test distance vision and near vision (CN II).
2. Test color vision.
3. Test visual fields via confrontation (CN II).
4. Assess extraocular muscle mobility: cover-uncover test, corneal light reflex, and six cardinal fields of gaze (CNs III, IV, VI).
5. Assess direct and consensual light reflexes and accommodation (CN III).
6. Inspect the eyelids, eyebrows, palpebral fissures, and position of eyes.
7. Inspect and palpate the lacrimal apparatus.
8. Inspect the conjunctiva, sclera, cornea, iris, pupils, and lens.
9. Assess the corneal reflex.
10. Conduct funduscopic assessment: retinal structures, macula.

Ears

1. Test gross hearing: voice-whisper test or watch-tick test (CN VIII).
2. Inspect and palpate the external ear.
3. Assess ear alignment.
4. Conduct otoscopic assessment: canal, landmarks, and tympanic membrane.
5. Perform Weber and Rinne tests.

Nose and Sinuses

1. Inspect the external surface of the nose.
2. Assess nostril patency.
3. Test olfactory sense (CN I).
4. Conduct internal assessment with nasal speculum: mucosa, turbinates, and septum.
5. Inspect, percuss, and palpate frontal and maxillary sinuses.

Mouth and Throat

1. Note breath odor.
2. Inspect the lips, buccal mucosa, gums, hard and soft palates.
3. Inspect the teeth; count the teeth.
4. Inspect the tongue; ask the patient to stick out the tongue (CN XII).
5. Inspect the uvula; note movement when the patient says "ah" (CNs IX, X).
6. Inspect the tonsils; note grade.
7. Inspect the oropharynx.
8. Test gag reflex (CNs IX, X).
9. Test taste (CN VII).
10. Palpate the lips and mouth if indicated.

Neck

1. Inspect the musculature of the neck.
2. Inspect range of motion (assess strength against hand) and shoulder shrug (CN XI).
3. Palpate the musculature of the neck.
4. Inspect and palpate the trachea.
5. Palpate the carotid arteries (one at a time).
6. Inspect the jugular veins for distension; estimate jugular venous pressure (JVP) if indicated.
7. Inspect and palpate the thyroid (use only one approach, either anterior or posterior).
8. Auscultate the thyroid and carotid arteries.
9. Inspect and palpate the lymph nodes: preauricular, postauricular, occipital, submental, submandibular, anterior cervical chain, posterior cervical chain, tonsillar, and supraclavicular.

Upper Extremities

1. Inspect nailbed color, shape, and configuration; palpate nailbed texture.
2. Assess capillary refill on nailbed.
3. Inspect muscle size and palpate muscle tone of hands, arms, and shoulders.
4. Palpate the joints of fingers, wrists, elbows, and shoulders.
5. Assess range of motion and strength of fingers, wrists, elbows, and shoulders.
6. Test position sense.
7. Palpate radial and brachial pulses.
8. Palpate the epitrochlear node.

Move behind the patient. Untie the gown so that the entire back is exposed. The gown should cover the shoulders and the anterior chest.

Back, Posterior and Lateral Thoraxes

1. Palpate the thyroid (posterior approach).
2. Inspect and palpate the spinous processes; inspect range of motion of the cervical spine.
3. Note thoracic configuration, symmetry of shoulders, and position of scapula.
4. Palpate the posterior thorax and lateral thorax.
5. Perform posterior thoracic expansion.
6. Perform tactile fremitus on the posterior thorax and lateral thorax.
7. Percuss the posterior thorax and lateral thorax.
8. Perform diaphragmatic excursion.
9. Palpate the costovertebral angle (CVA); percuss the CVA with your fist.
10. Auscultate the posterior thorax and lateral thorax, perform voice sounds if indicated.

Move in front of the patient. Drape the patient's gown at waist level (females may cover their breasts).

Anterior Thorax

1. Inspect shape of the thorax, symmetry of the chest wall, presence of superficial veins, costal angle, angle of ribs, intercostal spaces, muscles of respiration, respirations, and sputum.
2. Palpate the anterior thorax.
3. Perform anterior thoracic expansion.
4. Perform tactile fremitus.
5. Percuss the anterior thorax.
6. Auscultate the anterior thorax; perform voice sounds if indicated.

Heart

1. Auscultate cardiac landmarks: aortic, pulmonic, mitral, and tricuspid areas and Erb's point.

Ask the female patient to uncover her breasts.

Female Breasts

1. Inspect the breasts with the patient in these positions: arms at side, arms raised over the head, hands pressed into hips, hands in front and patient leaning forward.
2. Palpate the supraclavicular and infraclavicular lymph nodes.
3. Palpate the breasts with the patient's arms first at her side and then raised over her head.
4. Palpate the anterior, posterior, central, and lateral axillary lymph nodes.
5. Teach breast self-examination.

Male Breasts

1. Repeat the sequence used for female breasts. Having the patient lean forward is usually unnecessary unless gynecomastia is present.

Assist the patient into a supine position with the chest uncovered. Drape the abdomen and legs. Stand on the right side of the patient.

Jugular Veins

As the patient changes from a sitting to a supine position for the remainder of the breast assessment, observe the jugular veins when the patient is at a 45° angle. Assess again when the patient is supine.

1. Inspect the jugular veins for distension; estimate JVP if indicated.

Female and Male Breasts

1. Palpate each breast. The arm on the same side of the assessed breast should be raised over the head.
2. Compress the nipple to express any discharge.

Heart

1. Inspect cardiac landmarks for pulsations.
2. Palpate cardiac landmarks for pulsations, thrills, and heaves.

3. Palpate the apical impulse.
4. With the diaphragm of the stethoscope, auscultate the cardiac landmarks; count the apical pulse.
5. With the bell of the stethoscope, auscultate the cardiac landmarks.
6. Turn the patient on the left side and repeat auscultation of cardiac landmarks.

Return the patient to a supine position. Cover the patient's anterior thorax with the gown. Uncover the abdomen from the symphysis pubis to the costal margin.

Abdomen

1. Inspect contour, symmetry, pigmentation, and color.
2. Note scars, striae, visible peristalsis, masses, and pulsations.
3. Inspect the rectus abdominis muscles (supine and with head raised) and respiratory movement of the abdomen.
4. Inspect the umbilicus.
5. Auscultate bowel sounds.
6. Auscultate for bruits, venous hum, and friction rub.
7. Percuss all four quadrants.
8. Percuss liver span and liver descent; percuss liver with fist if indicated.
9. Percuss the spleen, stomach, and bladder.
10. Lightly palpate all four quadrants.
11. Note any muscle guarding.
12. Deeply palpate all four quadrants.
13. Palpate the liver, spleen, kidney, aorta, and bladder.
14. Assess superficial abdominal reflexes.
15. Perform hepatojugular reflux if indicated.

Inguinal Area

1. Inspect and palpate the inguinal lymph nodes.
2. Inspect for inguinal hernias.
3. Palpate the femoral pulses.
4. Auscultate the femoral pulses for bruits.

Cover the exposed abdomen with the gown. Lift the drape from the bottom to expose the lower extremities.

Lower Extremities

1. Inspect for color, capillary refill, edema, ulcerations, hair distribution, and varicose veins.
2. Palpate for temperature, edema, and texture.
3. Palpate the popliteal, dorsalis pedis, and posterior tibial pulses.
4. Inspect muscle size and palpate muscle tone of the legs and feet.
5. Palpate the joints of the hips, knees, ankles, and feet.
6. Assess range of motion and strength of the hips, knees, ankles, and feet.
7. Test position sense.
8. Assess for clonus.

Drape the lower extremities. Assist the patient to a sitting position and note the ease with which the patient sits up. Have the patient dangle the legs over the edge of the examination table.

Neurological System

1. Assess light touch: hands, lower arms, abdomen, feet, legs, and face (CN V).
2. Assess superficial pain (sharp and dull): hands, lower arms, abdomen, feet, legs, and face (CN V).
3. Assess two-point discrimination: fingers, dorsum of hand, tongue, lips, feet, and torso.
4. Assess vibration sense: toes and fingers.
5. Assess stereognosis, graphesthesia, and extinction.
6. Assess cerebellar function: finger to nose, rapid alternating hand movements, touch thumb to each finger, running heel down shin, and foot tapping.
7. Assess deep tendon reflexes: biceps, triceps, brachioradialis, patellar, and achilles.
8. Assess plantar reflex and Babinski's reflex.

Ask the patient to stand barefoot on the floor. If the patient is unsteady, use caution when performing these tests. Remain physically close to the patient at all times.

Musculoskeletal System

1. Assess mobility: casual walk, heel walk, toe walk, tandem walk, backwards walk, stepping to the right and left, and deep knee bends (one knee at a time). Note any indications of discomfort.

Stand behind the patient.

2. Assess range of motion of the spine.

Open the patient's gown to expose the back. Ask the patient to bend forward at the waist.

3. Inspect the spine for scoliosis.

Close the patient's gown. Stand in front of the patient.

Neurological System

1. Perform the Romberg test; assess pronator drift.
2. Assess the ability to hop on one foot, run heel down shin, and draw a figure eight with foot.

Assist the female patient back to the examination table. Ask her to assume the lithotomy position. Drape the patient. Sit on a stool in front of the patient's legs.

Female Genitalia, Anus, and Rectum

1. Inspect pubic hair distribution, presence of parasites, and skin color and condition: mons pubis, vulva, clitoris, urethral meatus, vaginal introitus, sacrococcygeal area, perineum, and anal mucosa.
2. Palpate the labia, urethral meatus, Skene's glands, vaginal introitus, and perineum.

3. Insert the vaginal speculum.
4. Inspect the cervix: color, position, size, surface characteristics, discharge, and shape of cervical os; inspect the vagina.
5. Collect specimens for cytological smears and cultures.

Stand in front of the patient's legs.

6. Perform bimanual assessment of the vagina, cervix, fornices, uterus, and adnexa.
7. Perform rectovaginal assessment.
8. Palpate the anus and rectum.
9. If stool is on the glove, save it to test for occult blood.

Assist the patient to a sitting position. Offer her some tissues to wipe the perineal area. Ask her to redress. You can answer her questions when she is dressed.

Ask the male patient to stand. Sit on a stool in front of the patient. Have the patient lift the gown to expose the genitalia.

Male Genitalia

1. Inspect hair distribution, penis, scrotum, urethral meatus, and inguinal area.
2. Palpate the penis, urethral meatus, and scrotum.
3. Palpate the inguinal area for nodes and hernias.
4. Auscultate the scrotum if indicated.
5. Teach testicular self-examination.

Ask the patient to bend over the examination table. If the patient is bedridden, the knee-chest or left lateral position may be used. Expose the buttocks. Stand behind the patient.

Male Anus, Rectum, and Prostate

1. Inspect the perineum, sacrococcygeal area, and anal mucosa.
2. Palpate the anus and rectum.
3. Palpate the prostate.
4. If stool is on the glove, save it to test for occult blood.

Re-cover the buttocks. Ask the patient to stand up and redress. You can answer his questions when he is dressed.

The patient has the opportunity to regain composure and formulate questions about the assessment while getting redressed. It is often difficult for patients to discuss future plans when wearing an examination gown. For this reason, give the patient a few minutes to redress in privacy before proceeding with the assessment. Always thank the patient for his or her time and explain what can be expected next.

When completing the assessment, ensure that you return the patient to the state you found him or her in at the beginning of the assessment. For example, for the bedridden patient, ensure that the side rails are up (if appropriate) and that the call bell is readily accessible. Ask the patient if there is anything else that can be done to make him or her comfortable.

Now that you have all of this information, what do you do with it and how do you make sense of it? Refer back to Chapter 1, which discussed how to make the leap from assessment data to formulating a nursing diagnosis and nursing care plan.

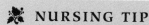

NURSING TIP

Assessing the Comatose Patient

For the comatose patient, the family and prior health care records can provide valuable information for the health history. Do not let the patient's condition deter you from conducting a thorough physical assessment. Omit components of the assessment that require volition and patient cooperation; complete the remainder of the assessment as indicated. Remember to assess neurological status thoroughly. Consider assessing: doll's eyes, corneal reflex, grasp reflex, snout reflex, glabellar reflex, sucking reflex, Babinski's reflex, clonus, superficial and deep pain response.

NURSING TIP

Communicating Bad News

Be sensitive when communicating bad or unexpected news to the patient, significant other(s), or caregiver. Talk to the patient in a quiet, private room. Be specific and straightforward. Speak in terms that will be understood. Give the patient time to process the information, alone if desired. Convey the same high level of respect that you have shown throughout the interview and assessment process. Finally, allow time for questions.

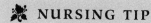

NURSING TIP

Assessing the Bedridden Patient

The bedridden patient is usually capable of cooperating for the health history and physical assessment. Components of the physical assessment that require the patient to be out of bed can be omitted. Cerebellar function of the lower extremities can still be assessed by having the patient run the heel of each foot down each shin and draw a figure eight with each foot on the bed or in the air.

Frequently, assessing the bedridden patient requires the assistance of a second person to help hold the patient in a side-lying position while a posterior assessment is conducted. If the patient can tolerate a sitting position, the second person can help hold the patient in this position while an assessment of the head, face, neck, and anterior thorax is conducted. Always use extra caution to protect the patient against falls.

LABORATORY AND DIAGNOSTIC DATA

The laboratory and diagnostic data that are obtained from the patient vary according to presenting symptoms and clinical assessment. Order only those tests that are necessary. Consider the risks, time, discomfort, cost, limitations, and contraindications of each test. Actively involve the patient in preparing for each test and incorporate clinical teaching when appropriate. Remember that technology can never replace the art of listening to what your patient is saying and the skill with which you perform physical assessments.

DOCUMENTATION

The documentation of the health and physical assessments is the legal record of the patient encounter. It also serves as the medium among health professionals for communicating about the patient's condition. The patient record represents a description of the patient's status and the care delivered to the patient. The documentation may be read by a multitude of professionals: nurses; doctors; dieticians; respiratory, physical, speech, and occupational therapists; risk managers; utilization reviewers; quality assurance personnel; accreditation organizations; lawyers; insurance companies; and, ultimately, the patient! Because all of these people have access to the patient's chart, you must document everything in a professional and legally acceptable manner. Table 24–1 outlines general principles to guide your documentation. Table 24–2 provides specific assessment-oriented "do's" and "don'ts" for documentation. Each institution also has its own documentation system. If you perform computerized charting in your workplace, always safeguard your access code to protect yourself.

CONCLUSION

Today's nurse is a sophisticated professional prepared to meet the demands of the health care market. Hospitalized patients have a greater acuity and are being discharged at a faster rate to the home environment. The home health nurse is therefore seeing a greater variety of patients who are sicker. Nurses in advanced practice settings are providing care to patients who are positioned at different points on the health-illness continuum. Because the entire plan of care is based on patient assessment, all nurses must possess adequate assessment skills. This text has supplied the information to assist the novice and the experienced nurse in acquiring, refining, and perfecting health and physical assessment skills. The pathophysiological basis for the physical assessment findings empowers the nurse to fully understand the patient's clinical state and make appropriate decisions. Ultimately, the patients are the benefactors of your knowledge, wisdom, and experience.

Table 24-1 General Documentation Guidelines

1. Ensure that you have the correct patient record or chart and that the patient's name and identifying information is on every page of the record.
2. Document as soon as the patient encounter is concluded to ensure accurate recall of data (follow institution's guidelines on frequency of charting).
3. Date and time each entry.
4. Sign each entry with your full legal name and with your professional credentials, or per your institution's policy.
5. Do not leave space between entries.
6. If an error is made while documenting, use a single line to cross out the error, then date, time, and sign the correction (check institutional policy); avoid erasing, crossing out, or using correction fluid.
7. Never correct another person's entry, even if it is incorrect.
8. Use quotes to indicate direct patient responses (e.g., "I feel lousy").
9. Document in chronological order; if chronological order is not used, state why.
10. Use legible writing.
11. Use a permanent ink pen. (Black is usually preferable because of its ability to photocopy well.)
12. Document in a complete but concise manner by using phrases and abbreviations as appropriate (see abbreviation list on inside back cover).
13. Document telephone calls that relate to the patient's case.
14. Remember, from a legal standpoint, if you didn't document it, it wasn't done.

Table 24-2 Assessment-Specific Documentation Guidelines

1. Record all data that contribute directly to the assessment (i.e., positive assessment findings and pertinent negatives).
2. Document any parts of the assessment that are omitted or refused by the patient.
3. Avoid using judgmental language such as "good," "poor," "bad," "normal," "abnormal," "decreased," "appears to be," and "seems."
4. Avoid evaluative statements (e.g., "patient is uncooperative," "patient is lazy"); cite instead specific statements or actions that you observe (e.g., "patient said 'I hate this place' and kicked trash can").
5. State time intervals precisely (e.g., "every 4 hours," "bid," instead of "seldom," "occasionally").
6. Do not make relative statements about findings (e.g., "mass the size of an egg"); use specific measurements (e.g., "mass 3 cm × 5 cm").
7. Draw pictures when appropriate (e.g., location of scar, masses, skin lesion, decubitus, deep tendon reflex, etc.).
8. Refer to findings using anatomic landmarks (e.g., left upper quadrant [of abdomen], left lower lobe [of lung], midclavicular line, etc.).
9. Use the face of the clock to describe findings that are in a circular pattern (e.g., breast, tympanic membrane, rectum, vagina).
10. Document any change in the patient's condition during a visit or from previous visits.
11. Describe what you observed, not what you did.

CASE STUDY

The Patient with Pneumonia

❖ HEALTH HISTORY

TODAY'S DATE	January 21
BIOGRAPHICAL DATA	
Patient Name	Maria Rivera
Address	12 Rock Street, Apt. 1 B, Miami, FL 33158
Phone Number	(305) 111-2222
Date of Birth	March 21, 1925
Birthplace	Tegucigalpa; Honduras, Central America
Social Security Number	121-21-2121
Occupation	Retired secretary
Insurance	Medicare
Usual Source of Health Care	None; last trip to hl care facility was 10 yr ago
Source of Referral	Friend (Nelly) told her about the "wonderful" nurses at this practice
Emergency Contact	Nelly Perera (friend): (305) 222-1111
Source and Reliability of Information	Pt, reliable
PATIENT PROFILE	73 yo WHF
CHIEF COMPLAINT	"I feel lousy. I'm having a hard time breathing. I haven't been checked out in so long. Please give me a good going over so I know that I'm all right."
HISTORY OF PRESENT ILLNESS	In usual state of good hl until 4 d PTA; began to feel very tired, had "stuffy nose"; didn't have energy to do housework, visit friends, or go to volunteer work or church; persistent, hacking, nonproductive cough c̄ chills; felt "warm" but never took temp; felt "achy" & took ASA 325 mg po q 6 h × 2 d; 2 d PTA SOB developed; felt "winded" preparing meals, walking; rest improved SOB but did not make it go away; states hardly slept all night & became frightened this AM when coughed up "red stuff"; denies chest pain, N, V, D, diaphoresis, H/A; states "I don't have time to be ill; I miss my church meetings & volunteer work."

continued

PAST HEALTH HISTORY

Medical
Told she had HTN 10 yr PTA; took "some med" for 2 mo but never had Rx refilled b/c "I felt fine so I didn't take it any more"; "stiffness" in fingers that makes needlepointing difficult

Surgical
Denies

Medications
MVI q AM; ASA 325 mg po q 1–2 d for "aches & pains"; doesn't share drugs c̄ friends; believes in taking as few meds as possible

Communicable Diseases
Denies TB, HSV, gonorrhea, syphilis, hepatitis, ⊕ HIV, AIDS

Allergies
NKA

Injuries/Accidents
Fell in apt 6 mo ago on throw rug; hip hurt × 1 wk but never sought tx; fell & hit head getting out bathtub 3 mo ago; suffered head bruise, H/A × 2 d, & sore wrist × 10 d; no tx sought

Disabilities/Handicaps
Denies

Blood Transfusions
Denies

Childhood Illnesses
Doesn't recall

Immunizations
Up to date when emigrated to U.S. 45 yr ago; doesn't recall date of last tetanus

FAMILY HEALTH HISTORY

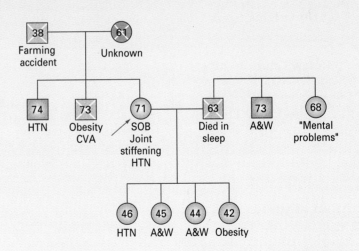

LEGEND
- ◯ Living female
- ◻ Living male
- ⊗ Deceased female
- ⊠ Deceased male
- ↗ Points to patient

A&W = Alive & well
CVA = Cerebrovascular accident
HTN = Hypertension
SOB = Shortness of breath

Denies family hx of heart dz, CVA, HTN, TB, DM, CA, kidney dz, blood disorders, epilepsy, migraine H/A, gout, thyroid dz, liver dz, asthma, allergic disorders, alcoholism, mental illness, drug addiction, AIDS, HIV dz, violent rx.

SOCIAL HISTORY

Alcohol Use
Denies

Tobacco Use
Denies

continued

Drug Use	Denies
Sexual Practice	Monogamous relationship c̄ husband of 40 yr; husband died 11 yr ago; not currently sexually active
Travel History	∅ travel outside Miami × 20 yr; made annual trip to visit family in Honduras for 25 yr prior to this
Work Environment	Secretary × 42 yr; retired age 60; volunteers c̄ ladies auxiliary at local hospital 20 hr/wk in gift shop
Home Environment	Lives in modern 1 BR apt by self (ground level); states it is "nice" & well maintained; no CO or smoke detectors; has kitten; walks to grocery store & church; takes bus to hospital; doesn't know neighbors; considers neighborhood safe
Hobbies/Leisure Activities	Needlepointing (limited due to stiff fingers), church socials, watching TV
Stress	Inability to get to church services, socials, & meetings; inability to get to hospital work ("they count on me to interpret & work at gift shop"); worries about children who live in other states
Education	Completed 1 yr of college in Honduras
Economic Status	States she is "OK"; receives SS & small pension
Military Service	Denies
Religion	Roman Catholic; attends weekly mass at Hispanic church; devotion to God is important focus in life
Ethnic Background	Hispanic from Central America; speaks English & Spanish fluently; naturalized citizen for 33 yr
Roles/Relationships	Has many friends at hospital & church; talks on phone q wk c̄ children
Characteristic Patterns of Daily Living	Rises at 0630, bathes, dresses, & eats breakfast; 0730 catches bus for hospital (5 d/wk); 0800–1200 works at hospital; 1200 eats bag lunch at hospital c̄ friends then goes home, rests/takes nap, does housework or calls friends, prepares & eats dinner; 1800 goes to church for meeting or social gathering, returns home, watches TV; 2230 goes to bed
HEALTH MAINTENANCE ACTIVITIES	
Sleep	8 hr/night; sleeps through the night s̄ difficulties
Diet	Rx low-salt diet not followed; salts food to taste; fries tortillas in vegetable oil; fries most dinners; snacks on potato chips; likes to eat while watching TV; does not know wt ("my clothes still fit")
Exercise	Walks 2 blocks to grocery store qd; walks 4 blocks to church qd
Stress Management	Eats when stressed or bored; states it "works like a charm"
Use of Safety Devices	Denies

continued

Health Check-Ups	Can't recall last time eyes or ears checked; can't recall last PAP smear; denies getting flu shot
REVIEW OF SYSTEMS	
General	States she is usually very healthy; last wk was difficult since she isn't used to being sick
Psychological	Denies irritability, nervousness, tension, ↑ stress ($\bar{x}$ for past wk), difficulty concentrating, mood changes, suicidal thoughts, depression
Skin, Hair, and Nails	Denies rashes, itching, Δ in skin pigmentation, ecchymoses, Δ in skin texture, sores, lumps, odors, sweating, acne, alopecia, hirsutism, Δ in nails; denies sunbathing & use of sunblock
Head	Denies CHI; severe H/A q 2–3 wk that occur in AM, treats $\bar{c}$ ASA 325 mg po (× 9 mo)
Eyes	Denies photophobia, ↑ tearing, diplopia, eye drainage, bloodshot eyes, eye pain, blind spots, flashing lights, halos around objects, glaucoma, cataracts; wears bifocal glasses; vision gets blurry occasionally & can't always read signs
Ears	Denies hearing deficits, hearing aid, ear pain, d/c, vertigo, earaches, infection; tinnitus occurs q few days ("I just ignore it")
Nose and Sinuses	Denies frequent URIs, d/c, itching, hay fever, postnasal drip, stuffiness, sinus pain, nasal polyps, obstruction, Δ in sense of smell; nosebleed 1 × month, applies pressure to nose & lies down
Mouth	Denies toothache, tooth abscess, dentures, bleeding/swollen gums, difficulty chewing, sore tongue, Δ in taste, lesions, Δ in salivation, bad breath; sputum as per HPI
Throat/Neck	Denies hoarseness, Δ in voice, frequent sore throats, difficulty swallowing, pain/stiffness, goiter
Breasts	Denies pain, tenderness, d/c, lumps, dimpling; doesn't perform BSE ("I'm too old for that!")
Respiratory	Refer to HPI, denies frequent URIs
Cardiovascular	Denies PND, CP, orthopnea, heart murmur, palpitations, syncope, edema, cold hands/feet, leg cramps, MI, valvular dz, intermittent claudication, varicose veins, thrombophlebitis, anemia; HTN as per PHH
Gastrointestinal	Denies Δ in appetite, N, V, D, constipation, melena, hematemesis, Δ in stool color, flatulence, belching, regurgitation, heartburn, dysphagia, abd pain, jaundice, hemorrhoids, hepatitis, PUD, gallstones; hard, brown stool 2 ×/wk $\bar{c}$ straining ("I've always been a little slow in that department")
Musculoskeletal	Denies back pain, redness, swelling, bone deformity, weakness, broken bones, dislocations, sprains, gout, arthritis, herniated disc; fingers are "stiff" q AM; exercises hands on bus ride to hospital & they feel better by lunchtime; c/o muscle aches qd

continued

Neurological	Denies Δ in balance, incoordination, loss of mvt, Δ in sensory/perception, Δ in speech, Δ in smell, loss of memory, tremors, involuntary mvt, ↓ LOC, sz, weakness; dizziness q few d ("I just sit down when it happens")
Urinary	Denies Δ in urine color & volume, voiding habits, dysuria, hesitancy, urgency, frequency, nocturia, polyuria, dribbling, reduced force of stream, bedwetting, incontinence, suprapubic pain, kidney stones, UTI; voids clear yellow urine 6–7 × qd
Female Reproductive	Denies vaginal d/c, Δ in libido, vaginal bleeding; menarche 15 yo; menopause 52 yo, "I got through the change OK. It was no fun but it's over"; OB hx: 4 pregnancies c̄ 4 vaginal deliveries s̄ complications
Nutrition	Doesn't know wt ("I don't have a scale & I don't want to know"), prepares own meals, denies food allergies; prefers diet of beef, beans, rice, & tortillas but will "eat anything"
Endocrine	Denies bulging eyes, fatigue, Δ in size of head/hands/feet, heat/cold intolerance, ↑ sweating, ↑ thirst, ↑ hunger, Δ in body hair distribution, swelling in ant neck, DM
Lymph Nodes	Denies enlargement, tenderness
Hematological	Denies easy bleeding/bruising, anemia; doesn't know blood type

PHYSICAL ASSESSMENT

General	WDWN Hispanic ♀ who looks her stated age and in mild resp distress
	HT: 5'5" (163.6 cm)
	WT: 220 lb (100 kg)
	T: 100.5°F po (38.5°C)
	P: 98
	R: 26
	BP: 168/103 (Ⓛ arm sitting)
	  168/102 (Ⓛ arm lying)
	  162/100 (Ⓡ arm sitting)

Skin, Hair, and Nails	Light tan in color s̄ lesions, rashes, ecchymoses, edema, bleeding; very warm to touch c̄ diaphoresis, smooth texture, ↓ turgor; hair shiny black c̄ even distribution, s̄ infestations; nailbeds pale, firm c̄ 3 sec cap refill, no clubbing
Head	Normocephalic s̄ lesions, masses, depressions, or tenderness; face symmetrical s̄ involuntary mvt or swelling; scalp shiny & intact s̄ lesions or masses; TMJ articulates smoothly s̄ clicking or crepitus
Eyes	Acuity by Snellen chart c̄ eyeglasses: OD 20/30, OS 20/25, able to read newspaper s̄ difficulty c̄ bifocals, color vision intact, visual fields by confrontation intact, eyebrows full & symmetrical, eyelashes evenly distributed & s̄ inflammation, Ø ptosis or lid lag, lacrimal apparatus s̄ inflammation or d/c, corneal light reflex symmetrical s̄ strabismus, cover-uncover test s̄ deviation, EOM mvt intact, Ø nystagmus, conjunctiva pink, Ø foreign bodies, Ø tearing, sclera white s̄ exudate, PERRLA (3 mm) Funduscopic: ⊕ red reflex, discs flat c̄ sharp margins, vessels in A-V ratio of 2:3 c̄ arteriolar tortuosity & narrowing, A-V nicking noted, background uniformly pink s̄ hemorrhages or exudate

continued

Ears Gross hearing intact by watch tick test; pinna s̄ masses, lesions, nodules, inflammation, or tenderness; EAC clear s̄ inflammation; TMs shiny & mobile c̄ visible landmarks; Weber midline; Rinne AC>BC

Nose and Sinuses Ø deformities, bleeding, lesions, masses, swelling; nares patent, nontender; septum midline s̄ perforation; mucosa pink, moist s̄ swelling; sinuses nontender, resonant

Mouth and Throat Breath fresh; lips pink s̄ swelling or lesions; gums & mucosa pink & moist; 30 teeth in good repair; tongue midline, well papillated, & s̄ fasciculations, lesions, swelling, or bleeding; hard & soft palates intact s̄ lesions or masses; pharynx pink s̄ exudate; uvula midline & rises c̄ phonation; 1+/4+ tonsils; ⊕ gag reflex

Neck Supple s̄ masses or spasms & c̄ full ROM, neck symmetrical s̄ masses or tenderness, lymph nodes nonpalpable, trachea midline, thyroid nontender s̄ enlargement, Ø bruits, Ø JVD at 90°, 45°, & supine

Breasts Light tan c̄ striae over both breasts; areola & nipples dark in pigmentation; uniform consistency; Ø thickening, edema, vascularity, erosion, fissures, lesions, masses, retraction, d/c; Ⓛ breast >Ⓡ breast (breasts assessed in sitting position only due to SOB); nonpalpable lymph nodes

Thorax and Lungs AP: transverse diameter = 1:1, chest wall symmetrical, costal angle <90°, angle of the ribs c̄ sternum = 45°, Ø bulging of ICS or retractions, using trapezius & sternocleidomastoid muscles, resp reg & shallow c̄ sl nasal flaring, rust-colored sputum noted on expectoration, thoracic expansion 2 cm ant & 2 cm post, tactile fremitus = bilaterally x̄ ↑ in LLL, lungs resonant x̄ for dullness in LLL, diaphragmatic excursion 3 cm on Ⓡ (unable to measure on Ⓛ), coarse inspiratory crackles in LLL that clear c̄ coughing, clear in other lobes though slightly ↓ in RLL, ⊕ voice sounds in LLL

Heart Precordium s̄ pulsations/heaves/thrills, apical pulse 100, apical impulse 1 cm at 5th ICS 2 cm to Ⓛ of MCL, S_1 & S_2 present s̄ murmur/gallop/rub, ⊕ S_4 mitral area

Abdomen Lg convex, symmetrical c̄ striae, light tan s̄ dilated veins, scars, incisions, ⊕ bowel sounds in 4 quadrants, Ø bruits, venous hum, friction rub; tympanic, abd soft, Ø masses/tenderness to light/deep palpation; remainder of assessment deferred due to pt's inability to tolerate supine position any longer 2° to SOB

Peripheral Vasculature Ø edema or ulcerations, ⊖ Homan's sign, pulse reg & strong, Ø pulsus paradoxus, Ø bruits

	Carotid	Brachial	Radial	Femoral	Popliteal	Dorsalis Pedis	Posterior Tibial
R	2+	2+	2+	2+	2+	2+	2+
L	2+	2+	2+	2+	2+	2+	2+

Scale: 0–4+

Musculoskeletal Spine s̄ scoliosis/lordosis, muscles s̄ atrophy = in size bilaterally c̄ adequate tone, Ø involuntary mvt, extremities c̄ full ROM x̄ for fingers, weak hand grip, redness & swelling of distal interphalangeal joints (Heberden's nodes), s̄ masses, crepitus

continued

Neurological	Mental Status: appropriate affect, mood, & behavior, A, A & O × 3, thought processes & memory intact
	CN II–XII: intact, CN I deferred.
	Sensory: light touch, pain, position & vibration senses, intact; stereognosis, graphesthesia, & 2-point discrimination intact
	Motor: ⊖ pronator drift
	Cerebellar: ⊖ Romberg, gait smooth & steady, tandem walk steady, draws figure 8 c̄ each foot, finger-to-nose & rapid alternating hand movements intact
	Reflexes:

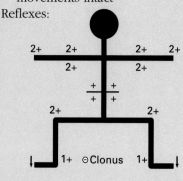

Scale = 4+

Genitalia and Rectum	Deferred; pt unable to assume supine position for extended period of time due to SOB

LABORATORY DATA

Blood Work

	Pt's Values	Normal Range
RBC	3.3 M/mm³	3.6–5.0 M/mm³
WBC	17.1 k/mm³	4–11 k/mm³
HCT	35%	35%–47%
HGB	10.5 g/dl	12–16 g/dl

Sputum Culture	Pneumoccal pneumonia

DIAGNOSTIC DATA

Chest X-Ray	Impression: LLL consolidation consistent with pneumonia
Hand X-Ray	Impression: osteoarthritis in all fingers

REVIEW QUESTIONS AND ACTIVITIES

1. Conduct a nursing grand rounds at your facility to discuss ethical dilemmas encountered by the staff during health histories or physical assessments.

2. Read your state Nurse Practice Act and then discuss the legal implications for your assessment practice.

3. Formulate all of the nursing diagnoses that can be derived from the case study. Develop care plans for three of them.

4. The following statements are documented in a physical assessment. Decide which are stated correctly and suggest ways to alter those statements that are worded incorrectly.
   a. Denies SOB, CP, DOE
   b. Refused rectal exam
   c. Good capillary refill
   d. Pea-sized lump in left upper quadrant of right breast
   e. Percussed abdomen
   f. Seems to be depressed

5. Which of the following assessments are you capable of performing on a comatose patient?
   a. Corneal reflex
   b. Snellen test
   c. Cerebellar function
   d. Stepping reflex

   The correct answer is (a).

6. Which of the following is the correct sequence for a complete physical assessment?
   a. Skin, eyes, neck, mouth, and throat
   b. Abdomen, inguinal area, lower extremities, neurological system
   c. Neurological system, musculoskeletal system, inguinal area, anus, and rectum
   d. Anterior thorax, neck, upper extremities, breasts

   The correct answer is (b).

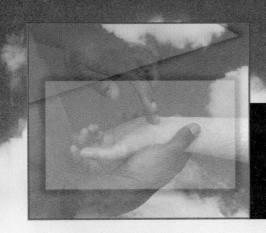

References and Bibliography

CHAPTER 1
The Nursing Process

REFERENCES

American Nurses Association (1980). *Nursing: A social policy statement*. Kansas City, MO: Author.

American Nurses Association (1991). *Standards of clinical nursing practice*. Washington, DC: Author.

Gordon, M. (1997). *Manual of nursing diagnosis: 1997–1998*. St. Louis, MO: Mosby-Yearbook, Inc.

North American Nursing Diagnosis Association (1996). *Nursing diagnoses: Definitions & classification 1997–1998*. Philadelphia: Author.

BIBLIOGRAPHY

Buchanan, L. M. (1994). Therapeutic nursing intervention knowledge development and outcome measures for advanced practice. *Nursing and Health Care, 15*(4), 190–195.

Carlson, J. H., Craft, C. A., McGuire, A. D., & Popkess-Vawter, S. (1991). *Nursing diagnosis: A case study approach*. Philadelphia: Saunders.

Carpenito, L. J. (1997). *Nursing diagnosis: Application to clinical practice* (7th ed.). Philadelphia: Lippincott.

Carroll-Johnson, R. M., & Paquette, M. (Eds.). (1994). *Classification of nursing diagnoses: Proceedings of the tenth conference*. Philadelphia: Lippincott.

Cox, H. C., Lubno, M. A., Ridenour, N. A., Svidaromont, K. L., Slater, M. M., Newfield, S. A., and Hinz, M. D. (1993). *Clinical applications of nursing diagnosis: Adult, child, women's, mental health, gerontic and home health considerations* (2nd ed.). Philadelphia: F. A. Davis.

Crummer, M. B., & Carter, V. (1993). Critical pathways: The pivotal tool. *Journal of Cardiovascular Nursing, 7*(4), 30–37.

Daly, J. M., McCloskey, J. C., & Bulechek, G. B. (1994). Nursing interventions classification use in long-term care. *Geriatric Nursing: American Journal of Care for the Aging, 15*(1), 41–46.

Davis, B. D., Billings, J. R., & Ryland R. K. (1994). Evaluation of nursing process documentation. *Journal of Advanced Nursing, 19*(5), 960–968.

Doenges, M. E., Moorhouse, M. F., & McCoy, S. M. (1995). *Application of nursing process and nursing diagnosis: An interactive text*. (2nd ed.) Philadelphia: F. A. Davis.

Frisch, N. (1993). Home care nursing and psychosocial-emotional needs of clients: How nursing diagnosis helps to direct and inform practice. *Home Healthcare Nurse, 11*(2), 64–65, 70.

Gebbie, K. M., & Lavin, M. A. (1975). *Classification of nursing diagnoses: Proceedings of the first national conference*. St. Louis: Mosby.

Heafey, M. L., Edwards, P. A., & McLaughlin, T. F. (1994). Developing care plans for psychosocial nursing diagnoses. *Ostomy Wound Management, 40*(3), 18–22, 24–26.

Jankin, J. (1994). Research validation of nursing diagnoses: How much progress? *Nursing Diagnosis, 5*(1), 46.

McFarland, G. K., & McFarlane, E. A. (1996). *Nursing diagnosis & intervention: Planning for patient care*. (3rd ed.) St. Louis: Mosby.

Moss, M. T. (1994). Nursing tools: A global perspective . . . Three tools form a triangular analytical instrument: outcomes management, case management, and critical pathways. *Nursing Management, 25*(6), 64 A–B.

Townsend, M. C. (1997). *Nursing diagnoses in psychiatric nursing: A pocket guide for care plan construction* (4th ed.). Philadelphia: F. A. Davis.

Tripp, S. L., & Stachowiak, B. (1992). Health maintenance, health promotion: Is there a difference? *Public Health Nursing, 9*(3), 155–161.

Webb, C., & Mason, G. (1993). Nursing diagnosis in sick children's nursing. *Journal of Clinical Nursing, 2*(5), 279–286.

White, A. K. (1993). The nursing process: A constraint on expert practice. *Journal of Nursing Management, 1*(5), 245–252.

Young-Meyer, V. (1993). A two-level approach to nursing process. *Journal of Nursing Staff Development, 9*(5), 230–235.

Zink, M. R. (1994). Nursing diagnosis in home care: Audit tool development. *Journal of Community Health Nursing, 11*(1), 51–58.

CHAPTER 2
The Patient Interview

REFERENCES

Aromando, L. (1995). *Mental health and psychiatric nursing: Clinical rotation guide*. (2nd ed.) Springhouse, PA: Springhouse Corporation.

Bradley, J. C., & Edinberg, M. A. (1990). *Communication in the nursing context* (3rd ed.). East Norwalk, CT: Appleton & Lange.

Cormier, W. H., & Cormier, L. S. (1991). *Interviewing strategies for helpers: Fundamental skills and cognitive behavioral interventions* (3rd ed.). Pacific Grove, CA: Brooks/Cole.

Greenstone, J. L., & Leviton, S. C. (1993). *Elements of crisis intervention: Crises and how to respond to them.* Pacific Grove, CA: Brooks/Cole.

Ivey, A. (1994). *Intentional interviewing and counseling: Facilitating client development in a multicultural society* (3rd ed.). Pacific Grove, CA: Brooks/Cole.

Morrison, E. (1992). When staff are attacked. *Journal of Psychosocial Nursing, 30*(7), 13.

Northouse P. G., & Northouse, L. L. (1992). *Health communication: Strategies for professionals.* (2nd ed.) Stamford, CT: Appleton & Lange.

BIBLIOGRAPHY

Barnes, L. P. (1994). Useful tools in patient teaching: Interviewing skills. *American Journal of Maternal Child Nursing, 19*(5), 289.

Braverman, B. G. (1990). Eliciting assessment data from the patient who is difficult to interview. *Nursing Clinics of North America, 25*(4), 743–750.

Cornell, D. (1993). Say the words: Communication techniques. *Nursing Management, 24*(3), 42–44.

Dyehouse, J. M. (1992). Abuse of women in the health care system. In C. M. Sampselle (Ed.), *Violence against women: Nursing research, education, and practice issues* (pp. 219–234). New York: Hemisphere Publishing.

Eliopoulos, C. (1990). *Health assessment of the older adult* (2nd ed.). Reading, MA: Addison Wesley.

Fry, A. (1994). Affective communication with people with visual disabilities. *Nursing Times, 90*(44), 42–43.

Johnson, J. R. (1994). The communication training needs of registered nurses. *Journal of Continuing Education in Nursing, 25*(5), 213–218.

Lukas, S. (1993). *Where to start and what to ask: An assessment handbook.* New York: W. W. Norton.

Marshall, S. L., & While, A. E. (1994). Interviewing respondents who have English as a second language: Challenges encountered and suggestions for other researchers. *Journal of Advanced Nursing, 19*(3), 566–571.

Mezey, M. (1994). *Health assessment of the older individual.* New York: Springer Publishing Co.

Morrison, J. (1995). *The first interview: Revised for DSM-IV.* New York: Guilford.

Ornstein, P., Cuchetti, D., Levine, J., & Freiman, L. (1968). Some parameters of verbal behavior that reliably differentiate novice from experienced psychotherapists. *Journal of Abnormal Psychology, 73*, 240.

Professional growth. Asking questions effectively . . . How to improve your interviewing skills. (1995). *Nursing95*(3), 839–885.

Sampselle, C. M. (1990). The influence of feminist philosophy on nursing practice. *Image, 22*(4), 243–247.

Sands, J. K. (1992). Essential interviewing strategies: Covering all the bases. *Healthcare Trends and Transition, 38*(3), 18, 21, 22.

Smith, M. E., & Hart, G. (1994). Nurses' responses to patient anger: From disconnecting to connecting. *Journal of Advanced Nursing, 20*(4), 643–651.

Taylor, M. W. (1991). Listening: A key management tool. *Pediatric Nursing, 17*(4), 390, 422.

Thornburg, L. (1994). When interviewing the disabled, focus on their abilities. *Journal of Long Term Care Administration, 22*(1), 14–16.

Wainrub, B. R. (1992). *Gender issues across the life cycle.* New York: Springer Publishing Co.

Wright, L., & Leahey, M. (1994). *Nurses and families: A guide to family assessment and intervention.* (2nd ed.). Philadelphia: F. A. Davis.

CHAPTER 3
The Complete Health History

REFERENCES

Brown, D. (1994, July 24). Triumphant in the desert, stricken at home. *Washington Post*, A, 1:2.

Dodd, R. Y. (1992). The risk of transfusion-transmitted infection (Editorial). *New England Journal of Medicine, 327*(6), 419–420.

BIBLIOGRAPHY

Buchwald, D., Caralis, P. V., Gany, F., et al. (1993). The medical interview across cultures. *Patient Care, 27*(7), 141–144, 146, 148.

Charmaz, K. (1991). *Good days, bad days: The self in chronic illness and time.* New Brunswick, NJ: Rutgers University Press.

Fred, H. L., Hinthorn, D. R., Larson, E. B., et al. (1994). Diagnostic pearls for 10 common problems. *Patient Care, 28*(1), 70–72, 75, 79–80.

Gehring, P. E. (1991). Physical assessment begins with a history. *RN, 54*(11), 26–32.

Kerr, S. D. (1992). A comparison of four nursing documentation systems. *Journal of Nursing Staff Development, 8*(1), 26–31.

Milner, I. B., Axelrod, B. N., Pasquantonio, J., & Sillanpaa, M. (1994). Is there a Gulf War syndrome? *Journal of the American Medical Association, 271*(9), 661.

Morrissey, J. (1994). Obtaining a "reasonably accurate" health history. *Plastic Surgical Nursing, 14*(1), 27–30.

Moyers, B. (1993). *Healing and the mind.* New York: Doubleday.

Murphy, S. A. (1991). Human responses to catastrophe. *Annual Review of Nursing Research, 9*, 57–76.

Owen, K. (1994). Listen to what patients don't say. *RN, 57*(1), 96.

Sayers, L. (1992). Prejudice pre-empted . . . allowing stereotypical views to govern the assessment of patients. *Nursing Times, 88*(37), 46–48.

Selye, H. (1946). The general adaptation syndrome and diseases of adaptation. *Journal of Clinical Endocrinology, 6*(2), 117–230.

Selye, H. (1974). *Stress without distress.* Philadelphia: Lippincott.

Skinn, B., & Stacey, D. (1994). Establishing an integrated framework for documentation: Use of a self-reporting health history and outpatient oncology record. *Oncology Nursing Forum, 21*(9), 1557–1566.

Tiernan, P. J. (1994). Independent nursing interventions: Relaxation and guided imagery in critical care. *Critical Care Nurse, 14*(5), 47–51.

Topf, M. (1992). Effects of personal control over hospital noise on sleep. *Research in Nursing & Health, 15*(1), 19–28.

Watson, R. R. (1992). *Exercise and disease.* Boca Raton, FL: CRC Press.

CHAPTER 4
Developmental Assessment

REFERENCES

Aguilera, D. C. (1994). *Crisis intervention theory and methodology* (7th ed.). Baltimore: Mosby.

Aldwin, C. M. (1992). Aging, coping, and efficacy: Theoretical framework for examining coping in life-span developmental context. In M. L. Wykle, E. Kahana, & J. Kowal (Eds.), *Stress and health among the elderly* (pp. 96–113). New York: Springer Publishing Company.

Antonovsky, A. (1987). *Unraveling the mystery of health: How people manage stress and stay well.* San Francisco: Jossey-Bass Publishers.

Antonovsky, A. (1993). The structure and properties of the sense of coherence scale. *Social Science Medicine, 36*(6), 725–733.

Brandt, J., Spencer, M., & Folstein, M. (1988). The Telephone Instrument for Cognitive Status. *Neuropsychiatry, Neuropsychology, and Behavioral Neurology, 1,* 11–17.

Brazelton, T. B. (1996). *Neonatal behavioral assessment scale* (3rd ed.). Philadelphia: Lippincott.

Carey, W. B., & McDevitt, S. (1978). Revision of the Infant Temperament Questionnaire. *Pediatrics, 61,* 735–739.

Carnevali, D. L., & Patrick, M. (1993). *Nursing management for the elderly* (3rd ed.). Philadelphia: Lippincott.

Coplan, J. (1983). Evaluation of the child with delayed speech or language. *Pediatric Annals, 14*(3), 202–208.

Darling-Fisher, C., & Leidy, N. K. (1988). Measuring Eriksonian development in the adult: The Modified Erikson Psychosocial Stage Inventory. *Psychological Reports, 62,* 747–754.

Erikson, E. (1974). *Dimensions of a new identity.* New York: W. W. Norton.

Folstein, M. F., Folstein, S. E., & McHugh, P. R. (1975). "Mini-Mental State": A practical method for grading the cognitive state of patients for the clinician. *Journal of Psychiatric Research, 12,* 189–198.

Freud, S. (1946). *The ego and the mechanism of defense.* New York: International Universities Press.

Fullard, W., McDevitt, S., & Carey, W. (1984). Assessing temperament in one to three year old children. *Journal of Pediatric Psychology, 9,* 205–217.

Gallagher, D. (1986). The Beck Depression Inventory and older adults: Review of its development and utility. In T. L. Brink (Ed.), *Clinical gerontology: A guide to assessment and intervention* (pp. 149–163). New York: Haworth Press.

Gilligan, C. (1982). *In a different voice: Psychological theory and women's development.* Cambridge, MA: Harvard University Press.

Grey, M. (1993). Stressors and children's health. *Journal of Pediatric Nursing, 8*(2), 85–91.

Hegvik, R., McDevitt, S., & Carey, W. (1982). The Middle Childhood Temperament Questionnaire. *Journal of Developmental Behavior in Pediatrics, 3,* 197–200.

Jackson, D. B., & Saunders, R. B. (1993). *Child health nursing: A comprehensive approach to the care of children and their families.* Philadelphia: Lippincott.

Kohlberg, L. (1981). *The philosophy of moral development: Moral stages and the idea of justice.* New York: Harper & Row.

Lazarus, R. S. (1981). Little hasards can be hasardous to your health. *Psychology Today, 15*(7), 58–62.

Lazarus, R. S., & Folkman, S. (1984). *Stress, appraisal and coping.* New York: Springer Publishers.

Leidy, N. K., & Darling-Fisher, C. S. (1995). Reliability and validity of the modified Erikson psychosocial stage inventory in diverse samples. *Western Journal of Nursing Research, 17*(2), 168–187.

Levinson, D. J., Darrow, C. N., & Klein, E. B. (1986). *The seasons of a man's life* (2nd ed.). New York: Ballantine.

McDowell, I., & Newell, C. (1987). *Functional disability and handicap. Measuring health: A guide to rating scales and questionnaires.* New York: Oxford University Press.

Miller, L. H., Smith, A. D., & Mehler, B. L. (1991). *The stress audit.* Brookline, MA: Biobehavioral Associates.

Murray, R. B., & Zentner, J. P. (1993). *Nursing assessment and health promotion strategies through the life span* (5th ed.). Norwalk, CT: Appleton & Lange.

Neinstein, L. S. (1991). *Adolescent health care: A practical guide* (2nd ed.). Baltimore: Williams & Wilkins.

Piaget, J. (1952). *The origins of intelligence in children.* New York: International Universities Press.

Powell, M. L. (1981). *Assessment and management of developmental changes and problems in children* (2nd ed.). St. Louis: Mosby.

Rahe, R. H. (1975). Epidemiological studies in life change and illness. *International Journal of Psychiatry, 6*(1–2), 133–146.

Resnick, N. M. (1994). Geriatric medicine and the elderly patient. In L. M. Tierney, Jr., S. J. McPhee, & M. A. Papadakis (Eds.), *Current medical diagnosis and treatment* (33rd ed., pp. 41–60). Norwalk, CT: Appleton & Lange.

Sarason, J. G., Johnson, J. H., & Siegal, J. M. (1978). Assessing the impact of life changes: Development of life experiences survey. *Journal of Consulting Clinical Psychology, 46*(5), 932–946.

Saunders, A., & Remsberg, B. (1984). *The stress-proof child: A loving parent's guide.* New York: Holt, Rinehart, & Winston.

Schiedel, D., & Marcia, J. (1985). Ego identity, intimacy, sex role orientation, and gender. *Developmental Psychology, 21,* 149–160.

Tombaugh, T. N., & McIntyre, N. J. (1992). The Mini-Mental State Examination: A comprehensive review. *Journal of the American Geriatric Society, 40,* 922–935.

Ullmann, R. K., Sleator, E. K., & Sprague, R. L. (1991). *ACTeRS profile* (2nd ed). Champaign, IL: MetriTech, Inc.

Weinberger, M., Hiner, S. L., & Tierney, W. M. (1987). In support of hassles as a measure of stress in predicting health outcomes. *Journal of Behavioral Medicine, 10,* 19–31.

Wong, D. L. (1995). *Whaley and Wong's nursing care of infants and children* (5th ed.). Baltimore: Mosby.

Wykle, M. L., Kahana, E., & Kowal, J. (Eds.) (1992). *Stress and health among the elderly.* New York: Springer Publishing Company.

BIBLIOGRAPHY

Antonovsky, A. (1991). The structural sources of salutogenic strength. In C. L. Cooper & R. Payne (Eds.), *Personality and stress: Individual differences in the stress response* (pp. 67–104). New York: John Wiley & Sons.

Camp, B. W., & Kosleske, E. B. (1995). Adolescence. In W. W. Hay, Jr., J. R. Groothuis, A. R. Hayward, & M. J. Levin (Eds.), *Current pediatric diagnosis and treatment* (12th ed., pp. 129–153). Norwalk, CT: Appleton & Lange.

Erikson, E. H. (1950). *Childhood and society.* New York: W. W. Norton.

Erikson, E. H. (1968). *Identity: Youth and crisis.* New York: W. W. Norton.

Gallo, J. J., Reichel, W., & Andersen, L. M. (1995). *Handbook of geriatric assessment* (2nd ed.). Gaithersburg, MD: Aspen Publishers, Inc.

Howard, B. T. (1990). Growing together: The toddler years need not be turbulent. *Contemporary Pediatrics*, 7(6), 21–40.

Jung, C. (1968). *The archetypes and the collective conscious.* Princeton: Princeton University Press.

Levinson, D. (1977). The mid-life transition: A period of adult psychosocial development. *Psychiatry*, 40, 99–112.

Neugarten, B., Moore, J. W., & Lowe, J. C. (1965). Age norms, age constraints, and adult socialization. *American Journal of Sociology*, 70, 710–717.

Peck, R. C. (1955). Psychological developments in the second half of life. In J. E. Anderson (Ed.), *Psychological aspects of aging*. Washington, DC: American Psychological Association.

Schaie, K. W. (1977). Toward a stage theory of adult cognitive development. *Journal of Aging and Human Development*, 8(2), 129–138.

Wender, P. H. (1987). *The hyperactive child, adolescent, and adult.* New York: Oxford University Press.

CHAPTER 5
Cultural Assessment

REFERENCES

The American Academy of Nursing Expert Panel on Culturally Competent Nursing Care (1992). AAN expert panel report: Culturally competent health care. *Nursing Outlook*, 40(6), 277–283.

Burk, M. E., Wieser, P. C., & Keegan, L. (1995). Cultural beliefs and health behaviors of pregnant Mexican-American women: Implications for primary care. *Advances in Nursing Science*, 17(4), 37–52.

Carnevali, D. L., & Patrick, M. (Eds.) (1993). *Nursing management for the elderly* (3rd ed). Philadelphia: Lippincott.

Geissler, E. M. (1994). *Pocket guide to cultural assessment.* Baltimore: Mosby-Year Book, Inc.

Giger, J. N., & Davidhizar, R. E. (1995). *Transcultural nursing: Assessment and intervention.* St. Louis: Mosby.

Johnson, K. E., & Rogers, S. (1994). When cultural practices are health risks: The dilemma of female circumcision. *Holistic Nursing Practice*, 8(4), 70–78.

Kluckhorn, K., & Strodtbeck, F. (1961). *Variations in value orientation.* Evanston, IL: Row, Peterson.

Korbin, J. (1977). Anthropological contributions to the study of child abuse. *Child Abuse and Neglect*, 1(1), 7–24.

Kreps, G. L., & Kunimoto, E. N. (1994). *Effective communication in multicultural health care settings.* Thousand Oaks, CA: Sage Publications.

Leininger, M. M. (1994). *Transcultural nursing: Concepts, theory, research, and practice* (2nd ed.). Columbus, OH: McGraw Hill and Greyden Press.

McDonald, D. D. (1994). Gender and ethnic stereotyping and narcotic analgesic administration. *Research in Nursing & Health*, 17, 45–49.

Meleis, A., Lipson, J., & Paul, S. (1992). Ethnicity and health among five Middle Eastern immigrant groups. *Nursing Research*, 41(2), 98–103.

Office of Disease Prevention and Health Promotion. (1994). *Clinician's handbook of preventive services.* Washington, DC: U.S. Department of Health and Human Services, Public Health Service.

Spector, R. (1996). *Cultural diversity in health and illness* (4th ed.). Norwalk, CT: Appleton & Lange.

Schensul, J. J., & Guest, B. H. (1994). Ethnics, ethnicity, and health care reform. In A. Dula & S. Goering (Eds.), *"It just ain't fair": The ethics of health care for African Americans* (pp. 24–36). Westport, CT: Praeger Publishers.

Sprott, J. E. (1993). The black box in family assessment: Cultural diversity. In S. L. Feetham, S. B. Meister, J. M. Bell, & C. L. Gilliss (Eds.), *The nursing of families: Theory, research, education, practice* (pp. 189–199). Norwalk, CT: Sage Publications.

Stevens, P. E. (1992). Who gets care? Access to health care as an arena for nursing action. *Scholarly Inquiry for Nursing Practice: An International Journal*, 6(3), 183–198.

Stevens, P. E. (1994). Lesbians' health-related experiences of care and noncare. *Western Journal of Nursing Research*, 16(6), 639–659.

Thomas, R. K. (1993). *Health care consumers in the 1990s.* Ithaca, NY: American Demographics Books.

U.S. Department of Commerce, Bureau of the Census (1992). *Statistical abstract of the United States: 1992 (112th ed.).* Washington, DC: U.S. Government Printing Office.

Wenger, A. F. Z. (1993). Cultural meaning of symptoms. *Holistic Nursing Practice*, 7(2), 22–35.

Wilson, H. S., & Kneisl, C. R. (1996). *Psychiatric nursing* (5th ed.). Reading, MA: Addison-Wesley.

Wong, D. L. (1995). *Whaley and Wong's nursing care of infants and children* (5th ed.). Baltimore: Mosby.

BIBLIOGRAPHY

Andrews, M. M., & Boyle, J. S. (1995). *Transcultural concepts in nursing care* (2nd ed). Philadelphia: Lippincott.

Baj, P. A. (1995). Integrating the Russian emigre nurse into U.S. nursing. *Journal of Nursing Administration*, 25(3), 43–47.

Brookins, G. (1993). Culture, ethnicity, and bicultural competence: Implications for children with chronic illness and disability. *Pediatrics*, 91(5), 1056–1062.

Browning, M. A., & Woods, J. H. (1993). Cross-cultural family-nurse partnerships. In S. L. Feetham, S. B. Meister, J. M. Bell, & C. L. Gilliss (Eds.), *The nursing of families: Theory, research, education, practice* (pp. 177–188). Norwalk, CT: Sage Publications.

Burner, O. Y., Cunningham, P., & Hattar, H. S. (1990). Managing a multicultural nursing staff in a multicultural environment. *Journal of Nursing Administration*, 20(6), 30–34.

Bushy, A. (1992). Cultural considerations for primary health care: Where do self-care and folk medicine fit? *Holistic Nursing Practice*, 6(3), 10–18.

Charonko, C. (1992). Cultural influences in "noncompliant behavior and decision making." *Holistic Nursing Practice*, 6(3), 73–77.

Cookfair, J. M. (1996). *Nursing care in the community* (2nd ed.). Baltimore: Mosby-Year Book.

D'Avanzo, C. E., Frye, B., & Froman, R. (1994). Stress in Cambodian refugee families. *Image: Journal of Nursing Scholarship*, 26(2), 101–105.

Day, N. A. (1990). Training providers to serve culturally different AIDS patients. Special issue: AIDS: Clinical perspective. *Family and Community Health*, 13(2), 46–53.

Eliason, J. J., & Randall, C. E. (1991). Lesbian phobia in nursing students. *Western Journal of Nursing Research*, 13(3), 363–374.

Frye, B. A., & D'Avanzo, C. D. (1994). Cultural themes in family stress and violence among Cambodian refugee women in the inner city. *Advances in Nursing Science, 16*(3), 64–77.

Germain, C. P. (1992). Cultural care: A bridge between sickness, illness, and disease. *Holistic Nursing Practice, 6*(3), 1–9.

Gunter, L. M. (1991). Cultural diversity among older Americans. In E. M. Baines (Ed.), *Perspectives on gerontological nursing* (pp. 215–230). Newbury Park, NJ: Sage Publications.

Hardy, A. M. (1992). AIDS knowledge and attitudes for January-March, 1991. Provisional Data from the National Health Interview Survey. *Advance Data from Vital and Health Statistics, 21*(6). Hyattsville, MD: National Center for Health Statistics.

Hansen, M. M., & Resic, L. K. (1990). Health beliefs, health care, and rural Appalachian subcultures from an ethnographic perspective. *Family Community Health, 13*(1), 1–10.

Higgins, P. G., & Dicharry, E. K. (1991). Measurement issues addressing social support with Navajo women. *Western Journal of Nursing Research, 13*(2), 242–255.

Jackson, D. B., & Saunders, R. B. (1993). *Child health nursing: A comprehensive approach to the care of children and their families.* Philadelphia: Lippincott.

Jandt, F. E. (1995). *Intercultural communication.* Thousand Oaks, CA: Sage Publications.

Kulwicki, A., & Cass, P. S. (1994). An assessment of Arab American knowledge, attitudes, and beliefs about AIDS. *Image: Journal of Nursing Scholarship, 26*(1), 13–17.

Leininger, M. M. (1994). Transcultural nursing education: A worldwide imperative. *Nursing and Health Care, 15*(5), 254–257.

Leininger, M. M. (Ed.). (1991). *Culture care diversity and universality: A theory of nursing.* New York: National League for Nursing Press.

McDonald, D. D. (1994). Gender and ethnic stereotyping and narcotic analgesic administration. *Research in Nursing and Health, 17*, 45–49.

Meleis, A. I., Arruda, E. N., Lane, S., & Bernal, P. (1994). Veiled, voluminous, and devalued: Narrative stories about low-income women from Brazil, Egypt, and Colombia. *Advances in Nursing Science, 17*(2), 1–15.

Mikhail, B. I. (1994). Hispanic mothers' beliefs and practices regarding selected children's health problems. *Western Journal of Nursing Research, 16*(6), 623–638.

Neill, K. M. (1993). Ethnic pain styles in acute myocardial infarction. *Western Journal of Nursing Research, 15*(5), 531–547.

Olness, K. (1992). Cultural issues in primary pediatric care. In R. A. Hoekelman, S. B. Friedman, N. M. Nelson, & H. M. Seidel (Eds.), *Primary Pediatric Care* (2nd ed.). Baltimore: Mosby-Year Book.

Pachter, L. M. (1994). Culture and clinical care: Folk illness beliefs and behaviors and their implications for health care delivery. *Journal of the American Medical Association, 271*, 690–694.

Rojas, D. (1994). Leadership in a multicultural society: A case in role development. *Nursing and Health Care, 15*(5), 258–261.

Rosella, J. D., Regan-Kubinski, M. J., & Albrecht, S. A. (1994). The need for multicultural diversity among health professionals. *Nursing and Health Care, 15*(5), 242–246.

Schlesinger, A. M. (1991). *The disuniting of America: Reflections on a multicultural society.* Knoxville, TN: Whittle Direct Books.

Stevens, P. E. (1994). Protective strategies of lesbian clients in health care environments. *Research in Nursing and Health, 17*, 217–229.

Stevens, P. E., Hall, J. M., & Meleis, A. I. (1992). Narratives as a basis for culturally relevant holistic care: Ethnicity and everyday experiences of women clerical workers. *Holistic Nursing Practice, 6*(3), 49–58.

Torres, S. (1993). Cultural sensitivity: A must for today's primary care provider. *Advance for Nurse Practitioners, 1*(4), 16–18.

Tripp-Reimer, T. (1992). Cultural assessment. In J. Bellack & B. Edlund (Eds.), *Nursing assessment and diagnosis.* Boston: Jones and Bartlett.

Tripp-Reimer, T., Brink, P., & Saunders, J. (1984). Cultural assessment: Content and process. *Nursing Outlook* (2nd ed.), *32*(2), 78–82.

U.S. Department of Health and Human Services: Public Health Services. (1990). *Healthy people 2000* (DHHS Pub [PHS] 91-50212). U.S. Government Printing Office.

Witte, K., & Morrison, K. (1995). Intercultural and cross-cultural health communication: Understanding people and motivating healthy behaviors. In R. L. Wiseman (Ed.), *Intercultural communication theory* (pp. 216–246). Thousand Oaks, CA: Sage Publications.

CHAPTER 6
Spiritual Assessment

REFERENCES

Andrews, M. M., & Hanson, P. A. (1989). Religious beliefs: Implications for nursing practice. In J. S. Boyle & M. M. Andrews (Eds.), *Transcultural concepts in nursing care.* Glenville, IL: Scott, Foresman and Co.

Bhikkhu, M. (1991). Buddhist ethics in the practice of medicine. In C. Wei-haun Fu & S. A. WaWryTko (Eds.), *Buddhist ethics and modern society: An international symposium.* New York: Greenwood Press.

Carter, S. L. (1993). *The culture of disbelief: How American law and politics trivialize religious devotion.* New York: Basic Books.

Ellwood R. S., Jr. (1995). *Many peoples, many faiths* (5th ed.). Englewood Cliffs, NJ: Prentice-Hall, Inc.

Guzzetta, C., & Dossey, B. (1993). Guiding critical care nurses on the body-mind-spirit journey. *Critical Care Nurse, 13*(4), 104–111.

Holst, L. E. (Ed.). (1985). *Hospital ministry: The role of the chaplain today.* New York: Crossroad.

Labun, E. (1988). Spiritual care: An element in nursing care planning. *Journal of Advanced Nursing, 13*(3), 314–320.

Linn, E. (1986). *I know just how you feel: Avoiding the clichés of grief.* Incline Village, NV: The Publisher's Mark.

NANDA (1996). *Nursing diagnoses: Definitions & classification, 1997–1998.* Philadelphia: Author.

Soeken, K. L., & Carson, V. J. (1987). Responding to the spiritual needs of the chronically ill. *Nursing Clinics of North America, 2*(3), 603–611.

Sullivan, L. E. (1988). Healing. In Mercea Eliade (Ed.), *The encyclopedia of religion.* New York: Macmillan.

BIBLIOGRAPHY

Brooke, V. (1987). The spiritual well-being of the elderly. *Geriatric Nursing, 8*(4), 194–195.

Ellerhorst-Ryan, J. (1985). Selecting an instrument to measure spiritual distress. *Oncology Nursing Forum, 12*(2), 93–99.

Feldman, David M. (1986). *Health and medicine in the Jewish tradition.* New York: Crossroad.

Haase, J. E. (1992). Simultaneous concept analysis of spiritual perspective, hope, acceptance and self-transcendence. *Image: The Journal of Nursing Scholarship, 24*(2), 141–147.

Harvey, V. A. (1964). *A handbook of theological terms.* New York: Macmillan.

Jacobsen, B. S., et al. (1992). Why me? Causal thinking, affect, and expectations in myocardial infarction patients. *Journal of Cardiovascular Nursing, 6*(2), 57–65.

McCormick, R. A. (1987). *Health and medicine in the Catholic tradition.* New York: Crossroad.

Rahman, Fazlur. (1987). *Health and medicine in the Islamic tradition.* New York: Crossroad.

Shelly, J. A., & Fish, S. (1988). *Spiritual care: The nurse's role* (3rd ed.). Downer's Grove, IL: InterVarsity Press.

Thurkauf, G. E. (1989). Understanding the beliefs of Jehovah's Witnesses. *Focus on Critical Care, 16*(1), 199–204.

Wheeler, M. S., & Cheung, A. H. S. (1996). Minority attitudes toward organ donation. *Critical Care Nurse, 16*(1), 30–34.

CHAPTER 7
Nutritional Assessment

REFERENCES

American Academy of Pediatrics, Committee on Nutrition. (1982). The promotion of breastfeeding. *Pediatrics, 69,* 654–661.

American Psychiatric Association. (1994). *Diagnostic and statistical manual of mental disorders* (4th ed.). Washington, DC: Author.

Frisancho, A. R. (1981). New norms of upper limb fat and muscle areas for assessment of nutrition status. *American Journal of Clinical Nutrition, 34,* 2540.

Jensen, G. L. (1996). The rural elderly: Living the good life? *Nutrition Reviews, 54*(1, Pt. II), S17–S21.

Minister of Supply and Services. (1992). *Canada's food guide to healthy eating.* Cat. No. H39-252/1992E.

U.S. Department of Health and Human Services, Public Health Services, Office of Disease Prevention and Health Promotion. (1994). *Clinician's handbook of preventive services: Put prevention into practice.* Washington, DC: U.S. Government Printing Office.

U.S. Departments of Agriculture and U.S. Health and Human Services. (1990). *Nutrition and your health: Dietary guidelines for Americans* (3rd ed.) (Home and Garden Bulletin No. 232). Washington, DC: U.S. Government Printing Office.

U.S. Departments of Agriculture and U.S. Human Services. (1992). *The food guide pyramid: A guide to daily food choices* (Leaflet No. 572). Washington, DC: U.S. Government Printing Office.

BIBLIOGRAPHY

Anderson, K. (Ed.). (1994). *Mosby's medical, nursing, and allied health dictionary* (4th ed.). St. Louis: Mosby.

Behrman, R. (Ed.). (1996). *Nelson: Textbook of pediatrics* (15th ed.). Philadelphia: Saunders.

Carnevali, D., & Patrick, M. (Eds.). (1993). *Nursing management for the elderly* (3rd ed.). Philadelphia: Lippincott.

Cook-Fuller, C. (Ed.). (1995). *Nutrition 95/96.* Guilford, CT: Dushkin Publishing Group, Inc.

Dudek, S. (1997). *Nutrition handbook for nursing practice* (3rd ed.). Philadelphia: Lippincott.

Dyment, P. (1991). How to make the sports physical exciting. *Contemporary Pediatrics, 10,* 93–106.

Eschleman, M. (1996). *Introduction to nutrition and diet therapy* (3rd ed.). Philadelphia: Lippincott.

Fischbach, F. (1996). *A manual of laboratory and diagnostic tests* (5th ed.). Philadelphia: Lippincott.

Goroll, A., Lawrence, A., & Mulley, A. (1995). *Primary care medicine: Office evaluation and management of the adult patient.* Philadelphia: Lippincott.

Hoekelman, R. (Ed.). (1996). *Primary pediatric care* (3rd ed.). St. Louis: Mosby.

Kim, M., McFarland, G., & McLane, A. (1995). *Pocket guide to nursing diagnoses* (6th ed.). St. Louis: Mosby.

Lutz, C., & Przytulski, K. (1994). *Nutrition and diet therapy.* Philadelphia: F. A. Davis.

McFarland, G., & McFarlane, E. (1993). *Nursing diagnosis and intervention* (2nd ed.). St. Louis: Mosby.

Nelson, J., Mosness, K., Jensen, M., & Gastineau, C. (1994). *Mayo Clinic diet manual* (7th ed.). St. Louis: Mosby.

Stutts, M. (1994). Pica: Some pregnant women really do eat dirt. *Pulse: East Caroline School of Nursing, Fall,* 10–11.

Thompson, J., McFarland, G., Hirsch, J., & Tucker, S. (1993). *Mosby's clinical nursing* (3rd ed.). St. Louis: Mosby.

Wardlaw, G., Insel, P., & Seyler, M. (1992). *Contemporary nutrition: Issues and insights.* St. Louis: Mosby.

Wong, D. (1996). *Whaley and Wong's essentials of pediatric nursing* (5th ed.). St. Louis: Mosby.

Wong, D. (1996). *Whaley and Wong's clinical manual of pediatric nursing* (4th ed.). St. Louis: Mosby.

Youngkin, E., & Davis, M. (1994). *Women's health: A primary care clinical guide.* Connecticut: Appleton and Lange.

U.S. Department of Agriculture. (1993). *Nutrition: Eating for good health* (Bulletin No. 685). Washington, DC: U.S. Government Printing Office.

CHAPTER 8
Physical Assessment
Techniques

BIBLIOGRAPHY

DeGowin, E. L. (1994). *DeGowin and DeGowin's beside diagnostic examination.* New York: Macmillan.

Fay, M. (1992). Safety issues of latex products. *AANA Journal, 60*(3), 214–216.

Hogstel, M. O., & Keen-Payne, R. (1993). *Practical guide to health assessment through the lifespan.* Philadelphia: F. A. Davis.

Holbrook, J., & Schneiderman, H. (1990). Honing physical diagnostic skills. *Patient Care, 24*(7), 123–141.

Martin, S. M. (1994). Stethoscope or staphoscope? *American Journal of Nursing, 94*(8), 56.

Mezey, M. D. (1993). *Health assessment of the older individual.* New York: Springer.

Pugliese, G. (1992). Universal precautions: Now they're the law. *RN, 55*(9), 63, 65–66, 69.

Reding, M. (1992). Sound effects: The art and science of stethoscopy. *Emergency Medical Services, 21*(3), 17–21.

Reitz, D. (1994). Study shows low compliance with universal precautions. *OR-Manager, 10*(1), 13–14.

Sayer, L. (1988). Prejudice pre-empted . . . allowing stereotypical views to govern the assessment of patients. *Nursing Times, 88*(37), 46–48.

White, J. E., Nativio, D. G., Kobert, S. N., & Engberg, S. J. (1992). Content and process in clinical decision-making by nurse practitioners. *Image: The Journal of Nursing Scholarship, 24*(2), 153–158.

CHAPTER 9
General Assessment and Vital Signs

BIBLIOGRAPHY

Behrman, R. (Ed.). (1996). *Nelson textbook of pediatrics* (15th ed.). Philadelphia: Saunders.

Chamberlain, J. et al. (1991). Comparison of a tympanic thermometer to rectal and oral thermometers in a pediatric emergency department. *Clinical Pediatrics, 4,* 24–29.

Chameides, L. (Ed.). (1994). *Textbook of pediatric advanced life support.* Dallas, TX: American Heart Association.

Davis, K. (1993). The accuracy of tympanic temperature measurement in children. *Pediatric Nursing, 19*(3), 267–272.

Edelman, C., & Mandle, C. (1994). *Health promotion through the lifespan* (3rd ed.). St. Louis: Mosby-Year Book.

Guyton, A. C., & Hall, J. (1995). *Textbook of medical physiology* (9th ed.). Philadelphia: Saunders.

McArdle, W., Katch, F., & Katch, V. (1996). *Exercise physiology* (4th ed.). Philadelphia: Lea & Febiger.

Steismyer, J. (1993). A four step approach to pulmonary assessment. *American Journal of Nursing, 93*(8), 22–28.

Thermoscan®, Inc. (1992). *Tympanic thermometry: Clinical summary on the accuracy and efficiency of tympanic thermometry.* Pub. No. 1092-068 P-R 0493. San Diego, CA: Author.

Thompson, J., McFarland, G., Hirsch, J., & Tucker, S. (1993). *Mosby's clinical nursing* (4th ed.). St. Louis: Mosby.

Wong, D. (1996). *Whaley and Wong's essentials of pediatric nursing* (5th ed.). St. Louis: Mosby.

CHAPTER 10
Skin, Hair, and Nails

BIBLIOGRAPHY

American Cancer Society, Inc. (1994). *Cancer facts and figures* [On-line]. Internet address: bcic/acsz/gifs/fact-map.GIF.

Andreoli, T., Bennett, J., Carpenter, C., Plum, F., & Smith, L. (1993). *Cecil: Essentials of medicine* (3rd ed.). Philadelphia: Saunders.

Collins, R. D. (1987). *Differential diagnosis in primary care* (2nd ed.). Philadelphia: Lippincott.

Fitzpatrick, T., Johnson, R., Palano, M., Suurmond, D., & Wolff, K. (1992). *Color atlas and synopsis of clinical dermatology* (2nd ed.). New York: McGraw-Hill.

Habif, T. P. (1996). *Clinical dermatology: A color guide to diagnosis & therapy* (3rd ed.). St. Louis: Mosby.

Ham, R. J., & Sloane, P. D. (1996). *Primary care geriatrics: A case-based approach* (3rd ed.). St. Louis: Mosby-Year Book.

Holzberg, M. (1990). Nails. In H. K. Walker, W. D. Hall, & J. W. Hurst (Eds.), *Clinical methods: The history, physical, and laboratory examinations* (3rd ed., pp. 536–539). Boston: Butterworth.

McFarland, G. K., & McFarlane, E. A. (1996). *Nursing diagnosis & intervention: Planning for patient care* (3rd ed.). St. Louis: Mosby.

McKay, M. (1990). An overview of the skin and appendages. In H. K. Walker, W. D. Hall, & J. W. Hurst (Eds.), *Clinical methods: The history, physical, and laboratory examinations* (3rd ed., pp. 515–517). Boston: Butterworth.

Netter, F. H. (1989). *Atlas of human anatomy.* Summit, NJ: CIBA-GEIGY Corporation.

Rosen, T., & Martin, S. (1981). *Atlas of black dermatology.* Boston: Little, Brown and Company.

Papa, C. (1990). Hair. In H. K. Walker, W. D. Hall, & J. W. Hurst (Eds.), *Clinical methods: The history, physical, and laboratory examinations* (3rd ed., pp. 532–535). Boston: Butterworth.

Papa, C. (1990). Skin. In H. K. Walker, W. D. Hall, & J. W. Hurst (Eds.), *Clinical methods: The history, physical, and laboratory examinations* (3rd ed., pp. 520–529). Boston: Butterworth.

Underwood, P., & Armour, A. (1993). Cases of Lyme disease reported in a military community. *Military medicine, 152*(2), 116–119.

Uphold, C. R., & Graham, M. V. (1993). *Clinical guidelines in family practice.* Gainesville, FL: Barmarrae Books.

Willms, J. L., Schneiderman, H., & Algranati, P. S. (1994). *Physical diagnosis: Bedside evaluation of diagnosis and function.* Baltimore: Williams & Wilkins.

CHAPTER 11
Head and Neck

BIBLIOGRAPHY

Barker, L. R., Burton, J. R., & Zieve, P. D. (1995). *Principles of ambulatory medicine* (4th ed.). Baltimore: Williams & Wilkins.

Baumel, B., & Eisner, L. S. (1991). Diagnosis and treatment of headache in the elderly. *Medical Clinics of North America, 75*(3), 661–675.

Carnevali, D. L., & Patrick, M. (1993). *Nursing management for the elderly* (3rd ed.). Philadelphia: Lippincott.

Green, D. B. (1992). Orofacial and craniofacial pain: Primary care concerns. *Postgraduate Medicine, 88*(8), 57–64.

Hoffert, M. J. (1994). Treatment of migraine: A new era. *American Family Physician, 49*(3), 633–638.

Holdcroft, C. (1993). Sumatriptan: New relief for migraine headaches. *Nurse Practitioner: American Journal of Primary Health Care, 18*(7), 11, 14.

Hole, J. W., Jr. (1995). *Human anatomy and physiology* (7th ed.). Dubuque, IA: William C. Brown.

Kane, R. L., Ouslander, J. G., & Abrass, I. B. (1994). *Essentials of clinical geriatrics* (3rd ed.). New York: McGraw-Hill.

McCance, K. L., & Huether, S. E. (1994). *Pathophysiology: The biologic basis for disease in adults and children* (2nd ed.). St. Louis: Mosby.

Weiss, J. (1993). Assessment and management of the client with headaches. *Nurse Practitioner: American Journal of Primary Health Care, 18*(4), 44, 47, 51–54.

Yeomans, A. C. (1990). Assessment and management of hypothyroidism. *Nurse Practitioner: American Journal of Primary Health Care, 15*(11), 8–16.

CHAPTER 12
Eyes, Ears, Nose, Mouth, and Throat

BIBLIOGRAPHY

Boyd-Monk, H. (1990). Assessing acquired ocular diseases. *Nursing Clinics of North America, 25*(4), 811–822.

Carnevali, D. L., & Patrick, M. (1993). *Nursing management for the elderly* (3rd ed.). Philadelphia: Lippincott.

DeGowin, R. L. (1994). *DeGowin & DeGowin's diagnostic examination* (6th ed.). New York: McGraw-Hill.

Donnenfeld, E. D., Kaufman, H. E., & Schwab I. R. (1993). Conjunctivitis: Update on diagnosis and treatment. *Patient Care, 27*(10), 22–25, 29–30, 32.

Faherty, B. (1992). Chronic blepharitis: Easy nursing interventions for a common problem. *Journal of Ophthalmic Nursing & Technology, 11*(1), 20–22.

Frankel, C. A. (1992). Strabismus. In R. A. Hoekelman, S. B. Friedman, N. M. Nelson, & H. M. Seidel (Eds.), *Primary pediatric care* (2nd ed., pp. 1068–1074). St. Louis: Mosby.

Godley, F. A. (1992). Chronic sinusitis: An update. *American Family Physician, 45*(5), 2190–2199.

Gordon, D. M. (1971). *Fundamentals of ophthalmoscopy.* Kalamazoo, MI: The Upjohn Company.

Herr, R. D. (1991). Acute sinusitis: Diagnosis and treatment update. *American Family Physician,* 2055–2062.

Hole, J. W., Jr. (1990). *Human anatomy and physiology* (5th ed.). Dubuque, IA: William C. Brown.

Kallman, H., & Keightley, S. (1987). The aging eye. *Postgraduate Medicine, 81*(2), 108–135.

Kane, R. L., Ouslander, J. G., & Abrass, I. B. (1994). *Essentials of clinical geriatrics* (3rd ed.). New York: McGraw-Hill.

McCance, K. L., & Huether, S. E. (1994). *Pathophysiology: The biologic basis for disease in adults and children* (2nd ed.). St. Louis: Mosby.

Polk, S. E. (1994). Making sense of swimmer's ear. *Advance for Nurse Practitioners, 2*(7), 25–27.

Schachat, A. P. (1995). Common problems associated with impaired vision: Cataracts and age-related macular degeneration. In L. R. Barker, J. R. Burton, & P. D. Zieve (Eds.), *Principles of ambulatory medicine* (4th ed., pp. 1415–1428). Baltimore: Williams & Wilkins.

Schachat, A. P. (1995). The red eye. In L. R. Barker, J. R. Burton, & P. D. Zieve (Eds.), *Principles of ambulatory medicine* (4th ed., pp. 1428–1436). Baltimore: Williams & Wilkins.

Wilder, B. E. (1993). A comprehensive overview of allergic rhinitis. *Advance for Nurse Practitioners, 1*(8), 9–12, 28.

CHAPTER 13
Breasts and Regional Nodes

REFERENCES

American Cancer Society, Inc. (1994). *Cancer facts and figures* [On-line]. Internet address: bcic/acsz/gifs/fact-map.GIF.

Love, S., & Lindsey, K. (1995). *Dr. Susan Love's breast book* (2nd ed.). Reading, MA: Addison-Wesley.

BIBLIOGRAPHY

American Cancer Society, Inc. (1994). *Cancer facts and figures* [On-line]. Internet address: bcic/acsz/gifs/fact-map.GIF.

Andreoli, T., Bennett, J., Carpenter, C., Plum, F., & Smith, L. (1993). *Cecil: Essentials of medicine* (3rd ed.). Philadelphia: Saunders.

Brinton, L. A., et al. (1995). Oral contraceptives and breast cancer risk among younger women. *Journal of the National Cancer Institute, 87*(11), 827–835.

Ciatto, S., Rosselli del Turco, M., Catarzi, S., Cataliotti, L., Cardona, G., Teglia, C., Pacini, P., & Caridi, G. (1991). Causes of breast cancer misdiagnosed at physical examination. *Neoplasm, 38*(5), 523–531.

Collins, R. D. (1987). *Differential diagnosis in primary care* (2nd ed.). Philadelphia: Lippincott.

Fitzpatrick, T., Johnson, R., Palano, M., Surmond, D., & Wolff, K. (1997). *Color atlas and synopsis of clinical dermatology* (3rd ed.). New York: McGraw-Hill.

Ham, R. J., & Sloane, P. D. (1996). *Primary care geriatrics: A case-based approach* (2nd ed.). St. Louis: Mosby-Year Book.

Love, S., & Lindsey, K. (1995). *Dr. Susan Love's breast book* (2nd ed.). Reading, MA: Addison-Wesley.

McFarland, G. K., & McFarlane, E. A. (1996). *Nursing diagnosis and intervention: Planning for patient care* (3rd ed.). St. Louis: Mosby.

Mitchell, G.W., & Bassett, L.W. (1990). *The female breast and its disorders.* Baltimore: Williams & Wilkins.

National Institutes of Health. (1994). *What you need to know about breast cancer* (NIH Publication No. 89-1556). Washington DC: U.S. Government Printing Office.

Netter, F. H. (1989). *Atlas of human anatomy.* Summit, NJ: CIBA-GEIGY Corporation.

Uphold, C. R., & Graham, M. V. (1993). *Clinical guidelines in family practice.* Gainesville, FL: Barmarrae Books.

Willms, J. L., Schneiderman, H., & Algranati, P. S. (1994). *Physical diagnosis: Bedside evaluation of diagnosis and function.* Baltimore: Williams & Wilkins.

CHAPTER 14
Thorax and Lungs

BIBLIOGRAPHY

Cotes, J. E., & Steel, J. (1987). *Work-related lung disorders.* Oxford, England: Blackwell Scientific Publications.

Elliott, M. W., Adams, L., Cockcroft, A., Maorae, K. D., Murphy, K., & Guz, A. (1991). The language of breathlessness: Use of verbal descriptors by patients with cardiopulmonary disease. *American Review of Respiratory Disease, 144*(4), 826–832.

Glauser, F. L. (Ed.). (1983). *Signs and symptoms in pulmonary medicine.* Philadelphia: Lippincott.

Irwin, M. J. (1991). Assessing color changes for dark skinned patients. *Advancing Clinical Care, 6*(6), 8–11.

Kersten, L. D. (1989). *Comprehensive respiratory nursing: A decision making approach.* Philadelphia: Saunders.

Kuhn, J. K., & McGovern, M. (1992). Respiratory assessment of the elderly. *Journal of Gerontological Nursing, 18*(5), 40–43.

Murray, J. F., & Nadel, J. A. (1994). *Textbook of respiratory medicine* (2nd ed.). Philadelphia: Saunders.

Parkes, W. R. (1994). *Occupational lung disorders* (3rd ed.). Oxford: Butterworth-Heinemann.

Timmer, S., & Rosenman, K. (1993). Occurrence of occupational asthma. *Chest, 104*(3), 816–820.

U.S. Environmental Protection Agency Office of Respiratory Health. (1992). *Effects of passive smoking: Lung cancer and other disorders.* Washington, DC: Office of Health and Environmental Assessment, Office of Research.

CHAPTER 15
Heart and Peripheral Vasculature

REFERENCES

Guyton, A. C., & Hall, J. (1995). *Textbook of medical physiology* (9th ed.). Philadelphia: Saunders.

New York Heart Association Criteria Committee. (1964). *Diseases of the heart and blood vessels: Nomenclature and criteria for diagnosis* (6th ed.). Boston: Little, Brown.

BIBLIOGRAPHY

After a heart attack. (1993). Dallas: American Heart Association.

Alspach, J. G. (Ed.). (1991). *Core curriculum for critical care nursing* (4th ed.). Philadelphia: Saunders.

Bright, L. D., & Georgi, S. (1992). Peripheral vascular disease: Is it arterial or venous? *American Journal of Nursing, 92*(9), 34–47.

Brody, J. A. (1987). *Jane Brody's nutrition book.* New York: Bantam Books.

Congestive heart failure: What you should know. (1993). Dallas: American Heart Association.

Cox, C. W. (1994). After thrombolytic therapy: Avoiding a disabling complication. *Nursing 94, 24*(6), 32K–32L.

Estes, M. E. Z. (1989). Chagas' disease. *Critical Care Nurse, 9*(7), 48–50, 52–54, 57–60+.

Fagius, D. B., & Stunkard, J. (1994). Uncovering the secrets of snaps, rubs, and clicks. *Nursing 94, 24*(7), 45–52.

Fahey, V. A. (Ed.). (1994). *Vascular nursing* (2nd ed.). Philadelphia: Saunders.

Gawlinski, A., & Jensen, G. A. (1991). The complications of cardiovascular aging. *American Journal of Nursing, 91*(11), 26–32.

Hickey, A. (1994). Catching deep vein thrombosis in time. *Nursing 94, 24*(10), 34–42.

Kinney, M. R., Packa, D. R., Andreoli, K. G., & Zipes, D. P. (1991). *Comprehensive cardiac care* (7th ed.). St. Louis: Mosby-Year Book.

Koziol-McLain, J., Lowenstein, S. R., & Fuller, B. (1991). Orthostatic vital signs in emergency department patients. *Annals of Emergency Medicine, 20*(6), 606–609.

Schlant, R. C., Alexander, R. W., O'Rourke, R. A., Roberts, R., & Sonnenblick, E. H. (Eds.). (1994). *Hurst's the heart* (8th ed.). New York: McGraw-Hill.

Sex and heart disease. (1990). Dallas: American Heart Association.

Solomon, J. (1991). Managing a failing heart. *RN, 54*(8), 46–51.

Understanding angina. (1994). Dallas: American Heart Association.

Yacone-Morton, L. (1991). Perfecting the art: Cardiac assessment. *RN, 54*(12), 28–35.

CHAPTER 16
Abdomen

BIBLIOGRAPHY

Alspach, J. G. (Ed.). (1991). *Core curriculum for critical care nursing* (4th ed.). Philadelphia: Saunders.

Altman, D. F. (1990). Changes in gastrointestinal, pancreatic, biliary, and hepatic function with aging. *Gastroenterology Clinics of North America, 19*(2), 227–234.

Beare, P. G., & Myers, J. L. (1994). *Principles and practices of adult health nursing* (2nd ed.). St. Louis: Mosby-Yearbook.

Black, J. M., & Jacobs, E. M. (1993). *Luckmann and Sorensen's medical surgical nursing: A psychophysiologic approach* (4th ed.). Philadelphia: Saunders.

Burkhart, C. (1992). Guidelines for rapid assessment of abdominal pain indicative of acute surgical abdomen. *Nurse Practitioner, 17*(6), 39–49.

Creager, J. G. (1992). *Human anatomy and physiology* (2nd ed.). Dubuque, IA: William C. Brown.

Gaedeke Norris, M. K. (1992). Assessing albumin values. *Nursing 92, 22*(1), 84.

Harald, E. A., & Kaufman, K. (1994). Understanding the gastrointestinal system. Part 1. *Nursing 94, 24*(7), 71–72.

Jess, L. W. (1993). Acute abdominal pain: Revealing the source. *Nursing 93, 23*(9), 34–42.

Kinney, M. R., Packa, D. R., & Dunbar, S. B. (1993). *AACN's clinical reference for critical care nursing.* St. Louis: Mosby-Yearbook.

Lehne, R. A. (1994). *Pharmacology for nursing care.* Philadelphia: Saunders.

Sigardson-Poor, K. M., & Haggerty, L. M. (1990). *Nursing care of the transplant recipient.* Philadelphia: Saunders.

Snell, R. S. (1995). *Clinical anatomy for medical students* (5th ed.). Boston: Little, Brown and Company.

Thompson, J. M., McFarland, G. K., Hirsch, J. E., & Tucker, S. M. (1997). *Mosby's clinical nursing* (4th ed.). St. Louis: Mosby.

Wagner, M. M. (1990). The patient with abdominal injuries. *Nursing Clinics of North America, 25*(1), 45–55.

Wardell, T. L. (1991). Assessing and managing a gastric ulcer. *Nursing 91, 21*(3), 34–42.

Woodtli, M. A., & Van Ort, S. (1993). Nursing diagnoses and functional health patterns in patients receiving external radiation therapy: Cancer of the digestive organs. *Nursing Diagnosis, 4*(1), 15–25.

Young, L. M. (1993). Managing the patient with liver failure. *MedSurg Nursing, 2*(4), 275–281.

CHAPTER 17
Musculoskeletal System

BIBLIOGRAPHY

Apley, A. G., & Solomon, L. (1982). *Apley's system of orthopedics and fractures* (6th ed.). Boston: Butterworth.

Black, J., & Matassarin-Jacobs, E. (1993). *Luckman and Sorenson's medical-surgical nursing: A psychophysiological approach* (4th ed.). Philadelphia: Saunders.

Brozenec, S., & Russell, S. (Eds.) (1994). *Core curriculum for medical-surgical nursing.* Pitman, NJ: Jannetti Publications Inc.

Carpenito, L. J. (1997). *Nursing diagnosis: Application to clinical practice* (5th ed.). Philadelphia: Lippincott.

Fecht-Gramley, M. E. (1994). Emergency: Recognizing compartment syndrome. *American Journal of Nursing, 94*(10), 41.

Hipp, J. A., Springfield, D. S., & Hayes, W. C. (1995). Predicting pathologic fracture risk in the management of metastatic bone defects. *Clinical Orthopaedics & Related Research, 312,* 120–135.

Lappe, J. M. (1994). Bone fragility: Assessment of risk and strategies for prevention. *Journal of Obstetric, Gynecologic, & Neonatal Nursing, 23*(3), 260-268.

Liscum, B. (1992). Osteoporosis: The silent disease. *Orthopaedic Nursing, 11*(4), 21–25.

Maher, A. B., Salmond, S. W., & Pellino, T. A. (1994). *Orthopedic nursing.* Philadelphia: Saunders.

McCaffery, M., & Beebe, A. (1989). *Pain: Clinical manual for nursing practice.* St. Louis: Mosby.

Mourad, L. (1991). *Orthopedic disorders: Mosby's clinical nursing series.* St Louis: Mosby.

Mourad, L. A. (1995). *Plans of care for specialty practice: Orthopedic nursing.* Albany, NY: Delmar Publishers.

Mourad, L. A., & Droste, M. M. (1993). *The nursing process in the care of adults with orthopedic conditions.* Albany, NY: Delmar Publishers Inc.

Weinstein, S. L., & Buckwalter, J. A. (1995). *Turek's Orthopedics: principles and their applications* (5th ed.). Philadelphia: Lippincott.

Williams, P., et al. (1989). *Gray's anatomy* (37th ed.). Edinburgh, Scotland: Churchill Livingstone.

CHAPTER 18
Mental Status and Neurological Techniques

BIBLIOGRAPHY

Adams, R. D., & Victor, M. (1993). *Principles of neurology.* New York: McGraw Hill.

Bannister, Sir Roger. (1992). *Brain and Bannister's clinical neurology.* Oxford, England: Oxford University Press.

Beare, P. G., & Myers, J. L. (1994). *Principles and practice of adult health nursing* (2nd ed.). St. Louis: Mosby.

Beck, C. K., & Shue, V. M. (1994). Interventions for treating disruptive behavior in demented elderly people. *Nursing Clinics of North America, 29*(1), 143–156.

Caine, R. M. (1993). The cutting edge in neuroscience. *Critical Care Nurse, 13*(Suppl. 5), 6–7.

Chenitz, W. C., Stone, J. T., & Salisbury, S. A. (1991). *Clinical gerontological nursing.* Philadelphia: Saunders.

Cammermeyer, M., & Appledorn, C. (1990). *Core curriculum for neuroscience nursing* (3rd ed.). Chicago: American Association of Neuroscience Nurses.

Formen, M. D. (1992). Adverse psychologic responses of the elderly to critical illness. *AACN Clinical Issues in Critical Care Nursing, 3*(1), 64–72.

Geary, S. M. (1995). Nursing management of cranial nerve dysfunction. *Journal of Neuroscience Nursing, 27*(2), 102–108.

Glick, O. J. (1993). Normal thought processes: An overview. *The Nursing Clinics of North America, 28*(4), 715–728.

Guin, P. R., & Freudenberger, K. (1992). The elderly neuroscience patient: Implications for the critical care nurse. *AACN Clinical Issues in Critical Care Nursing, 3*(1), 98–105.

Gunderson, C. H. (1990). *Essentials of clinical neurology.* New York: Raven Press.

Guyton, A. C., Hall, J. (1995). *Textbook of medical physiology* (9th ed.). Philadelphia: Saunders.

Haerer, A. F. (1992). *DeJong's the neurologic examination.* Philadelphia: Lippincott.

Hall, G. R., Buckwalter, C. C., Stolley, J. M., Gerdner, L. A., Garand, L., Ridgeway, S., & Crump, S. (1995). Standardized care plans managing Alzheimer's patients at home. *Journal of Gerontological Nursing, 21*(1), 37–47.

Hicky, J. V. (1992). *The clinical practice of neurological and neurosurgical nursing* (3rd ed.). Philadelphia: Lippincott.

Lower, J. (1992). Rapid neuro assessment. *American Journal of Nursing, 12*(6), 38–48.

Mason, P. J. B. (1992). Neurodiagnostic testing in critically injured adults. *Critical Care Nurse, 12*(6), 64–75.

Morris, J. C. (1994). Differential diagnosis of Alzheimer's disease. *Clinics in Geriatric Medicine, 10*(2), 257–276.

Pellegrino, T. R. (1990). A faster, focused neurologic exam. *Emergency Medicine, 22*(16), 71–95.

Phipps, M. A. (1991). Assessment of neurologic deficits in stroke. *Nursing Clinics of North America, 26*(4), 957–969.

Pryse-Phillips, W. E. M., & Murray, T. J. (1992). *Essential neurology.* New York: Medical Examination Publishing Co.

Rocca, W. A. (1994). Frequency, distribution, and risk factors for Alzheimer's disease. *The Nursing Clinics of North America, 29*(1), 101–112.

Waxman, S. G., & deGroot, J. (1992). *Correlative neuroanatomy.* Norwalk, CT: Appleton & Lange.

Wykle, M. L., & Morris, D. L. (1994). Nursing care in Alzheimer's disease. *Clinics in Geriatric Medicine, 10*(2), 351–366.

Yi, E. S., Abraham, I. L., & Holraoyd, S. (1994). Alzheimer's disease and nursing: New scientific and clinical insights. *The Nursing Clinics of North America, 29*(1), 85–100.

CHAPTER 19
Female Genitalia

REFERENCE

American Cancer Society, Inc. (1994). *Cancer facts and figures* [On-line]. Internet address: bcic/acsz/gifs/fact-map.GIF.

BIBLIOGRAPHY

Catterson, M., & Zadoo, V. (1993). Prevalence of asymptomatic chlamydial cervical infection in active duty army females. *Military Medicine, 158*(9), 618–619.

Collins, R. D. (1987). *Differential diagnosis in primary care* (2nd ed.). Philadelphia: Lippincott.

Evers, J. L., & Heineman, M. J. (1990). *Gynecology: A clinical atlas.* St. Louis: Mosby.

Ham, R. J., & Sloane, P. D. (1996). *Primary care geriatrics: A case-based approach* (3rd ed.). St. Louis: Mosby-Year Book.

Long, W. N. (1990). An overview of the female genitalia and breasts. In H. K. Walker, W. D. Hall, & J. W. Hurst (Eds.), *Clinical methods: The history, physical, and laboratory examinations* (3rd ed., pp. 801–802. Boston: Butterworths.

Markenson, G., Raez, E., & Colavita, M. (1992). Female health care during Operation Desert Storm: The eighth evacuation hospital experience. *Military Medicine, 157*(11), 610–613.

McFarland, G. K., & McFarlane, E. A. (1996). *Nursing diagnosis and intervention: Planning for patient care* (3rd ed.). St. Louis: Mosby.

Netter, F. H. (1989). *Atlas of human anatomy.* Summit, NJ: CIBA-GEIGY Corporation.

Uphold, C. R., & Graham, M. V. (1993). *Clinical guidelines in family practice.* Gainesville, FL: Barmarrae Books.

Willms, J. L., Schneiderman, H., & Algranati, P. S. (1994). *Physical diagnosis: Bedside evaluation of diagnosis and function.* Baltimore: Williams & Wilkins.

CHAPTER 20
Male Genitalia

BIBLIOGRAPHY

Aronson, M. D., & Phillips, R. S. (1993). Screening young men for chlamydial infection. *Journal of the American Medical Association, 270*(17), 2097–2098.

Brock, G., & Lue, T. F. (1992). Impotence: A patient's goal-directed approach. *Monographs in Urology, 13*(5), 45–52.

Hooten, T. M. (1994). Newer therapies for urethritis. *Contemporary Internal Medicine, 6*(1), 12–23.

Husmann, D. A., & Cain, M. (1994). Microphallus: Eventual phallic size is dependent on the timing of androgen administration. *The Journal of Urology, 152,* 734–739.

Mandell, G. L., Douglas, R. G., & Bennett, J. E. (1992). *Principles and practice of infectious disease: Handbook of antimicrobial therapy.* Philadelphia: Saunders.

O'Donnell, L., San Doval, A., Vornfett, R., & O'Donnell, C. (1994, May/June). STD prevention and the challenge of gender and cultural diversity: Knowledge, attitudes, and risk behaviors among black and hispanic inner-city STD clinic patients. *Sexually Transmitted Diseases,* 137–148.

Reiter, R. E., & Linehan, W. M. (1993). Evaluating intrascrotal masses. *Internal Medicine, 14*(6), 49–56.

Walsh, P. C., Retik A. P., Stamey, T. A., & Vaughan, E. D. (1992). *Campbell's urology* (6th ed.). Philadelphia: Saunders.

Yachia, D., Beyar, M., Aridogan, A., & Dascalu, S. (1993). The incidence of congenital penile curvature. *The Journal of Urology, 150,* 1478–1479.

CHAPTER 21
Anus, Rectum, and Prostate

BIBLIOGRAPHY

Berger, R. E., & Hanno, P. M. (1992). The fine points of prostatitis care. *Patient Care, 261*(14), 91–107.

Garnick, M. B. (1993). Prostate cancer: Screening, diagnosis, and management. *Annals of Internal Medicine, 118*(10), 804–818.

Haubrich, W. S., Schaffner, F., & Berk, J. E. (1994). *Gastroenterology.* Philadelphia: Saunders.

Kemp, E. D. (1992). Prostate cancer. *Postgraduate Medicine, 92*(1), 67–89.

Matzen, R. N., & Lang, R. S. (1993). *Clinical preventive medicine.* St. Louis: Mosby.

Meares, E. M., & Sant, G. R. (1992). *Differential diagnosis of prostate disorders.* New York: Gower Medical Publishing.

Plenta, K. J. (1993). Risk factors for prostate cancer. *Annuals of Internal Medicine, 118*(10), 793–803.

Shapiro, A., Lebensart, P. D., Pode, D., & Bloom, R. A. (1994). The clinical utility of transrectal ultrasound and digital rectal examination in the diagnosis of prostate cancer. *The British Journal of Radiology, 67*(799), 668–671.

Sleisenger, M. H., & Fordtran, J. S. (1993). *Gastrointestinal disease.* Philadelphia: Saunders.

Walsh, P. C. (1992). *Campbell's urology.* Philadelphia: Saunders.

Yamada, T., Alpers, D. H., Owyang, C., Powell, D. W., & Silverstien, F. E. (1995). *Textbook of gastroenterology* (2nd ed.). Philadelphia: Lippincott.

CHAPTER 22
Pregnant Patient

BIBLIOGRAPHY

Artal, R., & Subak-Sharpe, G. (1992). *Pregnancy and exercise.* New York: Delacorte Press.

Benson, R. C., & Pernoll, M. L. (1994). *Handbook of obstetrics and gynecology* (9th ed.). New York: McGraw-Hill.

Bobak, I. M., Jensen, M. D., & Lowdermilk, D. L. (Assoc. Eds.). (1993). *Maternal and gynecologic care: The nurse and the family* (5th ed.). St. Louis: Mosby.

Cherry, S. H., & Merkatz, I. R. (Eds.). (1991). *Complications of pregnancy: Medical, surgical, gynecologic, psychosocial and perinatal* (4th ed.). Baltimore: Williams & Wilkins.

Cnattingius, S., Forman, M. R., Berendes, H. W., & Isotalo, L. (1992). Delayed childbearing and risk of adverse perinatal outcome: A population-based study. *Journal of the American Medical Association, 268*(7), 886–890.

Committee on Infectious Diseases and Committee on Fetus and Newborn (1992). Guidelines for prevention of Group B Streptococci (GBS) infection by chemoprophylaxis. *Pediatrics, 90*(5), 775–778.

Cunningham, F. G., MacDonald, P. C., Gant, N. F., Leveno, K. J., & Gilstrap, L. C., III. (1993). *Williams obstetrics* (19th ed.). Norwalk, CT: Appleton & Lange.

Czeizel, A. E., & Dudas, I. (1992). Prevention of the first occurrence of neural-tube defects by periconceptional vitamin supplementation. *New England Journal of Medicine, 327*(26), 1832–1835.

Czeizel, A. E., Dudas, I., Fritz, G., Tecsoi, A., Hanck, A., & Kunovits, G. (1992). The effect of periconceptional multi-vitamin-mineral supplementation on vertigo, nausea, and vomiting in the first trimester of pregnancy. *Archives of Gynecology and Obstetrics, 251*(4), 181–185.

Freeman, R. K., & Hauth, J. C. (Eds.). (1992). *Guidelines for perinatal care* (3rd ed.). Washington, DC: The American College of Obstetricians and Gynecologists (ACOG).

Fuchsia, A. R., Fuchs, F., & Stublefield, P. G. (1993). *Preterm birth, causes, prevention, and management* (2nd ed.). New York: McGraw-Hill.

Gabbe, S. G., Niebyl, J. R., & Simpson, J. L. (Eds.). (1991). *Obstetrics: Normal and problem pregnancies* (2nd ed.). New York: Churchill Livingstone.

Gigante, J., Hickson, G. B., Entman, S. S., & Oquist, N. L. (1995). Universal screening for Group B Streptococcus: Recommendations and obstetricians' practice decisions. *Obstetrics & Gynecology, 85*(3), 440–443.

Knuppel, R. A., & Drukker, J. E., (1993). *High risk pregnancy: A team approach* (2nd ed.). Philadelphia: Saunders.

Krutzen, E., Olofsson, P., Back, S. E., & Nilsson-Ehle, P. (1992). Glomerular filtration rate in pregnancy: A study in normal subjects and in patients with hypertension, preeclampsia and diabetes. *Scandinavian Journal of Clinical Laboratory Investigation, 52*(5), 387–392.

Larsen, T., Larsen, J. F., Petersen, S., & Greisen, G. (1992). Detection of small-for-gestational-age fetuses by ultrasound in a high risk population: A randomized controlled study. *British Journal of Obstetrics Gynaecology, 99*(6), 469–474.

Magee, M. S., Walden, C. E., Benedetti, T. J., & Knopp, R. H. (1993). Influence of diagnostic criteria on the incidence of gestational diabetes and perinatal morbidity. *Journal of the American Medical Assocation, 269*(5), 609–615.

Mattson, S., & Smith, J. E. (Eds.). (1993). *Core curriculum for maternal newborn nursing.* Philadelphia: Saunders.

May, K. A., & Mahlmeister, L. R. (1994). *Maternal and neonatal nursing, family-centered care* (3rd ed.). Philadelphia: Lippincott.

Mills, J. L., Holmes, L. B., Aarons, J. H., Simpson, J. L., Brown, Z. A., Jovanovic-Peterson, L. G., Conley, M. R., Graubard, B. I., Knopp, R. H., & Metzger, B. E. (1993). Moderate caffeine use and the risk of spontaneous abortion and intrauterine growth retardation. *Journal of the American Medical Assocation, 269*(5), 593–597.

Milunsky, A., Ulcickas, M., Rothman, K. J., Willett, W., Jick, S. S., & Jick, H. (1992). Maternal heat exposure and neural tube defects. *Journal of the American Medical Association, 268*(7), 882–885.

Niswander, K. R., & Evans, A. T. (1991). *Manual of obstetrics* (4th ed.). Boston: Little, Brown and Company.

Schmidt, J., Boilanger, M., & Abbott, S. (1989). Peripartum cardiomyopathy. *JOGNN, 18,* 465–472.

Scott, J. R., Philip, J. P., DiSaia, P. J., Hammond, C. B., & Spellacy, W. N. (Eds.). (1994). *Danforth's obstetrics and gynecology* (7th ed.). Philadelphia: Lippincott.

Sharp, K., Brindle, P. M., Brown, M. W., & Turner, G. M. (1993). Memory loss during pregnancy. *British Journal of Obstetrics and Gynaecology, 100*(3), 209–215.

The American College of Obstetricians and Gynecologists (ACOG). (1989). *Standards for obstetric-gynecologic services* (7th ed.). Washington, DC: Author.

Valdivieso, V., Covarrubias, C., Siegel, F., & Cruz, F. (1993). Pregnancy and chlolelithiasis: Pathogenesis and natural course of gallstones diagnosed in puerperium. *Hepatology, 17*(1), 1–4.

Wilailak, S., Suthutvoravut, S., Cherng-sa-ad, P., Herabutya, Y., & Chaturachinda, K. (1992). Assessment of fetal well-being: Fetal movement count versus non-stress test. *International Journal of Gynaecology and Obstetrics, 39*(1), 23–27.

CHAPTER 23
Pediatric Patient

REFERENCES

Boynton, R. W., Dunn, E. S., & Stephens, G. R. (1994). *Manual of ambulatory pediatrics.* Philadelphia: Lippincott.

Gerchufsky, M. (1994). Lead poisoning. *Advance for Nurse Practitioners, 2*(11), 19–37.

Hahn, M. S., & Mastrangelo, R. (1995). Pediatric focus: Feeding baby. *Advance for Nurse Practitioners, 3*(4), 17–22.

Jones, K. F., Berg, J. H., & Coody, D. (1994). Update in pediatric dentistry. *Journal of Pediatric Health Care, 8*(4), 160–167.

Norris, J. (1985). Taking temperatures: The changing state of the art. *Contemporary Pediatrics, 2*(1), 22–39.

Stein, H. A., Slatt, B. J., & Stein, R. M. (1994). *The ophthalmic assistant: Fundamentals and clinical practice* (6th ed.). St. Louis: Mosby.

U.S. Department of Health and Human Services, Public Health Service - CDC, (1997). Washington, DC: Author.

BIBLIOGRAPHY

Behrman, R. E., & Kliegman, R. M. (1996). *Nelson essentials of pediatrics* (2nd ed.). Philadelphia: Saunders.

Devlin, B. K., & Reynolds, E. (1994). Child abuse: How to recognize it, how to intervene. *American Journal of Nursing, 94*(3), 26–31.

Emery, A. E., & Rimoin, D. L. (1992). *Principles and practice of medical genetics.* New York: Churchhill Livingstone.

Frankenburg, W. K. & (1990). *Denver II screening manual.* Denver, CO: Denver Developmental Materials, Incorporated.

Gessner, I. H., & Victorica, B. E. (1993). *Pediatric cardiology.* Philadelphia: Saunders.

Giger, J. N., & Davidhizar, R.E. (1995). *Transcultural nursing.* St. Louis: Mosby.

Hay, W. W., Groothuis, J. R., Hayward, A. R., & Levin, J. J. (1995). *Current pediatric diagnosis and treatment.* Norwalk, CT: Appleton and Lange.

Hazinski, M. F. (1992). *Nursing care of the critically ill child.* St. Louis: Mosby.

Johnson, K. B. (1993). *The Harriet Lane handbook.* St. Louis: Mosby.

McCance, K. L., & Huether, S. E. (1994). *Pathophysiology: The biologic basis for disease in adults and children* (2nd ed.). St. Louis: Mosby.

Monteleone, J. A. (1994). *Child maltreatment.* St. Louis: G. W. Medical.

Murphy, M. A., & Hagerman, R. J. (1992). Attention deficit hyperactivity disorder in children: Diagnosis, treatment and follow-up. *Journal of Pediatric Health Care, 6*(1), 2–11.

Oski, F. A. (1994). *Principles and practice of pediatrics.* Philadelphia: Lippincott.

Park, M. K. (1988). *Pediatric cardiology for practitioners.* Chicago: Year Book Medical Publishers.

Phillips, C. F. (1991). Keeping up with the changing immunization schedule. *Contemporary Pediatrics, 8*(1), 20–45.

Plotkin, S. A., & (1990). Haemophilus influenzae type b conjugate vaccines: Immunization of children at 15 months of age. *Pediatrics, 86*(5), 749–795.

Queen, P. M., & Lang, K. E. (1993). *Handbook of pediatric nutrition.* Gaithersburg, MD: Aspen.

Reece, R. M. (1994). *Child abuse: Medical diagnosis and management.* Philadelphia: Lea & Febiger.

U.S. Department of Health and Human Services. (1991). *Healthy people 2000.* Boston: Jones and Bartlett.

U.S. Preventive Task Force. (1993). Screening for adolescent idiopathic scoliosis. *Journal of the American Medical Association, 269*(20), 2664–2672.

Wong, D. L. (1996). *Whaley and Wong's essentials of pediatric nursing* (5th ed.). St. Louis: Mosby.

CHAPTER 24
The Complete Health and Physical Assessment

BIBLIOGRAPHY

Benjamin, M., & Curtis, J. (1992). *Ethics in nursing* (3rd ed.). New York: Oxford University Press.

Betta, P. A. (1991). Documenting to stay out of the courtroom. *Imprint, 38*(2), 39–40.

Burnard, P., & Chapman, C. M. (1993). *Professional and ethical issues in nursing: The code of professional conduct* (2nd ed.). London: Scutari Press.

Eggland, E. T., & Heinemann, D. S. (1994). *Nursing documentation: Charting, recording and reporting.* Philadelphia: Lippincott.

Ellenbecker, C. H., & Shea, K. (1994). Documentation in home health care practice. *Nursing Clinics of North America, 29*(3), 494–506.

Fiesta, J. (1993). Failure to assess. *Nursing Management, 24*(9), 16–17.

Fischbach, F. T. (1991). *Documenting care: Communication, the nursing process and documentation standards.* Philadelphia: F. A. Davis.

Iyer, P. W. (1991). Six more charting rules to keep you legally safe. *Nursing 91, 21*(7), 34–39.

Langel, B. C., Brewer, S. G., & Olszewski, C. (1991). Developing quality documentation. *Nursing Management, 22*(11), 48–50, 52.

Marrelli, T. M. (1992). *Nursing documentation handbook.* St. Louis: Mosby-Year Book.

Philipsen, N., & McMullen, P. (1993). Charting basics 101 . . . legal issues. *Nursing Connections, 6*(3), 62–64.

Rushton, C. H., & Hogue, E. E. (1993). Confronting unsafe practice: Ethical and legal issues. *Pediatric Nursing, 19*(3), 284–286, 288.

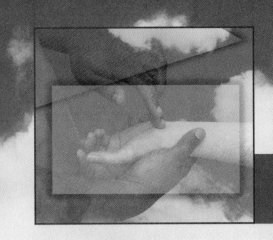

Glossary

A

Accommodation   Visual focusing from a far to a near point as pupils constrict and eyes converge.

Acculturation   Informal process of adaptation through which the beliefs, values, norms, and practices of a dominant culture are learned by a new member born into a different culture.

Acini   *See* **Alveoli (of the Breast)**.

Acrocyanosis   Normal phenomenon in light-skinned newborns whereby the hands and feet are blue and the rest of the body is pink.

Acromegaly   Abnormal enlargement of the skull, bony facial structures, and bones of the extremities, caused by excessive secretion of growth hormone.

Action Response   Attempt to stimulate patients to make some change in their thinking and behavior.

Active Listening   Act of perceiving what is said both verbally and nonverbally.

Actual Nursing Diagnosis   Statement describing human responses that have been validated by the nurse.

Adnexa   Fallopian tubes, ovaries, and their supporting ligaments.

Advance Directive   Document (Living Will or Durable Medical Power of Attorney) outlining what should be done if a patient is too ill to self-direct medical care.

Adventitious Breath Sound   Added breath sound that is superimposed on normal breath sounds.

Afterload   Initial resistance that the ventricles must overcome in order to open the semilunar valves to propel the blood into both the systemic and the pulmonary circulation.

Ages and Stages Developmental Theory   Belief that individuals experience much the same sequential physical, cognitive, socioemotional, and moral changes during the same age periods, each of which is termed a developmental stage.

Ageusia   Loss of the sense of taste.

Aggravating Factors   Events that worsen the severity of the patient's chief complaint.

Agonal Respirations   Irregularly irregular respirations that signal impending death.

Agnosia   Inability to recognize the form and nature of objects or persons.

Agnostic   Person who is unsure if God exists.

Agraphia   Loss of the ability to write.

Air Trapping   Abnormal respiratory pattern with rapid, shallow respirations and forced expirations; the lungs have insufficient time to fully exhale and air becomes trapped, leading to over-expansion of the lungs.

Albinism   A generalized whiteness of the skin, hair, and eyebrows, which is caused by a congenital inability to form melanin.

Albumin   Substance that transports nutrients, blood, and hormones and helps maintain osmotic pressure.

Alexia   Loss of the ability to grasp the meaning of written words and sentences; also known as word blindness.

Allen Test   Test used to assess for the patency of the radial and ulnar arteries.

Alleviating Factors   Events that decrease the severity of the patient's chief complaint.

Alopecia   Partial or complete loss of hair.

Alveoli (of the Breast)   Milk-producing glands located in the lobules; also called acini.

Alveoli (of the Lung)   Smallest functional unit of the respiratory system; where gas exchange occurs.

Amblyopia   Permanent loss of visual acuity resulting from certain uncorrected medical conditions.

Amenorrhea   Absence of menses.

Anal Canal   Terminal 3 to 4 cm of the large intestine.

Anal Columns   Longitudinal folds of mucosa in the superior portion of the anal canal.

Anal Fissure   Linear tear in the epidermis of the anal canal.

Anal Incontinence   Involuntary release of rectal contents.

Anal Orifice   Exit to the gastrointestinal tract; located at the seam of the gluteal folds.

Anal Sinuses   Pockets in the anal canal that lie superior to the anal valves; they secrete mucus when compressed by feces.

Anal Valves   Folds in the anal canal that are formed by joining anal columns.

Analgesia   Absence of normal sense of pain.

Anemia   Decreased number of red blood cells.

Anencephaly   Condition where the cerebral cortex or cranium does not develop.

Anergy   Diminished reaction to antigens.

Aneroid Manometer   Blood pressure measurement equipment with a calibrated dial and indicator that points to numbers representing blood pressure.

Anesthesia   Absence of touch sensation.

Angina   Myocardial ischemia that manifests as chest, neck, or arm pain.

Angle of Louis (Manubriosternal Junction or Sternal Angle)   Junction of the manubrium and the sternum.

Animism Belief that all things in nature have souls.

Anisocoria Difference in pupil sizes.

Anoderm Epithelial tissue that lies in the lower 2 cm of the anal canal.

Anorectal Abscess Undrained collection of perianal pus of the tissue spaces in and adjacent to the anorectum.

Anorectal Fistula Hollow, fibrous tract lined by granulation tissue and filled with purulent or serosanguineous discharge; it has an opening inside the anal canal or rectum, and one or more orifices in the perianal skin.

Anorectum Area where the anal canal fuses with the rectum.

Anosmia Loss of the sense of smell.

Anterior Axillary Line Vertical line drawn from the origin of the anterior axillary fold along the anterolateral aspect of the thorax.

Anterior Chamber Space anterior to the pupil and iris.

Anterior Triangle Area of the neck formed by the mandible, the trachea, and the sternocleidomastoid muscle; contains the anterior cervical lymph nodes, the trachea, and the thyroid gland.

Anthropometric Measurements Measurements of the human body, including height, weight, and body proportions.

Anticipatory Guidance Approach covering health promotion and education; designed to inform at-risk individuals of physical, cognitive, psychological, and social changes that occur and what their nutritional needs are.

Antigen Skin Testing Test of immune function.

Apex (of the Heart) Lower portion of the heart.

Apex (of the Lung) Top of the lung.

APGAR Scoring Method to assess newborn's status; a score of 0–10 rates the newborn's color, reflex irritability, muscle tone, respiratory effort, and heart rate.

Aphasia Impairment or absence of language function.

Aphonia Total loss of voice.

Apnea Lack of respirations for 10 or more seconds.

Apneustic Respirations Prolonged gasping in inspiration followed by a very short, inefficient pause that can last 30 to 60 seconds.

Apocrine Glands Sweat glands that are associated with hair follicles.

Appendicular Skeleton Limbs, pelvis, scapula, and clavicle.

Apraxia Inability to convert intended speech into the motor act of speech; inability to perform purposeful acts or to manipulate objects.

Arcus Senilis Hazy, gray ring about 2 mm in size and located just inside the limbus; most commonly found in older individuals.

Areola Pigmented area approximately 2.5 to 10 cm in diameter that surrounds the nipple.

Arrector Pili Muscle Muscle that causes contraction of the skin and hair, resulting in "goose bumps."

Arrhythmia Irregular heart rhythm; also known as dysrhythmia.

Ascites Excess accumulation of fluid in the abdominal cavity.

Assessment First step of the nursing process; the orderly collection of objective and subjective data on the patient's health status.

Associated Manifestations Signs and symptoms that accompany a patient's chief complaint.

Astereognosis Inability to recognize the nature of objects by touch.

Asystole Absence of pulse.

Ataxic Respirations *See* **Biot's Respirations**.

Atheist Person who does not believe in God.

Atherosclerosis Development of plaques along the coronary arteries.

Atlas First cervical vertebra.

Atrial Kick Final phase of ventricular diastole, when the atria contract to complete the final 20% to 30% of ventricular filling.

Atrioventricular (A-V) Node One of the heart's pacemakers that delays the impulse from the atria before it goes to the ventricles; inherent rate is 40 to 60 beats per minute.

Atrioventricular (A-V) Valves Valves that prevent blood from entering the ventricles until diastole and prevent retrograde blood flow during systole; composed of the tricuspid and mitral valves.

Atrophy Reduction in muscle size.

Attention Deficit Hyperactivity Disorder (ADHD) Condition in which a child demonstrates periods of inattention, impulsiveness, and hyperactivity for a period of 6 or more months.

Augmentation Mammoplasty Surgical breast augmentation.

Auricle External flap of the ear; also called the pinna.

Auscultation Process of active listening to sounds within the body to gather information on a patient's health status.

Axial Skeleton Facial bones, skull, auditory ossicles, hyoid bone, ribs, sternum, and vertebrae.

Axillary Nodes Nodes composed of four groups: central axillary, pectoral (anterior), subscapular (posterior), and lateral.

Axis Second cervical vertebra.

B

Ballottement Palpation technique to identify an organ or fluid.

Baroreceptors Receptors that are located in the walls of most of the great arteries and that sense hypotension and initiate reflex vasoconstriction and tachycardia to bring the blood pressure back to normal.

Barrel Chest Abnormal thorax configuration where the ratio of the anteroposterior diameter to the transverse diameter of the chest is approximately 1:1.

Bartholin's Glands (Greater Vestibular Glands) Located in the cleft between the labia minora and the hymenal ring; these glands secrete a clear, viscid, odorless, alkaline mucus that improves the viability and motility of sperm along the female reproductive tract.

Base (of the Heart) Uppermost portion of the heart.

Base (of the Lung) Bottom of the lung.

Bell's Palsy Idiopathic facial palsy of CN VII resulting in asymmetry of the palpebral fissures, nasolabial folds, mouth, and facial expression on the affected side.

Bilingualism Habitual use of two different languages, particularly when speaking.

Biot's (or Ataxic) Respirations Irregularly irregular respiratory pattern caused by damage to the medulla.

Blepharitis Inflamed, scaly, red-rimmed eyelids, sometimes with loss of the eyelashes.

Blood Pressure Vital sign collected to assess cardiac output and vascular resistance; it measures the force exerted by the flow of blood pumped into the large arteries.

Borborygmi Loud, audible, gurgling bowel sounds.

Bouchard's Node Bony enlargement of the proximal interphalangeal joint of the finger.

Bow Legs *See* **Genu Varum**.

Bradycardia Pulse rate under 60 beats per minute in a resting adult.

Bradypnea Respiratory rate under 12 breaths per minute in a resting adult.

Braxton Hicks Contractions Uterine contractions that are irregular and painless; also known as false labor.

Breasts Pair of mammary glands located on the anterior chest wall and extending vertically from the second to the sixth rib and laterally from the sternal border to the axillae.

Bregma Junction of the coronal and sagittal sutures.

Bronchial (or Tubular) Breath Sound Breath sound that is high in pitch and loud in intensity and that is heard best over the trachea; has a blowing/hollow quality; heard longer in expiration than inspiration.

Bronchophony Voice sound where the patient says the words "ninety-nine" or "one, two, three" to determine if the lung is filled with air, fluid, or a solid.

Bronchovesicular Breath Sound Breath sound that is moderate in pitch and intensity and that is heard best between the scapula and the first and second intercostal spaces lateral to the sternum; its quality is a combination of bronchial and vesicular breath sounds; heard equally in inspiration and expiration.

Bruit Blowing sound that can be auscultated when the blood flow becomes turbulent because blood is rushing past an obstruction.

Brushfield's Spots Small, white flecks located around the perimeter of the iris, and associated with Down syndrome.

Bulbar Conjunctiva Covering of the anterior surface of the sclera.

Bulbourethral Glands Pea-sized glands located below the prostate; secretions are emptied from here at the time of ejaculation.

Bursae Sacs filled with fluids.

C

Cachexia Extreme malnutrition in which the patient exhibits wasting.

Callus Thickening of the skin due to prolonged pressure.

Canthus Nasal or temporal angle where the eyelids meet.

Caput Medusae Venous pattern of congested veins around the umbilicus, attributed to obstruction of the portal vein and seen in liver dysfunction.

Caput Succedaneum Swelling over the occipitoparietal region of the skull that occurs during delivery of the newborn.

Carbohydrate Major source of energy for various functions of the body; supplies fiber and assists in the utilization of fat.

Cardiomegaly Enlargement of the heart.

Carotenemia Orange-yellow coloration of palmar and plantar surfaces caused by elevated levels of serum carotene.

Caruncle Round, red structure in the inner canthus; contains sebaceous glands.

Castration Anxiety Young boys' fear of having the penis cut off or mutilated.

Cataract Opacity in the lens of the eye that gives the pupil a pearly gray appearance.

Cephalocaudal Head-to-toe approach.

Cephalhematoma Localized subcutaneous swelling over one cranial bone that occurs during delivery of the newborn.

Cerumen Waxlike substance produced in the ear canal.

Cervix Inferior aspect of the uterus.

Chadwick's Sign A blue, soft cervix, normally during pregnancy.

Chalazion Chronic inflammation of the meibomian gland in the upper or lower eyelid.

Chancre Reddish, round ulcer or small papular lesion with a depressed center and raised, indurated edges.

Chancroid Tender, ulcerated, exudative, papular lesion with an erythematous halo, surrounding edema, and a friable base.

Chandelier's Sign Cervix motion tenderness on palpation.

Characteristic Patterns of Daily Living Patient's normal daily routines; includes meal, work, and sleeping schedules and patterns of social interactions.

Chemosis Swelling of the palpebral conjunctiva.

Cherry Angioma Bright-red, circumcised areas that may be flat or raised and that darken with age.

Cheyne-Stokes Respirations Crescendo/decrescendo respiratory pattern interspersed between periods of apnea.

Chief Complaint Symptom or problem that causes the patient to seek health care.

Chloasma *See* **Melasma**.

Cholesterol Lipid found only in animal products; it is transported in the body by high-density lipoproteins (HDLs) and low-density lipoproteins (LDLs).

Choroid Vascular tissue of the posterior uveal tract lining the inner surface of the globe of the eye, beneath the retina; provides nutrition to the retina and helps absorb excess light.

Ciliary Body Extension of the uveal tract that produces aqueous humor.

Circadian Rhythm Normal fluctuation of body temperature, pulse, and blood pressure during a 24-hour period.

Click Extrasystolic heart sound that is high pitched and can radiate in the chest wall.

Clitoris Cylindrical, erectile body located at the superior aspect of the vulva, between the labia minora; it contains erectile tissue and has a significant supply of nerve endings.

Clonus Rhythmic oscillation of involuntary muscle contraction.

Clubfoot *See* **Metatarsus Varus**.

Clustering Placing similar or related data into meaningful groups.

Coarse Crackle Discontinuous adventitious breath sound that is caused by air passing through moisture in large airways that suddenly reinflate; it resembles a low-pitched crackling or gurgling sound.

Cochlea Snail-shaped structure in the bony labyrinth of the inner ear.

Code of Ethics Codified beliefs and lists of mandatory or prohibited acts.

Collaborative Intervention Physician-prescribed orders that are implemented by nurses.

Collaborative Problem Patient problem for which the nurse works jointly with the physician and other health care workers to monitor, plan, and implement treatment.

Colloquialism Word or phrase particular to a community and used in informal conversation and writing.

Coloboma Defect of the choroid and retina resulting when development in utero is interrupted.

Colostrum A thin, milky secretion expressed by the breast during pregnancy and for a few days after parturition; it is rich in antibodies and colostrum corpuscles.

Complete Health History Comprehensive history of the patient's past and present health status; includes physical, emotional, psychological, developmental, cultural, and spiritual data.

Condyloma Acuminatum Genital wart.

Cones Retinal structures in the macular region that are responsible for color vision.

Confabulation Fabrication of answers, experiences, or situations unrelated to facts.

Conservation The understanding that altering the physical state of an object does not change the basic properties of that object.

Constructional Apraxia Inability to reproduce figures on paper.

Cooper's Ligaments Ligaments that extend vertically from the deep fascia through the breast to the inner layer of the skin, and provide support for the breast tissue.

Corn Conical area of thickened skin.

Cornea Transparent covering of the iris.

Costal Angle Angle formed by the intersection of the costal margins at the sternum.

Costal Margin Medial border created by the articulation of the false ribs.

Cough Stimulation of afferent vagal endings that helps to clear the airway of extraneous material by producing a sudden, forceful, and noisy expulsion of air from the lungs.

Cradle Cap Seborrheic dermatitis manifesting as greasy-appearing scales on an infant's scalp.

Craniosynostosis Abnormal shape of the skull due to premature ossification of one or more suture lines before brain growth is complete.

Craniotabes Softening of the skull.

Creatinine Substance found in muscle and excreted in the urine.

Crepitus Subcutaneous emphysema; beads of air escape from the lungs and create a crackling sound when palpated.

Crescendo Heart murmur configuration that proceeds from soft to loud.

Critical Pathway Map in the case management patient care delivery system that shows the outcome of predetermined patient goals over a period of time.

Cross-Cultural Nursing Care Nursing care that is provided within the cultural context of a patient who is a member of a culture or subculture other than that of the nurse.

Cryptorchidism Condition in which a testicle has not descended into the scrotum.

Cullen's Sign Bluish discoloration encircling the umbilicus and indicative of blood in the peritoneal cavity.

Cult Organized group centered around religious devotion to a set of beliefs or to a person.

Cultural Beliefs Explanatory ideas and knowledge about various aspects of the world in which members of a given culture place their faith and confidence.

Cultural Diversity State of different combinations of cultural and subcultural minorities (e.g., ethnic, racial, national, religious, generational, marital status, socioeconomic, occupational, health status, and preference in life partner orientations) coexisting in a given location.

Cultural Identity Subjective sense of cultural definition or cultural orientation with which an individual self-identifies.

Cultural Norms Often unwritten but generally understood prescriptions for acceptable behavior by members of a cultural group.

Cultural Relativism Belief that no culture is either inferior or superior to another; that behavior must be evaluated in relation to the cultural context in which it occurs; and that respect, equality, and justice are basic rights for all racial, ethnic, subcultural, and cultural groups.

Cultural Rituals Highly structured and prescribed patterns of behavior used by a cultural group to respond to or in anticipation of specific life events such as birth, death, illness, healing, marriage, and worship.

Cultural Values Fundamental, often unshakable and unchanging set of principles on which the cultural beliefs, behaviors, and customs of all members of the culture are based.

Culturally Competent Nursing Care Nursing care that is provided by nurses who use cross-cultural nursing models and research to identify health care needs and to plan and evaluate the care provided within the cultural context of their patients.

Culture Learned and socially transmitted orientation and way of life of a group of people that is based on shared values, beliefs, customs, and norms of behavior and that determines how members of the group think, act, and relate to and with others as well as how they perceive and respond to all aspects of their life.

Culture Shock Disorientation and uncertainty that results from the expenditure of mental, emotional, and physical energy during the process of adjusting to a new cultural group; it can lead to frustration, anger, alienation, or depression.

Custom Frequent or common practice carried out by tradition; culturally learned behaviors associated with a specific culture, including communication patterns, family and kinship relations, work patterns, dietary and religious practices, and health behaviors and practices.

Cutaneous Hypersensitivity Stimulus detecting specific zones of peritoneal irritation.

Cyanosis Blue coloration of the skin or nails that occurs when more than 5 g/dl of hemoglobin is deoxygenated in the blood.

Cystocele Bulging of the anterior vaginal wall.

Cystourethrocele Bulging of the anterior vaginal wall, bladder, and urethra into the vaginal introitus.

D

Dacryoadenitis Acute inflammation of the lacrimal gland.

Dacryocystitis Inflammation of the lacrimal duct.

Decerebrate Rigidity Rigidity and sustained contraction of the extensor muscle.

Decorticate Rigidity Hyperflexion of the arms and hyperextension, internal rotation, and plantar flexion of the legs.

Decrescendo Heart murmur configuration that proceeds from loud to soft.

Deep Palpation Palpating the body's internal structures to a depth of 4 to 5 cm to elicit information on organs and masses, including position, size, shape, mobility, and consistency.

Defecation Expulsion of feces from the rectum.

Defining Characteristics Signs, symptoms, or statements made by the patient that validate the existence of the health problem or situation.

Dehydration Lack of fluid in the tissues.

Dermatome Skin area innervated by afferent spinal nerves from a specific nerve root.

Dermis Corium, or the second layer of the skin.

Descriptor or Qualifier Adjective that describes or qualifies the human response.

Desquamation Shedding of old skin cells as new cells are pushed up from the lower layers of the epidermis.

Development Patterned and predictable increases in the physical, cognitive, socioemotional, and moral capacities of individuals that enable them to successfully adapt to their environments.

Developmental Dislocation of the Hip Dislocated hip found in infants and related to familial factors, maternal hormones, firstborn children, and breech presentations.

Developmental Stage One of multiple sequential age periods during which individuals experience the same physical, cognitive, socioemotional, and moral changes.

Developmental Task Specific physical or psychosocial skill that must be achieved during each developmental stage.

Diaphragmatic Excursion Technique used to assess the patient's depth of ventilation.

Diaphragmatic Hernia Protrusion of intestines into the thoracic cavity.

Diaphysis Central shaft of the long bone.

Diastasis Recti Separation of the rectus muscle of the abdominal wall.

Diastole Pressure in the arteries when the heart is at rest.

Direct Fist Percussion Using the ulnar aspect of a closed fist to strike the patient's body to elicit tenderness over specific body areas.

Direct Inguinal Hernia Protrusion of the bowel and/or omentum directly through Hesselbach's triangle.

Direct (or Immediate) Auscultation Active listening to body sounds via the unaided ear.

Direct (or Immediate) Percussion Striking of an area of the body directly with the index or middle finger pad or fist to elicit sound.

Distress Negative stress that is harmful and unpleasant.

Dislocation Complete dislodgement of a bone from its joint cavity.

Disuse Atrophy Decrease in muscle mass and strength as a result of immobility.

Dogma Beliefs that are essential to the identity of a religion.

Down Syndrome Congenital chromosomal aberration marked by slanted eyes with inner epicanthal folds; a short, flat nose; a protruding, thick tongue and mental retardation.

Ductus (Vas) Deferens Tube that permits sperm to exit from the epididymis and pass from the scrotal sac upward into the abdominal cavity.

Dullness Descriptor for a percussable sound that is moderate in intensity, moderate in duration, of high pitch, thudlike, and normally located over organs.

Duration (of Percussion) Time period over which a sound is heard.

Dysarthria Disturbance in muscular control of speech.

Dyscalculia Inability to perform calculations.

Dysdiadochokinesia Inability to perform rapid, alternating movements.

Dysesthesia Abnormal interpretation of a stimulus such as burning or tingling from a stimulus such as touch or superficial pain.

Dysmenorrhea Pain or cramping during menses.

Dysmetria Impairment of judgment of distance, range, speed, and force of movement.

Dyspareunia Painful sexual intercourse.

Dysphagia Difficulty swallowing.

Dysphonia Difficulty in making laryngeal speech sounds.

Dyspnea Subjective feeling of shortness of breath.

Dysrhythmia *See* **Arrhythmia**.

Dyssynergy Lack of coordinated action of the muscle groups.

E

Ecchymosis A red-purple discoloration of varying size caused by extravasation of blood into the skin; a black-and-blue mark.

Eccrine glands Sweat glands that are not associated with hair follicles.

Echolalia Involuntary repetition of a word or sentence that was uttered by another person.

Eclampsia Seizure associated with pregnancy-induced hypertension.

Ecogram Diagram of a patient's relationships with family members and significant friends, peers, neighbors, and work associates, noting those with whom the person has the most frequent contact and their relative importance to the patient.

Ectodermal Galactic Band *See* **Milk Line**.

Ectopic Pregnancy Nonviable, extrauterine pregnancy.

Ectropion (of the Eye) Turning outward or eversion of the eyelid, usually the lower.

Ectropion (or Eversion, of the Cervix) Reddish circle around the cervical os.

Edema Accumulation of fluid in the intercellular spaces, leading to swelling of the extremities, usually the feet and hands.

Ego Personality component that is conscious, rational, emerges during the first year of life, and seeks realistic and acceptable ways to meet needs.

Egocentrism Viewing the world in terms of only the self and interpreting one's own actions and all other events in terms of the consequences for the self.

Egophony Voice sound where the patient says the letter "ee" to determine if the lungs are filled with air, fluid, or a solid.

Ejaculatory Ducts Ducts located posterior to the urinary bladder; they eject sperm into the prostatic urethra prior to ejaculation.

Electra Complex Girls' sexual attraction toward their fathers and rivalry with their mothers.

Electrocardiogram (EKG) Record of the electrical activity of the heart.

Eleidin Translucent substance that aids in the formation of keratin.

Emergency Health History History taken from the patient or other sources when the patient is experiencing a life-threatening state.

Enculturation Informal process through which the beliefs, values, norms, and practices of a culture are learned by members born into that culture.

Enophthalmos Backward displacement of the globe of the eye.

Entropion Turning inward or inversion of the eyelid, usually the lower.

Epidermis Multilayered outer covering of the skin, consisting of four layers throughout the body, except for the palms of the hands and soles of the feet, where there are five layers.

Epididymis Comma-shaped organ that lies along the posterior border of each testis; consists of a tightly coiled tube where sperm maturation occurs.

Epimysium Connective tissue sheath covering the muscle belly.

Epiphyses Ends of the long bone.

Episodic Health History History taken from the patient for a specific problem or need.

Epispadias Congenital abnormality in which the urethral meatus lies on the dorsal surface of the penis.

Epstein's Pearls Small, hard, white cysts found on a newborn's hard palate and gum margins.

Eructation Belching.

Escutcheon Characteristic triangular pattern of coarse, curly hair that develops over the mons pubis at puberty.

Esophoria Latent misalignment of the eye; nasal, or inward, drift.

Esotropia Inward deviation of the eye.

Ethnic Group Classification of individuals based on their unique national or regional origin and social, cultural, and linguistic heritage.

Ethnic Identity Subjective sense of ethnic definition or social orientation with which an individual self-identifies.

Ethnocentrism Condition that occurs when individuals or groups of people perceive their own cultural group and cultural values, beliefs, norms, and customs to be superior to all others and have disdain for the expression of any way of life but their own.

Eupnea Normal breathing; respirations are 12 to 20 per minute for the resting adult.

Eustachian Tube Auditory tube that serves as an air channel connecting the middle ear to the nasopharynx to allow equalization between the air pressure in the ear and in the atmosphere.

Eustress Positive stress that challenges, provides motivation, and prevents stagnation.

Evaluation Last step of the nursing process; the patient's progress in achieving the outcomes is determined.

Exophoria Latent misalignment of the eye; temporal, or outward, drift.

Exophthalmos Abnormal protrusion of the globe of the eye.

Exotropia Outward deviation of the eye.

F

Faith Orientation to a belief structure.

Fallopian Tubes Site of fertilization; they extend from the cornu of the uterus to the ovaries and are supported by the broad ligaments.

False Ribs Rib pairs 8–10.

Fat-Soluble Vitamins Vitamins stored in dietary fat and absorbed in the fat portions of the body's cells.

Fats Substances that supply essential fatty acids, which form a part of the structure of all cells.

Femoral Hernia Protrusion of the omentum and/or bowel through the femoral wall.

Fetoscope Special stethoscope for hearing fetal heart beats.

Fine Crackle Discontinuous adventitious breath sound that is caused by air passing through moisture in small airways that suddenly reinflate; it resembles a high-pitched crackling sound.

Fissure Groove separating the different lobes of the lungs.

Flatness Descriptor for a percussable sound that is soft in intensity, short in duration, of high pitch, and normally located over muscle or bone.

Flatulence Passage of excess gas via the rectum.

Floating Ribs Rib pairs 11 and 12; they do not articulate at their anterior ends.

Fluid Wave Abnormal finding elicited during palpation and indicating fluid in the peritoneal cavity.

Folk Illness Illness believed to be caused by disharmony, an imbalance, or as a punishment.

Folk Practitioner Healer or other individual who is not part of the scientific care system but is believed to have special knowledge or power to prevent, treat, or provide resources needed to heal folk illnesses.

Follow-Up Health History *See* **Interval Health History**.

Food Guide Pyramid Guideline to improve daily diet using the concepts of proportion and moderation.

Fourchette Transverse fold of skin of the posterior aspect of the labia minora; also known as frenulum.

Fornices Pouchlike recesses around the cervix.

Fovea Centralis Center of the macula; the area of sharpest vision.

Frenulum (of the Mouth) Tissue that connects the tongue to the floor of the mouth.

Friability Susceptibility to bleeding from the cervix.

Functional Health Patterns Groups of human behavior that facilitate nursing care; there are 11 patterns (refer to Table 1-3 on page 5).

Fundus Superior aspect of the uterus.

G

Gallop Extra heart sound; an S_3 is a ventricular gallop, whereas an S_4 is an atrial gallop.

Ganglion Benign, cystic growth.

Genogram Pictorial representation of the patient's family health history.

Genu Valgum Inward deviation toward the midline at the level of the knees; also known as knock knees.

Genu Varum Outward deviation away from the midline at the level of the knees; also known as bow legs.

Glans Penis Bulbous end of the penis.

Glasgow Coma Scale International scale used in grading neurological response.

Glaucoma Disease in which intraocular pressure is elevated.

Glycosuria Glucose in the urine.

God Concept of a diety or personal, present being.

Goiter Enlargement of the thyroid gland.

Goniometer Device used to measure the angle of the skeletal joint during range of motion; it is a protractor with two movable arms.

Granulation Tissue Inflamed tissue, new vessels, and white blood cells at the base of a wound in the process of healing.

Granulomatous Reaction (in the Breast) Development of small, nodular, inflammatory lesions and capsular membranes over the breasts.

Graphanesthesia Inability to identify numbers, letters, or shapes drawn on the skin.

Graphesthesia Ability to identify numbers, letters, or shapes drawn on the skin.

Growth Increase in body size and function to the point of optimum maturity.

Gynecomastia Enlargement of male breast tissue; may occur normally in adolescent and elderly males.

H

Hallux Valgus Lateral deviation of the big toe and medial deviation of the first metatarsal; also known as bunion.

Hammer Toe Flexion of the proximal interphalangeal joint and hyperextension of the distal metatarsophalangeal joint.

Harlequin Color Change Condition in which one-half of a newborn's body is red or ruddy and the other half appears pale.

Health Maintenance Activities Practices that a person incorporates into a lifestyle and that can promote healthy living.

Heave Lifting of the cardiac area secondary to an increased workload and force of left ventricular contraction; also known as a lift.

Heaven Blissful resting place for souls after death, according to Christianity.

Heberden's Node Bony enlargement of the distal interphalangeal joint of the finger.

HELLP Syndrome Complication of pregnancy-induced hypertension; the acronym represents hemolysis, elevated liver enzymes, and low platelets.

Hematemesis Vomiting of blood.

Hematocrit Measurement to determine the percentage of red blood cells to the volume of whole blood.

Hemiparesis Unilateral weakness or paralysis; also known as hemiplegia.

Hemiplegia *See* **Hemiparesis**.

Hemoglobin Measurement of the iron component that transports oxygen in the blood.

Hemorrhoids Dilatation of hemorrhoidal veins in the anorectum.

Heretic Person who rejects the official teachings or dogma of a religion or belief system.

High-Density Lipoprotein Substance that carries cholesterol away from the heart and arteries and toward the liver; the "good" cholesterol.

Hirsutism Excessive body hair.

History of the Present Illness Chronological account of the patient's chief complaint and the events surrounding it.

Holistic Nursing Care that addresses all aspects of a person's health and well-being.

Holosystolic Murmur that is heard throughout all of systole; also known as pansystolic.

Homan's Sign Pain in the calf when the foot is dorsiflexed; sign of venous thrombosis of the deep veins of the calf.

Hordeolum Infection of a sebaceous gland in the eyelid.

Human Response Patterns Groups of human behavior that facilitate nursing care; there are nine patterns (refer to Table 1-4 on pages 6 and 7).

Hydrocele Fluid collection within the tunica vaginalis of the testis.

Hydrocephalus Enlargement of the head without enlargement of the facial structures; it is due to increased accumulation of cerebrospinal fluid within the ventricles of the brain.

Hymen Avascular, thin fold of connective tissue surrounding the vaginal introitus; it may be annular or crescentic in shape.

Hypalgesia Diminished sensitivity to pain.

Hyperalgesia Increased sensitivity to pain.

Hyperemesis Gravidarum Excessive nausea and vomiting during pregnancy.

Hyperesthesia Abnormal acuteness to the sensitivity of touch.

Hyperglycemia Increase in serum glucose.

Hyperkinetic Increased movement.

Hyperopia Farsightedness.

Hyperpnea Breath that is greater in volume than the resting tidal volume.

Hyperresonance Descriptor for a percussable sound that is very loud in intensity, long in duration, of very low pitch, boomlike, and normally not found in the healthy adult.

Hypertelorism Abnormal width between the eyes.

Hypertension Blood pressure remaining consistently above 140 mm Hg systolic or 90 mm Hg diastolic in an adult.

Hyperthermia Generalized or localized excessive warming of the skin; body temperature that exceeds 38.5°C, or 101.5°F.

Hypertrophy Increase in muscle size due to an increase in the bulk of muscle fibers.

Hypesthesia Diminished sense of touch; also known as hypoesthesia.

Hyphema Condition in which there is blood in the anterior chamber of the eye.

Hypoesthesia *See* **Hypesthesia**.

Hypogeusia Diminution of taste.

Hypoglycemia Decrease in serum glucose.

Hypokinetic Decreased movement.

Hypospadias Congenital abnormality in which the urethral meatus lies on the ventral surface of the penis.

Hypotension Blood pressure that is lower than what is needed to maintain adequate tissue perfusion and oxygenation.

Hypothermia Generalized or localized cooling of the skin; body temperature that is below 34°C, or 93.2°F.

Hypotonicity Decrease in normal muscle tone (flaccidity).

I

Id Personality component that is inborn, unconscious, and driven by biological instincts and urges to seek immediate gratification of needs such as hunger, thirst, and physical comfort.

Iliopsoas Muscle Test   Technique used to assess for an inflamed appendix.

Immediate Auscultation   *See* **Direct Auscultation**.

Immediate Percussion   *See* **Direct Percussion**.

Implementation   Fourth step of the nursing process; the execution of the nursing interventions that were devised during the planning stage to help the patient meet predetermined outcomes.

Impotence   Inability to achieve or maintain an erection.

Independent Nursing Interventions   Actions that the nurse is legally capable of implementing based on education and experience.

Indirect Fist Percussion   Using the closed ulnar aspect of the fist of the dominant hand to strike the nondominant hand to elicit tenderness over specific body areas.

Indirect Inguinal Hernia   Portions of the bowel and/or omentum that enter the inguinal canal through the internal ring and exit at the external ring.

Indirect (or Mediate) Auscultation   Active listening to body sounds via some amplification or mechanical device, such as a stethoscope or Doppler transducer.

Indirect (or Mediate) Percussion   Using the plexor to strike the pleximeter to elicit sound.

Infarction (Myocardial)   Necrosis of cardiac muscle due to decreased blood supply.

Injection   Redness around the cornea.

Inspection   Use of one's senses to consciously observe the patient; in physical assessment, vision, hearing, smell, and touch are used.

Insufficiency   *See* **Regurgitation**.

Integumentary System   Skin and cutaneous tissue.

Intensity (of Percussion)   Relative loudness or softness of sound; amplitude.

Intercostal Space   Area between the ribs.

Intermediary   Individual who serves to assist with communication between the patient and another individual, usually a member of the health care team.

Interpleural Space   *See* **Mediastinum**.

Interval (or Follow-Up) Health History   History that builds on the patient's last health care visit and documents resolution or nonresolution of a problem or health care need.

Intervention   Nursing action designed to achieve patient outcomes.

Intussusception   Formation of a sausage-shaped mass in the upper abdomen resulting when the ileocecal region of the intestine telescopes into the ileum.

Iris   Most anterior portion of the uveal tract; provides a distinctive color for the eye.

Ischemia (Myocardial)   Local and temporary lack of blood supply to the heart; may progress to an infarction if left untreated.

Isoelectric Line   Electrical resting period after the T-wave on the EKG.

Isthmus (of the Uterus)   Constricted area between the body of the uterus and the cervix.

Isthmus (of the Thyroid)   Narrow portion of the thyroid gland that connects the two lobes and lies over the tracheal rings.

J

Jaundice   Yellow-green to orange cast or coloration of skin, sclera, or mucous membranes; caused by an elevated bilirubin level.

Joining Stage   Introduction or first stage of the interview process, during which the nurse and patient establish rapport.

Joint   Union between two bones.

K

Keratosis   Lesions on the epidermis characterized by overgrowth of the horny layer.

Kilocalorie   Amount of heat required to raise 1 gram of water 1 degree centigrade; also called calorie.

Knock Knees   *See* **Genu Valgum**.

Korotkoff Sounds   Sounds generated when the flow of blood through the artery is altered by the inflation of a blood pressure cuff around the extremity.

Kussmaul's Respirations   Respirations characterized by extreme increased rate and depth, as in diabetic ketoacidosis.

Kwashiorkor   Severe deficiency of protein; means "disease of the displaced child."

Kyphosis   Excessive convexity of the thoracic spine; known as "humpback."

L

Labia Majora   Two longitudinal folds of adipose and connective tissue that extend from the clitoris anteriorly and gradually narrow to merge and form the commissure of the perineum posteriorly.

Labia Minora   Two thin folds of skin that enclose the vulval vestibule and extend to form the prepuce, or hood, of the clitoris anteriorly and a transverse fold of skin that forms the fourchette posteriorly.

Labyrinth   Bony and membranous system of interconnecting tubes in the inner ear; essential for hearing and equilibrium.

Lacrimal Apparatus   Lacrimal gland and ducts.

Lactiferous Ducts   Openings at the nipple through which milk and colostrum are excreted.

Lagophthalmos   Condition in which the patient is unable to completely close the eyelid.

Lanugo   Fine, downy hair present during gestational life and that gradually disappears toward the end of pregnancy; it remains in smaller quantities over the temples, back, shoulders, and upper arms after birth.

Lentigo   Areas of hyperpigmentation resulting from the inability of melanocytes to produce even pigmentation of the skin; known as "liver spots."

Lens   Crystalline structure of the eye that changes shape to refract light from various focusing distances.

Lesion   Circumscribed, pathological change in tissue.

Lichenification   Localized thickening, hardening, and roughness of the skin; can be a result of chronic pruritus.

Life Event/Transitional Developmental Theory   Belief that development occurs in response to specific events, such as new roles (e.g., parenthood), and life transitions (e.g., career changes).

Life Review Reflection on the experiences, relationships, and events of one's life as a whole, viewing successes and failures from the perspective of age, and accepting one's life and accompanying life choices and outcomes in their entirety.

Lift *See* **Heave**.

Ligament Strong, fibrous, connective tissue that connects bones to each other at a joint.

Light Palpation Superficial palpation; depressing the skin 1 cm to elicit information on skin texture and moisture, masses, fluid, muscle guarding, and tenderness.

Lightening Descent of the presenting fetal part into the pelvis.

Limbus Junction of the sclera and cornea.

Linea Nigra Darkening of the abdominal linea alba during pregnancy.

Linear Raphe Linear ridge in the middle of the hard palate.

Lipoma Non-mobile, fatty mass with a smooth, circular edge.

List Leaning of the spine.

Listening Response Attempt made by the nurse to accurately receive, process, and respond to the patient's messages.

Lobes (of the Breast) Glandular breast tissue arranged radially in the form of 12 to 20 spokes.

Lobules (of the Breast) Grapelike bunches that are clustered around several lactiferous ducts; each lobe is composed of 20 to 40 lobules that contain milk-producing glands called alveoli or acini.

Long-Term Outcome Goal that a patient strives to achieve and having a time frame of weeks or months.

Lordosis Excessive concavity of the lumbar spine.

Low-Density Lipoprotein Substance that carries cholesterol toward the heart; the "bad" cholesterol.

Lunula White, crescent-shaped area at the proximal end of each nail.

Lymphatic Drainage Yellow, alkaline drainage originating in the lymph vessels and composed primarily of lymphocytes.

M

Macromineral Major mineral needed by the body in large amounts.

Macrosomia Newborn weighing more than 4,000 grams.

Macula Tiny, darker area in the temporal area of the retina.

Major Defining Characteristics Signs and symptoms that must be present in the patient to use a specific NANDA-approved diagnostic label.

Manubriosternal Junction *See* **Angle of Louis**.

Manubrium Upper bone of the sternum; it articulates with the clavicles and the first pair of ribs.

Marasmus Form of protein calorie malnutrition.

Mast cells Body's major source of tissue histamine, which triggers the body's reaction to invasive allergens.

Mastectomy Excision, or surgical removal, of the breast.

Matrix Undifferentiated epithelial tissue from which keratinized cells arise to form the nail plate.

McBurney's Point Anatomic location that is approximately at the normal location of the appendix in the right lower quadrant; point of increased tenderness in appendicitis.

Meconium Dark-green, sticky, stool-like material excreted from the rectum of the newborn within the first 24 hours after birth.

Mediastinum (Interpleural Space) Area between the lungs.

Mediate Auscultation *See* **Indirect Auscultation**.

Mediate Percussion *See* **Indirect Percussion**.

Medullary Cavity Interior of the diaphysis; contains the bone marrow.

Melanocytes Cells that produce pigmented substances that provide color to the hair, skin, and choroid of the eye.

Melasma Irregular pigmentation on the face due to pregnancy; also known as chloasma.

Melena Black, tarry stool.

Menarche Onset of menstruation.

Menopause Cessation of menstruation.

Menorrhagia Heavy menses.

Mercury Manometer Blood pressure measurement equipment that uses a calibrated column of mercury that corresponds to blood pressure values.

Metatarsus Varus Condition in which the toes and foot are inverted and medially adducted; known as clubfoot.

Microcephaly Small brain with a resultant small head.

Micromineral Trace mineral needed by the body in small amounts.

Microphallus Small penis for developmental stage.

Mid-Arm Circumference Anthropometric measurement that provides information on skeletal muscle mass and adipose tissue.

Mid-Arm Muscle Circumference Anthropometric measurement derived from mid-arm circumference; provides information on skeletal muscle mass and adipose tissue.

Midaxillary Line Vertical line drawn from the apex of the axilla; it lies midway between the anterior and the posterior axillary lines.

Midclavicular Line Vertical line drawn from the midpoint of the clavicle.

Midspinal (or Vertebral) Line Vertical line drawn from the midpoint of the spinous processes.

Midsternal Line Vertical line drawn from the midpoint of the sternum.

Milia Plugged sebaceous glands manifesting as small, white papules and appearing on the infant's head, especially on the cheeks and nose.

Milk Line Ectodermal galactic band that develops from the axilla to the groin during the fifth week of fetal development.

Mineral Inorganic element that regulates body processes and builds body tissue; classified into macrominerals and microminerals.

Minor Defining Characteristics Signs and symptoms that need not be present in the patient to use a specific NANDA-approved diagnostic label but add validity to the diagnosis.

Minority Group Members Individuals who are considered by themselves and others to be members of a minority because they have a different racial, ethnic, cultural, gender, socioeconomic, or sexual orientation than the members of the dominant cultural group.

Molding Condition in which the newborn's parietal bone overrides the frontal bone as a result of increased pressure during delivery.

Mongolian Spots Various, irregularly sized areas of deep bluish pigmentation on the upper back, shoulders, buttocks, and lumbosacral area of newborns of African, Latino, and Asian descent.

Monosaturated Fats Fatty acids that contain one double bond between carbon atoms.

Monotheism Belief in one all-powerful, omnipresent, and omnipotent god.

Mons Pubis Pad of subcutaneous fatty tissue lying over the anterior symphysis pubis.

Montgomery's Tubercles Sebaceous glands present on the surface of the areola.

Multicultural Identity Unique combination of cultural influences that result from membership in a variety of subcultures within the primary culture.

Multiculturalism The act of living and functioning in two or more cultures simultaneously.

Murphy's Sign Abnormal finding elicited during abdominal palpation in the right upper quadrant and revealing gallbladder inflammation; characteristically, the patient will abruptly stop inspiration and complain of sharp pain.

Myopia Nearsightedness.

N

Nabothian Cysts Small, round, yellow lesions on the cervical surface.

Nail Bed Vascular bed located beneath the nail plate.

Nail Plate Tissue that covers and protects the distal portion of the fingers and toes.

Nail Root Nail portion that is posterior to the cuticle and attached to the matrix.

NANDA North American Nursing Diagnosis Association; the professional nursing organization that sets the standards for the development, clinical testing, and approval of nursing diagnoses.

Naturalistic Illness Illness believed to be caused by an imbalance or disequilibrium between essentially impersonal factors, for example, hot and cold.

Nevi Pigmented moles that may be flat or elevated.

Nipple A round, hairless, pigmented protrusion of erectile tissue approximately 0.5 to 1.5 cm in diameter located in the center of the breast.

Nirvana Buddhist belief of the perfect blessedness and peace of the soul.

Nitrogen Component of amino acids.

Nocturia Excessive urination at night.

Nonverbal Communication Communicating a message without using words.

Nulliparous Descriptor for a woman who has not given birth.

Nursing Care Plan Patient care record that uses the nursing process as its framework.

Nursing Diagnosis "A clinical judgment about individual, family, or community responses to actual and potential health problems/life processes" (NANDA, 1996, p. 8).

Nursing Process Dynamic, five-step process that uses information in a meaningful way through the use of problem-solving strategies to place the patient, family, or community in an optimal health state; includes assessment, nursing diagnosis, planning, implementation, and evaluation.

Nutrient Substance found in food that is nourishing or useful to the body.

Nutrition Processes of the human body that metabolize and utilize nutrients.

Nystagmus Involuntary oscillation of the eye.

O

Obesity Weight greater than 120% of ideal body weight.

Object Permanence Ability to form a mental image of an object and to recognize that, although removed from view, the object still exists.

Objective Data Data that are tangible or visible and can be corroborated by others; unbiased data not based on opinion or feeling.

Obturator Sign Differential technique for assessing appendicitis, indicative of an irritated obturator internus muscle.

Oedipus Complex Boys' sexual attraction toward their mothers and feelings of rivalry toward their fathers.

Oogenesis Development and formation of an ovum.

Optic Disc Round area on the nasal side of the retina, where retinal fibers join to form the optic nerve.

Orchitis Acute onset of testicular swelling.

Orthopnea Difficulty breathing except in an upright position.

Orthostatic Hypotension Hypotension that occurs when changing from a supine to an upright position.

Ossicles Three tiny bones in the middle ear that play a crucial role in the transmission of sound: the malleus, the incus, and the stapes.

Osteoporosis Disease characterized by reduced bone mass.

Otitis Media Inflammation or infection of the middle ear.

Ovaries Pair of almond-shaped glands, approximately 3 to 4 cm in length, in the upper pelvic cavity; oogenesis and hormonal production are the ovaries' principal function.

P

PES Acronym for problem, etiology, and signs/symptoms; the nursing diagnosis comprises these elements.

Pack/Year History Term used to describe the quantity of cigarettes smoked over a period of time.

Pagan Person without religion.

Paget's Disease Malignant neoplasm, which is usually unilateral in its involvement and presents as persistent eczematous dermatitis of the areola and nipple.

Pallor Lack of color.

Palpation Touching the patient in a diagnostic manner to elicit specific information.

Palpebral Conjunctiva Mucous membrane covering the interior surface of the eyelid.

Palpebral Fissure Opening between the eyelids.

Palpitation Irregular and rapid heart beat, or sensation of fluttering of the heart.

Pansystolic *See* **Holosystolic**.

Papilla Small projection on the dorsal surface of the tongue and containing opening to taste buds.

Papillary Layer Upper layer of the dermis; composed primarily of loose connective tissue, small elastic fibers, and an extensive network of capillaries that serve to nourish the epidermis.

Paranasal Sinuses Air-filled cavities in the cranial bones and lined with mucous membranes.

Paraphimosis Condition in which the retracted foreskin develops a fixed constriction proximal to the glans penis.

Paresthesia An abnormal sensation, such as numbness, pricking, or tingling.

Parietal Pericardium Pericardial layer that lies close to the fibrous tissues.

Parietal Pleura Lining of the chest wall and the superior surface of the lung.

Parous Descriptor for a woman who has given birth to one or more neonates.

Past Health History History that covers the patient's health from birth to the present.

Pastoral Care Care and response needed when a person is in spiritual crisis.

Patient Goal Broad, unmeasurable statement directed toward removal of related factors or patient response to an adverse condition.

Patient Outcome Measureable statement of the expected change in patient behavior.

Patient Profile Demographics that may be linked to health status.

Peau d'Orange Thickening or edema of the breast tissue or nipple; may present itself as enlarged skin pores that give the appearance of an orange rind.

Pectus Carinatum Abnormal thorax configuration in which there is a marked protrusion of the sternum; known as "pigeon chest."

Pectus Excavatum Abnormal thorax configuration in which there is a depression in the lower body of the sternum; known as "funnel chest."

Penis Cylindrical male organ of copulation used to introduce spermatozoa into the vagina.

Penis Envy Young girls' desire to have a penis.

Percussion Striking one object against another to cause vibrations that produce sound.

Pericarditis Inflammation of the pericardium.

Perineum External surface located between the fourchette and the anus.

Peripheral Vascular Resistance Opposing force against which the left ventricle must contract to pump blood into the aorta; also known as systemic vascular resistance.

Periungual Tissue Tissue that surrounds the nail plate and the free edge of the nail.

Perseveration Repetitive motion that may manifest as continual lip licking, chewing, or tapping.

Personalistic Illness Illness that is believed to occur either because an individual committed some offense and is being punished, or as a result of acts of aggression (sometimes unintentional) by other individuals.

Pertinent Negatives Manifestations that are expected in the patient with a suspected pathology but that are denied or absent.

Pes Cavus Foot with an exaggerated height to the arch.

Pes Planus Foot with a low longitudinal arch; also known as "flatfoot."

Pes Valgus Foot that is turned laterally away from the midline.

Pes Varus Foot that is turned inward toward the midline.

Petechiae Reddish purple skin discoloration that is less than 0.5 cm in diameter and does not blanch.

Phimosis Constriction of the distal penile foreskin that prevents normal retraction over the glans.

Phoria Latent misalignment of an eye.

Physiological Cup Pale, central area of the optic disc.

Physiological Weight Loss Tendency of a neonate to lose approximately 10% of birth weight within a few days after birth and regain it by 2 weeks of age.

Pica Craving for substances other than food (e.g., dirt, clay, starch, ice cubes).

Pinguecula Yellow nodule on the nasal, or temporal, side of the conjunctiva.

Pinna External flap of the ear; also called the auricle.

Pitch (of Percussion) Highness or lowness of a sound.

Planning Third step of the nursing process; involves the prioritization of nursing diagnoses, formulation of patient goals, and selection of nursing interventions.

Pleura Serous sac that encases the lung.

Pleural Friction Fremitus Palpable grating that feels more pronounced on inspiration when there is an inflammatory process between the pleura.

Pleural Friction Rub Continuous adventitious breath sound caused by inflamed parietal and visceral pleura; it resembles a creaking or grating sound.

Pleximeter Stationary finger of the nondominant hand used in indirect percussion.

Plexor Middle finger of the dominant hand; used to strike the pleximeter to elicit sound in indirect percussion.

Polycythemia Elevated number of red blood cells.

Polydactyly Extra digits on the hand or foot.

Polytheism Belief in many gods of different levels of power and status.

Posterior Axillary Line Vertical line drawn from the posterior axillary fold.

Posterior Chamber Space immediately posterior to the iris.

Posterior Triangle Area of the neck between the sterno-cleidomastoid and the trapezius muscles, with the clavicle at the base; contains the posterior cervical lymph nodes.

Prayer Means to communicate with a higher, spiritual power.

Precordium Anterior area of the body that lies over the heart, its great vessels, the pericardium, and some pulmonary tissue.

Preload Resting force on the myocardium as determined by the pressure in the ventricles at the end of diastole.

Prepuce Foreskin covering the glans penis.

Presbycusis Hearing loss commonly found in older individuals.

Presbyopia Impaired near vision occurring in middle-aged or older individuals.

Priapism Abnormal prolonged penile erection unrelated to sexual desire.

Prioritize Ranking the patient's nursing diagnoses; the most critical concerns should be dealt with first.

Proprioception Position sense.

Prostate Glandular organ that lies anterior to the wall of the rectum and encircles the urethra; an accessory male sex organ.

Protein Group of complex nitrogenous compounds, each containing amino acids.

Proteinuria Presence of protein in the urine.

Prurigo Itchy skin eruptions of unknown cause.

Pruritus Severe itching.

Pterygium Triangular, yellow thickening of the bulbar conjunctiva, extending from the nasal side of the cornea to the pupil.

Ptosis Drooping of the eyelid.

Ptyalism Excessive secretion of saliva.

Puddle Sign Percussion technique that distinguishes abdominal fluid from a tumor.

Pulse Palpable expansion of an artery in response to cardiac functioning; used to determine heart rate, rhythm, and estimated volume of blood being pumped by the heart.

Pulse Deficit Apical pulse rate greater than radial pulse rate; occurs when some heart contractions are too weak to produce a palpable pulse at the radial site.

Pulse Pressure Difference between systolic and diastolic pressures.

Pulsus Paradoxus Pathological decrease in systolic blood pressure by 10 mm Hg or more on inspiration.

Puncta Opening at the inner canthus of the eye and through which tears drain.

Pupil Opening in the center of the iris; regulates the amount of light entering the eye.

Purpura Condition characterized by the presence of confluent petechiae or confluent ecchymosis over any part of the body.

Q

Qualifier *See* **Descriptor**.

Quality (of Percussion) Timbre; how a sound is perceived musically.

Quickening First fetal movements felt by the pregnant woman.

R

Race Classification of individuals based on shared inherited biological traits such as skin color, facial features, and body build.

Rash Cutaneous skin eruption that may be localized or generalized.

Reason for Seeking Health Care Problem or health care need that brought the patient to seek health care.

Rebound Tenderness Pain elicited during deep palpation, frequently associated with peritoneal inflammation or appendicitis.

Recommended Dietary Allowance Recommended amount of nutrients to be eaten daily; recommendations differ according to sex, age, and pregnancy or lactation status.

Rectal Prolapse Protrusion of the rectum through the anal orifice.

Rectocele Bulging of the posterior vaginal wall with a portion of the rectum.

Rectouterine Pouch Deep recess formed by the outer layer of the peritoneum; the lowest point in the pelvic cavity, encompassing the lower posterior wall of the uterus, the upper portion of the vagina, and the intestinal surface of the rectum.

Rectovaginal Septum Surface that separates the rectum from the posterior aspect of the vagina.

Rectum Lower portion of the large intestine; passes downward in front of the sacrum.

Reepithelialization Reformation of epithelium over denuded skin.

Regurgitation Backward flow of blood through a diseased heart valve; also known as insufficiency.

Reincarnation Belief that, after death, a person lives another life on earth in another body.

Related Factors "Conditions/circumstances that contribute to the development/maintenance of a nursing diagnosis" (NANDA, 1996, p. 90).

Religion Organized system of beliefs that is usually centered around the worship of a supernatural force or being and that, in turn, defines the self and the self's purpose in life.

Resonance Descriptor for a percussable sound that is loud in intensity, moderate to long in duration, low in pitch, hollow, and normally located in healthy lungs.

Respiration Breathing act that supplies oxygen to the body and occurs in response to changes in the concentration of oxygen, carbon dioxide, and hydrogen in the arterial blood.

Reticular Layer Lower layer of the dermis that is formed by a dense bed of vascular connective tissue; it also includes nerves and lymphatic tissue.

Retina Innermost layer of the eye.

Retromammary Adipose Tissue Tissue that composes the bulk of the breast.

Reversibility The understanding that an action does not need to be experienced before one can anticipate the results or consequences of the action.

Review of Systems The patient's subjective response to a series of body-system–related questions; serves as a double-check that vital information is not overlooked.

Rhonchal Fremitus Coarse, palpable vibration produced by the passage of air through thick exudate in the large bronchi or the trachea.

Rinne Test Method of evaluating hearing loss by comparing air and bone conduction of tuning fork vibrations.

Risk Nursing Diagnosis Statement describing "human response to health conditions/life processes which may develop in a vulnerable individual, family, or community . . . supported by risk factors that contribute to increased vulnerability" (NANDA, 1996, p. 89).

Ritual Solemn, ceremonial act that reinforces faith.

Rod Retinal structure responsible for peripheral vision and dark/light discrimination.

Rosving's Sign Technique to elicit referred pain indicative of peritoneal inflammation.

S

Saturated Fats Lipids derived from animal or vegetable sources.

Scapular Line Vertical line drawn from the inferior angle of the scapula.

Schismatic Person who shares the essential beliefs or dogma of a religion but who is separated from the group because of political or other disagreements.

Scientific Illness Illness in which the presence of pathology is the defining characteristic.

Sclera Opaque covering of the eye; appears white.

Scoliosis Lateral curvature of the thoracic and/or lumbar vertebrae.

Scrotum Pouchlike supporting structure of the testes.

Sebaceous Glands Sebum-producing glands that are found almost everywhere in the dermis except for the palmar and plantar surfaces.

Seborrhea Dandruff.

Sebum Oily secretion that is thought to retard evaporation and water loss from the epidermal surface.

Seizure Transient disturbance of cerebral function caused by an excessive discharge of neurons.

Semicircular Canals Anterior, posterior, and lateral canals in the bony labyrinth of the inner ear that provide balance and equilibrium.

Seminal Vesicles Paired pouches located posteriorly to and at the base of the bladder; fluid from here forms 60% of the volume of semen.

Septum (of the Heart) Wall that divides the left side of the heart from the right side.

Sequelae Aftermath.

Serum Iron Amount of transferrin-bound iron.

Shifting Dullness Abnormal finding elicited during percussion and corresponding to positive identification of ascites.

Short-Term Outcome Goal that a patient strives to achieve in a relatively brief time frame (hour, day, or week).

Sibilant Wheeze Continuous adventitious breath sound caused by narrowing of large airways or obstruction of a bronchus; it resembles a musical sound.

Sighing Normal respiration interrupted by a deep inspiration and followed by a deep expiration.

Sign Objective finding.

Sin Deliberate and conscious act against the teachings of a belief system.

Sinoatrial (SA) Node Normal pacemaker of the heart; intrinsic adult rate is approximately 70 beats per minute.

Skene's Glands (Paraurethral Glands) Glands that open in a posterolateral position to the urethral meatus and provide lubrication to protect the skin.

Skinfold Thickness Anthoropometric measurement to determine body fat stores and nutritional status.

Smegma White, cottage cheese-type substance sometimes found under the female labia minora or the male foreskin.

Snap High-pitched sound that is heard in early diastole; usually occurs in mitral stenosis.

Snellen Chart Chart used for testing distance vision; contains letters of various sizes with standardized numbers at the end of each line of letters.

Social History Information that is related to the patient's lifestyle and can have an impact on health.

Sonorous Wheeze Continuous adventitious breath sound caused by narrowing of large airways or obstruction of a bronchus; it resembles a snoring sound.

Soul Essential, spiritual part of a person; thought to continue after physical death.

Spasticity Increase in muscle tension on passive stretching, especially rapid or forced stretching of a muscle.

Spermatic Cord Connective tissue sheath made up of arteries, nerves, veins, lymphatic vessels, and the cremaster muscle.

Spermatocele Well-defined cystic mass on the superior testes.

Spermatogenesis Production of sperm.

Sphygmomanometer Gauge used to measure blood pressure; consists of a blood pressure cuff with an inflatable bladder, connecting tubes, bulb air pump, and a manometer.

Spider Angioma Bright-red, star-shaped vascular marking that often has a central pulsation; it blanches in the extensions when pressure is applied.

Spinnbarkeit Elasticity of cervical mucus during ovulation.

Spirit Soul, being, or supernatural force.

Spiritual Distress State in which a person feels that the belief system, or her or his place within it, is threatened.

Spiritual Well-Being State in which a person is satisfied with the way in which particular circumstances fit into the belief system.

Spirituality A person's concern for the meaning and purpose of life.

Sputum Substance that is produced by the respiratory tract and can be expectorated or swallowed; it is composed of mucus, blood, purulent material, microorganisms, cellular debris, and, occasionally, foreign objects.

Squamocolumnar Junction Cervical area between the squamous epithelial surface and the columnar epithelial surface.

Standard Precautions Practices health care providers use to prevent the exchange of blood and body fluids when coming into contact with a patient; outlined by the Centers for Disease Control (CDC).

Steatorrhea Pale-yellow, greasy, fatty stool.

Stenosis Narrowing or constriction (e.g., diseased heart valve).

Stensen's Ducts Openings from the parotid glands; located just opposite the upper second molars.

Stereognosis Ability to identify objects by manipulating and touching them.

Sternal Angle *See* **Angle of Louis**.

Stork Bites *See* **Telangiectatic Nevi**.

Strabismus True deviation of gaze due to extraocular muscle dysfunction.

Stratum Corneum Horny layer, or outer layer of the epidermis.

Stratum Germinativum Basal cell layer, or deepest layer of the epidermis.

Stratum Granulosum Epidermal layer where skin cell death occurs; it overlays the stratum spinosum.

Stratum Lucidum Additional skin layer found exclusively on the palmar and plantar surfaces.

Stratum Spinosum Epidermal layer that overlays the stratum germinativum and consists of layers of polyhedral cells.

Stress Physiologically defined response to changes that disrupt the resting equilibrium of an individual.

Striae Atrophic lines or scars commonly found on the abdomen, breasts, thighs, or buttocks.

Striae Gravidarum Stretch marks that occur in pregnancy.

Stridor Continuous adventitious breath sound caused by a partial airway obstruction in the larynx or trachea; it resembles a crowing sound.

Subculture Within a larger cultural group, a smaller group whose members share most of the beliefs and ways of life of the larger cultural group but differ on others.

Subcutaneous Tissue Superficial fascia, composed of loose areolar connective tissue and/or adipose tissue, depending on its location in the body; it lies below the dermis.

Subjective Data Information perceived by the patient to be real; such data cannot always be verified by an independent observer.

Subluxation Partial dislodgement of a bone from its place in the joint cavity.

Sulcus Terminalis Midline depression separating the anterior two-thirds from the posterior one-third of the tongue.

Superego Personality component that represents the internalization of the moral values formed as children interact with their parents and significant others.

Supernumerary Nipples (Extra Nipples) Extra nipples or breast tissue along the milk line resulting from incomplete atrophy of the galactic band.

Suprasternal Notch Visible and palpable depression in the midsternal line superior to the manubrium.

Sutures Immovable joints connecting the cranial bones.

Sweat Glands Glands that produce perspiration; composed of two types: eccrine and apocrine glands.

Symptom Subjective finding.

Syncope Fainting; transient loss of consciousness due to decreased oxygen or glucose supply to the brain.

Syndactyly Fusion between two or more digits on the hand or foot.

Synovial Effusion Excessive synovial joint fluid.

Systemic Vascular Resistance *See* **Peripheral Vascular Resistance**.

Systole Phase in the cardiac cycle during which the myocardial fibers contract and tighten to eject blood from the ventricles; correlates with the first Korotkoff sound.

T

Tachycardia Pulse rate greater than 100 beats per minute in an adult.

Tachypnea Respiratory rate greater than 20 breaths per minute in an adult.

Tactile (or Vocal) Fremitus Palpable vibration of the chest wall that is produced by the spoken word.

Tail of Spence Upper outer quadrant of the breast that extends into the axilla.

Tangential Lighting Light that is shone at a right angle on the patient to accentuate shadows and highlight subtle findings.

Tarsal Plates Connective tissue that gives shape to the upper eyelid.

Taxonomy Classification system.

Telangiectatic Nevi Marks appearing on the back of the neck, lower occiput, upper eyelids, and upper lip of the newborn that are flat, deep, irregular, and pink in light-skinned children and deep-red in dark-skinned children; also known as "stork bites."

Temperature Vital sign collected to assess core body heat.

Tendons Epimysium ends that attach a muscle to a bone.

Terminal Hair Coarse body hair in the axillary and pubic areas as well as the eyebrows, eyelashes, scalp, and, in men, the chest and face.

Termination Stage Last segment of the interview process, during which information is summarized and validated.

Testes Pair of ovoid glands located in the scrotum.

Thenar Eminence Rounded prominence at the base of the thumb.

Thoracic Expansion The extent and symmetry of chest wall expansion.

Thrill Vibrations related to turbulent blood flow that feel similar to what one feels when a hand is placed on a purring cat.

Tilts Set of blood pressures taken in supine, sitting, and standing positions.

Torticollis Lateral deviation of the neck; intermittent or sustained dystonic contraction of the muscles on one side of the neck.

Total Iron-Binding Capacity Amount of iron with which transferrin can bind.

Transferrin Protein that regulates iron absorption.

Triceps Skinfold Anthropometric measurement used to determine body fat stores and nutritional status.

Triglyceride Substance that accounts for most of the fat stored in the body's tissues.

True Ribs *See* **Vertebrosternal Ribs**.

Tubular Breath Sound *See* **Bronchial Breath Sound**.

Turbinate (or Concha) Projection from the lateral wall of the nose and covered with mucous membranes that greatly increase the surface area within the nose.

Turgor Elasticity of the skin; it reflects the skin's state of hydration.

Tussive Fremitus Palpable vibration produced by coughing.

Tympany Descriptor for a percussable sound that is loud in intensity, long in duration, of high pitch, drumlike, and normally located over a gastric air bubble.

U

Uvula Fingerlike projection hanging down from the center of the soft palate.

Urethra Duct from the urinary bladder to the urethral meatus; carries urine and, in the male, semen.

Uterus Inverted pear-shaped, hollow, muscular organ in which the impregnated ovum develops into a fetus.

V

Vagina Pink, hollow, muscular tube extending from the cervix to the vulva, located posterior to the bladder and anterior to the rectum.

Vaginal Introitus Entrance to the vagina, situated at the inferior aspect of the vulval vestibule.

Value Orientation Patterned principles (about time, human nature, activity, relations, and people-to-nature) that provide order and give direction to an individual's thoughts and behaviors related to the solution of commonly occurring human problems.

Varicocele Bluish mass resulting from abnormal dilatation of the veins of the pampiniform plexus of the spermatic cord.

Vellus Hair Fine, faint hair that covers most of the body.

Venous Hum Continuous, medium-pitched sound originating in the inferior vena cava and associated with obstructed portal circulation.

Venous Star Linear or irregularly shaped blue vascular pattern on the skin; does not blanch when pressure is applied.

Vernix Caseosa Protective integumentary mechanism of the newborn; consists of sebum and shed epithelial cells.

Vertebra Prominens The long spinous process of the seventh cervical vertebra.

Vertebrosternal (or True) Ribs Rib pairs 1–7; they articulate via the costal cartilage to the sternum.

Vertigo Dizziness or lightheadedness.

Vesicular Breath Sound Breath sound that is low in pitch and soft in intensity and is heard best over the peripheral lung; has a breezy, gentle rustling quality; heard longer on inspiration than expiration.

Vestibule Boat-shaped area between the labia minora and containing the urethral meatus, the openings of the Skene's glands, the hymen, the openings of the Bartholin's glands, and the vaginal introitus.

Vestibule (of the Ear) Part of the inner ear located between the cochlea and the semicircular canals.

Visceral Pericardium Pericardial layer that lies against the actual heart muscle.

Visceral Pleura Lining of the external surface of the lungs.

Visual Analog Scale Numerical scale used to rate pain from 0 to 10.

Vital Signs Measurements, including temperature, pulse, respirations, and blood pressure, that provide an index of the patient's physiological status.

Vitamin Organic substance needed to maintain the function of the body.

Vitiligo Patchy, symmetrical areas of white on the skin.

Vitreous Humor Gelatinous material that fills the center cavity of the eye and helps maintain the shape of the eye and the position of the internal structures.

Voice Sounds Techniques used to assess whether the lungs are filled with air, fluid, or a solid.

W

Water-Soluble Vitamin Vitamin soluble in water; is not stored in the body and is excreted in the urine.

Weber Test Tuning fork test to evaluate hearing loss and determine whether the loss is conductive or sensorineural.

Wellness Nursing Diagnosis Diagnosis that represents the patient's striving for a higher level of health and wellness.

Wharton's Ducts Openings from the submaxillary glands; located on either side of the frenulum.

Whispered Pectoriloquy Voice sound where the patient whispers the words "ninety-nine" or "one, two, three" to determine if the lungs are filled with air, fluid, or a solid.

Working Stage That segment of the interview process during which the majority of data are collected.

X

Xanthelasma Creamy, yellow plaque on the eyelid and secondary to hypercholesterolemia.

Xerosis Excessive dryness of the skin.

Xiphoid Process Cartilaginous process at the base of the sternum; it does not articulate with the ribs.

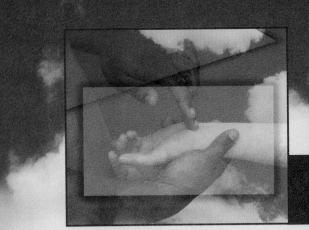

Index

Note: Page numbers in *italics* indicate illustrations; page numbers followed by "t" indicate tables.